# **health** *in the new millennium*

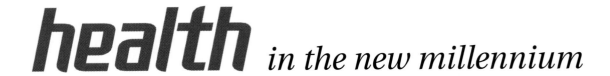

# health *in the new millennium*

**Jeffrey S. Nevid**
St. John's University

**Spencer A. Rathus**
Montclair State University

**Hannah R. Rubenstein**

**WORTH PUBLISHERS**

**Health in the New Millennium**



Manufactured in the United States of America

Library of Congress Catalog Card Number: 97-062009

ISBN: 1-57259-171-4

ISBN: 1-57259-509-4 (comp.)

Printing: 1 2 3 4 5—01 00 99 98

Executive Editor: Kerry Baruth

Development and Production Editor: Judith Wilson

Manuscript Editor: Betty Gatewood

Design: Malcolm Grear Designers

Art Director: George Touloumes

Production Manager: Stacey B. Alexander

Layout: Fernando Quiñones, Lee Ann Mahler

Picture Editor: June Lundborg Whitworth

Graphics Art Manager: Demetrios Zangos

Illustrations: J/B Woolsey Associates

Cover Photograph: Rod Walker/Workbook/Co-op Stock

Composition and Prepress: Progressive Information Technologies

Printing and Binding: R. R. Donnelley & Sons Company



**Worth Publishers**

33 Irving Place

New York, NY 10003

*To Judith Wolf-Nevid, always with love.*

*J.S.N.*

*To my children—Jill, Allyn, Jordan, and Taylor.*

*S.R.R.*

*For my son Samuel Jesse, who grew inside me as this project took shape, his soon-to-be-born sibling, who reminds me daily of the importance of healthy habits, and my husband, Fred, whose wisdom and support make it all possible.*

*H.R.R.*

# About the Authors

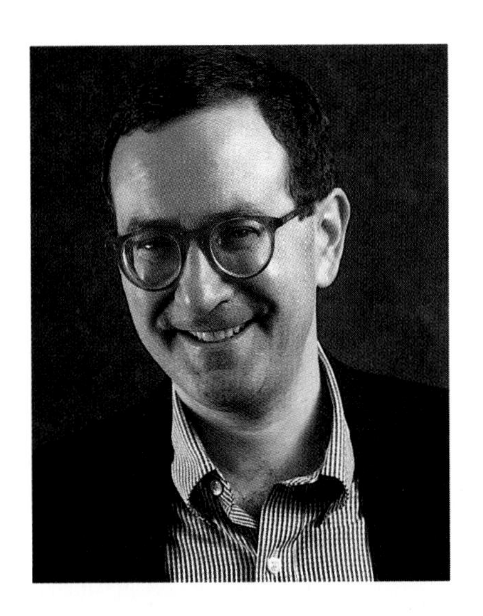

**Jeffrey S. Nevid** is a professor and health researcher at St. John's University in New York. He received his Ph.D. from the State University of New York at Albany and completed an NIMH postdoctoral fellowship in evaluation research at Northwestern University. His most recent research, which was supported by the National Heart, Lung, and Blood Institute of the NIH, involved the development of a culturally specific smoking cessation program for Hispanic smokers. His research has appeared in such journals as *American Journal of Health Promotion, Health Psychology, Journal of Occupational Medicine, Sex Roles, Journal of Social Distress and the Homeless, Behavior Therapy,* and the *Journal of Consulting and Clinical Psychology.* He has co-authored several books with Spencer Rathus and is the author of several books on AIDS and STDs: *A Student's Guide to AIDS and Other Sexually Transmitted Diseases, 201 Things You Should Know about AIDS and Other STDs,* and *Choices: Sex in the Age of AIDS.*

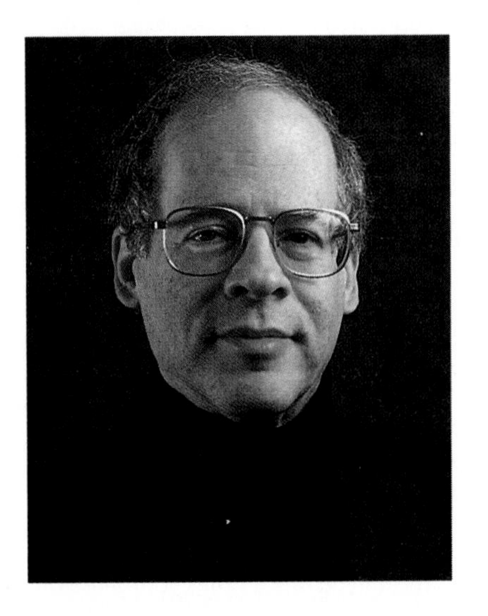

**Spencer A. Rathus** received his Ph.D. from the State University of New York at Albany and is on the faculty of Montclair State University in New Jersey. His research interests have included treatment of obesity and eating disorders, smoking cessation, human growth and development, methods of therapy, and sexual dysfunctions. He is the originator of the Rathus Assertiveness Schedule and has authored several books, including *Psychology in the New Millennium* and *The World of Children.* He has co-authored *AIDS: What Every Student Needs to Know* with Susan Boughn, *The Right Start* with Lois Fichner-Rathus, *Human Sexuality in a World of Diversity* with Jeffrey S. Nevid and Lois Fichner-Rathus, and *Adjustment and Growth* and *Behavior Therapy* with Jeffrey S. Nevid.

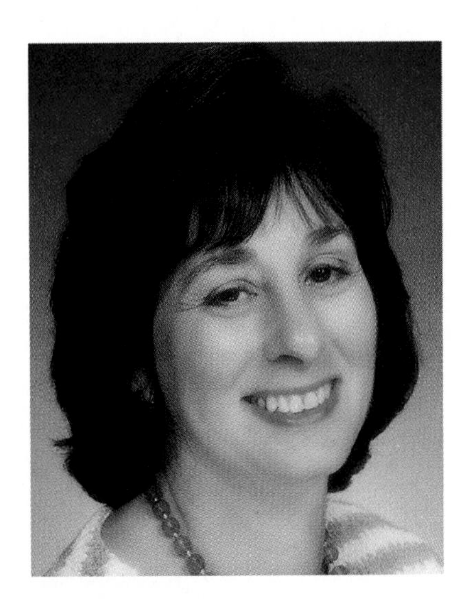

**Hannah R. Rubenstein** received her M.A. in communications and is a writer and editor with 16 years experience in scholarly and academic publishing. Her specialities include health communications and sociology. Formerly on the staffs of several major publishing houses, she now heads her own communications firm, Hedgehog Productions.

# Contents in Brief

# Contents

# Feature Boxes

## PREVENTION



## Health*Check*

## WORLD OF *diversity*

## Take **Charge**

# Preface

We stand at the edge of the new millennium. Revolutions are taking place all around us. New nations are forming. Virtual reality vies for our attention with "real" reality. New vaccines, drugs, and surgical techniques have vanquished many diseases and promise hope for others.

What will the new millennium mean for our health? For our longevity? For our access to health care services in a changing health care system? For an environment threatened by old and new hazards, including global warming and overpopulation? How will technology affect health care and the ways in which we obtain and use health information? How can we prepare ourselves and our students for the health challenges that await us? This book can help to find the answers.

## THEMES OF THE TEXT

This book is written at the threshold of the new millennium to provide students with the skills they need to meet challenges to their health and optimize their physical and psychological well-being. **Health in the New Millennium** offers the necessary breadth and currency of coverage. We examine topics including fitness, nutrition, mental health, and infectious and chronic diseases in a way that distills the most important information and makes it accessible and interesting to readers. Within each topic, we emphasize self-empowerment, prevention, an understanding of the health impact of human diversity, and the importance of thinking critically. Learning and interest are enhanced throughout by the latest educational technology made possible by our development of the **Smart Textbook**™.

### Self-Empowerment

We live in an era when advances in medical technology and treatment seem to rush at us fast and furiously. Imaging techniques like MRI, once the stuff of science fiction, have become routine. New forms of surgery such as laparoscopy and laser surgery have transformed some operations into "minor" outpatient procedures.

With so much attention focused on medical advances, it is easy to lose sight of the critical role of our own behavior in the promotion of wellness and longevity. Then too, many people, especially young adults, take their health for granted. Health risks like heart disease and cancer may seem a long way off, so the perceived risks of less-than-healthy choices do not appear to be compelling. This book invites students to examine their health-related behavior and attitudes and to begin making healthful changes. For example, they can control two of the major risk factors for cancer and heart disease—smoking and diet. Similarly, many students underestimate their risk of contracting AIDS or of becoming one of the more than 60 million Americans infected with other sexually transmitted diseases. Or they believe that the responsibility for safeguarding their health lies with their health care provider (assuming they have one), not with themselves.

This text raises students' awareness of the importance of developing healthful habits *now* and encourages them to become active managers of their own health care. Throughout this book, we provide students with the tools they need to change their behavior. The ***Take Charge*** feature at the end of every chapter gives specific suggestions for making strides toward a healthier life, for example, "Taking the Distress out of Stress" (Chapter 3), "Quitting Smoking" (Chapter 14), "Protecting Yourself from Infectious Diseases" (Chapter

15), and "Turning Off Your Anger Alarm" (Chapter 21).

### Prevention

Despite the very real threats of infectious disease, the major killers in our society are chronic, noncommunicable diseases, especially cardiovascular diseases, cancer, and diabetes. What new developments in prevention and treatment of these killer diseases lie beyond the horizon? *Meanwhile, what will we do for ourselves to prevent them?*

Prevention is a key aspect of the personal health course. We integrate specific prevention strategies throughout the text. For example, research is clear about the effects of diet on many aspects of our health. This book provides dietary strategies that will help students take full advantage of a diet richer in fruits and vegetables and lower in fat. Of course, there is no question about the harmful health effects of tobacco. We outline specific methods for quitting smoking, including behavior modification and nicotine replacement. We present the latest research on heart disease and cancer and offer concrete advice on reducing the risk factors that we can control.

Further, we highlight many topics in ***Prevention*** features, such as "Preventing Accidents" (Chapter 1), "Suicide Prevention" (Chapter 4), "Preventing Obesity" (Chapter 6), "Combating Drinking and Driving" (Chapter 13), "Preventing Lyme Disease" (Chapter 15), "Rape Prevention" (Chapter 21), and "Keeping Your Home Safe from Carbon Monoxide Poisoning" (Chapter 22).

### Health and Human Diversity

Our health is influenced by factors associated with our ethnic and cultural backgrounds, our gender, and our age. This book promotes understanding of, and respect for, the differences among groups of people and raises students' awareness of the health risks and problems faced by various groups. We also discuss ways of eliminating the barriers that have prevented traditionally disadvantaged groups from obtaining access to high-quality health care.

Issues highlighted in ***World of Diversity*** features include "Women and Health Research—A History of Exclusion" (Chapter 1), "Social Class, Gender, Ethnicity, and Psychological Health" (Chapter 4), "Ethnic Food—Eating Out, Eating Smart" (Chapter 5), "Fitness Is for Everyone—Exercise and the Physically Challenged" (Chapter 7), "You've Come a Long Way, Baby? On Women and Smoking" (Chapter 14), "Combating High Blood Pressure among African Americans" (Chapter 17), and "Toxic Communities and Environmental Racism" (Chapter 22).

### Critical Thinking

We are barraged with health information from many sources—professional journals, print media, radio and TV, and the Internet. Hardly a day goes by without some report of an important development in health. While we present the latest, most accurate health information, we recognize that one of the most important aspects of teaching is to help students develop and apply critical thinking skills whenever—and however—they receive health information. We begin in Chapter 1 to teach students how to sort the well-researched wheat from the faddish chaff and continue with special **Critical Thinking** questions throughout the book.

## TECHNOLOGY TO ENRICH LEARNING—A NEW KIND OF TEXTBOOK FOR THE NEW MILLENNIUM

**Health in the New Millennium** is a new kind of textbook—a **Smart Textbook**™.[1] It literally brings a world of health information to the student's fingertips. The **Smart Textbook**™ serves as a "launching pad" or remote-control device for accessing relevant material from the accompanying CD-ROM. As students read the text, icons indicate the kinds of multimedia materials that are stored on the CD-ROM. By typing in the code, students can directly access the desired video clip, health-related document, self-assessment exercise, application, self-scoring quiz, or **Talking Glossary**™ item.[2]

The health-related information on the CD-ROM was selected from leading universities, federal health agencies, health organizations, and periodicals. Were we to include all of this information between the covers of the book, it would swell to thousands of pages.

[1] For information about **The Smart Textbook**™ contact **textcom@aol.com** or **textcom2@aol.com.**

[2] For students without access to computers, a paper version of the self-scoring quizzes and self-assessment exercises is included.

## ACKNOWLEDGMENTS

First, we owe a great deal of gratitude to the many scholars, practitioners, and researchers whose contributions to the health sciences are represented in these pages. We are indebted to the many researchers who have generously allowed us to reprint their work.

We also wish to thank our professional colleagues who so carefully reviewed our manuscript and helped us to refine and strengthen the material:

Gail B. Arnold, University of Massachusetts—Boston
Rosemary C. Clark, City College—San Francisco
Kenton Conner, Miami University
Sam Crowther, Marietta College
Neil E. Gallagher, Towson University
Sharon A. Garcia, Diablo Valley College
Valerie Goodwin-Colbert, Southwestern College
Donna R. Gray, Middlesex County College
Heather Hahn, New Mexico State University
Shelia C. Harbet, California State University—Northridge
D. Craig Huddy, Appalachian State University
Ray Johnson, Central Michigan University
R. Mark Kelley, Southeastern Louisiana University
Stan Ledington, Walla Walla College
Michael Lee, Joliet Junior College
Carol Lyke, Chabot College
Sally McGill, Cañada College
Linda L. Rankin, Idaho State University
Patty Reagan, University of Utah
Kerry J. Redican, Virginia Polytechnic Institute and State University
Juan Robles, California State University—Hayward
Henry Ross, Texas A & M University—Commerce
N. Heather Savage, Mississippi University for Women
Gayle Strang, Rockford College
James H. Tanaka, Solano Community College
Susan Yeager, Mesa State College

We also express our appreciation to our long-term colleagues, Professor Beverly Drinnin, Des Moines Area Community College, and Professor Gary Piggrem, DeVry Institute of Technology, for preparing the supplements that enrich our text. We also wish to acknowledge the extraordinary contributions of the many talented people at Worth Publishers who consistently "raise the bar" in college publishing. To all of the people at Worth whose devoted efforts made this book come to life, thank you. We extend special appreciation and thanks to our acquisitions editor, Kerry Baruth, who brought our book to Worth and helped shape its development; to our extremely dedicated and gifted developmental editor, Judith Wilson, and her multitalented editorial assistant, Yuna Lee; to our managing editor Suzanne Thibodeau; to our Marketing Manager, John Britch; to our manuscript editor, Betty Gatewood; to our supplements editor, Maja Lorkovic; to our photo researcher, June Whitworth; to our director of photo research, Cindy Joyce. We also wish to acknowledge the unique talents of art director George Touloumes and his associates, who framed our words in this stunningly beautiful design by Malcolm Grear Designers. Special thanks are also due to the creative team of John Philp and Michelle Evans, who produced, scripted, shot, and edited the video clips for the accompanying CD-ROM. Last, but certainly not least, we wish to thank Worth president Susan Driscoll for her unstinting support of this project and belief in our work.

We also wish to acknowledge that portions of the material in this text are reprinted from *Human Sexuality in a World of Diversity* by Spencer A. Rathus, Jeffrey S. Nevid, and Lois Fichner-Rathus, published by Allyn & Bacon, Inc. Portions of the material on the accompanying CD-ROM first appeared in *Choices: Sex in the Age of STDs* by Jeffrey S. Nevid, also published by Allyn & Bacon, Inc. The authors gratefully appreciate the cooperation of Allyn & Bacon, Inc., in permitting them to use this material.

We extend a special thanks to our spouses and family members without whose support and understanding this book would never have materialized.

Finally, we thank you for choosing **Health in the New Millennium.** We hope that this book and its supplements provide you with an excellent resource for good health and good teaching and learning experiences.

New York, New York
e-mail: JNevid@aol.com

Short Hills, New Jersey
e-mail: PsychLinks@aol.com

West Simsbury, CT

# To the Student

This is your book. It is about your health and the health of those you care about. As we take a glimpse of the new millennium, we see that things will never be as they were before. At the forefront of these changes are advances in technology that affect our health care—and our access to health-related information. Today, 24-hour-a-day cable news channels and the Internet add to the flow of information from network TV, radio, newspapers, magazines, and—yes—textbooks. Information is thrust our way at a relentless pace.

Much health-related information comes to you in the form of opinion and speculation. A friend, a TV report, or someone's home page on the web touts a new diet that will supposedly help you shed pounds, boost your energy, and fight cancer and heart disease. This textbook gives you the tools to evaluate such claims. It offers you the latest research findings, strategies for critical thinking, and advice as to how to explore and evaluate information from any source.

This text is itself a product of the revolution in information technology. It is the first **Smart Textbook**™, a textbook that is also a launching pad for a variety of multimedia presentations on the accompanying CD-ROM. Text-related material on the CD-ROM is identified by icons in the margins of the text. To access this material—a video clip, a ***Close-up*** feature containing additional health-related information, a ***HealthCheck*** self-assessment, a ***Take Charge*** health application, or a self-study quiz—double-click the **Smart Text** icon appearing on your computer desktop (after installing the program). Then, after the program loads, type in the code for the particular item appearing under the text icon. That's all there is to it. One CD-ROM feature we think you'll find especially useful is the ***Talking Glossary***™. Have trouble pronouncing some tongue-twisting medical or scientific terms? Just type in the code and hear the word correctly pronounced. We also think you'll like the video clips. Two young video professionals, John Philp and Michelle Evans, developed and shot these video features, including several *New Millennium* features that highlight recent developments in the health sciences. Check out "The Quest," the first feature in Chapter 1 that begins their personal journey.

This text puts your health in your own hands. You may have little or no background in biology or health sciences. You may not be planning a career as a health professional. Nevertheless, this text shows you how to be in the driver's seat when it comes to making choices about your health. It helps you develop a healthy diet, manage your weight, and control stress. It helps you evaluate the kind of exercise program that may be right for you and how and when to begin to exercise. It gives you tools in the form of prevention strategies you can use to reduce your risk of chronic and infectious diseases, including sexually transmitted diseases. It provides strategies to help you quit smoking, drink responsibly, and adopt drug-free alternatives for healthy living. It gives you information to protect yourself from unwanted pregnancies and to plan a healthy pregnancy. It helps you become an active health consumer so you can make informed decisions about *who* will provide your health care and *how to* benefit the most from the health care you receive. This textbook provides you with the information and strategies you need to make these decisions.

As we enter the new millennium, we also find that not everyone belongs to the same health care system. Many Americans have access to some of the most sophisticated health care in the world, yet others are rarely referred to such health care or simply cannot afford it. This text considers the differences among Americans as well as the similarities, and how *all* Americans can enhance their health in the new millennium.

We wish you good reading and good health! If you would like to share your thoughts about this book or give us suggestions for the next edition, you can reach us at the following address:

Worth Publishers
33 Irving Place
New York, NY 10003

Or you can contact us by e-mail:

JNevid@aol.com PsychLinks@aol.com

# A Guide to health in the new millennium

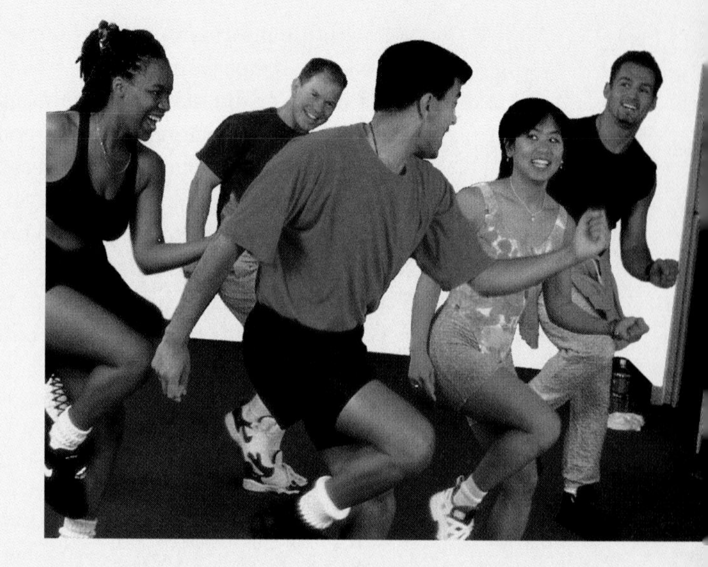

A textbook is more than a storehouse of information. **Health in the New Millennium** is a teaching and learning device that offers a set of learning aids to expand understanding, stimulate interest, encourage critical thinking, and, most importantly, help students learn about health.

*Items marked with a yellow crescent indicate features found on the accompanying CD-ROM. They are described on the following pages.*

## SPECIAL FEATURES

### Did You Know That?

***Did you know that?*** *sections at the beginning of each chapter offer thought-provoking and often surprising facts that involve students and encourage them to read on.*

### Think about it!

***Think about it!*** *features throughout each chapter ask students to apply the major ideas to their own experiences.* ***Think about it!*** *features promote active learning and critical thinking.*

**DID YOU KNOW THAT**

- Stress can be good for you? p.54
- Our bodies produce natural painkillers that are chemically similar to the narcotic morphine? p.58
- Video games help children with cancer manage the side effects of chemotherapy? p.60
- The ability to raise the temperature in a finger may help relieve migraine headaches? p.61
- The emotional stress of divorce can weaken the immune system? p.69
- Stress can make you more vulnerable to the common cold? p.69
- Humor may be good medicine for handling stress? p.72

***think about it!***

Smart Quiz
Q0503

- What kinds of dietary fats are there? How do fats contribute to your health? How are fats harmful to your health?
- Do you consume enough fats? Too much? What are your favorite food sources of fats?
- What is cholesterol? What are some of the connections between diet and cholesterol levels in the bloodstream?

**critical thinking** Has this chapter changed your ideas about the role of fat in nutrition and health? If so, how?

## Prevention Section

***Prevention** features offer specific strategies for optimizing health and reducing the risk of disease and accidents.*

PREVENTION

*Ensuring Food Safety*

While food is needed to sustain life, it can also endanger life. Ensuring food safety is not merely the responsibility of federal and local governments; we all must take measures to ensure our own and our family's safety. The foods we eat can become contaminated by various harmful substances, including disease-causing bacteria and other microorganisms, as well as poisonous substances or **toxins** that can be deposited in our bodies and lead to serious illnesses, including cancer.

**Food-Borne Illnesses** Food can serve as a channel for transmission of disease-causing bacteria and other microorganisms. The term *food poisoning* is used to refer to food-borne illnesses and reactions to toxins produced by food-borne bacteria. Symptoms vary with the type of illness and the amount of the infected material ingested, but they commonly include gastrointestinal complaints like diarrhea and abdominal cramping, fever, vomiting, and exhaustion. Tens of millions of cases of food-borne diarrheal diseases worldwide are reported annually.

Though food-borne illnesses can cause significant distress, they are usually brief and not life-threatening for otherwise healthy people. Yet they can cause serious problems for the very young, the old, or people with compromised immune systems. In all, the government estimates that 7 million people in the U.S. suffer from food-borne illnesses each year. Nine thousand people die from them.[63]

Close-up
Preventing food-borne illness
T0505

Life-threatening food-borne illness can be caused by *Salmonella* and *E. coli* bacteria. *Salmonella* are normally pres- ...ock but can cause gastrointestinal ...hough most *Sal-* ... cause

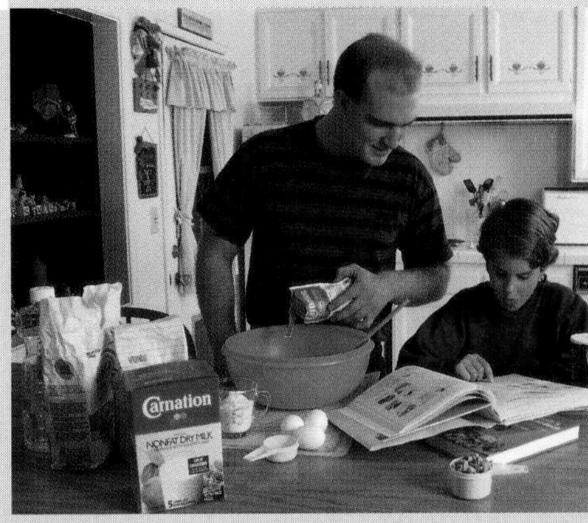
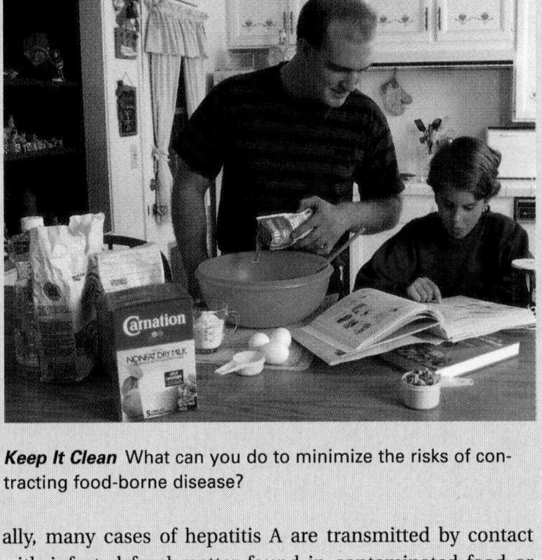

***Keep It Clean*** What can you do to minimize the risks of contracting food-borne disease?

ally, many cases of hepatitis A are transmitted by contact with infected fecal matter found in contaminated food or water. Hepatitis A may be unsymptomatic or produce such symptoms as nausea, fever, abdominal discomfort, vomiting, and jaundiced (yellowish) skin. It is largely because of the risk of hepatitis A that restaurant employees are required to wash their hands after using the toilet. Ingesting raw, contaminated shellfish is also a frequent means of transmission of hepatitis A and other viruses and bacteria. Never eat shellfish such as oysters, clams, or mussels unless it is cooked thoroughly.

If you develop symptoms of a food-borne illness, contact your doctor or health care provider. This is esp... tant for children and older people, who may be... tible to the effects of dehydration. Drink liquid... bodily fluid lost through diarrhea or vomiting.

**Environmental Contaminants** Harmfu... or toxic substances in the environment can ... They

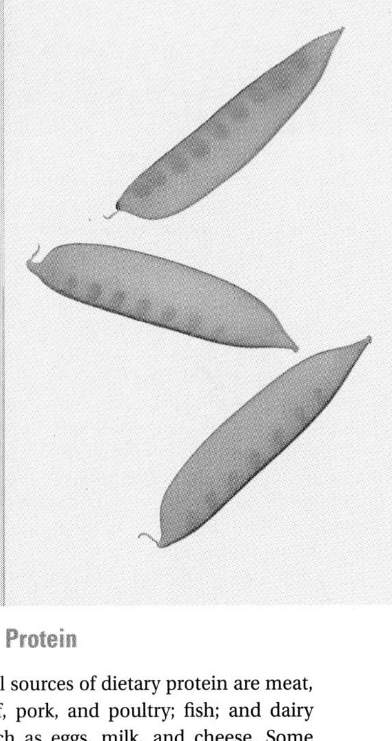

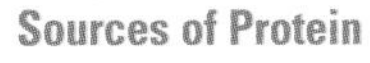

### Sources of Protein

The principal sources of dietary protein are meat, such as beef, pork, and poultry; fish; and dairy products such as eggs, milk, and cheese. Some vegetable matter, such as legumes (beans, chickpeas, and lentils) and grains are also rich sources of protein. We get about two-thirds of our protein from animal sources in the form of meat and animal by-products, such as milk and cheese. The rest comes from a combination of cereal grains, beans, and other sources.

Most Americans consume more than enough protein in their diets to meet their nutritional needs. Any ... that we

**Nutrition** The process by which plants and animals ingest and utilize food.

**Nutrients** Essential substances in food that our bodies need but are incapable of producing on their own.

**Proteins** Organic molecules that form the basic building blocks of body tissues.

**Amino acids** Organic compounds from which proteins are made.

**Essential amino acids** Amino acids essential to survival that must be obtained ...food we eat since the body is unable

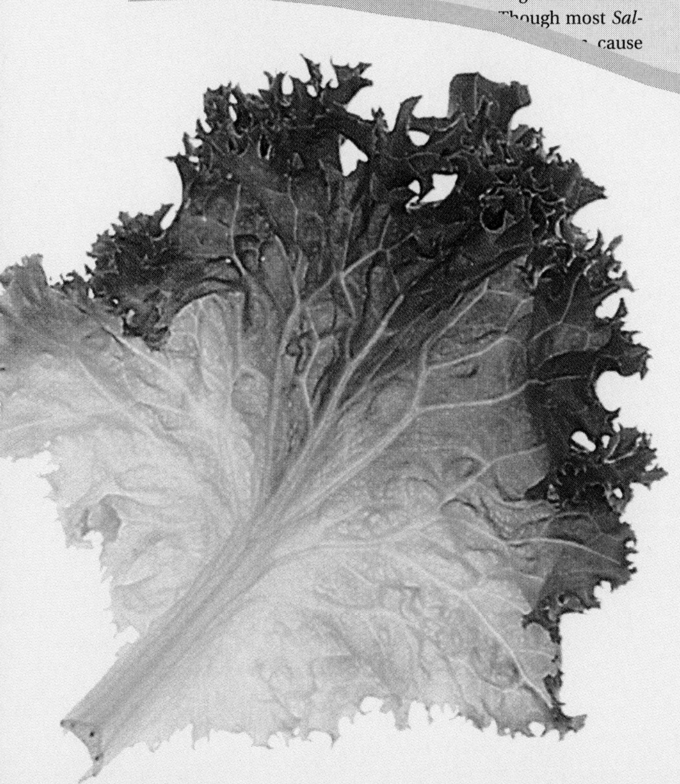

## Glossaries

*Key terms are highlighted in the text and defined in the margin. On the **Smart Text™ CD-ROM**, a **Talking Glossary™** helps students master difficult or unusual pronunciations.*

## World of Diversity Boxes

***World of Diversity** gives insights into how ethnicity, culture, gender, and age affect health around the world. Students will gain a more complete understanding of global health issues and of the larger context of their personal health status.*

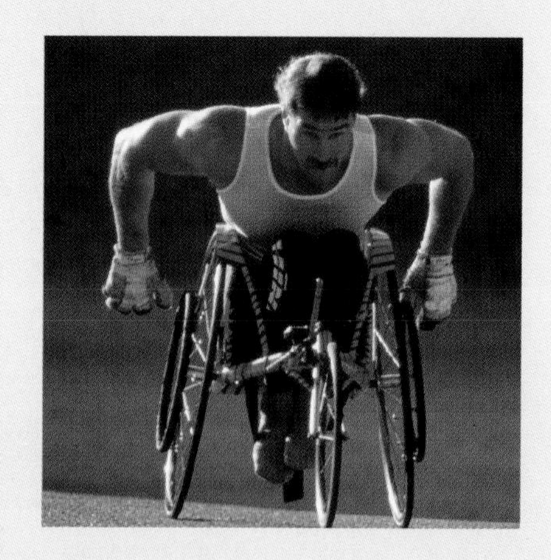

WORLD OF ***diversity***

### Smoking and Ethnic Minorities

Antismoking campaigns have been less effective in promoting smoking cessation among people of color than among whites. Cigarette companies have also targeted much of their advertising effort toward minority communities, especially African-American and Hispanic-American communities. Smoking is also associated with lower socioeconomic status, and people of color tend to be overrepresented in these lower strata. Taken together, it is not surprising that cigarette smoking is more prevalent among some ethnic minorities, especially African-American men, Native Americans, and some Hispanic-American subgroups such as Puerto Ricans.

Smoking, especially among men, is a worldwide health problem of staggering proportions. The World Health Organization estimates that more than 60% of men in China, Indonesia, Korea, and the Philippines smoke, compared with 28% of men in the United States.[43] Across Latin America and East Asia, about one in two men smokes.[44] In China alone, 300 million people smoke, which is more than the entire U.S. population!

Let us take a closer look at smoking among minority groups in the United States.

#### African Americans

African-American men have the highest smoking rates among the major racial/ethnic groups in the U.S. (see Figure 14.5). Yet African-American women smoke at a rate similar to that of the general female population. African-American men also have the

and unemployment, affect African Americans disproportionately, especially those living in depressed inner-city neighborhoods. Not surprisingly, smoking is a major contributor to shorter life expectancy among African-American men in inner-city neighborhoods.[47]

According to the National Cancer Institute, if antismoking campaigns are to achieve widespread success among African Americans, especially those of lower socioeconomic status, several barriers will need to be overcome:[48]

- Reliance on cigarettes as a way of coping with the stresses and social disadvantages associated with lower socioeconomic status and pervasive discrimination.
- Less use of primary health care providers, who might serve to encourage smoking cessation and provide helpful advice. Limited access to health care in general and to smoking-related services and resources in particular.

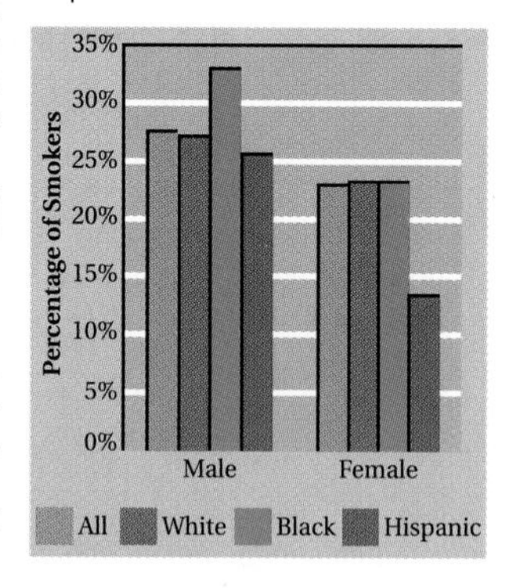


**Figure 14.5** ***Percentages of Adults Who Smoke by Gender and ...nic Group*** Smoking is ... black men

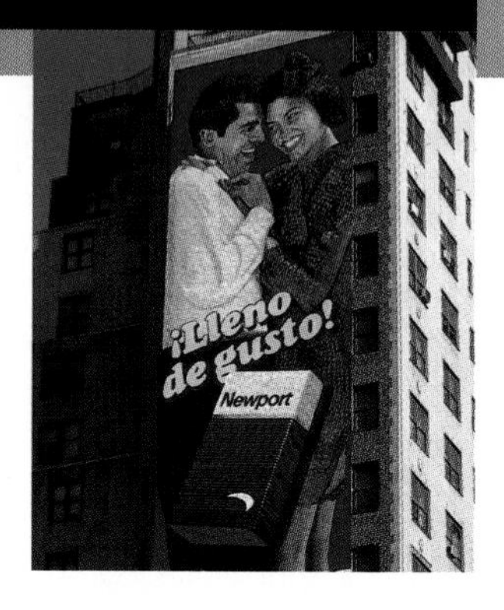


- Attitudes in African-American communities that may encourage smoking.
- Considering smoking to be less critical than other pressing social problems such as drugs, unemployment, racism, and crime.
- Powerful advertising tailored to African-American consumers that not only glamorizes and legitimizes smoking but also downplays the health risks. (Billboard advertisements are particularly prominent in minority communities.)

#### Hispanic Americans

Overall, Hispanic men smoke about as much as non-Hispanic white men, while Hispanic women smoke less than non-Hispanic white women and Hispanic men (see Figure 14.5).[49] Smoking has declined among Hispanic groups overall, but it has remained stable among some Hispanic subgroups and has increased among others, such as young Puerto Ricans.

Acculturation affects smoking patterns among Hispanic Americans, especially Hispanic women.[50] Traditional Hispanic-American cultures discourage smoking among women but not among men, which may explain the

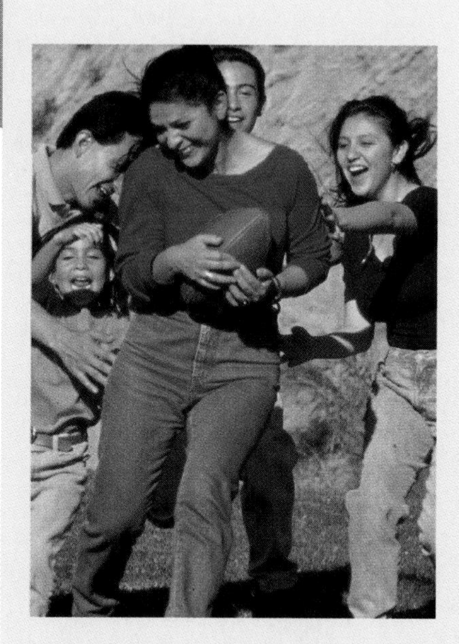

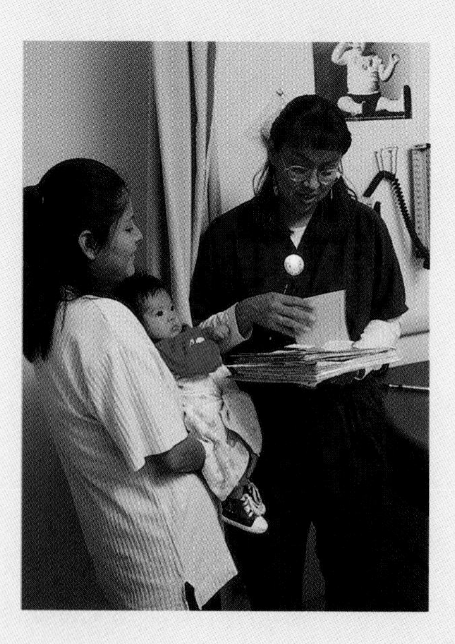

## HealthChecks

***HealthCheck** self-assessment questionnaires encourage students to pause and evaluate their own health-related behavior and attitudes.*

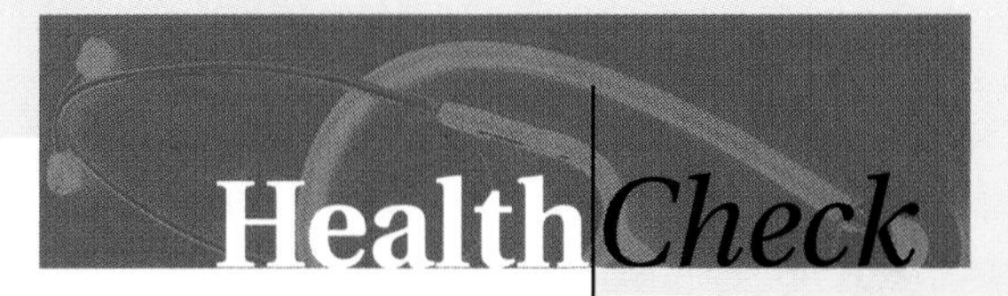


### Are You an Optimist or a Pessimist?

Do you see a silver lining behind every cloud, or do clouds darken your horizon? Do you believe that things will work out well or do you expect the worst? The Life Orientation Test can help you gain some insight into whether you tend to see the glass as half full or half empty.[19]

*Use the following scale to indicate your response to the following items. Write your response in the spaces provided below. Then check the scoring key in Appendix B at the back of the book.*

4 = strongly agree
3 = agree
2 = neutral
1 = disagree
0 = strongly disagree

____ 1. In uncertain times, I usually expect the best.
____ 2. It's easy for me to relax.
____ 3. If something can go wrong for me, it will.
____ 4. I always look on the bright side of things.
____ 5. I'm always optimistic about my future.
____ 6. I enjoy my friends a lot.
____ 7. It's important for me to keep busy.
____ 8. I hardly ever expect things to go my way.
____ 9. Things never work out the way I want them to.
____10. I don't get upset too easily.
____11. I'm a believer in the idea that "every cloud has a silver lining."
____12. I rarely count on good things happening to me.

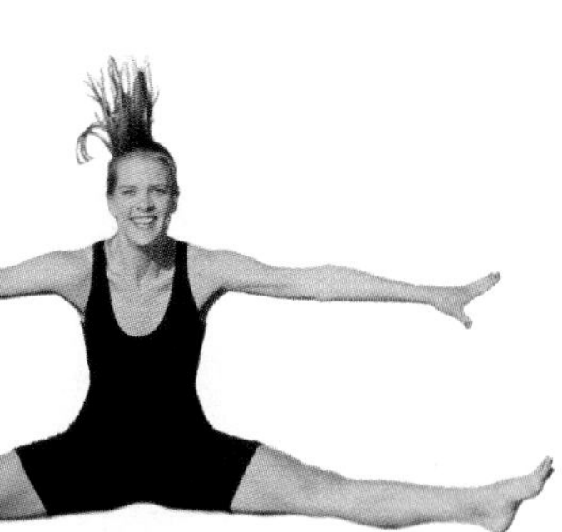

***Optimism*** Optimism is strongly connected to psychological and physical health, even to the ability to bounce back from major surgery.

HealthCheck

### How Much Do You Know about Cold and Flu Remedies?[38]

The over-the-counter cold remedy industry is a $2 billion a year enterprise. That's a lot of pills and potions. The following ***HealthCheck*** will help you become more aware of treatment options and will help you prepare for the next time the cold bug strikes or you get the flu. After answering each item, check your knowledge by turning to the answer key at the end of this chapter.

**True or False**

T F **1.** Antibiotics kill cold and flu viruses within a day or two.

T F **2.** Treating a common cold will shorten its duration.

T F **3.** It is always best to treat the common cold.

T F **4.** You should use a multisymptom cold remedy that treats as many symptoms as possible.

T F **5.** By using a cold remedy, you not only reduce your suffering but can help prevent a recurrence.

T F **6.** An antihistamine is good for clearing your stuffy nose, while a decongestant is good for stopping a runny nose.

T F **7.** Fortunately, most antihistamines on the market today do not induce drowsiness, so they are safe to use when driving.

T F **8.** You should not use nasal sprays or drops for longer than a few days.

T F **9.** Chicken soup is of absolutely no value in treating a common cold.

T F **10.** Always check the ingredients on cold remedies, especially if you have sensitivities to certain chemicals.

T F **11.** Any of the major over-the-counter pain relievers or analgesics—acetaminophen, aspirin, ibuprofen—work about equally well in relieving the pain and fever of a cold.

T F **12.** All cough medicines have the same effects.

T F **13.** Feed a cold; starve a fever.

## Take Charge

*Each chapter ends with a **Take Charge** feature that offers suggestions on how to actively apply the important health information presented in the chapter. Many **Take Charge** features provide detailed road maps to help students translate their learning into healthy lives. **Take Charge** is a source of useful and specific information on many practical health matters.*

24

# Practicing Self-Care

Take Charge

The ***Take Charge*** features in this textbook help you apply the material in the chapter to your own life. This first ***Take Charge*** feature focuses on an important element of achieving wellness, practicing self-care.

Though there is no guarantee that practicing self-care will keep you free of disease or infirmity, the odds are in your favor that it will help you live a longer, healthier, and fuller life. Practicing self-care involves taking steps to prevent disease and maintain vigor and vitality as you age. Much of the information contained in this textbook is focused toward these ends:

- Keeping fit and remaining active mentally and physically
- Adopting a healthful diet and sticking to it
- Controlling stress, getting sufficient sleep, and coping with emotional problems
- Avoiding harmful substances, such as tobacco, illicit drugs, and excessive alcohol
- Protecting yourself from infectious agents and environmental hazards.

People who practice self-care are knowledgeable and active consumers of health care. They understand that they have both a right and a responsibility to take an active part in managing their health care. They get regular medical checkups and screening tests. They approach the choice of health care providers seriously and carefully scrutinize health insurance plans and the facilities and institutions that provide health care services (see Chapter 23).

A good starting point is choosing a **primary care physician,** the person primarily responsible for your medical care on an ongoing basis.

### Choosing a Primary Care Physician

Many people spend more time picking out a new television or stereo system than selecting a primary care physician. They may assume (wrongly) that all physicians are equally competent. Or they may not think that they have the knowledge or competence to make an informed choice. True enough, the average consumer may not be able to judge medical competence. No, medical boards do not routinely evaluate physicians' skills. Even well-informed patients may not know whether their doctors' skills are sharp or whether they keep up with the latest medical developments. Some doctors do get report cards. In some states, such as New York and Pennsylvania, expert panels issue ratings of heart surgeons based on their surgical performance in relation to the severity of the cases they treat. Some consumer groups have applauded these efforts and believe that they have weeded out some sloppy practitioners. Yet the rating system has drawn fire from doctors who believe it is unfair and confusing.[40] Another concern is that doctors may shy away from treating the sickest patients if they believe that negative outcomes might jeopardize their ratings.

Despite the difficulty of judging medical competence, there is much that health consumers can do to make better-informed decisions about their health care providers:

1. *Get recommendations.* Ask around. Seek recommendations from those whose opinions you trust. Be aware, however, that what is important to one person, such as the availability of weekend hours, may be relatively unimportant to another. Other professionals with whom the doctor works, such as nurses and fellow physicians, may not be reliable sources of information as they may hesitate to say negative things about a colleague. However, should you hear any negative comments from the doctor's colleagues, consider it a sign to look

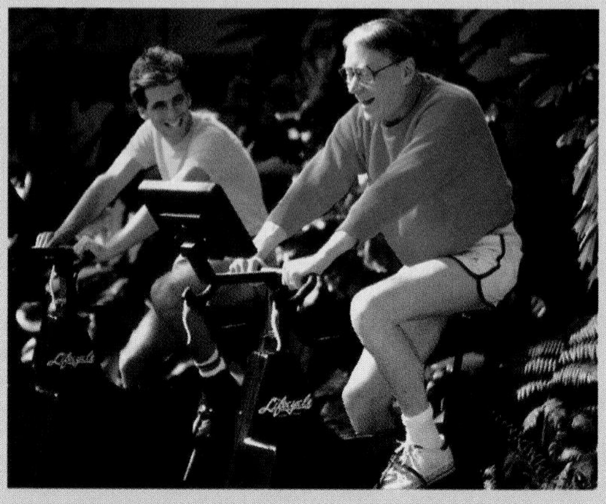

***Striving for Wellness*** What changes in your lifestyle and habits can you make to optimize your health and well-being?

**Primary care physician** A physician who provides a patient with regular, ongoing medical care and makes recommendations to

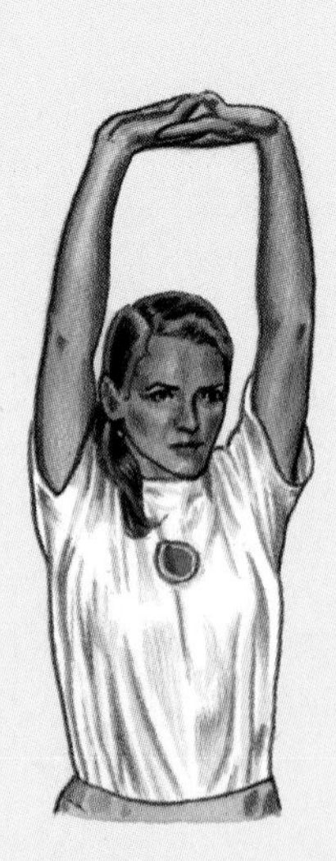

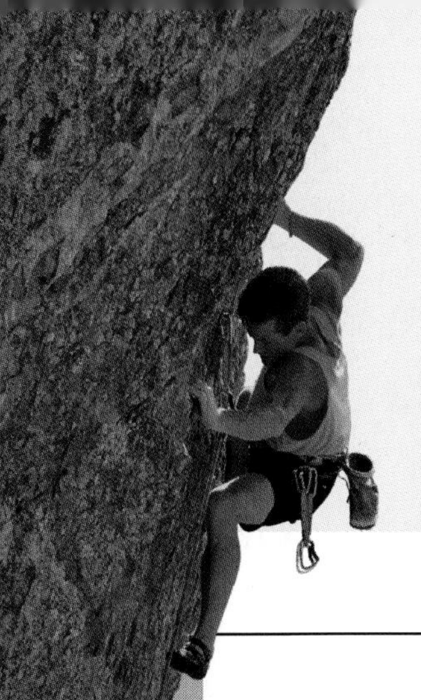

## Summing Up

*Located at the end of each chapter,* ***Summing Up*** *encourages active review by using a question-and-answer format that corresponds to the section headings within the chapter.*

# SUMMING UP

## Questions and Answers

### WHAT IS HEALTH?

**1. What is health?** Physical health is the soundness of your body. We can also speak of such other aspects or dimensions of health as psychological health, spiritual health, social health, and environmental health.

**2. What is wellness?** Wellness refers to a state of optimum health, which is characterized by active efforts to maximize one's health and well-being.

### STRIVING FOR WELLNESS

**3. What are the factors involved in making changes in health behavior?** Factors involved in changing health behavior include predisposing factors (e.g., beliefs, attitudes, knowledge, expectancies, values), enabling factors (e.g., skills or abilities, physical and mental capabilities, and availability and accessibility of resources), and reinforcing factors (praise and support from self and others; internal reinforcement).

**4. What are some general guidelines for making healthy behavior changes?** These include setting reasonable goals, approaching goals gradually, identifying specific behaviors you want to change, tracking problem behavior, acquiring information you need to know, adopting an internal locus of control, challenging negative thinking, not giving up when you give in, and making healthy habits a part of your lifestyle.

### HEALTHY PEOPLE 2000—INTO THE NEW MILLENNIUM

**5. What is *Healthy People 2000*?** This is the title of a government work, published in 1990, that established three main health goals and set some 300 specific objectives for the nation by the year 2000. The major goals are to increase the span of healthy life, to reduce health disparities among Americans, and to achieve access to preventive services for all Americans.

**6. How is the nation doing in meeting these objectives, according to the 1995 midcourse review?** It's a mixed picture. Progress is being made in about two-thirds of the objectives on which we have collected data. For example, there has been a decline in deaths from heart disease, cancer, and stroke—the three leading causes of death. On the other hand, there has been a small *decline* in the health-related quality of life, and health differences between white people and people from ethnic minority groups persist.

### HUMAN DIVERSITY AND HEALTH—NATIONS WITHIN THE NATION

**7. What are some ethnic differences in health?** Poorer, less educated groups of people have shorter life expectancies than better-educated groups. There are disproportionate numbers of deaths from AIDS among African Americans and Hispanic Americans. African Americans are most likely to have hypertension and sickle-cell anemia. The outcome in cancer is worse for African Americans, apparently because of later diagnosis and treatment. Hispanic Americans are less likely to receive regular medical care than either African Americans or non-Hispanic white Americans.

**8. What are some gender differences in health?** Women live longer than men do, in part because men are less likely to seek preventive health care and early diagnosis of troubling symptoms. Women are less likely than men to develop heart disease (before menopause) but more likely to develop arthritis and osteoporosis.

### CRITICAL THINKING AND HEALTH

**9. What is critical thinking?** Critical thinking is a tool we can use to evaluate information about health. It is characterized by skepticism and by thoughtful analysis of arguments.

**10. What are some features of critical thinking?** These include analyzing definitions of terms and premises of arguments; evaluating evidence; and avoiding oversimplification and overgeneralization.

## References and Suggested Readings

### SMART REFERENCES FROM SCIENTIFIC AMERICAN


**Zorpette, G. Dentistry: Electric Smile Aid.** *Scientific American,* 274(5) (May 1996), 26. **R0101**


### SUGGESTED READINGS


**Kunz, J. R. M., and Finkel, A. J. (Eds).** *The American Medica Family Medical Guide* (Revised and Updated). House, 1987. A flowcha


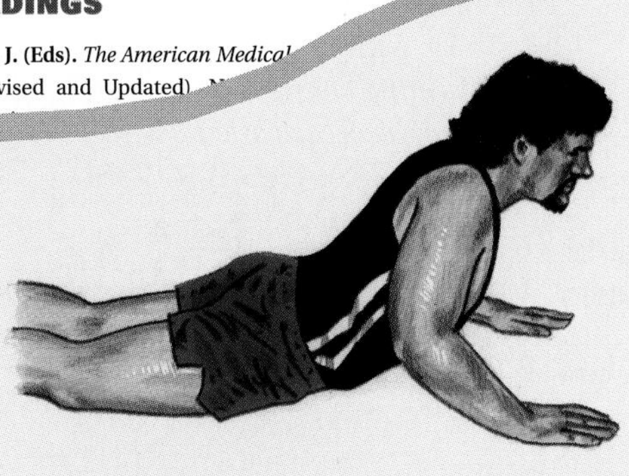

# THE SMART TEXTBOOK

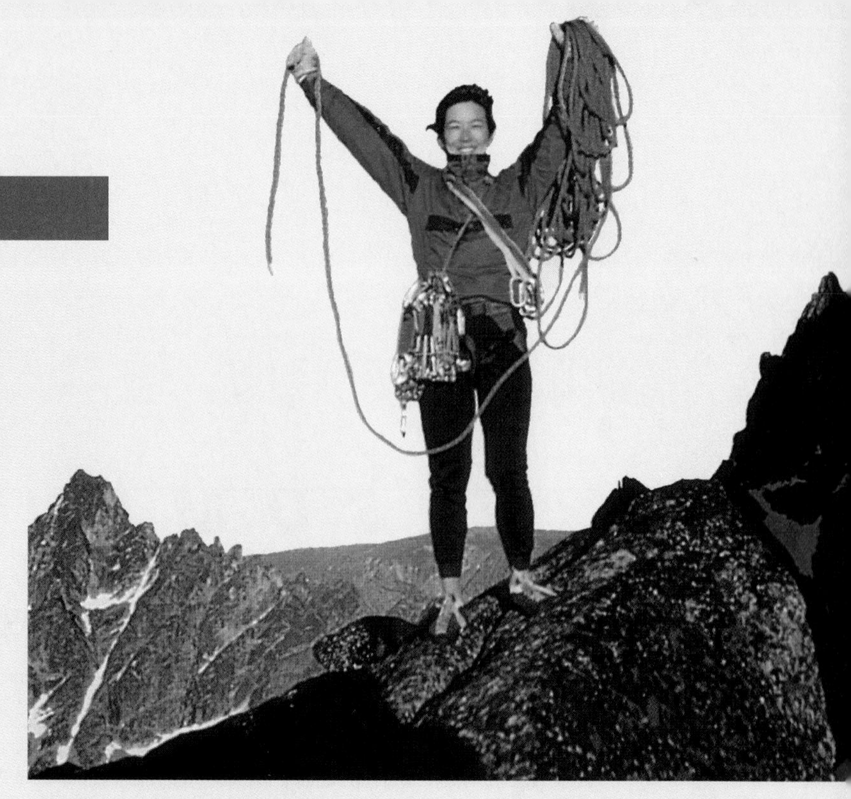

**Health in the New Millennium** is the first ever **Smart Textbook™**—a textbook thoughtfully integrated with its companion CD-ROM to provide the ultimate learning experience. Created by the authors using a patent-pending technology, it offers students the opportunity to access a seamless flow of information without breaking stride. The textbook guides students through contemporary coverage, enhanced with the latest research, of the topics that concern them most, including wellness, sexuality, pregnancy and contraception, diet and exercise, psychological disorders, and the effects of alcohol and drugs. Special icons in the text indicate when to go to the CD-ROM for additional information.

**The CD-ROM** The CD-ROM component contains a number of innovative learning features:

**Video**
Anti-aging drugs: Hope or hype?
**V1904**

- ***Health Videos*** Our 23 video segments highlight important topics in **Health in the New Millennium.** Some segments feature interviews with major figures in health, focusing on issues and new technologies related to topics including AIDS, obesity, psychotherapy, and cardiovascular medicine. Other videos feature students' perspectives on taking charge of their health.

**Smart Quiz**
**Q0504**

- ***Smart Quizzes*** These self-scoring tests help students assess their understanding as they progress through the text.

**Take Charge**
Become assertive
**C0202**

- ***Take Charge*** Similar to the corresponding sections in the textbook, these applications help students analyze and improve their health-related attitudes and behaviors. Among the many topics included are *"Coping with Loneliness," "Your Asthma Can be Controlled,"* and *"Preventing HIV and AIDS: What You Can Do."*

**Talking Glossary**
Carotenoids
**G0504**

- ***Talking Glossary™*** This unique feature allows students to hear pronunciations of selected key terms.

**HealthCheck**
Fitness and heart disease IQ test
**H0701**

- ***HealthCheck*** Additional self-assessment tools developed by federal health agencies, the authors, and other sources help students clarify their thinking about topics that are important to them, for example, *"Fear of Fat Scale," "Can Your Kitchen Pass the Food Safety Test?"(FDA), "Are You Having an Identity Crisis?"* These are also available in paper form in the ***Paper CD.***

**Close-up**
Stress and cancer
**T0301**

- ***Close-up*** A world of health information is brought home with over 300 health documents from government, professional, and academic sources such as the CDC; National Cancer Institute; National Institute on Aging; National Heart, Lung, and Blood Institute; and the FDA. Some of these resources include: *"FDA Highlights: Women's Health," "Taking a Shot at Allergy Relief,"* and *"DDT and Breast Cancer."*

**Smart Reference**
Chewing the fat
**R0501**

- ***Smart References*** A selection of health-related articles from the nation's leading popular science magazine, **SCIENTIFIC AMERICAN,** extend understanding.

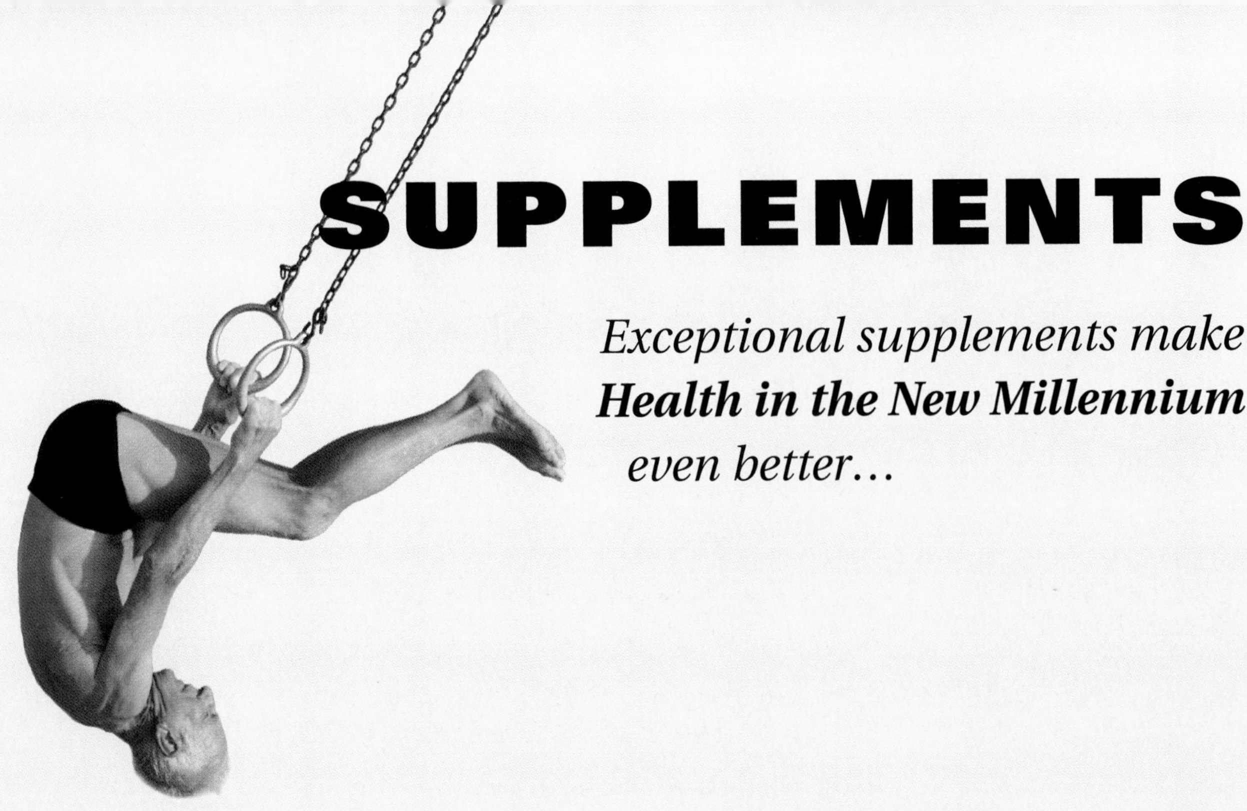

# SUPPLEMENTS

*Exceptional supplements make* ***Health in the New Millennium*** *even better...*

- The **Smart Textbook™ CD-ROM** Encourages students to delve into videos, additional readings, self-questionnaires, quizzes, and the **Talking Glossary™** to enhance their understanding of material covered by the text. Instructors can use the CD-ROM to enhance class presentations.

- **Paper CD** Shrink-wrapped with each text, contains quizzes and ***HealthCheck*** questionnaires from the CD-ROM for students who don't have a CD-ROM drive or who wish to study away from their computers.

- **Health Website** An online Worth resource specifically geared toward students and instructors in health courses; provides cross-links to other health resources on the net, downloads the latest health information, and offers a special ***"Ask the Authors"*** mailbox for inquiries from course instructors.

- **Scientific American Frontiers Videos** Features health segments from the popular, nationally broadcast television series hosted by Alan Alda; available for classroom use.

- **Study Guide** By Beverly A. Drinnin of Des Moines Area Community College; incorporates a variety of features and exercises designed to help students master concepts presented in the text, including summary, fill-in-the-blank, short-answer, matching, and true-false exercises; "Issues to Think About"; crossword puzzles of key terms; and other activities. Answers to all questions, with text page references, are located at the back.

- **Instructor's Resources** Also by Beverly Drinnin of Des Moines Area Community College; contains brief overviews of each text chapter, extended class outlines that include references to other supplementary material, suggested class discussion topics and student activities, and a film and video list.

- **Test Bank** By Gary Piggrem of DeVry Institute of Technology; contains approximately 170 multiple-choice questions per chapter (textbook heading, page number, level of difficulty, question type, and correct answer provided for each question). Instructors can custom-design their own tests with the ***Computerized Test-Generation System,*** available for Windows and Macintosh systems.

- **Transparencies** Approximately 100 illustrations from the textbook are provided on acetate transparencies.

**health** *in the new millennium*

# Health in the New Millennium

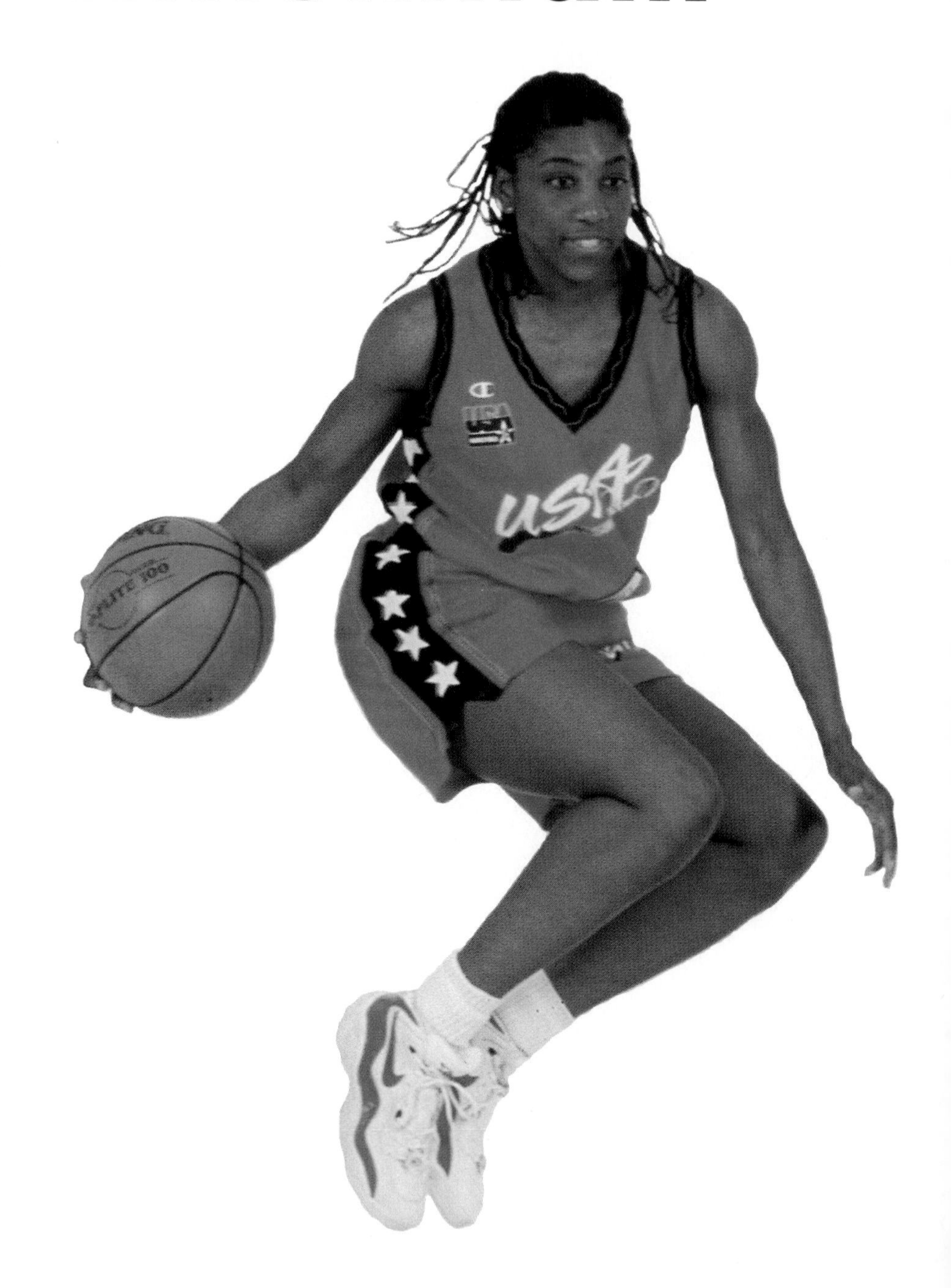

## DID YOU KNOW THAT

- There are nearly 1 million *preventable* deaths in the United States each year? p.14
- It is unhealthy to be poor? p.17
- Women have historically been excluded from many medical research studies? p.18
- Hispanic Americans visit doctors less often than either African Americans or non-Hispanic white Americans? p.18
- You can obtain listings and abstracts of scientific studies from major medical journals by using your home computer? p.22
- Medical boards do not routinely evaluate physicians' skills? p.24
- You should look for a doctor who is board-certified, not just board-eligible, in his or her specialty? p.25
- Brushing your teeth too hard can eventually strip the enamel from your teeth, causing heat and cold sensitivities and damaging your gums? p.26

*We live at a time of great technological advances in medicine and the wider scientific community. Doctors today can thread a tiny balloon into a clogged artery and then inflate it to clear away blockages that might otherwise lead to a heart attack. They can use viruses to ferry cancer-killing drugs directly to malignant tumors. They can transplant donated organs, giving recipients a new lease on life. New technologies even offer promise of correcting genetic defects by substituting healthy genes for defective or missing genes. Other advances offer hope of slowing down or even reversing some of the effects of aging.*

*Technological advances raise hopes of curing or preventing many of the illnesses and maladies that afflict us today and shorten our life spans. Throughout this text we introduce you to the latest medical advances that promise to shape health care in the new millennium. Yet this book is really more about you than about medical science. It is about your role in protecting and enhancing your own personal health by taking charge of your health-related behavior.*

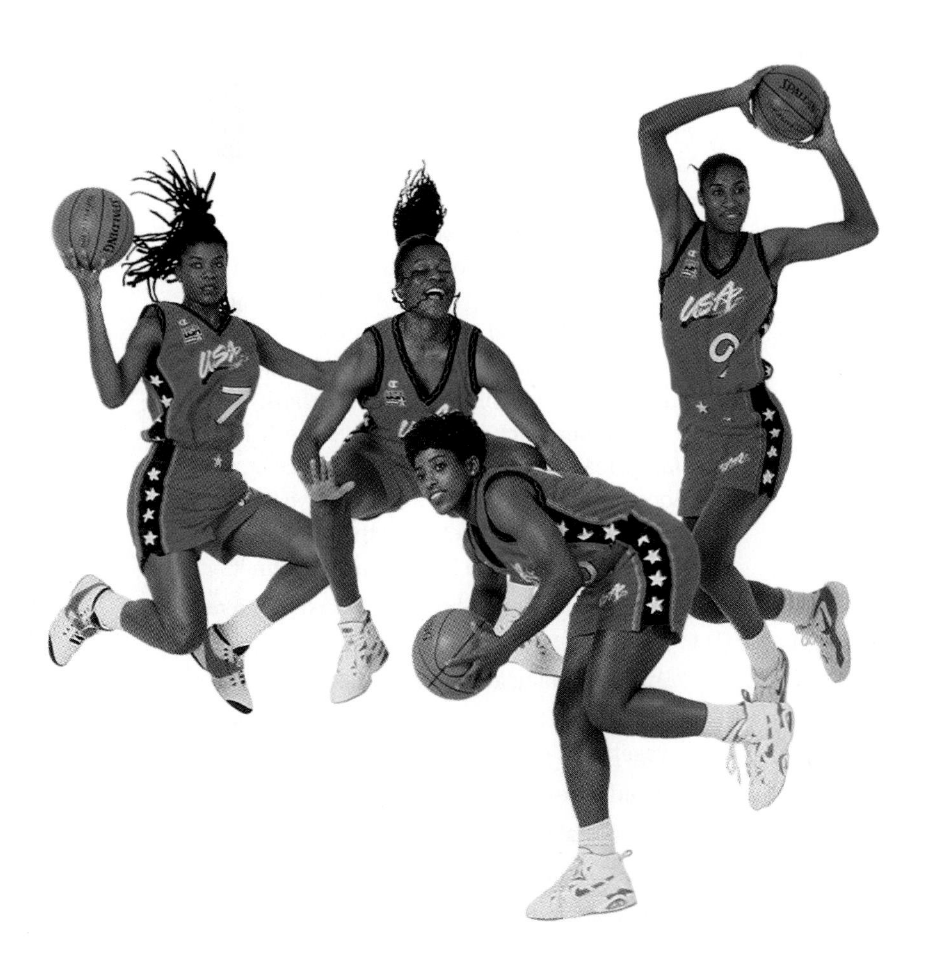

# 1

The best way to safeguard your health and increase your chances of leading a healthier and longer life is to adopt a healthy lifestyle. Factors such as proper diet, weight control, regular exercise, and avoidance of harmful substances, such as tobacco and drugs, play critical roles in determining health and longevity. They are pivotal in determining your risk of many diseases, including the nation's leading killers: heart disease, cancer, and stroke. Preventive health practices such as keeping vaccinations up to date are other examples of health-enhancing behaviors. So too is early detection, such as making sure to have regular medical checkups. Early detection can detect serious diseases at their most curable stages. Avoiding unsafe sexual practices can protect you against sexually transmitted diseases, including AIDS. Washing your hands regularly, especially after using the bathroom, can keep potentially dangerous microbes at bay. Taking precautions when hiking in the woods, or even when playing in the backyard, can help protect you and your family from Lyme disease.

This book focuses on ways of taking charge of your health. The ***Take Charge*** sections at the end of each chapter describe specific ways of putting the information contained in the chapter to work for you in enhancing your health. Taking charge of your health includes the following:

- *Becoming more aware of health risks.* A health risk is a factor that increases the chances of developing a disease. Some factors, like genetics, you cannot control—at least not yet. Some you can control, like diet and exercise patterns. Knowing the health risks associated with specific health problems can alert you to the steps to take to reduce these risks. For example, the risks of certain birth defects are tied to a lack of folic acid, a B vitamin (see Chapter 5). Pregnant women can greatly reduce the risk of these birth defects by consuming sufficient amounts of the vitamin (400 mcg daily).
- *Keeping informed.* Health developments are reported at a dizzying pace. Some information challenges long-held assumptions, such as the belief that vigorous, aerobic exercise is the only form of exercise that has health benefits. (See Chapter 7 for a discussion of the health benefits of regular moderate exercise.) Other developments reflect new directions in prevention and treatment, such as the finding that low daily doses of aspirin can reduce the risk of heart attacks in people with heart disease (see Chapter 17). However, not all information that reaches us through the popular media is trustworthy. We need to develop critical thinking skills—discussed later in the chapter—to evaluate what we read and hear.
- *Practicing preventive behaviors.* A key aspect of health promotion is prevention. Preventive health care involves undergoing regular cancer screening examinations, performing self-examinations (breast self-exams for women and testicular self-exams for men), keeping vaccinations current, practicing healthy behaviors such as exercising regularly and following a nutritionally sound diet, and avoiding unsafe behaviors such as reckless driving, smoking, and excessive drinking. Throughout this text you'll find features on prevention that suggest steps you can take to safeguard your health.

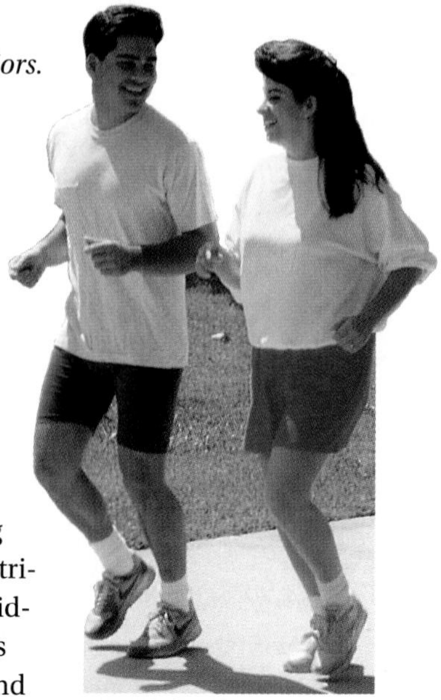

***Practicing Healthy Behaviors*** Adopting healthy habits, including regular exercise, can help protect your health and prevent disease.

- *Becoming a knowledgeable consumer of health care services.* Do you have a primary care physician? Do you have health insurance, and if so, do you know whether it provides adequate coverage? Are you a member of an HMO, and if so, do you know how to obtain health care services? Do you know what limits might apply on the use of specialist services or emergency care? In this chapter's ***Take Charge*** feature, we offer suggestions about choosing a physician. In Chapter 23 we focus on the health care system and the importance of becoming an active health care consumer.
- *Changing your health behavior.* Take a moment to answer a few questions: *Do you . . .*

  Avoid smoking and other tobacco use?

  Eat at least five servings of fresh fruits and vegetables daily?

  Avoid excessive use of alcohol?

  Limit intake of dietary fat?

  Avoid unsafe sexual practices?

  Avoid illicit drugs?

Use prescription drugs wisely?

Have a carbon monoxide detector and a smoke detector in your home?

Maintain your weight within a healthy level?

Always wear seat belts in the car?

This is but a small sample of health-enhancing behaviors. If you answered "no" to any of these questions, we invite you to take stock of your behavior again at the end of the semester to see if we haven't persuaded you by then to make healthful changes in your behavior.

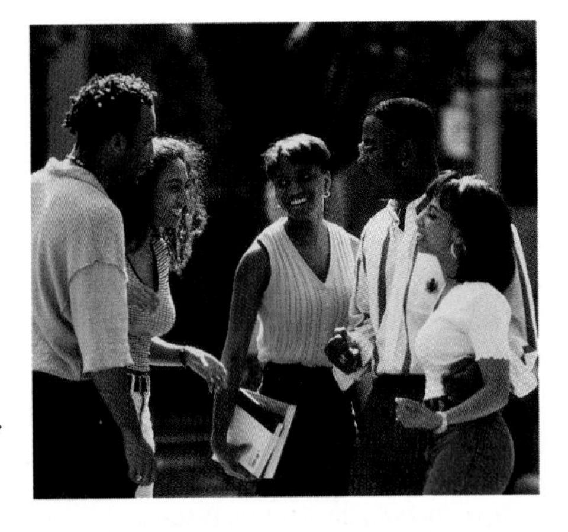

***How's Your Social Health?*** Your ability to relate well to others is an important component of your overall health.

## WHAT IS HEALTH?

Many people think of **health** as the absence of disease. True, people who are healthy are free of disease. But health involves more. It involves vitality, vigor, and general physical and mental well-being. Perhaps the best definition of health was one espoused by the ancient Greeks: *a sound mind in a sound body.* Having a "sound body" or physical health is an important component of your overall health. Yet people are more than physical beings. They are also psychological, social, even spiritual beings. Thus we can also speak of these other dimensions of health: psychological health, social health, and spiritual health. We can also speak about a dimension of health that relates to the relationship between the individual and his or her physical environment.

**Video**
The quest
**V0101**

### Dimensions of Health

**Physical health** refers to soundness of body. It involves such aspects of your physical being as your weight and body shape, the sharpness of your senses, the ways in which your body functions, and the presence—or absence—of disease or infirmity.

**Psychological health** or "soundness of mind" involves the ability to think clearly, to adjust to life's demands, to solve problems, to pursue goals, and to maintain your emotions on an even keel. People who are psychologically healthy are not free of negative emotions, like anxiety and depression. Yet their emotional responses are appropriate to the situations they face. They may feel anxious when taking an important test, or sad when they experience loss or disappointment. However, their emotional responses are not prolonged or so severe that their ability to function becomes impaired. Nor are they prone to angry outbursts that affect their relationships with others or lead to aggressive behavior.

Our physical health is intertwined with our psychological health. Physical illness may affect us emotionally, leading to depression or anxiety, or make it difficult to maintain an active social life. Emotional factors can also impair physical health. Chronic anger or hostility can increase the risks of developing coronary heart disease or suffering a heart attack. Lingering depression or anxiety can make us vulnerable to physical health problems by impairing the body's immune system.[1]

**Social health** is the ability to relate effectively to other people as family members, lovers, friends, fellow students or workers, professors or supervisors. People need people to lead healthy and fulfilling lives. To paraphrase the sixteenth-century English poet John Donne, *No man, and no woman, is an island, entire of itself.* Social stressors such as divorce, unemployment, marital discord, and lack of social support can impair the immune system, increasing our vulnerability to physical illness.[2] Lack of social reinforcement can also be a prelude to depression. On the other hand, people may be better able to handle the challenges of coping with a serious physical or mental illness if they have supportive relationships with friends and loved ones.

**Health** Soundness of body and mind; a state of vigor and vitality that permits one to function effectively physically, psychologically, and socially.

**Physical health** Soundness of body.

**Psychological health** Soundness of mind, characterized by a cluster of characteristics such as accurate perceptions, clear thinking, emotional stability, and adaptive behavior.

**Social health** The ability to relate effectively to family members, intimate partners, friends, and work associates.

**Spiritual health** refers to the attainment of transcendental meaning, a connectedness to a higher order or purpose beyond yourself. For some, this involves a commitment to a particular religion. For others, it involves a commitment to aesthetic values, such as the enjoyment or creation of music, poetry, or visual arts. For still others, spirituality involves a commitment to serving the needy or the larger community. Spiritual experience permits people to transcend the ordinary events of daily life. It imbues their lives with meaning and purpose.

Unlike other dimensions of health that pertain to the individual, **environmental health** involves the relationship between the individual and the environment. We depend on the environment to sustain us. Yet the environment can also threaten our health and our very survival. The relationship we have with the environment works both ways: We affect the environment, for better or for worse, and the environment affects us. If we are to thrive in the new millennium, we need to be committed to preserving, protecting, and cleaning up the environment.

What do you envision when you think of the environment? Is it vast tracts of wilderness and deep, rolling oceans? Or do you think of endangered species and shore birds coated in oil from oil spills? Do you conjure up visions of billowing summer storm clouds and refreshing rain, or do you imagine crowded sidewalks and acid rain? All these—the beauty and the horror—affect environmental health. Factors that threaten environmental health include extremes of temperature, pollution, exposure to lead and other toxic substances, and ultraviolet radiation from the sun.

### Health and Wellness

**Wellness** refers to a state of maximal or optimum health. People who achieve wellness have developed a lifestyle that enhances their health, protects them from disease, and maximizes their physical, psychological, spiritual, and social well-being. They follow a healthy diet, keep their weight within a recommended range, get sufficient sleep, keep physically fit, find meaning in life, develop and maintain healthy relationships, avoid using harmful substances, and take steps to protect themselves from disease-causing agents.

**Spiritual health** The attainment of a meaningful life by connecting to social, religious, or aesthetic experiences beyond oneself.

**Environmental health** The relationship between organisms and their physical environment that allows them to survive and flourish.

**Wellness** A state of optimum health, characterized by active efforts to maximize one's physical health and well-being.

Figure 1.1 shows many of the factors that influence health and wellness—physical, psychological, spiritual, social, environmental, and sociocultural. Sociocultural factors that figure prominently in health and wellness include socioeconomic status, availability of health care and health insurance, and cultural patterns in diet.

**think about it!**

- **How would you describe your own physical, psychological, spiritual, and social health?**
- **To what extent does your environment either sustain or threaten your health?**
- **What is the difference between health and wellness? Are you doing what you can to optimize your health? If not, why not?**

Smart Quiz Q0101

## STRIVING FOR WELLNESS

Striving for wellness involves making changes in your lifestyle and behavior that enhance your health and well-being and improve the quality of your life.

### Factors Involved in Changing Health Behavior

When asked about quitting smoking, the writer Mark Twain quipped that it was easy. He'd done it a dozen times. The fact is that changing unhealthy habits and behaviors is never easy. Like Twain, even people who succeed in making healthy changes in behavior often return to their former unhealthy ways. Making changes in your health behavior, and maintaining these changes, depends on several factors, including predisposing factors, enabling factors, and reinforcing factors.

**Predisposing Factors** These are factors that either promote or hinder change, including beliefs, attitudes, knowledge, expectancies, and values. Holding the belief that smoking is dangerous only to people with a family history of lung

**Figure 1.1** ***Factors Affecting Health and Wellness***

**Sociocultural factors in health**

Gender
Ethnic identity
Socioeconomic status
Level of education
Prejudice and discrimination
Social climate in the workplace, sexual harassment
Health-related cultural and religious beliefs and practices
Health promotion programs in the workplace or the community
Health-related legislation
Availability of health insurance
Availability of and accessibility to health care providers

**Psychological factors in health**

Clarity and accuracy of one's perception of the world and of oneself
Self-esteem
Self-acceptance
Problem-solving ability
Ability to think clearly and logically
Ability to think creatively
Openness to new ideas
Seeking (or avoiding) information about health risks
Maintaining curiosity and interest in life
Self-confidence (beliefs that "I can" or "I can't")
Psychological hardiness (psychological attributes associated with resiliency to stress)
Optimism vs. pessimism
Internal vs. external locus of control
Coronary-prone (Type A) personality
Emotional stability
Presence or absence of severe psychological disorders (e.g., schizophrenia, bipolar disorder)

**Physical factors in health**

Family history of illness
Age
Exposure to infectious pathogens (e.g., bacteria and viruses)
Immune system functioning
Inoculations
Medication history
Congenital disabilities, perinatal complications
Physiological conditions (e.g., hypertension, serum cholesterol level)
Diet (intake of calories, fats, fiber, vitamins, etc.)
Consumption of alcohol and other drugs
Cigarette smoking (or use of smokeless tobacco products)
Level of physical activity
Sleep patterns

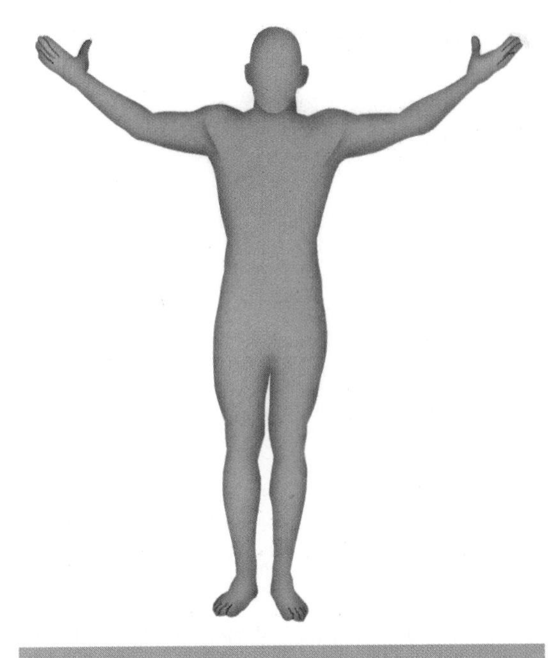

**Environmental factors in health**

Water safety and quality
Solid waste treatment and sanitation
Belonging or contributing to groups that protect the environment
Air, water, and soil pollution
Indoor air pollution
Radiation
Ozone depletion
Natural disasters (earthquakes, floods, hurricanes, drought, extremes of temperature, tornadoes)
Radon
Presence of toxic chemicals in foods, the workplace, and the larger environment
Architecture (e.g., accessibility for disabled people, injury-preventive design, nontoxic construction materials, air quality, noise insulation)

**Spiritual factors in health**

Connectedness with what is beyond oneself
Belief in the meaning or order of the universe
Identification with a religious tradition
Attainment of a sense of meaning or purpose in life
Appreciation of the beauty in the arts and the environment
Commitment to family and community
Involvement in one's community
Perceiving oneself as part of the larger scheme of things

**Social factors in health**

Interpersonal/social skills
Relationships with other students, professors, and co-workers
Friendship patterns
Romantic relationships
Relationships with family members
Availability and use of social support (as opposed to peer rejection or isolation)
Major life changes such as death of a spouse or divorce

cancer can increase the likelihood of smoking in people without a family history of the disease. Young people who think that smoking is "cool" or glamorous (after all, many movies today feature Hollywood stars smoking on screen) are more likely to take up smoking than are their peers who hold more negative attitudes toward smoking.

Knowledge can encourage change. Millions of people in the U.S. quit smoking after the Surgeon General in 1964 first reported on the dangers of smoking. Knowledge about the risk factors in diseases such as heart disease and cancer can lead people to make the kinds of changes in their habits and behavior that reduce their risks of these diseases. Unfortunately, knowledge may not be enough to encourage healthy changes in behavior. Most smokers today know the dangers of smoking but continue to smoke. Most sexually active people know the dangers of unprotected sex, but many fail to practice safer sex.

Psychologists recognize that expectations play an important role in change. Young people who expect that drinking alcoholic beverages will make them more popular, sexier, or outgoing are more likely to use alcohol than their peers who don't hold these expectations.

A person's values—the importance one places on things—are an important determinant of change. Young people who value their popularity over their future health would be more likely to succumb to peer pressures to smoke than would those who place a greater value on health.

**Enabling Factors** Enabling factors promote change. These include skills or abilities, physical and mental capabilities, and availability and accessibility of resources. You are more likely to begin an exercise program, or stick with one, if it is convenient and accessible (a gym around the corner rather than half an hour's drive away), if you have developed the skills and abilities needed to accomplish the task (you can follow the steps in an aerobics dance class or serve a tennis ball), and possess the physical and mental capabilities needed to perform the behavior (the strength, coordination, endurance, and concentration, for example). Access to health care services is another enabling factor. People who lack health insurance or access to health care facilities may not receive the preventive care they need.

**Reinforcing Factors** Reinforcing factors include the praise and support you receive from others and from yourself that encourages healthy behavior. If you shrug off the healthy changes you make in your behavior (e.g., starting a beginners' exercise class) by saying to yourself, "it's no big deal," you'll be less likely to keep at it than if you give yourself credit for getting started. You're also more likely to continue making healthy changes if you receive reinforcing comments from friends or loved ones than if your efforts go unnoticed. To maintain your commitment over time, however, reinforcement must become internalized. Whether it is losing weight, quitting smoking, or maintaining an exercise routine, you need to feel that what you are doing will ultimately benefit *you*—to feel better about yourself and to live a healthier life.

Now let's turn to you. Are you on the road to wellness or still stuck in the driveway? The questionnaire in the ***HealthCheck*** on page 10 encourages you to examine your health behaviors.

## Making Changes

Throughout this book we encourage you to make healthy changes in behavior, including changes in diet, exercise patterns, stress management, and relationships with others. Here we offer some general guidelines for making healthful changes in behavior:

**Set Reasonable Goals** Strive toward achieving attainable goals. For most of us mere mortals, that may mean taking a brisk walk or swimming 30 minutes several times a week, not training to qualify for the next Olympics. If you are overweight, set a goal for yourself of achieving a healthy weight (see Chapter 6), not an unrealistic weight or dangerously thin weight.

**Approach Goals Gradually** Nibble, don't bite. For instance, begin an exercise program slowly, working up gradually to meet your training goals. Don't overtax your muscles or your endurance. Develop a timetable for approaching your health goals step by step. Sign a contract with yourself that specifies specific goals each week you expect to achieve. Keep the contract handy or post it on the refrigerator as a daily reminder.

**Identify Specific Behaviors You Want to Change** Rather than saying to yourself, "I need to follow a healthier diet," identify the specific food choices that constitute a healthy diet. Lay out a specific menu plan that meets the nutritional guidelines described in Chapter 5. Rather than say,

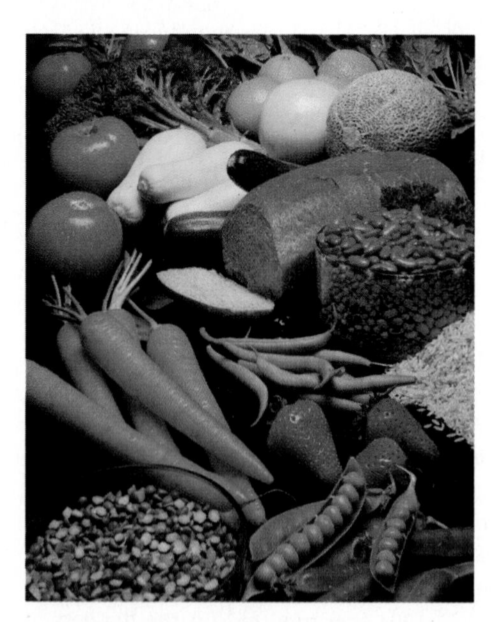

***Making Healthy Choices*** What changes in your diet and lifestyle can you make to lead a healthier life?

"I need to do more exercise," set specific exercise goals for yourself: "I plan to work out on the treadmill for 30 minutes three times a week. . . . I plan to go to an aerobics class twice a week."

**Track Your Problem Behavior** Want to change unhealthy habits, like excessive snacking? Track the problem behavior for a week a two, noting where it took place, when it occurred, who you were with, and how you felt before and after. Notice any patterns that emerge, such as a tendency to overeat when you have unstructured time on your hands. Develop a plan of action based on what you've learned. For example, you might begin filling in those empty hours with interesting activities.

**Acquire Information You Need to Know** Use this textbook and other resources (the library, your instructor, the Internet, etc.) to obtain the information you need to make healthful changes in behavior. Chapter 5, for example, will inform you about nutritional guidelines for designing a healthy diet. Chapter 7 will help get you started in designing an exercise program you can live with. Other chapters provide information about stress management (Chapter 3), building healthy relationships (Chapter 8), practicing safer sexual behaviors (Chapter 16), controlling your anger (Chapter 21), and protecting yourself from infectious diseases (Chapters 15 and 16) and chronic diseases such as heart disease (Chapter 17) and cancer (Chapter 18).

Finding information is one thing. Thinking critically about the information you find is another. Later in the chapter we focus on developing critical thinking skills to help you carefully evaluate health information and health claims.

**Adopt an Internal Locus of Control** Who's in charge here? The answer can be *you*, if you decide it will be you. People with an internal locus of control believe that they are in control of what happens to them, for better or for worse. In contrast, people with an external locus of control tend to see their fates as being out of their hands. If you are more of an "external," consider an attitude shift in the other direction. Begin asking yourself, how can I make a difference? What can I do to enhance my health? True, there are no guarantees of good health and long life. But *you* can help shift the odds in your favor and move ahead on the road to wellness by making wise choices about diet, drinking, smoking, exercise, and so on.

**HealthCheck**
Locus of control scale
H0101

**Challenge Negative Thinking** Negative thoughts and beliefs can undermine your confidence and motivation. Replace negative thoughts like "I just can't succeed. . . . Nothing ever changes" with rational alternatives: "Think positive. . . . Take it a step at a time. . . . I can do this." Negative beliefs about yourself ("I'm stupid"), the world ("This school is awful"), and the future ("Nothing will ever work out for me") can become a recipe for depression and hopelessness. Identify and correct negative beliefs (see Chapter 4) to gain better control over your moods and help keep you motivated to achieve your health goals.

**Don't Give Up When You Give In** Don't give up on yourself if you have an occasional slip. You might miss an exercise session or lose a battle with a chocolate eclair. Becoming discouraged whenever you experience a setback can lead you to give up your health goals. Recognize that an occasional slip is inevitable. After all, no one is perfect. The best response to a slip is to pick yourself up and get back on track.

**Make Healthy Habits a Part of Your Lifestyle** Make your exercise routine a regular part of your weekly schedule. Climb stairs rather than use the elevator to get to class or work. Park at the farther end of the lot, and practice walking briskly to class or to the mall. Make unhealthy behavior difficult or impossible. You can't reach for the chocolate cheesecake in your refrigerator if you have left it at the supermarket (that is, not bought it).

### think about it!

- **Identify the predisposing factors, enabling factors, and reinforcing factors that affect your health behavior. To what extent do these factors encourage healthy changes? To what extent do they hinder healthy changes? What can you do to control these factors?**
- **Select a health behavior you want to change, such as modifying your eating behavior, developing a regular exercise routine, or quitting smoking. How might you use the guidelines for change to develop and implement a behavior change plan to achieve your goal?**

**Smart Quiz**
Q0102

# Health Check

## Striving for Wellness—How Do You Measure Up?

All of us want to be healthy and achieve wellness, but many of us have not taken stock of our health habits. This questionnaire is designed to help you examine your health habits with respect to each of the dimensions of health and related health concerns, such as exercise and fitness, accident prevention, and so on.

Read each of the following items. Circle the number that best corresponds to your honest response. Add up your scores for each category. Then use the guidelines that follow to interpret your scores.

| **Physical Health** | *Rarely or Never* | *Sometimes* | *Usually* | *Always* |
|---|---|---|---|---|
| 1. I take care of my health. | 1 | 2 | 3 | 4 |
| 2. I try to keep my body healthy and fit. | 1 | 2 | 3 | 4 |
| 3. I am screened regularly for the health problems that are likely to affect people with my family history. | 1 | 2 | 3 | 4 |
| 4. I am free of chronic or disabling diseases. | 1 | 2 | 3 | 4 |
| 5. I feel I am basically in good health. | 1 | 2 | 3 | 4 |
| 6. I am not bothered by allergies. | 1 | 2 | 3 | 4 |
| 7. I do not lose much time at work or school because of illness. | 1 | 2 | 3 | 4 |
| 8. I get at least 7 to 8 hours of sleep at night and wake up feeling rested and refreshed. | 1 | 2 | 3 | 4 |

**Physical health score** ________

| **Exercise and Physical Fitness** | *Rarely or Never* | *Sometimes* | *Usually* | *Always* |
|---|---|---|---|---|
| 1. I participate in moderately intense physical activity, like walking briskly or working around the house, for at least 30 minutes a day. | 1 | 2 | 3 | 4 |
| 2. I participate in vigorous exercise like running, lap swimming, speed walking, or aerobics dance classes for at least 20 to 30 minutes a day at least three times a week. | 1 | 2 | 3 | 4 |
| 3. I lead an active life. | 1 | 2 | 3 | 4 |
| 4. I am about as physically fit as most people my age. | 1 | 2 | 3 | 4 |
| 5. I spend much of leisure time involved in active sports or physical activities like bicycling, hiking, swimming, gardening, or playing competitive sports. | 1 | 2 | 3 | 4 |
| 6. I have good physical endurance. | 1 | 2 | 3 | 4 |
| 7. I participate in muscle-strengthening exercises at least several times a week. | 1 | 2 | 3 | 4 |
| 8. I have enough energy to get through the day without feeling fatigued. | 1 | 2 | 3 | 4 |

**Exercise and fitness score** ________

| **Alcohol, Tobacco, and Other Drug Use** | *Rarely or Never* | *Sometimes* | *Usually* | *Always* |
|---|---|---|---|---|
| 1. I avoid smoking cigarettes. | 1 | 2 | 3 | 4 |
| 2. I avoid all other tobacco use, including pipe smoking, cigar smoking, and smokeless tobacco. | 1 | 2 | 3 | 4 |
| 3. I avoid drinking beer or wine, or if I do drink, I avoid drinking more than 1 or 2 drinks a day. | 1 | 2 | 3 | 4 |
| 4. I avoid drinking in situations in which it would be unsafe to drink. | 1 | 2 | 3 | 4 |
| 5. I avoid binge drinking (drinking five or more drinks in a sitting). | 1 | 2 | 3 | 4 |
| 6. I avoid use of illicit drugs. | 1 | 2 | 3 | 4 |
| 7. I avoid socializing with people who use illicit drugs or drink to excess. | 1 | 2 | 3 | 4 |
| 8. I avoid using alcohol or other drugs to cope with problems or to make me feel more socially confident. | 1 | 2 | 3 | 4 |

**Alcohol, tobacco, and other drug use score** ________

| Preventive Health Practices | Rarely or Never | Sometimes | Usually | Always |
|---|---|---|---|---|
| 1. I regularly visit my doctor for routine checkups. | 1 | 2 | 3 | 4 |
| 2. I have my blood pressure and blood cholesterol checked regularly. | 1 | 2 | 3 | 4 |
| 3. I practice monthly testicular/breast self-exams. | 1 | 2 | 3 | 4 |
| 4. If I engage in sexual intimacy, I practice safer sex. | 1 | 2 | 3 | 4 |
| 5. I avoid excessive exposure to the sun. | 1 | 2 | 3 | 4 |
| 6. I use sunscreen whenever I am out in the sun for more than a few minutes. | 1 | 2 | 3 | 4 |
| 7. I wash my hands after using the bathroom. | 1 | 2 | 3 | 4 |
| 8. I keep my vaccinations up to date. | 1 | 2 | 3 | 4 |

**Preventive health practices score** ________

| Accident Prevention | Rarely or Never | Sometimes | Usually | Always |
|---|---|---|---|---|
| 1. I have a working smoke detector in my home. | 1 | 2 | 3 | 4 |
| 2. I have a working carbon monoxide detector in my home. | 1 | 2 | 3 | 4 |
| 3. I keep household chemicals safely stored. | 1 | 2 | 3 | 4 |
| 4. I wear seat belts whenever I drive or ride in a car. | 1 | 2 | 3 | 4 |
| 5. I make sure that children are securely buckled in a car safety seat or seat belt when riding in a car. | 1 | 2 | 3 | 4 |
| 6. I obey traffic rules when driving. | 1 | 2 | 3 | 4 |
| 7. I wear safety helmets and other recommended safety equipment when bicycling or rollerblading. | 1 | 2 | 3 | 4 |
| 8. I read and follow instructions for proper use of household cleansers, solvents, pesticides, and electrical devices. | 1 | 2 | 3 | 4 |

**Accident prevention score** ________

| Nutrition and Weight Control | Rarely or Never | Sometimes | Usually | Always |
|---|---|---|---|---|
| 1. I limit my intake of fat, including saturated fat. | 1 | 2 | 3 | 4 |
| 2. I limit my intake of high-cholesterol foods such as eggs, liver, and meat. | 1 | 2 | 3 | 4 |
| 3. I follow a nutritionally balanced diet. | 1 | 2 | 3 | 4 |
| 4. I eat five or more servings of fruits and vegetables daily. | 1 | 2 | 3 | 4 |
| 5. I limit the amount of salt and sugar I consume. | 1 | 2 | 3 | 4 |
| 6. I eat food that is broiled or steamed, not fried or sauteed. | 1 | 2 | 3 | 4 |
| 7. I eat high-fiber foods several times a day. | 1 | 2 | 3 | 4 |
| 8. I am careful to keep my weight within a healthy range. | 1 | 2 | 3 | 4 |

**Nutrition and weight control score** ________

| Psychological Health | Rarely or Never | Sometimes | Usually | Always |
|---|---|---|---|---|
| 1. I am able to concentrate on my work at school or on the job. | 1 | 2 | 3 | 4 |
| 2. I have a clear direction in life. | 1 | 2 | 3 | 4 |
| 3. I generally like myself. | 1 | 2 | 3 | 4 |
| 4. I am able to relax and unwind. | 1 | 2 | 3 | 4 |
| 5. I am hopeful about the future. | 1 | 2 | 3 | 4 |
| 6. I enjoy a challenge. | 1 | 2 | 3 | 4 |
| 7. I am able to express my feelings. | 1 | 2 | 3 | 4 |
| 8. I am able to manage the stress in my life. | 1 | 2 | 3 | 4 |

**Psychological health score** ________

*Continued on next page*

| Spiritual Health | *Rarely or Never* | *Sometimes* | *Usually* | *Always* |
|---|---|---|---|---|
| 1. I find meaning in life. | 1 | 2 | 3 | 4 |
| 2. I have a sense of connectedness to something larger than myself, whether it be organized religion, nature, or social causes. | 1 | 2 | 3 | 4 |
| 3. I believe every life has a purpose. | 1 | 2 | 3 | 4 |
| 4. I enjoy the arts—painting and sculpture, dance, good music, or good books. | 1 | 2 | 3 | 4 |
| 5. I believe that I have a worthwhile place in my community. | 1 | 2 | 3 | 4 |
| 6. I try to help people in need without expecting anything in return. | 1 | 2 | 3 | 4 |
| 7. I try to do things that will be of lasting value. | 1 | 2 | 3 | 4 |
| 8. I feel a need to make a difference in people's lives. | 1 | 2 | 3 | 4 |

**Spiritual health score** ______

| Social Health | *Rarely or Never* | *Sometimes* | *Usually* | *Always* |
|---|---|---|---|---|
| 1. I have close friends. | 1 | 2 | 3 | 4 |
| 2. I am able to develop trusting relationships with others. | 1 | 2 | 3 | 4 |
| 3. I can express feelings of liking and love to other people as well as feelings of disappointment and anger. | 1 | 2 | 3 | 4 |
| 4. When there is a problem I can't handle on my own, I usually have or find someone to talk to about it. | 1 | 2 | 3 | 4 |
| 5. I have good relationships with family members. | 1 | 2 | 3 | 4 |
| 6. I am the kind of person who is there for people when I am needed. | 1 | 2 | 3 | 4 |
| 7. I am able to assert myself in a responsible way and not allow others to take advantage of me. | 1 | 2 | 3 | 4 |
| 8. I am respectful of the feelings of others. | 1 | 2 | 3 | 4 |

**Social health score** ______

| Environmental Health | *Rarely or Never* | *Sometimes* | *Usually* | *Always* |
|---|---|---|---|---|
| 1. I keep informed about environmental issues such as the depletion of the ozone layer, the destruction of the rain forests, and acid rain. | 1 | 2 | 3 | 4 |
| 2. I recycle paper, bottles, and aluminum cans. | 1 | 2 | 3 | 4 |
| 3. I am aware of the safety and quality of the water I use. | 1 | 2 | 3 | 4 |
| 4. I participate in or contribute to environmental causes. | 1 | 2 | 3 | 4 |
| 5. I make sure any refuse I produce is properly disposed of. | 1 | 2 | 3 | 4 |
| 6. I avoid use of pesticide sprays in the house or yard, or if I do use them, I am careful to follow all safety instructions. | 1 | 2 | 3 | 4 |
| 7. I wash all fruits and vegetables before eating them. | 1 | 2 | 3 | 4 |
| 8. I make an effort to conserve water use and electricity. | 1 | 2 | 3 | 4 |

**Environmental health score** ______

**Interpreting Your Scores**

**Scores of 24 to 32:** *Congratulations! Give yourself credit for taking charge of your health. You appear to have developed healthy habits and to be moving toward optimal health. Still, there may be room for improvement. Ask yourself what more you can do to move further along on the road to wellness.*

**Scores of 16 to 23:** *You appear to have developed some healthy habits but have considerable room for improvement. Examine responses that are less than "always," especially those that are "sometimes" or "rarely or never." Consider ways of changing your health behavior to improve your score.*

**Scores below 16:** *On balance, it appears you have more negative health habits than positive ones. Unhealthy behaviors can increase your risk of illness and accidents. This book can help you succeed in making healthy changes in behavior. You might also benefit from seeking assistance from your instructor, college health service, or family physician.*

## HEALTHY PEOPLE 2000—INTO THE NEW MILLENNIUM

The *Healthy People 2000* project was initiated by the federal government to promote health and prevent disease among all Americans.[3] The project brought together government health officials, health experts, representatives of voluntary and professional health organizations, business representatives, and individuals. The result was a 1990 publication outlining the nation's major health goals to be achieved by the turn of the new millennium. Three broad health-promotion goals were identified:

**Close-up**
Health, U.S.
**T0101**

- *To increase the span of healthy life for all Americans.* Adding years to the life span is not enough. The goal is to add healthy, fulfilling years. While the average life expectancy is 76 years, the average number of *healthy* years is only 64.[4] For African Americans, the figure is even lower—56 years. Many people thus survive for a number of years in a state of declining health with a poor quality of life.
- *To reduce the health discrepancies among Americans.* There are many nations within our nation. Some **ethnic groups** are more vulnerable to certain diseases than others because of differences in lifestyle, access to health care, and possible genetic factors. Women typically outlive men. One reason is that women seek advice for health problems sooner than men do.
- *To achieve access to preventive services for all Americans.* Some groups, especially ethnic minorities, have less access to preventive health care than others do. Partly because of limited access, they tend to suffer more health problems and stand a greater risk of early death. Thus, one of the major health goals is to remove barriers that limit access to these services.

TABLE 1.1

**Leading Causes of Death in the U.S.A.—1995[7]**

More than 2 million people die each year in the United States and an estimated 1 million are in the process of dying. The leading causes of death overall are heart disease, cancer, and strokes.

| Cause | Deaths |
|---|---|
| Heart disease | 739,000 |
| Cancer | 538,000 |
| Stroke | 158,000 |
| Lung disorders (other than lung cancer) | 105,000 |
| Accidents | 90,000 |
| Pneumonia and flu | 84,000 |
| Diabetes | 59,000 |
| AIDS | 43,000 |
| Suicide | 31,000 |
| Liver disease | 25,000 |

### Midcourse Update

*Healthy People 2000* set 300 specific health objectives. In 1995, a midcourse review was conducted.[5] It showed optimistically that the nation was moving toward more than two-thirds of the objectives on which data have been collected.

Here is some good news based on health data compiled during 1995.[6] In that year there was:

- A decline in deaths from heart disease, cancer, and stroke—the three leading causes of death (see Table 1.1). This is in part because of improvements in medical care, but also because of changes in lifestyle, such as quitting smoking (50% of adults smoked in 1955 vs. about 25% today) and reduced fat intake in our diets. We are also exercising more and watching our weight more closely.
- A record low infant mortality rate (7.5 deaths per 1,000 live births).
- Continued increase in the number of women obtaining early prenatal care (81% began care during the first trimester).
- A decline in the birth rate for unmarried women (to 44.9 per 1,000 unmarried women aged 15 to 44).
- Continued decline in the birth rate for teenage mothers (to 56.9 per 1,000 women aged 15 to 19).
- A decline in the homicide rate.
- Continued increase in life expectancy (75.8 years overall; however, there were continuing differences according to race and gender. Life expectancy for white males was 73.4 years and 65.4 years for African-American males; 79.6 years for white females and 74 years for African-American females).

**Close-up**
Nation's health improving
**T0102**

**Ethnic group** A group of people who are united by their cultural heritage, race, language, and common history.

## Meeting the Nation's Health Goals for the Year 2000

| | Baseline | Update | Target | Progress |
|---|---|---|---|---|
| **HEALTH HABITS** | | | | |
| People exercising regularly | 22% | 24% | 30% | YES |
| Overweight people | 26% | 34% | 20% | NO |
| People with high-fat diets | 36% | 34% | 30% | YES |
| People smoking cigarettes | 29% | 25% | 15% | YES |
| Youth beginning to smoke | 29% | 25% | 15% | YES |
| Alcohol-related automobile deaths (per 100,000 people) | 9.8 | 6.8 | 8.5 | YES |
| Alcohol use among youth aged 12–17 | 25.2% | 18% | 12.6% | YES |
| Marijuana use among youth aged 12–17 | 6.4% | 4.9% | 3.2% | YES |
| Teen-age pregnancies (per 1,000 people) | 71.1 | 74.3 | 50.0 | NO |
| Suicides (per 100,000 people) | 11.7 | 11.2 | 10.5 | YES |
| Homicides (per 100,000 people) | 8.5 | 10.3 | 7.2 | NO |
| Assault injuries (per 100,000 people) | 9.7 | 9.9 | 8.7 | NO |
| **PROTECTING HEALTH AND SAFETY** | | | | |
| People with clean air in their communities | 49.7% | 76.5% | 85% | YES |
| People using automobile safety restraints | 42% | 67% | 85% | YES |
| Work-related deaths (per 100,000 people) | 6 | 5 | 4 | YES |
| Work-related injuries (per 100,000 people) | 7.7 | 7.9 | 6.0 | NO |
| Children with high blood lead level | 234,000 | 93,000 | 0 | YES |
| **HEALTH CARE AND ITS RESULTS** | | | | |
| Low-birth-weight babies | 6.9% | 7.1% | 5.0% | NO |
| Pregnant women with first-trimester care | 76% | 77.7% | 90% | YES |
| Deaths from coronary heart disease (per 100,000 people) | 135 | 114 | 100 | YES |
| Stroke deaths (per 100,000 people) | 30.4 | 26.4 | 20.0 | YES |
| Cholesterol levels (average) | 213 | 205 | 200 | YES |
| Cancer deaths (per 100,000 people) | 134 | 133 | 130 | YES |

**Figure 1.2** ***National Health Goals*** In 1995, the United States Public Health Service issued an interim report on progress toward meeting national health goals set in 1990. These are some of the results.

- A leveling off in the death rate from AIDS (1996 saw even more progress: an actual decrease in the death rate from AIDS, due to the availability of new combinations of drug therapies).

Figure 1.2 depicts the progress we have made or have failed to make in meeting the nation's health goals for the turn of the new millennium.

Yet there remains much to be done if the *Healthy People 2000* goals are to be met. For example, there are nearly 1 million preventable deaths in the United States each year, as shown in Table 1.2. Moreover, although Americans are living longer, there has been a small *decline* in the health-related quality of life. Health differences between whites and people of color persist, as shown by their different life expectancies. In addition, the percentage of Americans with private health insurance *declined* (from 77% of people under age 65 in 1986 to 72% in 1992).

TABLE 1.2

**Annual Preventable Deaths in the United States[8]**

Elimination of tobacco use could prevent 400,000 deaths each year from cancer, heart and lung diseases, and stroke.

Improved diet and exercise could prevent 300,000 deaths from conditions like heart disease, stroke, diabetes, and cancer.

Control of underage and excess drinking of alcohol could prevent 100,000 deaths from motor vehicle accidents, falls, drownings, and other alcohol-related injuries.

Immunizations for infectious diseases in children and adults could prevent 63,000 to 100,000 deaths.

Eliminating firearms from public possession could prevent 35,000 deaths.

Safer sex or sexual abstinence could prevent 30,000 deaths from sexually transmitted diseases (STDs).

Other measures for preventing needless deaths include improved worker training and safety to prevent accidents in the workplace, wider screening for breast and cervical cancer, and control of high blood pressure and elevated blood cholesterol levels.

PREVENTION

## *Preventing Accidents*

Nearly four of ten emergency room visits result from accidents.[9] Accidents are also the fifth leading cause of death in the United States, accounting for 90,000 deaths annually, most of which involve motor vehicle accidents. Yet accidental falls account for twice as many injury-related emergency room visits, about 23%, compared with 12% for motor vehicle accidents. Accidentally being struck by people, objects, or falling objects accounts for another 11% of accident-related ER visits; cuts or punctures by sharp objects for 9%; and violence for 5%.

Most accidents are preventable. What can you do to prevent them? Here are some suggestions:

- *Buckle up.* Make sure to always use your seat belt when driving or riding in a car. Make sure all children are securely buckled and young ones placed in a children's car safety seat.
- *Keep household chemicals and prescription drugs out of the reach of children.* See Chapter 22 for additional suggestions for preventing accidental poisonings.
- *If you have young children, child-proof your home.* Secure all windows with window guards. Cover all exposed electrical outlets.
- *Avoid using a cellular phone while driving.* Using a cell phone while driving quadruples your chances of getting into an accident.[10] When you're driving, *drive.*

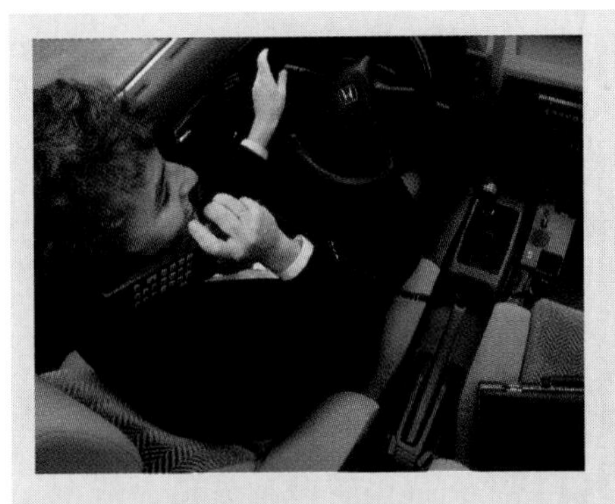

***What's Wrong With This Picture?*** Drivers are four times more likely to have an accident when they are speaking on a car phone than when they are not.

- *Never drink and drive or allow someone else to drink and drive.* Alcohol use is implicated in about 50% of all motor vehicle fatalities. Promote the idea of zero tolerance for drinking and driving.
- *Drive safely.* Obey traffic laws. Remember: The posted speed limit is the maximum allowable speed, not the minimum.
- *Practice safe swimming and boating.* Many deaths resulting from drowning and boating accidents can be prevented by following safety guidelines. Obey all swimming restrictions. Avoid swimming alone or in isolated areas. Obtain proper training for operating a boat or other water equipment. Never mix drinking and boating.
- *Think safety first.* Anticipate accidents before they occur and take steps to prevent them from happening.

### *think about it!*

- **How can you help bring the nation into a healthy new millennium? That is, what can *you* do to help the nation meet the goals of *Healthy People 2000*?**
- **There are 1 million preventable deaths in the United States each year. What can you do to prevent yourself and the people you care about from becoming part of these statistics?**

Smart Quiz Q0103

## HUMAN DIVERSITY AND HEALTH—NATIONS WITHIN THE NATION

The population of the United States is becoming increasingly diverse, so much so that the use of the term "minority" as applied to nonwhite groups is becoming something of a misnomer. By the turn of the millennium or shortly thereafter, non-Hispanic white Americans (white Americans of Euro-

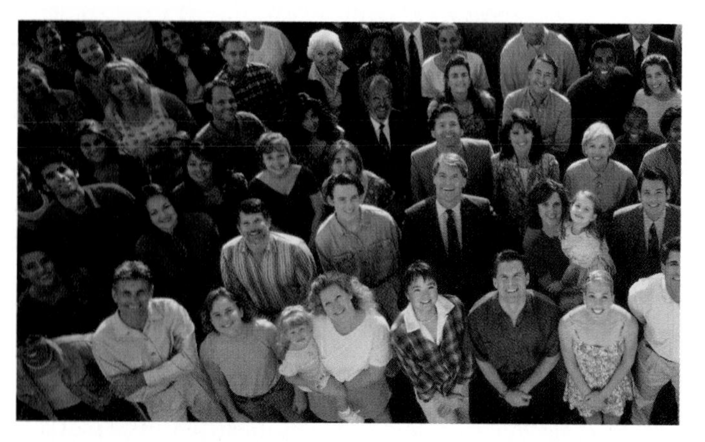

***Increasing Ethnic Diversity in the U.S.*** As a nation, we are a mosaic composed of people representing many different ethnicities and cultural backgrounds.

pean ancestry) are expected to constitute a minority of residents in the state of California. Presently, African Americans constitute the largest nonwhite ethnic group in the United States (12% of the population), followed by nonwhite Hispanic Americans (nearly 10%), Asian Americans/Pacific Islanders (3%), and Native Americans (nearly 1%). If present trends continue, non-Hispanic whites will be in the minority nationwide sometime during the twenty-first century. Figure 1.3 shows the expected changes in the ethnic distribution of the U.S. population by the year 2050. Increasing ethnic diversity is mirrored in the college student population as well, as you can see in Figure 1.4.

When it comes to health, there are nations within the nation. Wide differences exist in the U.S. in both the health status and life expectancy of the majority white population and ethnic minority groups.[11] Differences too exist in the health status and longevity of men and women in our society. Throughout this text we focus on ethnic and gender differences in health status and utilization of health care services. Here we offer a preview.

## Ethnicity

Life expectancy of African Americans is five to eight years shorter than that of non-Hispanic white Americans. Why? It appears that differences in income level and education, rather than race per se, may be largely responsible.[12] Better-educated and wealthier people tend to take better care of themselves (they exercise more, are less often obese, are less likely to smoke, and consume less fat in their diet) than do poorer or less-educated people. African Americans tend to be poorer and less well educated than white Americans. African Americans also tend to have less access to health care than do white Americans.[13] African Americans are also more likely to be exposed to life stressors that can have a negative impact on health, such as overcrowded housing, poverty, and crime.

Genetic factors also play a role in ethnic group differences in health. The incidence of **sickle-cell anemia** is highest among African and Hispanic Americans. The incidence of **Tay-Sachs disease** is greatest among Jews of East European origin.

African Americans are also five to seven times more likely than white Americans to have **hypertension**.[14] However, African Americans are also

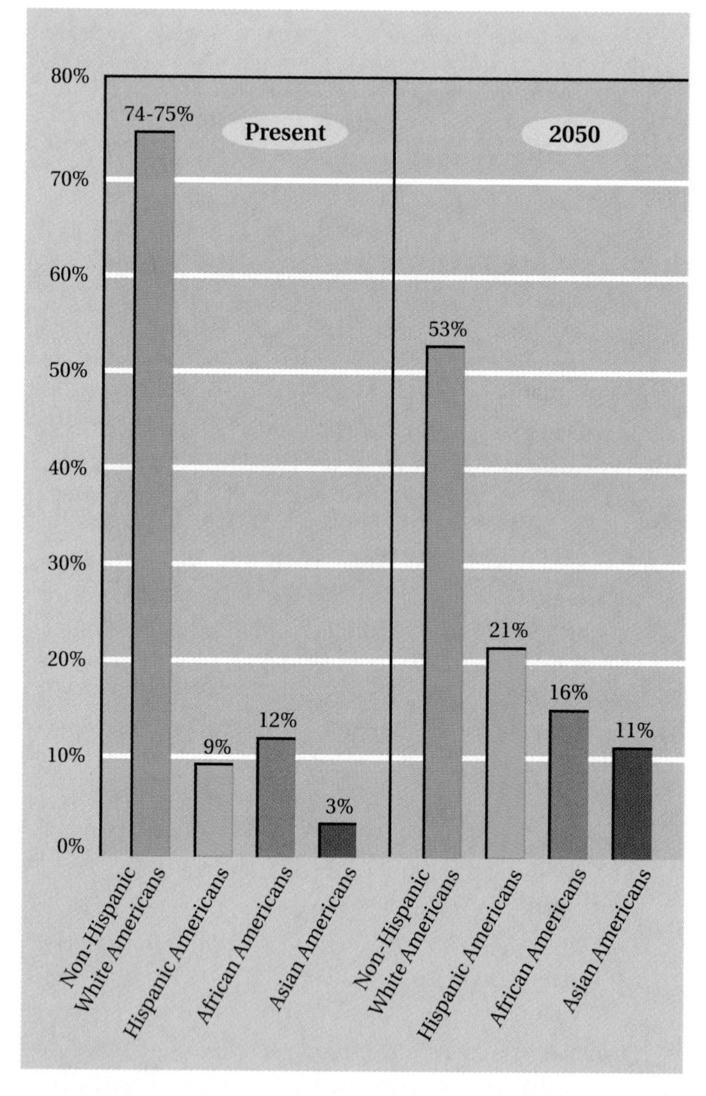


**Figure 1.3** ***Projected Changes in the Ethnic Makeup of the United States*** By the year 2050, the number of non-Hispanic white Americans will grow, but they will make up a much smaller percentage of the population than they do now. The percentage of Asian Americans is expected to more than triple by 2050, making them the most rapidly growing ethnic group in the United States.

## Socioeconomic Status—The Rich Get Richer and the Poor Get . . . Sicker

WORLD OF *diversity*

**Socioeconomic status (SES)** and health have been intimately connected throughout history. Generally speaking, people higher in SES enjoy better health and lead longer lives.[33] Again, the question is *why*. Several factors may be involved.

One factor is educational level. Lower educational levels are associated with lower incomes and SES. Less educated people tend to possess more risk factors for serious disease, such as smoking, inactivity, and obesity.[34] Health-promotion efforts designed to help people change these unhealthy habits have been less successful in reaching people at lower educational levels. Living in poorer neighborhoods may also foster obesity because junk food is heavily promoted and many residents overeat as a way of coping with stress.[35]

Moreover, stress places individuals at greater risk of physical illness ranging from gastrointestinal disorders to heart attacks.[36] People at lower SES levels are more likely to suffer the effects of stress for two reasons. First, the poor are more likely to encounter more significant life stressors, such as financial hardship, overcrowded housing, and neighborhood crime. Second, the poor are less likely to have the resources to cope with stress.[37]

Then, too, individuals who are unhealthy may be downwardly mobile, perhaps because disability or infirmity prevents them from functioning more effectively in the workplace. Let us also not forget that poorer people typically have less access to health care.[38] The problem is compounded by the fact that people of low SES are less likely to receive health education messages about the importance of regular health checkups and early medical intervention when symptoms arise.

more likely to have hypertension than black Africans are. Though not discounting possible genetic factors, this evidence leads researchers to believe that environmental factors found among many African Americans—such as stress, diet, and smoking—contribute to their increased risk of high blood pressure.

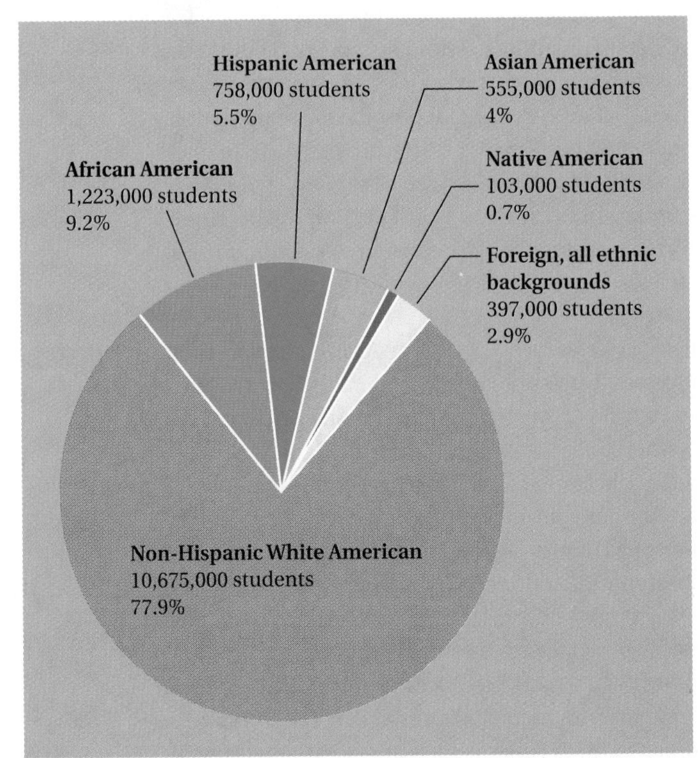


**Figure 1.4** ***Ethnic Diversity in the United States College Population*** The percentages of Hispanic Americans and Asian Americans have had the most rapid rates of increase in recent years.

African Americans are more likely than white Americans to suffer heart attacks and strokes and to die from them.[15] Early diagnosis and treatment might help reduce the racial gap.[16] African Americans with heart disease are also less likely than white Americans to obtain procedures such as bypass surgery, even when it appears that they would benefit equally from the procedure.[17]

African Americans are also more likely than white Americans to die from cancer.[18] This, health experts say, is largely due to their lower socioeconomic status.[19] Consider racial differences in breast cancer. Though white women are more likely to develop breast cancer, black women have a higher death rate from the disease.[20] Cancer is more curable when it is detected early. Women who carry private health insurance are more likely to undergo regular cancer screenings that can detect breast cancer in its earlier stages than women without health insurance coverage or who have Medicaid coverage (public health insurance for people of low socioeconomic

**Close-up**
Health care for underserved
T0103

**Sickle-cell anemia** An inherited blood disorder that afflicts mainly African Americans. Deformed sickle-shaped blood cells obstruct small blood vessels, decreasing their capacity to carry oxygen.

**Tay-Sachs disease** A fatal neurological disorder that primarily afflicts Jews of Eastern European origin.

**Socioeconomic status (SES)** Relative position in terms of education and economic standing.

**Hypertension** High blood pressure.

WORLD OF *diversity*

## Women and Health Research—A History of Exclusion

**Close-up**
Women's health T0104
Women's health forum T0105
Women's health initiative T0106
Women's issues T0107

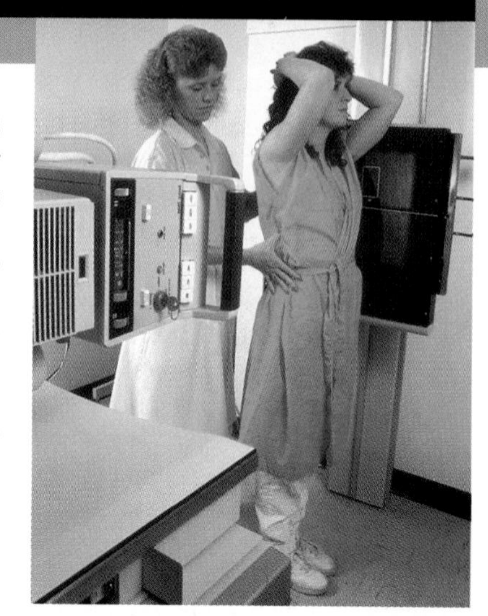

Women have long been underrepresented in health research and have even been excluded from participating. Historically, women's health research focused on issues of fertility and reproduction. Other health research has focused disproportionately on men. Despite this imbalance, new drugs tested on men, once approved, were prescribed to women without comparable trials of effectiveness or safety.

Women have been excluded from medical research for at least two reasons: concerns about pregnancy during a research trial, and concerns that women's changing hormone levels during menstrual cycles might distort the results. Today it is generally accepted that there are no valid reasons for excluding women from health research. In most cases, females and males respond similarly to therapy; however, there are exceptions. For example, women need lower dosages of some medications, and some therapies, such as estrogen replacement, are specific to women.

The federal government is now sponsoring one of the largest clinical trials ever undertaken focused on women's health issues. This 15-year project, called the Women's Health Initiative (WHI), focuses on ways of preventing several major chronic diseases that are some of the leading causes of death and disability among women: heart disease, breast and colorectal (colon and rectal) cancer, and osteoporosis in postmenopausal women.[27] The study, which will involve 164,500 women, attempts to redress many of the inequities in women's health research as well as provide practical information to women and their physicians about strategies to prevent these chronic diseases.

status).[21] People who are more affluent are more likely to carry private health insurance. Black women, who on the average are poorer than white women, are less likely to have private health insurance. African Americans are also more likely than non-Hispanic white Americans to die from homicide, infant death, diabetes, and AIDS.[22]

Hispanic Americans are at greater risk than non-Hispanic white Americans of developing such diseases as AIDS and adult-onset diabetes. Yet Hispanic Americans generally have lower cancer rates and death rates due to cancer than either African Americans or non-Hispanic white Americans.

Mexican Americans, the largest group of Hispanic Americans, have higher rates of heart disease than non-Hispanic whites. The major reason, researchers say, is that Mexican Americans tend to receive less health-related information and have less access to health care services. Health officials hope that risks can be lowered by changes in diet and exercise patterns and improved access to preventive health services.[23]

Hispanic Americans, overall, visit physicians less often than do African Americans and non-Hispanic White Americans. The reasons include lack of health insurance, difficulty speaking English, misgivings about medical technology, and—for illegal aliens—fear of deportation.[24] One consequence of the lack of health care is that Hispanic-American preschoolers are less likely than their African American and non-Hispanic white counterparts to be immunized against childhood diseases.

**Cross-Cultural Factors** Also consider some cross-cultural differences in health. Death rates from cancer are higher in nations such as the Netherlands, Denmark, England, Canada, and—yes—the United States, where the population has a high daily fat intake.[25] Death rates from cancer are much lower in nations such as Thailand, the Philippines, and Japan, where the daily fat intake is markedly lower. Don't assume that the difference is racial just because Thailand, the Philippines, and Japan are Asian nations! The diets of Japanese Americans are similar in fat content to those of other Americans—and so are their death rates from cancer.

Because of dietary differences associated with American culture, especially high fat intake,

Japanese-American men living in California and Hawaii are two to three times more likely to become obese than Japanese men who live in Japan.[26]

### Gender

The life expectancy of African Americans is five to eight years shorter than that of white Americans. Similarly, men's life expectancies are seven years shorter, on the average, than women's. A survey of 1,500 physicians suggests that the gender difference in life expectancy is due, at least in part, to women's greater willingness to seek health care.[28] Men often let symptoms go until a problem that could have been prevented or readily treated becomes serious or life-threatening. Some men, according to the survey, have a "bulletproof mentality." Says a representative of the Men's Health Network: "In their twenties, they're too strong to need a doctor; in their thirties, they're too busy, and in their forties, too scared." Consequently, women are much more likely to examine themselves for signs of breast cancer than men are to examine their testicles for any unusual lumps.

Men and women are also at different risks for various kinds of health problems. Men are at higher risk than women for some diseases, including coronary heart disease, the nation's leading killer. Women are apparently protected by high levels of estrogen until menopause. After menopause, women's risk of heart disease increases dramatically. Gender differences even out by around age 65. Women are at higher risk for many nonfatal chronic conditions, such as **arthritis** and **osteoporosis.** Severe or moderately reduced bone density affects 7 out of 10 women over age 50. Arthritis affects a third of women aged 45 to 64 years and half of women aged 65 years and above.

Talking Glossary
Osteoporosis
G0101

Increased rates of smoking among women since the 1940s have resulted in a burgeoning death rate among women due to smoking-related illnesses. Between the early 1970s and the early 1990s, the death rate for lung cancer almost tripled among women. The death rate for **chronic obstructive pulmonary disease** or **COPD,** a category that includes two smoking-related diseases, **chronic bronchitis** and **emphysema,** more than doubled for women between 1979 and 1993.[29]

Women, particularly poor women, are much more likely than men to be victims of violent crime committed by an intimate (a current or former partner) or relative. The victimization rate of women by intimates is nearly seven times as high for women as for men. For women in the lowest income group, the rate is more than four times that for women in the highest income group.[30]

The physician's gender can also make a difference in women's health status and survival. A study of more than 90,000 women found that women whose internists or family practitioners are women are more likely to have screenings for cancer (mammograms and Pap tests) than women whose internists or family practitioners are men.[31] Female physicians are also more likely than male physicians to conduct breast examinations properly.[32]

**think about it!**

- **To what ethnic group(s) do you belong? What health problems are more likely to occur among people of your ethnic group? What are you doing to prevent or detect these problems?**
- **What health problems are more likely to occur among people of your gender? What are you doing to prevent or detect these health problems?**

Smart Quiz
Q0104

## CRITICAL THINKING AND HEALTH

We are flooded with so much information about health that it is difficult to sort fact from fiction. Some reports contradict each other. Others contain half-truths, or draw misleading or unsupported conclusions. In some cases, we are bewildered because health professionals and other authorities do not agree among themselves. Becoming a critical thinker means never taking claims at face value. It means looking carefully at both sides of the argument.

**Critical thinking** can help us to evaluate claims, arguments, and widely held

**Arthritis** Inflammation of a joint, typically accompanied by pain, stiffness, and swelling.

**Osteoporosis** A condition of generalized bone loss that makes bones brittle and subject to breakage.

**Chronic obstructive pulmonary disease (COPD)** General term applying to chronic lung diseases, especially emphysema and chronic bronchitis, which result in impaired lung function.

**Chronic bronchitis** An inflammation of the lining of the bronchial tubes, producing chronic coughing.

**Emphysema** A lung disease involving destruction of the walls of the air sacs (alveoli) in the lungs.

**Critical thinking** The adoption of a questioning attitude characterized by a careful weighing of evidence and thoughtful analysis of the claims and arguments of others.

beliefs. Critical thinking has several meanings. One aspect of critical thinking is being skeptical of things that are presented in print or uttered by authority figures or celebrities, or passed along by friends. Another aspect of critical thinking is thoughtful analysis of claims and arguments. It means scrutinizing definitions of terms, evaluating the premises of arguments and their logic. It also means finding *reasons* to support your beliefs, rather than relying only on feelings or "gut impressions."

Throughout the book we raise issues that demand critical thinking. These issues may stimulate you to analyze and evaluate your beliefs and attitudes about the health choices available to you in the light of scientific evidence. For example, in Chapter 5 we consider the controversy over the use of megadoses of certain vitamins. In Chapters 13 and 17 we turn to other controversies that have pitted even experts against each other: Should people take a drink or two of alcohol daily to help protect their hearts? Should they take a daily low dose of aspirin toward the same end? Then there are the issues that invoke moral values that concern each of us on a deeper, more personal level: Should I have children? Where do I stand on the issue of abortion? Should doctors be permitted to help people end their lives painlessly by administering lethal drugs? Critical thinkers know that while scientific knowledge can help inform their decisions, many decisions need to be approached by considering their moral and ethical implications.

## Features of Critical Thinking

Critical thinkers weigh premises, consider evidence, and decide whether arguments are valid and logical. Here are suggestions for thinking critically about health information.

1. *Be skeptical.* Politicians, religious leaders, and other authority figures attempt to convince you of their points of view. Maintain a skeptical attitude and consider the evidence for yourself.
2. *Examine definitions of terms.* Some statements are true when a term is defined in one way but not true when it is defined in another. Consider the statement, "Stress is bad for you." If we define stress in terms of hassles and work or family pressures that stretch our ability to cope to the max, then there is perhaps substance to the statement. However, if we define stress (see Chapter 3) more broadly to include any factors that impose a demand on us to adjust, including events such as a new marriage or the birth of a child, then perhaps certain types of stress can be a good thing.
3. *Examine the assumptions or premises of arguments.* Consider the statement, "Abortion is murder." The current edition of *Webster's New World Dictionary* defines murder as "the unlawful and malicious or premeditated killing of one human being by another." The statement can be true, according to this dictionary, only if the victim is held to be a human being (and if the act is unlawful and malicious or premeditated). Pro-life advocates argue that embryos and fetuses are human beings. Pro-choice advocates claim that they are not, at least not until they are capable of surviving on their own. So the argument that abortion is murder rests in part on the assumption that the embryo or fetus is a human being.
4. *Recognize that correlation is not causation.* In Chapter 5 we consider evidence showing that people whose diets contained the highest amounts of vitamin E had the lowest rates of mortality from heart disease. In other words, a correlation (a statistical association) was shown to exist between death rates from heart disease and dietary intake of vitamin E. Does this mean that vitamin E plays a *causal role* in lowering the death rate from heart disease? We can't say. We cannot ascertain from a correlational relationship whether the variables are causally connected. It is possible that other ingredients in foods containing high levels of vitamin E deserve the credit. Or perhaps people who consume high levels of vitamin E in their diets engage in other healthy behaviors that explain their good fortune. To determine cause and effect, scientists need to conduct experimental studies in which they manipulate the variable of interest (vitamin E in this case) and study its effects while controlling for other factors such as diet and lifestyle.
5. *Consider the kinds of evidence on which conclusions are based.* Some conclusions, even seemingly "scientific" conclusions, are based on anecdotes and personal endorsements. They are not founded on sound research.
6. *Do not oversimplify.* Consider the statement, "Alcoholism is inherited." In Chapter 13, we

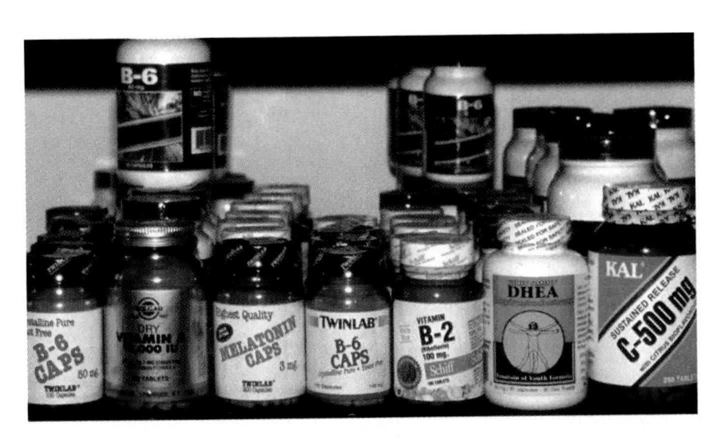


***Safe or Sorry?*** Just because products are sold in a health food store doesn't mean they are healthy for you. Some may even be harmful. Critical thinkers carefully examine health claims and arm themselves with information to make informed decisions regarding their health.

review evidence suggesting that genetic factors may create a predisposition to alcoholism, at least in males. But the origins of alcoholism, as well as of cancer, heart disease, and many of the other health problems we discuss in this text, are more complex, reflecting a complicated interplay of biological and environmental factors. Consider that people may inherit a predisposition to heart disease but might possibly avert its development if they adopt a healthy lifestyle in which they watch their diet, exercise regularly, and learn to manage stress effectively. On the other hand, people may develop heart problems if they smoke, don't exercise, and follow a high-fat diet, even if there is no history of the disease in their families. In only a few cases are diseases the product of a single defective gene.

7. *Do not overgeneralize.* In Chapter 21, we consider evidence showing that teenage parents and single parents, parents from lower income levels, and undereducated parents are more likely than other parents to abuse or neglect their children. Does this mean that all parents having such characteristics abuse or neglect their children? In Chapter 22 we consider the health risks posed by certain chemicals in our environment. Some of these chemicals can be very dangerous, even deadly at high levels of exposure. But does this mean that they pose a significant risk to the average person who is likely to be exposed to only very small levels of these chemicals in everyday life?

## PREVENTION

### *Avoiding Harmful Self-Help Books—Of Elvis, UFOs, and Quick Fixes*[39]

*Eight Weeks to Optimum Health; Chicken Soup for the Soul; Dr. Atkins' New Diet Revolution; The Road Less Traveled; The 7 Habits of Highly Effective People; Our Bodies Our Selves; The 8-Week Cholesterol Cure; Treating Type A Behavior and Your Heart . . .*

These are barely a shelfful of the self-help books that have flooded the marketplace in recent years. Many of us who are shy, anxious, heavy, stressed, or confused scan the bookstores and the checkout racks of supermarkets in hope of finding the book that will provide the answer. How are we to know what to buy? How can we be informed consumers of these works? Unfortunately, there are no easy answers. Anecdotes about how John lost 60 pounds in 60 days and how retiring Joni blossomed into a social butterfly in a month have a powerful allure, especially when we are needy. It's important to keep in mind that a price we pay for freedom of speech is that nearly anything can wind up in print. Authors can make extravagant claims with little fear of imprisonment. They can lie about the effectiveness of a new fad diet as easily as they can lie about communicating with the departed Elvis Presley or being kidnapped by the occupants of a UFO.

How can you protect yourself? We don't have all the answers. We *do* have some helpful hints:

1. *First, don't judge the book by its cover or its title.* Good books as well as bad books can have catchy titles and interesting covers. Dozens, perhaps hundreds, of books are competing for your attention. It is little wonder, then, that publishers try to do something sensational with the covers.
2. *Avoid books that make extravagant claims.* If it sounds too good to be true, it probably is. No method helps everyone who tries it. Very few methods work overnight. Yet people want the instant cure. The book that promises to make you fit in ten days will outsell the book that says it will take ten weeks. Responsible health professionals do not make lavish claims.
3. *Check authors' educational credentials.* Be suspicious if the author's title is just "Dr." placed before the name. The degree could be a phony doctorate bought through the mail. It could be issued by a religious cult rather than a university or professional school. It is better if the "doctor" has an M.D., Ph.D., Psy.D., or Ed.D. after her or his name, rather than "Dr." in front of it.
4. *Check authors' affiliations.* There are no guarantees, but health professionals who are affiliated with medical schools, colleges, and universities may have more to offer than those who are not.

5. *Consider authors' complaints about the conservatism of professional groups to be a warning.* Do the authors boast that they are ahead of their time? Do they berate professional health organizations as being pigheaded or narrow-minded? If so, be suspicious. Yes, great discoveries are sometimes met with opposition. But most health professionals are open-minded. They just ask to see *evidence* before they jump on the bandwagon. Enthusiasm is no substitute for research and evidence.
6. *Check the evidence reported in the book.* Bad books usually make much of anecdotes, unsupported stories about fantastic results with a few individuals. Responsible health professionals check the effectiveness of techniques with large numbers of people. They assign them at random to experimental or control groups. They carefully measure the outcomes. They use qualified language; they say "It appears that . . ." or "It may be that . . ."
7. *Check the reference citations for the evidence.* Legitimate health research is reported in the journals you will find in the reference sections in this textbook. These journals report only research methods and outcomes that seem to be scientifically valid. If there are no reference citations, or if the list of references seems suspicious, you should be suspicious, too.
8. *Ask your instructor for advice.* Ask for advice on what to do, whom to talk to, what to read.
9. *Read textbooks and professional books, like this textbook, rather than self-help books.* Roam the college bookstore for texts in fields that interest you. Try the suggested readings at the ends of textbook chapters.
10. *Consult with a respected health professional.* Stop by and chat with faculty in health, physical education, and psychology departments. Talk to someone in your college or university health center.

There are no guarantees. There are few, if any, quick fixes to nagging health problems. Do your homework. Become a sophisticated consumer of health advice.

## Thinking Critically about Online Health Information

With today's online services, a world of health information is literally at your fingertips. If you have access to the Internet, you can obtain information relating to:

- Listings and abstracts (brief descriptions) of scientific studies published in leading health and medical journals. Much of this information is provided free of charge.
- Information about medications, medical treatments, and medical conditions.
- Consumer-oriented material, such as the latest health-related reports from *Consumer Reports.*
- Access to electronic encyclopedias that contain entries for thousands of health-related terms.
- Listings of thousands of medical service providers, including leading hospitals, clinics, and health organizations.
- Forums and "chat lines" that bring together people who have shared medical concerns or interests.
- Vendors who supply a range of medical products and services.
- Information provided by federal health agencies, including the National Cancer Institute and the National Institute on Aging.
- Information from leading national health organizations, such as the American Heart Association, the American Diabetes Association, and the American Lung Association.

**Close-up**
Internet resources
**T0108**

Most people gain access to the Internet and the World Wide Web through commercial online services such as America Online, MSN, Prodigy, or CompuServe. Once you are connected to one of these services, a menu structure will appear that will guide you to find relevant information by clicking on a series of icons that increasingly narrow the focus of your search. You can search the Internet by using a search engine provided by your online provider. You enter the key terms you want to search and then the search engine retrieves a listing of relevant entries. Say you were interested in exploring material relating to hypertension and stress. You could enter the term "hypertension." This would retrieve every site that is indexed to hypertension, perhaps thousands. To narrow your

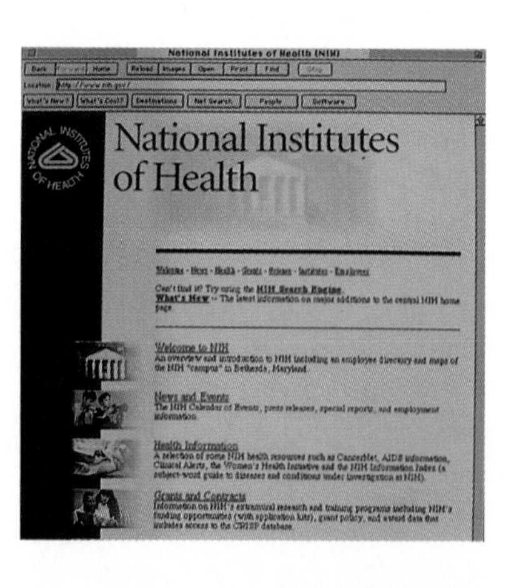


***Health Net*** With access to the Internet, a world of health information is literally at your fingertips. The homepage of the National Institutes of Health, for example, is a springboard to a wealth of health information and research. However, not all information posted on the web is accurate or reliable.

scope, limit the search by inputting the key terms "hypertension and stress." In this case, only sites containing references to both terms, hypertension and stress, would be retrieved. Once you've landed on an Internet site, you may see "hypertext links" (connections to other sources of information) that can be clicked to bring you to related information that may be of interest.

A more direct way of accessing a particular Internet or World Wide Web site is to type its address in the window provided on your online service. These addresses are becoming as commonplace as telephone numbers. They all share the same prefix: http://. Examples of health-related Internet sites are listed in Table 1.3 at the end of this chapter.

Many health-related resources have recently come online. For example, the Health Education and Wellness Program of Columbia University in New York offers an online service called Healthwise. A team of professional and peer educators answer users' questions to help them make more informed health choices. Readers can also obtain health-related information and access to other Internet health sites by visiting the Worth Publishers website at www.worthpublishers.com.

**Close-up** Health online T0109

The Internet holds a vast repository of health-related information. Anyone can post information on the net, so the casual browser may not know how to distinguish accurate, scientifically based information from misinformation. *The beauty—and the risk—of the Internet is that it is freely available to anyone to post just about anything, from credible scientific information to advertising hype to complete malarkey.* Don't believe everything you get from the net: Think critically!

1. *Check out the credentials of the source.* Who is posting the material? Is it a well-respected medical or scientific institution or an individual or group of individuals with no scientific credentials or perhaps even with an axe to grind with the scientific or medical establishment?

   The most reliable sources are scientific journals that are subject to peer review, a process by which other scientists carefully scrutinize each potential contributor's work before publication. In addition to scientific journals, the more reliable sources of health and medical information are those that are frequently updated, such as websites maintained by government agencies such as the National Institutes of Health and its many divisions, as well as those sponsored by leading health organizations, like the American Medical Association, the American Heart Association, the American Lung Association, and the American Dental Association.
2. *Look for citations.* Scientists back up what they say with citations to the original scientific sources. The endnotes in the appendix of this book, for example, represent the sources your authors have used in preparing this textbook. If the authors cite findings from the scientific literature, you should expect them to supply some of the references they use, such as noting the journals or other periodicals in which the studies were published (including the year, volume, and page numbers). Having this information allows the reader to check the original sources to see if the statements made are accurate. In some cases, however, scientific organizations like the National Institutes of Health and leading medical schools and medical centers prepare information for the general public that is no less reliable but not annotated with source notes or references.
3. *Beware of any product claims.* Many commercial organizations use the Internet to promote or sell health-related products. Don't assume that product claims are scientifically valid. Think of them as electronic advertising, basically an Internet version of a television commercial. Don't be misled by the offer of a money-back guarantee; often there are strings attached.

Recognize too that information from the Internet is no substitute for consulting your personal physician about any health-related concerns. Be sure to check first with your physician before making any changes in your lifestyle or health-related habits based on information obtained from the net. In the ***think about it*** sections, like the one below, we include items that encourage you to think critically about issues that affect your health.

### think about it!

- **Are you a critical thinker? Why or why not?**

**critical thinking** **How would you go about determining the accuracy of health information obtained from a doctor, a website, or a magazine article?**

**Smart Quiz** Q0104

# Practicing Self-Care

## Take Charge

The ***Take Charge*** features in this textbook help you apply the material in the chapter to your own life. This first ***Take Charge*** feature focuses on an important element of achieving wellness, practicing self-care.

Though there is no guarantee that practicing self-care will keep you free of disease or infirmity, the odds are in your favor that it will help you live a longer, healthier, and fuller life. Practicing self-care involves taking steps to prevent disease and maintain vigor and vitality as you age. Much of the information contained in this textbook is focused toward these ends:

- Keeping fit and remaining active mentally and physically
- Adopting a healthful diet and sticking to it
- Controlling stress, getting sufficient sleep, and coping with emotional problems
- Avoiding harmful substances, such as tobacco, illicit drugs, and excessive alcohol
- Protecting yourself from infectious agents and environmental hazards.

People who practice self-care are knowledgeable and active consumers of health care. They understand that they have both a right and a responsibility to take an active part in managing their health care. They get regular medical checkups and screening tests. They approach the choice of health care providers seriously and carefully scrutinize health insurance plans and the facilities and institutions that provide health care services (see Chapter 23).

A good starting point is choosing a **primary care physician,** the person primarily responsible for your medical care on an ongoing basis.

### Choosing a Primary Care Physician

Many people spend more time picking out a new television or stereo system than selecting a primary care physician. They may assume (wrongly) that all physicians are equally competent. Or they may not think that they have the knowledge or competence to make an informed choice. True enough, the average consumer may not be able to judge medical competence. No, medical boards do not routinely evaluate physicians' skills. Even well-informed patients may not know whether their doctors' skills are sharp or whether they keep up with the latest medical developments. Some doctors do get report cards. In some states, such as New York and Pennsylvania, expert panels issue ratings of heart surgeons based on their surgical performance in relation to the severity of the cases they treat. Some consumer groups have applauded these efforts and believe that they have weeded out some sloppy practitioners. Yet the rating system has drawn fire from doctors who believe it is unfair and confusing.[40] Another concern is that doctors may shy away from treating the sickest patients if they believe that negative outcomes might jeopardize their ratings.

**Primary care physician** A physician who provides a patient with regular, ongoing medical care and makes recommendations to specialists when the need arises.

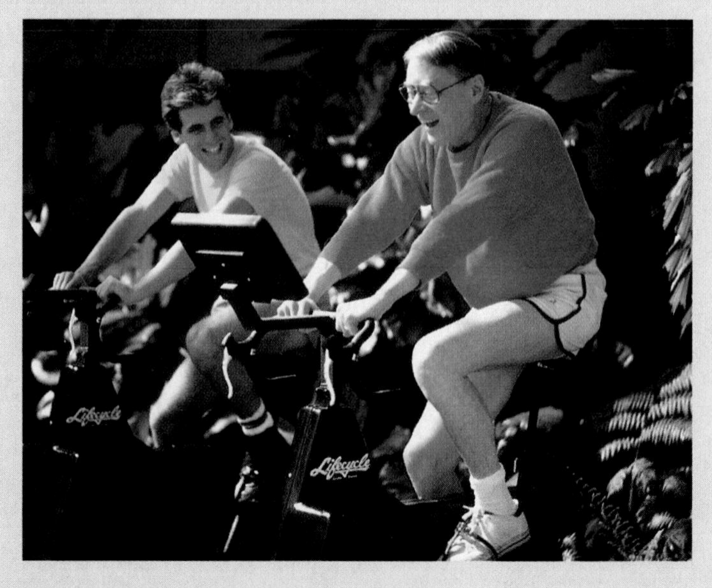

***Striving for Wellness*** What changes in your lifestyle and habits can you make to optimize your health and well-being?

Despite the difficulty of judging medical competence, there is much that health consumers can do to make better-informed decisions about their health care providers:

1. *Get recommendations.* Ask around. Seek recommendations from those whose opinions you trust. Be aware, however, that what is important to one person, such as the availability of weekend hours, may be relatively unimportant to another. Other professionals with whom the doctor works, such as nurses and fellow physicians, may not be reliable sources of information as they may hesitate to say negative things about a colleague. However, should you hear any negative comments from the doctor's colleagues, consider it a sign to look

elsewhere for a primary health care provider. A helpful suggestion is to ask other medical professionals whom they would choose for themselves or their family.[41] You can also call your local medical center or medical school and ask for the appropriate unit or department, either pediatrics or internal medicine. Ask to speak to the head nurse on the unit. Explain that you are seeking a primary care physician and would like a recommendation for two or three doctors in your area. Nurses interact with a large number of doctors and may be able to give you an unbiased recommendation. Once you have established a relationship with a primary care physician, he or she can help you find other specialists you may need.

2. *Set up an appointment.* Selecting a primary care physician is one of the most important health care decisions you may ever make. This is the person in whom you place your trust for overseeing your health care and monitoring changes in your health status from year to year. Before making a choice, make an appointment for a brief interview or for a routine physical exam or consultation for a relatively minor medical problem. Then consider whether the physician makes the grade on the following key factors:
   - *Empathy.* Empathic physicians relate to their patients in a warm and supportive manner. They express understanding and concern for their problems and complaints. They have what used to be called a "good bedside manner." Ask yourself the following questions:

     Does the physician seem genuinely interested in you as a person, or as just another case?

     Does the physician take the time to get to know something about your background and health concerns? Or does the physician seem impatient or curt in his or her responses?

     Does the physician seem to be the kind of person who will be available to you in times of medical need?
   - *Availability.* Ask about office hours, coverage for medical emergencies, weekend and evening availability, and backup coverage during vacations. Ask whether he or she offers opportunities for phone consultation and how quickly you can expect a return call.
   - *Ability to communicate medical information in language you can understand.* Steer clear of a doctor who speaks only in "doctorese." Likewise, avoid someone who is vague in giving answers or who doesn't take the time or have the ability to explain medical information in a way that you can clearly understand. You can't make informed choices about your medical treatment if you don't understand the options available to you.
   - *Credentials.* Don't be shy about asking the doctor about his or her professional background. Pose questions such as the following:

     From what medical school did you graduate?

     Where did you complete your residency training, and in what area or areas?

     In which specialty areas are you board-certified?

     Nearly two-thirds of the nearly 700,000 physicians in the United States are **board-certified.**[42] Board certification has increasingly become a minimum standard that doctors must meet to obtain hospital privileges and be accepted in managed care plans. Studies demonstrate that board-certified doctors tend to provide better care than noncertified physicians. Also inquire about the hospitals with which the doctor is affiliated. More prestigious hospitals tend to weed out doctors with questionable records. You may also want to select a doctor who practices in a hospital in your area that is known to have a good reputation.

     You can check your doctor's credentials by using the American Medical Association's *Directory of Physicians in the U.S.*, a book that contains information about each doctor's medical and residency training, hospital affiliations, teaching positions, and board certification. Many public libraries have copies of the directory. You can also find out whether your doctor is board-certified in his or her specialty area by calling the American Board of Medical Specialties at 800-776-CERT. Don't be misled by the designation "board-eligible." This means that the doctor has completed the required residency training in a specialty area but has not yet taken the required exam to become certified or may well have flunked it.

     You might also call the hospitals with which the doctor is affiliated to check on the doctor's standing in the hospital and to check that the hospital itself is accredited by the national accrediting body, the Joint Commission on Accreditation of Healthcare Organizations.
   - *Costs and insurance coverage.* Ask about the doctor's fees for a typical office visit and annual physical exam. Are the fees reasonable for your area? Find out whether you would be expected to pay for each visit and later be reimbursed by your insurance carrier, or whether the doctor will bill the insurance company directly and have you pay only for the difference between the charges and the amount of reimbursement received. Members of **health maintenance organizations (HMOs)** are typically limited to physicians who are part of their

**HealthCheck**
Selecting a physician
H0102

**Board-certified** A physician who has met the criteria required for certification in a medical specialty area by a recognized medical specialty board.

**Health maintenance organization (HMO)** A prepaid managed care plan that offers medical services through affiliated doctors and hospitals or freestanding clinics. Costs are usually based on a fixed amount of money per enrolled member.

HMO network, and fees are usually fixed by the particular plan. Some plans allow members to select physicians outside the network, though at higher cost.

3. *Consider a trial period.* Don't expect to obtain all the information you need to make a fully informed decision based on an initial interview or office visit alone. Knowledge is usually acquired over time. Consider a trial period of perhaps three to six months to see how well your doctor lives up to expectations.

## Putting Prevention First

Prevention is an important element of self-care. Preventive care means:

- Pregnant women receive good prenatal and postnatal care.
- Infants, children, and adults receive immunizations.
- Sexually active people take steps to avoid unwanted pregnancies and sexually transmitted diseases.
- All of us work toward creating safe environments in which to work and live.

Preventive care also means having regular physical examinations and screening tests and replacing abusive patterns of behavior with healthier habits, as shown in Table 1.4.

## Practicing Dental Self-Care

Tooth decay and eventual tooth loss due to gum disease are caused by bacteria that form plaque. Fight back against the bacteria in your mouth by brushing twice a day with a fluoridated toothpaste that carries the American Dental Association Seal of Acceptance and by flossing at least daily. Though many toothpastes are on the market today, there is no evidence that any one fluoridated toothpaste is better than any other. When brushing, use up-and-down strokes with toothbrush positioned at about a 45-degree angle to remove plaque and food particles. Use a soft-bristled brush, and don't brush hard the way you might if you were sanding a plank of wood. Brushing too vigorously, especially with a hard brush, can eventually strip the enamel (protective covering) of the tooth, producing sensitivity to heat and cold and damaging the gums. Brush longer (about two minutes each time), not harder. And remember to see your dentist for a twice-yearly checkup.

## Keeping a Home Health Record

Keeping your medical records in a home medical file is an important aspect of self-care. Include in the record all information relating to your medical history—medical visits, medications taken and adverse reactions (if any), results of lab tests and special diagnostic tests like CT scans and X-rays—as well as any other medical or personal information your doctor may need to know. Why is it important to keep a home health record? For one thing, knowing whether you have had allergic reactions to certain medications may prevent you from inadvertently taking the same medication again. For another, keeping X-rays and records of diagnostic or screening tests gives your doctor a baseline against which to assess your present health. Here are some items that should go into your home health record:[43]

1. *Any allergic reactions or other adverse reactions to medications.* Keep a record of any allergic response or other adverse response you may have had to any medication, prescription or over-the-counter. Include the name of the medication, the dosage level, the length of time you took the medication, the type of reaction you had, and what you did about it.
2. *Vaccination record.* Keep a record of all vaccinations (including tetanus shots) you received, noting the type of vaccine, the date or dates of vaccination, and any adverse reactions you may have experienced. Having an up-to-date record may prevent you from having to undergo a vaccination you don't need.
3. *Insurance claim forms.* Keep a copy of your insurance claim forms. Claim forms typically include a record of diagnosis and treatments provided. This information can help you reconstruct earlier medical problems and the course of treatments you received.

**Take Charge**
Healthy teeth
**C0101**

4. *Copies of all lab tests.* Results of previous tests such as X-rays, MRIs, ultrasound tests, urinalysis, blood work, and EKGs may be used as a yardstick or baseline for evaluating changes in your health. Ask for copies of any lab analyses or diagnostic tests.
5. *Hospitalization records.* Keep a copy of your hospitalization records, including invoices for services rendered and the discharge report. If you had an operation, ask for copies of the surgeon's and pathologist's reports.

**Smart Reference**
Electric smile aid
**R0101**

6. *Obtain a copy of your medical record.* Ask your primary care physician for a copy of your medical record. If it is too bulky to copy in its entirety, ask for a detailed, written summary. Most states require doctors to release your medical records to you, although in some cases they may be permitted to withhold certain records if disclosing them would cause the patient psychological harm.
7. *Build a medical family tree.* Create a document showing the medical history of each member of your family—age, or if deceased, age at death and cause of death, and history of serious illnesses, hospitalizations, and major surgeries. Include your parents, grandparents, uncles and aunts, siblings, and children.
8. *Keep your records in a secure place.* Keep all your records in the same place, preferably in a secure cabinet, but accessible in case of emergency (not in the bank safe deposit box).

## Keeping Abreast of Health Developments

Knowledge about health and illness is constantly expanding. People who take charge of their health keep abreast of scientific

**TABLE 1.4**

**Replacing Patterns of Abuse with Healthier Habits**

| Body System | Patterns of Abuse | Predicted Problems | Healthier Habits |
|---|---|---|---|
| *Cardiovascular (heart and blood vessels)* | Lack of regular exercise; lack of proper diet; lack of stress control; smoking | Heart disease; hypertension; increased risk of heart attack and stroke | Regular aerobic exercise; avoiding smoking and excessive drinking; keeping stress under control; adopting a healthy, low-fat diet (Chapters 3, 5, 7, 14, and 17) |
| *Respiratory (lung function)* | Lack of regular exercise; smoking; exposure to secondary smoke and environmental pollutants | Shortness of breath; diminishing lung capacity; progressive pulmonary disease; cancer | Building cardiorespiratory endurance through regular aerobic exercise; avoiding smoking (Chapters 7 and 14) |
| *Central nervous system (CNS: brain and spinal cord)* | Reckless behavior; substance abuse; lack of stress control; lack of attention to mental health problems | Paralysis resulting from accidents caused by reckless behavior; impaired learning ability or memory; loss of motivation and social withdrawal; difficulties functioning | Practicing stress-management techniques like relaxation or meditation; becoming more aware of signs of psychological distress and seeking help for mental health problems (Chapters 3 and 4) |
| *Gastrointestinal (stomach and intestines)* | Lack of proper diet; inadequate fluid intake; lack of exercise; poor elimination habits | Constipation, recurrent diarrhea, gas, bloating; hemorrhoids; cancer | Eating a balanced diet with plenty of high-fiber fruits and vegetables; avoiding excess alcohol intake; avoiding smoking; exercising regularly (Chapters 5, 7, and 14) |
| *Urinary (kidneys, bladder, ureters, urethra)* | Inadequate fluid intake; poor personal hygiene; high-risk sexual behavior; neglect of symptoms | Concentrated urine; urinary tract infections; difficulty urinating or pain or burning during urination | Avoiding high-risk sexual practices; promptly reporting any pain or burning upon urination, urinary discharges, genital sores, or other changes to your primary health care provider (Chapter 16) |
| *Skeletal (bones and spinal column)* | Lack of proper diet, especially lack of calcium; lack of regular exercise; reckless behavior | Discomfort; loss of bone mass; trauma; stress fractures | Maintaining adequate calcium intake and intake of other essential vitamins and minerals; avoidng unreasonable risks; using seat belts when riding in a car and safety equipment when biking or rollerblading; exercising regularly to strengthen bones, especially weight-bearing exercise (Chapters 5 and 7) |
| *Muscular (muscles and connective tissue)* | Lack of proper diet; lack of regular exercise; reckless behavior | Weakness; muscle atrophy; cramps; strains; sprains; tears; loss of range of motion | Regular muscle-strengthening exercises; warming up before vigorous exercise (Chapter 7) |
| *Reproductive (ovaries, testes,external and internal organs)* | Poor hygiene; lack of proper diet; failure to use effective contraception; unsafe sexual practices | Infections; amenorrhea; infertility; unwanted pregnancy; death | Avoiding high-risk sexual practices; using effective contraception to prevent unwanted pregnacies; maintaining regular medical checkups (for women, a twice-yearly pelvic exam and Pap smear; for men, an annual physical exam); promptly reporting any physical symptoms involving the genitals or reproductive tract to your primary physician (Chapters 9, 10, 16, 18, and 23) |
| *Endocrine (hormones and ductless glands)* | Lack of proper diet; exposure to infections; exposure to radiation; lack of stress control | Disorders of the thyroid, parathyroid, and pituitary glands, ovaries and testes; oversecretion of stress hormones (Chapter 3) | Maintaining a proper diet; keeping stress under control; getting sufficient sleep. (Chapters 3 and 5) |

developments in the health field. Armed with this information, they are in a better position to safeguard their personal health and the health of their families and make better-informed choices about treatment alternatives available to them.

This chapter is the beginning of a new stage in your quest for optimum health. There is much to learn from this course, and from life itself. We invite you to proceed with us as we continue our journey.

Smart Quiz
Q0105

# SUMMING UP

## Questions and Answers

### WHAT IS HEALTH?

**1. What is health?** Physical health is the soundness of your body. We can also speak of such other aspects or dimensions of health as psychological health, spiritual health, social health, and environmental health.

**2. What is wellness?** Wellness refers to a state of optimum health, which is characterized by active efforts to maximize one's health and well-being.

### STRIVING FOR WELLNESS

**3. What are the factors involved in making changes in health behavior?** Factors involved in changing health behavior include predisposing factors (e.g., beliefs, attitudes, knowledge, expectancies, values), enabling factors (e.g., skills or abilities, physical and mental capabilities, and availability and accessibility of resources), and reinforcing factors (praise and support from self and others; internal reinforcement).

**4. What are some general guidelines for making healthy behavior changes?** These include setting reasonable goals, approaching goals gradually, identifying specific behaviors you want to change, tracking problem behavior, acquiring information you need to know, adopting an internal locus of control, challenging negative thinking, not giving up when you give in, and making healthy habits a part of your lifestyle.

### HEALTHY PEOPLE 2000—INTO THE NEW MILLENNIUM

**5. What is *Healthy People 2000*?** This is the title of a government work, published in 1990, that established three main health goals and set some 300 specific objectives for the nation by the year 2000. The major goals are to increase the span of healthy life, to reduce health disparities among Americans, and to achieve access to preventive services for all Americans.

**6. How is the nation doing in meeting these objectives, according to the 1995 midcourse review?** It's a mixed picture. Progress is being made in about two-thirds of the objectives on which we have collected data. For example, there has been a decline in deaths from heart disease, cancer, and stroke—the three leading causes of death. On the other hand, there has been a small *decline* in the health-related quality of life, and health differences between white people and people from ethnic minority groups persist.

### HUMAN DIVERSITY AND HEALTH—NATIONS WITHIN THE NATION

**7. What are some ethnic differences in health?** Poorer, less educated groups of people have shorter life expectancies than better-educated groups. There are disproportionate numbers of deaths from AIDS among African Americans and Hispanic Americans. African Americans are most likely to have hypertension and sickle-cell anemia. The outcome in cancer is worse for African Americans, apparently because of later diagnosis and treatment. Hispanic Americans are less likely to receive regular medical care than either African Americans or non-Hispanic white Americans.

**8. What are some gender differences in health?** Women live longer than men do, in part because men are less likely to seek preventive health care and early diagnosis of troubling symptoms. Women are less likely than men to develop heart disease (before menopause) but more likely to develop arthritis and osteoporosis.

### CRITICAL THINKING AND HEALTH

**9. What is critical thinking?** Critical thinking is a tool we can use to evaluate information about health. It is characterized by skepticism and by thoughtful analysis of arguments.

**10. What are some features of critical thinking?** These include analyzing definitions of terms and premises of arguments; evaluating evidence; and avoiding oversimplification and overgeneralization.

## References and Suggested Readings

### SMART REFERENCES FROM SCIENTIFIC AMERICAN

**Zorpette, G. Dentistry: Electric Smile Aid.** *Scientific American,* 274(5) (May 1996), 26. **R0101**

### SUGGESTED READINGS

**Kunz, J. R. M., and Finkel, A. J. (Eds).** *The American Medical Association Family Medical Guide* (Revised and Updated). New York: Random House, 1987. A complete, authoritative guide to family health, featuring flowcharts that show you what to do in response to many common medical problems, from rash with fever to cramps and painful knees.

**Carlson, K. J., Eisenstat, S. A., and Ziporyn, T.** *The Harvard Guide to Women's Health.* Cambridge, MA: Harvard University Press, 1996. A comprehensive guide to women's health concerns.

**American Medical Association.** *Complete Guide to Women's Health.* New York: Random House, 1996. An authoritative and comprehensive guide to health concerns of women.

**American Red Cross and Handal, K. A.** *The American Red Cross Health & Safety Handbook.* Boston: Little Brown, 1992. An authoritative guide to handling every type of first aid emergency, from allergic reactions to wounds.

**U.S. Department of Health and Human Services.** *Healthy People 2000: National Health Promotion and Disease Prevention Objectives.* Washington, DC: U.S. Government Printing Office, 1991. Charting America's goals for health promotion and disease prevention by the year 2000.

TABLE 1.3

**Health-Related Internet Sites**

| Health Resource | Who They Are/What They Do | Internet Address[1] (use http:// as a prefix) |
|---|---|---|
| National Institutes of Health (NIH) | Gateway to information on the latest biomedical research, spanning 24 institutes | www.nih.gov |
| Food Nutrition Information Center (FNIC) | A service provided by the U.S. Department of Agriculture (USDA) designed to help people look for information and educational materials on food and nutrition | www.nal.usda.gov/fnic |
| American Heart Association (AHA) | Information on fighting heart disease and stroke | www.amhrt.org |
| American Cancer Society (ACS) | Information about cancer and its treatment | www.cancer.org |
| Food & Drug Administration (FDA) | Information about food safety | www.fda.gov |
| Environmental Protection Agency (EPA) | Citizen information about threats to the environment; EPA publications, programs, and initiatives | www.epa.gov |
| Centers for Disease Control and Prevention (CDC) | Federal agency that provides information about diseases and health risks | www.cdc.gov |
| National Center for Health Statistics (NCHS) | A division of CDC that provides statistical - information about diseases and health care | www.cdc.gov/nchswww/nchshome.htm |
| Healthy Devil Online, Duke University | Information on health issues, including STDs, mental health, women's health, nutrition, and drinking and smoking | h-devil-www.mc.duke.edu/h-devil |
| National Center for Infectious Disease (NCID) | Information on infectious diseases ranging from STDs to Lyme disease | www.cdc.gov/ncidod/about.htm |
| National Women's Resource Center | Consortium of federal agencies addressing women's physical and mental health | www.nwrc.org |
| American Social Health Association (ASHA) | Information, frequently asked questions, and materials relating to AIDS and other STDs | sunsite.unc.edu/ASHA |
| American Psychological Association (APA) | Information on psychology for the general public | www.apa.org |
| American Psychiatric Association (APA) | Information on mental health, including online pamphlets on topics including depression, phobias, and Alzheimer's disease | www.psych.org |
| National Committee for Quality Assurance (NCQA) | Evaluates and accredits HMOs | www.ncqa.org |
| Go Ask Alice! (Go Ask Alice! is a feature of Healthwise, a service offered by the Health Education and Wellness Program of Columbia University) | Questions and answers about health-related issues including sexual health and relationships, alcohol and drugs, and fitness and nutrition | www.columbia.edu/cu/healthwise/alice.html (Healthwise website: www.columbia.edu/cu/healthwise) |

[1]Internet addresses sometimes change; these were the current addresses at the time of publication.

# The Healthy Personality

## DID YOU KNOW THAT

- An average student may have higher self-esteem than a highly respected scientist? p.36
- People with healthy personalities do not see their health as a matter of luck or chance? p.39
- An identity crisis is a normal aspect of healthy personality development? p.40
- Optimists tend to recover faster from coronary artery bypass surgery than pessimists do? p.41
- Many lottery winners who quit their jobs after striking it rich feel aimless and dissatisfied? p.42
- Some cells in your body are several feet long? p.44
- Hispanic-American women who are acculturated to life in the United States are more likely to be heavy drinkers than less well-acculturated Hispanic-American women? p.47

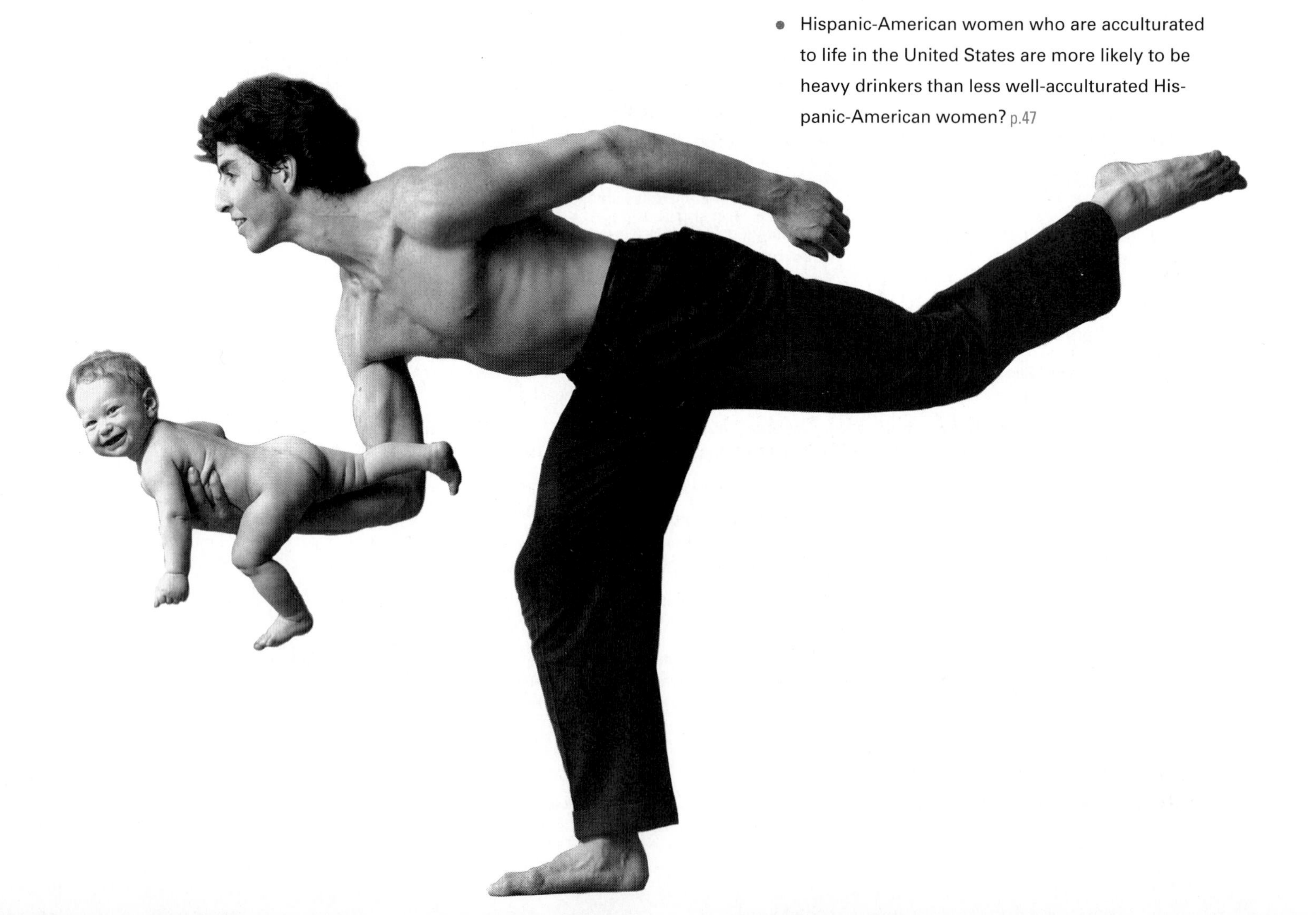

*Sirens wail. Ambulances shriek up to the doors. Stretchers are brought inside. The emergency room at Dallas's Parkland Memorial Hospital teems with life, and with problems. Because of the volume of patients, beds line the halls. People who do not require immediate care cram the waiting rooms. Many hours may pass before they are seen. People who are not considered in imminent danger may wait for 10 to 12 hours.*

*Does all this sound forbidding? Perhaps, but good things are happening at Parkland as well. One is that physicians are attempting to pay attention to people's psychological needs as well as to their physical needs. Dr. Ron Anderson has been influenced by his own clinical experience and by Native American wisdom about healing and wellness. For example, he teaches his medical students that science does not replace* caring *about people. Caring about patients is not an outdated ideal found only in rural practices. Rather, caring is a powerful weapon in the modern war against disease.*

*TV journalist Bill Moyers[1] describes Anderson on rounds with students:*

> *I listen as he stops at the bedside of an elderly woman suffering from chronic asthma. He asks the usual questions: "How did you sleep last night?" "Is the breathing getting any easier?" His next questions surprise the medical students: "Is your son still looking for work?" "Is he still drinking?" "Tell us what happened right before the asthma attack." He explains to his puzzled students: "We know that anxiety aggravates many illnesses, especially chronic conditions like asthma. So we have to find out what may be causing her episodes of stress and help her find some way of coping with it. Otherwise she will land in here again, and next time we might not be able to save her. We cannot just prescribe medication and walk away. That is medical neglect. We have to take the time to get to know her, how she lives, her values, what her social supports are. If we don't know that her son is her sole support and that he's out of work, we will be much less effective in dealing with her asthma."*

# 2

Note some key concepts noted by Moyers:

- "Anxiety aggravates many illnesses."
- "We have to find out what may be causing . . . stress and . . . find some way of coping with it."
- "We cannot just prescribe medication and walk away."
- "We have to take the time to get to know [patients], how [they] live, [their] values, what [their] social supports are."

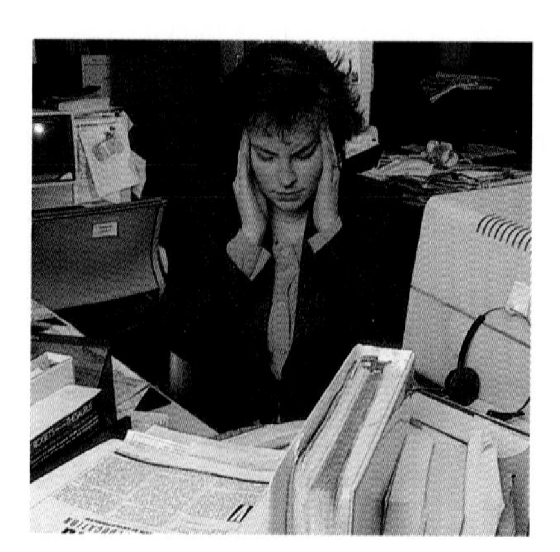

***Problems at Work?*** Psychological health involves the ability to derive satisfaction from one's work, social relationships, and leisure activities. Difficulties at work may compromise both our psychological and physical health.

Anxiety is a psychological problem, but it is intertwined with biological health problems. Stress is also a psychological factor, but it affects the body. Your attitudes and beliefs, emotions, and behavior patterns are all psychological factors, yet each of them also affects your body. Health professionals need to get to know the people they treat to learn how psychological factors affect their physical health.

We can speak of your biological or physical health. So, too, can we speak of your psychological health. Psychological health is important in its own right. **Psychological health** means many things, among them being aware of your needs, values, and goals. It also means finding—and creating—meaning in life. Psychological health means being able to meet the challenges of life and to derive fulfillment and satisfaction from one's work, interpersonal relationships, and leisure pursuits.

Part and parcel of psychological health is the development of a healthy personality. Just as you have a body—a physical or biological self—you also have a psychological self, or personality. Your **personality** is made up of the traits, thoughts, feelings, and behavior that distinguish you from other people. A healthy personality is characterized by traits such as self-esteem, self-confidence, and ego identity, to name a few.

Overall, psychological health means a sense of well-being—of psychological wellness. Psychological health is the sense that things are right with ourselves, with who we are as individuals.

In this chapter, we explore the healthy personality. We consider characteristics associated with a healthy personality and factors that contribute to its development. Since psychological factors affect every aspect of life, including physical health, we will first help you learn more about your psychological self—your needs, goals, and values.

**Psychological health** The possession of a sound mind, emotional stability, and ability to function effectively and to achieve a sense of fulfillment and satisfaction in one's life.

**Personality** The constellation of traits, attitudes, dispositions, and behavioral patterns that constitutes our individuality.

**Need** A state of want, or a condition arising from a deficiency status, such as hunger or thirst.

## GETTING TO KNOW YOURSELF—WHAT ARE YOUR NEEDS, VALUES, AND GOALS?

The ancient Greek philosopher Socrates offered a simple prescription for wisdom: "Know thyself." Most of us probably feel we know ourselves fairly well. We know what we like to eat, what music we like to listen to, and what movies we enjoy. We may have a good handle on our likes and desires. Yet how many of us have sorted out the deeper dimensions of our personalities—our needs, values, and goals? Self-knowledge helps us evaluate our progress toward achieving psychological health.

### Needs

What are your most important needs? To achieve status and financial security? To make a difference in the world? To achieve something that no one has ever achieved before? To eat, drink, and be merry?

When you experience a **need,** you feel motivated to do something to satisfy it. Psychologists have identified many needs, including needs for achievement and for other people. Perhaps the best-known psychological model of needs was offered by Abraham Maslow, who believed that needs are ordered in the form of a hierarchy.

**HealthCheck** Sensation-seeking scale H0201

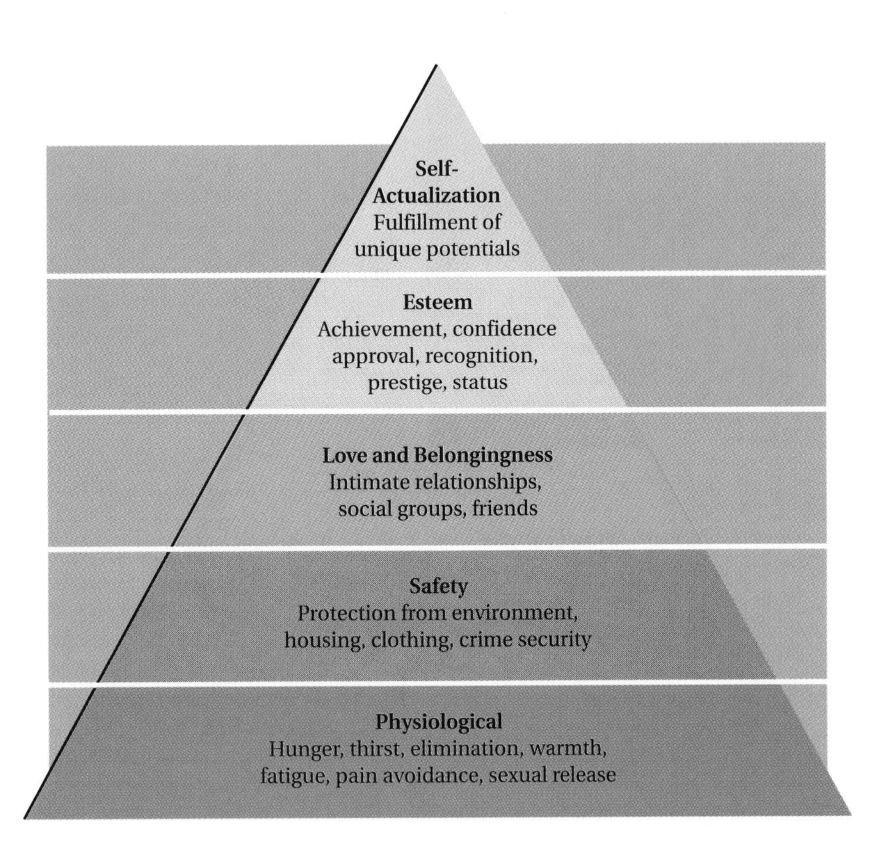


**Figure 2.1** ***Maslow's Hierarchy of Needs*** According to Maslow, we are motivated to first satisfy lower needs before progressing to meet higher needs. Do you agree? Why or why not? Where might you place yourself in this pyramid?

**Maslow's Hierarchy of Needs** Maslow believed that needs are ordered from basic biological needs such as hunger and thirst to psychological needs such as self-esteem and self-actualization (see Figure 2.1). According to Maslow, we first attempt to meet basic needs. Once these are satisfied, we strive to meet higher-level needs. In other words, once our bellies are full, we don't merely snooze until we have hunger pangs again.

The highest need in Maslow's hierarchy is **self-actualization.** Self-actualization is the need to become all that we are capable of being. Self-actualization motivates us to try to fulfill our unique potentials. Since no two people are alike, self-actualization can take many forms. It can be creating art, becoming an accomplished athlete, theologian, military officer, teacher, or parent. Maslow was an optimist. He believed that people are genuinely good and if given the opportunity, they will strive to achieve the higher goals relating to love, esteem, and self-actualization.

In a relatively affluent society like ours, most people can satisfy basic physiological and safety needs. The struggles for love and belongingness often take center stage in our lives. Not all of us climb to the top of the hierarchy. Many people are frustrated in their efforts to achieve acceptance and love. Not all of us achieve self-actualization. Maslow believed that achieving the full measure of psychological health and wellness required that all five levels of need be satisfied.

How about you? Are you a self-actualizing person? Self-actualization does not depend on how much money you make or how many friends you have. It is more closely related to your approach to life, to whether you are open to experiences and opportunities that help you fulfill your potential. The ***HealthCheck*** (next page) may give you a clearer idea about your self-actualizing tendencies.

**Close Up**
Characteristics of self-actualizing people
**T0201**

**Need for Achievement** Some students persist in their studies despite distractions. Some people strive relentlessly to get ahead, to "make it," to earn vast sums of money, to invent, to achieve the impossible. Such people are said to have a strong need for achievement.

People with a strong **need for achievement** earn higher grades than people of comparable ability but with a lower need for achievement. They are more likely to earn high salaries and be promoted than less motivated people with similar opportunities. Most college graduates with strong needs for achievement take positions characterized by

**Self-actualization** A tendency to strive to realize one's potential.

**Need for achievement** A psychological need to accomplish extrinsic goals, such as success and esteem.

## Health Check

### Do You Strive to Be All That You Can Be?[2]

Are you a self-actualizer? Do you strive to be all that you can be? Maslow attributed the following characteristics to the self-actualizing person. How many of them describe you? Why not undertake some self-evaluation?

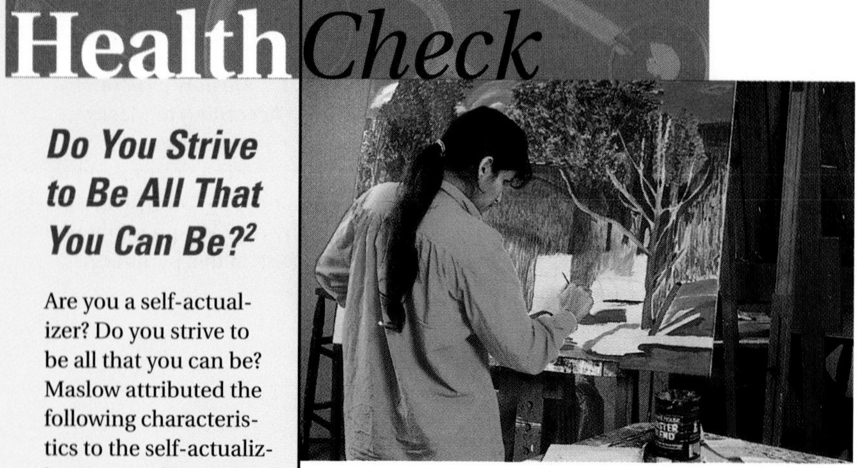

**YES NO**

____ ____ 1. *Do you fully experience life in the present—the here and now?* (Self-actualizers do not focus excessively on the lost past or wish their lives away as they stride toward distant goals.)

____ ____ 2. *Do you make growth choices rather than fear choices?* (Self-actualizers take reasonable risks to develop their unique potentials. They do not bask in the dull life of the status quo. They do not "settle.")

____ ____ 3. *Do you seek to acquire self-knowledge?* (Self-actualizers look inward; they search for values, talents, and meaningfulness. The questionnaires in this book offer a good jumping-off point for getting to know yourself. It might also be enlightening to take an "interest inventory"—a test frequently used to help make career decisions—at your college testing and counseling center.)

____ ____ 4. *Do you strive toward honesty in interpersonal relationships?* (Self-actualizers strip away the social facades and games that stand in the way of self-disclosure and the formation of intimate relationships.)

____ ____ 5. *Do you behave self-assertively and express your ideas and feelings, even at the risk of occasional social disapproval?* (Self-actualizers do not bottle up their feelings merely to avoid disapproval.)

____ ____ 6. *Do you strive toward new goals? Do you strive to be the best that you can be in a chosen life role?* (Self-actualizers do not live on the memory of past accomplishments, nor do they make halfhearted efforts.)

____ ____ 7. *Do you seek meaningful and rewarding life activities?* Do you experience moments of actualization that Maslow referred to as **peak experiences?** (Peak experiences are times of rapture filled with personal meaning. Examples might include completing a work of art, falling in love, redesigning a machine tool, solving a complex problem in math or physics, or having a baby. Again, we differ as individuals; one person's peak experience might be a bore to another.)

____ ____ 8. *Are you open to new experiences?* (Self-actualizers do not hold themselves back for fear that novel experiences might shake their views of the world or their views of right and wrong. Self-actualizers are willing to revise their expectations, values, and opinions.)

The more "yes" responses to these items, the closer you are to achieving self-actualization. Self-actualization is a continuing process of growth and realization, more a road to be followed than a final destination. The question is, where along this road are you?

risk, decision making, and the chance of great success.[3] For example, they may enter business management or sales or establish businesses of their own. People with a strong need for achievement prefer challenges and are willing to take reasonable risks to achieve their goals.

**Peak experience** A moment of intense joy and personal satisfaction arising from self-actualization.

The need for achievement can be driven by different forces.[4] Some students are mainly driven by *performance goals*. They aim to achieve tangible rewards such as a good job, entry into graduate school, the approval of their parents or professors—or averting their criticism. Other students are motivated by *learning goals*. They want to enhance their knowledge and skills. Performance

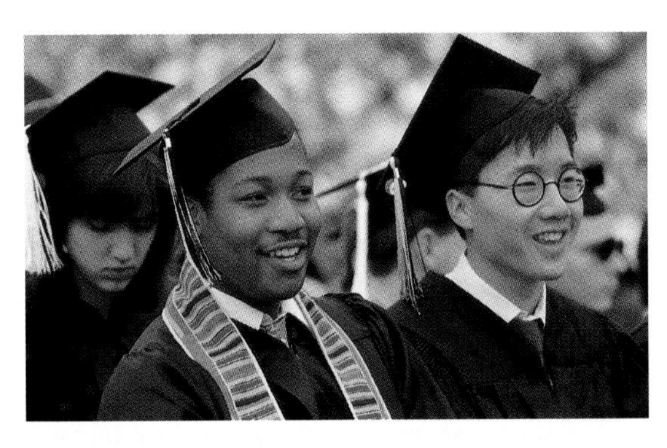

***Achievement Motivation*** College graduates with a strong need for achievement seek career opportunities that may be somewhat risky but promise high rewards and opportunities for personal decision making.

goals are usually reinforced through external rewards such as money and prestige. Learning goals usually lead to internal rewards such as self-satisfaction. Many of us aim to meet both performance and learning goals. It's not that one set of goals is superior; both can have value to the individual.

## Values

We hear much talk of values. Politicians make noises about supporting family values, although the meaning of "family values" seems to vary from politician to politician. What are values? How are values linked to health?

**Values** are our ideas about what is important in life. They are the standards by which we define good and bad. They underlie our preferences and guide our choices. Just as on a cold day you probably place greater value on a good pair of gloves than on air-conditioning, our values may change with the seasons of our lives. What we valued when young, such as freedom to experiment with alternative lifestyles, may diminish in importance as we grow older. We may come to place greater values on family stability and financial security. Some people value money above anything else; to others, money has a low priority. What do you value?

**HealthCheck**
Values clarification
H0202

Our values are shaped largely by our experiences and by the important people in our lives—particularly our parents, teachers, and other role models. For many people, cultural and religious values provide a solid anchor in a changeable world.

Differences in values are sources of conflict between people. Much twentieth-century conflict arose between people who valued the individual above the state and those who valued the state above the individual. Parents and children often experience clashes in values. Parents may value grades above popularity at a time when children are coming under great peer pressure to be liked and to conform. Reflect on your situation: Have you experienced conflicts in values with your parents? Over what issues? Were they resolved? If so, how? If not, how painful is the experience of clashing values?

Our values also affect our health-related behavior. To the extent that we value our health, we are likely to adopt healthful behaviors. We will eat a balanced, low-fat diet, exercise regularly, and avoid harmful practices such as smoking. However, health values sometimes take a back seat to other things, especially among adolescents and young adults. Young people often perceive themselves to be invulnerable.[5] Although older people are at greater risk of serious health problems like heart disease and cancer, the habits we establish early in life may either increase or decrease our risks of these problems later on. We know, for example, that childhood obesity is a strong predictor of adult obesity, and obesity is a major risk factor for heart disease and premature death. We also know that addiction to tobacco almost always occurs before age 30. Moreover, young adults are at greater risk than older adults of dying from accidents.

Perhaps it is time for you to take stock of your values. Where does *a healthy life* fall in your scheme of things?

## Goals

Our **goals** are the flip sides of our needs. We are motivated to satisfy our needs. The satisfaction of a need becomes a goal. If you have a strong need for friendship, for example, your goal will involve making new friends or joining groups. If you are motivated by a need for achievement, you will set goals such as high grades and income.

Setting goals involves reflecting on your needs, determining what is most important, and deciding how to get from where you are to where you want to be. Set goals that are realistic but somewhat challenging. You may want to write a great novel or play shortstop for the Atlanta Braves, but is this realistic? Then again, if you have the talent and desire, why not strive to reach the top in your field—whether it is

**Values** The worth or importance placed on objects or goals; standards of worth.

**Goals** The ends toward which we strive that result in satisfaction of needs.

writing, baseball, or something else? There is nothing wrong with trying hard and finding out how far you can go in life.

Don't sell yourself short. Don't set goals that are far beneath your potential. If you set your goals low, you will probably achieve them, but how satisfying will that be? How will it boost your self-esteem? Your educational choices affect the opportunities that will be available to you later. Settling for sure things prevents you from learning how far your desires and abilities may take you.

Investigate career opportunities in a field that interests you. Learn about the courses and practical experiences you'll need to achieve your career goals. Lay out a plan to get from here to there step by step. Such a plan may include seeking advice from a career-counseling center.

Smart Quiz
Q0201

**think about it!**

- **What are your most important psychological needs?**
- **Are you a self-actualizer? Why or why not?**
- **How are your own values related to your health-related behavior?**

**critical thinking** **Agree or disagree and support your answer: Psychological health is an important part of our overall health and well-being.**

## THE HEALTHY PERSONALITY

Who are you? Are you optimistic or pessimistic? Are you independent or group-minded? Are you one of your favorite people or do you get down on yourself? Are you hard-driving or easy-going? No two of us are quite alike. Your personality is distinct, but is it healthy? Though professionals may argue about the particular constellation of traits that constitute a healthy personality, there is general agreement the following traits enter into the composite: self-esteem, self-confidence, self-direction, self-assertiveness, psychological hardiness, ego identity, a sense of humor, and meaningfulness.

**Self-esteem** A sense of self-worth or self-approval.

**Self-concept** One's perception of oneself.

**Ideal self** The mental image corresponding to what we believe we ought to be like.

### Self-Esteem—How Do You Compare to Your Ideal Self?

**Self-esteem** is the core component of the healthy personality. Self-esteem refers to our sense of self-worth. Psychologically healthy people have positive self-esteem. They value themselves and consider themselves worthy of success. They also recognize their deficits and limitations. Thus they have a positive but realistic view of themselves.

Self-esteem is an important feature of our **self-concept,** the totality of perceptions we have about ourselves in terms of the physical, psychological, emotional, intellectual, and spiritual parts of our being. Our self-concept encompasses our impressions of ourselves as well as our evaluation of what others think of us.

**The Ideal Self** Even people with high self-esteem may fall short of their ideal selves. Our **ideal self** is our concept of what we ought to be. The greater the *differences* between your perception of your *actual* self and your *ideal* self on important traits, the *lower* your self-esteem is likely to be. The *closer* your self-perceptions are to your ideal self, the *higher* your self-esteem is likely to be. Therefore, an average student may have higher self-esteem than a respected scientist. Self-esteem depends on the difference between one's self-concept and one's ideal self on highly valued traits. The average student may not value scholarship or intellectual achievement as much as the scientist does. Then, too, even scientists who are held in high regard by colleagues may impose such perfectionistic standards on themselves that their self-esteem suffers.

If you have relatively low self-esteem, don't give up the ship. The chapter's ***Take Charge*** section focuses on ways of enhancing self-esteem.

**Self-Esteem and Healthful Behavior** Self-esteem plays a critical role in the choices we make about our health. Those with high self-esteem are less likely to abuse their health by drinking to excess, ignoring guidelines for safer sex, or denying the signs of illness.

Our self-esteem rises when we are good to ourselves. Eliminating unhealthful habits enhances self-esteem. Virtually all former smokers feel better about themselves than they did when they were smoking. So do people who eat a balanced diet and exercise regularly.

# Health Check

## Examining Your Self-Concept[6]

What do you *really* think of yourself? Are you pleased with the person you see in the mirror? Or do you put yourself down at every opportunity? One way to measure your self-concept is to evaluate yourself according to a set of traits, such as those listed here.

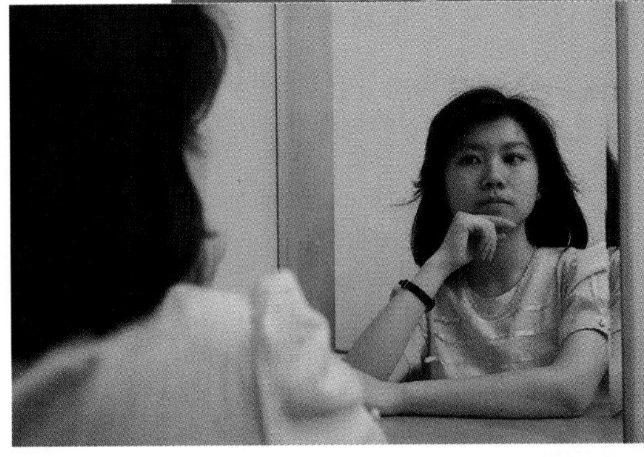

*Place a checkmark next to the number that best corresponds to how you see yourself on each of the traits by using the following code:*

1 = extremely
2 = rather
3 = somewhat
4 = equally ____ and ____; not sure
5 = somewhat
6 = rather
7 = extremely

| | 1 | 2 | 3 | 4 | 5 | 6 | 7 | |
|---|---|---|---|---|---|---|---|---|
| Fair | ___ | ___ | ___ | ___ | ___ | ___ | ___ | Unfair |
| Independent | ___ | ___ | ___ | ___ | ___ | ___ | ___ | Dependent |
| Religious | ___ | ___ | ___ | ___ | ___ | ___ | ___ | Irreligious |
| Unselfish | ___ | ___ | ___ | ___ | ___ | ___ | ___ | Selfish |
| Self-Confident | ___ | ___ | ___ | ___ | ___ | ___ | ___ | Lacking Confidence |
| Competent | ___ | ___ | ___ | ___ | ___ | ___ | ___ | Incompetent |
| Important | ___ | ___ | ___ | ___ | ___ | ___ | ___ | Unimportant |
| Attractive | ___ | ___ | ___ | ___ | ___ | ___ | ___ | Unattractive |
| Educated | ___ | ___ | ___ | ___ | ___ | ___ | ___ | Uneducated |
| Sociable | ___ | ___ | ___ | ___ | ___ | ___ | ___ | Unsociable |
| Kind | ___ | ___ | ___ | ___ | ___ | ___ | ___ | Cruel |
| Wise | ___ | ___ | ___ | ___ | ___ | ___ | ___ | Foolish |
| Graceful | ___ | ___ | ___ | ___ | ___ | ___ | ___ | Awkward |
| Intelligent | ___ | ___ | ___ | ___ | ___ | ___ | ___ | Unintelligent |
| Artistic | ___ | ___ | ___ | ___ | ___ | ___ | ___ | Inartistic |
| Tall | ___ | ___ | ___ | ___ | ___ | ___ | ___ | Short |
| Obese | ___ | ___ | ___ | ___ | ___ | ___ | ___ | Skinny |

Add other traits of importance to you:

| | 1 | 2 | 3 | 4 | 5 | 6 | 7 | |
|---|---|---|---|---|---|---|---|---|
| ________ | ___ | ___ | ___ | ___ | ___ | ___ | ___ | ________ |
| ________ | ___ | ___ | ___ | ___ | ___ | ___ | ___ | ________ |
| ________ | ___ | ___ | ___ | ___ | ___ | ___ | ___ | ________ |

Now consider your *ideal self.* Place an X instead of a checkmark next to the number that corresponds to *how you would like to be* for each trait. Ratings for some dimensions might overlap, indicating a match between how you see yourself (your self-concept) and your self-ideal. Next, look at the discrepancies between your ratings of your self-concept and your ideal self. Traits with a low discrepancy score are likely to contribute to self-esteem, while those with larger discrepancy scores are likely to lower self-esteem. In general, the closer your self-perceptions are to your ideal self, the higher your self-esteem is likely to be.

## Self-Confidence

Psychologically healthy people are self-confident.[7] They believe in their ability to get things done, such as completing a college course (in personal health, for instance) or doing a back flip off a diving board. Self-confident people are more likely to face the challenges of life rather than retreat from them. They are also likely to grasp opportunities, such as gaining a foothold in a new career, or taking up a new sport or hobby, and to make healthful changes in their behavior, such as quitting smoking, controlling their weight, and exercising. It is not that they know more about the positive or negative consequences of their behavior. It is because they have greater confidence in their ability to make healthful changes that they undertake them. Thus they are more likely to try to change their behavior. They are also more likely to stick to their efforts, even when they confront obstacles in their path.

***To Climb Any Mountain*** Self-confidence is a key aspect of psychological health. People who have a strong belief in their abilities are willing to overcome challenges rather than retreat from them.

Self-confidence is a strong predictor of positive health outcomes. It predicts who will recover most successfully from a heart attack and who will be better able to cope with the pain of arthritis. During childbirth, women with more self-confidence are more likely to waive pain-killing medication.[8] People with self-confidence are less likely to relapse once they have quit smoking or lost weight.[9]

Self-confidence is generally higher among people who are free of psychological disorders such as anxiety disorders or depression.[10] Life is not necessarily a bowl of cherries for people with self-confidence. But if they should need psychological help for emotional problems, they are more likely than people lacking self-confidence to benefit from psychotherapy.[11]

Self-confidence and success go hand in hand. People with self-confidence are more likely to succeed in accomplishing the tasks that they undertake. Yet success also boosts self-confidence.[12] This is one reason that "success experiences" are so important to children and adults alike.

**Psychological hardiness** A cluster of traits, characterized by commitment, challenge, and control, that buffer the effects of stress.

**Internal locus of control** The perception that the control over rewards and punishments resides within the individual.

**External locus of control** The perception that one's future is determined by forces beyond one's control.

## Psychological Hardiness

Some people seem to be more resistant to illness than others. They also seem to snap back more quickly when they do become ill. Psychologists have identified a constellation of traits, labeled **psychological hardiness,** that may explain why some people are more resilient than others. Psychologically hardy people continue to function in the face of stresses that might push others to the sidelines. Much of the research on psychological hardiness was conducted by Suzanne Kobasa[13] and her colleagues. She studied business executives who resisted illness despite high levels of stress. These highly driven but hardy executives were even less likely to have heart attacks than highly driven, less hardy executives. The hardy executives differed from their nonhardy counterparts in three key ways:

1. They were highly *committed.* They involved themselves deeply in their undertakings.
2. They sought *challenges.* They saw change as interesting, not as a threat. Hardy people are more resistant to stress because they *choose* to face it.
3. They saw themselves as being *in charge* of their lives. Life may be uncertain. The ultimate end may be inevitable. Yet psychologically healthy people feel in control of their lives. They have an **internal locus of control,** believing they are in control of the rewards and punishments of life. They believe that rewards are brought about by their own actions, not by forces beyond their control. People who believe that their fortunes, for better or worse, are at the mercy of luck or the whims of others have an **external locus of control.**

Because they believe they hold the keys to success, people with an internal locus of control are more likely to apply themselves to meet their health challenges. Similarly, they are willing to credit themselves for their successes. People with an external locus of control are likely to attribute successes in health to luck, the doctor, or the medicine.

Like self-confidence, locus of control plays an important role in physical health. Some health outcomes may be beyond our control. We may be exposed to harmful pathogens or inherit a health problem. Yet if we believe our health is largely determined by our own behavior, we are more likely to take steps to prevent disease and enhance our well-being. For example, we are more likely to watch what we eat.

Professional advice or treatment may be required for a health problem. Nevertheless, people with an internal locus of control actively seek advice and choose to follow it. Those with an internal locus of control do not surrender responsibility for their own health to professionals. When they are in doubt, they seek second and third opinions.

People with healthy personalities do *not* see their health as a matter of luck or chance. They see themselves as responsible for their fates. What about you? Are you the master of your fate? Or do you see your prospects as subject to the whims of others or blind luck?

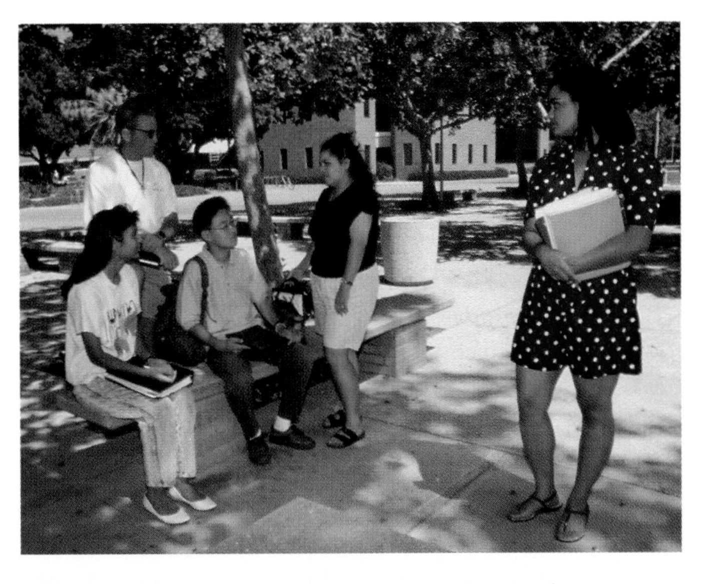

***Shyness*** People who are shy experience anxiety or fear that keeps them on the sidelines of social situations. By learning to manage their social anxiety, people can overcome shyness and learn to become more self-assertive.

## Self-Direction—Making Your Own Way in the World

Psychologically healthy people have a sense of self-direction, or **autonomy.** They steer their own course through life. They consider their personal needs, values, and goals in reaching decisions as well as the ideas of other people. They are open to listening to advice from other people, but do what they believe is right. Self-direction is related to **individuation.** That is, autonomous people have developed a psychological identity that is separate from that of others, including their parents and other powerful role models.

**Talking Glossary**
Individuation
G0201

**Take Charge**
Making the most of college
C0201

Self-directed people recognize that their parents and teachers are not always right. They come to rely on their own resources when things go wrong, rather than expecting their parents or others to rescue them.

## Self-Assertiveness—Express Yourself

**Self-assertiveness** is the expression of one's genuine feelings and beliefs. An assertive person communicates who she or he is as a person. Assertiveness means taking an active rather than a passive approach to life. Assertiveness is learned behavior that can be acquired at any stage of life.

Assertiveness is not aggressiveness. Assertive people are not bossy or belligerent. They don't have a chip on the shoulder. They don't put other people down. Assertive people express positive feelings as well as grievances. They respect the rights and feelings of others, even when they disagree with them.

**Take Charge**
Become assertive
C0202

**Shyness** One roadblock to self-assertion is **shyness.** Shy people are bashful or retiring. They feel afraid or uncomfortable when they approach others. This alerts us to one of the difficulties encountered by shy adults as well as children: The anxiety or fear they experience in social interactions leads to avoidance. Their fears may be so intense that they fail to develop intimate relationships.

Fortunately, most people can overcome shyness by practicing assertive behavior. Psychologists help shy people by showing them how to cope with a series of increasingly more challenging social encounters. Clients learn to manage their anxiety at each step, rather than let it prevent them from participating.

**Autonomy** Self-direction or independence.

**Individuation** The process of developing a psychological identity separate and distinct from others.

**Self-assertiveness** Expression of one's feeling and beliefs in a way that is true to oneself.

**Shyness** A quality of timidness or reserve around other people.

Some general guidelines for assertive behavior can help to overcome shyness.

1. *Challenge irrational beliefs.* Tell yourself that it is not your primary duty in life to make everyone else happy all of the time. Tell yourself that the world won't end if someone doesn't like you. You cannot expect that everyone will approve of you all the time.
2. *Establish eye contact with others.* Look people directly in the eye when you talk to them. (Do not maintain a fixed stare, which may be interpreted as an aggressive challenge.)
3. *Start sentences with, "I feel . . . "* Become accustomed to expressing *how* you feel about things, not just *what* you think about them.
4. *Join campus social organizations.* You may find it more comfortable to interact with others to achieve common goals than to be in unstructured social interactions.
5. *Practice, practice, practice.* Give yourself plenty of opportunity to practice assertive behavior. Don't get down on yourself if you stumble at times.
6. *Accentuate the positive.* Share your positive feelings with others, as well as the negative. When you are pleased or appreciative, speak up.
7. *Don't apologize unnecessarily.* Don't start conversations by saying things like, "I'm sorry. I know I really shouldn't bother you with this, but . . . " You have a right to your feelings.

## Ego Identity—Who Are You? What Do You Stand For?

Psychologically healthy people have **ego identity.** Ego identity is a firm sense of who we are and what we stand for. Ego identity is based on understanding or creating our personal needs, values, and goals. Achievement of ego identity is a key developmental task of adolescence and young adulthood.

According to the **psychoanalyst** Erik Erikson, the development of ego identity often involves periods of serious self-questioning and self-doubting which he called **identity crises.** To Erikson, an identity crisis is an opportunity for personal growth, a time for serious reflection, even though the use of the term "crisis" implies that it may be a stressful experience. Therefore, an identity crisis is a normal aspect of healthy personality development.

People who fail to develop ego identity do not develop clear values and goals. As a result, they may drift without direction. They may be especially vulnerable to negative peer influences, such as illicit drug use. One important aspect of ego identity that typically occurs during adolescence or early adulthood is the development of *role identity,* of establishing a public identity or role through a process that involves choosing and developing a commitment to an occupational or life role. To the college student, this issue may involve an identity crisis over which college major or career path to pursue.

**Close-up**
Factors in identity formation
T0202

**HealthCheck**
Identity crisis quiz
H0203

**Ego identity** The sense of who one is and what one stands for.

**Psychoanalyst** A practitioner of psychoanalysis, the method of therapy that focuses on probing the childhood roots of emotional problems.

**Identity crises** In Erikson's view, periods of serious soul-searching and self-examination that contribute to achieving ego identity.

**Optimism** The tendency to look on the more favorable aspects of events or future possibilities.

## Optimism—Do You See the Cup as Half Empty or as Half Full?

Psychologically healthy people are optimists.[14] They believe their prospects are bright and the future holds promise. Because they are hopeful, optimists are more likely than pessimists to make the most of every opportunity and to bounce back from disappointments.

Researchers find that **optimism** is also strongly connected to health outcomes. In one study, college students were given an optimism scale, the Life Orientation Test (LOT). (See nearby ***HealthCheck.***) The students were asked to track their physical symptoms for one month. Students scoring higher on the optimism scale reported fewer physical symptoms such as dizziness, fatigue, muscle soreness, and blurred vision during the month.[15]

Consider a study of people in chronic pain. During flare-ups of pain, people who held more pessimistic thoughts reported more severe pain and distress.[16] Examples of these pessimistic thoughts included, "No one cares about my pain," "It isn't fair I have to live this way," and "I can no longer do anything." Optimistic women are also less likely than pessimistic women to experience postpartum depression (a type of

# HealthCheck

## Are You an Optimist or a Pessimist?

Do you see a silver lining behind every cloud, or do clouds darken your horizon? Do you believe that things will work out well or do you expect the worst? The Life Orientation Test can help you gain some insight into whether you tend to see the glass as half full or half empty.[19]

*Use the following scale to indicate your response to the following items. Write your response in the spaces provided below. Then check the scoring key in Appendix B at the back of the book.*

4 = strongly agree
3 = agree
2 = neutral
1 = disagree
0 = strongly disagree

____ 1. In uncertain times, I usually expect the best.
____ 2. It's easy for me to relax.
____ 3. If something can go wrong for me, it will.
____ 4. I always look on the bright side of things.
____ 5. I'm always optimistic about my future.
____ 6. I enjoy my friends a lot.
____ 7. It's important for me to keep busy.
____ 8. I hardly ever expect things to go my way.
____ 9. Things never work out the way I want them to.
____10. I don't get upset too easily.
____11. I'm a believer in the idea that "every cloud has a silver lining."
____12. I rarely count on good things happening to me.

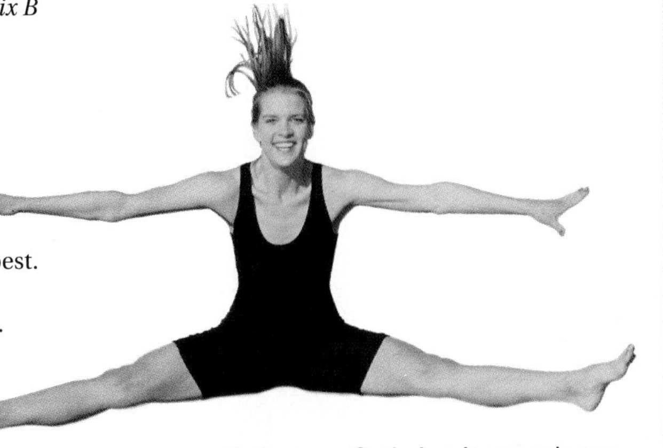

***Optimism*** Optimism is strongly connected to psychological and physical health, even to the ability to bounce back from major surgery.

depression that affects some women after giving birth).[17]

Holding optimistic attitudes is even linked to faster, more successful recovery from surgery. Consider a study of people recovering from coronary artery bypass surgery. Optimists were up and about their rooms more quickly than pessimists. Optimists also had fewer postoperative complications and returned more quickly to their normal lives.[18]

### Sense of Humor

Possessing a sense of humor helps people withstand stress and is linked to higher self-esteem. In one study, students with a good sense of humor had better self-concepts and higher self-esteem than other students.[20] They tended to find things to smile about even when things were not going well. Humor not only serves as a buffer to stress, but may also enhance our ability to appreciate life's fortunate events.

### Meaningfulness—Finding or Creating Purpose in Life

To psychologically healthy people, life is not just a matter of somehow muddling through each day. Rather, each day offers opportunities to find meaning and purpose.

There are many different kinds of meaning in life, many different purposes. For some people, meaning takes on the spiritual quality of connecting themselves spiritually to something larger—whether it be a specific religion, God, or the cosmos.

Others find meaning in their community. Their community may consist of people who share a common ethnic identity and cultural heritage. The development of ethnic pride can help boost self-esteem. Or their community may be their religious congregation. Some take great civic pride in their neighborhoods and in community service. Many people find meaning and fulfillment in love and family.

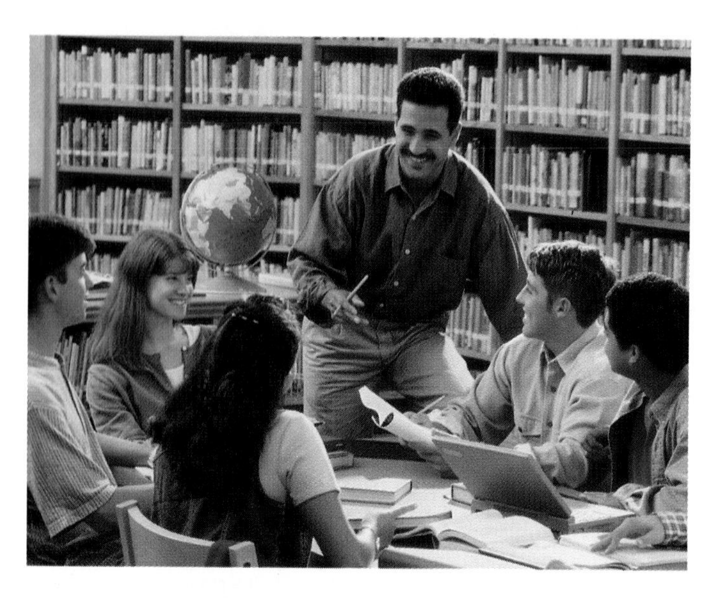

*How Meaningful Is Your Life?* Psychologically healthy people have a sense of meaning or purpose to their lives. We may find meaning in different ways, but having a sense of purpose makes our lives richer and more fulfilling.

**think about it!**

- **Do you have high or low self-esteem? Why?**
- **What is the relationship between self-confidence and success?**
- **Are you psychologically hardy? Why or why not?**
- **Can you describe your ego identity? Who are you? What do you stand for?**

**critical thinking** **Agree or disagree and support your answer: Having a healthy personality can help you cope with stress and disappointment.**

Smart Quiz
Q0202

Still others find meaning in their work, which not only brings home the bacon, but also satisfies internal motives. Work provides an opportunity to engage in stimulating and satisfying activities. Our identities and social roles become wrapped up in our work. We do not think, "I teach." We think, "I *am* a teacher." Or "I *am* a nurse." "I *am* an architect." Not too surprisingly, many lottery winners quit their jobs only to encounter feelings of aimlessness and dissatisfaction.[21]

In sum, these traits—self-esteem, self-confidence, self-direction, psychological hardiness, self-assertiveness, ego identity, optimism, sense of humor, and meaningfulness—are part and parcel of the healthy personality. They help us appreciate what is good in life and help us cope with what is not.

Do not be concerned if you do not possess all these traits or if some are weaker than others. Think of yourself as a work in progress. Knowing the components of a healthy personality will give you psychological goals toward which you can strive. Appreciate your positive qualities and work on the rest. You needed a challenge, didn't you?

**Central nervous system** One of the two major parts of the nervous system; consists of the brain and spinal cord.

**Peripheral nervous system** One of the two major parts of the nervous system; consists of the nerves that connect the brain and spinal cord to the internal organs, skin, and muscles.

**Neurons** Nerve cells.

## FACTORS THAT CONTRIBUTE TO THE HEALTHY PERSONALITY

Many factors contribute to psychological health and wellness: biological factors, psychological factors, and sociocultural factors.

### Biological Factors—Is Biology Destiny?

Our nervous system gives rise to our thoughts, feelings, and behavior. The nervous system is made up of two major parts. The **central nervous system** consists of the brain and spinal cord. The **peripheral nervous system** connects the central nervous system to other parts of the body and to the world outside (see Figure 2.2). The peripheral nervous system receives and transmits sensory messages (nerve impulses from the sense organs such as the eyes and ears) to the central nervous system, and carries nerve impulses from the brain and spinal cord to the muscles, causing them to contract, and to glands, causing them to secrete hormones. Health professionals are interested in the links between the nervous system and our psychological and physical health.

Video
Image-guided surgery
V0201

The nervous system, including the brain and spinal cord, is made up of nerve cells called **neurons.** We are each born with some 12 billion neurons, which is all we will ever have. Neurons carry messages in the form of electrical impulses between the brain and spinal cord and the muscles, glands, and other organs of the body. Some neu-

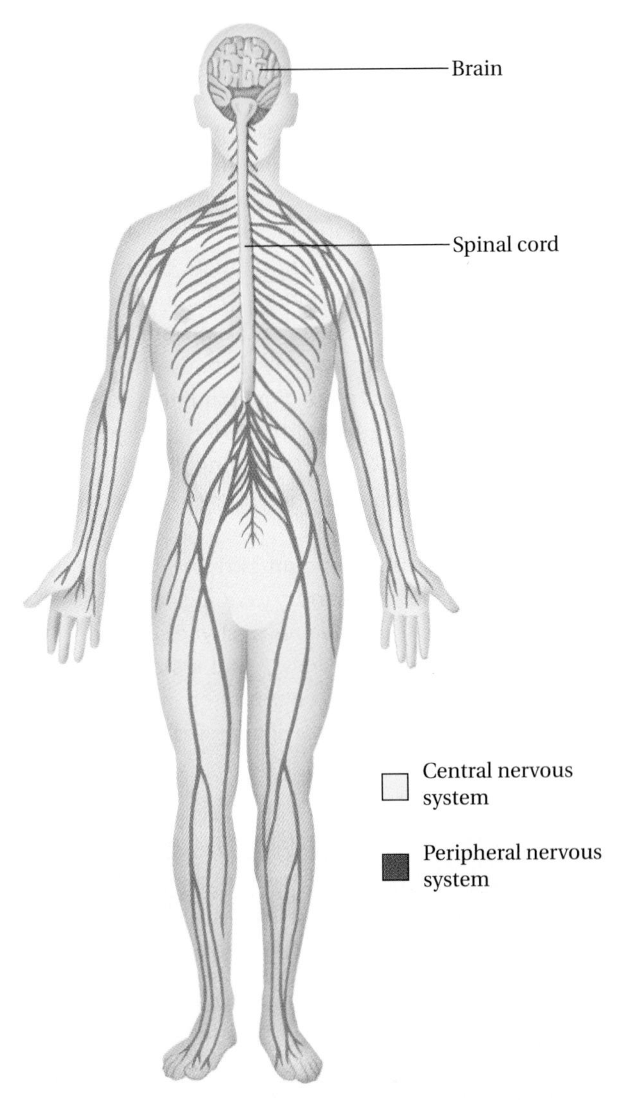


**Figure 2.2** ***Parts of the Nervous System*** The nervous system is composed of two major parts, the central nervous system and the peripheral nervous system. The central nervous system is composed of the brain and spinal cord. The peripheral nervous system connects the central nervous system to the sense organs, muscles, and glands.

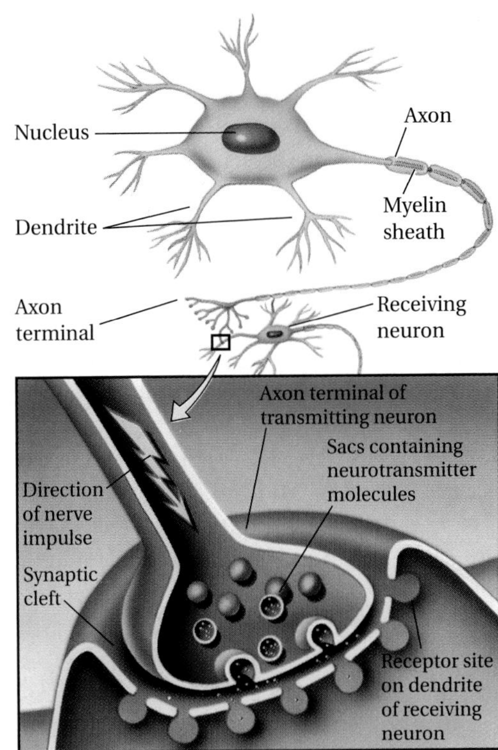


**Figure 2.3** ***Anatomy of a Neuron*** Nerve cells consist of cell bodies (somas), axons, and dendrites. Receptor sites on dendrites receive messages (nerve impulses) from adjacent neurons, which are then transmitted along the axon to axon terminals. Neurotransmitter molecules released from axon terminals carry nerve impulses across the synaptic cleft to receptor sites on neighboring neurons. Neurotransmitter molecules that are not taken up by receptor sites on the receiving neuron are decomposed in the synaptic cleft or reabsorbed by the transmitting neuron. Axons are covered by a myelin sheath, a layer of fatty substance called myelin, which insulates them and facilitates transmission of nerve impulses.

rons carry signals that regulate the heart rate, others are involved in the release of glucose from the liver, while still others mediate sexual response and other bodily functions. Neurons in the brain allow us to think, to dream, and to experience the world around us through the processing of messages from our sensory organs.

**Talking Glossary**
Soma, Dendrites, Axon **G0202**
Neurotransmitters, Synaptic cleft **G0203**

Each neuron consists of a cell body, or **soma, dendrites,** and an **axon** (see Figure 2.3). The soma houses the cell nucleus and metabolizes oxygen to fuel the work of the cell. Dendrites are fibers that project from the cell body and receive messages from adjacent neurons. A single axon projects trunklike from the cell body, terminating in small branching structures called **terminals.** At the tips of axon terminals are swellings called **terminal knobs,** or bulbs, which contain sacs of chemical substances called **neurotransmitters** Neurotransmitters ferry messages from one neuron to another

**Soma** A cell body.

**Dendrites** The rootlike structures at the end of neurons that receive nerve impulses from adjoining neurons.

**Axon** The thin, tubelike part of the neuron along which the nervous impulse travels for transmission to the adjoining neuron.

**Terminals** The small branching structures at the tips of axons.

**Terminal knobs** The structures at the end of axon terminals containing sacs of neurotransmitters.

**Neurotransmitters** Chemical substances that transfer impulses from one neuron to another.

across the **synaptic cleft,** which is the tiny, fluid-filled space between neurons. Sacs in the axon terminals release molecules of neurotransmitters into the synaptic cleft. Neurotransmitters "dock" at receiving stations on the dendrites of the receiving neurons. These docking stations are called **receptors** or receptor sites. Neurotransmitters that do not dock either decompose in the synaptic cleft or are reabsorbed by the transmitting neuron. This process prevents the receiving cell from continuing to fire. Once the receiving neuron fires, it propagates the electrical impulse along its axon and then transmits it to other neurons.

Messages are received by dendrites, conducted electrically along the axon, then transmitted to other neurons. Neurotransmitters each have a distinctive chemical structure that allows them to fit into only one kind of port, or receptor site, on the receiving neuron. Consider an analogy to a lock and key. Only the right key (neurotransmitter) is capable of opening the lock, which causes the receiving neuron (called a *postsynaptic* neuron) to "fire," which forwards the nerve impulse or message.

Neurons are microscopic in width. The axons of neurons in your brain may be only a few thousandths of an inch long. Other axons, such as those that run from your spinal cord to your toes, are several feet long. Many axons are covered with a fatty substance called **myelin,** which insulates them from the surrounding body fluid. Myelin makes transmission of neural impulses more efficient. In the disease **multiple sclerosis,** myelin is replaced by tough fibrous tissue that throws off the timing of messages and impairs muscular control. If the neurons that regulate breathing are affected, death may result from suffocation.

When neurotransmitter systems are in balance, they help keep our thinking processes organized and our moods on an even keel. However, excesses or deficits of neurotransmitters have been linked to a wide variety of psychological disorders, including depression, eating disorders, Alzheimer's disease, and schizophrenia.

Health professionals are also concerned with the influences of hormones and genes on our physical and psychological functioning. **Hormones** are chemical substances secreted by glands into the bloodstream. The hormone *prolactin,* for example, stimulates production of milk. *Oxytocin* is a hormone that stimulates labor in pregnant women. Sex hormones stimulate development of the sex organs and regulate the menstrual cycle. Stress hormones enhance our resistance to stress. Excesses and deficiencies in hormone levels are connected with many physical and psychological disorders. For example, excess thyroid hormones are linked to anxiety and restlessness. Thyroid deficiencies are linked to sluggishness, weight gain, and—in children—mental retardation.

**Genes** are the basic units of heredity. Genetic factors are involved in many psychological traits, such as intelligence, sociability, shyness, emotional stability, aggressiveness, and leadership. Genes are even involved in determining our interest in the arts and our feelings of happiness.[22] Each

**Synaptic cleft** The gap or junction between neurons through which nerve impulses pass.

**Receptors** The sites on receiving neurons where neurotransmitters "dock."

**Myelin** A fatlike substance that coats the axons of certain neurons and helps smooth transmission of nervous impulses.

**Multiple sclerosis** A disease involving degeneration of the myelin that covers the axons of certain neurons.

**Hormones** Chemical substances secreted by glands into the bloodstream.

**Genes** The basic units or building blocks of heredity that contain the genetic code.

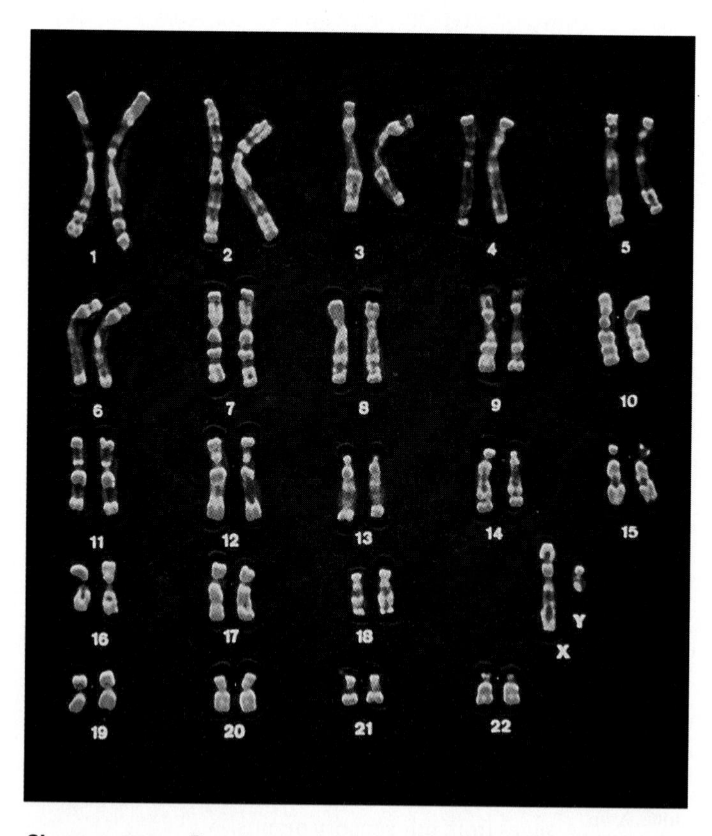


***Chromosomes*** People normally have 46 chromosomes arranged in 23 pairs. Each parent contributes one member of each pair. The unnumbered pair shown here are the sex chromosomes, in this case a male set composed of one X and one Y chromosome. Females have two X sex chromosomes.

**Talking Glossary**
Chromosomes, Deoxyribonucleic acid
G0204

human cell carries about 100,000 genes. Genes are located within the cell's chromosomes. **Chromosomes,** rod-shaped structures housed in the nucleus of the cell, consist of large molecules of **deoxyribonucleic acid (DNA).** Normal human cells contain 46 chromosomes organized into 23 pairs, each of which carries more than 1,000 genes. A child normally inherits one member of each pair of chromosomes from each parent. Thus a child inherits 50% of its genes from each parent. Generally speaking, genetic factors provide a *range* for the expression of various traits; environmental factors such as learning experiences help determine how *or if* these traits are expressed.

**Close-up**
Human Genome Project
T0203

Genetic factors play a role in a range of psychological disorders, including anxiety disorders, addictive disorders, mood disorders, and schizophrenia. Moreover, genetic factors can increase risks for many physical health problems, including coronary heart disease and cancer.

**Changing the Unchangeable—Is Biology Destiny?** What can we do about counterproductive traits, such as shyness and nervousness, that appear to be at least partly inherited? Is it healthful to accept biology as destiny and say, "That's me—that's my personality"? Or is it more healthful to try to change self-defeating behavior patterns, such as social withdrawal and tendencies to avoid challenging situations?

And what of people who inherit tendencies toward obesity or coronary heart disease? Should they throw up their hands and say, "What will be will be"? Or should they eat properly and exercise to maximize their chances of averting these health problems? (We think you know the answer.) Almost all traits are the result of a complex (and not entirely measurable) interaction between "nature" and "nurture." Each trait generally has a range of expression that can be influenced, at least to some extent, by environment.

By focusing on changing their health *behavior,* for example, by following the suggestions for enhancing self-esteem discussed later in the chapter, people can take greater control over their lives and not simply accept their traits as "part of their nature."

## Psychological Factors

Parents help their children develop needs for achievement by encouraging them to think and act independently from an early age. Parents of children with strong needs for achievement encourage them to persist in their schoolwork and make decisions for themselves.[23] They expose their children to new, stimulating experiences. Openness to experience is an important aspect of the self-actualizing individual.

Parents of children with a strong need for achievement show warmth and praise their children for their accomplishments. Children of such parents frequently set high standards for themselves. They associate their achievements with self-worth. They come to attribute their achievements to their own efforts rather than to chance or to the intervention of others.[24] Thus, they also develop an internal locus of control.

Psychologist Carl Rogers has written extensively on the development of self-esteem. He notes that our self-esteem at first mirrors the value placed on us by others. For this reason, Rogers believed it is crucial for parents to show **unconditional positive regard** for their children. That is, parents should accept their children as having worth and value regardless of their behavior at any particular moment. Unfortunately, many parents show **conditional positive regard** toward their children. They bestow approval only when their children behave "properly." Children given conditional positive regard come to think of themselves as worthwhile only when they behave in approved ways. Consequently, they may develop a distorted self-concept, denying or disowning the distinctive parts of themselves that differ from what others value. Their self-esteem may become shaky, as it comes to depend on what other people think of them.

Erik Erikson believed that people who uncritically adopt the values of their parents and other role models are foreclosing their abilities to develop their own ego identities. Erikson did not advocate seeking conflict with parents and dismissing their values. He did believe, however, that it is psychologically healthiest to adopt values only after we have carefully examined them and found them to fit our own individual identities.

Rogers does not suggest that parents accept all of their children's *behavior.* Parents can reject and

**Chromosomes** Rod-shaped structures in the cell's nucleus that consist of molecules of DNA.

**Deoxyribonucleic acid (DNA)** The molecule that makes up genes and chromosomes.

**Unconditional positive regard** Unconditional acceptance of the intrinsic merit or worth of another person regardless of the person's behavior at the moment.

**Conditional positive regard** Judging a person's value in terms of the acceptability of the person's behavior at a given time.

correct children's misbehavior without damaging their self-concepts. However, parents need to make it clear that the behavior is being rejected, not the child.

Psychologists Maslow and Rogers note that because each of us has unique feelings, desires, and needs, we cannot completely abide by the wishes of others and still be true to ourselves. The path to psychological health is paved with awareness and acceptance of all parts of ourselves, warts and all. Rogers encouraged people to be aware of their genuine feelings, accept them as their own, and act in ways that are consistent with their own personalities.

Early childhood experiences have major influences on our personalities. Children whose basic needs are met in a loving and a secure family environment are likely to develop traits such as warmth, confidence, and self-esteem. Children exposed to neglect or abuse, however, may not develop self-esteem or care deeply about other people. Instead, they may develop antisocial tendencies.

## Sociocultural Factors

Sociocultural factors also affect our self-concept and self-esteem. Carl Rogers noted that our self-concepts tend to reflect the ways in which other people see us. Thus, members of the dominant culture in the United States are likely to have a positive sense of self. They share in the expectations of personal achievement and respect that are typically accorded groups who ascend to power. But members of disadvantaged groups that have been subjected to discrimination and poverty may come to develop poorer self-concepts and lower self-esteem than members of the dominant culture.[25]

Sociocultural factors also affect the development of autonomy. Cross-cultural research reveals that people in the United States and many northern European nations tend to be individualistic or self-directed. **Individualists** tend to define themselves in terms of their personal identities. They give priority to their personal goals. When asked to complete the statement "I am," they are likely to respond in terms of their personality traits ("I am outgoing," "I am artistic") or occupations ("I am a nurse," "I am a systems analyst").[26] In contrast, many people from cultures in Africa, Asia, and Central and South America tend to be collectivistic. **Collectivists** tend to define themselves in terms of the groups to which they belong and to give priority to the goals of their group. They feel most complete in terms of their social relationships with others.[27] When asked to complete the statement "I am," they are more likely to respond in terms of their family role, religion, or ethnicity ("I am a father," "I am a Buddhist," "I am a Japanese").[28] These are general tendencies of course; differences exist within cultures as well as between cultures.

The seeds of individualism and collectivism are found in the culture in which a person grows up. The capitalist system fosters individualism. It assumes that individuals are entitled to amass personal fortunes and that the process of doing so creates jobs and wealth for large numbers of people. The individualist perspective is found in the self-reliant heroes and antiheroes in Western media—from Homer's Odysseus to Clint Eastwood's gritty cowboys and Walt Disney's Pocahantas. The traditional writings of the East have exalted people who resisted personal temptations to do their duty and promote the welfare of the group.

Note, too, that neither individualism nor collectivism in its extreme form is desirable. Extreme forms of individualism, such as personal greed or selfishness, can tear the social fabric. Extreme collectivism can stifle creativity, innovation, and personal striving.

**Individualists** People who define themselves in terms of their own personal identities.

**Collectivists** People who define themselves in terms of belonging to certain groups.

### think about it!

Smart Quiz Q0203

- **Explain how biological factors are related to psychological health.**
- **What child-rearing practices contribute to psychological health?**
- **Are you an individualist or a collectivist? Are your views connected with your psychological health?**

**critical thinking Agree or disagree and support your answer: Biology is destiny.**

## Making It in the United States—Acculturation and Psychological Health among Hispanic Americans

WORLD OF *diversity*

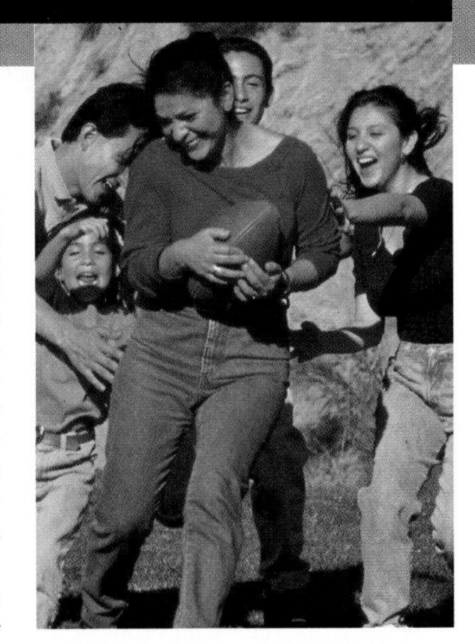

Should Mexican Americans teach their children Spanish in the home? Should African-American children be acquainted with the music and art of African peoples? Should women from traditional Islamic societies lift the veil and enter the workplace alongside American Murphy Browns? Immigrants are pressured to become **acculturated**—that is, to learn about and adopt the values and behavior patterns of the dominant culture in the United States. How do the stresses of acculturation affect their psychological health?

Consider the challenges faced by Hispanic Americans. There are two general theories of the relationships between acculturation and psychological health.[29] One, dubbed the *melting pot theory,* holds that people adjust better to living in the host culture by becoming more like the people who make up the dominant culture. From this perspective, Hispanic Americans might adjust better by replacing Spanish with English and adopting the values and customs associated with mainstream American culture. The second, *bicultural theory,* holds that people adjust best by maintaining their traditional values and beliefs while also striving to adapt to the host culture. That is, adaptability combined with a supportive cultural tradition and a sense of ethnic identity foster psychological health.

Health professionals measure acculturation among Hispanic Americans according to factors such as their preferences for using English or Spanish, their preferences for types of food and styles of clothing, and their self-perceptions of ethnic identity. Using such measures, researchers have found the following relationships between acculturation and psychological health among groups of Hispanic Americans:

- Highly acculturated Hispanic-American women are more likely than relatively unacculturated women to be heavy drinkers.[30] Traditional Latin American cultures impose greater cultural constraints on drinking among women than men. Mainstream U.S. culture has less rigidly defined gender roles, so it is not surprising to find a loosening of these traditional constraints among Hispanic-American women who adopt dominant U.S. attitudes and values.
- Acculturated Mexican Americans born in the United States have higher incidences of depression, phobias, and substance abuse than people born in Mexico.[31]
- Highly acculturated Hispanic-American high school girls are more likely than less acculturated girls to show scores on an eating inventory associated with anorexia.[32] (Anorexia nervosa is an eating disorder characterized by excessive fear of fat and weight loss—see Chapter 6.) Perhaps acculturation makes girls more vulnerable to striving to meet the contemporary American ideal of the ultrathin female.
- Other studies find higher levels of anxiety and depression among low-acculturated Mexican Americans.[33] Are relatively unacculturated Mexican Americans more anxious and depressed because they remain invested in Mexican culture? Or are they anxious and depressed because they typically lack language proficiency and have more difficulty gaining an economic foothold in the U.S.? Mexican-American women who remain more invested in Mexican culture also show generally lower levels of self-esteem and encounter more stress in adapting to life in the United States.

Some studies thus suggest acculturation is connected with psychological health problems. Others link psychological health problems with *failure* to become acculturated. Still other researchers have found that *bicultural* Hispanic Americans—those who identify both with their traditional culture and their host society—are most psychologically healthy. Some outcomes require very careful interpretation. For example, does the finding that acculturated Hispanic-American women are more likely to drink argue in favor of placing greater social constraints on women? Not necessarily. The point seems to be that a loosening of restraints is a double-edged sword. New freedoms may lead to psychological health problems in anyone—male or female, Hispanic or non-Hispanic.

Adjustment to a new society appears to depend on many factors. These include economic opportunity, language proficiency, and a supportive network of acculturated people from one's own background.

**Acculturated** The state of adapting to a host culture.

# Enhancing Self-Esteem

## Take Charge

Self-esteem is at the heart of the healthy personality. In a nutshell, when self-esteem is low, it is usually because we see ourselves as falling short of some ideal. Yet self-esteem is not a fixed quality. We can change it. How? Ways of building self-esteem include developing **competencies**—skills and abilities that allow us to achieve our goals and thus enhance our sense of self-worth. But building self-esteem also involves challenging perfectionistic standards and learning to accept ourselves if we fall somewhat short of our ideal.

### Develop Competencies

Our self-esteem is related to our competencies, or life skills, which include academic skills such as reading and writing; artistic skills such as drawing or playing the piano; athletic skills such as walking a balance beam and throwing a football; social skills such as knowing how to express one's feelings; job-related skills; and many others. The more capabilities we have, especially in areas that matter to us, the better we feel about ourselves.

There are many reasons for individual differences in competencies. For example, there are genetic differences in musical talent and athletic ability. Some of us take lessons in music or sports. Some of us receive warmth and encouragement from parents and teachers. Others have cold, demanding teachers who can never be pleased. Cultural factors play a role. One is unlikely to become competent in, say, football if one belongs to a cultural group that does not practice or value the sport.

Competencies can be acquired through training and practice. You may not be able to throw a baseball at 90 miles per hour unless you have a certain genetic advantage in arm strength and coordination. However, most skills can be developed within a normal range of genetic variation. Most people can learn to ski, although only a few are gifted enough to become Olympians. Most skills valued in our society are achievable by most people.

How can *you* develop the skills or competencies you need to improve yourself? Are you unhappy because you are overly dependent on other people for financial or emotional support? You can work on enhancing social or vocational skills to become more independent. Are you stuck in a career path leading nowhere? Do you lack the skills you need to compete successfully in another line of work? Speak to a vocational counselor or career advisor to help determine what skills you need and how you can get them.

Health-related competencies include accurate knowledge of your body and skills in safeguarding your health and in relating to health professionals. As you progress through this book, you will expand your knowledge about health, learning ways to prevent disease and to optimize wellness.

**Competencies** Skills or abilities needed to perform tasks.

### Strive toward Realistic, Attainable Goals

Carl Rogers believed that striving to meet meaningful goals can yield happiness. Although we may never qualify for the track team, most of us can gradually build our jogging or running abilities to the point where we can lope along at a good speed for half an hour or more. Although we may never play for the New York Philharmonic, most of us can learn to play the piano well enough to enjoy good music and entertain our friends.

Part of boosting self-esteem is setting realistic goals. This does not mean that we should not strive to be the best that we can be. It does mean that we should evaluate our goals in light of our true needs and capabilities.

**Build Your Self-Confidence** Success breeds success. Smaller successes have a way of leading to larger, more meaningful successes. You can build self-confidence by choosing tasks that are consistent with your interests and abilities and working at them. To boost your confidence and encourage you to move forward, start with small, achievable goals. Treat disappointments as opportunities to learn from mistakes, not as signs of inevitable failure.

**Challenge Your Perfectionism** One of the hurdles in striving toward realistic, achievable goals is perfectionism. Psychologist Albert Ellis notes that some of us are unwilling to tackle areas of life unless we can be perfect in them. It would be nice to be competent in everything we do, but it's unreasonable to expect that we can be.

Are you a perfectionist? Perfectionists set unrealistic goals that prevent them from appreciating what they have achieved and keep their self-esteem in the cellar.[34] Even if you can't break a 4-minute mile, you may be able to put a few 8- to 10-minute miles back to back—and feel happier with yourself as well. You may even be able to whip up a dynamite vegetable lasagna.

If you're down on yourself, you probably blame yourself for falling short of your self-ideals. Ask yourself whether your self-appraisal is fair. Do other people see you the same way? Are you your own worst critic? Do you blow up minor flaws in your personality into catastrophes? Do you dwell on imperfections that are apparent to you alone? Do you minimize your achievements? Do you always focus on what remains to be done rather than on what you have accomplished?

Try a shift in your frame of reference. View yourself as if you were another person. Add up your pluses and minuses. Ask yourself: Would you be as hard on someone else who possessed your attributes? Would you be as unforgiving?

Take it a step further. Counsel yourself. Advise yourself in the way you would advise someone else who exaggerated her or his faults.

Taking a more realistic view of yourself doesn't mean that you'll come out unblemished. Self-esteem requires the ability to accept yourself, warts and all. It requires the ability to see your weaknesses as challenges to be met, not as impossible hurdles.

***Challenge Your Need for Approval*** Self-approval begins with the approval of others. Albert Ellis notes that some of us find it nearly impossible to survive without the approval of other people. However, if we are true to ourselves, we will follow our own stars and not become a slave to other people's approval.

Ellis believes that excessive needs for social approval set the stage for low self-esteem.[35] He suggests that we challenge the need for approval:

**Video**
Albert Ellis
**V0201**

- Ask yourself: *How realistic is it to expect that everyone I meet will respect me and like me? And what if they don't? Is it truly so awful if occasionally someone disagrees with me or thinks poorly of me?*
- Replace an irrational need for approval with more rational expectations. Think: *Sure, it would be nice to be liked by everyone, but it is not reasonable to assume that everyone will. Nor is it the end of the world if people sometimes criticize me or are so blind they can't appreciate my finer points. The sun will still rise in the morning. The electric bill will still come on time.*

**Smart Quiz**
**Q0204**

On the other hand, it would hurt your authors' self-esteem if you did not fully approve of this perfect chapter.

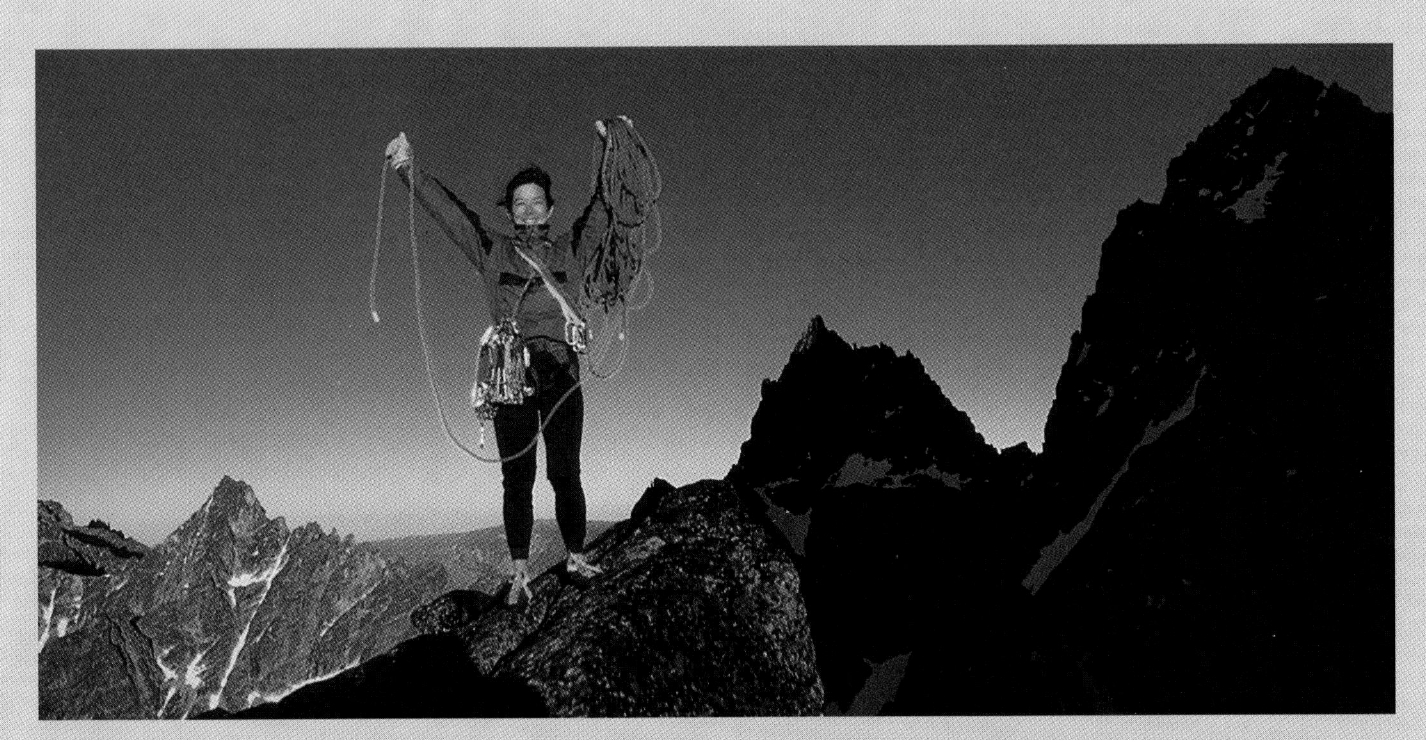

***Self-Esteem*** Self-esteem is a hallmark of the healthy personality. People can help build self-esteem by developing skills or competencies that enable them to achieve their goals, by striving toward realistic, attainable goals, and by learning to accept themselves even if they fall short of perfection.

# SUMMING UP

## Questions and Answers

1. **What is psychological health?** Psychological health means being aware of your needs, possessing traits such as self-esteem, and finding—or creating—meaning in life.

### GETTING TO KNOW YOURSELF—WHAT ARE YOUR NEEDS, VALUES, AND GOALS?

2. **What are our needs?** Our needs are our source of motivation. Maslow created a hierarchy of needs that runs from basic biological needs such as hunger and thirst to psychological needs such as self-esteem and self-actualization. People with a high need for achievement accomplish more than people with similar abilities but a lower need for achievement.

3. **What are our values?** Our values define what is important to us, what is good and bad. We are likely to adopt healthful behaviors according to the value we place on our health.

4. **What are our goals?** Our goals help satisfy our needs. We seem to fare best when our goals are challenging but reachable.

### THE HEALTHY PERSONALITY

5. **What is the connection between psychological health and self-esteem?** Our self-esteem is our sense of self-worth. Psychologically healthy people have positive self-esteem. Our self-esteem depends on how our self-concepts fit with our ideal selves.

6. **What is the connection between psychological health and self-confidence?** Psychologically healthy people have self-confidence. They believe in their ability to meet their needs. Self-confident people are more likely to face the challenges of life rather than retreat from them.

7. **What is the connection between psychological health and psychological hardiness?** Psychologically hardy people continue to function in the face of stresses that often sideline other people. Psychologically hardy people are committed to their undertakings, seek challenges, and see themselves as being in charge of their own lives.

8. **What is the connection between psychological health and self-direction?** Psychologically healthy people steer their own course through life.

9. **What is the connection between psychological health and self-assertiveness?** Psychologically healthy people express their genuine feelings and beliefs.

10. **What is the connection between psychological health and ego identity?** Ego identity is a firm sense of who we are and what we stand for. The development of ego identity often involves a period of serious self-questioning and self-doubting which Erikson dubbed an identity crisis.

11. **What is the connection between psychological health and optimism?** Psychologically healthy people believe the future holds promise. Optimists are more likely than pessimists to take advantage of opportunities and to bounce back from disappointments.

12. **What other traits define the healthy personality?** Psychological health also involves a sense of humor and meaningfulness. For some people, meaning is spiritual. Other people find meaning in their community, their family, or their work.

### FACTORS THAT CONTRIBUTE TO THE HEALTHY PERSONALITY

13. **What biological factors contribute to the healthy personality?** The healthy personality largely involves the functioning of the nervous system, hormones, and genes. Imbalances in neurotransmitters are connected with serious psychological disorders such as depression and schizophrenia. Stress hormones enhance our resistance to stress. Genetic factors are involved in traits ranging from intelligence to sociability to happiness.

14. **What psychological factors contribute to the healthy personality?** Psychological factors such as a need for achievement, unconditional positive regard, ego identity, and a basic sense of optimism and trust all contribute to the healthy personality.

15. **What sociocultural factors contribute to the healthy personality?** Members of disadvantaged groups who have experienced discrimination and poverty may have poorer self-concepts and lower self-esteem than members of the dominant culture. Factors such as individualism and collectivism are also related to personality development.

## Suggested Readings

**Goleman, D., and Gurin, J. (Eds.).** *Mind Body Medicine: How to Use Your Mind for Better Health.* Yonkers, NY: Consumer Reports Books, 1993. A compendium of information on mind-body connections for health, including contributions from many leading authorities on psychological aspects of health.

**Seligman, M. E. P.** *Learned Optimism.* New York: Simon & Schuster, 1990. Techniques for changing negative attitudes into optimistic, health-enhancing attitudes, from a leading psychologist.

**Gilligan, C.** *In a Different Voice.* Cambridge, MA: Harvard University Press, 1982. An influential book that examines differences between men and women with respect to issues of autonomy and intimacy.

**Steinem, G.** *Revolution from Within: A Book of Self-Esteem.* Boston: Little, Brown, 1992. A leading feminist discusses her personal search for and attainment of self-esteem.

**Peterson, C., and Bossio, L.** *Health and Optimism: New Research on the Relationship between Positive Thinking and Physical Well-Being.* New York: The Free Press, 1991. An examination of the pathways between optimism and health.

# Stress and Your Health

**DID YOU KNOW THAT**

- Stress can be good for you? p.54
- Our bodies produce natural painkillers that are chemically similar to the narcotic morphine? p.58
- Video games help children with cancer manage the side effects of chemotherapy? p.60
- The ability to raise the temperature in a finger may help relieve migraine headaches? p.61
- The emotional stress of divorce can weaken the immune system? p.69
- Stress can make you more vulnerable to the common cold? p.69
- Humor may be good medicine for handling stress? p.72
- Deep breathing can help to relieve stress. p.75

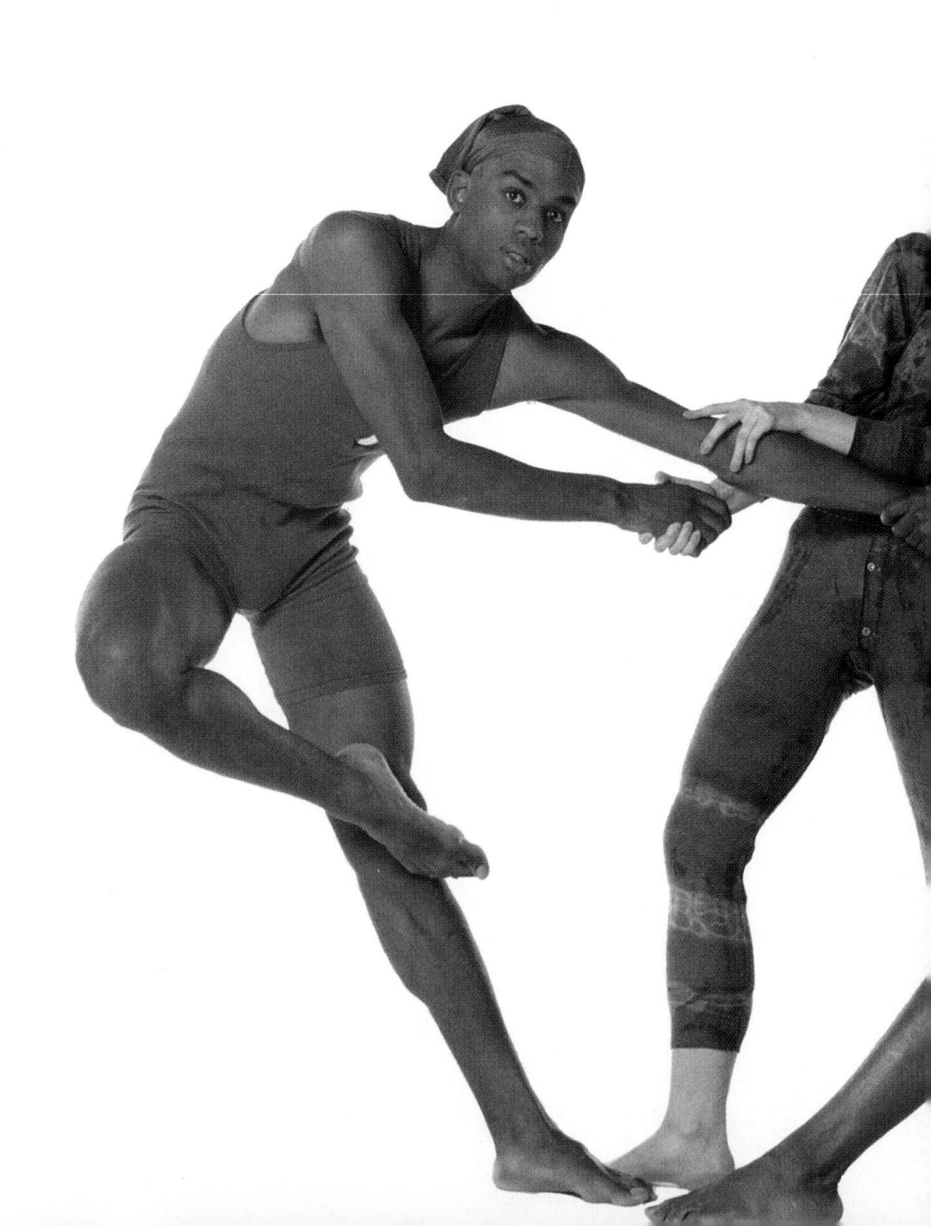

# 3

*Which straw will break the camel's back? The final one, of course. Stressors, like straws, can accumulate gradually until there is one too many. Although a heavy load of stress may not literally break our backs, it can tax our coping ability and our immune systems.*

*In physics, stress is the pressure or force placed upon a body, for example, when a spring is stretched. With people,* **stress** *refers to pressures to adjust or adapt. Stresses on people include job strain, academic demands, parental responsibilities, even the neighbor's stereo.*



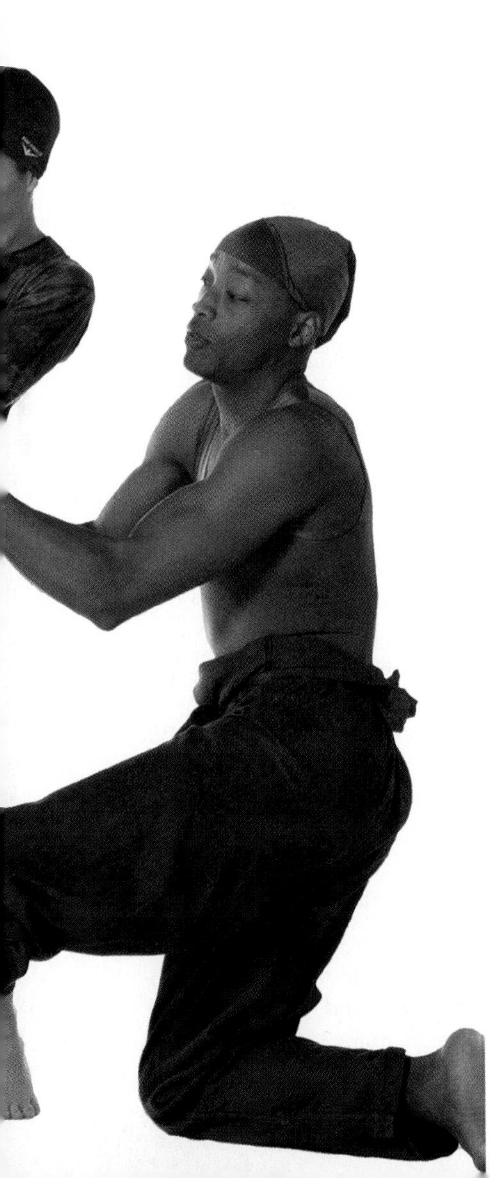

***Eustress*** Not all stress is bad. Joyous events that impose a demand to adjust, like the birth of a child, can be sources of good stress, or eustress. However, even eustress can strain our ability to cope.

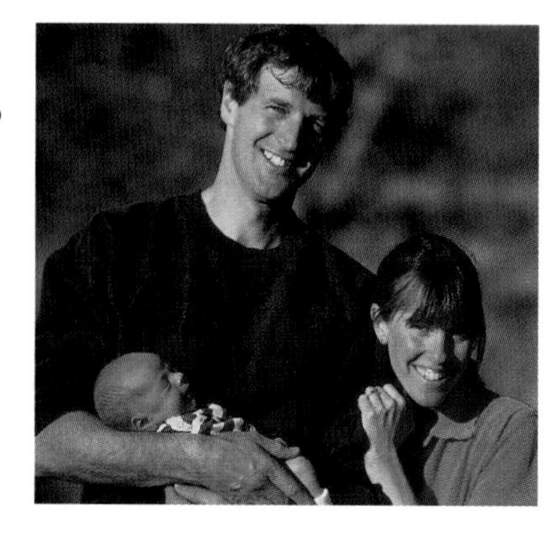

Although some **stressors** threaten our well-being, most people are remarkably resilient to stress. People actually need some stress to keep active, alert, and energized. Without it, we can become stagnant and bored. Positive stress is called **eustress.** Exercise, hard but rewarding work, and joyous events such as graduating from school, getting married, or having a baby are examples of eustress. Intense or prolonged stress, even eustress, can overtax our ability to adjust and lead to health problems such as those in Table 3.1. Learning to manage stress is one of the keys to achieving and maintaining wellness.

Talking Glossary
Eustress
G0301

**TABLE 3.1**

**Stress-Related Health Problems**

| Biological Problems | Psychological Problems |
|---|---|
| Tension or migraine headaches | Fatigue |
| Painful menstruation | Depression |
| Allergic reactions | Anger |
| Back pain, especially low back pain | Resentment |
| High blood pressure | Short temper |
| Skin inflammations (such as hives and acne) | Irritability |
| Rheumatoid arthritis (painful inflammation of the joints) | Anxiety |
| Nausea and vomiting | Feeling overwhelmed |
| Sleep problems | Difficulty concentrating |
| Upset stomach or indigestion | Alcohol or substance abuse |
| Shortness of breath | |
| Ulcers | |
| Regional enteritis (inflammation of the intestine, especially the small intestine) | |
| Ulcerative colitis (inflammation and open sores of the colon, or large intestine) | |
| Asthma | |
| Cardiac problems, such as tachycardia (rapid heartbeat), arrhythmia (irregularity in the rhythm of the heart), angina pectoris (recurrent pain in the chest and the left arm, caused by sudden decrease in the blood supply to the heart), and cardiospasm (sudden contractions of the heart muscle) | |
| Frequent urination or diarrhea | |
| Overeating | |
| Skin rashes | |

# SOURCES OF STRESS

Many different kinds of stressors affect our well-being. These include daily hassles, life changes, frustration, conflict, and pain.

## Daily Hassles

**Daily hassles** are stressors that affect us regularly.[1] No doubt you will recognize most, if not all, of the following daily hassles:

1. *Household hassles.* Household hassles, such as making meals, shopping, and housecleaning, are significant sources of stress. These especially affect women, who typically shoulder a full-time job and a disproportionate burden of household and child care responsibilities. As a result, many working women are tired all the time, emotionally drained, and resentful of those men who believe that household tasks and child care are "woman's work." These feelings can lead to marital strain and depression.
2. *Health hassles.* Minor illnesses, difficulty contacting a health professional, and side effects of medications are examples.
3. *Time-pressure hassles.* Having too little time to do the things you need to do can be a major source of stress. At the other extreme is having too much "empty time" on our hands, which can lead to feelings of boredom and apathy. College students often feel pressure to study and to socialize. Procrastination—putting off tasks and decisions until the last minute—can also be a source of stress. Time-pressure hassles can be reduced by making a list of what you want to accomplish, creating a schedule for doing it, and sticking to the schedule.
4. *Inner-concern hassles.* Examples are feelings of loneliness, fears of social confrontations, and doubts about the value of what we are doing with our life.

**Stress** In human terms, stress refers to pressures that require a person to adjust.

**Stressors** Sources of stress.

**Eustress** "Good stress," which motivates and energizes us.

**Daily hassles** Minor annoyances of daily life that are common sources of stress.

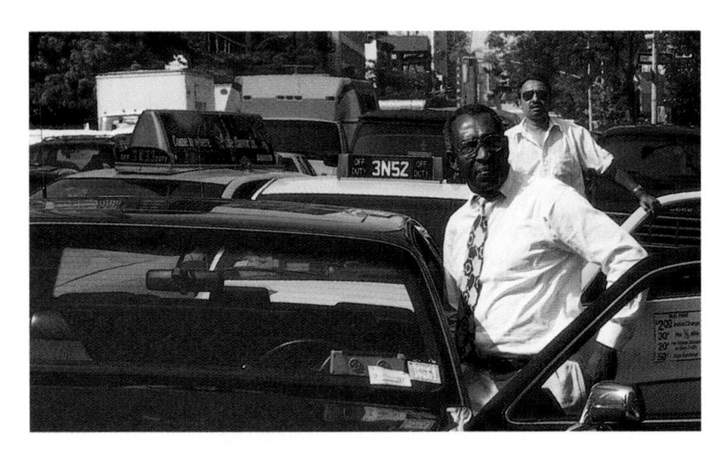


***Hassles*** Daily hassles, including traffic jams, are a major source of stress. What hassles do you regularly face? What can you do about them to reduce your stress burden?

5. *Environmental hassles.* Air and noise pollution, traffic congestion, neighborhood deterioration, and fear of crime are sources of environmental stress. Fear of crime can be an especially serious stressor, especially for those in crime-plagued neighborhoods.
6. *Financial-responsibility hassles.* Debts and other financial worries can be a source of enormous pressure and **chronic stress.**
7. *Work hassles.* Also called **job stress,** work hassles include dissatisfaction on the job, job strain, and problems with supervisors and coworkers. Other daily hassles, such as time pressure, can converge in the work arena.
8. *Future-security hassles.* Job security, investments, taxes, and getting by in retirement can be recurrent concerns.
9. *Interpersonal hassles.* Continuing difficulties with relatives, partners, teachers, and so on, can be chronic sources of stress.

## Life Changes

**Life changes** also create stress. Daily hassles occur regularly and are all negative. Life changes occur intermittently and may be beneficial and desirable, for example, getting married or receiving a promotion.

We all face change. Leaving school, getting a job, moving to another town, becoming spouses and parents, and experiencing illness and loss are life changes. Each transition challenges us to cope with a new situation. Some people navigate change with confidence and relatively low levels of **distress.** Other people are more vulnerable to life changes, perhaps because they lack skills or confidence. Feelings of optimism and of being in control help us meet the challenges.

The stress of a life change depends on its meaning to the individual and on the ability to cope with it. For example, the stress of pregnancy is related to a couple's desire for a baby and their readiness to care for it. A possibly stressful event is less taxing for people who find it meaningful and feel equipped for it. Similarly, you are more likely to perceive your job as stressful if you feel rushed or overwhelmed by the demands of others than if you feel in control of how and when you do your work.[2]

## Frustration

We experience **frustration** when our efforts to achieve our goals are thwarted. The seeds of frustration are obvious enough. Adolescents are frustrated when they are told they are too young to drive, date, wear makeup, drink, spend money, or hold a job. A student may be frustrated by lack of money for college or by fear of leaving home. We can frustrate ourselves by setting our goals too high or making unreasonable demands on ourselves, such as expecting perfection.

## Conflict

**Conflict** is a state of tension brought about by competing motives. People in conflict feel "damned if they do and damned if they don't." Students may feel torn about whether to pursue further training in graduate school or enter the job market. The longer they remain in conflict, the greater the stress and frustration.

The way out of conflict is to make decisions. To make decisions we need to:

- Sort out our competing values and needs, and identify meaningful, attainable goals.
- Make plans to obtain those goals.
- Try out the plans.
- Evaluate the results.

**Chronic stress** Persistent or recurrent stress.

**Job stress** Pressures, demands, or dissatisfaction associated with work.

**Life changes** Positive or negative changes in life circumstances that are stressful because they impose on us a demand to adjust.

**Distress** Emotional or physical pain or suffering.

**Frustration** The negative feeling state experienced when one's efforts to pursue one's goals are thwarted.

**Conflict** A state of tension resulting from two opposing motives occurring simultaneously.

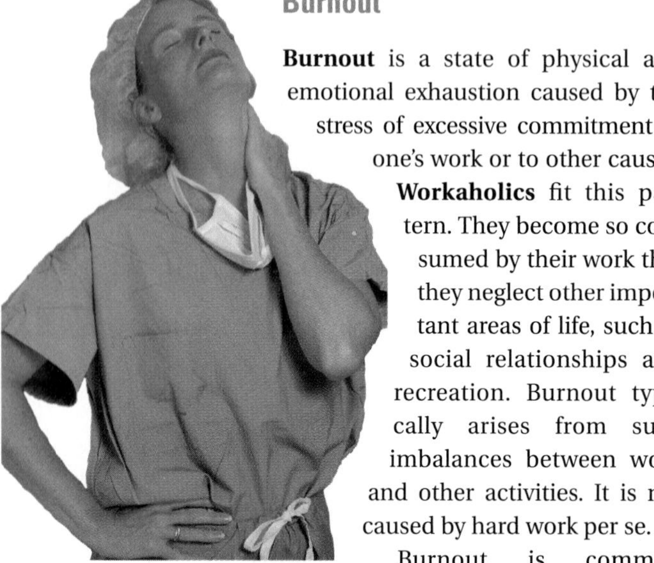

*Burnout* Burnout is common among health care workers in hospitals who face overbearing workloads and the emotional strain of dealing with illness and death.

## Burnout

**Burnout** is a state of physical and emotional exhaustion caused by the stress of excessive commitment to one's work or to other causes. **Workaholics** fit this pattern. They become so consumed by their work that they neglect other important areas of life, such as social relationships and recreation. Burnout typically arises from such imbalances between work and other activities. It is not caused by hard work per se.

Burnout is common among health professionals with impossible workloads. In addition to attempting to help people with health problems such as substance or spousal abuse, they may face mountains of paperwork. Health professionals who began their careers with enthusiasm and idealism can become apathetic toward their work and the people they serve.[3]

Burnout is also common in people with high levels of *role conflict, role overload,* or *role ambiguity.* People in role conflict, such as working mothers, face competing demands for their time. They feel pulled in several directions at once. Their efforts to meet competing demands eventually lead to burnout. People with role overload find it hard to say no. They take on more and more responsibilities until they burn out. People with *role ambiguity* are uncertain as to what others expect of them. Thus, they work hard at trying to be all things to all people.

**Warning Signs of Burnout** Burnout develops slowly. The initial signs may not appear for years, but may include the following:

- Loss of energy and feelings of exhaustion, both physical and mental.
- Increased irritability and shortness of temper.
- Stress-related problems, such as depression, headaches, backaches, or general malaise.
- Difficulty concentrating at work or feeling disengaged from one's work.
- Loss of motivation and concern in someone who was previously enthusiastic and committed.
- Lack of satisfaction or a sense of accomplishment in one's work.
- Feeling that one has nothing left to give.

**HealthCheck**
Burnout quiz
**H0301**

**Burnout** Physical and mental fatigue or exhaustion caused by excessive work-related stress.

**Workaholics** People who are consumed by their work to the exclusion of personal relationships and leisure pursuits.

**Type A personality** A personality type characterized by impatience, time urgency, competitiveness, and hostility.

## Type A Personality Pattern

Your personality style may also be a source of stress. Are you the type of person other people describe as hard driving, competitive, and impatient? Does waiting in line or getting stuck in traffic lead you to pull your hair out or pound your fists? If so, your personality type would probably fit the profile of a **Type A personality.** Possessing this personality profile could pose a threat to your health, perhaps even to your life. Evidence shows the Type A personality pattern is associated with a modestly higher risk of coronary heart disease.[4]

Type A's are impatient, competitive, and aggressive. They have a strong sense of time urgency and are constantly in a rush. They feel pressured and keep one eye glued to the clock. They are often early for appointments. They tend to talk, walk, and eat fast. They quickly become impatient and even hostile toward others who work slowly or fail to meet their expectations. They are intense, even at play. On the tennis court, they are not content to bat the ball around for enjoyment. Instead they scrutinize every stroke, constantly polishing their form and demanding constant self-improvement. By contrast, Type B's are relaxed, easy-going, and take life at a slower pace.

The nearby ***HealthCheck*** "Are You a Type A?" can help you determine whether you fit the Type A profile. Certainly not all people with the Type A personality suffer health consequences. Moreover, some of the characteristics of the Type A profile, especially hard-driving ambitiousness, may be associated with potential for material success. Perhaps the important question to consider is whether these characteristics are balanced with the ability to relax and "smell the roses," even as you are striving to climb the corporate ladder.

## Health Check

### Are You a Type A?[5]

People with the Type A behavior pattern are impatient, competitive, and aggressive. They feel rushed, under pressure; they keep one eye glued to the clock. They are prompt and often arrive early for appointments. They walk, talk, and eat rapidly. They grow restless when others work slowly.

Type A people don't just stroll out on the tennis court to bat the ball around. They scrutinize their form, polish their strokes, and demand consistent self-improvement. This questionnaire may help you determine whether you fit the Type A profile.[6]

*Write a checkmark under the* ***Yes*** *if the behavior pattern described is typical of you. Place a checkmark under the* ***No*** *if it is not. Work rapidly and answer all items. Then check the scoring key in Appendix B at the back of this book.*

| Do You: | Yes | No |
|---|---|---|
| 1. Strongly emphasize important words in your ordinary speech? | ___ | ___ |
| 2. Walk briskly from place to place or meeting to meeting? | ___ | ___ |
| 3. Think that life is by nature dog-eat-dog? | ___ | ___ |
| 4. Get fidgety when you see someone complete a job slowly? | ___ | ___ |
| 5. Urge others to complete what they're trying to express? | ___ | ___ |
| 6. Find it exceptionally annoying to get stuck in line? | ___ | ___ |
| 7. Envision all the things you have to do even when someone is talking to you? | ___ | ___ |
| 8. Eat while you're getting dressed, or jot notes down while you're driving? | ___ | ___ |
| 9. Catch up on work during vacations? | ___ | ___ |
| 10. Direct the conversation to things that interest you? | ___ | ___ |
| 11. Feel as if things are going to pot because you're relaxing for a few minutes? | ___ | ___ |
| 12. Get so wrapped up in your work that you fail to notice beautiful scenery? | ___ | ___ |
| 13. Get so wrapped up in money, promotions, and awards that you neglect expressing your creativity? | ___ | ___ |
| 14. Schedule appointments and meetings back to back? | ___ | ___ |
| 15. Arrive early for appointments and meetings? | ___ | ___ |
| 16. Make fists or clench your jaws to drill home your views? | ___ | ___ |
| 17. Think that you have achieved what you have because of your ability to work fast? | ___ | ___ |
| 18. Have the feeling that uncompleted work must be done *now* and fast? | ___ | ___ |
| 19. Try to find more efficient ways to get things done? | ___ | ___ |
| 20. Struggle always to win games instead of having fun? | ___ | ___ |
| 21. Interrupt people who are talking? | ___ | ___ |
| 22. Lose patience with people who are late for appointments and meetings? | ___ | ___ |
| 23. Get back to work right after lunch? | ___ | ___ |
| 24. Find that there's never enough time? | ___ | ___ |
| 25. Believe that you're getting too little done, even when other people tell you that you're doing fine? | ___ | ___ |

## PREVENTION

### *Preventing Burnout*

People may become burned out when they are overextended. Yet burnout is not inevitable. Here are some suggestions for preventing burnout:

1. *Establish Your Priorities.* Make a list of the things that are truly important to you. If your list starts and ends with work, rethink your values. Ask yourself some key questions: Am I making time for the relationships and activities that bring a sense of meaning, fulfillment, and satisfaction to life? Getting in touch with what's truly important to you may help you reorder your values and priorities.
2. *Set Reasonable Goals.* People at risk of burnout drive themselves to extremes. Set realistic long-term and short-term goals for yourself and don't push yourself beyond your limits.
3. *Take Things One Day at a Time.* Work gradually toward your goals. Burning the candle at both ends is likely to leave you burned (out).

4. *Set Limits.* People at risk of burnout often have difficulty saying "no." They are known as the ones who get things done. Yet the more responsibilities they assume, the greater their risk of burnout. Learn your limits and respect them. Share responsibilities with others. Delegate tasks. Cut back on your responsibilities before you have difficulty coping.
5. *Share Your Feelings.* Bottiing up negative feelings like anger, frustration, and sadness is stressful. Share your feelings with people you trust.
6. *Build Supportive Relationships.* Developing and maintaining relationships helps buffer us against the effects of stress.
7. *Do Things You Enjoy.* Balance work and recreation. Do something you enjoy every day. Breaks clear your mind and recharge your batteries.
8. *Take Time for Yourself.* Counterbalance the demands that others place on your shoulders by setting some time aside for yourself. Make it part of your weekly schedule. Learn to say "No" or "Later."
9. *Don't Skip Vacations.* People who are headed for burnout often find reasons to skip vacations. This is a mistake: vacations provide time off from the usual stresses.
10. *Be Attuned to Your Health.* Be aware of stress-related physical symptoms such as fatigue, headache, or backache, reduced resistance to colds and the flu, and psychological symptoms such as anxiety, depression, irritability, or shortness of temper. Consider changes in health as signals to examine the sources of stress in your life and do something about them. Consult health professionals about any symptoms that concern you. Get regular checkups to help identify developing health problems.

Smart Quiz Q0301

### think about it!

- **In what ways are the stresses in your life harmful for you? Good for you?**
- **What daily hassles and life changes have you been experiencing? What are you doing about them?**
- **What kinds of frustrations and conflicts do you experience in your own life?**
- **To what extent might your personality type be a source of stress in your life? What do you think you might do about it?**

## PAIN—WHAT IT IS, WHAT TO DO ABOUT IT

Pain is a formidable stressor. It impairs our ability to function and to cope. Athletes report that pain damages their ability to perform even when the injury itself does not weaken them. For some of us, pain is occasional and passes quickly. Headaches, backaches, and toothaches are but a small sample of the types of pain that most of us encounter from time to time. For others, pain is a constant companion. Millions of people experience intense, chronic pain from conditions such as arthritis, digestive disorders, and cancer.

### What Is Pain?

While pain can be unpleasant and even excruciating, it is necessary for survival. Pain alerts us to danger and prompts us to seek the source of the problem. Acute pain, such as stabbing pain in the chest, is a signal to seek immediate medical attention. Doing so can save your life.

When you stub your toe, nerves in your toe send pain messages through the spinal column to the brain. It is in the brain that discomfort is registered. We can trace the development of pain to the point of contact (see Figure 3.1). Hormones called **prostaglandins** are released into the bloodstream to help transmit pain messages to the brain. Prostaglandins also increase the blood flow to the affected area, leading to **inflammation** (redness or swelling). Inflammation serves the purpose of drawing infection-fighting white blood cells to combat organisms that might try to enter the body at the site of injury. **Analgesic drugs** such as aspirin and ibuprofen work by inhibiting the production of prostaglandins, thus reducing pain as well as inflammation and fever.

Talking Glossary Prostaglandins G0302

Talking Glossary Analgesic drugs G0303

According to the **gate theory of pain,** a gate in the nervous system opens and closes to allow pain messages through to the brain or shut them out. **Endorphins** are types of neurotransmitters that are released in response to pain. They help shut the gate. The word endorphin is a contraction of the words *endogenous* (meaning "coming from within") and *morphine.* Morphine is a narcotic drug that deadens pain by locking into and blocking receptor sites on brain cells that transmit pain messages. Pain messages are thus locked out. Endorphins are natural painkillers produced in the brain that apparently work in the same way as morphine.

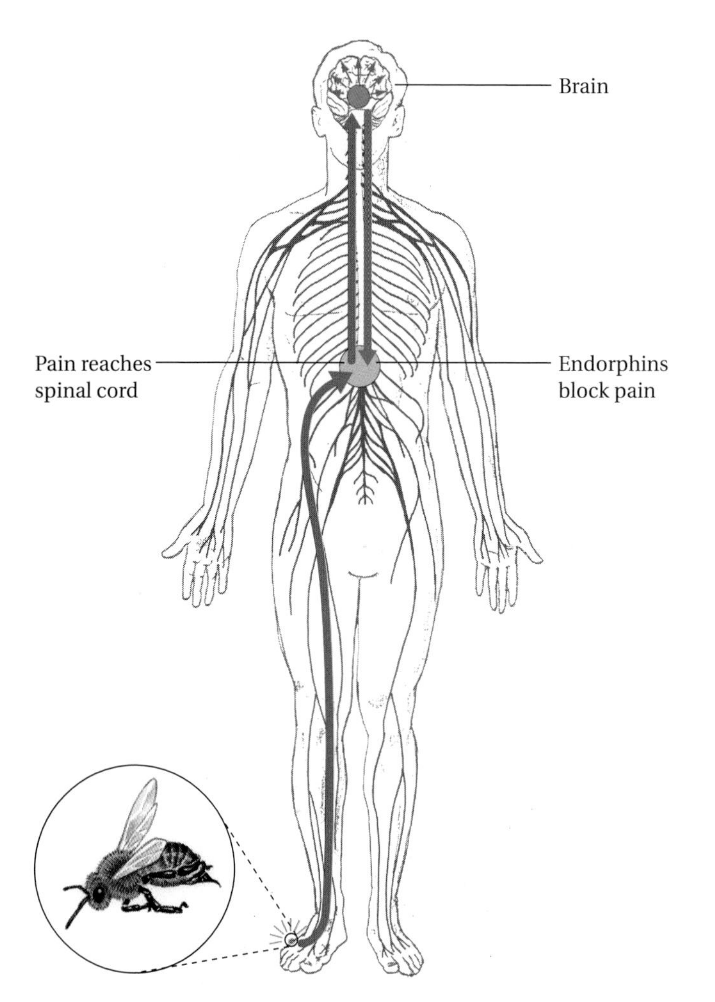


**Figure 3.1** ***Pain: How We Sense It, How It Is Relieved*** Pain signals originate at the point of contact. Various chemicals, including prostaglandins, play a role in facilitating the transmission of pain messages to the brain. Prostaglandins also increase circulation to the injured area, resulting in the redness or swelling associated with inflammation. The brain responds to pain messages by releasing chemicals called endorphins. Endorphins apparently relieve pain by blocking pain signals from reaching the brain.

The brain is a marvel of engineering. We are alerted to danger by the first pangs of pain. Otherwise, we might not pull our hand away from a hot object in time to prevent burns. Then the release of endorphins gradually diminishes pain.

But in some injuries and chronic diseases, endorphins are not enough to shut the gate. For some 11 million Americans, the pain of injuries or chronic disease is a constant unwelcome companion.[7] Chronic pain can last for months or years. It drains the pleasure from life, saps vitality, and can cause depression. People in pain may not be able to think about anything else. Sources of chronic pain include nagging back problems, migraines, temporomandibular joint (TMJ) pain (pain in the jaw), and diseases such as cancer.

## Managing Pain

Never ignore persistent pain. Consult a health professional. Most pain can be relieved by treatment of the underlying condition. Chronic or intermittent pain, such as backaches or headaches, can often be alleviated by analgesic drugs such as aspirin and ibuprofen and perhaps bed rest.

**Drug Therapy** Aspirin, ibuprofen, and other analgesics available over the counter (without prescription) can relieve intermittent pain such as headaches, backaches, and menstrual cramps. Analgesic drugs are not always effective in relieving pain, however, and some people cannot tolerate them.

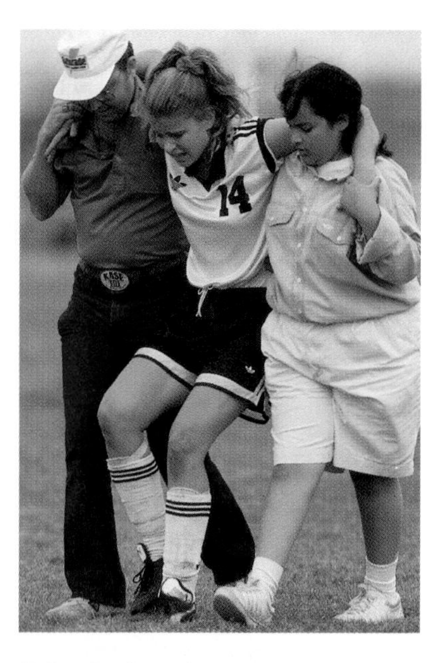

***Pain*** Coping with pain is a major source of stress. What are the various ways that help people manage pain?

When chronic pain is brought on by serious illnesses such as cancer, the stronger pain-deadening action of narcotic drugs like morphine may help. These are available only by prescription and are highly addictive. Moreover, the dangers of overdosing on them or combining them with other drugs can be serious, even life-threatening. In general, narcotics such as morphine and Demerol are prescribed only for post-surgical pain or the treatment of terminal or incapacitating illness.

**Get Accurate Information** Don't take pain lying down! And don't avoid thinking about it. If your personal health care provider doesn't have the answers, you can consult with a pain specialist at a medical center or hospital. One of the most effective psychological methods for managing pain is obtaining factual and

**Prostaglandins** Hormones that play a role in the transmission of pain messages to the brain.

**Inflammation** A swelling or redness that occurs around an injured area.

**Analgesic drugs** Drugs that combat pain, such as aspirin and ibuprofen.

**Gate theory of pain** Explains that the perception of pain involves a gating mechanism in the central nervous system that allows or blocks pain messages to the brain.

**Endorphins** Naturally occurring hormones that directly stimulate pleasure centers in the brain.

thorough information. People who face uncomfortable and frightening medical procedures, such as chemotherapy for cancer, often find that being informed about why a procedure is recommended, how it will feel, and the nature of side effects helps them cope.

**Distraction and Fantasy** Psychologists have discovered that distraction or fantasy helps to manage pain. Suppose you've injured your arm and are waiting to be seen in an emergency room. You can distract yourself by focusing on the immediate environment—counting ceiling tiles, checking out the clothing of health professionals, fantasizing about a vacation, or dwelling on the patterns on the soles of your shoes.

Children with cancer have reduced the side effects of chemotherapy by playing video games.[8] While nausea-inducing cancer drugs are administered intravenously, the children focus on combating monsters on the video screen.

**Change Your Thoughts** What you say to yourself about pain can affect how much pain you feel and how well you cope in general. Stressful beliefs include exaggerated appraisals of pain ("This is the worst thing in the world"), helplessness ("I can't cope with this anymore"), and hopelessness ("What's the use of trying? This pain will never end"). Changing your thinking may not eliminate pain, but it can help you cope more effectively. Here are some suggested alternatives to stressful beliefs:

Change *"This is the worst thing in the world"* to *"Yes, this is bad, but there are things that are worse."*

Change *"I can't cope with this anymore"* to *"I can deal with this. I've dealt with pain like this before, and I can do it again."*

Change *"What's the use of trying? This pain will never end"* to *"Don't give in to hopelessness. Focus on what you need to do to cope with this pain. It will come to an end. In a few days (weeks) you will be looking back at this and congratulating yourself for getting through it."*

**Relaxation training** Techniques aimed at helping people learn to relax.

**Meditation** A form of focused attention that leads to a relaxed state of mind and body.

**Biofeedback training (BFT)** The use of physiological monitoring equipment to help people develop the ability to gain some control over internal functions.

**Electromyographic (EMG) biofeedback** Changes in muscle tension in selected muscles are relayed to the user in the form of audio or video signals.

**Relaxation, Meditation, and Biofeedback** Relaxation training and meditation are emerging as important adjuncts to pain management. In some cases, these techniques are so successful that people in chronic pain are able to dispense with traditional drug therapy altogether.

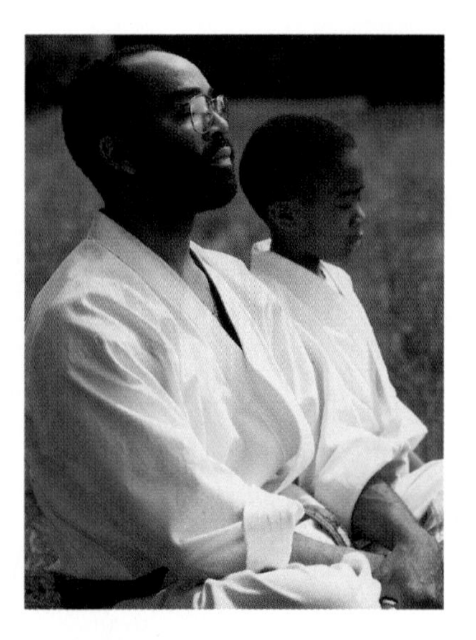

***Meditation*** Meditation is a popular means of combating pain and relieving stress by inducing feelings of relaxation.

**Relaxation training** involves a number of techniques to help people relax. Muscle relaxation helps relieve pain that stems from muscle tension, such as tension headaches and some forms of backache. Even when pain stems from other sources, relaxation can help people calm down, get their minds off their pain, and avoid tensing up.

**Meditation** is a form of focused attention that produces a relaxed, contemplative state. One study showed that people in persistent pain reduced their pain symptoms through a stress reduction program that included regular meditation.[9] Though there are many forms of meditation, they all involve a narrowing of attention through some form of repetition: repeating a word, thought, or phrase; focusing on a burning candle or, as followers of yoga do, focusing on the design on a vase or a mandala. Some people meditate by repeating a brief prayer.

Meditation may lead to greater self-acceptance, which improves our ability to cope better with stressors, including pain.[10] Meditative techniques have wider applicability to stress management, as we see later in the chapter.

In another relaxation technique, **biofeedback training (BFT),** people use devices to learn to relax their muscles and calm their nervous systems. In one form of BFT, **electromyographic (EMG) biofeedback,** electrodes placed on the forehead or elsewhere on the body monitor muscle tension. The device produces a tone that changes as muscle tension increases or decreases. By learning to lower the tone, the person develops the ability to relax the forehead muscles, which can reduce headache pain.

**Talking Glossary**
Electromyographic feedback
G0304

In **thermal biofeedback,** devices that measure temperature are attached to the body, generally around a finger. As the temperature in the fingers rises, the device beeps more slowly. The temperature rises because of increased blood flow to the extremities. This change in blood flow that raises the temperature of a finger can help relieve **migraine headaches**. These intense, throbbing headaches involve a dysregulation in the blood flow to the brain. Some people can raise the temperature by simply imagining the finger growing warmer.

**Social Support—Don't Go It Alone** Those who have social support may be better able to cope with pain than those who go it alone. A supportive shoulder helps them get through the day. Moreover, when other people care about us, we take better care of ourselves. For example, we may be more likely to follow the advice of health care providers. Doing enjoyable things with others also distracts us from pain.

**One Day at a Time . . .** People with chronic pain often find that some days are worse than others. On good days, pain may seem to be off in the wings. On bad days, they may barely be able to meet minimal responsibilities. On those days, it may make sense for them to go easy on themselves, to reduce their self-expectations. Unrealistic expectations set us up for failure, which can compound pain and discomfort.

**Keep Abreast of New Developments** New technologies and approaches to pain management are being introduced to clinical practice each year. **Electrostimulation,** the use of electrical impulses to block or interfere with the transmission of pain signals, offers hope to many chronic pain sufferers. On the horizon are drugs that may block pain receptors in the brain and analgesic drugs that offer more potent pain relief without the adverse effects and addiction potential associated with narcotics.

Smart Quiz
Q0302

### think about it!

- What kinds of pain do you or people you know experience?
- Does pain ever interfere with your (or their) activities? How?
- What do you (or they) do to cope with pain?

## WHAT STRESS DOES TO THE BODY

Much of what we know about the body's response to stress is the result of the work of the famed stress researcher Hans Selye, known affectionately as "Dr. Stress." Selye found that the body responds in a similar manner to various stressors—a car veering toward us, pain, or strong emotions.

### The General Adaptation Syndrome

Selye labeled the body's response to stress the **general adaptation syndrome,** or **GAS**. The GAS is also known as the *stress response*. Selye found that under persistent stress, our bodies are like clocks with alarm systems that do not shut off until their energy is depleted—sometimes dangerously so. The GAS has three phases:

**The Alarm Reaction** When people encounter a stressor, the nervous system sets off an **alarm reaction** that mobilizes the body's resources. Imagine that the car in front of you swerves out of control. The car's movement is a stressor that demands your immediate action. You slam on the brakes and swerve yourself. Afterward you note that beads of sweat are dripping down your forehead. Your heart is pounding. These are features of the alarm reaction.

During the alarm reaction, we experience strong physiological and psychological arousal. Our muscles tense and we are flooded with strong emotions such as terror, fright, anxiety, rage, or anger. The alarm reaction mobilizes the body's defenses to prepare for action.

The alarm reaction can be set off by a seemingly small provocation or by an imminently threatening event. The strength of the reaction depends on the degree to which the event is perceived as threatening. One person's alarm system may be set off when she or he is introduced to a new person. Another person's alarm (also

**Thermal biofeedback** Temperature devices called thermistors relay changes in temperature in selected areas of the user's body.

**Migraine headache** A type of severe headache characterized by piercing or throbbing sensations on one side of the head.

**Electrostimulation** The use of electric current to block pain signals.

**General adaptation syndrome (GAS)** Describes the body's three-stage response to persistent or intense stress.

**Alarm reaction** The body's initial response to stress; activation of the sympathetic nervous system and release of stress hormones.

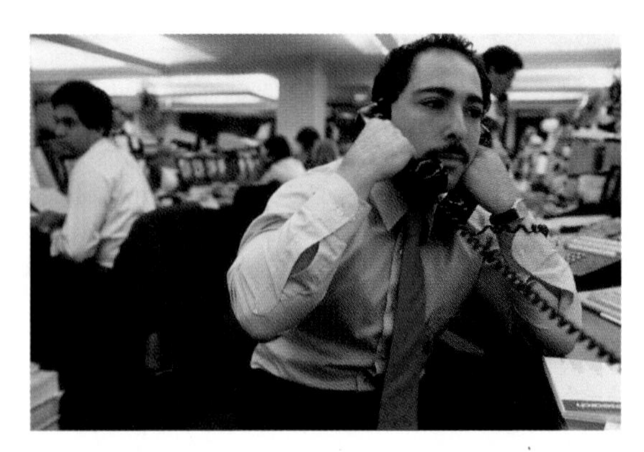

***Stressed Out?*** Though some people thrive on higher levels of stress than others, we all have our limits. Are you overstressed? If so, what can you do about it?

called the **fight-or-flight reaction**) may be triggered by taking a test. In such cases, the stress reaction is invoked by a psychological stressor (fear of rejection or failure) rather than a physical stressor, but the body's response is the same.

The alarm reaction is wired into the nervous system. This wiring is a legacy we inherited from our earliest ancestors, who faced many stressors that threatened their lives. For them, the alarm may have been triggered by the sight or sound of a predator lurking in the bushes. The alarm reaction did not last long; they either fought off the predator or fled. If they survived, the "alarm" was turned off and the body returned to normal.

A sensitive alarm system may have kept our ancestors alive. Today, however, it can be a handicap. The stresses of modern life can be recurring or enduring. The daily grinds of academic or work life and stressors at home may excite our alarm systems day after day, year after year. Our ancestors did not have to juggle school and jobs to make ends meet. They didn't have to battle traffic to get to work or school.

**Fight-or-flight reaction** Corresponds to the alarm reaction; mobilization of the body's resources to fend off a threat by fighting or fleeing.

**Resistance stage** The body attempts to conserve its resources in an attempt to cope with prolonged stress. Also called the *adaptation stage.*

**Exhaustion stage** The final stage of the response to prolonged stress, characterized by depletion of bodily resources and a lowering of resistance to illness.

**Homeostasis** The maintenance of a steady state.

**Somatic nervous system** The part of the peripheral nervous system that involves the voluntary control of skeletal muscles and feeds information from the sense organs to the brain.

**The Resistance Stage** When a stressor is intense and persistent, the body progresses to the **resistance stage** (or *adaptation stage*). In this stage, the body tries to renew spent energy and repair damage. It seeks to restore the normal biological state. In the resistance stage, bodily arousal remains high, but not as high as during the alarm reaction. Prolonged arousal may be expressed in the form of emotions such as anger, fatigue, irritability, and impatience.

**The Exhaustion Stage** If stressors persist, the body's resources become seriously depleted. The body now enters the final stage of the GAS—the **exhaustion stage.** Now the heart rate and respiration rate *decrease* to conserve bodily resources.

Some of us are hardier than others, but relentless, intense stress can eventually exhaust any of us. If stress endures, we may develop what Selye called "diseases of adaptation." These diseases range from allergic reactions to coronary heart disease, and can be fatal. Figure 3.2 illustrates the body's reaction to stress.

The stress reaction affects **homeostasis,** the body's tendency to maintain a steady state, for example, maintaining body temperature or blood sugar levels. Our bodies require a state of equilibrium or balance to function smoothly. When prolonged stress interferes with our homeostatic balance, we become more vulnerable to stress-related disorders.

**Talking Glossary**
Homeostasis
G0305

## The Role of the Nervous System

The body's response to stress is regulated by the nervous system. The nervous system consists of the body's electrical circuitry. Control mechanisms in the brain regulate everything from the rate at which your heart beats, to the movements of your eyes as you scan these words, to your higher mental processes, such as thinking and reasoning. You'll recall from Chapter 2 that the nervous system consists of two parts, the central nervous system (brain and spinal cord) and the peripheral nervous system. The peripheral nervous system is further divided into two major divisions, the autonomic nervous system (ANS) and the somatic nervous system.

**Somatic Nervous System** The **somatic nervous system** is responsible for transmitting messages between your brain and your sense organs (eyes, ears, tongue, nose, and skin). The somatic nervous system enables us to perceive the world. It also causes your muscles to contract in response to your intentional commands and regulates the

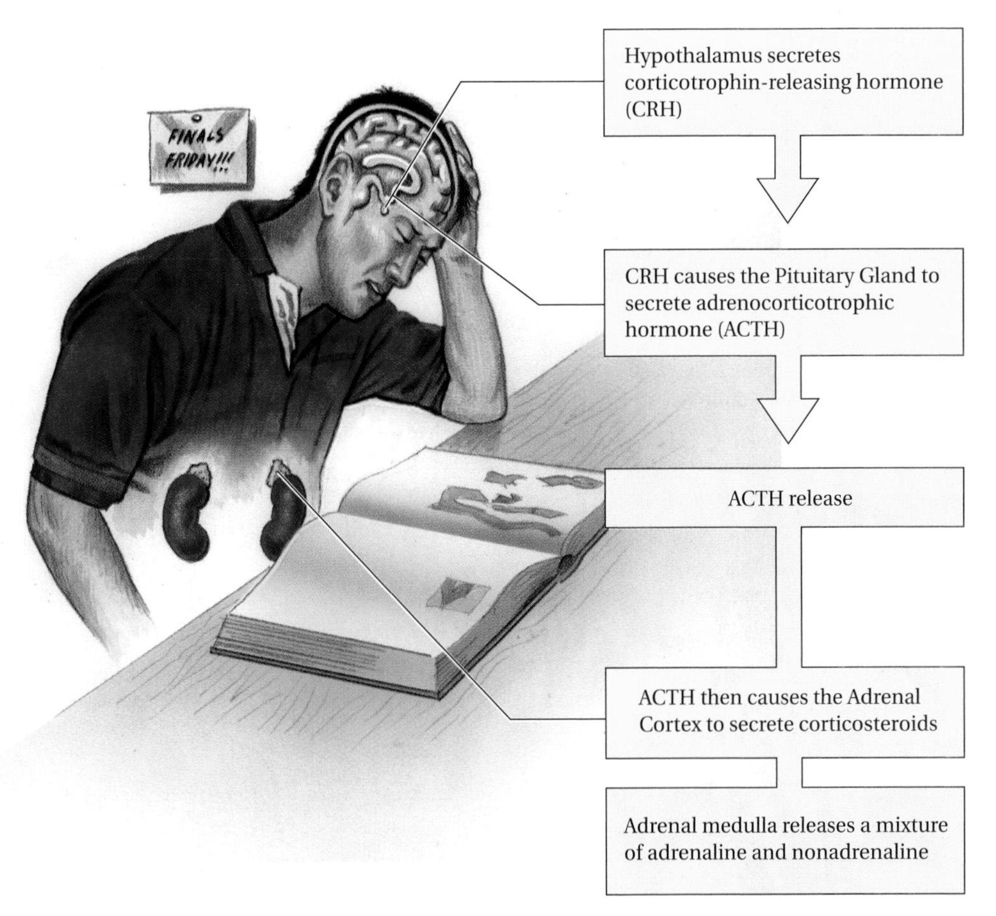

FINALS FRIDAY!!!
Hypothalamus secretes corticotrophin-releasing hormone (CRH)
CRH causes the Pituitary Gland to secrete adrenocorticotrophic hormone (ACTH)
ACTH release
ACTH then causes the Adrenal Cortex to secrete corticosteroids
Adrenal medulla releases a mixture of adrenaline and nonadrenaline

**Figure 3.2** ***The Body's Response to Stress*** Under stress, the body responds by releasing stress hormones (adrenaline and noradrenaline) from the adrenal medulla and corticosteroids from the adrenal cortex. These hormones help the body prepare to cope with immediate stress. Under control of the sympathetic nervous system, the stress hormones increase heart rate, respiration, and blood pressure, suppress digestion, and dilate the pupils. Secretion of corticosteroids leads to the release of stored reserves of energy. If stress persists, continued secretion of corticosteroids can suppress the immune system response by inhibiting the production of antibodies.

subtle movements that maintain posture and balance. Nerve impulses travel from the brain to the spinal cord and through the somatic nervous system to the muscles that control body movement.

**The Autonomic Nervous System** The **autonomic nervous system (ANS)** controls involuntary bodily activities like heartbeat, respiration, digestion, and dilation of the pupils of the eyes. Because it works automatically, the ANS regulates these vital bodily processes without your having to think about them. Your ANS is at work even when you are asleep.

The autonomic nervous system is subdivided into two branches, the **sympathetic branch** and the **parasympathetic branch** (see Figure 3.3, next page). These two branches have largely opposite effects. The sympathetic nervous system accelerates bodily processes such as heart rate and respiration. The parasympathetic nervous system slows them down. The sympathetic system is most active when we are engaged in vigorous physical activities or experience strong emotions (which is why we sense our hearts beating faster when we are anxious). The parasympathetic system fosters processes, such as digestion, that replenish bodily resources.

**The ANS and the Stress Response** During the alarm reaction of the GAS, the sympathetic nervous system takes control. It accelerates heart and respiration rates, which help the body to contend with the stressor—to flee or, if need be, to fight. During the exhaustion stage, the parasympathetic nervous system dominates and many bodily processes slow down in the effort to replenish spent resources.

## The Role of the Endocrine System

The autonomic nervous system also regulates the **endocrine system.** The endocrine

**Autonomic nervous system (ANS)** The part of the peripheral nervous system that "automatically" controls processes such as heart rate, respiration, and endocrine functioning.

**Sympathetic branch** The branch of the autonomic nervous system that accelerates bodily processes and releases stores of energy needed for physical exertion; activated as part of the alarm reaction to stress.

**Parasympathetic branch** The branch of the autonomic nervous system involved in processes such as digestion that preserve and replenish energy stores.

**Endocrine system** The system of glands that secrete hormones directly into the bloodstream, rather than by means of ducts.

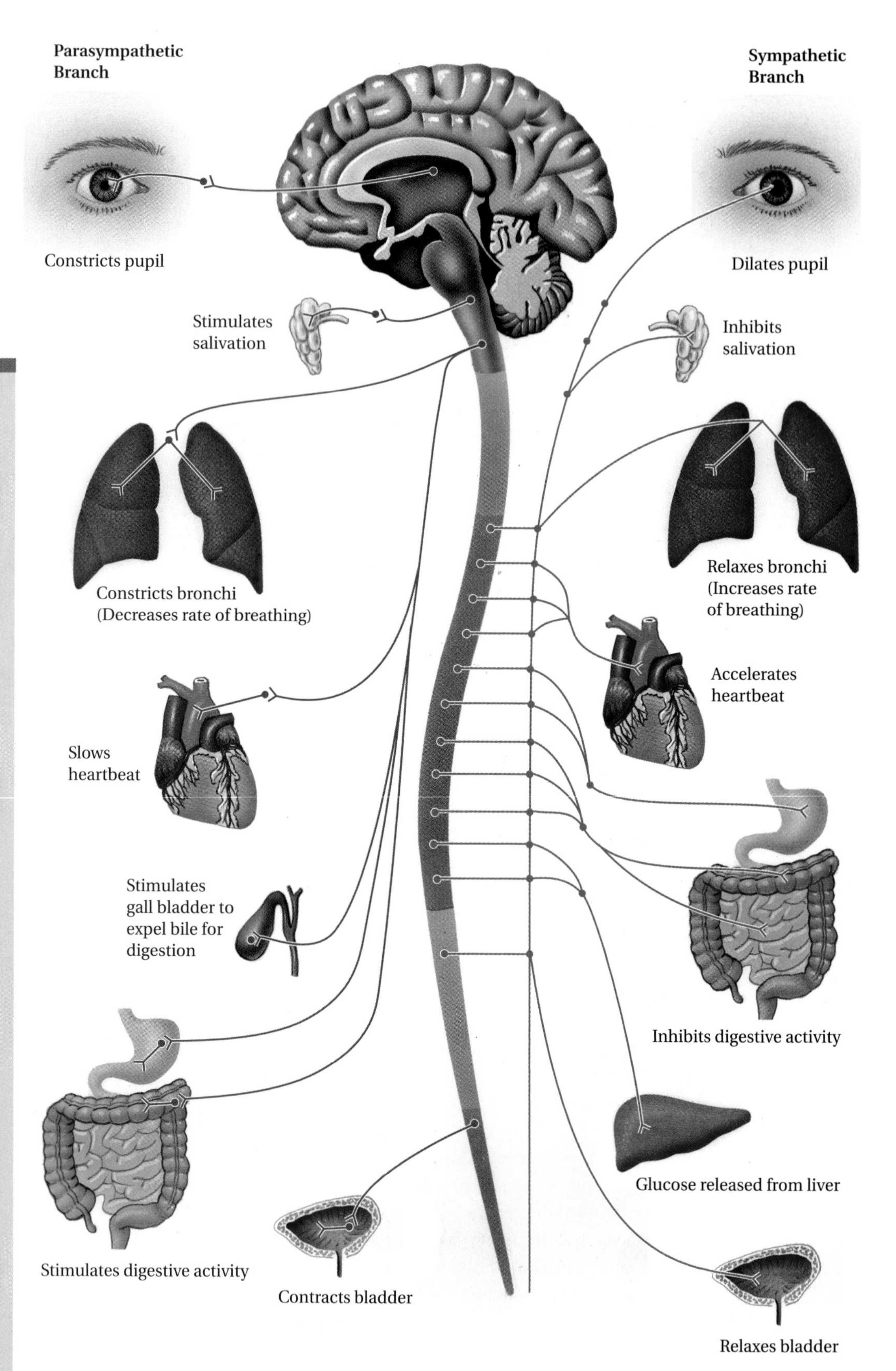


**Figure 3.3** ***Two Branches of the Autonomic Nervous System*** The autonomic nervous system is divided into the sympathetic and parasympathetic branches, which have generally opposite effects. The sympathetic branch speeds up heart rate and respiration, helping the body cope with stressful demands, while the parasympathetic branch slows down these responses and helps restore bodily resources by stimulating digestive processes.

**Hormones** Substances secreted by endocrine glands that are involved in the regulation of a wide range of bodily processes, including reproduction and growth.

**Hypothalamus** A structure in the lower middle part of the brain, involved in regulating a range of processes, including motivation, emotion, and body temperature.

**Corticotrophin-releasing hormone (CRH)** A substance produced by the hypothalamus that causes the pituitary gland to release adrenocorticotrophic hormone (ACTH).

**Pituitary gland** A brain structure dubbed the "master gland" because of its key role in many processes, including growth and reproduction.

**Adrenocorticotrophic hormone (ACTH)** A hormone produced by the pituitary gland; activates the adrenal cortex to secrete corticosteroids.

**Adrenal glands** Endocrine glands that lie just above the kidneys and produce various stress hormones.

**Adrenal cortex** The outer part of the adrenal glands, which produces corticosteroids.

**Corticosteroids** Steroids or steroidal hormones that help the body cope with stress by making stored energy available.

**Adrenal medulla** The inner part of the adrenal glands; produces adrenaline and noradrenaline.

**Adrenaline** Also called *epinephrine.* A hormone produced by the adrenal medulla; accelerates heart and respiration rate and leads to the release of energy reserves.

**Noradrenaline** A hormone produced by the adrenal medulla; has chemical properties similar to adrenaline. In the nervous system, noradrenaline functions as a neurotransmitter.

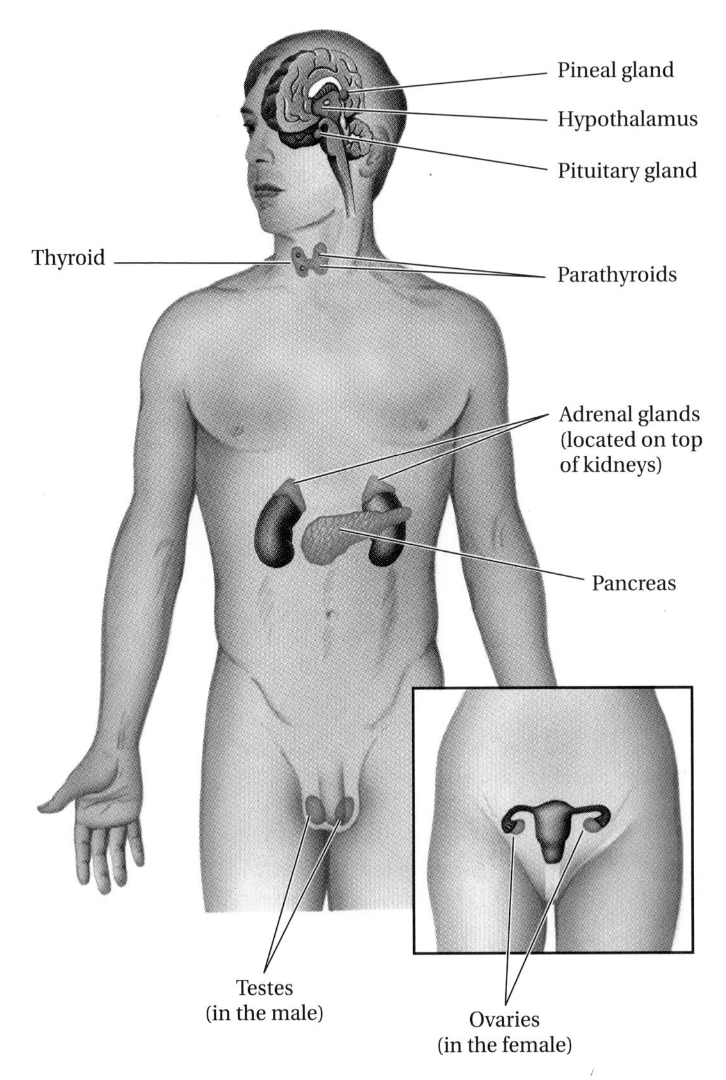


**Figure 3.4** ***Major Glands of the Endocrine System*** The endocrine system consists of ductless glands that release hormones directly into the bloodstream.

system contains ductless glands that secrete hormones directly into the bloodstream (see Figure 3.4). The word *hormone* is derived from Greek roots meaning "to set in motion." **Hormones** are chemical substances that regulate and coordinate the functions of organs and body cells.

A small structure in the brain, the **hypothalamus,** helps coordinate the body's response to stress. The hypothalamus secretes so-called releasing hormones that cause other glands to secrete their own hormones. The process is akin to a series of falling dominoes.

**Talking Glossary**
Corticotrophin-releasing hormone, Adrenocorticotrophic hormone
**G0306**

Under stress, the hypothalamus secretes **corticotrophin-releasing hormone (CRH).** CRH in turn stimulates the **pituitary gland,** which lies just below the hypothalamus. The pituitary is sometimes referred to as the "master gland" because it plays a role in many bodily processes. Pituitary hormones spur growth of muscles and bones. They stimulate the production of sperm in the male and ova (egg cells) in the female.

In response to CRH, the pituitary gland secretes **adrenocorticotrophic hormone (ACTH).** ACTH is taken up by receptor sites in the **adrenal glands,** which are a pair of small endocrine glands located just above the kidneys. ACTH stimulates the outer layer of the adrenal glands, the **adrenal cortex,** to release stress hormones called **corticosteroids** (or *cortical steroids*). Corticosteroids help the body manage stress by making stored nutrients more available to meet the increased demands for energy the body may face in coping with a stressor.

**Talking Glossary**
Corticosteroids
**G0307**

The sympathetic nervous system also activates the inner layer of each adrenal gland, the **adrenal medulla,** to secrete a cocktail of stress hormones, consisting of **adrenaline** and **noradrenaline.** Adrenaline and noradrenaline work together to accelerate the heartbeat to pump more oxygen to the muscles and to cause the liver to release stores of energy in the form of glucose (sugar). Glucose makes energy available to fuel the intense muscle activity that might be needed to fight or flee from a threat. The "racing heart" we experience under stress is caused by this surge of adrenaline and noradrenaline.

**Talking Glossary**
Adrenal medulla
**G0308**

During the resistance or adaptation stage, the body attempts to restore homeostasis—its steady state. The parasympathetic branch of the ANS slows the heart rate and breathing rate. Whether the body succeeds in restoring homeostasis depends on whether the stressor is removed or is coped with effectively.

## think about it!

- **Have you experienced the alarm reaction of the general adaptation syndrome? What triggered it? How did it feel? What was the outcome?**
- **What is the role of the nervous system in the general adaptation syndrome? What is the role of the endocrine system?**

**critical thinking** **Agree or disagree and support your answer: Stress can be healthy or unhealthy.**

**Smart Quiz**
**Q0303**

# Health Check

## Are You Overstressed?

Some people thrive on higher levels of stress than others. An event that threatens one person may be an exciting challenge to another. Yet any of us can become overstressed if pressures mount up. How can you know if you are overstressed? The answers to these questions may offer some insight.

| YES | NO | |
|---|---|---|
| ____ | ____ | 1. Are you cutting back on sleep or leisure activities because of work or other demands? |
| ____ | ____ | 2. Are you experiencing headaches or other aches and pains without any apparent physical cause? |
| ____ | ____ | 3. Are you unusually fatigued or tired much of the time? |
| ____ | ____ | 4. Do people tell you that you need a vacation? |
| ____ | ____ | 5. Are you feeling tense, uptight, or stressed much of the time? |
| ____ | ____ | 6. Do you lie awake at night worrying about how you are going to accomplish everything you need to do the next day? |
| ____ | ____ | 7. Are you unable to unwind at the end of the day? |
| ____ | ____ | 8. Are you drinking more alcohol than usual? |
| ____ | ____ | 9. Do you feel there is too much pressure on you at home? At work? Both? |
| ____ | ____ | 10. Do you have too little time for yourself? |
| ____ | ____ | 11. Is it difficult to remember the last time you enjoyed yourself? |
| ____ | ____ | 12. Do people expect too much from you? |
| ____ | ____ | 13. Are you expecting too much from yourself? |
| ____ | ____ | 14. Are you facing difficult financial or health problems? |
| ____ | ____ | 15. Do you find yourself snapping at people too much? |

If you answered "yes" to several of these items, you may be experiencing a stress overload. You might ask yourself: What can I do to eliminate the avoidable stressors in my life? How can I better handle the sources of stress I cannot avoid?

## STRESS AND HEALTH

Stress is a fact of life. But when it overtaxes our ability to adjust, it can affect our psychological and physical health.

### Stress and Psychological Health

Stress can lead to negative emotions and psychological disorders.

**Anxiety** We experience anxiety when we face a threat. You may feel anxious if a midterm exam is coming up and you haven't yet cracked your textbook. You may feel anxious before a big date or a dental or medical examination. The physical symptoms of anxiety—"butterflies" in the stomach, rapid heartbeat, and sweating—are all features of the alarm reaction, the body's initial response to stress. They are caused by the stress hormones adrenaline and noradrenaline.

Anxiety can be adaptive if it motivates us to prepare for the stressor—to study for a test or to consult a health professional about a troubling symptom. Other ways of handling anxiety can be counterproductive, such as deciding to escape one's troubles by going out drinking. Use anxiety as a cue to examine the stressors in your life and plan ways of coping.

**Depression** Prolonged stress can tax our coping abilities to the point that we lack the energy to tackle everyday challenges. Our moods are dampened, and we can become depressed. Various stressors, especially the loss of a loved one, prolonged unemployment, illness, marital problems, pressures at work, and poverty, increase the risk of depression. Although there is a genetic component to many psychological disorders, including depression, stress appears to interact with this genetic vulnerability, making the development of depression more likely. Feelings of anxiety and depression can also impair the functioning of the immune system, leaving us more vulnerable to physical disorders.[11]

**Anger** Minor annoyances, hassles, or frustrations may give rise to anger. Stress may cause us to "fly off the handle." The "final straw" may trigger an angry outburst. Afterward, we might wonder why we reacted so strongly. We are most likely to feel angry when we blame others for thwarting us in our efforts to attain our goals. Anger tends to compound rather than solve problems and contributes to further stress. Anger can trigger arguments and alienate the important people in our lives.

Other psychological reactions to stress take the form of stress-related psychological disorders, such as adjustment disorders and posttraumatic stress disorder.

**Adjustment Disorders** It is normal to feel sad when we experience loss or have a disappointing experience at work or school. But when our emotional distress is excessive or when it interferes with our ability to function, we may be experiencing a type of psychological disorder called an **adjustment disorder.** If you break up with your fiancee and find that your mood is thrown into a tailspin, you may be experiencing an adjustment disorder. Or your grades fall off as you become preoccupied with the failed relationship. It may seem impossible to keep up at work or at school.

Adjustment disorders may be overcome when the stress is removed or the person learns to cope more effectively with it. When problems in coping with stress persist, adjustment disorders may lead to other psychological disorders, such as depression.

Adjustment disorders are treatable. Do you need help adjusting to a stressful change in your life? If so, consider consulting a health professional in your college counseling center or elsewhere.

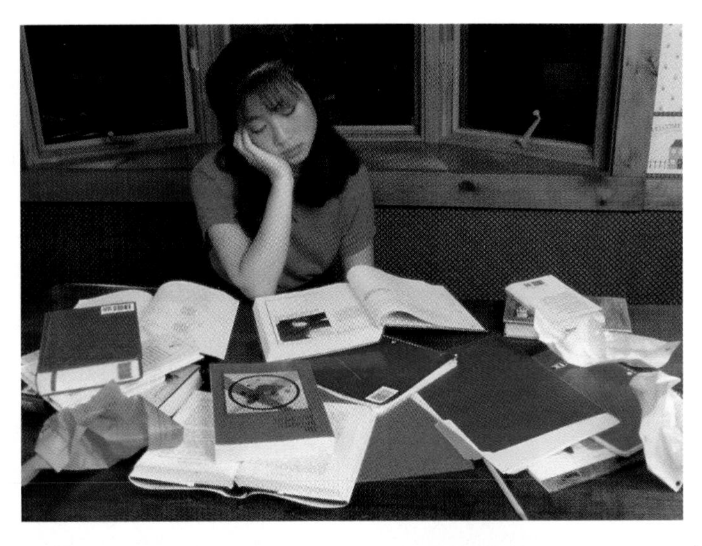

***Just Losing Concentration or Adjustment Disorder?*** Difficulties in keeping your mind on your studies could be a sign of an adjustment disorder, a maladaptive reaction to a stressful life event.

**Posttraumatic Stress Disorder (PTSD)** Psychological disorders may also arise following exposure to traumatic events such as combat and warfare, natural catastrophes, crimes of violence, and the violent death of another person. People may be diagnosed with **posttraumatic stress disorder (PTSD)** when they:

- *Reexperience the traumatic event in the form of intrusive memories, images, dreams, or nightmares.* For example, some combat veterans report "flashbacks" to the battlefield.
- *Avoid situations that remind them of the experience.* The rape survivor may avoid the part of town where the rape took place. The combat veteran may avoid his service buddies so that he need not talk about his combat experiences.
- *Have high levels of bodily arousal.* The person may feel keyed up or on edge and have difficulty relaxing or getting to sleep. He or she may seem always on guard and jumpy in response to sudden noises.
- *Experience emotional numbing.* The person may have difficulty feeling love or other strong emotions.
- *Cannot function or have significant emotional distress.*

**Adjustment disorder** A psychological disorder characterized by a maladaptive reaction to an identifiable stressor or stressors.

**Posttraumatic stress disorder (PTSD)** A psychological disorder involving a maladaptive reaction to a traumatic experience. Onset may be delayed until months or years after the traumatic event.

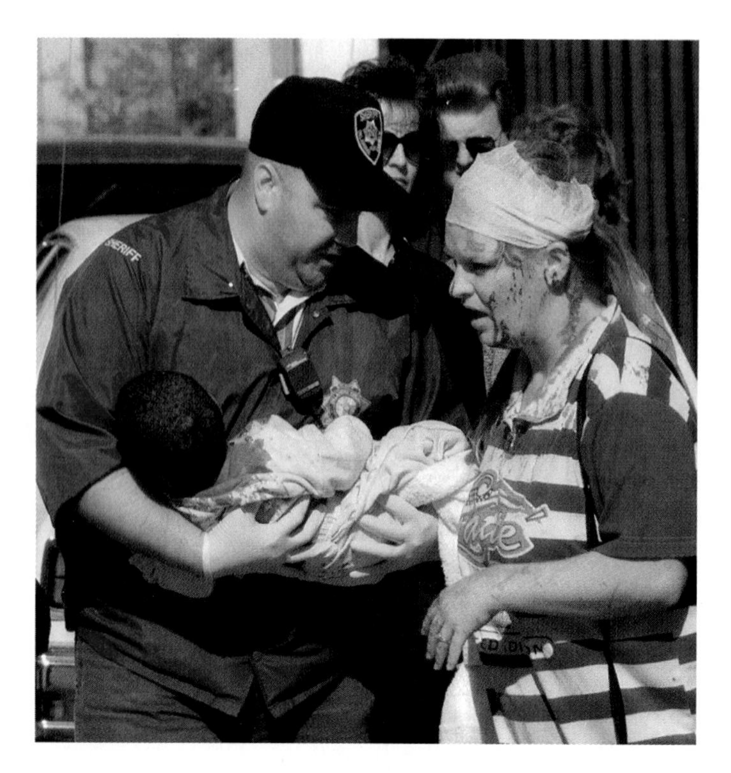

***Psychological Effect of Trauma***
Exposure to traumatic events, such as the Oklahoma City bombing, can have long-lasting psychological effects on survivors. Stress-related problems may linger for years in the form of posttraumatic stress disorder (PTSD).

The person may have difficulty meeting responsibilities as worker, student, spouse, or parent. She or he may be bothered by feelings of depression or anxiety.

Not everyone who experiences a traumatic event develops PTSD, but many do. Firefighters regularly come across fires, accidents, stabbings, shootings, suicides, medical emergencies, bombs, and hazardous material explosions. One firefighter in six can be diagnosed with PTSD.[12] Or consider the effects of exposure to horrific trauma among survivors of a mass killing in a cafeteria in Killeen, Texas, in 1991. A gunman killed 24 people, including himself, as the police cornered him. One in five male survivors, and one in three female survivors, developed PTSD.[13] Vulnerability to PTSD depends on factors such as the severity of the trauma, individual differences in biological reactivity and coping ability, and social support.

**Psychoneuroimmunology** The scientific study of interrelationships among stress and the body's nervous system, immune system, and endocrine system.

**Immune system** The body's system for identifying and eliminating disease-causing agents, such as bacteria and viruses, and for disposing of diseased, mutated, or worn-out cells.

**White blood cells** Specialized immune cells in the blood, these are the front-line soldiers in the body's war against invading pathogens.

**Antibody** A specialized type of protein produced by white blood cells; attaches itself to invading microbes and other foreign bodies, inactivates them, and marks them for destruction.

## Stress and Physical Health

Links between stress and physical health have been documented for many disorders, including hypertension, cancer, heart disease, and asthma. Let us consider some of the relationships between stress and physical health.

**Talking Glossary**
Psychoneuroimmunology
G0309

**Stress and the Immune System** Evidence from the field of **psychoneuroimmunology** supports Selye's belief that stress can impair health. Psychoneuroimmunology studies the interrelationships among the nervous system, the endocrine system, the **immune system,** and the effects of stress.

One way that stress may damage our health is by impairing the immune system, the body's line of defense against disease.[14] The immune system attacks and disarms disease-causing agents, such as bacteria and viruses, that invade the body. The soldiers in this battle are **white blood cells.** Specialized types of white blood cells conduct search-and-destroy missions to locate and eradicate microbial invaders. They also rid the body of diseased and worn-out cells. Some white blood cells produce specialized proteins called **antibodies.** Antibodies attach to invading microbes, inactivate them, and mark them for destruction by immune system cells. (The workings of the immune system are discussed further in Chapter 15.)

Many stressors, such as divorce, unemployment, sleep deprivation, and college tests, can impair the immune system. A weakened immune system increases vulnerability to common illnesses like colds and flu and perhaps even to chronic diseases, such as cancer. Chronic stresses and worries may also lengthen healing time for wounds.[15]

**Stress and Chronic Diseases** High levels of stress associated with life changes are linked to an increased risk of chronic health problems, including the two major killers in the United States: heart disease and cancer.[16] In the case of cancer, scientists suspect that stress may gradually weaken or compromise the immune system, making it less capable of ridding the body of cancerous cells. Other evidence comes from findings that exposure to high levels of stress can accelerate the onset of experimentally induced cancer in laboratory animals.[17]

**Close-up** Stress and cancer T0301

Prolonged stress may also compromise the cardiovascular system, increasing the risk of heart disease or strokes. Evidence shows that people who encounter a great deal of pressure on the job are at increased risk of developing heart disease.[18] Workers with high-strain jobs—jobs in which they have little decision-making latitude but have high standards of performance—also show higher rates of coronary heart disease. Waiters and waitresses, telephone operators, and cooks hold high-strain jobs (see Figure 3.5). Workers in these high-strain jobs stand about 1½ times greater risk of developing coronary heart disease as those in low-strain jobs.[19]

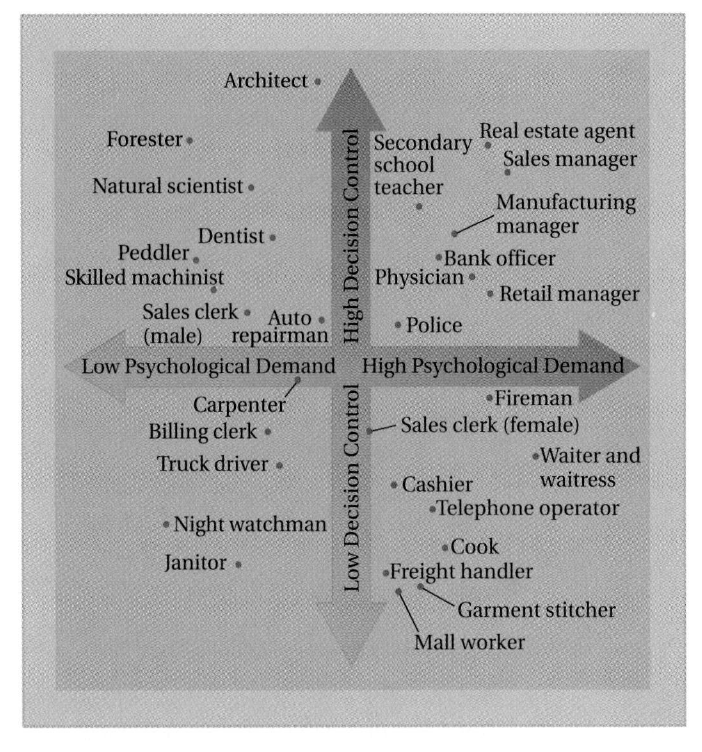


**Figure 3.5** ***Job Strain Model*** Workers holding high-strain jobs, which are characterized by little control and high demand (the bottom right quadrant) are at increased risk of developing coronary heart disease.

**Stress and Illness** Stress appears to increase vulnerability to the common cold. High levels of stress dampen the body's production of immunoglobulin A, an antibody that fends off cold viruses that enter through the nose and mouth.[20] This may explain why many people develop colds during times of stress, such as around the time of final examinations.

Corticosteroids—cortical steroids—may also play a role in the linkage between stress and illness. Cortical steroids are released as part of the alarm reaction to stress. They help the body cope with stress by increasing the availability of stored nutrients to provide extra fuel. But if the source of stress persists, continued secretion of these steroids at high levels may suppress the production of antibodies, including those that fight cold viruses. Long-term use of prescribed steroidal anti-inflammatories can also lead to impaired immunological functioning, as can unsanctioned use of synthetic steroids by body builders and other athletes.

**think about it!**

- **Have you experienced any of the psychological effects of stress?**
- **What are the effects of stress on the immune system?**

**critical thinking** **Why might people be more likely to catch a cold or become ill in other ways when they are under stress? Explain.**

**Smart Quiz** Q0304

# Taking the Distress out of Stress

## Take Charge

The aim of stress management is not to eliminate stress from our lives—indeed, some stress is actually good for us—but rather to help us manage the stress we encounter and help us cope more effectively with the effects of stress. First, however, let us consider some ineffective ways of reacting to stress.

### Poor Ways of Managing Stress

Ineffective ways of handling stress involve pretending that it does not exist, dulling it at any cost, and acting out aggressively.

**Withdrawal** Some people withdraw quickly from stressful situations rather than putting in reasonable time and effort to master them. One man who wanted to become a firefighter withdrew from the fire training academy three days into the training program, citing the high level of stress. (He later regretted his decision and was able to get reinstated.)

Temporary withdrawal can be an adaptive response to stress. Most of us need breaks, or vacations, from the stresses of everyday life. Withdrawal may also be adaptive if there is no other way to handle a difficult situation. However, beating a hasty retreat at the first sign of stress prevents us from learning to cope with the normal demands of life.

**Denial** Denial prevents us from acknowledging stressors. People with serious illnesses like heart disease or cancer may attribute their symptoms to minor problems, which they assume will pass if left alone. The person with a heart condition may dismiss chest pain as "no big deal" or as a sign of indigestion. Denial may minimize the emotional impact of threatening stressors for a time, but the eventual consequences can be devastating, even lethal.

**Substance Abuse** Some people turn to alcohol or other drugs to help them cope with stress. Drugs may temporarily blot out emotional distress but do nothing to help resolve underlying problems. Moreover, alcohol or drug abuse leads to yet another set of stressful problems.

**Close-up**
Alcohol and stress
**T0302**

**Aggression** Aggression is a maladaptive way of coping with the stress of interpersonal conflicts or social provocations. Lashing out verbally tends to beget a similar response, which only aggravates the stressful situation. Physical violence is illegal and dangerous. Health professionals can help those who have difficulty controlling their tempers.

Now let us consider better ways to deal with stress.

### More Effective Ways of Managing Stress

**Keep Stress at Manageable Levels** Do things run smoothly in your daily life? Do you have enough time to "stop and smell the roses"? Or do you find yourself running frantically from place to place just to keep up with the many demands on your time? Does it seem that no matter how hard you try, there is still much more that needs to be done? If so, you may be facing more stress than you can handle. Here are some ways to turn down the level of stress in your life:

1. *Don't bite off more than you can chew.* Don't take on more tasks than you can reasonably accomplish given the other demands on your time. Don't sacrifice family or personal needs to cram more work-related activities into your busy schedule.
2. *Reduce daily hassles.* What can you do to reduce daily hassles? Might you be able to change your schedule to avoid the morning traffic jam? Can you car pool? Being stuck in traffic may be more tolerable if you are not the one behind the wheel and can use the time to catch up on your reading. What other daily hassles can you eliminate?
3. *Reduce the duration of stress.* Some stressors may be unavoidable, but you may be able to lessen their impact by reducing their duration. Perhaps you can divide your exposure to them into manageable doses. Take more frequent breaks. If possible, take things more slowly and stretch deadlines when stressful burdens become too taxing. For example, reduce the impact of studying for exams by starting to study earlier than you normally would. You can then afford some study breaks. We're not suggesting that you compromise your work ethic, but that you work out a manageable workload. Your final products may even be better in quality.

4. *Develop time-management skills.* Organize your time more efficiently. Use a monthly calendar. Fill in appointments and important events (like upcoming exams, doctor's visits, family get-togethers, etc.). Make sure there's a time for everything you need to do.
5. *Use prioritized to-do lists.* Start each day with a list of things you feel you need to do. Then prioritize them, using a three-point code. Assign a 1 to things you absolutely must get done today. Assign a 2 to things you'd like to get done today, but don't absolutely need to do. Give a 3 to things you'd like to get done if time allows. Also, break down large tasks into small, manageable ones. Don't try to finish off that term paper in just one or two marathon sittings. Divide the project into smaller tasks and tackle them one by one.

**Become More Aware of Your Body's Response to Stress** Become aware of how your body reacts to stress. Does your back hurt more than usual? Is that nagging headache becoming a daily occurrence? Are you biting your nails? Are you exhausted at the end of the day? These physical and psychological symptoms may signal that you've reached or exceeded your stress threshold.

Close-up
Headache
T0303

**Preserve Your Physical Resources** Maintain your body's ability to cope with stress. Follow a nutritionally balanced diet. Get enough sleep. Have regular medical checkups. Avoid tobacco and other harmful substances. Keep active and fit.

**Know What to Expect** Stressors are more manageable when you're prepared. Knowing that a final exam is coming in three or four weeks puts you on notice that you need to adjust your study routine to prepare for it. In the case of unexpected stressors, like power blackouts, you can prepare in general by having flashlights and candles in the house. Knowing what to expect allows you to develop coping strategies. People with accurate knowledge of medical procedures they are about to undergo tend to cope with them more effectively than people who remain in the dark. When you face a particular stressor, find out who can help you learn about it.

**Reach Out and Be Touched by Someone** Social support buffers the effects of stress. Studies with medical students and dental students, two highly stressed groups, show that students who had more friends had better immune system functioning than those with fewer friends.[21] Hospitalized people who receive significant levels of emotional support have speedier recoveries than people with weaker emotional-support networks.[22]

Social support can even ease the effects of large-scale disasters. After the Three-Mile Island nuclear accident in Pennsylvania in 1979, those residents with solid networks of social support reported less stress than residents who had to go it alone.[23]

People with social support may even live longer, as suggested by studies in Tecumseh, Michigan,[24] and Alameda County, California.[25] The Tecumseh study followed 2,754 adults from 1967 through 1979. The mortality rate during this time was significantly lower for men who were married, who attended meetings of voluntary associations, and who participated regularly in social leisure activities. The California study tracked 7,000 adults over a 9-year period. People with weak social ties had a death rate two to five times higher than those with stronger social ties.

How can you broaden your own social support network? The Social Support Inventory (see Table 3.2) offers suggestions for getting the kinds of social support that people rely upon, especially in times of stress.

TABLE 3.2

**Social Support—What It Is, How to Get It**

| Type of Support | What It Is | How to Get It |
|---|---|---|
| Emotional concern | Having others available who will listen to your problems and express understanding, sympathy, caring, and reassurance. | Develop friendships and maintain relationships with present friends and family members. Make contact with trusted advisors in your community, such as your local priest, minister, or rabbi. Get involved in clubs, social organizations, or community activities that provide opportunities to expand your social network. |
| Instrumental aid | Material assistance and services to support adaptive behavior in times of stress. | Learn about the resources in your community that assist people in times of need. Become acquainted with government support programs and the work of voluntary support agencies. |
| Feedback | Honest response from others that tells us how we're doing when we're under stress. | Develop a give-and-take relationship with several people whose opinions you trust. |
| Socializing | Interacting with others in our free time is an important source of social support. | Invite friends and family members to get together with you regularly, perhaps for enjoyable activities like dinner, sports, or shows. |

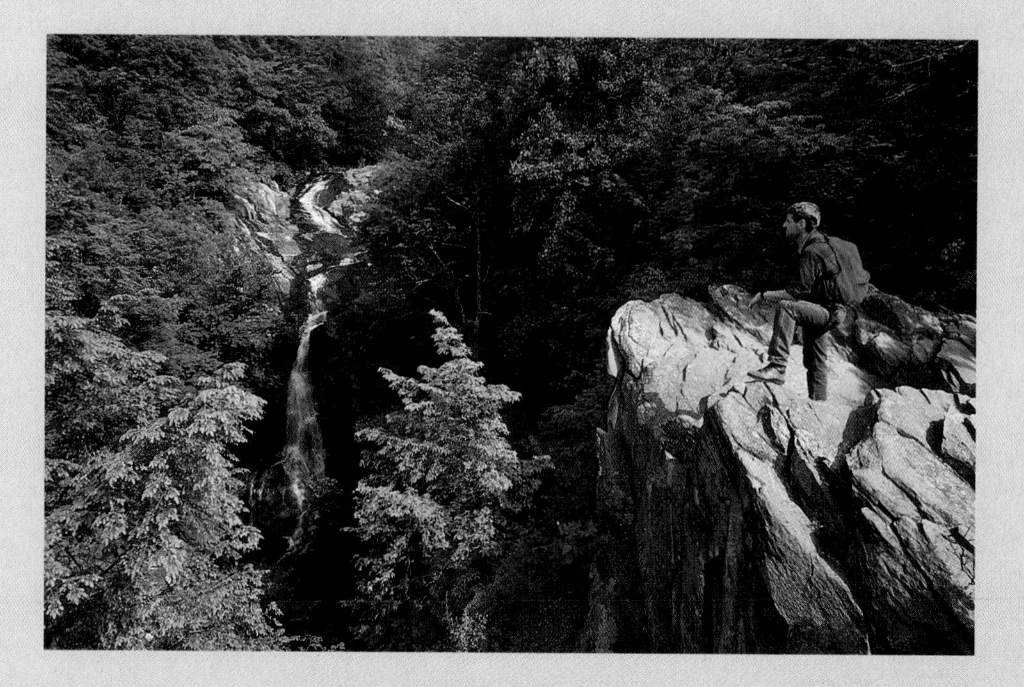

***Managing Stress*** How many different ways of combating stress can you think of? How many of these ways are you practicing?

**Work It Out by . . . Working Out** Exercise not only enhances health; it can also directly combat stress. Many people work off the tensions of the day with a vigorous game of racquetball, a run around the park, or a dozen laps in the pool.

How does exercise help us cope with stress? Regular exercise can help strengthen body systems, such as the cardiovascular system, that are affected by stress. Vigorous exercise also raises the levels of endorphins in the bloodstream, which counters stress by inducing feelings of well-being. Exercise also reduces uncomfortable responses to stress, such as muscle tension and anxiety, for at least a few hours,[26] thus restoring a more relaxed state of mind and body. Even mild levels of exercise—a gentle swim, a brisk walk—can relieve stress.

Choose a physical activity that you enjoy. Pushing yourself to do something you dislike will only increase the stress you experience.

**Change Stressful Thoughts to Stress-Busting Thoughts** What are you telling yourself about the events that distress you? Are you sizing things up correctly, or are you blowing them out of proportion? Do you react to disappointing experiences by feeling disillusioned and hopeless? Do you refuse to compromise? Do you feel miserable when you fall short of your expectations?

These dysfunctional thoughts only aggravate stress. Don't focus only on the negative parts of your experiences. Avoid thinking in all-or-nothing, black-and-white terms. Allow for shades of gray.

Table 3.3 gives examples of a common category of stressful thoughts and some alternatives that can help keep things in perspective.

**Express Your Feelings** When something is bothering you, don't keep it inside. Talk it over with someone you trust. Or write down your feelings in a personal journal. Expressing your feelings is especially helpful in coping with stressful or traumatic events. Keeping disturbing thoughts and feelings to yourself may place additional stress on your autonomic nervous system and can impair your immune system. Researchers find that talking or writing about stressful experiences actually has positive effects on the immune system.[28]

**Try a Little Humor—It's Good Medicine** Humor can help buffer the effects of stress. The notion that humor eases life's burdens is an ancient one. Indeed, we can find references to humor's tonic effect in the biblical adage, "A merry heart doeth good like a medicine" (Proverbs 17:22). Humor can get our minds off our troubles, at least for a time, and make stress more bearable. In one study, stress had less of an impact on college students who had a good sense of humor, especially those who were able to laugh in the face of adversity.[29] You might try a dose of something amusing tonight, a comedy perhaps.

**Do Something That You Enjoy** Stress is more manageable when you do something each day that brings you joy—perhaps leisure reading, watching or participating in a sports event, working on the car, or cruising the web.

**Change "I Can'ts" into "I Can's"** Self-confidence enhances our ability to withstand stress. People with self-confidence also bounce back more easily from failure. If you believe you can accomplish what you set out to do, you are likely to marshal your resources and apply yourself until you reach your goal. If you doubt yourself, you may give up when you encounter the first setback. Start with small, achievable goals to boost your confidence and encourage you to move forward. Treat disappointments as opportunities to learn from your mistakes, not as signs of failure.

TABLE 3.3

**Thoughts That Blow Stressors Out of Proportion and Rational Alternatives That Help Keep Things in Perspective**[27]

| Thoughts That Blow Stressors Out of Proportion | Rational Alternative Thoughts That Help Keep Things in Perspective |
|---|---|
| Oh my God, it's going to be a mess! I'm losing all control! | This is annoying and upsetting, but I haven't lost all control and I'm not going to. |
| This is awful. It'll never end. | It's bad, but it doesn't have to get the best of me. Upsetting things do come to an end, even if it's hard to believe right now. |
| I just can't stand it when ................. gives me that look. | Life is more pleasant when everyone is pleased with me, but I have to be myself. So people are going to disagree with me from time to time. |
| There's no way I can get up there and perform/give that speech! I'll look like an idiot. | I'm not perfect, but that doesn't mean I'm going to look like an idiot. And if someone thinks I look bad, it doesn't mean I *am* bad. And if I am bad, so what? I can live with that, too. I don't have to be perfect every time. So stop being such a worrywart and get up and have some fun. |
| My heart's beating a mile a minute! How much of this can I take? | Take it easy! Just slow down—stop and think. Take a few deep breaths. Focus on the problem, not on my beating heart. |
| What can I do? I'm helpless! It's just going to get worse and worse. | Take it easy. Just stop and think for a minute. Just because there's no obvious solution doesn't mean that I won't be able to do anything about it. There's no point to getting so upset. Why don't I just take it from minute to minute for the time being. Break down the problem into smaller steps. Think of one small thing to do first. |

**Increase Your Psychological Hardiness** Psychologically hardy people handle stress more effectively because they see themselves as *choosing* to live challenging lives. They think of stress as making life interesting, not as intensifying pressure. They feel in control of the stress they encounter. They seek to solve problems, not to avoid them. **Psychological hardiness** is a buffer against stress, a mental shock-absorber that makes stress more manageable.

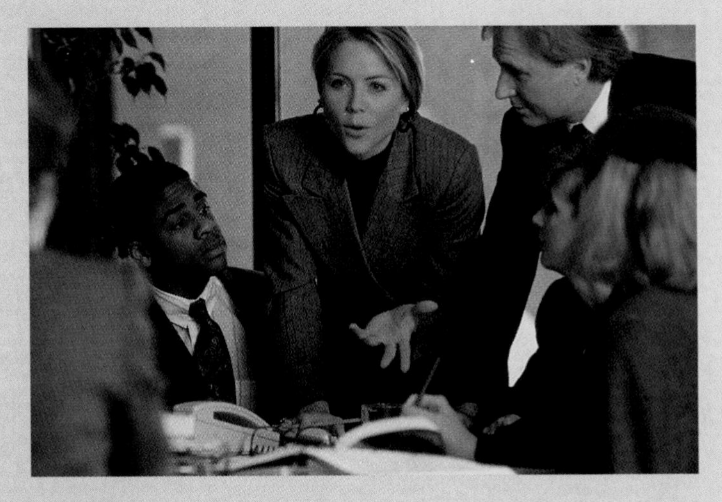

***Psychological Hardiness*** Psychologically hardy people are better able to handle stress because they feel in control of the stress in their lives and view stressful challenges as making their lives more interesting.

Psychologist Salvadore Maddi[30] offers the following suggestions for increasing our psychological hardiness:

1. *Situation Reconstruction: "It Could Be Worse, but Can You Make It Better?"* In situational reconstruction, you imagine how your situation could be worse and ways in which it could be made better. This helps us put stressful situations into perspective, and not as the absolute calamities we may take them to be. It also encourages us to use our problem-solving skills to find ways of improving our situation.
2. *Focusing: "What's Really Bothering You?"* Sometimes you feel distressed or unhappy but can't put your finger on the reason. In focusing, you attend to the negative body sensations associated with the feeling state, such as tightness in the chest. You think back to other times when you've experienced these sensations. In one case a young woman focused on the churning in her stomach. She recalled that this sensation had begun during her early school years when she failed to do her homework and feared being reproached by her teachers. Now the sensation arose when she feared she wouldn't have enough time to do her term papers or study for exams. Her recognition of the source of her problem raised her awareness that she faced a specific challenge, not a nameless feeling. She felt a greater sense of control and committed herself to resolving the underlying source of

**Psychological hardiness** A cluster of traits believed to buffer the effects of stress, consisting of commitment, challenge, and control.

stress by developing more efficient studying and writing schedules.

3. *Compensatory Self-Improvement: "If Not Love, then Perhaps Tennis?"* Mark became depressed after his efforts to win a woman's affections were rebuffed. She decided to end the relationship once and for all. He could do nothing to change her mind and felt helpless. A counselor suggested that perhaps what he needed was to take up aerobics. Aerobics, he wondered? How could that help him heal these emotional wounds? Nonetheless, he enrolled in an aerobics class. He felt awkward and clumsy at first, but after a while he learned the routines and gradually worked himself into condition. He began feeling better about himself and made some new acquaintances in the class, including some women he began dating. He felt he was taking charge of his life rather than just allowing things to happen to him. The lesson: If your efforts to achieve a certain goal keep knocking up against a roadblock, try your hand at something else. You just might succeed. Tennis, anyone?

**Meditate** Meditation induces a relaxed state in which the person's connection with the environment is transformed. Worry, planning, and routine concerns are suspended. Consciousness is narrowed to repetitive, relaxing stimuli. The sympathetic nervous system calms down. The body's alarm reaction is toned down or shut off.

One of the most widely practiced forms of meditation is **transcendental meditation (TM),** a form of Indian meditation that was introduced to the U.S. in 1959 by Maharishi Mahesh Yogi. The distinguishing feature of TM is the repetition of *mantras*—relaxing sounds like *ieng* and *om.*

TM produces what has been called a **relaxation response,**[31] a physical state characterized by a reduced metabolic rate (gauged by a reduction in oxygen consumption) and by a lowering of blood pressure in people with **hypertension** (high blood pressure).[32] Meditators also produce more **alpha waves,** brain waves connected with states of relaxation.

Learning to relax by using meditation can be healthy even for those with normal blood pressure. Here are some guidelines to help you learn a straightforward meditation technique:

1. *Avoid eating for about an hour before meditation.* Avoid caffeine, the stimulant found in coffee and tea, for at least two hours beforehand.
2. *Put yourself in a hushed, calming environment.* Dim the lights. Take the phone off the hook. Shut off the TV and radio.
3. *Get into a relaxed position, but don't feel obliged to hold a fixed posture.* You can scratch or yawn if you feel the urge.
4. *Accept a passive mental attitude.* Don't attempt to force a meditative state. Tell yourself, "What happens, happens." Permit yourself to relax. Take what you get. Don't *strive* to make it happen.
5. *Find a focusing device.* Many people use their breathing as a focusing device. Focus on your breathing while you sit before a serene object, like a plant or painting. You may count your breaths or repeat the word "one" or "relax" on every outbreath. Or you could focus on a resonant word, or mantra, like *ah-nam, rah-mah,* or *shi-rim.* Repeat the mantra aloud on each outbreath for a number of times. Then say it more softly. Then just think it. Allow your thinking to become more "passive" so that you "perceive" the mantra rather than actively think it. Again, embrace a "what happens, happens" attitude. The mantra may become softer or louder in your mind. It may fade away, then reappear.
6. *Let your mind drift.* (You won't get lost.) If unsettling thoughts arrive while you're meditating, just allow these thoughts to "pass through." Attempts to squelch them might make you feel more tense.[33]
7. *Incorporate meditation into your daily routine.* Practice meditation for about 10 to 20 minutes at a time twice a day. Try to incorporate your meditation breaks into your daily routine.

**Relax** There are many other relaxation techniques. Health professionals at your college or university counseling center can introduce you to them.

One method, called **progressive muscle relaxation,** was developed by Edmund Jacobson. Jacobson noticed that people tend to tense their muscles when they are under stress, although they may not be aware of it. Since muscle contractions are associated with emotional tension, Jacobson reasoned that relaxing muscles can reduce states of tension. Many of the people he worked with, however, didn't have a clue as to how to relax their muscles.

Jacobson taught people first to tense, then to relax specific muscle groups in the body. The method is "progressive" in that people progress from one group of muscles to another, literally from head to toe.

You can get a feel for this technique by practicing on a particular muscle group, for example, the muscles in your right hand. First, make a fist with your right hand; tighten until you feel the tension. After tensing for a few seconds, unclench your fist and let go of tensions completely. Study the difference between the states of tension and relaxation. Notice how the muscles in your hand seem to unwind and let go of the tension. As you gain experience with the technique, you may find that you can relax your muscles by "just letting them go" without first having to tense them.

**Transcendental meditation (TM)** An adaptation of an Indian meditation technique involving the repetition of a mantra with each outbreath.

**Relaxation response** A state of relaxation brought about by meditation that is characterized by a slowing down of metabolism and a lowering of blood pressure in people with hypertension.

**Hypertension** Elevated blood pressure that is a major risk factor in heart disease and stroke.

**Alpha waves** A brain wave pattern associated with states of relaxation.

**Progressive muscle relaxation** A form of relaxation training that achieves the reduction of muscle tension through a series of tensing and relaxing exercises involving selected muscle groups.

**Breathe (Through Your Diaphragm, That Is)** Has anyone ever told you to take a few deep breaths when you were feeling stressed or anxious? When we are tense, our breathing becomes shallow. We may hyperventilate, or breathe more rapidly than usual. When we breathe we exchange oxygen for carbon dioxide. But when we hyperventilate, we breathe off too much carbon dioxide, which can cause feelings of dizziness or lightheadedness. Breathing slowly and deeply from the **diaphragm** tones down the body's response to stress and restores a correct balance between oxygen and carbon dioxide in our bloodstream.

**Diaphragmatic breathing** can be learned by practicing some simple skills:

1. Breathe through the nose only.
2. Take the same amount of time to inhale and exhale.
3. Make inhaling and exhaling continuous and leisurely. You can count silently to yourself ("one thousand one, one thousand two, one thousand three," etc.) as you breathe in and out. Or you may use a particular resonant-sounding word, like "relax" on each outbreath (elongate the x-sound as you breathe out).
4. Lie on your back in bed. Place your hands lightly on your stomach. Breathe deeply and slowly in such a way that your stomach rises as you inhale and lowers as you exhale. You can also practice the technique while sitting upright in a comfortable chair. Place your right hand lightly on your stomach (or your left hand if you are left-handed). Place your other hand on your upper chest. Breathe so that you can see your stomach move outward each time you inhale and inward each time you exhale. If the hand positioned on your upper chest remains still while your hand monitoring your abdomen moves outward and inward with each inbreath and outbreath, you are breathing diaphragmatically.

As you become more familiar with this technique, you may be able to breathe diaphragmatically by simply focusing your attention on taking deep, slow breaths, without monitoring the movements of your abdomen and chest with your hands. Many people find it helpful to use their relaxation word on each outbreath as a cue to restore the relaxation effect.

When you are tense, anxious, or in pain, diaphragmatic breathing may help distract you from your discomfort. Monitoring your breaths can also help block out disturbing thoughts.

**Reduce Type A Behavior** People with the Type A personality pattern continually pressure themselves to accomplish as much as possible in as little time as possible. Can Type A's learn to reduce or relieve their sense of time urgency and learn to take things slower? Researchers say "yes."[34] These stress-busting suggestions may be helpful to you even if you are not a bona fide Type A personality.

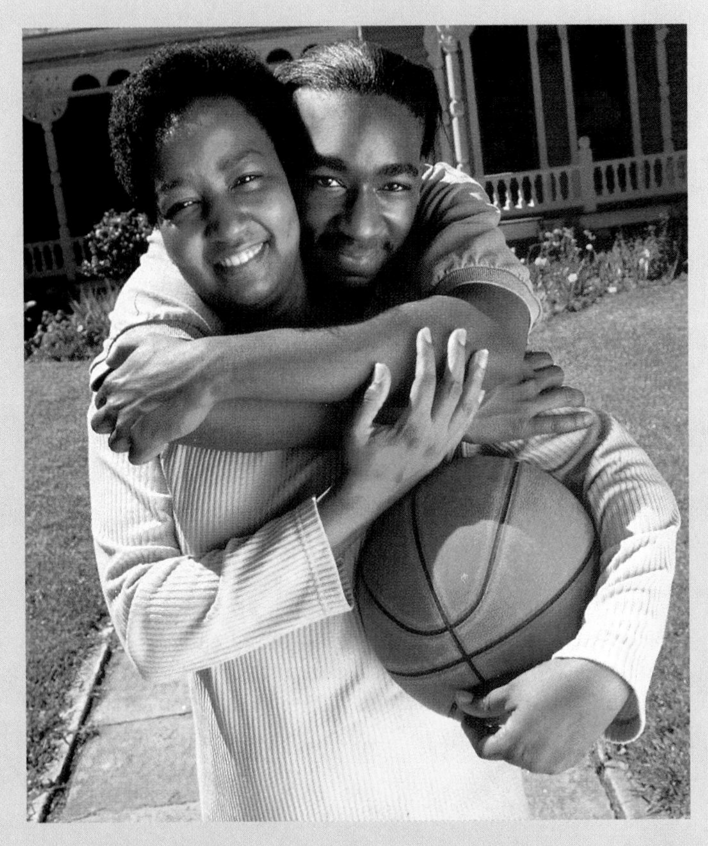

***Reducing Type A Behavior*** Spending more time socializing with friends and family members can help relieve stress, and not just for people with Type A personalities.

- *Spend more time socializing with friends and family.*
- *Take a few minutes each day to think about your earlier life experiences.* Examine old photographs of friends and family.
- *Cultivate enjoyable leisure activities.* Read for pleasure's sake. (Avoid books on succeeding in business or climbing the corporate ladder.) Take extension courses you enjoy and that are not career-related. Take up a hobby or learn to play a musical instrument.
- *Immerse yourself in cultural activities.* Spend time visiting museums and art galleries. Examine works of art for their beauty, not their prices. Attend the theater, ballet, or concerts. Or take in a movie.
- *Rediscover the art of writing letters to friends and family members.*
- *Lighten up on yourself.* Don't impose impossible schedules on yourself. Don't attempt to do too many things at once.

**Diaphragm** A muscular wall separating the chest cavity from the abdomen. For each inbreath, the diaphragm contracts, which causes the lungs to expand and take in air.

**Diaphragmatic breathing** Deep and regular breathing that can be monitored by the movement of the diaphragm with each inbreath and outbreath.

- *Enjoy mealtimes.* Relax while you eat. Make your meals an occasion. Ask friends or family members about their day. Listen to what they have to say without interrupting or finishing their sentences for them.
- *Slow down.* Remember that the posted speed limit tells you the maximum allowable driving speed, not the minimum. Walk around the campus for the sake of enjoying the day, not just to rush from one class to another. Read a newspaper or magazine for enjoyment.

***Reduce Hostility*** Chronic hostility seems to be the element of the Type A profile that is most clearly linked to heart disease. Hostility and anger are accompanied by heightened levels of the stress-related hormones epinephrine and norepinephrine, which over time may damage the heart and cardiovascular system. Here are some suggestions for reducing hostility:

1. *Change how you respond to annoying people.* Don't let them get you steamed. Tell yourself that the other person's behavior is just not worth getting hot and bothered about. Or just say what's on your mind assertively but not angrily. Let it out and let it go. Avoid discussions that lead only to pointless arguments. Avoid cursing or raising your voice. Keep your cool. (See Chapter 21 for further suggestions on controlling anger.)
2. *Form new friendships and nurture old ones.* Tell people you care about how you feel about them. Tell others that you are there to help them. Let others know that you appreciate their support and assistance.
3. *Get a pet and take time to stroke it and soothe it.* (Soothing works both ways.)
4. *Don't jump to conclusions that others mean you ill.* Don't expect others to live up to your expectations or hold them to blame when they don't.
5. *Appreciate beauty.*
6. *Participate in sports for the sake of playing, not winning at all costs.*
7. *Become more aware of how you hold anger in your facial muscles.* Look in a mirror when you're feeling angry and study your facial expressions. Learn to relax your anger muscles.
8. *Start the day with a cheerful "Good morning" to others.*

To sum up, stress is inescapable. Some stress keeps us alert and motivated, but too much stress can overtax our coping abilities and put us at risk of stress-related health problems. Stress may be a fact of life, but it is a fact we can learn to live with by averting unnecessary stressors, keeping stress at manageable levels, and toning down our body's alarm reaction to stress.

Smart
Quiz
Q0305

# SUMMING UP

## Questions and Answers

1. **What is stress?** Stress refers to pressures and demands to adjust or adapt. Yet without some stress we might become stagnant and bored. Positive stress is called eustress. Sources of stress include daily hassles, life changes, frustration, and conflict.

### SOURCES OF STRESS

2. **What are daily hassles?** Daily hassles are stressors that affect us regularly. They include household, health, time-pressure, inner-concern, environmental, financial-responsibility, work, and future-security hassles.

3. **What are life changes?** Life changes are intermittent changes that can be positive or negative, yet they, too, require adjustment.

4. **What is burnout?** Burnout is a state of physical and emotional exhaustion caused by the stress of overcommitment to work or other causes. Burnout is common among health professionals with impossible workloads.

5. **What is the Type A personality pattern?** People with the Type A personality pattern are highly driven, impatient, competitive, and hostile, and have a strong sense of time urgency. These traits may be a source of stress and pose a risk to their health.

### PAIN—WHAT IT IS, WHAT TO DO ABOUT IT

6. **What is pain?** Pain is a stressor that is a sign that something is wrong. Hormones called prostaglandins facilitate the communication of pain messages to the brain. Endorphins are natural painkillers.

### WHAT STRESS DOES TO THE BODY

7. **What is the general adaptation syndrome (GAS)?** The GAS is Selye's term for a three-stage response to stress. It consists of the alarm reaction, the resistance stage, and the exhaustion stage. The alarm reaction arouses us to cope with a threat.

8. **How does the nervous system respond to stress?** During the alarm reaction of the GAS, the sympathetic nervous system accelerates heart and respiration rates, which prepares the body to flee or, if need be, to fight. During the exhaustion stage, the parasympathetic nervous system attempts to restore body homeostasis.

9. **How does the endocrine system respond to stress?** The adrenal glands secrete stress hormones including steroids, adrenaline, and noradrenaline. Steroids help the body resist stress by combating allergic reactions and inflammation. Adrenaline and noradrenaline accelerate the heart rate and cause the liver to release stores of energy.

### STRESS AND HEALTH

10. **What is the connection between stress and psychological health?** Stress contributes to negative emotional responses such as anxiety, depression, and anger. Maladaptive reactions to stress may lead to psychological disorders such as adjustment disorders and posttraumatic stress disorder.

11. **What is the connection between stress and physical health?** Stress impairs the functioning of the immune system, leaving us prey to many illnesses, including the common cold.

12. **What are some relatively poor ways of responding to stress?** Poor ways of responding to stress include withdrawal, denial, substance abuse, and aggression.

13. **What are some better ways of responding to stress?** Better ways of responding to stress include becoming aware of your body's response to stress, knowing what to expect, obtaining social support, exercising, keeping things in perspective, expressing your feelings, developing a sense of humor, building self-confidence, increasing your psychological hardiness, meditating, relaxing, and reducing Type A behavior.

## Suggested Readings

**Benson, H., Stuart, E. M., and others.** *The Wellness Book: The Comprehensive Guide to Maintaining Health and Treating Stress-Related Illness.* New York: Fireside Books, Simon & Schuster, 1993. Herbert Benson, a leading expert on stress management, helps people gain greater control over their lives, combat stress, and improve well-being.

**Benson, H.** *The Relaxation Response.* New York: Morrow, 1975. A classic book on the principles and techniques of relaxation.

**Rathus, S. A., and Fichner-Rathus, L.** *Making the Most of College* (2nd ed.). Englewood Cliffs, NJ: Prentice-Hall, 1994. Advice about handling the stresses of adjusting to college.

**Greenberg, J.** *Comprehensive Stress Management.* Dubuque, IA: William C. Brown. A model for stress management, with special attention to particular types of stress, including occupational stress, college-related stress, and family stress.

## DID YOU KNOW THAT

- Virtually everyone is affected by psychological disorders? p.80
- Women are more likely than men to be depressed? p.81
- Among individuals at the same income levels, African Americans are no more likely than non-Hispanic white Americans to develop psychological disorders? p.81
- Some health professionals use bright light to treat depression—and it works? p.85
- Despite the myth to the contrary, people who threaten suicide are quite likely to be serious about taking their lives? p.93
- In many states, anyone can set up a practice as a psychotherapist? p.100

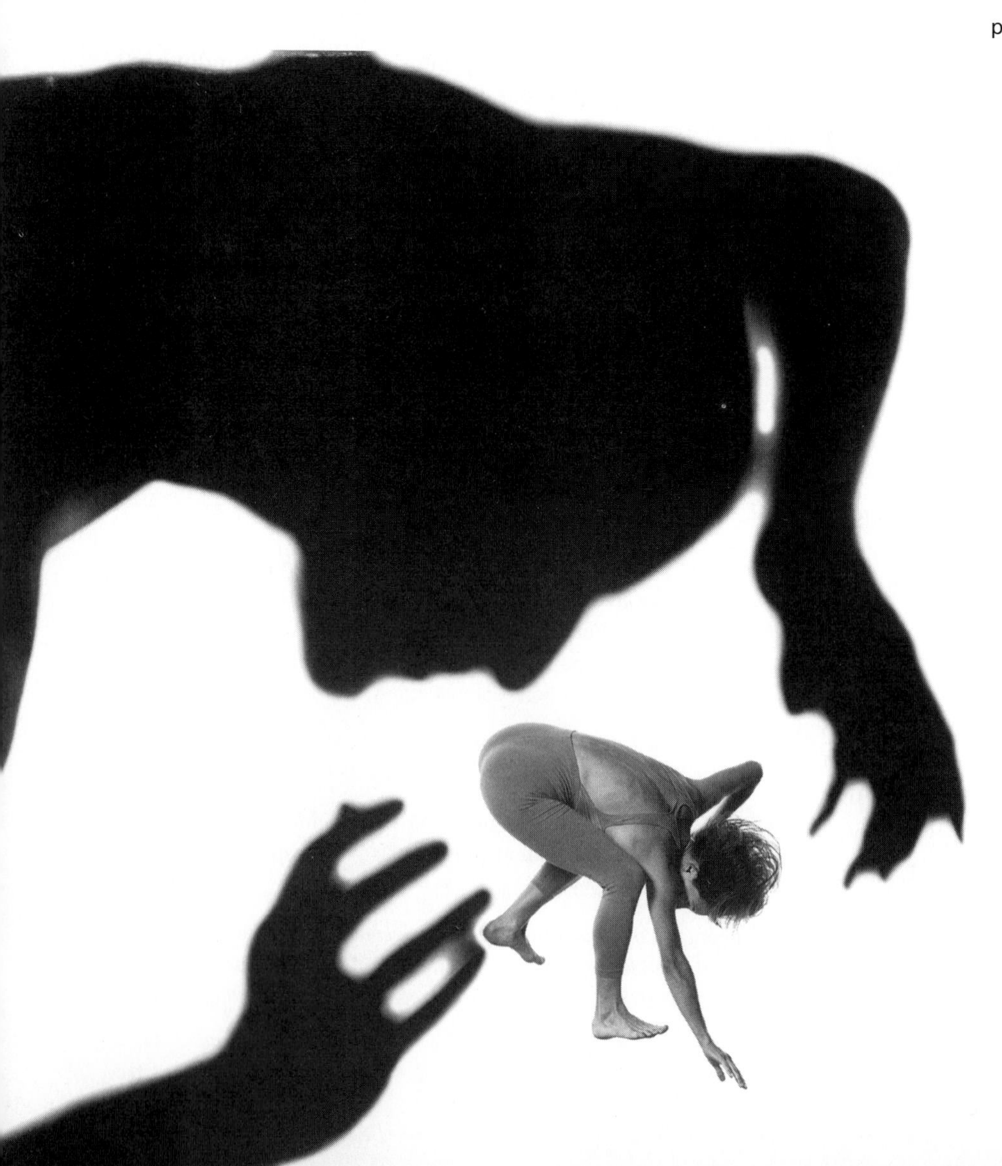

# 4 Psychological Disorders



*Linda was 23. Her husband Mark brought her into the emergency room because she had slit her wrists. When she was interviewed, her attention wandered. She seemed distracted by things in the air or something she might be hearing. It was as if she had an invisible earphone.*

*She explained that she had cut her wrists because the "hellsmen" had told her to. Then she seemed frightened. Later she said that the hellsmen had warned her not to reveal their existence. She had been afraid that they would punish her for talking about them.*

*Mark told the emergency room staff that Linda did not want to be near other people. So she had convinced Mark to rent a bungalow in the country. There she would make fantastic drawings of goblins and monsters during the days. Now and then she would become agitated and act as if invisible things were giving her instructions.*

*"I'm bad," Linda would mutter, "I'm bad." She would begin to jumble her words. Mark would then try to convince her to go to the hospital, but she would refuse. Then the wrist cutting would begin. Mark thought he had made the cottage safe by removing knives and blades. But Linda would always find something.*

*Then Linda would be brought to the hospital, have stitches put in, be kept under observation for a while, and medicated. She would explain that she cut herself because the hellsmen had told her that she was bad and must die. After a few days she would deny hearing the hellsmen, and she would insist on leaving the hospital.*

*Mark would take her home. The pattern continued.*[1]

*When the emergency room staff heard that Linda believed she had been following the orders of "hellsmen," they began to suspect that she had* schizophrenia, *a severe* psychological disorder.

# WHAT ARE PSYCHOLOGICAL DISORDERS?

Many of us are anxious or depressed now and then but do not have psychological disorders. Anxiety and depression are deemed abnormal, or signs of **psychological disorders,** when they are not appropriate to the situations we face. Yes, it is normal to be anxious before a job interview or a final exam. It is *not* normal to be anxious when one is looking out of a sixth-story window or about to receive a harmless vaccination. It is normal to feel down or depressed for a time because of a poor performance on a test. It is *not* normal to be depressed when things are going well.

The severity and persistence of the problem also indicate whether it is a psychological disorder. Although anxiety about a job interview is normal, feeling that your heart is pounding terrifyingly—and then avoiding the interview—is not. Nor is it normal to be depressed for many weeks or become so depressed that you can't meet your usual responsibilities.

Psychological disorders are also referred to as *mental disorders* and *mental illnesses.* They range from relatively mild disorders, such as **adjustment disorders** (discussed in Chapter 3), to more severe and enduring disorders like schizophrenia and **agoraphobia,** an anxiety disorder in which a person may become housebound because of fear of venturing out in public.

## Who Is Affected by Psychological Disorders?

In the United States, one adult in two experiences a diagnosable psychological disorder at some point in her or his life.[2] One in five is likely to have a psychological disorder in any given year. Even if we ourselves do not develop a psychological disorder, we are affected by disorders involving family members, friends, and coworkers. If we consider the economic costs of psychological disorders to the society at large, *then virtually all of us are affected.* Nearly all of us cover the costs of psychological treatment through taxes and health insurance.

One in five children and adolescents experiences a psychological disorder. Young people today are ten times more likely than their grandparents to develop severe depression.[3] The rising incidence of emotional disorders in young people—including depression, drug abuse, and stress-related disorders—may reflect life in a society with high rates of family disruption, substance abuse, and violence.

**Psychological disorder** A disturbance of psychological functioning resulting in emotional distress or impaired functioning (also called a *mental disorder* or *mental illness*).

**Adjustment disorder** A mild psychological disorder characterized by a maladaptive reaction to a stressful event or experience.

**Agoraphobia** A phobia characterized by fear of public places.

**Close-up**
Children's mental health
T0401

Hyperactivity
T0402

Psychological disorders also affect our physical health. Suicide, for example, is typically associated with depression and ranks as the ninth leading cause of death in the United States. It is the third leading cause of death among people aged 15 to 24. People with psychological disorders occupy one of every four hospital beds in the United States. The cost of caring for them, together with lost productivity, totals an estimated $150 billion a year,[4] that is, one dollar of every ten spent on health care in this country. In terms of treatment and lost productivity, the cost of depression equals the cost of heart disease, the leading cause of death in the United States.

**Close-up**
Mental health statistics
T0403

Psychotherapy, support groups, and drug therapy have helped millions to cope with psychological disorders. Unfortunately, many cases go untreated.[13] Some people are unaware that they have a psychological disorder. Others try to "tough it out." It doesn't make sense to try to walk with a broken leg, and it doesn't make sense to pretend that a psychological disorder doesn't exist or require treatment.

**Close-up**
You are not alone
T0404

## Psychological and Physical Health: An Interaction of Mind and Body

Mind and body are closely interlinked. Biological influences such as genetics and neurotransmitters are clearly involved in psychological disorders. Psychological health also affects physical health.

1. *Physical disorders can trigger or intensify psychological disorders.* The stress of illness can lead to or worsen psychological problems. Depression, for example, is common among people who are seriously ill with cancer, heart disease, HIV infection, or arthritis.
2. *Psychological disorders may present themselves as physical symptoms.* For example, a depressed person may complain of chronic fatigue and lack of appetite.
3. *Physical disorders can be affected by psychological factors.* Optimism and pessimism can have an important impact on recovery from illness. Maintaining a "fighting spirit" may well prolong life in people with heart disease, cancer, and HIV disease.

WORLD OF *diversity*

## Social Class, Gender, Ethnicity, and Psychological Health

The risk of psychological disorders varies in relation to sociocultural factors such as social class and ethnicity.

### Social Class and Psychological Health

The poorest among us are at greatest risk of developing severe psychological disorders, such as schizophrenia, regardless of race or ethnicity.[5] One explanation is that the stresses of poverty increase susceptibility to psychological disorders. Another explanation is that people who develop psychological disorders may lose jobs and drift downward in social class. There is probably some truth in both explanations. Nevertheless, psychological disorders affect the rich as well as the poor. No social class is immune.

### Gender and Psychological Health

Women are at higher risk than men of developing some psychological disorders, such as depression and agoraphobia. However, men are more likely to develop **antisocial personality disorder,** characterized by callousness and flagrant disregard of the rights of others. Men are also more likely to develop problems with gambling, alcohol abuse, and violent behavior. For some disorders, such as bipolar disorder (formerly manic-depression), the gender ratio is about equal. In any case, women are more likely to seek help for psychological problems than are men. Most patients who take medication for psychological disorders are women.[6]

**Close-up**
Mental illness in America
T0405

Social observers note that social inequality contributes to women's psychological problems. Yes, hormonal changes during the menstrual cycle and childbirth may play a role in women's greater vulnerability to depression. However, a panel convened by the American Psychological Association attributed most of the difference to stress.[7] Women are more likely to encounter stressors such as physical and sexual abuse, poverty, single parenthood, and sexism. Women also do most household and child care chores, even when both spouses work. Thus, working women often put in a double shift: one on the job and a second one at the home.[8] Also, women are more likely than men to shoulder the burdens of helping others deal with stress or cope with disabling illness.[9]

### Ethnicity and Psychological Health

When we examine ethnic differences in rates of psychological disorders, we need to take into account differences in income levels. Traditionally, disadvantaged minorities, such as African Americans, are more likely than whites to live in poverty. Poverty, as noted, is associated with a heightened risk of psychological disorders. However, among individuals at the same income levels, African Americans are no more likely to develop psychological disorders than non-Hispanic white Americans.[10]

Hispanic Americans, too, are no more likely than non-Hispanic white Americans of the same income level to develop anxiety disorders or problems with alcohol. They are more likely, however, to show evidence of current depression. We have scant information about psychological disorders among Asian Americans. The little we have suggests that Asian Americans are about as likely to suffer from psychological disorders as other ethnic groups. This flies in the face of the widespread belief that Asian Americans are relatively free of psychological problems.

A bleak picture emerges when we look at the prevalence of psychological disorders among Native Americans. They are among the poorest ethnic groups in the U.S. Like others facing economic hardship, they have high rates of depression and substance abuse.[11] They also have high rates of suicide, alcohol-related accidents, and alcohol-related diseases like cirrhosis of the liver.

Beyond poverty, the psychological health problems of Native Americans also reflect the legacy of colonization by European powers and the resulting destruction of their traditional ways of life. Confined to reservations, isolated from mainstream society, Native Americans were vulnerable to hopelessness and alienation, depression, and other psychological problems. A Native Canadian elder in northwestern Ontario explains:

> Before the White Man came into our world we had our own way of worshiping the Creator. We had our own church and rituals. When hunting was good, people would gather together to give gratitude. This gave us close contact with the Creator. There were many different rituals depending on the tribe. People would dance in the hills and play drums to give recognition to the Great Spirit. It was like talking to the Creator and living daily with its spirit. Now people have lost this. They can't use these methods and have lost conscious contact with this high power. . . . The more distant we are from the Creator the more complex things are because we have no sense of direction. We don't recognize where life is from.[12]

People of color—African Americans, Asian Americans, Hispanic Americans, and Native Americans—generally underuse psychological health services. They are more likely than white Americans to turn to religion or family for support and less likely to seek help from mental health facilities, in part because of cultural mistrust of such institutions.

**Antisocial personality disorder** A personality disturbance characterized by disregard of social norms and conventions, impulsivity, callousness, and failure to live up to interpersonal and vocational commitments.

Because of the overlap among psychological and physical health problems, psychologists and psychiatrists are often of help to people with physical as well as psychological disorders.

Smart Quiz
Q0401

**think about it!**

- **What are some of the connections between physical health and psychological health?**

**critical thinking** **Where does "normal" anxiety or depression end and a psychological disorder begin?**

**critical thinking** **Agree or disagree and support your answer: Nearly everyone is affected by psychological disorders.**

## TYPES OF PSYCHOLOGICAL DISORDERS

Let us have a closer look at several types of psychological disorders: anxiety disorders, mood disorders, and schizophrenia.

### Anxiety Disorders

Anxiety is a fact of life. There is always something to be anxious about—our health, our jobs, our families, the hole in the ozone layer, the state of the world. Anxiety can help us adapt by motivating us to study before an exam or to get a medical checkup. When anxiety is out of proportion to the situation or impairs our ability to function, however, it becomes a psychological disorder.

**Anxiety** An emotional state characterized by heightened arousal, feelings of nervousness or tension, and a sense of apprehension or foreboding about the future.

**Fear** Anxiety experienced in response to a specific threat or object.

**Anxiety disorders** Psychological disorders involving excessive or inappropriate anxiety reactions.

**Phobia** An excessive or irrational fear.

**Social phobia** Fear of social interactions.

**Specific phobias** Phobias involving specific objects or situations, such as fear of enclosed spaces (claustrophobia) or of small animals or insects.

**Acrophobia** Fear of heights.

**Claustrophobia** Fear of enclosed spaces.

**What Is Anxiety?** Anxiety has both psychological and physical components. Psychologically, **anxiety** is a feeling of uneasiness or apprehension that something bad is about to happen. Physically, anxiety is associated with activation of the sympathetic branch of the autonomic nervous system. Sympathetic activity leads to the release of the hormone adrenaline by the adrenal glands, which produces such physical symptoms as a pounding heart, trembling, sweating, elevated blood pressure and respiration rate, and a flushed face.

**Fear** is anxiety experienced in specific situations, as when experiencing turbulence on an airplane or confronting a hostile dog. **Anxiety disorders** are psychological disorders involving problems with excessive or inappropriate anxiety or fear. They include phobic disorders (phobias), panic disorder, generalized anxiety disorder, and obsessive-compulsive disorder. Posttraumatic stress disorder (see Chapter 3) is another anxiety disorder.

Close-up
Features of anxiety disorders
T0406
More on anxiety disorders
T0407

**Phobias** **Phobias** are irrational or excessive fears, such as **social phobia** (fear of social interaction or embarrassment in front of others, such as public speaking anxiety, stage fright, and dating anxiety) and **specific phobias** [fears of specific situations or objects, such as particular animals or insects; heights **(acrophobia);** enclosed spaces **(claustrophobia);** and open places (agoraphobia)]. People with claustrophobia may refuse to use elevators despite the inconvenience of climbing many flights several times a day. People with agoraphobia may become housebound or find it impossible to hold jobs or maintain a normal social life. People with phobias usually recognize that their fears are irrational or excessive but are still unable to bring themselves to face the objects of their fears. Phobias are the most common psychological disorder in the United States, affecting about 20 million people.[14]

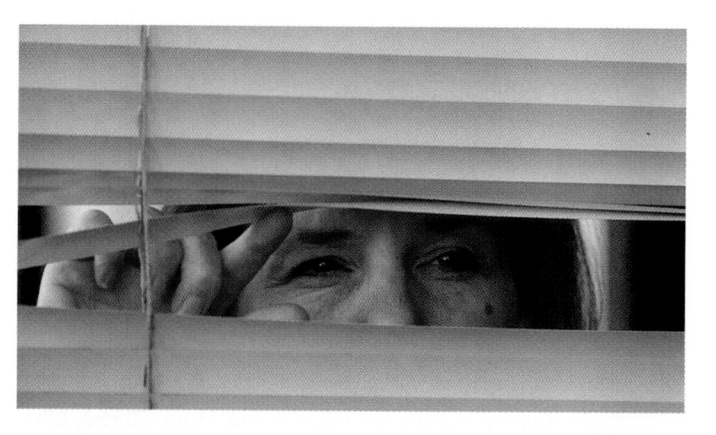

***Agoraphobia*** In its more severe forms, agoraphobia, or fear of venturing into open, public places, can lead people to become housebound.

# Health Check

## Are You Anxious?

This checklist will help you recognize the signs of anxiety. *Place a check in the column that indicates how often you have any of the following symptoms of anxiety.*

### Physical Features Connected with Anxiety

| Often | Sometimes | Rarely | |
|---|---|---|---|
| ____ | ____ | ____ | Jumpiness, jitteriness |
| ____ | ____ | ____ | Trembling or shaking of the hands or limbs |
| ____ | ____ | ____ | Sensations of a tight band around the forehead |
| ____ | ____ | ____ | Tightness in the pit of the stomach or chest |
| ____ | ____ | ____ | Heavy perspiration |
| ____ | ____ | ____ | Sweaty palms |
| ____ | ____ | ____ | Light-headedness or faintness |
| ____ | ____ | ____ | Dryness in the mouth or throat |
| ____ | ____ | ____ | Difficulty talking |
| ____ | ____ | ____ | Shortness of breath or shallow breathing |
| ____ | ____ | ____ | Heart pounding or racing |
| ____ | ____ | ____ | Tremulousness in one's voice |
| ____ | ____ | ____ | Cold fingers or limbs |
| ____ | ____ | ____ | Dizziness |
| ____ | ____ | ____ | Weakness or numbness |
| ____ | ____ | ____ | Difficulty swallowing |
| ____ | ____ | ____ | A "lump in the throat" |
| ____ | ____ | ____ | Stiffness of the neck or back |
| ____ | ____ | ____ | Choking or smothering sensations |
| ____ | ____ | ____ | Upset stomach or nausea |
| ____ | ____ | ____ | Hot or cold spells |
| ____ | ____ | ____ | Frequent urination |
| ____ | ____ | ____ | Diarrhea |
| ____ | ____ | ____ | Feeling irritable or "on edge" |

### Behavior Connected with Anxiety

| | | | |
|---|---|---|---|
| ____ | ____ | ____ | Avoiding certain situations out of fear |
| ____ | ____ | ____ | Clinging to or becoming dependent on others; relying on others for security |
| ____ | ____ | ____ | Agitated behavior |

### Thoughts Connected with Anxiety

| | | | |
|---|---|---|---|
| ____ | ____ | ____ | Thinking that something awful is going to happen, with no clear cause |
| ____ | ____ | ____ | Becoming keenly aware of your bodily sensations |
| ____ | ____ | ____ | Feeling threatened by people or events that are normally of little or no concern |
| ____ | ____ | ____ | Fearing loss of control |
| ____ | ____ | ____ | Fearing that you will not be able to cope with your problems |
| ____ | ____ | ____ | Thinking that the world is caving in on you |
| ____ | ____ | ____ | Thinking that things are getting out of hand |
| ____ | ____ | ____ | Thinking that things are swimming by too rapidly to take charge of them |
| ____ | ____ | ____ | Worrying about every little thing |
| ____ | ____ | ____ | Thinking the same disturbing thought over and over |
| ____ | ____ | ____ | Thinking that you must flee crowded places for fear of passing out or having a panic attack |
| ____ | ____ | ____ | Thinking that you are going to die, even when your doctor finds nothing medically wrong |
| ____ | ____ | ____ | Worrying that you are going to be left all alone |
| ____ | ____ | ____ | Having difficulty concentrating or focusing your thoughts |

*The more symptoms you checked, and the more often they occur, the more likely it is that anxiety is a problem for you. A health professional in your college counseling center can help you better understand the basis of your anxiety and the resources that are available to help you.*

### Panic Disorder

*All of a sudden, I felt a tremendous wave of fear for no reason at all. My heart was pounding, my chest hurt, and it was getting harder to breathe. I thought I was going to die.*

A person with panic disorder

**Close-up**
Features of panic T0408
Getting help for panic T0409
More on panic disorder T0410

People with **panic disorder** have sudden episodes of sheer terror called panic attacks. Such attacks have powerful physical symptoms: profuse sweating, choking sensations, nausea, numbness or tingling, flushes or chills, trembling, chest pain, shortness of breath, and pounding of the heart. People experiencing a panic attack may think they are about to die from a heart attack, go crazy, or lose control. The attack may last a few minutes or more than an hour.

Panic attacks, at least initially, seem to come "out of the blue." Yet they can become connected with situations in which they occur, such as shopping in a crowded department store or riding on a train. Agoraphobia may develop as the person avoids such public places out of fear of having another attack and being away from a secure place.

***Panic Attack*** Panic attacks are episodes of sheer terror accompanied by physical symptoms such as a pounding heart, dizziness, feelings of suffocation, and shortness of breath.

**Panic disorder** An anxiety disorder characterized by episodes of sheer terror, called panic attacks, and by the fear of such attacks occurring again.

**Generalized anxiety disorder** A disorder characterized by a high level of anxiety that is not limited to particular situations, and general feelings of worry, dread, and foreboding.

**Obsessive-compulsive disorder (OCD)** An anxiety disorder characterized by obsessions (nagging, intrusive thoughts or images) and/or compulsions (repetitive behaviors that the person feels compelled to perform).

**Mood disorders** Mood disturbances that affect a person's ability to function effectively or are unduly prolonged or severe.

**Dysthymia** A depressive disorder involving states of chronic, mild depression.

**Major depression** A severe form of depression characterized by downcast mood, negative thinking, and other related features, such as changes in sleeping patterns and appetite, and without a history of manic episodes.

### Generalized Anxiety Disorder

People with **generalized anxiety disorder** experience persistent, "free-floating" anxiety that is not specific to any object or situation. People with the disorder worry excessively, even about trifles. Symptoms include shakiness, inability to relax, fidgeting, sweating, and feelings of dread and foreboding.

### Obsessive-Compulsive Disorder

People with **obsessive-compulsive disorder (OCD)** have recurrent obsessions and/or compulsions. Obsessions are intrusive, nagging thoughts that the person feels unable to control. Compulsions are repetitive behaviors or rituals that the person feels compelled to perform. Those obsessed with the thought that their skin is contaminated by germs may spend hours each day compulsively washing their hands or showering. Others may spend hours each night checking and rechecking whether they have locked the doors and turned off the appliances.

People with obsessive-compulsive disorder may become trapped in a vicious cycle of obsessive thinking and compulsive behavior. Obsessive thoughts trigger anxiety. The anxiety is only temporarily relieved by the performance of the compulsive ritual, leading back to nagging thoughts and more compulsive behavior.

**Close-up**
More on OCD T0411

## Mood Disorders

Most of us have occasional ups and downs. We may feel unmotivated, lethargic, or just down in the dumps for a time. We feel sad if we have a setback at work or school or are rejected by Mr. or Ms. Right. In the case of **mood disorders,** we may feel down even when things are going right. Or we remain down long after others would have snapped back from misfortune. Some people with mood disorders have wild mood swings that, for no apparent reason, alternate between dizzying heights and abysmal depths.

### Depression

Depressive disorders involve severe or prolonged periods of downcast mood. One type of depressive disorder, **dysthymia,** involves relatively mild but chronic depression. Another type, **major depression,** involves more severe episodes of depression (see Table 4.1) characterized by often overwhelming feelings of sadness, hopelessness, worthlessness, and self-hate. Major depression is also associated with physical symptoms, such as changes in appetite and sleep and feelings of lethargy. People with major depression may not be able to get out of bed to face the day. They may feel helpless or be unable to make decisions, even about small things. They may be unable to concentrate. They may say they "don't care" anymore. They may have recurrent thoughts of suicide or attempt suicide.

**Smart Reference**
Multicultural studies of depression R0401

**Close-up**
Facts about depression T0412

## Health *Check*

### *Are You Depressed?*[16]

Many people suffer depression in silence out of ignorance or shame. They believe that depression is not a real problem because it does not show up on an X-ray or CAT scan. Or they may feel that asking for help is an admission of weakness and that they should bear it on their own. Depression is all too real, however. The feelings are real. The loss of appetite, the disruption of sleep patterns, the lethargy are real. Fortunately, depression can be treated successfully in most cases.

*This test was developed to help make people more aware of the warning signs of depression.*

| Yes | No | |
|---|---|---|
| ____ | ____ | 1. I feel downhearted, blue, and sad. |
| ____ | ____ | 2. I don't enjoy the things that I used to. |
| ____ | ____ | 3. I feel that others would be better off if I were dead. |
| ____ | ____ | 4. I feel that I am not useful or needed. |
| ____ | ____ | 5. I notice that I am losing weight. |
| ____ | ____ | 6. I have trouble sleeping through the night. |
| ____ | ____ | 7. I am restless and can't keep still. |
| ____ | ____ | 8. My mind isn't as clear as it used to be. |
| ____ | ____ | 9. I get tired for no reason. |
| ____ | ____ | 10. I feel hopeless about the future. |

*If you answered "yes" to at least five of the statements, including either item 1, 2, or 3, and if these complaints have persisted for at least two weeks, then professional help is strongly recommended. If you answered "yes" to the third statement, we suggest that you immediately consult a health professional. Contact your college or university counseling or health center. Or talk to your instructor.*

**TABLE 4.1**

**Symptoms of Major Depression**

Feeling down for most of the day, nearly every day.

Experiencing little or no pleasure from activities you formerly enjoyed.

Sleeping too much or too little.

Having little or no interest in things.

Changes in appetite or loss of appetite.

Gaining or losing a significant amount of weight without actively dieting.

Waking up in the early morning hours and being unable to fall back asleep ("early-morning awakenings").

Feeling fatigued, lacking energy, moving more slowly than usual, or having difficulty getting started in the morning or even getting out of bed.

Having difficulty concentrating or attending at school or work.

Feeling down on yourself or worthless.

Wanting to end it all.*

*All signs of depression should be taken seriously, especially thoughts of suicide. Depression is a treatable disorder. Contact a health professional for a full evaluation. If you believe that someone close to you is seriously depressed, help him or her make contact with a health professional.

**Seasonal Affective Disorder** **Seasonal affective disorder (SAD)** involves a repeated pattern of severe depression in the fall and winter, followed by elevations of mood in the spring and summer. SAD has been treated successfully with bright artificial light, a kind of substitute for natural sunlight, two to three hours a day through the winter season. Because of the success of this treatment, health professionals are paying more attention to the healing power of light. Exposure to light may also help alleviate some kinds of insomnia, help nighttime workers be more productive, and even improve the body's immune system.[15]

**Close-up**
Bipolar disorder
**T0413**

**Bipolar Disorder** Depression is *unipolar.* That is, the mood goes in a single direction: *down.* People with **bipolar disorder** (formerly called *manic-depression*) have mood swings between two "poles": mania and depression.

**Seasonal affective disorder (SAD)** A type of major depression involving episodes of severe depression during the fall and winter months, followed by elevated mood in spring and summer.

**Bipolar disorder** A mood disorder characterized by mood swings between severe depression and mania.

**Manic episodes** are periods of extreme excitability and elation that occur with no apparent reason. People in a manic episode may become extremely excited, argumentative, and show poor judgment. They may spend lavishly, drive recklessly, destroy property, or become involved in sexual escapades that appear out of character with their usual personalities. Even those who love them may find them abrasive. Other symptoms are pressured speech (talking too rapidly), rapid flight of ideas (flitting from topic to topic), and an inflated sense of self-worth (grandiosity). Manic people may even become delusional, as in believing that they have a special relationship with God. They may undertake tasks beyond their abilities, such as writing a symphony or giving away a fortune. They may have boundless energy and little need for sleep. Then, when the manic episode subsides, they may feel hopeless and despair. Some people with bipolar disorder commit suicide on the way down, to avert the depths of depression they have learned to expect.

### Schizophrenia

Talking Glossary
Schizophrenia
G0401

**Schizophrenia** is the disorder that most closely corresponds to the popular concept of "madness" or "lunacy." It is a **psychotic disorder,** a disorder that involves a break with reality. The break may involve **hallucinations,** such as "hearing voices" or seeing things that are not there, or **delusions,** false but unshakable beliefs about reality. Some common delusions include *delusions of persecution* (believing that one is being persecuted by demons or by the government) and *delusions of grandeur* (believing that one is Jesus or has superhuman powers). Schizophrenia should not be confused with "split" or multiple personality, a psychological disorder involving the appearance of two or more distinct personalities in the same individual.

People with schizophrenia show confused thinking characterized by a loosening of associations. Normally, our thoughts are connected; one thought follows another in a logical sequence. Those with schizophrenia often lack logical connections between their thoughts. They may form meaningless words or mindless rhymes. Their speech may be incoherent, jumping from topic to topic but communicating no useful information.

Schizophrenia typically affects young adults just at the point in their lives when they are beginning to make their way in the world. Though it typically follows a lifelong course, the use of antipsychotic medication, combined with rehabilitation services and psychological counseling, can help those with schizophrenia live more independently in the community.

**Manic episodes** Episodes of extremely inflated mood and excitability.

**Schizophrenia** An enduring psychotic disorder involving disturbances in thought processes, perception, emotion, and behavior.

**Psychotic disorder** A psychological disorder involving symptoms that indicate a break with reality, such as hallucinations and delusions.

**Hallucinations** False sense perceptions, such as "hearing voices" or seeing things that are not there.

**Delusions** False, unshakable beliefs.

Close-up
More on schizophrenia
T0414

**think about it!**

- **Have you ever "panicked"? Do you think you have a panic disorder? Why or why not?**
- **Have you ever known anyone who suffered from schizophrenia? How was this person's life affected? How is the person functioning today?**

**critical thinking** **How would you know whether you are anxious or depressed?**

Smart Quiz
Q0402

## CAUSES OF PSYCHOLOGICAL DISORDERS

Many factors play roles in the development of psychological disorders. They interact in complex ways that we are only beginning to understand.

### Biological Factors

The predominant biological factors in psychological disorders are genetics and neurotransmitters. Other biological factors involve complications of pregnancy and birth, and brain damage.

**Genetic Factors** Heredity plays a role in the development of many psychological disorders. Genetic factors create predispositions that make some people more likely to develop certain disorders, such as schizophrenia, bipolar disorder, and depression, especially when they encounter high levels of stress. Evidence for a genetic predisposition comes from several sources. We know that some psychological disorders run in families. Yet since families share a common environment as well as common genes, we need additional evidence to sort out the influences of nurture and nature. One source of evidence comes from studies demonstrating that family members who share a closer genetic relationship are also more likely to share disorders. In Figure 4.1 we see the relative risk of schizophrenia among family members. The risk is greater among closer blood relatives.

Twin studies provide still more insight. **Monozygotic (MZ) twins** (identical twins) share 100% of their genes. **Dizygotic (DZ) twins** (fraternal twins), like other brothers and sisters, share 50% of their genes. If genes are involved in a disorder, we would expect to find that MZ twins are more likely to share the disorder than DZ twins. MZ twins *are* in fact more likely than DZ twins to share anxiety disorders, mood disorders, and schizophrenia, which supports a role for genetics in these disorders. In fact, the risk of developing schizophrenia if one has an identical twin with schizophrenia is 48% on average. A fraternal (DZ) twin of a person with schizophrenia has only about a 17% chance of developing schizophrenia (see Figure 4.1). Note, however, that the agreement rate for identical twins is not perfect (it is less than 100%). Therefore, factors other than genetics also play a role in the development of schizophrenia. Some of these other factors are biological; others are environmental or psychological.

**Video**
Search for a schizophrenia gene
**V0401**

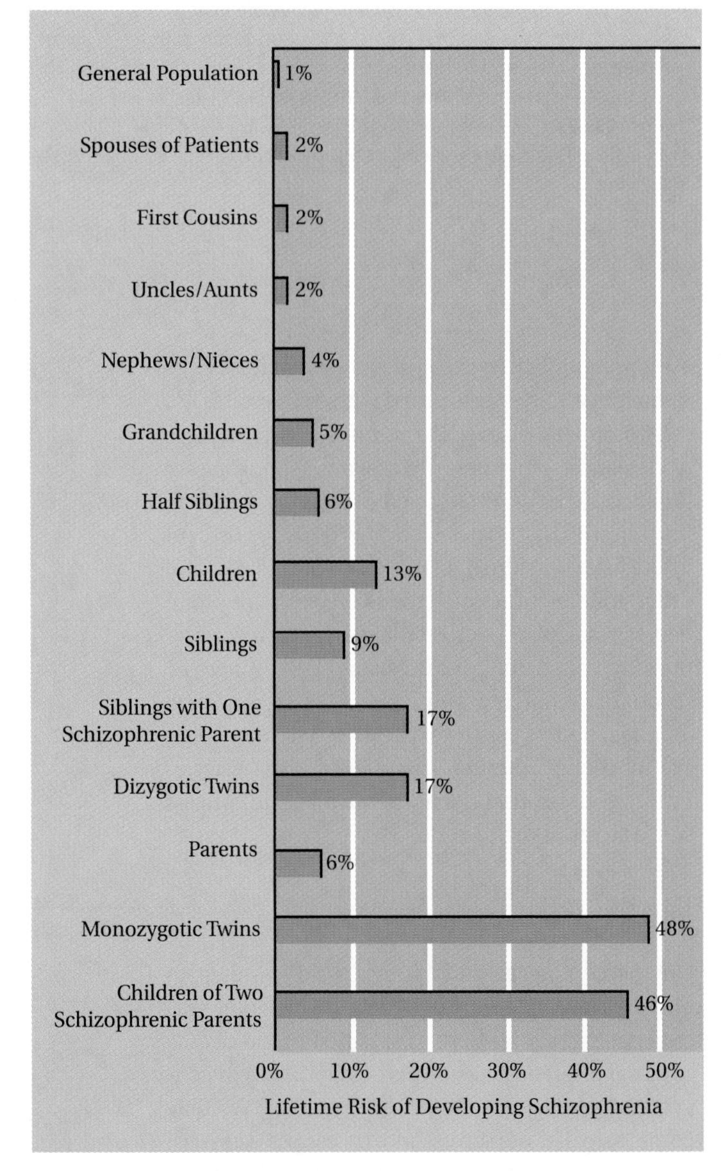


**Figure 4.1** ***Familial Risk of Schizophrenia*** Generally speaking, the closer the genetic relationship you have with someone who has schizophrenia, the greater the odds that you are at risk yourself. Even so, more than half of the identical twins of people with schizophrenia do not develop the disease themselves.

Adding further evidence of a genetic contribution to schizophrenia are studies of adoptees. For some psychological disorders, specifically bipolar disorder and schizophrenia, adoptees are more likely to share these conditions with their biological parents than the adoptive parents who raised them. This finding is powerful evidence indeed for a genetic contribution.[17]

**Disturbances in Neurotransmitters** Normal psychological functioning depends on the smooth transmission of messages between neurons. Neurotransmitters are the chemical messengers that ferry nerve impulses from one neuron to another. Sometimes too little or too much of a neurotransmitter is produced. Sometimes receptor sites do not accept neurotransmitters properly, or they allow too many to dock. Such disturbances play a role in the development of psychological disorders such as anxiety disorders, mood disorders, dementia, and schizophrenia.

**Alzheimer's disease,** for example, is a form of **dementia** that involves a progressive loss of memory and cognitive functioning. It is associated with a reduc-

**Monozygotic (MZ) twins** Twins that develop from the same fertilized egg cell and thus share identical genes. Also called *identical twins*.

**Dizygotic (DZ) twins** Twins that develop from two separate fertilized eggs and thus have half their genes in common, like any other two siblings. Also called *fraternal twins*.

**Alzheimer's disease** An irreversible brain disease involving gradual loss of mental abilities, especially memory, as well as personality changes.

**Dementia** A psychological disorder involving a deterioration of mental functioning involving memory, reasoning, use of language, judgment, and ability to carry out purposeful actions.

Talking Glossary
Acetylcholine
G0402

tion in the levels of the neurotransmitter **acetylcholine (Ach).** Depression has been linked to lower than normal levels of the neurotransmitters **noradrenaline** and **serotonin.** Drugs that help relieve depression, called **antidepressants**, increase the activity of these neurotransmitters in the brain. The most widely used antidepressant, Prozac, increases the availability of serotonin within the brain.

Talking Glossary
Gamma-aminobutyric acid (GABA)
G0403
Benzodiazepines
G0404

Panic disorder may involve faulty regulation of serotonin and noradrenaline.[18] In other anxiety disorders, the brain may not be sensitive enough to the neurotransmitter **gamma-aminobutyric acid (GABA).** GABA normally helps calm anxiety reactions. The **benzodiazepines**, a group of drugs that reduce anxiety (such as Valium and Librium) apparently work by increasing the brain's sensitivity to GABA. Schizophrenia has been linked to an overreactivity of brain receptors to the neurotransmitter **dopamine.**[19] Drugs used to treat schizophrenia block the actions of dopamine.

Most psychological disorders probably involve complex relationships among neurotransmitters rather than the actions of individual neurotransmitters per se. The brain is a highly complex electrochemical system. Changes in one part have a ripple effect on many others, the intricacies of which we are only beginning to unravel.

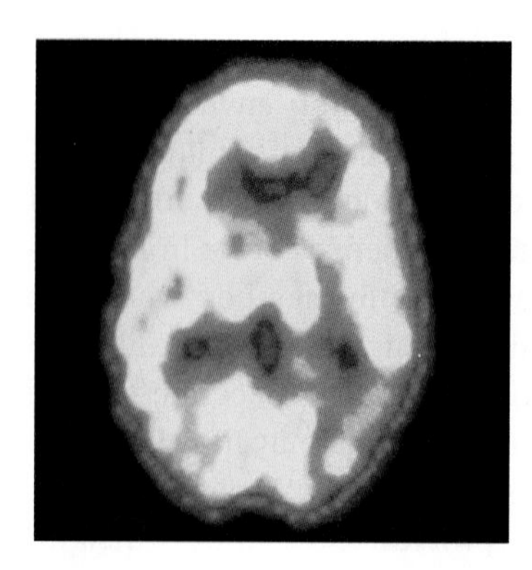
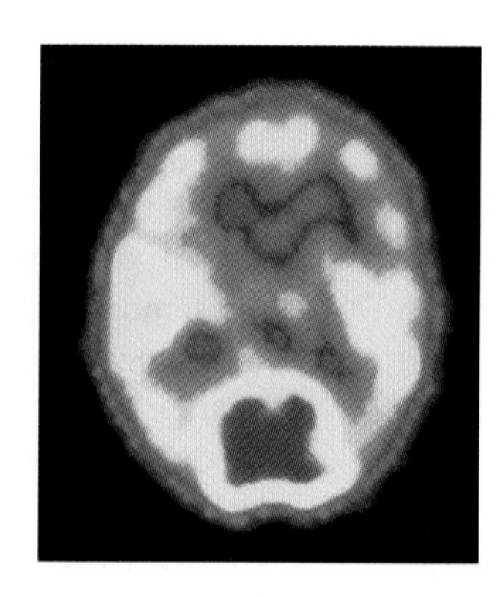

***PET Scans of Brain Activity*** Researchers use brain imaging techniques, such as PET scans (positron emission tomography), to explore abnormalities in the brains of people with psychological disorders. Here we see PET scans showing brain activity of a normal person (left) and schizophrenic person (right). Notice that the schizophrenic person shows less brain activity (darker areas) in the frontal part of the brain (top) than the normal person. This may offer clues to uncovering the biological bases of schizophrenia.

**Brain Damage** Brain damage occurring from an accident or stroke can have a wide range of effects. Sometimes these are barely noticeable; other times they are disabling or fatal. A **stroke** or cerebrovascular accident (CVA) occurs when a blood clot in a blood vessel cuts off the supply of blood to a part of the brain. The brain tissue served by that blood vessel dies. Strokes may lead to the loss of speech, sensation, and movement if the brain centers controlling these functions are affected (see Chapter 17). One form of dementia reflects the accumulated effects of many small strokes. Single strokes, however, are unlikely to cause the widespread decline in mental abilities associated with dementia.

Alzheimer's disease is the most common form of dementia. For some unknown reason, ropelike tangles of nerve tissue called plaques begin to form in the brain. These plaques destroy adjacent brain tissue, leading to the loss of memory and other mental functions (see Chapter 19). Brain damage has also been implicated in schizophrenia. Brain imaging studies using MRI (magnetic resonance imaging) and the CAT scan show enlarged hollow spaces in the brains of many people with schizophrenia. This suggests that deterioration of brain tissue may be involved in at least some forms of the disorder.

**Acetylcholine (Ach)** A neurotransmitter involved in the process of muscle contraction.

**Noradrenaline** A neurotransmitter linked to depression. Also called *norepinephrine.*

**Serotonin** A neurotransmitter involved in regulating motor functions that is also linked to depression.

**Antidepressants** Drugs that combat depression by altering the availability of neurotransmitters in the brain.

**Gamma-aminobutyric acid (GABA)** An inhibitory neurotransmitter believed to play a role in anxiety.

**Benzodiazepines** A class of minor tranquilizers, including such drugs as Valium, Librium, and Halcion.

**Dopamine** A neurotransmitter believed to play a role in schizophrenia.

**Stroke** Destruction of brain tissue resulting from the blockage of a blood vessel. Also called *cerebrovascular accident (CVA).*

## Psychosocial Factors

Our psychological functioning is the product of our learning experiences. Early in life, our self-concept and self-esteem are shaped or molded by external influences—our parents, families, teachers, and peers. If we are prized by others, we may come to prize ourselves and develop a sense of confidence that helps us to meet the challenges that await us in life. If, on the other hand, we are made to feel inadequate or unloved, we may develop a negative self-image that leaves us more vulnerable to psychological problems like anxiety and depression.

**Anxiety Disorders** Some phobias may be learned by the pairing of a previously neutral or benign stimulus with a traumatic or painful stimulus. Thus, a person who was bitten by a dog at a young age may develop a fear of dogs; someone who was once trapped in an elevator may acquire a fear of elevators or of confinement. When we acquire phobias as children, we may come to think of them as enduring traits and label ourselves "people who fear heights" or whatever. We then live up to the labels, avoiding the objects or situations we fear. Avoidance relieves our anxiety, which leads us to continue avoiding the feared object. Avoidance does not allow us to overcome our fear. The result is that our phobia is maintained indefinitely.

Cognitive ("thinking") factors are also involved in anxiety. People with panic attacks tend to misinterpret relatively minor bodily sensations as signs of imminent catastrophe, such as a heart attack. Their fearful thoughts begin to race, which triggers bodily sensations of anxiety, leading to more catastrophic thinking, and so on in a vicious cycle that can culminate in a full-blown panic attack (see Figure 4.2). People with panic disorder can be helped by learning that they can tolerate bodily sensations (like momentary light-headedness or heart palpitations) without panicking by learning to control their thoughts. They also learn to tone down their bodily arousal by practicing diaphragmatic breathing.[20]

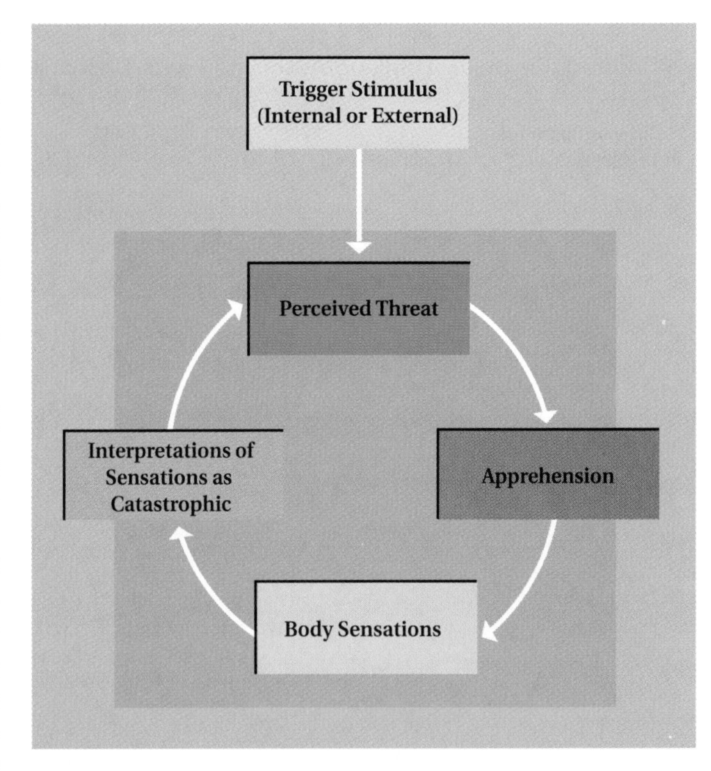


**Figure 4.2** ***The Panic Cycle*** A prominent model of panic disorder focuses on the interaction of physiological and cognitive factors. A triggering stimulus (sudden light-headedness or entering a crowded store) is perceived by panic-prone people as threatening. Perception of threat leads to apprehension (anxiety and worry), which leads to changes in bodily sensations (e.g., a tightening feeling in the chest). Cognitively, the person misinterprets these sensations as signs of impending catastrophe (a heart attack or loss of control), which intensifies perceptions of threat, further heightening anxiety, and so on in a vicious cycle that can quickly spiral into a full-blown panic attack.

**Mood Disorders** Cognitive factors—attitudes and beliefs—also contribute to depression. For example, perfectionists set themselves up for depression by setting unrealistic goals. When they inevitably fail to meet these unrealistic expectations, they react by getting down on themselves, which can lead to depression.[21] Depressed people also tend to be overly self-critical and pessimistic about the future.

Depressed people view the world and themselves through "blue-colored glasses." Psychiatrist Aaron Beck writes that depressed people filter their experiences through three types of negative, distorted beliefs: a nega-

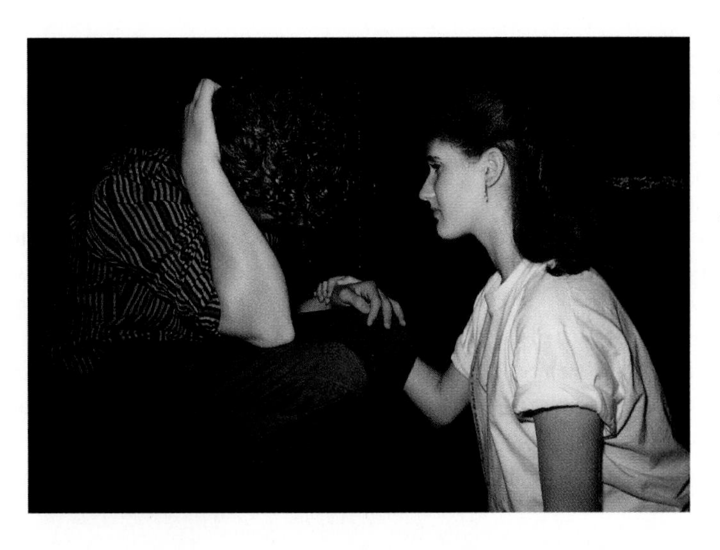

***"It's My Fault"*** Cognitive factors, such as tendencies to blame oneself for negative life events, are believed to be major contributors to depression.

TABLE 4.2

**Common Errors in Thinking Associated with Depression[22]**

| Type of Cognitive Distortion | Description | Examples |
|---|---|---|
| *All-or-Nothing Thinking* | Viewing events in dichotomous terms—as either all good or all bad. | Do you view a relationship that ended as a totally negative experience? Do you consider any performance less than perfect to be a failure? Is a B+ or even an A− tantamount to an F in your mind? |
| *Misplaced Blame* | Tendency to blame or criticize yourself for disappointments or setbacks while ignoring external circumstances. | Do you automatically assume that there is something inherently wrong with you when someone turns you down for a date or doesn't return your calls? Do others tell you that you are too hard on yourself or expect too much of yourself? |
| *Misfortune Telling* | The tendency to think that one disappointment will inevitably lead to another. | If you get a rejection letter from a job you applied for, do you assume that all the other applications you sent will meet the same fate? |
| *Negative Focusing* | Focusing your attention only on the negative aspects of your experiences. | Do you tend to dwell on the negative and overlook the positive? When you get a job evaluation, do you minimize the praise and recall only the criticism? |
| *Dismissing the Positives* | Trivializing or denying your accomplishments; minimizing your strengths or assets. | When someone compliments you, do you dismiss it as "no big deal"? Do you give yourself short shrift when sizing up your abilities? |
| *Jumping to Conclusions* | Drawing a conclusion that is not supported by the facts at hand. | If you meet someone new, do you naturally assume that he or she could not possibly like you? If you feel tightness in your chest, do you assume that it must be a sign of a heart attack? |
| *Catastrophizing* | Exaggerating the importance of negative events or personal flaws—making mountains out of molehills (magnification). | Do you react to a disappointing grade as if your whole life depended on it? |
| *Emotion-Based Reasoning* | Reasoning on the basis of your emotions rather than on evidence. | Do you think that things must really be hopeless because it feels that way? Do you believe that you must really have done something bad to feel so awful about yourself? |
| *"Shouldisms"* | Making unrealistic demands of yourself that you "should" or "must" be able to accomplish a certain task or reach a certain goal. | Do you think that you *must* be able to ace this course or else you're just a loser? Do you feel that you *should* be further along in your life than you are now? |
| *Name Calling* | Attaching negative labels to yourself or others as a way of explaining your own or someone else's behavior. | Do you think that people fail to meet your needs because they are selfish? Do you label yourself as lazy or stupid when you fall short of reaching your goals? |
| *Mistaken Responsibility* | Assuming that you are the cause of other people's problems. | Do you automatically assume that your partner is depressed or upset because of something you did (or didn't do)? |

tive view of the self ("I'm worthless"), a negative view of the environment ("This school is awful"), and a negative view of the future ("Nothing will ever work out for me"). He refers to these beliefs as the *cognitive triad of depression.* These beliefs set the stage for depression in the face of disappointments such as setbacks at work or romantic rejections. Persons with these beliefs are quick to blame themselves for disappointments and to treat minor setbacks as crushing defeats that reveal their personal shortcomings.

Beck considers this tendency to blow negative events out of proportion to be a type of error in thinking, or *cognitive distortion.* Table 4.2 lists a number of cognitive distortions along with some examples that might help you assess your own thinking styles. If some of these thinking errors hit home with you, we suggest you consider how you might rethink the ways in which you respond to unfortunate events. Later in the chapter we offer suggestions for replacing distorted thoughts with rational alternatives.

**Schizophrenia** The development of schizophrenia involves the interplay of biological factors with psychosocial stressors.[23] Schizophrenia is five times more common at the lowest rung of the socioeconomic ladder than at the highest, an indication that stress plays a role since poverty is associated with greater life stress.[24] Family factors such as poor communication styles within the family and poor parenting may increase the risk of developing the disorder among genetically vulnerable individuals. In contrast, a supportive and nurturing family atmosphere and a benign level of stress may reduce the risk that genetically vulnerable children will develop schizophrenia.

Smart Quiz
Q0403

### think about it!

- **What are neurotransmitters? How are they involved in psychological disorders?**
- **How are stress, "errors in thinking," and other psychological factors involved in psychological disorders?**
- **Do any of the "errors in thinking" described in Table 4.2 sound like your thoughts? If so, what will you do about them?**

**critical thinking** **If one of your parents had schizophrenia, do you think that you would develop the disorder? Why or why not?**

## SUICIDE

Did you know that many people entertain thoughts of suicide when they are under great stress? Even most college students in a recent poll (54%) reported thinking about suicide on at least one occasion.[25] Yet most people—fortunately!—do not act on suicidal thoughts. In the college sample, only about one in five of the students who had contemplated suicide had actually attempted it. Still, one in ten college students in this survey reported trying to take their lives.

Nearly one-quarter of a million Americans overall, including about 10,000 college students, attempt suicide each year.[26] About 30,000 of them succeed.

### Who Is at Risk?

Suicide cuts across every stratum of our society. Yet certain factors are related to an increased risk:

**Age** The overall suicide rate in the United States has changed relatively little since 1950. However, the rate among white men over the age of 65 has been rising. The suicide rate among teens rose steadily from the 1950s through the mid-1970s, when it began to level off. Adolescent suicides may seem especially hard to understand, since young people have "everything to live for." Obviously, many of them do not agree. The greatest suicide risk is among older adults, however. The suicide rate for people aged 65 and above is about 22 per 100,000 persons, a rate nearly double the average rate, which is 12.8[27] (see Figure 4.3).

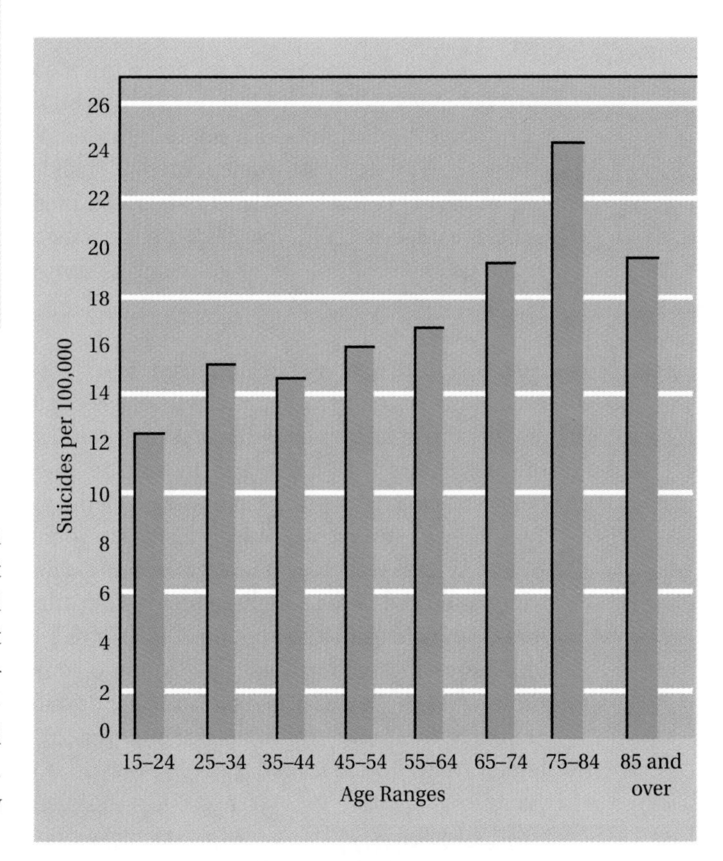


**Figure 4.3** ***Suicide Rates by Age*** People over the age of 65 are at greatest risk of suicide. However, suicide ranks as the second leading cause of death among college students.

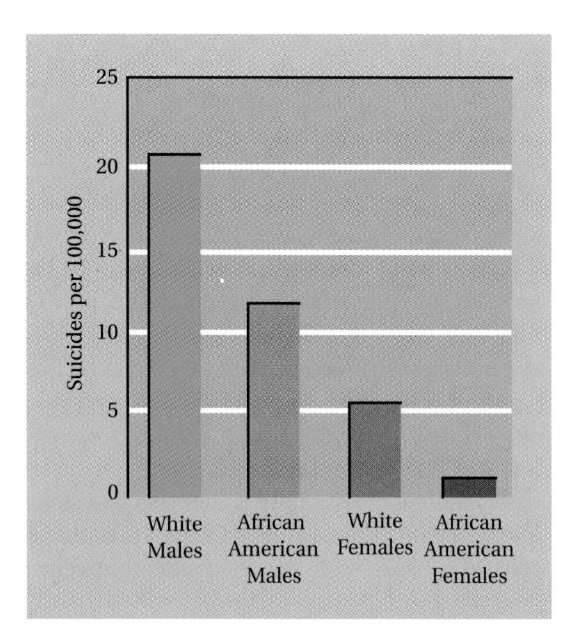


**Figure 4.4** ***Suicide Rates by Race and Gender*** Suicide is more common among men than women, and among white Americans than among African Americans.

**Gender** More women attempt suicide, but more men complete the act (see Figure 4.4). Men commit two to four times as many suicides as women.[28] Why do more women attempt suicide, but more men succeed? Men tend to use more lethal means, especially firearms. Women are more apt to use pills, poison, or other means that may be less lethal.

**Race** Non-Hispanic white Americans and Native Americans are more likely to take their lives than are African Americans or Hispanic Americans. Figure 4.4 shows the differences in suicide rates between African Americans and white Americans. Two of the groups most at risk of suicide are young Native Americans living on reservations and older white men.[29] Overall, about one in six Native American teenagers attempts suicide. This rate is four times the national average.[30] Among some tribes, the rate is even higher. The suicide rate among Native Americans for all age groups is 20% higher than the national rate.[31] How do we account for the high rate of suicide among Native Americans? One answer is the widespread sense of hopelessness that arises from lack of opportunity and segregation from the dominant culture. Such factors also set the stage for alcohol and drug abuse, which can be preludes to depression and suicide.

**Exit events** Life events involving loss of significant others through death, divorce or separation, termination of relationships, or relocation.

**Rational suicides** Suicides based on a reasoned choice in the face of terminal illness or intractable, severe pain.

## Why Do People Take Their Lives?

Most suicides are linked to depression, especially to feelings of hopelessness. UCLA suicide expert Edwin Shneidman points out that suicide is motivated by the attempt to end, once and for all, unendurable psychological pain.[32] Suicide attempts often follow stressful life events, especially **exit events.** Exit events involve loss of *social support,* as through death, divorce, separation, or a family member's leaving home. These events leave vulnerable people feeling stripped of crucial sources of social support. People who attempt suicide may also have limited problem-solving skills and be unable to find alternative ways of coping with psychological pain.

Not all suicides, of course, are related to depression. Some people with schizophrenia commit suicide. As we saw in the case that began this chapter, Linda attempted suicide because of a delusional belief that she deserved punishment and because "hellsmen" had ordered her to. Other people with schizophrenia wish to escape the voices that hound them.

Teenagers have been known to commit copycat suicides in the wake of widely publicized suicides in their communities. This tendency has been

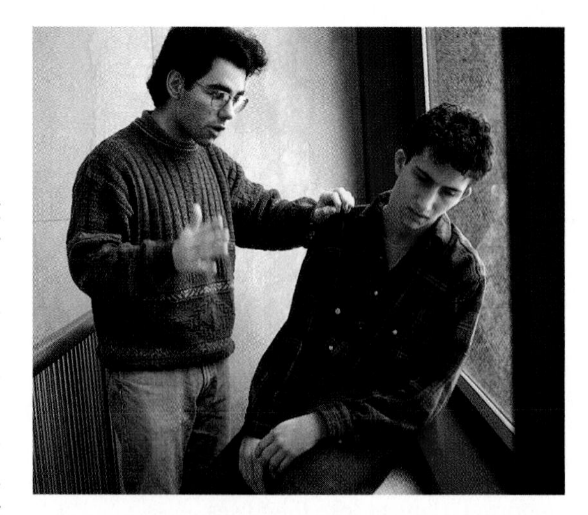

***Youth Suicide*** Young people who attempt suicide may see no other way of dealing with their problems. Having counselors and support persons available may help deter young people from ending their lives by helping them see alternative ways of resolving their problems and relieving the stress in their lives.

TABLE 4.3

**Myths About Suicide**

| Myth | Fact |
|---|---|
| People who threaten suicide are only seeking attention and aren't serious about killing themselves. | Not so. Researchers report that about 90 percent of people who kill themselves gave clear clues concerning their intentions prior to the act, such as disposing of all their possessions or securing a burial plot.[33] Most people who commit suicide have made previous unsuccessful attempts. |
| A person must be insane to attempt to commit suicide. | Most people who attempt suicide may feel hopeless, but they are not "insane" (that is, out of touch with reality). |
| Talking about suicide with a depressed person may prompt her or him to attempt it. | An open discussion of suicide with a depressed person does not prompt the person to attempt it. In fact, extracting a promise that the person will not attempt suicide before calling or visiting a mental health worker may well prevent a suicide. |
| If someone threatens suicide it is best to ignore it so as not to encourage repeated threats. | Though some people do manipulate others by making idle threats, it is prudent to treat every suicidal threat as genuine and take appropriate action (see nearby *Prevention* feature). |
| Drugs are behind most suicides. | Most suicides occur among people who suffer from depression, not drug abuse. |

called the "cluster effect." The sensationalism that attends a teenage suicide may make it seem a romantic or courageous statement to impressionable young people who are having problems.

So-called **rational suicides** have sparked a national debate. The debate has been fueled by highly publicized cases involving Jack Kevorkian, a physician who has helped terminally ill people end their lives. Consider the case of a terminally ill patient in unrelenting pain whose spouse has died and who feels like a burden to the family. Might suicide represent a rational response in this situation? Who is to say? Should other people, such as family members or health care providers, be permitted to assist someone who has made a "rational" decision to commit suicide? Individuals in pain may claim that they have the right to take their own lives. Society is conflicted over this issue (see Chapter 20).

PREVENTION

## *Suicide Prevention*[34]

You are having a heart-to-heart talk with one of your best friends on campus. Things haven't been going well. Your friend's grandmother died a month ago, and they were very close. Your friend's coursework has been suffering, and things have also been going downhill with the person he has been seeing regularly. But you are not prepared when your friend looks you straight in the eye and says, "I've been thinking about this for days, and I've decided that the only way out is to kill myself."

If someone tells you that he or she is considering suicide, you may feel frightened and flustered. You may feel that an enormous burden has been placed on you. It has. In such cases, encourage the person to consult a health professional, or consult a professional yourself as soon as possible. But if the person refuses to talk to anyone else and you feel that you can't break free for a consultation, there are a number of things you can do:

**Smart Reference**
Suicide prevention
R0402

1. *Draw the person out.* Schneidman suggests asking questions like "What's going on?" "Where do you hurt?" "What would you like to see happen?"[35] Questions like these may encourage people to express frustrated needs and provide some relief. They also give you time to assess the danger and think.
2. *Be empathetic.* Show that you understand how upset the person is. Take the person seriously—don't dismiss what he or she says.
3. *Suggest that measures other than suicide may solve the problem, even if they are not evident at the time.* Schneidman suggests that suicidal people can typically see only two solutions to their problems—either death or a magical answer. Therapists thus try to "widen the mental blinders" of suicidal people.
4. *Ask how the person intends to commit suicide.* People with concrete plans and a weapon are at greater risk. Ask if you may hold on to the weapon for a while.

5. *Suggest that the person go with you to obtain professional help now.* The emergency room of a general hospital, a campus counseling center or infirmary, or the local police can help. Some campuses and cities have suicide prevention centers with "hotlines" that can be called anonymously.
6. *Extract a promise that the person will not attempt suicide before seeing you again.* Arrange a concrete time and place to meet. Get professional help as soon as you are apart.
7. *Do not tell people threatening suicide that they're silly or crazy.* Do *not* insist on contact with specific people, like parents or a spouse. Conflict with these people may have led to the suicidal thinking. Above all, remember that your primary goal is to consult a health professional. Don't "go it alone" any longer than you must.

Smart Quiz Q0404

**think about it!**

- **What could you do if a friend confided that he or she intended to commit suicide?**

**critical thinking** **Agree or disagree and support your answer: It is normal to have suicidal thoughts now and then.**

**critical thinking** **Did you believe any of the myths about suicide presented in Table 4.3? Have you changed your mind? Why or why not?**

## TREATING PSYCHOLOGICAL DISORDERS

Many forms of treatment are available to people with psychological disorders. These include psychological and biological approaches.

### Psychotherapy

**Psychotherapy** involves the application of principles of psychology to help people overcome psychological disorders. Psychotherapy can also help people adjust to problems in living or develop as individuals. There are hundreds of different kinds of psychotherapy; we focus on the major types in use today.

**Psychodynamic Therapy** What comes to mind when you think of psychotherapy? If you think of someone lying on a couch and talking about childhood experiences, you are probably thinking of **psychoanalysis.**

Psychoanalysis is the form of therapy originated by Sigmund Freud. Today there are many different forms of therapy based on psychoanalysis, referred to collectively as *psychodynamic therapy.* All of these subscribe to Freud's belief that psychological problems are rooted in **unconscious** psychological conflicts that can be traced to early childhood. All assume that insight into these conflicts can help people resolve them and restore psychological health.

Freud believed that these unconscious conflicts are basically sexual or aggressive. Their true nature is kept hidden from consciousness by **defense mechanisms,** especially **repression.** For example, people may develop a fear of knives because of a repressed desire to harm themselves or others. The phobia has a strategic value; it keeps them from acting on these threatening impulses. Psychoanalysis is a sort of mental detective work intended to ferret out these unconscious conflicts and resolve them. This process is aided by **free association,** a process in which the client is instructed to say anything that comes to mind in the hope that eventually these associations will reveal emotionally laden issues that relate to unconscious material. Freud also emphasized the importance of **dream analysis,** which involves interpretation of the symbolic meaning of dreams (as opposed to their overt or manifest meaning) to shed light on unconscious conflicts. Dream symbols vary from person to person (flying on an airplane may symbolize erection to one client or freedom from parental authority to another), so the psychoanalyst may ask clients to free associate to the dream story in the hopes of discovering clues to its meaning.

Freud also believed that clients reenact with the therapist problem relationships they've had with parents and other significant figures, a process called **transference.** By analyzing the transference relationship, the therapist helps the client understand how problems with others intrude on their present relationships with significant others in their lives.

Traditional psychoanalysis is a lengthy, intensive process. It may require three to five sessions a week for many years. Modern psychodynamic approaches are briefer and focus less on sexual

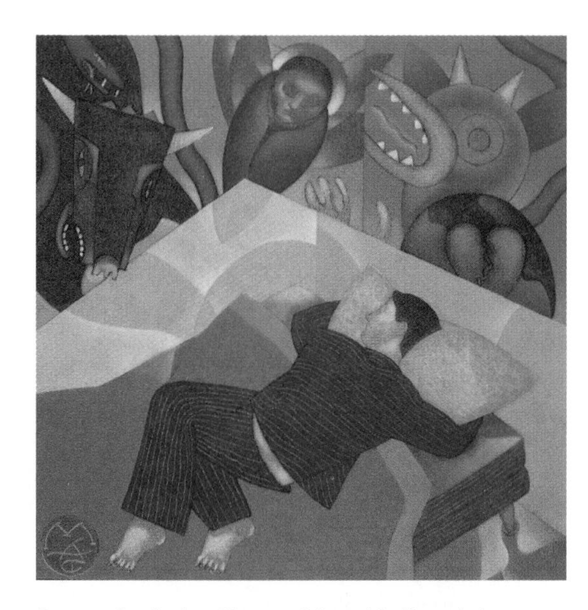

***Dream Analysis*** Sigmund Freud believed that dreams represent the "royal road to the unconscious." He held that uncovering the symbolic or hidden meaning of dreams can shed light on unconscious conflicts that underlie psychological problems.

and childhood issues. They focus more on a direct examination of the patient's defenses and how these defenses affect her or his ability to relate to others.

**Behavior Therapy** **Behavior therapy** assumes that psychological disorders are largely learned and can therefore be unlearned. Psychoanalysts try to help people gain insight into the root causes of their behavior. Behavior therapists focus on directly changing problem behavior in the here and now. Behavior therapy is relatively brief. It usually lasts no more than 10 to 20 sessions.

One behavior therapy technique, **systematic desensitization,** helps people overcome fears and phobias. The phobic person is first taught relaxation skills. She or he is then guided by the therapist to imagine confronting a series of increasingly frightening stimuli while remaining relaxed. Through this process, the bonds between frightening objects or situations and fear are gradually weakened.

Behavior therapists also use **gradual exposure,** which involves exposure in stages to increasingly frightening stimuli. By gradually confronting feared situations or objects directly, the person learns to tolerate them. **Assertiveness training** is a behavior therapy technique that helps inhibited or unassertive people express their feelings and stand up for their rights.

Behavior therapists typically assign homework to help clients sharpen their new skills. A depressed person may be asked to engage in pleasant activities; an inhibited person to start a conversation with a stranger or

**Psychotherapy** Therapy involving a systematic interaction between a patient and a therapist based on the application of psychological principles.

**Psychoanalysis** The type of therapy developed by Sigmund Freud that helps people achieve insight into unconscious processes and conflicts that are believed to give rise to psychological problems.

**Unconscious** Outside of awareness; in Freud's theory, unconscious conflicts of a sexual or aggressive nature lie at the root of psychological problems.

**Defense mechanism** According to Freud, a way in which the mind distorts reality to keep anxiety-evoking or troubling ideas or impulses away from consciousness.

**Repression** A defense mechanism, described as motivated forgetting, by which the unconscious mind banishes troubling ideas or impulses from awareness.

**Free association** A technique used in psychoanalysis in which the patient is encouraged to verbalize any thoughts that come to mind, free of any conscious efforts to censure or edit them.

**Dream analysis** A technique used in psychoanalysis that attempts to extract the symbolic meaning of dreams in a way that reveals unconscious material.

**Transference** A relationship a person develops with a therapist or other figure that represents a reenactment of an earlier conflicted relationship.

**Behavior therapy** A therapy based on the systematic application of learning techniques to help people change problem behaviors.

**Systematic desensitization** A behavior therapy technique for overcoming phobias by means of a series of imagined encounters with feared objects or stimuli while the person remains deeply relaxed.

**Gradual exposure** A behavior therapy technique for overcoming phobias involving actual exposure to increasingly fearful stimuli or situations.

**Assertiveness training** A behavior therapy program aimed at helping inhibited or unassertive people learn to express their feelings and stand up for their rights.

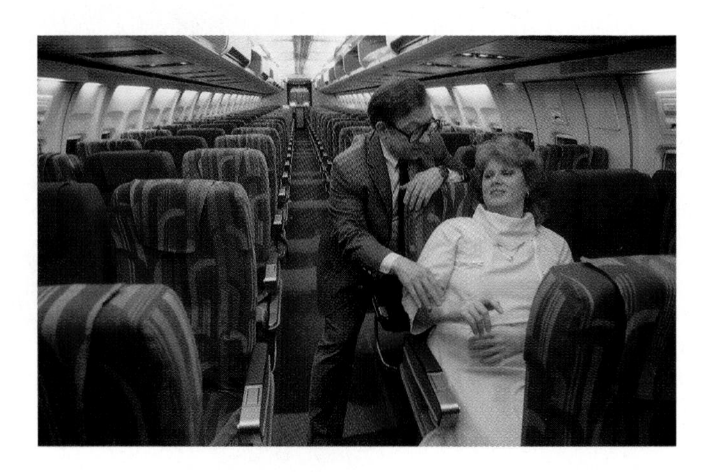

***Gradual Exposure*** This woman suffers from a fear of flying. Her therapist uses a gradual exposure approach by helping her manage fearful situations in a step-by-step process.

greet people on the elevator. Behavior therapists also use reinforcement-based strategies, in which rewards and punishments help people eliminate counterproductive behavior and acquire adaptive behavior. Parents may be trained to reward children for appropriate behavior and ignore problem behavior in order to weaken (extinguish) it. Or parents may use mild forms of punishment such as *time out,* in which children are removed from a rewarding environment and asked to "sit out" for a prescribed time when they misbehave. As we see in later chapters, behavior therapists also help people change problem behaviors such as overeating and smoking.

**Close-up**
Virtual therapy
T0415

Behavior therapists often incorporate techniques of cognitive therapy in a broader-based form of behavior therapy called cognitive-behavior therapy.

**Cognitive Therapy** Cognitive therapies focus on helping people change the types of thoughts and attitudes that can lead to psychological disorders. Like behavior therapy, cognitive therapy is relatively brief (10 to 20 sessions), and its concern is with what is happening in the present. It uses homework assignments to help people challenge distorted thinking and adopt rational thinking. Two of the major forms of cognitive therapy were developed by psychologist Albert Ellis and psychiatrist Aaron Beck.

**Take Charge**
Coping with panic
C0401

Ellis's **rational-emotive therapy** shows people how irrational beliefs, such as perfectionism and excessive needs for approval, can lead to the development of psychological problems like anxiety and depression. Beck's **cognitive therapy** focuses on identifying and correcting cognitive distortions. People are taught more adaptive, flexible, and realistic ways of thinking, as in the case of Christie:

*Christie, a 33-year-old real estate agent, had frequent episodes of depression. She would blame herself whenever a sale fell through and believed her future was bleak. Her therapist helped her recognize and challenge this depressing style of thinking by asking herself: "Am I always to blame? Does the evidence show that I alone was responsible? Might there be other reasons why this fell through?" With therapy, she learned to think logically when disappointments arose, telling herself, "Okay, I'm disappointed. I'm frustrated. I feel lousy. So what? It doesn't mean I'll never succeed. Let me discover what went wrong and try to correct it the next time. I have to look ahead, not dwell on past disappointments."*

The Authors' Files

**Rational-emotive therapy** A cognitive therapy that focuses on helping people dispute and correct irrational thinking.

**Cognitive therapy** A therapy that helps clients identify and correct dysfunctional thinking patterns.

**Eclectic therapy** In psychotherapy, the use of techniques or principles from different therapeutic approaches.

**Group therapy** Therapy in which clients are treated together.

**Family therapy** Therapy that helps troubled families learn to communicate better and resolve conflicts.

**Eclectic Therapy** **Eclectic therapy** uses techniques from several different therapeutic approaches. Depending on the person's needs, an eclectic therapist might use behavior therapy to help change problem behavior and psychodynamic techniques to help a person gain insight into underlying conflicts.

**Group Therapy** **Group therapy** brings people together in small groups to explore and cope with their problems. Group therapy is less costly than individual therapy. It is particularly helpful for interpersonal problems such as loneliness, shyness, and low self-esteem. Group members learn how others cope with similar problems and offer one another social support. The give-and-take of the group also improves social skills.

**Family Therapy** **Family therapy** helps troubled families communicate and resolve their differences. The family, not the individual, is the unit

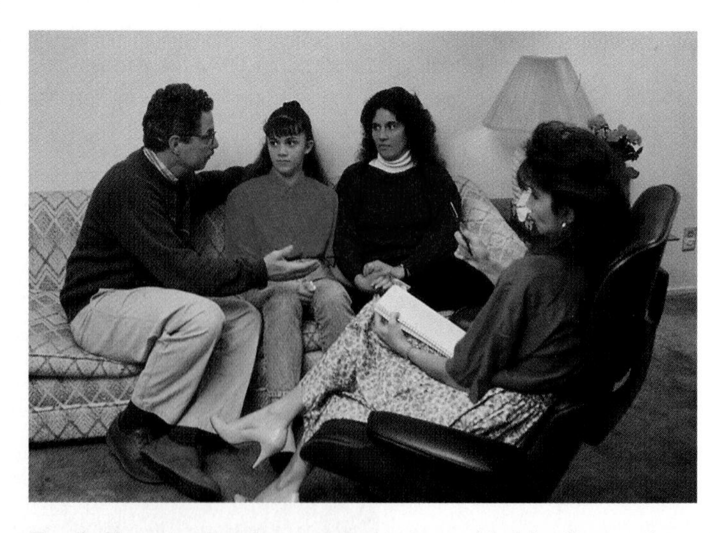

***Family Therapy*** Family therapists help troubled family members learn to communicate more effectively and become more accepting and supportive of each other.

of treatment. Most family therapists view the family unit as a complex social system in which individuals play certain roles. For instance, an "identified patient" is often considered the source of the family's problems. Family therapists show how the problems of the identified patient are symptomatic of a breakdown in the whole family system, not just the individual. They help dysfunctional families change the way members interact and relate to one another so that members become more accepting and supportive of each individual.

**Couples Therapy** **Couples therapy** helps couples build healthier relationships by enhancing communication skills and helping partners resolve conflicts. The therapist helps open channels of communication between partners and encourages them to share their feelings and needs in positive ways. Couples therapists also focus on disturbed role relationships, such as the tendency of one member to dominate the other. By correcting power imbalances, couples therapy seeks to enhance relationship satisfaction and lessen the potential for domestic violence.

## Biological Therapy

Two major forms of biological therapy are used to treat psychological disorders today: drug therapy and electroshock therapy.

**Drug Therapy** Remarkable gains have been made in treating a wide range of psychological disorders with psychotherapeutic drugs, called **psychotropics.** Psychotropic drugs include antidepressants (like Elavil and Prozac), antianxiety agents (like Valium and Xanax), and antipsychotic drugs (like Thorazine and Haldol). Antipsychotic drugs are used to treat schizophrenia. One person in eight in the United States aged 12 and over has used psychotropic drugs at some point. Nearly 1 in 50 currently uses them.[36] Table 4.4 on the next page shows some of the major psychotropic drugs.

Psychotropic drugs are not a cure, but they help relieve emotional distress and enable people to cope more effectively. When drugs are withdrawn, however, symptoms often return. Drugs such as lithium, which stabilizes the mood swings of many people with bipolar disorder, may need to be taken indefinitely.

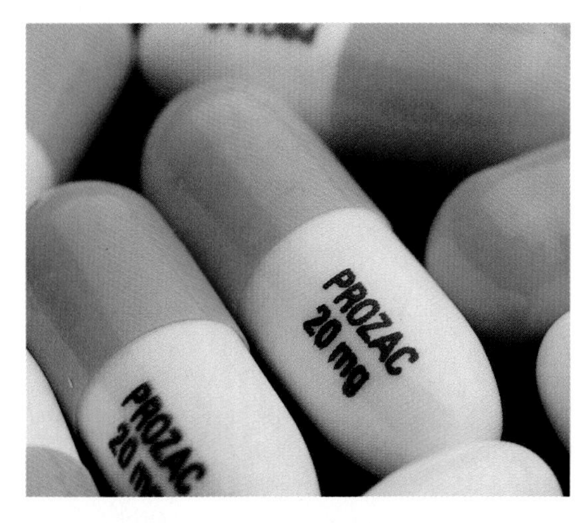


***Psychotropic Drugs*** Psychotropic drugs such as Prozac are not a cure but can help relieve psychological distress in people with psychological disorders and help them cope more effectively.

Psychotropic drugs can have side effects ranging from drowsiness (for antianxiety drugs) to muscular tremors and rigidity (for antipsychotic drugs). Prolonged use of antipsychotic drugs may also lead to a motor disorder, **tardive dyskinesia,** which is characterized by uncontrollable lip smacking, eye blinking, and grimacing. On the other hand, antipsychotic drugs have enabled many people with schizophrenia who were formerly hospitalized to return to community life. Some drugs, such as the antianxiety drug Valium, can lead to psychological and physical dependence (addiction). Valium can also be very dangerous, even deadly, if taken in an overdose or mixed with alcohol or other drugs.

Another limitation of psychotropic drugs is that while they relieve many symptoms of psychological disorders, they do not teach people how to resolve their underlying problems. Psychotherapy provides opportunities for anxious or depressed people to learn to change their thoughts, behavior, and ways of relating to others in healthy ways. The temporary relief that psychotropic drugs provide may be used as an opportunity to make lasting adaptive changes.

**Couples therapy** Therapy for married or unmarried couples that focuses on improving their relationships.

**Psychotropics** Psychoactive drugs used in the treatment of psychological or mental disorders.

**Tardive dyskinesia** A potentially irreversible disorder involving involuntary movement that arises from long-term use of certain antipsychotic drugs such as Thorazine and Mellaril.

TABLE 4.4

## Examples of Psychotropic Drugs

| Drug Class | Generic Name | Brand Name | Examples of Clinical Uses |
|---|---|---|---|
| **Antianxiety Agents (also called minor tranquilizers or anxiolytics)** | | | |
| *Benzodiazepines* | Diazepam | Valium | Temporary relief of anxiety and insomnia |
| | Chlordiazepoxide | Librium | |
| | Clorazepate | Tranxene | |
| | Oxazepam | Serax | |
| | Lorazepam | Ativan | |
| | Alprazolam | Xanax | |
| *Hypnotics* | Flurazepam | Dalmane | Temporary relief of insomnia |
| | Triazolam | Halcion | |
| **Antidepressants** | | | |
| *Tricyclic Antidepressants (TCAs)* | Imipramine | Tofranil | Depression, bulimia (eating disorder), panic disorder |
| | Desipramine | Norpramin | |
| | Amitriptyline | Elavil | |
| | Doxepin | Sinequan | |
| | Nortriptyline | Aventyl | |
| | Proptriptyline | Vivactil | |
| | Trimipramine | Surmontil | |
| *MAO Inhibitors (MAOIs)* | Phenelzine | Nardil | Depression |
| | Isocarboxazid | Marplan | |
| | Tranylcypromine | Parnate | |
| *Selective Serotonin Reuptake Inhibitors (SSRIs)* | Fluoxetine | Prozac | Depression, bulimia, obsessive-compulsive disorder |
| | Sertraline | Zoloft | |
| | Paroxetine | Paxil | |
| **Antiobsessional Drugs** | | | |
| *Selective Serotonin Reuptake Inhibitor* | Clomipramine | Anafranil | Obsessive-compulsive disorder |
| **Antipsychotic Drugs (also called neuroleptics or major tranquilizers)** | | | |
| *Phenothiazines* | Chlorpromazine | Thorazine | Schizophrenia and other psychotic disorders |
| | Thioridazine | Mellaril | |
| | Mesoridazine | Serentil | |
| | Perphenazine | Trilafon | |
| | Trifluoperazine | Stelazine | |
| | Fluphenazine | Prolixin | |
| *Butyrophenones* | Haloperidol | Haldol | Schizophrenia and other psychotic disorders |
| *Dibenzodiazepine* | Clozapine | Clozaril | Schizophrenia and other psychotic disorders, especially treatment-resistant schizophrenia |
| **Antimanic Drugs** | | | |
| *Antimanic Agents* | Lithium carbonate | Lithane | Manic episodes and stabilization of mood swings associated with bipolar disorder |
| | Carbamazapine | Tegretol | |
| | Divalproex | Depakote | |
| | Valproate | Depakene | |

**Electroshock Therapy** In **electroshock therapy (ECT)** a jolt of electricity strong enough to cause convulsions is passed through the head. The patient is put to sleep by general anesthesia so as not to experience any pain or discomfort and awakens shortly afterward with no memory of the procedure. The procedure typically involves a series of 6 to 12 treatments over several weeks. ECT is used almost exclusively in the treatment of severe depression, often in cases that have not responded to other forms of treatment. Although the procedure may sound barbaric, it often produces dramatic relief from severe depression and can be life-saving when depressed people are suicidal. ECT produces significant levels of improvement in 80 percent or more of cases of major depression overall and about half of cases of major depression that have failed to respond to antidepressant medication.[37] It is not clear how ECT works, but it may help normalize levels of neurotransmitters in the brain.

ECT is usually effective, but critics are concerned that it may wipe out large chunks of memory. Scientific reviews find that memory losses induced by ECT are temporary, except perhaps for memories of events that occurred shortly before or after ECT itself.[38] Still, because of its extreme nature, many health professionals view ECT as a treatment of last resort.

Smart Quiz Q0405

### think about it!

- What type of therapy would you prefer if you were seeking treatment for a psychological disorder? Why?
- What problems do you see in taking pills to cope with anxiety or depression that stems from academic or social difficulties?

## GETTING HELP

People seeking help for psychological problems face a bewildering array of choices. There are not only many different types of therapy, but also different types of therapists and helping professionals. Nor is professional treatment necessary for everyone. Many people with psychological disorders turn to clergy or trusted friends. **Self-help groups** or support groups, such as Alcoholics Anonymous, Overeaters Anonymous, and Gamblers Anonymous, also help many people experiencing psychological problems. When problems become overwhelming or persistent, or when people seem to be at risk of harming themselves or others, professional help is indicated.

### A Who's Who of Psychological Health Professionals

Different kinds of professionals treat psychological disorders, including physicians, psychologists, counselors, and social workers. Some people without psychological disorders also seek out health professionals to help them gain better insight into themselves or reach their full potentials.

**Psychiatrists** **Psychiatrists** are medical doctors (M.D.s or D.O.s) who complete residencies in psychiatry. Residencies last three to five years and provide training and experience in the diagnosis and treatment of psychological disorders. Psychiatrists use psychotherapy, and as licensed physicians, they can prescribe psychotropic drugs and use other medical techniques, such as ECT. Many psychiatrists also complete more extensive training in psychoanalysis or other psychotherapeutic approaches.

**Psychologists** Psychologists complete advanced graduate work in psychology, usually a doctoral degree (Ph.D., Ed.D., or Psy.D.). They may train in specialty areas within psychology, such as clinical or counseling psychology, that equip them to diagnose disorders and to treat them with psychotherapy. They complete internships in health care settings or university clinics and are licensed to practice in their states. **Clinical psychologists** also receive training in the use of psychological tests to diagnose psychological disorders and in research meth-

Take Charge
Finding a psychologist
C0402

**Electroshock therapy (ECT)** A therapy for severe depression involving the administration of brief pulses of electricity to the patient's brain.

**Self-help group** A group of people with a common psychological problem whose members help each other cope.

**Psychiatrists** Physicians who specialize in the practice of psychiatry.

**Clinical psychologists** Psychologists who specialize in the diagnosis and treatment of psychological disorders.

ods to enable them to conduct scientific studies in the field.

**Counselors** **Counselors** usually possess a master's degree in education or a health-related field (such as occupational therapy or rehabilitation counseling). Counselors work in many settings, including public schools, college testing and counseling centers, and hospitals and health clinics. Many specialize in academic, vocational, marital, or family counseling, or in career development or the treatment of milder psychological disorders, such as adjustment disorders. Pastoral counselors are religious personnel (ministers, etc.) who are trained to help parishioners cope with personal problems.

**Social Workers** Social workers usually hold a Master of Social Work (M.S.W.) degree and are licensed by the state in which they practice. **Clinical social workers** provide counseling or psychotherapy and help people obtain the services they need from community agencies and organizations. For example, they may help people with schizophrenia adjust to the community once they leave the hospital. Many social workers, like counselors, also specialize in marital or family therapy.

## Where to Turn for Help

In most areas, there are pages of clinics and health professionals in the telephone directory. Many people have no idea whom to call. They may thus turn to the professional with the largest advertisement. If you don't know where to go or whom to see, there are a number of things you can do to ensure receiving appropriate care:

1. *Get advice.* Ask your physician, instructor, college health service, or college counseling center for recommendations. Ask family members and friends for their recommendations. Consult your minister, priest, or rabbi. Contact the local community mental health center. Ask whether they offer help for your type of problem or can refer you to people who do.
2. *Contact professional organizations and ask for recommendations.* Call or write your state psychiatric association or psychological association for information. If they are not handy, try the American Psychiatric Association or American Psychological Association, both of which are in Washington, DC.

   Consult the yellow pages. Look under physicians, psychologists, or social workers, or try listings for "Social & Human Services." Be wary of large ads by professionals who claim to be experts in the treatment of many different kinds of problems.

   Don't be enticed by commercial come-ons like "Free Consultation!" Responsible professionals do not resort to gimmicks to entice patients. Many health professionals allow you to pay according to your ability, and treatment may be covered by insurance.
3. *Choose a licensed professional.* In many states, anyone can set up practice as a "therapist," even as a "psychotherapist." Neither of these is a *profession,* however. Legitimate therapists are licensed in their profession, such as medicine, psychology, counseling, or social work. Professionals clearly display their degrees, licenses, and other credentials. Do not hesitate to ask for such information; ethical professionals will always provide it. You can always check out credentials with the state licensing authority.
4. *Ask what type of therapy the person practices, e.g., psychoanalysis, family therapy, behavior therapy, and so forth, and whether this type of therapy is appropriate for your problems.*
5. *Ask the health professional to discuss her or his experience treating people with your problem and the results.* Do not be afraid to ask why this particular treatment plan is most appropriate to your case.
6. *Ask how long therapy is likely to take—and why.* Many problems can be managed with a few sessions; others take longer.
7. *Ask how much treatment will cost.* Ask whether the provider will take your income into account. Ask whether you will be charged for missed or canceled sessions.
8. *Ask about the types of insurance that the treatment provider accepts and whether your insurance will cover the costs.* Ask if the treatment provider will accept "assignment" or direct billing and payment through your insurance company. If you are eligible for Medicaid or Medicare, find out whether the

**Counselors** Professionals who counsel people with psychological problems and disabilities.

**Clinical social workers** Social workers trained to work with people with psychological problems.

treatment provider accepts these coverages. Find out if the treatment provider is a member of any health maintenance organization to which you may belong.

9. *After an initial evaluation of your problem, ask the therapist to discuss with you the diagnosis and treatment plan.*
10. *If the treatment recommendations do not sound right to you, explain your concerns as best you can.* An ethical professional will be willing to address your concerns.
11. *If medication is prescribed, ask how long it takes to start working.* Ask about the possible side effects and what side effects should prompt you to call with questions.
12. *If you remain in doubt, request a second opinion.* An ethical professional will support your interest in gaining additional points of view and will recommend other professionals who might render a second opinion, or you can select your own.

## think about it!

- **How do psychologists differ from psychiatrists?**
- **How can you find a qualified health professional to help you with psychological problems?**

Smart Quiz
Q0406

# Coping with Depression

Take Charge

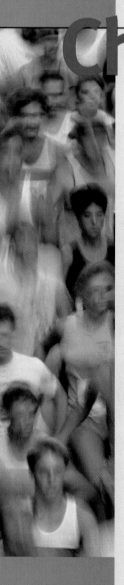

There is much we can do to improve our moods and adjust more effectively to the ups and downs of everyday life.

## Do Fun Things (Don't Sit Around and Mope!)

When we are feeling down, we tend to withdraw from the activities that usually lift our spirits. When others urge us to get out and do things, we may think that they are putting the cart before the horse. After all, don't we have to wait to feel better before we return to enjoyable activities? Not necessarily! Pleasant events are incompatible with feelings of depression. You can systematically use pleasant events to lift your mood—or enrich the quality of your daily life—through the following steps:

1. Think about and list those activities that you consider pleasant events.
2. Engage in at least three of the pleasant events on your list each day.
3. Record your pleasant activities in a diary. Add other activities and events that struck you as pleasant, even if they were unplanned.
4. Toward the end of each day, rate your response to each activity using a scale such as:

   + 3 Wonderful

   + 2 Very nice

   + 1 Somewhat nice

   0 No particular response

   − 1 Somewhat disappointing

   − 2 Rather disappointing

   − 3 The pits
5. After a week or so, check the activities and events in the diary that received positive ratings.
6. Repeat highly positive activities and continue to experiment with new ones.

## Think Rationally (Toss Out Mental Downers!)

Depressed people look at the world through blue-colored glasses. They tend to blame themselves for failures and problems, even when they are not at fault. Depressed people also make the cognitive errors of *magnifying* or *catastrophizing* their problems and *minimizing* their accomplishments.

Take stock of your thoughts and replace distorted thoughts with rational alternatives. For example, did you do poorly on a test? Though it's understandable to be disappointed, it is rational to recognize that it is not the end of the world. What might you say to yourself about the test result? "Well, this is really upsetting. I thought I was well prepared but I just seemed to forget what I knew when I walked into the room. It doesn't mean that I'll never succeed. But it does mean that I need to figure out how to cope with tests without drawing blanks. Perhaps I need to speak to the instructor about the problem."

Table 4.5 lists a number of depressing thoughts that often turn out to be irrational upon closer inspection. Column 2 shows the kind of cognitive error the thought represents, such as catastrophizing or "misfortune telling." Column 3 shows examples of rational alternatives—ways of talking sense to yourself. As you consider these examples, perhaps you can identify some nagging, mood-dampening irrational thoughts of your own.

You need not be stuck with depressing thoughts. You can learn to recognize and challenge them. In this way, you can exert control over your emotions.

## Exercise (Don't Sit Around!)

Vigorous physical activity, especially aerobic exercise like jogging, running, fast walking, swimming, or bicycle riding, can help combat depression.[39] Aerobic exercise actually increases the levels of neurotransmitters that may be deficient in depression.[40] Exercise may also lift our spirits for other reasons. For one thing, exercise can be a pleasant activity. For another, it may boost feelings of self-confidence and improve self-esteem.

## Assert Yourself (No More Doormat Imitations!)

When you're feeling down, you may feel inhibited around others. You may hold back from expressing your feelings or needs. Perhaps you just shy away from people. Asserting yourself and relating effectively to other people can improve your mood. Express your feelings and needs. If you want other people to know what's important to you, tell them. Expressing positive feelings—like telling people you like them or appreciate their efforts, or just cheerily saying "Good morning"—can help pave the way to healthy relationships.

### Put Meaning into Your Life (Stop *De*meaning Yourself!)

Is your life filled with drab, unmotivating activities? If so, it is no surprise that you're down in the dumps. We need meaningful activities to keep our motivation and spirits up. If daily life has become a grind, perhaps it's time to look inward to discover what is meaningful to you. Perhaps you find meaning in doing projects around the house. Perhaps you could develop hobbies or pursuits that hold a special interest for you. Perhaps you could get involved in your community by participating in civic, religious, or political organizations, or volunteering your time to charitable organizations or hospitals. Filling your life with meaningful activities is an excellent antidote for depression.

There is much we can do to lift our spirits and combat depression, but when depressed moods become severe or persist for more than a few weeks, we should consult a mental health professional for a thorough evaluation. Effective treatments for depression are available. Unfortunately, fewer than one in five people needing treatment seek professional help.

**Close-up**
Treatment for depression
**T0416**

**Smart Quiz**
**Q0407**

**TABLE 4.5**

**Thinking Rationally**

| Irrational Thought | Type of Cognitive Error | Rational Thinking |
|---|---|---|
| Things will never get better for me. | Misfortune telling | No one can predict the future. Just take it a day at a time. |
| My looks are hopeless. | Catastrophizing | I'm not a hopeless case. There are many things I can do to improve how I look and feel. |
| This is awful. I can't stand this. | Catastrophizing | I may feel overwhelmed, but I've handled situations like this before. |
| I guess I'm just a loser. | Name calling (Yes! You can call yourself self-defeating names.) | That's my negative self talking. I need to stop dumping on myself. |
| I've only lost six pounds. I'll never succeed in getting this extra weight off. | All-or-nothing thinking<br>Misfortune telling<br>Dismissing the positives | Six pounds is a start. Just keep with it. |
| I know things are really awful or I wouldn't feel so bad. | Emotion-based reasoning | My feelings stem from my perception of the situation, not from the reality itself. |
| I know that his/her problems are really my fault. | Mistaken responsibility | There are many reasons he/she has these problems that have nothing to do with me. |
| If this relationship doesn't work out, I will be devastated. | Catastrophizing | It would be disappointing, but I would get over it. |
| All I can think about are the negatives. | Negative focusing | It's not as bleak as it seems. |
| Someone my age should be doing better than I am. | "Shouldisms" | It's not helpful to compare myself with others. I'll just do my best. |
| I hurt those who get close to me. | Negative focusing<br>Mistaken responsibility | I've meant a lot to many people over the years. |
| I know she/he will think I'm dull. | Misfortune telling | How can I know for sure what someone else will think? |
| It's all my fault. | Misplaced blame | There's enough blame to go around. Better yet, can't I forget placing blame and think about solving the problem? |
| I just don't have the brains for college. | Name calling | I can accomplish a lot more than I give myself credit for. Thinking that way only makes me want to give up. |

# SUMMING UP

## Questions and Answers

### WHAT ARE PSYCHOLOGICAL DISORDERS?

1. **What are psychological disorders?** Psychological problems such as anxiety and depression are considered psychological disorders when their magnitude or persistence does not match the person's situation.

2. **How is psychological health connected with physical health?** Physical health problems can trigger psychological problems. Psychological factors such as optimism also affect physical health.

### TYPES OF PSYCHOLOGICAL DISORDERS

3. **What are anxiety disorders?** Anxiety disorders are characterized by feelings of apprehension and overactivity of the sympathetic branch of the autonomic nervous system. They include phobias, panic disorder, generalized anxiety disorder, obsessive-compulsive disorder, and posttraumatic stress disorder.

4. **What are mood disorders?** Mood disorders involve disturbances in mood that are either unusually severe or prolonged. Mood disorders include depressive disorders and bipolar disorder (formerly called manic-depression).

5. **What is schizophrenia?** Schizophrenia is a psychotic disorder, meaning that it is characterized by a break with reality. There may be gross confusion, delusions, and hallucinations.

### CAUSES OF PSYCHOLOGICAL DISORDERS

6. **What biological factors contribute to psychological disorders?** These include genetics, imbalances in neurotransmitter activity, and brain damage.

7. **What psychosocial factors contribute to psychological disorders?** These include self-esteem, early learning experiences, cognitive errors, and poverty and discrimination.

### SUICIDE

8. **Who is at risk for suicide?** Groups at highest risk of suicide include older white men and Native Americans. Men are more likely to "succeed" at suicide attempts than women because they tend to use more lethal means.

9. **Why do people commit suicide?** Most suicides result from feelings of hopelessness and despair. Teenagers have been known to commit copycat suicides (the "cluster effect").

### TREATING PSYCHOLOGICAL DISORDERS

10. **What kinds of psychotherapy are used to treat psychological disorders?** Some of the major types of psychotherapy are psychoanalysis, behavior therapy, and cognitive therapy. Other forms of therapy include group therapy, family therapy, and couples therapy. Psychoanalysis is relatively long-term and attempts to discover and work through the childhood roots of psychological disorders. Behavior therapy and cognitive therapy focus on the here and now. They attempt to change maladaptive behavior and thought patterns directly.

11. **What kinds of biological therapy are used to treat psychological disorders?** These include drug therapy and electroshock therapy (ECT). Drugs are available to treat many psychological disorders. Yet drugs are not cures and may produce adverse side effects. ECT may be used to treat major depression when antidepressant drugs fail to help.

### GETTING HELP

12. **What kinds of health professionals help people with psychological disorders?** Psychiatrists are physicians who can provide both biological therapy and psychotherapy. Psychologists usually have doctorates and practice psychotherapy. Counselors and social workers usually have master's degrees and provide counseling.

## References and Suggested Readings

### SMART REFERENCES FROM SCIENTIFIC AMERICAN

**Horgan, J. Mental Health: Multicultural Studies.** *Scientific American,* 275(5) (November 1996), 24. **R0401**

**Leutwyler, K. Neurobiology: Suicide Prevention.** *Scientific American,* 276(3) (March 1997), 18. **R0402**

### SUGGESTED READINGS

**Gorman, J.** *The Essential Guide to Psychiatric Drugs.* New York: St. Martin's Press, 1992. A practical guide to all types of psychiatric drugs, from antidepressants to tranquilizers and antipsychotics, it covers uses, dosages, side effects, withdrawal symptoms, and more information.

**American Psychiatric Association.** *DSM-IV: Diagnostic and Statistical Manual of Mental Disorders* (4th ed.). Washington, DC: 1994. The listing of recognized psychiatric disorders, containing information about their features, causes, and distinguishing characteristics.

**Burns, D.** *Feeling Good: The New Mood Therapy.* New York: Morrow, 1980. A highly readable and engaging approach to the principles of cognitive therapy, with many helpful suggestions that readers can apply to their own lives.

**Watson, D., & Tharp., R.** *Self-Directed Behavior: Self-Modification for Personal Adjustment.* Pacific Grove, CA: Brooks/Cole, 1993. Principles of behavior modification to help people have greater control over their behavior.

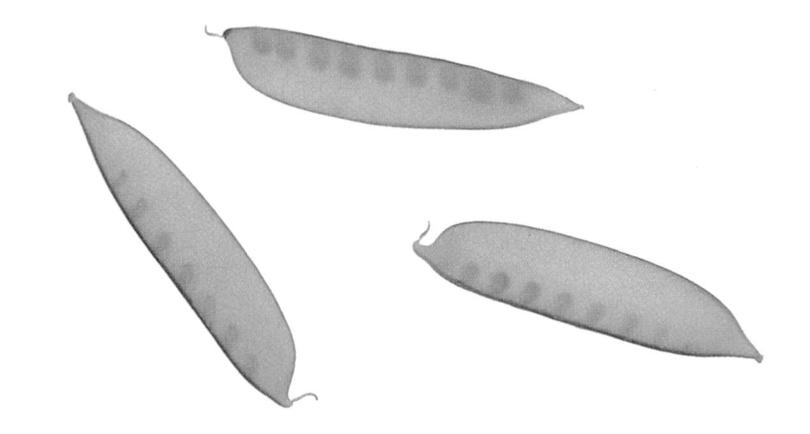

## DID YOU KNOW THAT

- Most Americans eat more than enough protein? p.108
- The starch in foods like potatoes and rice is made up of sugar molecules? p.109
- People who eat a fiber-rich diet have a lower risk of developing cardiovascular disease and some forms of cancer than people who eat a low-fiber diet? p.110
- Sugar is found in milk? p.110
- The average blueberry muffin has twice as much fat as a dish of ice cream or two Twinkies? p.112
- Your body makes all the cholesterol it needs? p.113
- Saturated fat in the diet actually plays a larger role in determining blood cholesterol levels than dietary cholesterol? p.114
- Most Americans get all the vitamins they need in their diets? p.119
- Megadoses of beta-carotene and vitamins C and E have *not* been shown to reduce the risk of cancer or heart disease? p.124
- Adequate calcium intake is important for bone health in adults as well as children? p.127
- Vegetarians have a lower incidence of cancer than meat eaters do? p.138

# Nutrition for Life

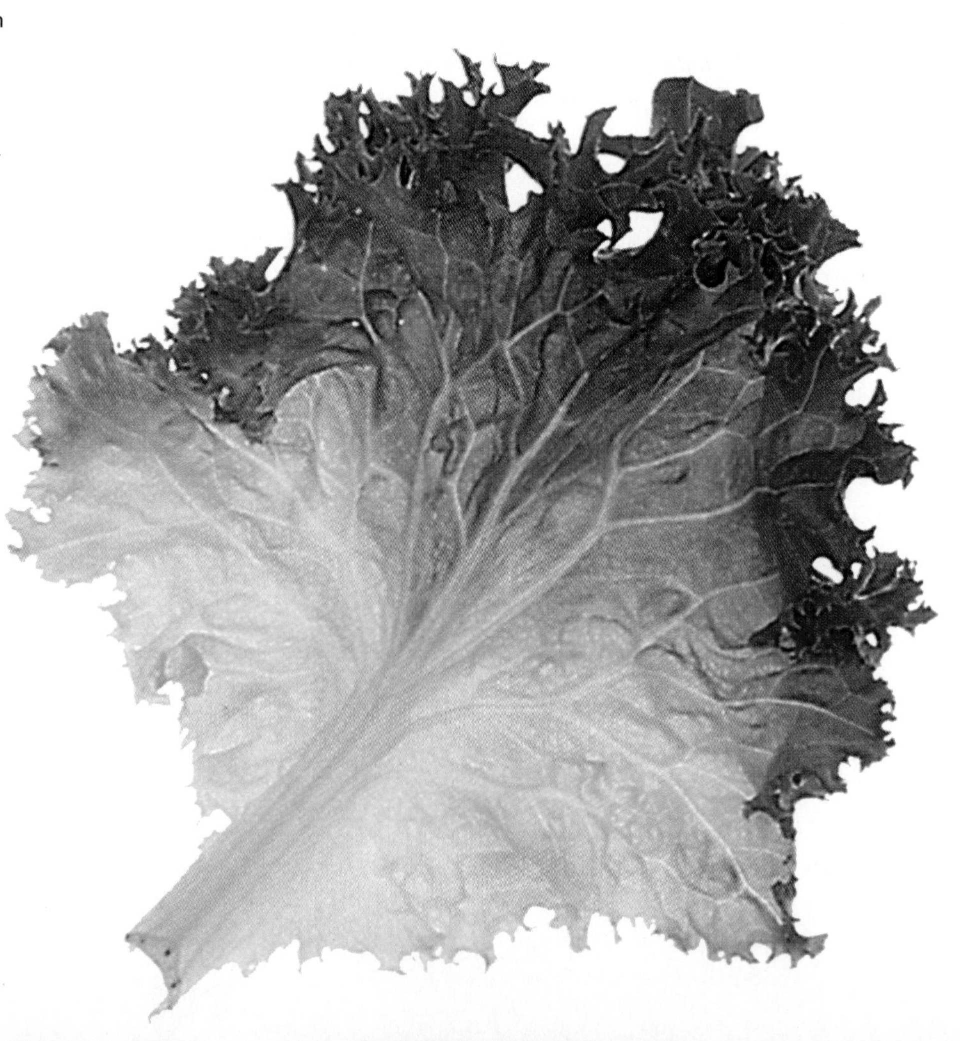

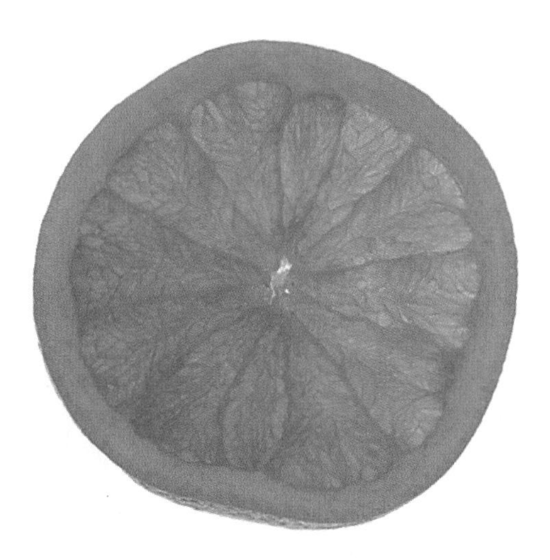

# 5

## PROTEINS

Sources of Protein

## CARBOHYDRATES

Starches

Dietary Fiber

**PREVENTION** Dietary Fiber and Disease Prevention

Sugars

## FATS

How Much Fat Should You Consume?

Types of Fat

**HEALTHCHECK** How Much Fat Is in Your Diet?

## VITAMINS

**WORLD OF DIVERSITY** Ethnic Food—Eating Out, Eating Smart

Types of Vitamins

Vitamin Deficiency Syndromes

Health Benefits of Vitamins

**PREVENTION** Should You Take Vitamin Supplements?

## MINERALS

Calcium

Iron

## WATER AND ELECTROLYTES

Sodium

**PREVENTION** Ensuring Food Safety

## Take Charge

Guidelines for Healthy Eating

*We really* are *what we eat: We convert our food into various body parts—bones, muscles, skin, blood, and other bodily tissues. Diet also plays a vital role in determining our risk of developing serious chronic diseases such as cancer, cardiovascular disease, and diabetes. A sensible diet—one low in fat and ample in fruits, vegetables, high-fiber grains, and low-fat sources of protein—can go a long way toward maintaining good health. As many as a third of all cancer deaths in the U.S. and a large proportion of deaths due to heart disease, the nation's leading killer, are linked to consumption of high-fat, high-calorie foods.*[1]

*The message that eating right is vital to health is beginning to get across. Americans have lowered their consumption of dietary fat and cholesterol over the past 30 years.*[2] *Yet there is still a long way to go, as fewer than a quarter of Americans follow a healthy diet. Far too many of us skimp on vegetables and grains and load up on high-fat foods like french fries, tacos, and burgers.*

*Today's consumer is often bewildered by research reports on nutrition. Some seem to report contradictory findings on the benefits or risks of certain foods. In this chapter we try to sort out the wheat from the chaff, so to speak, to help you make the best-informed choices about your diet.*

**Nutrition** (derived from the Latin root *nutri,* meaning "to feed") is the process by which organisms consume and utilize food. **Nutrients** are essential substances found in food. Some nutrients are fuels that furnish our bodies with energy when they are metabolized. Others serve as the basic building blocks of muscle, bone, and other body tissues. Five basic nutrients—proteins, carbohydrates, fats, vitamins, and minerals—are necessary to sustain life. We need to eat a variety of foods from each major food group to make sure that we get enough of these basic nutrients.

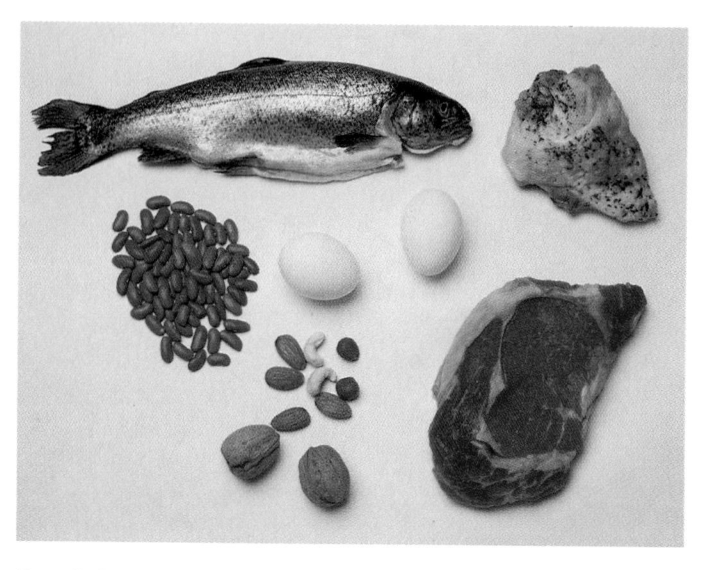

***Protein-Rich Foods*** There are many sources of protein in our diet, including fish, meat and poultry, nuts, beans, and dairy products.

## PROTEINS

**Proteins** are organic molecules that form the basic building blocks of muscle, bone, hair, blood, fingernails, antibodies, enzymes, hormones, and other body tissues. Proteins are composed of 22 different **amino acids,** 13 of which the body can produce from fats or carbohydrates. The other 9 that the body cannot make must be obtained from the diet. These 9 are called **essential amino acids;** they are vital to our diet.

### Sources of Protein

The principal sources of dietary protein are meat, such as beef, pork, and poultry; fish; and dairy products such as eggs, milk, and cheese. Some vegetable matter, such as legumes (beans, chickpeas, and lentils) and grains are also rich sources of protein. We get about two-thirds of our protein from animal sources in the form of meat and animal by-products, such as milk and cheese. The rest comes from a combination of cereal grains, beans, and other sources.

Most Americans consume more than enough protein in their diets to meet their nutritional needs. Any excess protein that we consume is converted into fat. Protein deficiencies are rare in the U.S. They are most commonly seen among children in impoverished countries. The physical signs of protein deficiency include stunted growth, poor muscular development, swelling, thin, fragile hair, and skin lesions.

**Nutrition** The process by which plants and animals ingest and utilize food.

**Nutrients** Essential substances in food that our bodies need but are incapable of producing on their own.

**Proteins** Organic molecules that form the basic building blocks of body tissues.

**Amino acids** Organic compounds from which proteins are made.

**Essential amino acids** Amino acids essential to survival that must be obtained from the food we eat since the body is unable to manufacture them on its own.

**Carbohydrates** Organic compounds forming the structural parts of plants that are important sources of nutrition for animals and humans.

**Complex carbohydrates** A class of carbohydrates that includes starches and fibers.

**Simple carbohydrates** A class of carbohydrates consisting of small molecules, including various sugars.

**think about it!**

- **How do proteins contribute to your health?**
- **Do you consume enough protein? Too much protein? How do you know?**
- **What are your favorite food sources of protein? Do these foods give you more than you want of other nutrients? Explain.**

Smart Quiz Q0501

## CARBOHYDRATES

**Carbohydrates** furnish the body with energy and give bulk to food. Carbohydrates are classified into two major categories: **complex carbohydrates,** including starches and fibers; and **simple carbohydrates,** including various sugars. Taken together, sugar and starches constitute the major sources of energy in our diet.

TABLE 5.1

**Dietary Sources of Starches and Fiber[3]**

| Foods Containing Starches | Foods Containing Dietary Fiber |
|---|---|
| Breads | Whole-grain breads |
| Breakfast cereals | Whole-grain breakfast cereals |
| Pasta, such as spaghetti and noodles | Whole-wheat pasta |
| Rice | Vegetables, especially those with edible skins, stems, and seeds |
| Dry beans and peas | Dry beans and peas |
| Starchy vegetables such as potatoes, corn, peas, and lima beans | Whole fruits, especially those with edible skins or seeds |
| | Dry fruits such as raisins and prunes |
| | Nuts and seeds |

## Starches

A complex carbohydrate, **starch** is actually a chain of sugar molecules. Common table sugar, by contrast, consists of only one or two sugar molecules. Starch is the form in which sugar (glucose) is stored in plant material. Because of the way the body breaks down starch, its chemical composition provides a steadier flow of energy than does dietary sugar. Sugar provides a quick spurt of energy but little else of nutritional value. Starchy vegetables such as potatoes, corn, green peas, and dry beans are abundant sources of energy and rich in vitamins and minerals. They are also low in fat and—despite the popular belief to the contrary—in calories. It's the sour cream or butter that people spread on baked potatoes, and the sauces added to pastas, that add excess calories. Some starches are also good sources of dietary fiber (see Table 5.1).

Nutritionists recommend that about 50 to 60% of our daily diet should consist of complex carbohydrates. Complex carbohydrates are found in breads and cereals; crucifers (cabbage-family vegetables) such as broccoli, cauliflower, and cabbage; citrus fruits; green leafy vegetables (spinach, romaine lettuce); legumes; pasta; root vegetables like potatoes and yams; and yellow fruits and vegetables, such as melon, squash, sweet potatoes, and carrots.

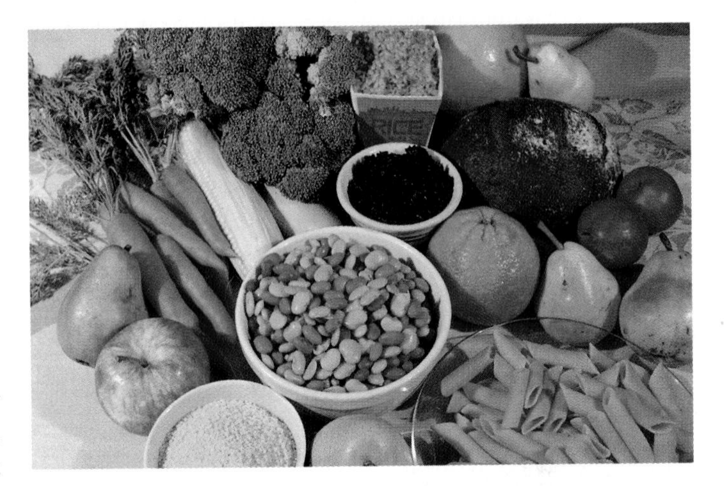

***High-Fiber Foods*** Dietary fiber is essential to good health. Fiber-rich foods include many kinds of fruits and vegetables, whole-grain breads and cereals, whole-wheat pasta, and brown rice.

## Dietary Fiber

**Dietary fiber** consists of complex carbohydrates that are found in the structural parts of plants, such as cellulose and pectin, that cannot be broken down by human digestive enzymes. Some forms of dietary fiber are actually broken down by bacteria that live in the digestive tract (not by human digestive enzymes) and converted into fat that the body absorbs, providing a small amount of available energy. Most fiber, however, passes through the digestive tract unchanged, providing bulk to the stool.

Different types of dietary fiber are found in varying amounts in different types of plant foods, such as vegetables and grains. Fibers that are readily dissolvable in water are called **soluble fibers.** Those that are not are called **insoluble fibers.** Solu-

**Starch** A complex carbohydrate that forms an important part of the structure of plants such as corn, rice, wheat, potatoes, and beans.

**Dietary fiber** Complex carbohydrates that form the structural parts of plants, such as cellulose and pectin, that cannot be broken down by human digestive enzymes.

**Soluble fibers** Types of dietary fiber that are dissolvable in water.

**Insoluble fibers** Types of dietary fiber that are not dissolvable in water.

ble fiber is found in many fruits and vegetables; in beans; and in grains such as oats and barley. Insoluble fiber is found mostly in dark, leafy vegetables; in the skins of fruits and vegetables; and in the bran (outer layer) of wheat and corn. Different types of fiber have different health benefits. Soluble fiber helps reduce blood cholesterol levels, while insoluble fiber produces softer, bulkier stools and promotes more rapid elimination of waste products through the intestines, which increases regularity and helps lower the risk of colon cancer. Eating a wide variety of vegetables, fruits, and grains is the best way of ensuring that you obtain the benefits of different types of fiber.

Whole grains are rich sources of dietary fiber. Whole grains consist of the entire edible parts of the grain, including the bran and germ where most of the fiber, and most of the vitamins and minerals, are found. Whole grains include cracked and whole wheat, bulgur, oatmeal, popcorn, whole cornmeal and ryes, scotch barley, and brown rice.

PREVENTION

### Dietary Fiber and Disease Prevention

Dietary fiber is helpful in both the prevention and treatment of various gastrointestinal problems, including constipation, **irritable bowel syndrome (IBS),** and **diverticulosis.** Fiber also provides bulk in the diet, which produces a feeling of fullness that may help weight-conscious people control how much they eat.

Talking Glossary
Diverticulosis
G0501

People who eat plentiful amounts of vegetables and grains that are rich in dietary fiber have low rates of life-threatening cardiovascular disease and colon cancer. Fiber helps speed the passage of waste material through the colon. It thus reduces the time that potentially carcinogenic materials in the waste remain in contact with the lining of the colon. Dietary fiber also appears to be good for the heart and circulatory system.

Some health experts believe that fiber may not deserve the credit for lowering the risk of cardiovascular disease and colon cancer. People who follow high-fiber diets tend to lead healthier lifestyles—to exercise more, watch their weight, and avoid smoking. Perhaps these habits explain their lower risk of these diseases. Recently, however, researchers who took into account healthy habits still found a protective effect for dietary fiber on the heart.[4] Though the story of dietary fiber and health is still being written, health experts believe it makes good health sense to consume more fiber-rich foods, such as many fruits and vegetables, legumes, and whole-grain cereals.

**Irritable bowel syndrome (IBS)** An oversensitivity of the digestive system, resulting in attacks of diarrhea, nausea, gas, and abdominal pain after eating certain foods or during times of stress.

**Diverticulosis** Inflammation of small pockets or sacs that may form in the wall of the colon and that become filled with stagnant feces, causing pain and discomfort. In severe cases, can be life-threatenting.

**Sugar** A simple carbohydrate present in different forms in many of the foods we eat.

Most health experts recommend that Americans consume 20 to 35 grams of dietary fiber a day (some experts recommend 25 grams minimum).[5] Currently, only half of all Americans consume more than 10 grams of fiber a day. Though most of us consume too little dietary fiber, some eat too much, which can interfere with the absorption of minerals and lead to other problems. Note too that fiber pills and supplements lack important nutritional components found in food sources of fiber, so they are not adequate substitutes.

You can meet your daily fiber requirements by following the guidelines for healthy nutrition of the U.S. Department of Agriculture (discussed later), which call for 2 to 4 servings of fruits, 3 to 5 servings of vegetables, and 6 to 11 servings of cereals and grains.[6] You can also increase your fiber intake by including in your diet many of the high-fiber foods listed in Appendix C.[7]

## Sugars

Most of us think of **sugar** in terms of table sugar, or *sucrose,* which is used in food preparation and to sweeten foods and beverages. Yet dietary sugars occur naturally in a wide variety of foods, including fruits, vegetables, and milk. *Lactose* is the form of sugar found in milk and milk products. *Maltose* is found in legumes and cereals, while *glucose* and *fructose* are sugars found in honey and fruits, respectively.

Sugars provide abundant energy but have little other nutritional value. Consuming large amounts of sugar may satisfy your hunger and keep you from eating other foods that are rich in the nutrients your body requires, such as vitamins and minerals. Sugar can also add excess calories that become converted into body fat, which can lead to obesity. Sugar also contributes to tooth decay. It's not just the amount of sugar that causes tooth decay, but also the form. Sugary foods that are

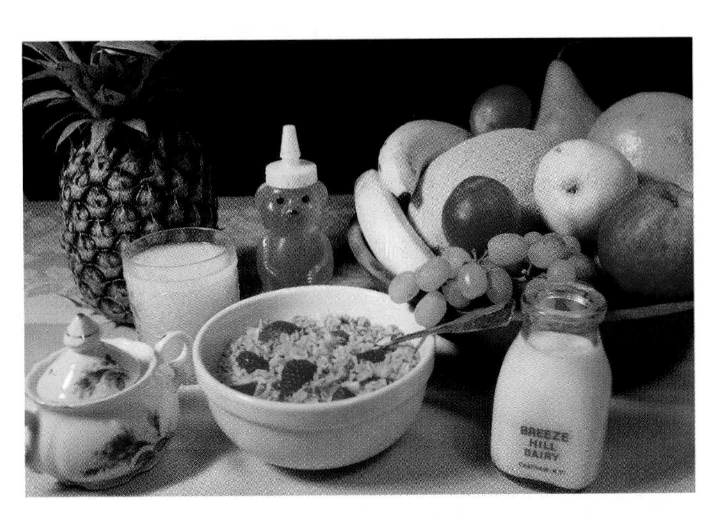


***Sugars, Anyone?*** Dietary sugars are found in many kinds of foods, such as fruits, vegetables, milk, syrup, molasses, and honey, as well as in table sugar.

chewy or sticky tend to stay on the teeth longer, thereby increasing the potential for decay. Sugary foods eaten between meals are also more likely to lead to decay than those consumed at mealtime.

Most of us are aware of the obvious sources of sugar, such as table sugar. Other sources of sugar, such as syrup, honey, and molasses, may be less obvious. Still less obvious are the sugars found in fruits and in many processed foods and baked goods.

On the whole, Americans consume too much sugar. To cut back, consider the following:[8]

- Use table sugar and other dietary sources of sugar, such as syrup, honey, and molasses, sparingly, if at all.
- Avoid drinking sugared soft drinks. The average 12-ounce can of cola contains a whopping 9 teaspoons of sugar.
- If you buy canned fruit, buy only fruit packed in water or juice, not in heavy syrup.
- Limit the baked goods, candies, sugared soft drinks, and sweet desserts you consume.
- Use seasonings and spices when cooking and preparing food, rather than sugar. Experiment with cinnamon, ginger, nutmeg, and other spices to enhance the natural flavors of food.
- Select fruit juice rather than fruit drinks. Fruit drinks typically have added sugar in addition to the natural sugar found in the juice. Better yet, eat fresh fruits rather than concentrated fruit juices, which tend to be high in natural sugars. See Appendix C for a listing of common foods to which sugar is added.

**think about it!**

- **Do you consume enough carbohydrates? What are your favorite food sources of carbohydrates?**

**critical thinking** **How do carbohydrates contribute to your health?**

**critical thinking** **Has this chapter changed your ideas about starches, sugar, or dietary fiber? If so, how?**

Smart Quiz
Q0502

## FATS

Although the word "fat" is usually connected with all things negative, in balanced amounts, **fats,** like other nutrients, play essential roles in the body. Fats nourish the skin, aid in the absorption of certain vitamins, help form cell membranes and hormones, help provide stamina, and serve to insulate the body from extremes of temperature.

Fats are the most concentrated sources of food energy or calories found in the diet. Each gram of fat provides about 9 calories, compared with 4 calories in each gram of protein or carbohydrate. So ounce for ounce, you will take in more than twice as many calories by eating fats as you would eating proteins or carbohydrates. It's easy to see why people with a high-fat diet often become obese.

Fats are present in at least small amounts in a wide range of foods. There is thus little cause for concern that you will *not* consume enough fat. Actually, all the fat your body needs during a day amounts to about *one tablespoon* of vegetable oil. Most Americans face the opposite concern—consuming excessive amounts of dietary fat. Fat accounts for about 35% of the calorie intake in the typical American diet, which is higher than the 30% level recommended by health officials. A high-fat diet is a major culprit in the two leading killers, heart disease and cancer. Eating less fat can lower the risk of heart disease and certain types of cancer, such as colon cancer and prostate cancer.

Close-up
Taking out the fat
T0501

The list of high-fat foods is practically endless. A small sampling includes cakes and cookies; fatty cuts of beef; poultry skin; lamb and pork products; dairy foods such as whole milk, sour cream, mayonnaise, cheese, yogurt, butter,

**Fats** Organic compounds that form the basis of fatty tissue of animals, including humans, and are also found in some plants.

and ice cream; nuts and seeds; lard, shortening, and oils used in cooking; margarine; and salad dressings. One reason why high-fat foods taste so good is that fats absorb and retain the natural flavors of foods, which enhances their taste.

Some sources of fat in our diet can be clearly seen, such as the "marble" in steak. But most of the fat we consume is not so obvious. Are you aware that the average blueberry muffin you pick up on the way to work may contain a whopping 34 grams of fat, almost as much as a dish of ice cream or two Twinkies?[9] Dieters may opt for a Caesar salad for lunch without realizing they are loading up on 38 grams of fat, more fat than they'd consume if they downed a burger and fries. Confused about fat in the foods you eat? Make it a habit to check the fat content on the nutritional labels that are required on all prepared foods. Substitute low-fat alternatives. A bagel, for instance, has but a fraction of the fat of a blueberry or raisin-bran muffin. Preparing a salad without egg and cheese and skimping on the dressing brings the fat content way down. But don't mistake low fat for low calories. Some low-fat or even fat-free snack foods, for example, are loaded with calories, largely because of added sugar. When reading food labels, check both fat and calories.

**Close-up**
Healthy chips and dips?
T0502

## How Much Fat Should You Consume?

According to health officials in both the U.S. and Canada, fat intake should not exceed 30% of daily calorie consumption. To figure out your own fat limit, take the number of calories you consume daily and multiply that figure by 0.3 (30%). Then divide by 9 (1 gram of fat contains 9 calories). The result equals the recommended maximum number of grams of fat you should consume daily. A quick conversion table for selected calorie levels is shown in Table 5.2.

**TABLE 5.2**

**Amount of Fat That Provides 30% of Calories at Specified Calorie Levels[10]**

| Calories per Day in the Diet | Amount of Fat (in grams) That Provides 30% of Calories |
|---|---|
| 1,500 | 50 |
| 2,000 | 67 |
| 2,500 | 83 |
| 3,000 | 100 |

How can you tell how much fat is contained in the foods you eat? Look at the side panels of packaged and prepared foods to see how much fat each serving contains. For foods without labels, use a diet guide that lists the fat content (along with the calories) of various foods.

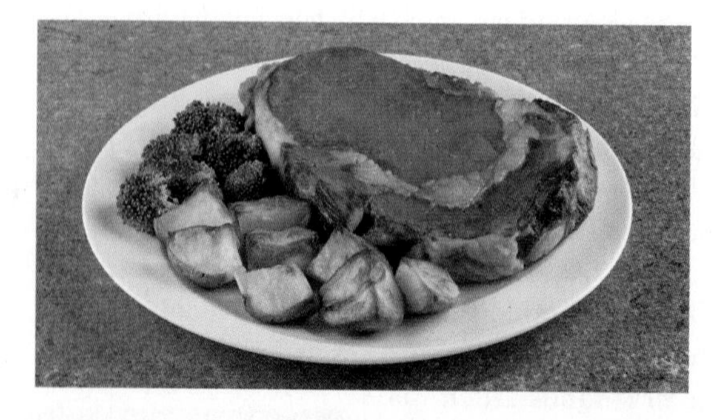

***Cutting Fat from Your Diet?*** Can you think of some ways of cutting back on your intake of dietary fat?

## Types of Fat

Fat consists of chemicals called *fatty acids.* There are three types of fatty acids: *saturated, monounsaturated,* and *polyunsaturated.* Each type differs in the amount of hydrogen it contains. Saturated fatty acids contain the most hydrogen, polyunsaturated the least. Monounsaturated and polyunsaturated fats are also referred to as unsaturated fats. Different kinds of dietary fat contain varying amounts and kinds of fatty acids. The greater the proportion of saturated fat, the harder the food is at room temperature. Most saturated fats are solid at room temperature, including butter, meat fat, cheese, and tropical oils such as coconut and palm oil.

The kinds of fatty acids contained in fat have important health implications. The body converts dietary sources of fat into blood cholesterol, the fatlike substance that can clog arteries and lead to heart disease and strokes. The greater the proportion of saturated fat, the greater the risk that the fat will raise blood cholesterol levels. Consumption of high levels of saturated fat, typically from such sources as meat and dairy products, also increases the risk of certain types of cancer, such as colon cancer.[11] Because of health concerns about fat,

**Close-up**
More on fats
T0503

especially saturated fat, millions of Americans have reduced their overall intake of dietary fat and have switched from foods high in saturated fats to those containing mostly monounsaturated or polyunsaturated fats. Major health organizations like the American Heart Association recommend limiting consumption of saturated fat to less than 10% of the total daily calorie intake.

People have also begun to choose leaner cuts of meat and to trim the visible fat from meat before cooking. Many have even given up eating meat entirely. Many have also switched from butter to low-fat margarine and from whole milk to low-fat or skim milk. Butter consumption in the U.S. fell by 43% from 1961 to 1989 as Americans became persuaded that the unsaturated fats found in margarine were a healthier choice than the saturated fats contained in the butter.[12] But . . .

**Smart Reference**
Chewing the fat
R0501

**Margarine—The Healthier Choice?** Some forms of margarine contain a type of fatty acid, **trans-fatty acid,** that raises blood cholesterol levels as much as the saturated fatty acids found in butter.[13] Trans-fatty acids are produced during the process of hydrogenation that transforms liquid vegetable oils into the familiar hardened form of margarine that is shaped into sticks (as well as vegetable shortening). Margarine manufacturers are looking for ways of hydrogenating liquid vegetable oils that will not produce trans-fatty acids. In the meantime, it may make sense to limit your use of hydrogenated margarine in stick or tub forms, or substitute squeezable liquid margarine in their place. Also limit your intake of partially hydrogenated vegetable oil that is added to many processed food products (check the list of ingredients on the label).

**Vegetable Oils** The vegetable oils we use in salad dressings and cooking contain varying proportions of saturated, monounsaturated, and polyunsaturated fats. The differences among them lie in their relative proportions of these fats. Some vegetable oils are high in saturated fat, such as coconut and palm oil, while others consist predominantly of monounsaturated fats (olive, canola, peanut, walnut, and avocado oils) or polyunsaturated fats (soybean, corn, safflower, sunflower, and cottonseed oils). It makes good health sense to stick to oils low in saturated fat.

The oil that has long given Italian cooking its distinctive flavor—olive oil—has gained in popularity as more people have become aware of the need to reduce saturated fat in their diet. Canola oil contains the lowest level of saturated fat of any of the oils. Its light flavor makes it a good choice in baked goods (olive or peanut oil may overpower the taste of bakery items) as well as in salad dressings and sauces.

We shouldn't think of vegetable oils, however, even the monounsaturated or polyunsaturated varieties, as health foods. All vegetable oils are 100% fat. Polyunsaturated and monounsaturated fats may be less unhealthy than saturated fats, but you should limit fats in general, not just saturated fats. Table 5.3 gives some suggestions for cutting fat from your diet.

Making healthy food choices does not require that you eliminate all sources of fat from your diet. Eating an occasional ice-cream bar or enjoying a steak dinner can still fit within a healthy diet, so long as you limit the overall amount of fat in your diet, especially saturated fat.

**Cholesterol** Few words have become as strongly linked in the public's perception of health risks as **cholesterol.** Just what is cholesterol? Is it bad for us?

**Talking Glossary**
Cholesterol
G0502

Cholesterol is a natural, fatlike substance found in body cells of humans and animals. The body makes use of cholesterol in the formation of hormones and cell membranes. Cholesterol is found in the lean and the fat of meat and in animal byproducts, such as eggs, milk, and other dairy products. Egg yolks and organ meats like liver and kidney meats contain the highest concentrations of dietary sources of cholesterol. One egg yolk, for example, contains about ten times the amount of cholesterol found in one ounce of meat, poultry, or fish. Cholesterol is not found in any foods derived from plants.

The body actually makes all the cholesterol it requires on its own. We do not need to consume additional cholesterol in our diets. Herein lies the problem: Since cholesterol is present in all animal tissue, including meat, poultry, dairy products, shellfish, and, in lesser amounts, fish, we may take in far more cholesterol from our diet than we could possibly use, which can increase the level of cholesterol circulating in our bloodstream. The body also converts dietary fat into blood cholesterol. The problem is that excess blood cholesterol can result in the formation of fatty deposits on artery

**Close-up**
Women and cholesterol
T0504

**Trans-fatty acid** A type of fatty acid produced in the hardening process of margarine that can raise blood cholesterol levels.

**Cholesterol** A natural, fatlike substance found in humans and animals.

walls, impeding the flow of blood to vital organs and increasing the risk of heart attacks and strokes.

Blood cholesterol is usually considered high when it exceeds 200 to 240 milligrams per deciliter of blood. The culprit in clogging arteries is the so-called bad form of cholesterol, **low-density lipoprotein (LDL).** A **lipoprotein** is a cluster of fat and protein that serves as a vehicle for transporting fats through the bloodstream. Another type of cholesterol, **high-density lipoprotein (HDL),** is dubbed "good" cholesterol. HDL actually helps lower the risk of cardiovascular disease. It clears away cholesterol deposits from artery walls and brings them to the liver, where they are processed and then excreted from the body.

Talking Glossary
Lipoprotein
G0503

There is no one-to-one relationship between diet and blood cholesterol levels. Some people can follow a diet rich in total fat, saturated fat, and cholesterol and still maintain normal levels of blood cholesterol. Others have elevated blood cholesterol levels even though they follow a low-fat, low-cholesterol diet. For the average person, however, blood cholesterol *is* directly affected by diet. For example, the average person who consumes an extra 200 milligrams of cholesterol per day (about as much cholesterol as found in one egg) can expect a rise in blood cholesterol of about 3 milligrams, which raises the risk of coronary heart disease (CHD) by about 6%.[16] Dietary changes can make a difference. Reducing dietary fat, especially saturated fat and cholesterol, can lower blood cholesterol levels. Health experts believe that for each 1% reduction in the total blood cholesterol levels, the risk of CHD declines by about 2%.[17]

Dietary cholesterol and saturated fat are often confused because both substances can raise the level of blood cholesterol, especially harmful LDL cholesterol. Saturated fat in the diet actually plays a stronger role in determining blood cholesterol levels than dietary cholesterol.[18] That doesn't mean that you should indulge in foods rich in cholesterol. Dietary cholesterol has a sizable though lesser effect than saturated fat on raising blood cholesterol levels.

**Low-density lipoprotein (LDL)** Cholesterol considered bad because it forms fatty deposits that can stick to artery walls and restrict the flow of blood to vital body organs, setting the stage for heart attacks and strokes.

**Lipoprotein** A compound or complex of fat and protein by which fats are transported through the bloodstream.

**High-density lipoprotein (HDL)** Cholesterol considered good because it sweeps away cholesterol deposits from artery walls for elimination from the body, thereby lowering the risk of cardiovascular disease.

TABLE 5.3

**Suggestions for Cutting Fat from Your Diet[14]**

- Choose tasty and nutritious low-fat foods.
- Add little butter, margarine, or oil when cooking or preparing food.
- Choose leaner cuts of meat and trim away visible fat.
- Use oil in place of shortening when baking.
- Switch from whole milk to skim milk or low-fat milk.
- Eat leaner cuts of beef and other meats in moderation. Avoid high-fat meat products such as butterfat, lard, suet, and chicken fat.
- Avoid tropical oils like coconut or palm oil.
- Use low-fat or fat-free yogurt or blender-whipped low-fat cottage cheese in recipes calling for sour cream or mayonnaise.
- Use light or fat-free cream cheese instead of regular cream cheese. Ditto for other types of cheese and for mayonnaise.
- Use low-fat or no-fat tomato sauces—check the nutritional labels.
- Use low-fat margarine rather than butter as a spread on toast or muffins. Better yet, because of the concerns raised over the presence of trans-fatty acids in hard margarine, use squeezable liquid margarine instead of stick margarine.
- Limit the number of egg yolks you consume, including those you use in cooking, to three per week. Use no more than one egg yolk when making a single serving of scrambled eggs. Increase the serving size by using additional egg whites.
- Substitute egg whites for whole eggs when baking. Use two egg whites for each whole egg called for in the recipe.
- Substitute vegetable sources of protein for meat sources.
- Substitute a low-fat for a high-fat snack food. Popcorn is a tasty low-fat alternative to potato chips or other fatty snacks.
- Steam, boil, or bake foods rather than fry them. If you do fry food, use a little vegetable oil instead of butter.
- Season foods with herbs and spices rather than butter and sauces.
- Remove the skin from chicken before cooking. Removing the skin from a half breast of roasted chicken reduces the fat content from 8 grams to 3 grams. It also reduces the calories by about 25%, from 195 to 140.
- Use a rack when cooking meat or chicken to allow the fats to drain off.
- Cook with a nonstick pan instead of fats.
- Avoid meat gravies. Use other seasonings instead.
- Use salad dressings sparingly and limit your use to low-fat or no-fat dressings.

These are some of the ways in which you can reduce dietary fat. Can you think of others?

## HealthCheck

### How Much Fat Is in Your Diet?[15]

Do the foods you eat provide more fat than is good for you? Answer the questions, then see how your diet stacks up.

| How often do you eat: | Seldom or never | 1 or 2 times a week | 3 to 4 times a week | Almost daily |
|---|---|---|---|---|
| 1. Fried, deep-fat fried, or breaded foods? | ☐ | ☐ | ☐ | ☐ |
| 2. Fatty meats such as bacon, sausage, luncheon meats, and heavily marbled steaks and roasts? | ☐ | ☐ | ☐ | ☐ |
| 3. Whole milk, high-fat cheeses, and ice cream? | ☐ | ☐ | ☐ | ☐ |
| 4. High-fat desserts such as pies, pastries, and rich cakes? | ☐ | ☐ | ☐ | ☐ |
| 5. Rich sauces and gravies? | ☐ | ☐ | ☐ | ☐ |
| 6. Oily salad dressings or mayonnaise? | ☐ | ☐ | ☐ | ☐ |
| 7. Whipped cream, table cream, sour cream, and cream cheese? | ☐ | ☐ | ☐ | ☐ |
| 8. Butter or margarine on vegetables, dinner rolls, and toast? | ☐ | ☐ | ☐ | ☐ |

*Several answers in the last two columns means you may have a high fat intake. Is it time to cut back on foods high in fat?*

Some foods, such as red meat, are rich in both fat and cholesterol. Eggs and organ meats are high in cholesterol but have moderate amounts of fat. Certain plant foods, such as palm or coconut oil and peanut butter, have high levels of saturated fat but no cholesterol. Health officials recommend limiting intake of foods rich in cholesterol, total fat, and saturated fat. Don't be misled by food manufacturers who boast that their products are low in cholesterol while conveniently ignoring their fat content.

The National Cholesterol Education Program recommends limiting dietary cholesterol to less than 300 milligrams per day. The average daily intake of dietary cholesterol among women in the U.S. is 304 milligrams, which only slightly exceeds the recommended level. Men, on the other hand, average 435 milligrams a day and so have to cut their intake by an average of 135 milligrams, or more than 30%, to meet the recommended guidelines.

How can you reduce your cholesterol intake? You can start by becoming aware of the cholesterol content of the foods in your diet and reducing your intake of those that are rich in cholesterol. Limiting the amount of meat and egg yolks you consume can go a long way toward reducing your cholesterol intake. Try reducing the size of your meat portions and substituting vegetable sources of protein for meat several times a week. Switch to low-cholesterol products (the cholesterol contents of products are now listed on food labels). Limit the number of egg yolks you use or substitute egg whites whenever possible. Or skip egg dishes altogether. Be aware of hidden sources of cholesterol, such as baked goods that are prepared with egg yolks or lard. Substitute grain products or popcorn when snacking.

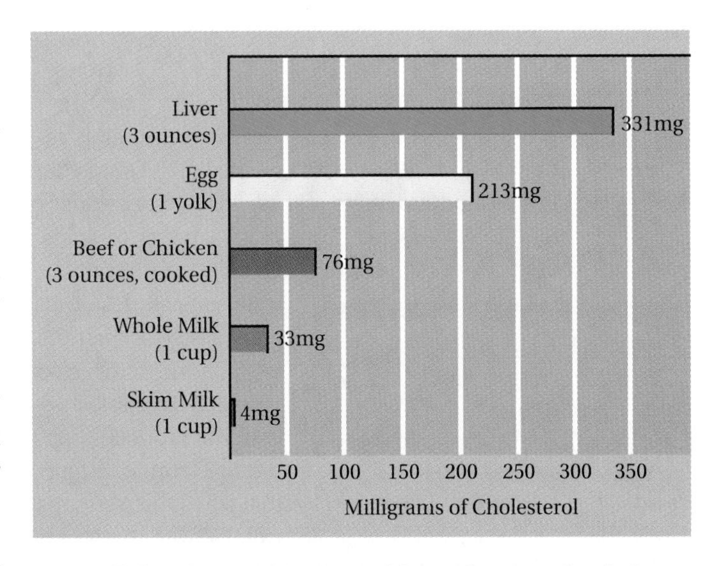


**Figure 5.1** ***Cholesterol Content of Some Common Foods*** Some of the highest cholesterol counts are found in organ meats, like liver, and in dairy products.

TABLE 5.4

**Foods High in Cholesterol and Saturated Fats, and More Healthful Foods**

| Foods High in Cholesterol and/or Saturated Fats | More Healthful Foods |
|---|---|
| Bacon and sausage | Beans |
| Beef | Bagels |
| Butter, lard | Breads |
| Cake | Cereals (most; read the contents) |
| Cheese | Chicken (white meat; skinless; broiled, baked, or barbecued) |
| Coconut | Egg whites |
| Crab | Fish (baked, broiled) |
| Cream (Half & Half) | Fruits |
| Croissants | Lean meats (broiled, in moderation) |
| Eggs (yolks) | Legumes |
| Frankfurters and luncheon meats | Nonfat milk and dairy products |
| French fries | Nonfat yogurt |
| Fried foods | Pasta |
| Ice cream (ice milk) | Peas |
| Lobster | Popcorn (no butter) |
| Organ meats (liver, etc.) | Taco sauce |
| Palm oil | Tomato sauces (meatless) |
| Pie | Turkey (without skin—watch the dressing and gravy) |
| Potato chips | Vegetables |
| Salad dressing (most) | Whole-grain products |
| Shrimp | |
| Whole milk | |

Table 5.4 lists some common foods that are high in both cholesterol and saturated fats, along with some healthful alternatives.

**Olestra—In Search of a Fat Substitute** The first fat substitute, olestra (brand name Olean) was approved by the Food and Drug Administration (FDA) in 1996 and introduced to the market in Pringles potato chips and some other salty snack foods. Synthesized from sugar and fatty acids, olestra gives foods the taste and texture of fat, but it has no calories or fat and passes through the body in an undigested state. The manufacturer of the product, Procter & Gamble, hopes that it will help Americans lower their fat intake (and, of course, boost sales of potato chips and other snacks). However, health experts claim that it can have unhealthy side effects. It can cause diarrhea and abdominal cramping and strip the body of important fat-soluble vitamins, including A, D, E, and K, and plant pigments called **carotenoids,** such as **beta-carotene,** which may have disease-preventive benefits. Carotenoids are found in various green and yellow vegetables and in yellow fruits and vegetable oils. They give fruits their yellow, orange, and red coloring.[19]

Procter & Gamble has taken steps to add to olestra some of the vitamins that may be lost but has not replaced the carotenoids. Nor do we know if adding vitamins to olestra can offset the loss of the dietary vitamins it depletes. Critics are also concerned that offering a fat substitute may encourage people to binge on snack foods, which are still high in calories and can add excess weight. The *University of California at Berkeley Wellness Letter,* a widely respected health newsletter, is not persuaded that olestra is a healthy choice. It urges Americans to "just say no" to olestra.[20]

**Carotenoids** Types of plant pigments (beta-carotene is one) that may have disease-preventive benefits.

**Beta-carotene** A type of carotenoid from which the body manufactures vitamin A, found in rich supply in carrots, sweet potatoes, and spinach.

**Vitamins** Organic substances required in minute amounts to serve a variety of vital roles in metabolism, growth, and maintenance of bodily processes.

**Talking Glossary**

Carotenoids G0504

Beta-carotene G0505

**think about it!**

- **What kinds of dietary fats are there? How do fats contribute to your health? How are fats harmful to your health?**
- **Do you consume enough fats? Too much? What are your favorite food sources of fats?**
- **What is cholesterol? What are some of the connections between diet and cholesterol levels in the bloodstream?**

**critical thinking** **Has this chapter changed your ideas about the role of fat in nutrition and health? If so, how?**

**Smart Quiz**

Q0503

## VITAMINS

**Vitamins,** found in small amounts in many foods, are organic compounds that are needed to maintain a variety of vital functions in the body. One important function they serve is to help regulate *metabolism,* the chemical process by which food is converted into energy and body tissue. Table 5.5 (pages 118–119) contains the recommended daily allowances, or RDAs, for essential vitamins and

WORLD OF *diversity*

## Ethnic Food–Eating Out, Eating Smart

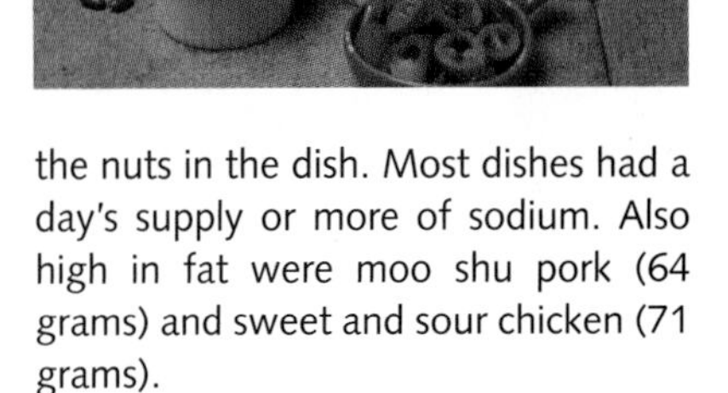

Many of us enjoy food from other countries and cultures, but how are we to know that what we are eating is really healthy for us? A leading consumer watchdog organization, the Center for Science in the Public Interest (CSPI), recently evaluated the nutritional value of offerings in a number of ethnic food restaurants, including Mexican, Italian, and Chinese restaurants.[21] Here is a summary of their main findings:

### Viva Mexican Food!

First the good news. The foundations of Mexican food, beans, rice, and tortillas, together with grilled fish or skinless chicken, can be quite healthy. So what's the bad news? Mexican dishes, at least those typically served in Mexican restaurants in the U.S. (as opposed to the food that Mexicans themselves consume) are so laden with fatty additions, like cheese, sour cream, and guacamole, that they are the food equivalent of a heart attack waiting to happen.

The CSPI sampled the fare in some popular Mexican restaurants like Chi Chi's, El Torito, and Chevy's. They found that many menu selections contained more total fat, more saturated fat, and more sodium than one should eat during an entire day. For instance, one beef burrito with beans, rice, sour cream, and guacamole registered 1,639 calories and exceeded the total daily values for fat, saturated fat, and sodium.* The worst offender, a main dish consisting of two chiles with beans and rice, contained 1,578 calories and tipped the scale at about 150% of the daily totals for fat, saturated fat, and sodium. And don't forget those tasty but oh-so-fatty appetizers, like nachos. A serving of 50 tortilla chips without cheese and guacamole contains 645 calories and accounts for about three-fourths of the daily fat value. But nachos (tortilla chips smothered in cheese and guacamole) logged in at 136% of the daily fat value and contained 1,362 calories. As the CSPI reviewers put it, if they're out of nachos, you might as well ask the waiter for a stick of butter and some salt.

Are there healthier alternatives for those who savor the taste of Mexican food? Fortunately, yes, but you have to be careful about the add-ons. Chicken fajitas, for instance, consisting of strips of chicken breast with sauteed peppers and onions, wrapped in flour tortillas, was the least fatty entree sampled by the CSPI staffers. But make sure to have it plain—no sour cream or guacamole, please. Or spread a tablespoon of salsa over it. Salsa adds flavor but little fat and sodium. A chicken or beef burrito is also a good alternative, but skip the cheese or sour cream. Sticking to rice and beans will save you calories and fat, but CSPI found that the typical restaurant serving of Mexican rice (3/4 cup) contained more than 800 milligrams of sodium, about a third of the daily maximum. The beans had almost as much. Then too, many restaurants offer refried beans that are cooked with fat, such as lard, bacon, or cheese. Order plain beans instead.

### Chinese Food: Eat It the Chinese Way, Not the American Way

Rice is the staple of the Chinese diet. The typical Chinese family prepares dishes that are mostly rice with a little added meat or fish. Americans who eat in Chinese restaurants prefer dishes with lots of meat (read "high fat") and rice on the side (or not at all). CSPI tested dishes from 20 Chinese restaurants in Washington, D.C., Chicago, and San Francisco. They found that fat content ranged from a respectable 19 grams (for stir-fried vegetables and Szechuan shrimp) to an incredible 76 grams (for kung pao chicken), which exceeds the recommended value for daily fat intake, largely as the result of the nuts in the dish. Most dishes had a day's supply or more of sodium. Also high in fat were moo shu pork (64 grams) and sweet and sour chicken (71 grams).

The CSPI offers a three-step solution to those who would sooner move to the North Pole than give up Chinese food:

1. *Increase your rice portion.* Follow the guideline of one cup entree to one cup rice. When you pile on the rice, it increases the number of portions but lowers the fat and sodium content of each portion.
2. *Order steamed vegetables.* Steamed vegetables are high in nutrition and low in fat, calories, and sodium. By adding steamed vegetables to your meal, you're likely to cut down on the meat portion.
3. *Practice the "forklift."* The Chinese typically transfer the entree from the sauce dish to a rice bowl before eating it. In this way, more of the sauce stays on the plate rather than winding up in the mouth.

Let us also suggest that you stick to white rice or brown rice (not fried rice) and avoid dishes that are breaded and deep fried.

### Italian Food—Mangia!

Ah, the many delights of Italian food, from exquisite pastas to the finest scallopine and parmigiana. But is it healthy? It certainly can be, as long as you watch the fat and cholesterol content. But beware: Many Italian dishes are laden with fat, probably none more than fettucine alfredo (noodles smothered in a cream- and cheese-based sauce), which has been called "a heart attack on a plate." According to the CSPI test, a dish of fettuccine alfredo contains as much saturated fat as *three pints* of Breyer's butter almond ice cream! Eggplant parmigiana contains as much fat as five egg rolls. Order a serving of fried calamari and you'll consume more cholesterol than a four-egg omelet. On the other hand, an entree (3.5 cups) of spaghetti with tomato sauce contains a respectable 17 grams of fat and some 849 calories. But switch to a meat sauce, and the fat content rises substantially to 25 grams and the calories to 918. Dishes laden with cheese pile on the fat, such as eggplant parmigiana (2.5 cups: 1,209 calories, 62 grams fat), cheese manicotti (1.5 cups: 695 calories, 38 grams fat), and lasagna (2 cups: 958 calories, 53 grams fat). Topping the list is—you guessed it—fettucine alfredo, at nearly 1,500 calories and an incredible 97 grams of fat for a 2.5-cup serving.

If you enjoy Italian food (as your authors do), here are some suggestions for making healthier choices:

1. *Eat more pasta, less meat.* As a side dish or entree, pasta is low in fat, sodium, and calories, and is delicious to boot! Avoid cream or meat sauces and stick to a good tomato sauce.
2. *Avoid dishes covered in cheese.* Cheese dripping over your rigatoni or eggplant, or baked into your manicotti or lasagna, may get your mouth watering, but watch out for the calories and fat it contains.
3. *Ask for vegetables.* Add vegetables to your entree. Not only are vegetables healthy for you, but they may help you feel full without eating as much meat or cheese. But ask the waiter to prepare your vegetables without butter, oil, or a cream sauce.

All in all, Mexican, Chinese, or Italian food, like other ethnic foods, can be healthy for you, as long as you make smart choices when dining out or preparing these dishes yourself.

* Daily values consisted of 65 grams of fat, 20 grams of saturated fat, and 2,400 milligrams of sodium.

## Recommended Dietary Allowances[23] [a,b,c]

| Category | Age (years) or Condition | Weight[d] (kg) | Weight[d] (lb) | Height[d] (cm) | Height[d] (in) | Protein (g) | Fat-Soluble Vitamins: Vitamin A (μg) | Vitamin D (μg) | Vitamin E (mg) | Vitamin K (μg) |
|---|---|---|---|---|---|---|---|---|---|---|
| *Infants* | 0.0–0.5 | 6 | 13 | 60 | 24 | 13 | 375 | 7.5 | 3 | 5 |
| | 0.5–1.0 | 9 | 20 | 71 | 28 | 14 | 375 | 10 | 4 | 10 |
| *Children* | 1–3 | 13 | 29 | 90 | 35 | 16 | 400 | 10 | 6 | 15 |
| | 4–6 | 20 | 44 | 112 | 44 | 24 | 500 | 10 | 7 | 20 |
| | 7–10 | 28 | 62 | 132 | 52 | 28 | 700 | 10 | 7 | 30 |
| *Males* | 11–14 | 45 | 99 | 157 | 62 | 45 | 1,000 | 10 | 10 | 45 |
| | 15–18 | 66 | 145 | 176 | 69 | 59 | 1,000 | 10 | 10 | 65 |
| | 19–24 | 72 | 160 | 177 | 70 | 58 | 1,000 | 10 | 10 | 70 |
| | 25–50 | 79 | 174 | 176 | 70 | 63 | 1,000 | 5 | 10 | 80 |
| | 51 + | 77 | 170 | 173 | 68 | 63 | 1,000 | 5 | 10 | 80 |
| *Females* | 11–14 | 46 | 101 | 157 | 62 | 46 | 800 | 10 | 8 | 45 |
| | 15–18 | 55 | 120 | 163 | 64 | 44 | 800 | 10 | 8 | 55 |
| | 19–24 | 58 | 128 | 164 | 65 | 46 | 800 | 10 | 8 | 60 |
| | 25–50 | 63 | 138 | 163 | 64 | 50 | 800 | 5 | 8 | 65 |
| | 51 + | 65 | 143 | 160 | 63 | 50 | 800 | 5 | 8 | 65 |
| *Pregnant* | | | | | | 60 | 800 | 10 | 10 | 65 |
| *Lactating* | 1st 6 months | | | | | 65 | 1,300 | 10 | 12 | 65 |
| | 2nd 6 months | | | | | 62 | 1,200 | 10 | 11 | 65 |

[a]The allowances, expressed as average daily intakes over time, are intended to provide for individual variations among most normal people as they live in the United States under usual environmental stresses. Diets should be based on a variety of common foods in order to provide other nutrients for which human requirements have been less well defined.

[b]Estimated safe and adequate daily intake for adults of other vitamins and minerals: biotin, 30–100 μg; pantothenic acid, 4.0–7.0 mg; copper, 1.5–3.0 mg; manganese, 2.0–5.0 mg; fluoride, 1.0–4.0 mg; chromium, 50–200 μg; molybdenum, 75–250 μg.

minerals. Table 5.6 (pages 120–121) lists the functions and dietary sources of vitamins, as well as the problems that can arise from getting too little or too much of these essential nutrients.

## Types of Vitamins

There are 13 known vitamins, which are divided into two major classes, *fat-soluble vitamins* and *water-soluble vitamins.* Fat-soluble vitamins—A, D, E, and K—are carried in the fats we eat and are stored in the liver and in fatty tissues in the body where they can accumulate until needed.[22] Water-soluble vitamins, such as the B vitamins and vitamin C, travel freely in the bloodstream, and excess amounts are excreted in the urine rather than stored in body tissues.

Some vitamins are synthesized by the body while others must be obtained directly from external sources, such as foods or supplements. Vitamin D, for example, is a vitamin that the body itself manufactures in response to ultraviolet light, such as sunlight. It is possible to get all the vitamin D you need by exposing yourself to sunlight or ultraviolet light. But factors such as cloud cover, season of the year, latitude, and coverage of the skin with clothing limit the amount of direct sunlight most people receive. Thus, most of us must obtain additional vitamin D from dietary sources or supplements. Some substances, called *provitamins,* are converted by the body into vitamins. Beta-carotene, for example, is classified as a provitamin because it is converted into vitamin A during metabolism.

In most cases, we can get all the vitamins we need through a balanced diet. Vitamin A, for example, is found in orange produce, such as sweet potatoes and carrots, and in deep green vegetables. Citrus fruits and juices are abundant sources of vitamin C. All the vitamin A and D we need can be obtained from fortified dairy products. Vitamin B is plentiful in vegetables, legumes,

**TABLE 5.5**

| Water-Soluble Vitamins | | | | | | | Minerals | | | | | | |
|---|---|---|---|---|---|---|---|---|---|---|---|---|---|
| Vitamin C (mg) | Thiamin (mg) | Riboflavin (mg) | Niacin (mg) | Vitamin $B_6$ (mg) | Folate (μg) | Vitamin $B_{12}$ (μg) | Calcium (mg) | Phosphorus (mg) | Magnesium (mg) | Iron (mg) | Zinc (mg) | Iodine (μg) | Selenium (μg) |
| 30 | 0.3 | 0.4 | 5 | 0.3 | 25 | 0.3 | 400 | 300 | 40 | 6 | 5 | 40 | 10 |
| 35 | 0.4 | 0.5 | 6 | 0.6 | 35 | 0.5 | 600 | 500 | 60 | 10 | 5 | 50 | 15 |
| 40 | 0.7 | 0.8 | 9 | 1.0 | 50 | 0.7 | 800 | 800 | 80 | 10 | 10 | 70 | 20 |
| 45 | 0.9 | 1.1 | 12 | 1.1 | 75 | 1.0 | 800 | 800 | 120 | 10 | 10 | 90 | 20 |
| 45 | 1.0 | 1.2 | 13 | 1.4 | 100 | 1.4 | 800 | 800 | 170 | 10 | 10 | 120 | 30 |
| 50 | 1.3 | 1.5 | 17 | 1.7 | 150 | 2.0 | 1,200 | 1,200 | 270 | 12 | 15 | 150 | 40 |
| 60 | 1.5 | 1.8 | 20 | 2.0 | 200 | 2.0 | 1,200 | 1,200 | 400 | 12 | 15 | 150 | 50 |
| 60 | 1.5 | 1.7 | 19 | 2.0 | 200 | 2.0 | 1,200 | 1,200 | 350 | 10 | 15 | 150 | 70 |
| 60 | 1.5 | 1.7 | 19 | 2.0 | 200 | 2.0 | 800 | 800 | 350 | 10 | 15 | 150 | 70 |
| 60 | 1.2 | 1.4 | 15 | 2.0 | 200 | 2.0 | 800 | 800 | 350 | 10 | 15 | 150 | 70 |
| 50 | 1.1 | 1.3 | 15 | 1.4 | 150 | 2.0 | 1,200 | 1,200 | 280 | 15 | 12 | 150 | 45 |
| 60 | 1.1 | 1.3 | 15 | 1.5 | 180 | 2.0 | 1,200 | 1,200 | 300 | 15 | 12 | 150 | 50 |
| 60 | 1.1 | 1.3 | 15 | 1.6 | 180 | 2.0 | 1,200 | 1,200 | 280 | 15 | 12 | 150 | 55 |
| 60 | 1.1 | 1.3 | 15 | 1.6 | 180 | 2.0 | 800 | 800 | 280 | 15 | 12 | 150 | 55 |
| 60 | 1.0 | 1.2 | 13 | 1.6 | 180 | 2.0 | 800 | 800 | 280 | 10 | 12 | 150 | 55 |
| 70 | 1.5 | 1.6 | 17 | 2.2 | 400 | 2.2 | 1,200 | 1,200 | 320 | 30 | 15 | 175 | 65 |
| 95 | 1.6 | 1.8 | 20 | 2.1 | 280 | 2.6 | 1,200 | 1,200 | 355 | 15 | 19 | 200 | 75 |
| 90 | 1.6 | 1.7 | 20 | 2.1 | 260 | 2.6 | 1,200 | 1,200 | 340 | 15 | 16 | 200 | 75 |

[c] Estimated minimum requirements of healthy adults: sodium, 500 mg; chloride, 750 mg; potassium, 2,000 mg.

[d] Weights and heights of reference adults are actual medians for the U.S. population of the designated age. The use of these figures does not imply that the height-to-weight ratios are ideal.

*Note:* The RDAs are the recommended levels set by the National Academy of Sciences for daily intake of essential nutrients. They are designed to prevent nutritional deficiencies and meet the nutrient needs of practically all healthy people in the United States, but are not meant to apply to people with special nutritional needs.

### Vitamins—Functions, Dietary Sources, Deficiency Syndromes, and Risks Associated with Excesses[24]

| Vitamins | Functions | Sources |
|---|---|---|
| **Fat-Soluble Vitamins** | | |
| *Vitamin A* | Involved in vision, growth, reproduction, immune system functioning, repair of body tissues, and maintenance of skin and mucous membranes. | Eggs, carrots, spinach, liver, red peppers, vegetable-based soups, and whole-milk products. |
| *Vitamin D* | Aids in bone formation and helps maintain proper balance of minerals through the absorption and metabolism of calcium and phosphorus. | Fortified foods (vitamin D milk), eggs and egg yolk, margarine, butter, sunlight, saltwater fish, fish oils, liver, and carrots. |
| *Vitamin E* | Traps free radicals, helping to protect cells from damaging effects of oxidation. | Vegetable oils, margarine, green leafy vegetables, wheat germ, oats, barley, peanuts, whole-grain cereals, shellfish, salmon, and some fruits such as apricots, apples, and peaches. |
| *Vitamin K* | Necessary for proper protein formation and regulation of blood coagulation. | Found in greater amounts in green leafy vegetables, such as spinach, kale, and broccoli, but also in meats, milk, eggs, other dairy products, and other vegetables such as cauliflower and cabbage. |
| **Water-Soluble Vitamins** | | |
| *Vitamin C* | Important for metabolism, formation of proteins and collagen, destruction of free radicals, immune system functioning, and healing. | Citrus fruits, red and green peppers, broccoli, spinach, tomatoes, collard greens, potatoes, liver, kidney, and in smaller amounts in fish, poultry, other meats, eggs, and dairy foods. |
| *Thiamine (Vitamin $B_1$)* | Involved in metabolism and nerve functioning. | Fortified and whole grains (whole-grain wheat and rye, oatmeal, brown rice), brewer's yeast, liver, green peas, and pork. |
| *Riboflavin (Vitamin $B_2$)* | Helps convert bodily fuels to energy and is important for healthy skin. | Meats, poultry, fish, dairy products, green leafy vegetables, beef, pork, lamb, and enriched breads. |
| *Niacin* | Plays an important role in metabolism and tissue respiration. | Meat (beef and lamb), poultry, milk, eggs, tuna, corn meal, rice, peanuts, and in various cereals, especially those made from wheat bran and whole-grain wheat. |
| *Vitamin $B_6$* | Important for enzymatic reactions and nerve functioning. | Meat, poultry, chicken, fish, liver, kidney, pork, eggs, rice, soy beans, nuts, bananas, potatoes, and whole-grain cereals. |
| *Folate* | Important for metabolism of amino acids, synthesis of DNA, and tissue growth. | Liver, yeast, dark-green and leafy vegetables, asparagus, cauliflower, legumes (dry beans and peas), mushrooms, whole wheat, and wheat germ. |
| *Vitamin $B_{12}$* | Important for metabolism, manufacture of red blood cells, and maintenance and growth of nerve cells. | Found only in animal-derived foods, including whole egg and egg yolk, meat, poultry, fish, dairy foods, organ meats (liver and kidney), eggs, and shellfish. |
| *Biotin* | Important for metabolism, fat synthesis, and breakdown of amino acids. | Found in a wide variety of foods including milk, liver, cauliflower, lentils, egg yolks, yeast, certain nuts such as peanuts and walnuts, and certain cereals. |
| *Pantothenic Acid* | Important for metabolism and steroid production. | Meat products such as liver, as well as milk, mushrooms, legumes, avocados, yeast, broccoli, and whole grains. |

TABLE 5.6

| Deficiency Syndromes | Risks of Excesses |
| --- | --- |
| Early deficiency may lead to night blindness and keratinization of hair follicles. Continued deficiency may lead to corneal lesions and irreversible blindness. | Excesses greater than 25,000 IU may lead to hair loss, blurred vision, headaches, vomiting, liver damage, bone abnormalities, and birth defects. |
| Deficiencies can lead to bone loss and rickets. Rickets has become quite rare as the result of the introduction of fortified milk. | Excesses are potentially toxic, especially for young children. Intake of amounts greater than 100 times the RDA may cause calcium deposits that affect muscle function, perhaps including the heart. Excessive amounts may also lead to vomiting, diarrhea, and weight loss. |
| Though quite rare, deficiencies may lead to anemia and nerve damage. | Toxicity is low, even at amounts 100 times the RDA. In unusual cases, very high doses may lead to headaches, nausea, fatigue, and muscular weakness. |
| Deficiencies are associated with hemorrhaging disorders. These are rare and mostly limited to cases of inadequate absorption or metabolism of the vitamin. Newborns, however, are at greater risk. | Syndromes associated with dietary excesses are negligible, even when large amounts of the vitamin are consumed over a period of time. |
| Scurvy, the deficiency syndrome associated with a lack of vitamin C, is believed related to deficiencies in the formation of collagen. Collagen, a fibrous protein, is the major structural component of skin, cartilage, tendon, and connective tissues. | Intake of greater than 20 to 80 times the RDA may lead to gastrointestinal distress, including diarrhea and stomach aches. |
| Deficiency syndromes include **beriberi** and **Wernicke-Korsakoff's syndrome,** seen most often in alcoholics with faulty diets. | Excesses of 100 to 200 times the RDA may lead to headaches, convulsions, paralysis, and heart arrhythmias. |
| Though rare in industrialized countries except for alcoholics with faulty diets, deficiencies can lead to lesions in the mouth and lips, skin problems, edema, and reduced production of blood cells and platelets. | No evidence of toxic effects from dietary excesses of riboflavin. |
| Deficiency syndromes include **pellagra,** a nutritional disorder characterized by skin eruptions, diarrhea, and neurological and psychological problems. Pellagra is typically found in developing countries where the diet is unbalanced. | Flushing, nausea, itching, and blurry vision may occur at amounts greater than 13 times the RDA. Even larger doses may lead to liver problems, jaundice, and gout. |
| Deficiencies can lead to skin disorders, neurological problems, and anemia. | Excesses of 200 times the RDA may lead to numbness of the mouth and hands, difficulty walking, and other neurological problems. |
| Deficiencies may lead to anemia, skin lesions, retarded growth, and problems in cell division and synthesis of DNA and RNA. | Very large doses may lead to convulsions among some people with epilepsy. |
| Deficiencies may lead to anemia, nervous system damage, and possible memory loss and dementia. | No dangers are known to be associated with excess dietary intake. |
| Deficiencies, though rare, may lead to appetite loss, nausea, vomiting, hair loss, muscle pain, depression, skin problems, and weakness. | No dangers are known to be associated with excess dietary intake. |
| Though rare, except under conditions of extreme malnutrition, deficiencies may result in damage to the skin, liver, adrenal glands, and nervous system. | Effects of dietary excess are negligible, though diarrhea and water retention may occur following very high doses. |

**Talking Glossary**
Beriberi, Wernicke-Korsakoff's syndrome
G0506

**Beriberi** A deficiency disorder caused by a lack of the vitamin thiamine. Characterized by difficulties with memory and concentration, fatigue, lethargy, insomnia, loss of appetite, and irritability.

**Wernicke-Korsakoff's syndrome** A deficiency syndrome resulting from a lack of the vitamin thiamine; appears most often in alcoholics who neglect their diets. Characterized by memory loss and confusion.

**Pellagra** A deficiency disorder caused by a lack of the vitamin niacin. Characterized by skin eruptions, diarrhea, neurological disturbances, and psychological problems involving anxiety, depression, and memory deficits for recent events.

***A "Fridge" Full of Vitamins*** Most of us can obtain all the vitamins we need by following a balanced diet that is rich in fruits, vegetables, and whole-grain foods.

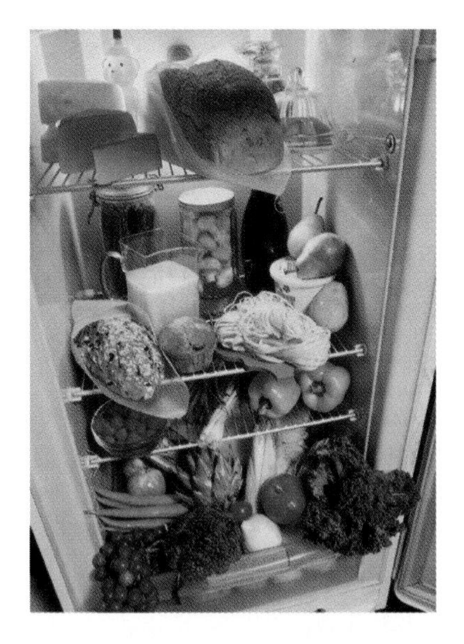

nuts, and whole-grain foods. Because many foods are fortified with vitamins, vitamin deficiencies are rare in our society, even among people who don't watch their diets. That's no excuse for not eating right, however, since poor nutrition may deprive you of other nutrients you may need to maintain your health.

## Vitamin Deficiency Syndromes

Deficiencies or underutilization of particular vitamins can lead to **vitamin deficiency syndromes.** Few of us today have to worry about **scurvy,** a disease caused by vitamin C deficiency that is characterized by sore gums, painful joints, and hemorrhaging. But it was not so for the European explorers who ventured around the world in the fifteenth and sixteenth centuries. The Spanish explorer Vasco de Gama reported losing more than 60% of his crew of 160 sailors to the disease during his voyage around the Cape of Good Hope in 1498. Scurvy was common among seamen on long voyages because their diets at sea lacked citrus fruits or other sources of vitamin C. It wasn't until the early 1600s that a lack of citrus fruits was linked to scurvy. By the early 1800s, the British navy had introduced the custom of issuing daily rations of lemon juice to all its sailors. Today, scurvy is generally limited in our society to two population groups, infants sustained exclusively on cow's milk and older people on limited diets.

**Vitamin deficiency syndromes** Deficiency disorders arising from deficiencies of various vitamins.

**Scurvy** A deficiency disorder resulting from a lack of vitamin C. Characterized by swollen and bleeding gums, weakness, loss of energy, and loosening of teeth.

**Rickets** A bone disorder in children resulting from a lack of vitamin D. Can lead to skeletal deformities and disturbances in growth.

**Osteoporosis** A bone disorder primarily affecting older people in which the bones become porous, brittle, and more prone to fracture.

**Antioxidants** Agents believed to contribute to health by reducing the buildup of free radicals in the body.

Another vitamin deficiency syndrome is **rickets,** a bone disease caused by a lack of vitamin D. The good news about rickets is that it has been virtually eliminated in the U.S. and Canada since milk began to be fortified with the vitamin. Fortification of other dietary staples, such as breads and infant formula, has greatly reduced or virtually eliminated other deficiency syndromes in technological societies such as the U.S. and Canada.

## Health Benefits of Vitamins

Vitamins may have health benefits beyond preventing vitamin deficiency syndromes. For many years now, we have heard claims that vitamin C can prevent the common cold. Vitamin E has long been considered by some to be a sexual energizer and a preserver of youth. Vitamin supplements, even megadoses, have become more popular than ever. Many people believe that the right mixture of vitamins can help them achieve optimal health, prevent cancer and other diseases, or thwart aging itself.

On one health front, evidence indicates that vitamin D can help reduce the risk of **osteoporosis.** Vitamin D may also reduce the risk of colon cancer.[25] Some scientists believe that vitamins A and D may even help reduce the risk of breast cancer. Supplementation of vitamin $B_6$ may help relieve symptoms of PMS and asthma in some cases. Vitamin $B_6$ may also enhance the functioning of the immune system.

Among the vitamin and provitamin substances receiving the most attention from health researchers are those (vitamins C and E and the plant pigment beta-carotene) that function in the body as **antioxidants.** These substances counteract the damaging effects of oxidation, a process that occurs during metabolism.

**Antioxidants—A Role in Preventing Disease?** You can see the corrosive effects of oxidation occurring outside the body in the form of rust, which is produced when oxygen and moisture come into contact with iron surfaces. Scientists believe that oxidation may also "corrode" the body. Oxidation occurs normally during metabolism and leads to the formation of metabolic waste products called **free radicals.** Free radicals are unstable molecules that can wreak havoc on cells by eating away their membranes and damaging their genetic material (DNA).

Damage caused by free radicals may hasten aging and contribute to the development of cancer and some 60 other age-related diseases such as cataracts, immunological disorders, heart disease, strokes, and rheumatoid arthritis.[26] Antioxidants are nutrients that counteract the damaging effects of oxidation by scavenging free radicals and rendering them harmless. Vitamins C and E and beta-carotene are the best known antioxidants. Rich sources of beta-carotene include dark yellowish and orange fruits, dark leafy green vegetables, apricots, pumpkins, carrots, squash, spinach, broccoli, and cantaloupes. Vitamin C is plentiful in citrus fruits, strawberries, and cantaloupes, among other sources. Various grains and vegetables, including vegetable oils, contain vitamin E.

Do antioxidant nutrients help ward off chronic diseases by protecting cells from the accumulative damage of free radicals? A number of studies show that people whose diets contain high levels of antioxidants have a lower than average incidence of cancer.[27] Antioxidants may also help prevent the clogging of blood vessels that can lead to heart attacks and strokes. Vitamin E may help protect the heart by preventing fatty deposits from adhering to artery walls.

Supporting the link between antioxidants and reduced risk of coronary heart disease (CHD), researchers in Finland reported that people whose diets contained the highest levels of vitamin E were least likely to die from CHD.[28] A study of 87,000 nurses in the United States found that nurses who ate five or more servings of carrots a week had a more than two-thirds lower risk of stroke than did those who consumed no more than one serving of carrots a month.[29] Carrots are a particularly rich source of beta-carotene.

But is it the beta-carotene or the vitamin E in the diet that is responsible for reducing the risks of chronic diseases like cancer and heart disease? Perhaps it is the mix of chemical substances naturally found in fruits and vegetables that is responsible for lowering the risk of these diseases. Plants contain more than 1,000 natural chemical substances called **phytochemicals,** many of which either alone or in combination may have disease-preventive benefits. Beta-carotene, for instance, is but one of more than 50 carotenoids found in fruits and vegetables. Carotenoids may need to work as a team in preventing disease, perhaps together with other phytochemicals.[30]

**Talking Glossary**
Phyto-chemicals
G0507

## PREVENTION

### *Should You Take Vitamin Supplements?*

Americans spend more than $3 billion annually on vitamin and mineral supplements.[31] About four in ten people take at least one vitamin or mineral supplement daily. A recent *Newsweek* survey found that seven of ten Americans take vitamin supplements at least occasionally.[32] The question is, should they?

You can obtain all the essential vitamins and minerals needed to meet RDA requirements from diet alone. Yet many of us fail to eat a balanced diet. We may skip meals or skimp on vitamin and mineral-rich foods, like fruits and vegetables. Fewer than one in ten adults in the U.S. consumes the recommended five or more servings of fruits and vegetables a day. Despite the best efforts of health and nutrition experts to get us to eat right, we are not likely to see any wholesale changes in the U.S. diet anytime soon. In light of this, a daily multivitamin may be advisable for those of us who don't eat what we should. Yet what about taking **megadoses** of certain vitamins, such as the antioxidant vitamins C and E, and the provitamin antioxidant beta-carotene?

Supporters of megadosing argue that the RDAs may be enough to prevent diseases like scurvy and rickets but not enough to protect against chronic diseases like heart disease and cancer. Megadosing advocates argue that greater amounts of antioxidant nutrients are needed to ward off the cumulative metabolic cell damage that occurs over time and that may underlie chronic diseases.

Advocates of vitamin E supplementation were buoyed by research findings of two separate studies involving more than 120,000 men and women.[33] These studies showed vitamin E supplements to be associated with a greatly reduced risk of heart disease. Among a sample of initially healthy women 34 to 59 years of age, those taking vitamin E supplements of 100 international units daily (3 times the RDA) for two years or more had a 40% lower risk of developing heart

**Free radicals** Metabolic waste products produced during normal oxidation that may damage cell membranes and genetic material.

**Phytochemicals** Naturally occurring plant chemicals.

**Megadoses** Extremely high doses of a drug or substance.

disease than those who took no supplements.[34] The other study, of men aged 40 to 75 who were initially free of coronary disease, showed a 36% lower risk among those consuming more than 60 units of vitamin E daily compared with those with a daily intake of less than 7.5 units.[35] A word of caution here: We can't be certain that the vitamin E was responsible for the reduced risk of heart disease in these studies. Because researchers did not control who received the supplements, it is possible some other dietary or lifestyle factor associated with people who happen to take vitamin E supplements may have been responsible for their reduced risk of disease.[36] Perhaps these people are more health-conscious in other ways—exercising regularly and limiting their fat intake. At present, we lack sufficient evidence to determine whether taking supplements of vitamin E or other antioxidants in pill form prevents heart disease or cancer, or has other health-enhancing or disease-preventive effects.[37] What we can say is that popping a pill is no substitute for eating right or for adopting other elements of a healthy lifestyle, such as exercising regularly, avoiding smoking, and monitoring your blood pressure.

The early hoopla that surrounded the possible health benefits of beta-carotene supplements faded in the mid-1990s when evidence from a long-term study of more than 22,000 doctors showed that these supplements did not reduce the risk of cancer or heart disease.[38] It is possible that beta-carotene or other antioxidants lose beneficial effects when they are removed from the foods in which they naturally occur. Beta-carotene supplements may actually harm some people. In one study, people at a high risk of lung cancer, including smokers and asbestos workers, who took beta-carotene supplements had a 28% higher rate of lung cancer than others who didn't take supplements.[39] It does not appear that beta-carotene poses a danger to nonsmokers, however.

Until more is known about the safety and benefits of long-term megadoses of antioxidant nutrients, most health experts warn against their widespread use. No government health agency or leading nutritional organization recommends taking doses of antioxidant vitamins that exceed the recommended daily allowances (RDAs).* Excess doses of certain vitamins can be harmful.[40] Megadoses of vitamin D, for example, can lead to calcium buildup in muscle tissue, including the heart. Megadoses of vitamin C (levels exceeding 1,000 mg daily) are a cause of kidney stones.[41] High doses of vitamin E (many nutritionists place the safe limit at around 1,000 IU daily) appear to be safe for most people. However, they may lead to bleeding in some people (especially those taking anticoagulants) and raise the blood pressure. Megadoses of beta-carotene, which the body converts into vitamin A, can yellow the skin and may increase the risk of lung cancer to smokers. Overdosing on vitamin A itself (daily intake exceeding 25,000 IU) can damage the liver. It may be harmful to take supplements in excess of the RDAs of vitamins A, D, or any mineral, or to take more than ten times the RDAs of other nutrients.

* In Canada, the recommended allowances are called the Recommended Nutrient Intakes (RNIs) and are generally similar to the U.S. RDAs.

**Nitrosamines** Cancer-causing chemical substances formed in the stomach following ingestion of nitrates and nitrites.

**Carcinogens** Cancer-causing substances.

**Vitamin C and Disease Prevention** As we have seen, vitamin C, like vitamin E, is an antioxidant that scavenges free radicals. This has led to speculation that vitamin C may have cancer-preventive effects,[43] perhaps by protecting cells from mutations caused by free radicals.

Food preservatives such as nitrates and nitrites that are found in ham, sausage, and other processed meats are converted in the stomach into **nitrosamines,** which are strong **carcinogens** (cancer-causing substances). Vitamin C blocks the formation of nitrosamines in the stomach, which raises the possibility that vitamin C may have an anticancer effect. (Vitamin E also blocks the formation of nitrosamines in the stomach.) However, we lack direct evidence of an anticancer effect of vitamin C (or vitamin E). People whose diets are rich in vitamin C do have a lower risk of some forms of cancer, such as oral, esophageal, gastric, and colorectal cancers.[44] But we do not know whether vitamin C or some other factor is responsible for this effect. Perhaps some other ingredient in vitamin-C-rich fruits and vegetables confers protection against cancer. Or perhaps people who consume higher levels of vitamin C also take better care of their health in other ways.

UCLA researchers recently reported a link between lower mortality and use of vitamin C.[45] They examined the records of more than 10,000 people whose dietary habits were studied in the early 1970s. The researchers found that people who had consumed higher levels of vitamin C (at least 50 or more milligrams daily) in the early 1970s were the ones least likely to die over the next ten years or so. The design of the research does not permit researchers to pinpoint cause and effect. We do not know whether it was vitamin C or some other element in their diets or lifestyles that played the causal role.

TABLE 5.7

## Beyond Beta-Carotene[42]

New claims for the health benefits of various natural remedies appear almost daily. In many cases, it is difficult for consumers to separate the hype from the facts. This table lists some substances that *may* have health benefits. (Notice the emphasis on the word *may:* None of these health benefits have been proven.) Some of these substances may prove to have legitimate health benefits; others may disappear from public attention as health claims fail to be supported by research. Some are dangerous when taken in high doses: Check with your physician or health care provider before taking any supplements. On the other hand, why not increase your intake of fruits and vegetables—including tomatoes, grapefruit, and dark green vegetables like broccoli and spinach—that contain possible disease-fighting substances that nutritionists are beginning to identify?

| Substance | How Obtained | Suspected Health Benefits |
|---|---|---|
| *Garlic* | Garlic cloves, garlic powder, or supplement tablets | May have antioxidant effects that protect against some forms of cancer. Also may inhibit growth of bacteria in the stomach, which may reduce the risk of stomach cancer since some forms of bacteria convert food into cancer-causing substances. May also retard growth of *H. pylori,* the bacterium that causes the great majority of stomach **ulcers.** *H. pylori* has been linked to an increased risk of stomach cancer. Garlic supplementation may reduce cholesterol levels, which may reduce the risk of heart attacks and strokes. Also suspected of reducing the risk of blood clots, which can clog arteries and lead to a heart attack or stroke. |
| *Flavenoids* | Red wine, onions, buckwheat, tea, and most fruits, such as grapes, apples, and cranberries. | Believed to enhance effects of vitamin C. May reduce the risk of some forms of cancer and cardiovascular disease. |
| *Carotenoids* | | Carotenoids may reduce risk of cardiovascular disease and some forms of cancer. Lutein and zeaxanthin are also linked to reduced risk of macular degeneration, the leading cause of blindness in people over the age of 65. |
| *Lycopene* | Tomatoes and tomato products, such as tomato sauce. Lycopene gives tomatoes their red color; also in red peppers, watermelon, guava, and pink grapefruit. | |
| *Lutein, Zeaxanthin* | Collard greens, kale, mustard greens, spinach, broccoli, sweet red peppers, romaine lettuce, okra, corn, hot chili peppers. | |
| *Alpha-carotene* | Carrots, pumpkins, cantaloupes, yellow corn. | |
| *Selenium* | Liver, mushrooms, garlic, fish, asparagus, shellfish, beef, chicken, eggs, whole grains. | May reduce risk of some forms of cancer. Believed to increase antioxidant effects of vitamin E. |
| *Fish Oils (fatty acids found in fish oils, better known as omega-3s)* | Various fish, especially salmon, sardines, mackerel, herring, bluefish, whitefish, and halibut, and in supplement form. | May have modest effects in reducing blood pressure in people with hypertension; may aid in the prevention or treatment of autoimmune diseases like lupus, kidney disease, and rheumatoid arthritis. However, the anticlotting tendencies of fish oils may increase the risk of bleeding and suppress immune functioning in healthy people. As a result of these concerns, health experts do not recommend fish-oil supplements. |
| *Melatonin* | A natural hormone produced in the brain, it is also available in the form of supplement pills. | May help relieve insomnia; some believe that it has anti-carcinogenic effects and may extend life. Possible adverse effects of long-term use of supplements is unknown. May also have short-term side effects, such as grogginess and mild depression. |
| *Ginseng* | Supplement pills. | May help boost immune functioning and improve resistance to stress; some believe it enhances virility. Long-term effects of supplementation are unknown. |
| *Chromium* | A mineral available in supplement form. | Touted as having fat-burning and muscle-building properties. Researchers warn of a possible cancer risk and chromosomal damage associated with use in high doses. |
| *Isoflavones* | Beans, grains, and soy products. | May reduce the risk of some forms of cancer and may slow bone loss in women following menopause. |
| *Indoles* | Cruciferous vegetables such as broccoli, brussels sprouts, cabbage, cauliflower, kale, and turnips. | May reduce the risk of some forms of cancer. |

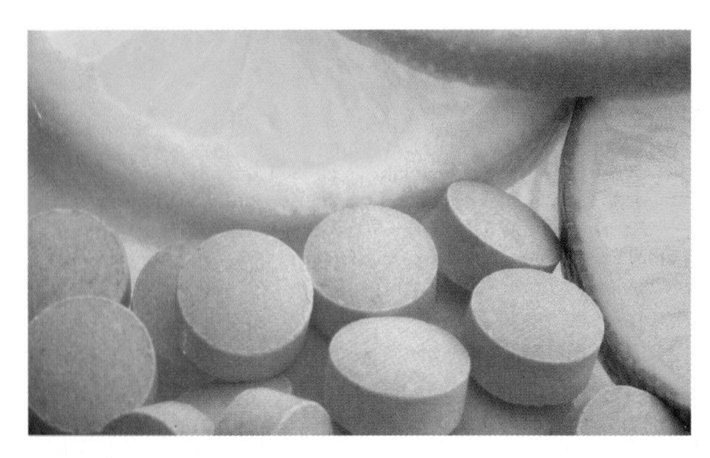

***Vitamin C*** Vitamin C is found in a variety of citrus fruits and in supplement form. Though research continues, we lack direct evidence that taking supplements can help stave off serious illness.

Other potential health benefits of vitamin C have been touted, such as the claim by the late Nobel Prize-winning chemist Linus Pauling that vitamin C can help ward off the common cold. Evidence supporting the claim is mixed. Some studies show no benefits for vitamin C in preventing or fighting colds. Others show limited benefits. Most authorities today agree that vitamin C supplements will not prevent the common cold; however, it may reduce the severity of cold symptoms and the duration of the cold by about a day.[46]

Researchers are investigating other possible health benefits of vitamin C. They suspect that vitamin C can bolster the disease-fighting capability of the immune system. Researchers also suspect that vitamin C may help safeguard the DNA, the genetic material found in chromosomes, in men's sperm.[47] Damaged DNA in sperm has turned up more often in men with low levels of vitamin C in their blood. Damaged DNA in sperm may increase the risk of birth defects in men's offspring. As an antioxidant, vitamin C may help lower the risk of cataracts by reducing damage to the lens of the eye caused by oxidation. Supplemental vitamin C may also reduce the risk of cardiovascular disease by increasing levels of HDL cholesterol and by reducing total cholesterol levels in people with elevated blood cholesterol.[48]

The story of vitamin C in promoting health and preventing disease is still being written. Vitamin C is not the only vitamin that may reduce blood cholesterol. Niacin, too, may help lower blood cholesterol in some people.[49] And vitamin E may reduce the risk of cardiovascular disease by preventing LDL cholesterol from forming plaque in artery walls.

**Folic acid** A B vitamin, also known as folate, that helps prevent neural tube defects and may play a role in preventing heart disease.

**Anencephaly** A fatal congenital defect in which a child is born without a brain or with only a rudimentary brain.

**Spina bifida** A congenital defect in which the child is born with a hole in the tube that surrounds the spinal cord.

**Folic Acid and Birth Defects—Did You Take Your Folic Acid Today?** The U.S. Public Health Service is leading the call for supplementation of **folic acid,** a B vitamin, also known as folate.[50] Why the concern about folic acid? Researchers find that consumption of 400 micrograms (0.4 milligrams) of folic acid during pregnancy can cut in half the risk of severe birth defects known as neural tube defects (NTDs).[51] Neural tube defects include **anencephaly,** in which the child is born without a brain and dies shortly after birth; and **spina bifida,** in which the child is born with a hole in the tube that surrounds the spinal cord. While most children born with spina bifida survive, they often develop mental retardation and other serious problems, including paralysis below the waist and difficulties with bladder or bowel control. NTDs kill or disable nearly 2,500 infants born each year in the U.S. Because NTDs develop early in pregnancy, often at a time before the woman even knows she is pregnant, the Public Health Service recommends that women of reproductive age who could possibly become pregnant (some 58 million by recent counts) should consume 400 micrograms daily of folic acid, which is more than twice the RDA for nonpregnant women. The recommendation applies to *all* sexually active women, even those using contraceptives, since not even the best contraceptive is foolproof.

**Talking Glossary**
Spina bifida
**G0508**

Folic acid is found in such foods as leafy green vegetables, orange juice, and beans. Since women typically consume about half the recommended level of folic acid in their diets, many health experts recommend that sexually active women of reproductive age take a daily multivitamin pill containing the recommended amount of folic acid just to be safe.[52] As of January 1998, all enriched foods including fortified cereals, bread, and pasta were required to be fortified with folic acid—the first new fortification of foods since 1943, when vitamins and iron were added to flour.[53] Most multivitamin pills contain 400 micrograms of folic acid. Yet health officials warn against taking folic acid in doses greater than 400 micrograms because of potential adverse effects.

TABLE 5.8

**Vitamins: Myths vs. Facts**

| Myth | Fact |
|---|---|
| Popping a vitamin pill can correct a poor diet. | Vitamin pills will not compensate for a poor diet. A multivitamin pill can ensure that you receive essential vitamins but will not provide the other nutrients you need for your health. |
| The more vitamins you take, the better. | Excess doses of vitamins can be harmful. Regularly taking just five times the recommended allowance (RDA) of vitamin D can lead to serious liver damage, for example. High doses of niacin (vitamin $B_3$) can also cause liver damage. |
| Vitamin supplements will help boost athletic performance. | Vitamins will not improve your game or increase your performance in sports. |
| Taking "stress vitamins" will help you cope better with emotional problems. | So-called stress vitamins help the body counter the effects of physical stress, such as changes in temperature. There is no evidence that vitamins help people cope with emotional stress. |
| "Natural" vitamins are better than synthetic vitamins. | There is no evidence that your body can tell the difference between natural and synthetic vitamins. |

Folic acid may yet have another important health benefit. Daily intake of 400 micrograms may reduce the risk of coronary heart disease (CHD) by more than 10% in men and 6% in women.[54] Folic acid reduces the levels of a substance in the blood linked to CHD. Low levels of folic acid in the diet are connected with an increased risk of death from CHD.[55]

Smart Quiz
Q0504

**think about it!**

- **What kinds of vitamins are there? How do vitamins contribute to your health?**
- **Do you consume enough vitamins? What are your sources of vitamins?**
- **What does research show about the connections between vitamins and health? (Consider vitamin deficiency syndromes, the common cold, heart disease, and cancer in your answer.)**

**critical thinking** **Agree or disagree and support your answer: Megadosing on vitamins is too much of a good thing.**

## MINERALS

**Minerals** are inorganic elements, like calcium, potassium, sodium, and magnesium, that are essential to health and obtained from food.[56] Like vitamins, minerals are involved in various vital functions in the body, such as the formation of bones and teeth, the transmission of nerve signals through the nervous system, and the manufacture of **hemoglobin** in red blood cells. Hemoglobin is a protein that gives blood its reddish color and that transports oxygen to body cells. Table 5.5 (pages 118–119) lists the RDAs for essential minerals. Table 5.9 (page 128) shows the functions, sources, deficiency syndromes, and risks of excesses of the essential minerals.

Talking Glossary
Hemoglobin
G0509

### Calcium

**Calcium** is the most plentiful mineral in the body. It is the major component of bones and teeth. Virtually all of the body's calcium—99%—is found in bone. Adequate calcium intake is important for bone health in adults as well as children. It is especially important in the prevention of osteoporosis, a bone disease

**Minerals** Inorganic elements obtained from the food we eat that are essential to survival.

**Hemoglobin** A protein in red blood cells that gives blood its reddish color and transports oxygen to body cells.

**Calcium** A mineral essential to the growth and maintenance of bones.

TABLE 5.9

**Minerals—Functions, Dietary Sources, Deficiency Syndromes, and Risks Associated with Excesses[57]**

| Minerals | Functions | Dietary Sources | Deficiency Syndromes | Risks of Excesses |
|---|---|---|---|---|
| *Calcium* | Involved in bone formation, nerve transmission, muscle contraction, and blood coagulation. | Dairy foods including milk, yogurt, and various cheeses; green leafy vegetables such as kale, collard greens, and broccoli; and various types of fish, particularly salmon (with the bones) and sardines. Many foods are fortified with calcium. | Deficiency may increase vulnerability to osteoporosis, a condition involving loss of bone density that makes bones become brittle and more likely to break. | Excess levels interfere with absorption of other minerals and can lead to constipation, increased risk of kidney stones, and problems with kidney function. |
| *Phosphorus* | Important for building bones, energy utilization, and cell reproduction. | Found in a wide variety of foods, including cereal grains, meat, milk, and poultry. | Deficiency syndromes, though rare, may lead to weakness, anorexia, and bone loss. | Excessive amounts can reduce calcium levels in the blood, leading to possible bone loss. |
| *Magnesium* | Important for many bodily processes, including bone mineralization and nerve functioning. | Nuts, legumes (dry beans and peas), cereal grains, bananas, cocoa, seafoods, most dark green vegetables, and milk. | Deficiencies may lead to nausea, muscle weakness, and irritability. | No evidence of harmful effects due to dietary excess in healthy people, although problems may occur in people with kidney disorders. |
| *Iron* | Essential for hemoglobin production (the reddish pigment in red blood cells that carries oxygen). | Meat, poultry, eggs, fish, cereals, fortified grain products, legumes, and green leafy vegetables. | Deficiencies may lead to anemia, weakness, impaired physical performance, and immunological problems. Children with iron deficiency may become lethargic, have reduced attention span, and develop learning problems. | Doses in excess of 100 mg can interfere with the absorption of zinc, which plays an essential role in metabolism and immune functioning. |
| *Zinc* | Involved in healing and growth, protein formation, immune function, DNA synthesis, and sensation of taste. | Variety of foods including meat, liver, poultry, seafoods, shellfish, egg yolks, whole-grain cereals, cocoa, and dry beans and peas. | Deficiencies may impair growth in children, lead to poor wound healing, reduced appetite, skin abnormalities, and impaired immune functioning. | Excesses may lead to gastrointestinal problems, including vomiting, nausea, and diarrhea. |
| *Iodine* | Aids the thyroid in regulating metabolism. | Iodized salt and seafoods. | Deficiencies may lead to thyroid enlargement, goiter, and, less commonly, mental retardation. | Very high doses may depress thyroid functioning. |
| *Selenium* | Destroys free radicals. | Seafoods, meats, grains. | May increase vulnerability to various diseases. | Excess doses from use of supplements may cause gastrointestinal distress. |

that primarily affects older persons, especially postmenopausal women (see Chapter 19). Bone matter is continuously renewed through reabsorption by the body and formation of new bone. The renewal process is why we need calcium throughout our lives—not just during our growth years.

**Meeting Your Calcium Needs** Calcium should be consumed from the foods you eat rather than from supplements, in part because absorption of the mineral is more consistent from dietary sources than from pills. Excess calcium should be avoided, as it can lead to constipation and other problems, such as increased risk of kidney stone formation and problems with kidney function. Excess calcium can also reduce absorption of other necessary minerals, such as iron and zinc. Because of the increased need for calcium during the growth years, the RDA calls for 1,200 milligrams of calcium daily up to the age of 24 and then 800 afterward. Yet women should consume 1,000 milligrams after menopause if they receive estrogen replacement therapy and 1,500 milligrams if they do not.[58] A consensus statement issued by a panel convened by the National Institutes of Health recommended even higher amounts for optimal daily intake: 1,200 to 1,500 milligrams daily for teenagers and young adults; 800 milligrams for men and 1,000 milligrams for women age 25 to 50; 1,000 milligrams for men 51 to 65; and 1,500 milligrams for men over 65 and for women over 50 not taking estrogen (1,000 milligrams for older women taking estrogen).[59]

**Dietary Sources of Calcium** Most dietary sources of calcium are dairy products. One 8-ounce cup of low-fat milk contains 300 milligrams of calcium, more than a third of the adult RDA of 800 milligrams. Other good sources of calcium include yogurt (452 milligrams in an 8-ounce container of plain nonfat), cheeses, fish (especially pink salmon and sardines), and green leafy vegetables, such as broccoli, collard greens, and kale. Many foods are also fortified with calcium. Bone material in our diets, such as the soft bones found in fish such as sardines and salmon, are also rich sources of calcium. Despite the availability of dietary sources of calcium, many Americans fail to consume enough of it and may need a calcium supplement.

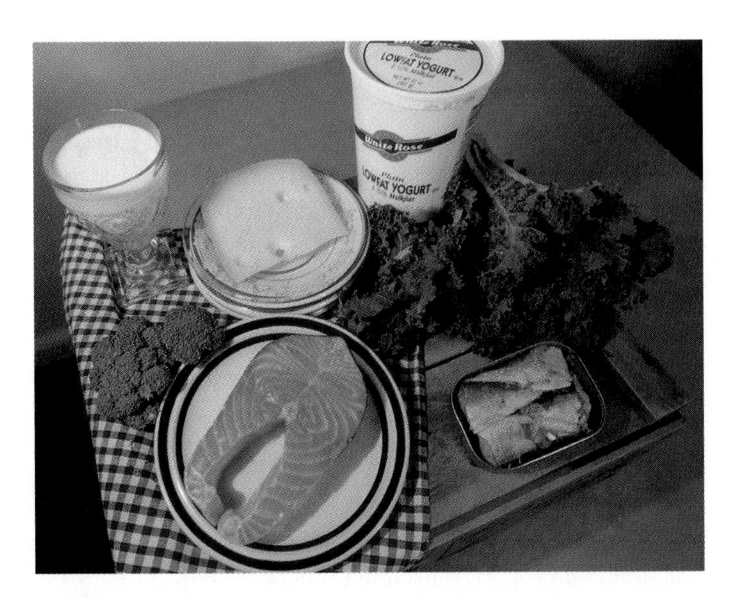


***Sources of Calcium*** Calcium is vital to healthy bones and teeth throughout our lives. Calcium-rich foods include sardines and salmon, broccoli and other green leafy vegetables, and milk and other dairy foods.

**TABLE 5.10**

**Calcium Content of Common Foods[60]**

| Food | Weight or Measure | Calcium (milligrams) |
|---|---|---|
| Plain skim and low-fat yogurts | 1 cup | 350–450 |
| Low-fat flavored and fruited yogurts | 1 cup | |
| Dry nonfat milk | $\frac{1}{4}$ cup | |
| Sardines, with bones | 3 ounces | |
| Some fruited yogurts | 1 cup | 250–350 |
| Skim and low-fat milks | 1 cup | |
| Whole milk, chocolate milk, buttermilk | 1 cup | |
| Swiss and Gruyere cheeses | 1 ounce | |
| Hard cheeses such as Cheddar and Edam | 1 ounce | 150–250 |
| Processed cheeses | 1 ounce | |
| Cheese spreads | 1 ounce | |
| Salmon, with bones | 3 ounces | |
| Collards | $\frac{1}{2}$ cup | |
| Cheese foods | 1 ounce | 50–150 |
| Soft cheeses such as mozzarella, blue, and feta | 1 ounce | |
| Cooked dried beans such as navy, pea, and lima | 1 cup | |
| Turnip greens, kale, dandelion greens | $\frac{1}{2}$ cup | |
| Ice cream and ice milk | $\frac{1}{2}$ cup | |
| Evaporated whole milk | 1 ounce | |
| Cottage cheese | $\frac{1}{2}$ cup | |
| Sherbet | $\frac{1}{2}$ cup | |
| Broccoli | $\frac{1}{2}$ cup | |
| Orange | 1 fresh | |
| Dates, raisins | $\frac{1}{4}$ cup | 20–50 |
| Egg | 1 | |
| Bread, whole-wheat or white | 1 slice | |
| Cabbage | $\frac{1}{2}$ cup | |
| Cream cheese | 1 ounce | |

Table 5.10 lists the calcium content of some common foods. Although milk and other dairy products are among the richest sources of calcium, some people need to avoid these because they cannot digest lactose, the type of sugar found in milk and other dairy products. They must satisfy their calcium needs in other ways or switch to milk products specially formulated for people who are lactose intolerant. Some lactose-intolerant people may need to take calcium supplements in order to obtain sufficient calcium from dietary sources.

### Iron

The metal **iron** forms part of the makeup of hemoglobin. An essential nutrient, iron is found in such foods as meats, eggs, cereals and grains (especially fortified cereal products), legumes, and green leafy vegetables. Iron deficiencies can lead to **anemia,** a condition in which there is too little hemoglobin in the blood to carry enough oxygen to body tissues. Short of anemia, iron deficiencies may result in weakness and reduced physical performance. Iron deficiencies are also linked to reduced immunological functioning. Iron deficiencies in children are associated with various behavioral problems, such as lethargy, short attention span, irritability, and learning disorders. Women need to be especially aware of their iron needs, as they tend to lose iron as the result of menstruation, pregnancy, and breast-feeding. Although there are no reports of iron toxicity from excess intake of dietary sources of iron alone, about 2,000 cases of iron poisoning are reported each year in the U.S., most involving children who swallow medicinal iron supplements.

Twenty-five percent of the iron in the American diet comes from fortified foods, such as enriched breads and breakfast cereals. The form of iron found in enriched foods is of a type that is better absorbed than iron in supplement form. However, some people may need to take additional iron supplements, including pregnant women; menstruating women, especially those who bleed heavily; infants, children, and adolescents whose rapid growth requires high iron intake; long-distance runners and other endurance athletes; dieters whose bodies may eliminate iron during intense, prolonged exercise or who may skimp on foods rich in iron.[61] Before taking any iron supplement, however, consult with your physician. Also, avoid taking high doses exceeding 100 milligrams (six times the RDA). High doses can hinder absorption of zinc, an essential mineral involved in metabolic and immune functioning.

**Iron** An essential mineral, a metallic element that forms part of the makeup of hemoglobin.

**Anemia** A condition involving a lack of hemoglobin in the blood, causing such symptoms as weakness, paleness, heart palpitations, shortness of breath, and lack of vigor.

**Sodium** A metallic element that functions as an electrolyte in the body.

**Electrolyte** A substance that conducts electricity.

**think about it!**

- Which minerals contribute to your health?
- What are your sources of these minerals? Do you consume enough of them? Too much?

Smart Quiz
Q0505

## WATER AND ELECTROLYTES

Water, often called the forgotten nutrient, is essential to life. Water serves a number of vital roles in the body, including transportation of nutrients, the removal of wastes through the blood system, and regulation of body temperature. One-half to perhaps four-fifths of our body weight is water. Each day we need to replenish the 4% or so of our body weight in water that we lose through sweating and the excretion of urine.

Much of the water we need is consumed in the beverages we drink. Yet water is also a major constituent of many solid foods. Many fruits and vegetables, for example, contain between 85 and 95% water. Water depletion can lead to various problems, including heat exhaustion, which can cause unconsciousness and heat stroke. More prolonged water depletion can lead to death.

### Sodium

Talking Glossary
Electrolyte
G0510

**Sodium** is an **electrolyte,** a substance that helps conduct electrical currents. In the body, sodium is involved in the conduction of electrical impulses (nerve signals) through the nervous system. Sodium and the other principal electrolytes in the body, potassium and chloride, are essential dietary nutrients. In addition to its role in the transmission of nerve signals, sodium is vital to muscle functioning. And by attracting water into blood vessels, it helps maintain normal blood volume and blood pressure.

Sodium is found naturally in a wide variety of foods and is added to many foods and beverages for taste. Most all of the sodium Americans consume in their diets is derived from sodium chloride, more commonly called table salt, which consists of about 40% sodium and 60% chloride. Other forms of sodium (sodium bicarbonate and monosodium glutamate) account for less than 10%

of our total dietary sodium intake. We also obtain virtually all of the chloride in our diets from salt.

Most Americans take in far more sodium than they need. A single teaspoon of table salt contains about 2,400 milligrams of sodium and is enough to satisfy the daily level of sodium recommended by the National Academy of Sciences. For some salt-sensitive individuals, excessive salt intake may contribute to hypertension (high blood pressure), a risk factor in heart disease and stroke.[62] Since you wouldn't know if you are salt sensitive until you develop hypertension, it makes good health sense to avoid excess salt intake.

Americans consume about a third of their daily intake of sodium in the form of salt added during cooking or eating. People who shake salt freely at the table may have no idea how much sodium they are adding to their food. Try this simple test to measure the amount of salt you normally add to your food. Cover a plate with wax paper or foil. Salt the plate as you would if it contained food. Collect the salt and measure it. If you used about a quarter of a teaspoon, you can figure that you regularly add 500 milligrams of sodium to your food at each meal. Sodium in the form of salt is added to so many foods that it is difficult to know how much sodium we normally consume. Salt is second only to sugar among the ingredients added by food manufacturers to processed foods. Sodium is added as a preservative and flavor enhancer, and it is especially common in bread and bakery products, cured and processed meats, canned soup and vegetables, soy sauce, and cheese.

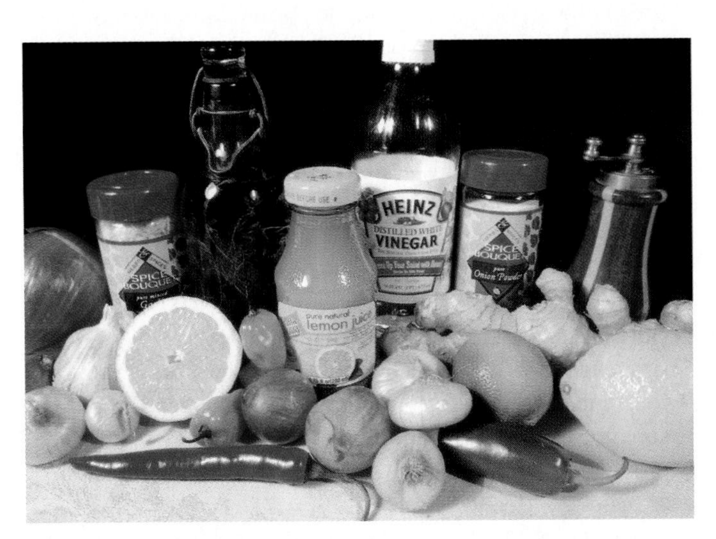


***Looking for That Lost Shaker of Salt?*** People who seek to cut back on salt can use a variety of other spices and condiments to season food.

**Cutting Back on Sodium** Here are some suggestions for cutting back your sodium intake:

1. *Read food labels carefully.* The government now requires packaged foods to list their sodium content per serving. Choose foods that are low in sodium.
2. *Do not add salt during cooking.* Find recipes that are low in sodium content. Also be careful when adding ingredients that are high in salt, such as canned soups and vegetables. Experiment with new spices and herbs in place of salt in your favorite recipes.
3. *Use table salt sparingly if at all.* Substitute other seasonings for salt, such as spices and herbs like garlic, basil, and onion powder. Substitute a squirt of lemon juice or a tablespoon of vinegar for a high-sodium salad dressing. Or switch to a low-sodium dressing. Always taste your food before salting. If you feel you must add salt, limit the amount to one shake.
4. *Balance your meals for sodium content.* Take into account the total sodium content of your meals throughout the day. If you eat a high-sodium food at a particular meal, select a low-sodium food to go along with it. If your lunch was packed with high-sodium foods, eat a dinner low in sodium to help balance things out.
5. *Avoid processed and convenience foods.* Processed and convenience foods typically contain high levels of sodium, except for those marked "low sodium" on the package. Frozen dinners and canned soups, for example, are typically loaded with sodium, as are cured meats and processed meats such as hot dogs and luncheon meats.
6. *Keep the sodium content of food in mind when ordering in a restaurant.* Ask your waiter to have your food prepared with little or no added salt. Avoid ordering foods that come with sauces, which are usually high in sodium, or ask to have the sauce on the side so that you can control how much you use.

## think about it!

**critical thinking** **What are your sources of water and electrolytes?**

- **How do water and electrolytes contribute to your health?**

**critical thinking** **Do you think you should be cutting back on your sodium intake? Why or why not?**

Smart Quiz
Q0506

PREVENTION

## Ensuring Food Safety

While food is needed to sustain life, it can also endanger life. Ensuring food safety is not merely the responsibility of federal and local governments; we all must take measures to ensure our own and our family's safety. The foods we eat can become contaminated by various harmful substances, including disease-causing bacteria and other microorganisms, as well as poisonous substances or **toxins** that can be deposited in our bodies and lead to serious illnesses, including cancer.

**Food-Borne Illnesses** Food can serve as a channel for transmission of disease-causing bacteria and other microorganisms. The term *food poisoning* is used to refer to food-borne illnesses and reactions to toxins produced by food-borne bacteria. Symptoms vary with the type of illness and the amount of the infected material ingested, but they commonly include gastrointestinal complaints like diarrhea and abdominal cramping, fever, vomiting, and exhaustion. Tens of millions of cases of food-borne diarrheal diseases worldwide are reported annually.

Though food-borne illnesses can cause significant distress, they are usually brief and not life-threatening for otherwise healthy people. Yet they can cause serious problems for the very young, the old, or people with compromised immune systems. In all, the government estimates that 7 million people in the U.S. suffer from food-borne illnesses each year. Nine thousand people die from them.[63]

Close-up
Preventing food-borne illness
T0505

Life-threatening food-borne illness can be caused by *Salmonella* and *E. coli* bacteria. *Salmonella* are normally present in the bodies of livestock but can cause gastrointestinal illness in humans who eat infected meat. Though most *Salmonella* infections are mild, some can cause repeated bouts of diarrhea that can drain the body of precious fluids and lead to death from dehydration if left untreated. In 1993, following a large-scale incident of food poisoning in which 300 persons became ill and several children died after eating fast-food hamburgers contaminated with *E. coli* bacteria, the U.S. Department of Agriculture instituted regulations requiring new labels on all packages of meat and poultry. These labels outline safe handling and cooking procedures aimed at minimizing the risk of bacterial infection. In 1996, the federal government announced sweeping changes in meat inspections.[64] No longer would government inspectors rely on the "sniff and poke" method of sniffing, touching, and visually inspecting meat and poultry to look for obvious signs of spoilage. Since the bacteria that cause many food-borne illnesses can't be seen, felt, or smelled, the government will now require meat and poultry producers to work with the Department of Agriculture in conducting laboratory tests to detect disease-causing bacteria in meat.

Smart Reference
Better red than dead?
R0502

**Toxins** Poisonous substances produced by plants, animals, or microorganisms.

**Hepatitis A** A type of hepatitis, or inflammation of the liver, caused by the hepatitis A virus.

*Botulism* is a rare form of food poisoning caused by a toxin produced by a type of *Clostridium* bacterium, which may be transmitted in smoked and preserved meat that has not been cooked to at least 100°C (212°F). The bacterium may also be found in some home-preserved vegetables and canned fruit and fish products. Severe abdominal pain and vomiting may result from botulism, as well as neurological problems, including paralysis and even death. Immediate medical attention is required to prevent or reverse muscle paralysis caused by the toxin.

Another potentially serious food-borne illness is the liver disease **hepatitis A.** Though it can also be transmitted sexually, many cases of hepatitis A are transmitted by contact with infected fecal matter found in contaminated food or water. Hepatitis A may be unsymptomatic or produce such symptoms as nausea, fever, abdominal discomfort, vomiting, and jaundiced (yellowish) skin. It is largely because of the risk of hepatitis A that restaurant employees are required to wash their hands after using the toilet. Ingesting raw, contaminated shellfish is also a frequent means of transmission of hepatitis A and other viruses and bacteria. Never eat shellfish such as oysters, clams, or mussels unless it is cooked thoroughly.

If you develop symptoms of a food-borne illness, contact your doctor or health care provider. This is especially important for children and older people, who may be more susceptible to the effects of dehydration. Drink liquids to replenish bodily fluid lost through diarrhea or vomiting.

**Environmental Contaminants** Harmful or toxic substances in the environment can get into our foods in various ways. They may be eaten by the animals or fish that wind up on our dinner plates, or be absorbed by the plants that provide us with fruits and vegetables, as in the case of pesticides. Aflatoxin, for example, is a naturally occurring chemical produced by molds. It grows on grains and nuts, including peanuts. In high doses, aflatoxin is a potent carcinogen. The Food and Drug Administration has judged products that contain very small amounts of aflatoxin, such as peanut butter, to be safe.

Close-up
Preventing iron poisoning
T0506

Pesticides are toxins that are used widely around the world to control pests that attack crops. Many pesticides are known or suspected carcinogens. Some, like DDT, have been banned in the U.S. but continue to be used elsewhere in the world. Imported foods contaminated with DDT and other pesticides may end up on our dinner tables.

Many people today buy *organically grown* fruits and vegetables because they are reportedly free of pesticides and chemical additives. Consumers should be aware that many so-called organically grown foods do contain residues of pesticides and other chemicals, sometimes because unscrupulous growers misrepresent their commercially prepared produce as "organically grown" because they know such foods command higher prices, and sometimes because pesticides and chemicals used in neighboring farms "wash over" and enter the soil used to grow "organic" fruits and vegetables. At the present time, there is no guarantee that food represented as "organically grown" in your health-food store or supermarket is indeed free of pesticide and chemical residue.

**Mercury,** a metallic element that is liquid at ordinary temperatures and evaporates into the air, has been discharged following industrial use into rivers and oceans, where it forms the compound *methyl mercury.* Eating mercury-contaminated fish can lead to serious neurological disorders and birth defects.

**Additives and Processing** Additives modify foods in various ways. Some lengthen their shelf life; others make them more appealing by altering or preserving their taste, color, or texture. Curing meat with salt and spices has gone on since ancient times. Today, some 3,000 substances are added to foods during production or processing. Federal regulations control the use of additives to ensure that they are safe for human consumption. Still, some additives can pose a risk to people when used regularly over a long period of time. Nitrates and nitrites, for example, retard spoilage (they kill bacteria that cause botulism) and give a reddish color to cured meat such as bacon, frankfurters, and sausages. But these chemicals are converted in the body into cancer-causing substances called nitrosamines. Though the risk of cancer from consuming nitrates and nitrites in the diet appears to be low, it would be prudent to limit your intake of cured meat products that contain these chemicals.

**Close-up**
Additives and cancer
T0507

Artificial sweeteners are another type of food additive. The sweetener saccharin has been linked to cancer in laboratory animals. The cancer risk increases with dosage levels, so it is wise to limit your intake of products containing saccharin (such as Sweet'N Low). The FDA requires a warning label on all products containing saccharin. Largely because of safety concerns regarding saccharin (and because it tends to leave a bitter aftertaste), soft-drink producers now sweeten their sugar-free beverages with another artificial sweetener called aspartame. Aspartame is also widely used by consumers as a sweetener (brand name Equal) for coffee, tea, or other beverages. Since suspicions have been raised about possible health risks associated with aspartame, it is prudent to limit your use of it also. Aspartame is known to be dangerous to people with a rare genetic disorder called **phenylketonuria.**

**Close-up**
Artificial sweeteners
T0508

Exposing food to low-dose radiation destroys insects and microorganisms, delays the ripening of fruit, and preserves vegetables such as potatoes and onions. Food manufacturers argue that irradiating food can help lengthen its shelf life and reduce the need for potentially harmful chemicals that are now used to preserve food. (Food that is irradiated does not become radioactive, just as people who get dental or medical X-rays do not become radioactive.) The FDA considers food irradiation to be safe for a variety of foods including herbs, fresh fruits, potatoes, pork, and poultry. However, there are no studies of the long-term effects of food irradiation.

**Food Allergies** People with **food allergies** are hypersensitive to certain foods or food additives. Consuming them can lead to unpleasant, even life-threatening, reactions. A boy with an allergic reaction to peanuts may cough and wheeze whenever he eats one. A man may break out into hives after eating a strawberry. A woman may develop a migraine headache hours after eating a product containing corn.[65]

Allergic reactions, including food allergies, are caused by an oversensitive immune response to the allergic substance or *allergen.* On exposure to the allergen, antibodies are produced that lead to the release of **histamines** (discussed further in Chapter 15). (*Anti*histamines are drugs that block the production of histamines, and help stop runny noses and other symptoms caused by histamines.) Many foods can elicit allergic reactions, including dairy products, soybeans, nuts, legumes, chocolate, shellfish, and wheat. Symptoms of food allergies can range from severe abdominal symptoms, such as pain, vomiting, and diarrhea; to skin problems, such as a rash or hives; to wheezing; and even to shock and loss of consciousness. If you suspect you have a food allergy, you should have a complete medical evaluation by an *allergist,* a medical doctor who specializes in the diagnosis and treatment of allergies. If the tests show that you have a particular food allergy, you may be placed on a diet that limits or eliminates your intake of the food.

**Mercury** A silver-white metallic element that is liquid at ordinary temperatures.

**Phenylketonuria** A genetic disorder involving inability to break down the amino acid *phenylalanine.* Abbreviated PKU.

**Food allergies** Hypersensitivities to certain foods.

**Histamines** Substances released during allergic reactions that stimulate secretion of mucus, dilate blood vessels, and produce allergy symptoms.

Some people are allergic to food additives, such as *sulfites*, which are used to prevent fresh fruit and vegetables from turning brown. The FDA requires the presence of sulfites to be listed on food product labels.

Close-up
More on sulfites
T0509

**Preventing Food-Borne Illness—What You Can Do** The government watchdog of the nation's food supply, the FDA, doesn't have nearly enough inspectors to ensure that every morsel of food sold in the U.S. meets government standards. There is much that we can do at home and when shopping to prevent the transmission of food-borne illnesses. Many cases of food poisoning are caused by improper food handling at home.[66] Allowing food to stand too long at room temperature can create an ideal breeding ground for disease-causing bacteria. Failing to cook food thoroughly enough or at high enough temperatures can fail to destroy potentially dangerous microbes, such as *Salmonella*. Cross-contamination may occur when a knife or cutting board is used to cut raw meat or chicken and then used again without washing to prepare vegetables.

Close-up
Meat and poultry safety
T0510

***First Rule of Food Safety*** Never taste any food that looks or smells "off," or anything even a little suspicious. When it comes to food safety, the saying to remember is "When in doubt, throw it out." Here are some specific tips to help ensure food safety:[67]

***Shopping Safely***

- Prevention of food poisoning starts with your trip to the supermarket. Pick up your packaged and canned foods first. Don't buy food in cans that are bulging or dented or in jars that are cracked or have loose or bulging lids. Look for the expiration date on the labels and never buy outdated food.
- Check the "use by" or "sell by" date on dairy products such as cottage cheese, cream cheese, yogurt, and sour cream. Pick the ones that will stay fresh longest. If you have a health problem, especially one that may have impaired your immune system, don't eat raw shellfish and use only pasteurized milk and cheese.

Close-up
Safe food to go
T0511
Egg safety
T0512
More on eggs
T0513

- Choose eggs that are refrigerated in the store. Before putting them in your cart, open the carton and make sure that none are cracked.
- Buy frozen foods and perishables such as meat, poultry, or fish last. Put these products in separate plastic bags so that drippings don't contaminate other foods in your shopping cart.
- Check for cleanliness at the meat or fish counter and the salad bar. For instance, cooked shrimp lying on the same bed of ice as raw fish could become contaminated.
- When shopping for shellfish, buy from markets that get their supplies from state-approved sources. Steer clear of vendors who sell shellfish from roadside stands or the back of a truck. Use an ice chest if it will take more than an hour to get your groceries home.

***Safe Storage***

- Refrigerate or freeze perishables right away. Refrigerator temperature should be 40 to 45°F, and the freezer should be zero. Check both "fridge" and freezer periodically with a good thermometer. Poultry and meat heading for the refrigerator may be stored as purchased in the plastic wrap for a day or two. Don't crowd the refrigerator or freezer so tightly that air can't circulate.
- Foods destined for the freezer should be tightly wrapped. Store leftovers in tight containers. Store eggs in their carton deep in the refrigerator, not on the door, where the temperature is warmer.

Close-up
Freezing foods
T0514

- Keep seafood in the refrigerator or freezer until preparation time.
- Check the leftovers in covered dishes and storage bags daily for spoilage. Throw out anything that looks or smells suspicious. One sign of spoilage is mold, which can grow even under refrigeration.
- Many items besides fresh meats, vegetables, and dairy products need to be kept cold. For instance, mayonnaise and ketchup should go in the refrigerator after opening.
- Check the labels on packages to determine how the contents should be stored. If you've neglected to refrigerate items, it's usually best to throw them out.

HealthCheck
Is your kitchen safe?
H0501

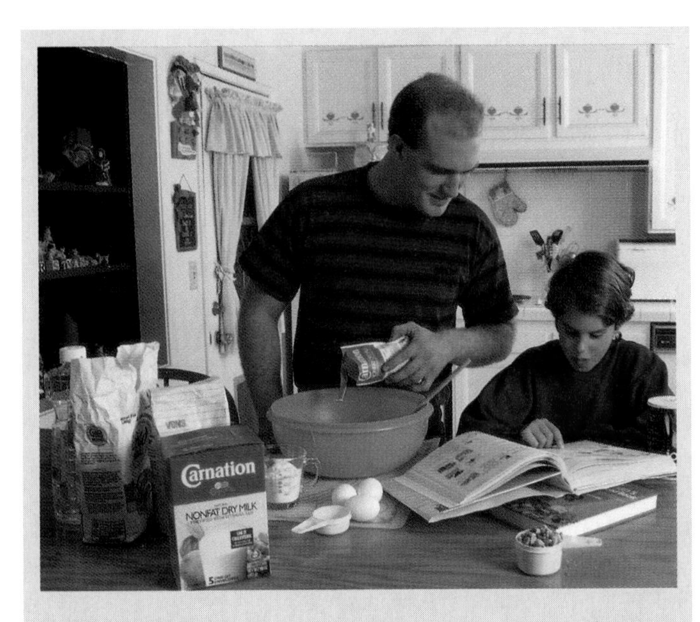


***Keep It Clean*** What can you do to minimize the risks of contracting food-borne disease?

### *Keep It Clean*

**Close-up**

Safety of fresh pork
**T0515**

Cutting board safety
**T0516**

Ground beef: Q & A
**T0517**

Summer food handling
**T0518**

- Keep everything clean. This rule applies to the areas where food is prepared and cooked.
- Rinse all fruits and vegetables thoroughly in cold water. The nasty and potentially dangerous *E. coli* bacteria, as well as other germs, may be present on the surface of fresh fruits and vegetables.[68]
- Wash your hands thoroughly before preparing a meal and after handling raw meat or poultry. Be sure that any open sores or cuts on the hands are completely covered. If the sore or cut is infected, stay out of the kitchen.
- Use clean utensils. Wash them in hot soapy water between cutting different foods.
- Clean the cutting board thoroughly after each use. Wash the lids of canned foods before opening to keep dirt from getting inside.
- Clean the blade of the can opener after each use. Food processors and meat grinders should be taken apart and cleaned as soon as possible after they are used.
- Do not put cooked meat on an unwashed plate or platter that has held raw meat.
- After the meal is prepared, wash all utensils, cutting boards, and countertops with hot soapy water.

### *Keep Temperature Right*

- Keep hot foods *hot* and cold foods *cold*. Ensure that meats are completely cooked.
- Meat and poultry should be cooked to 160°F, and juices should run yellow without any traces of pink or blood. This is especially important with hamburgers and other food made with ground meat (undercooked ground beef may harbor dangerous bacteria). Eggs should be cooked until the white is firm and the yolk begins to harden.
- Seafood should be thoroughly cooked. Fish is done when the thickest part becomes opaque and the fish flakes easily when poked with a fork. Shrimp can be simmered 3 to 5 minutes or until the shells turn red. Clams and mussels are steamed over boiling water until the shells open (5 to 10 minutes). Oysters should be sauteed, baked, or boiled until plump. This takes about 5 minutes.

**Close-up**

More on beef
**T0519**

Focus on chicken
**T0520**

Focus on hot dogs
**T0521**

- Protect seafood from cross-contamination after cooking. Eat it promptly.
- Disease-causing bacteria grow in temperatures between 40 and 140°F. Cooked foods that have been left in this temperature range for more than two hours should not be eaten.
- Get hot dishes from the stove to the table as quickly as possible. Reheated foods should be brought to a temperature of at least 165°F. Keep cold foods in the refrigerator or on a bed of ice till serving.
- After the meal, refrigerate leftovers as soon as possible. Leftovers should be used within three days. This rule is particularly important in the summer.

# Guidelines for Healthy Eating

## Take Charge

You don't have to be a nutritionist to eat correctly. The U.S. government has prepared seven dietary guidelines for healthy eating that are easy to follow even for people with limited knowledge of nutrition.[69] They emphasize balance, variety, and moderation:

1. Eat a variety of foods.
2. Maintain desirable weight.
3. Avoid too much fat, saturated fat, and cholesterol.
4. Eat foods with adequate starch and fiber.
5. Avoid too much sugar.
6. Avoid too much sodium.
7. If you drink alcoholic beverages, do so in moderation.

Several of these guidelines have been touched on in this chapter, such as avoiding too much fat, especially saturated fat, and cholesterol; eating ample quantities of complex carbohydrates (starches and fiber); and avoiding too much sugar and sodium. Since the kinds and amounts of nutrients vary among foods, you need to eat a variety of foods to ensure that your basic nutritional needs are met. The dietary guidelines also emphasize maintaining a desirable body weight. As we'll see in the next chapter, excess weight or obesity is linked to an increased risk of heart disease, diabetes, and some forms of cancer. The guidelines also encourage people who consume alcoholic beverages to drink in moderation. Women should consume no more than one drink a day, while men should not exceed two drinks a day. What counts as one drink is 12 ounces of regular beer, 8 ounces of wine, or 1.5 ounces of hard liquor.

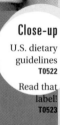


While not outright encouraging people to consume alcohol, the federal government issued an updated set of dietary guidelines in 1995 that for the first time recognized that moderate alcohol use may reduce the risk of heart attacks (see Chapter 13).

The Canadian government has issued a set of nutritional guidelines which largely parallel the U.S. guidelines. However, the Canadian guidelines encourage individuals to limit their caffeine intake as well as their salt and alcohol intake. The Canadian guidelines also emphasize the importance of physical activity, along with healthy eating, in maintaining a healthy body weight.

### Planning a Daily Menu—The Food Guide Pyramid

The *Food Guide Pyramid* was issued by the U.S. Department of Agriculture to help people plan healthful daily menus. It divides foods into five major food groups:

1. Grains, consisting of breads, cereals, rice, and pasta
2. Vegetables
3. Fruits
4. Milk, yogurt, and cheeses
5. Meat, poultry, fish, dry beans, eggs, and nuts.

A sixth group, consisting of fats, oils, and sweets, provides calories but little else of nutritional value. These foods should be eaten sparingly. A pyramid shape was selected because it is meant to encourage Americans to consume greater amounts of foods in the lower, wider bands of the pyramid (see Figure 5.2), specifically grains, fruits, and vegetables, and lesser amounts of foods at the higher, narrower bands—meats, dairy products, and especially fats. In 1995 the U.S. government issued a revised set of guidelines that cautioned people to limit their intake of high-fat processed meats, like sausage, salami, and organ meats.[70] The bulk of the diet should come from grain-based foods, which are rich sources of complex carbohydrates.

The *Food Guide Pyramid* also lists the recommended number of daily servings from each of the major food groups. These are not rigid daily requirements, but rather a general guide to planning healthy menus. The recommended servings are also helpful in planning menus that provide the appropriate number of calories per day to maintain a healthy weight. The recommended number of servings varies because nutrient and calorie needs vary from person to person, depending on such factors as age, sex, body size, and activity level. Active, growing teenagers probably need to consume the higher number of servings in each category to meet their daily calorie and nutritional needs. The lower to middle number of servings is probably appropriate for most women and for older sedentary adults, while the average to higher number of servings is appropriate for most men. The lower number of servings in each food group, combined with a moderate

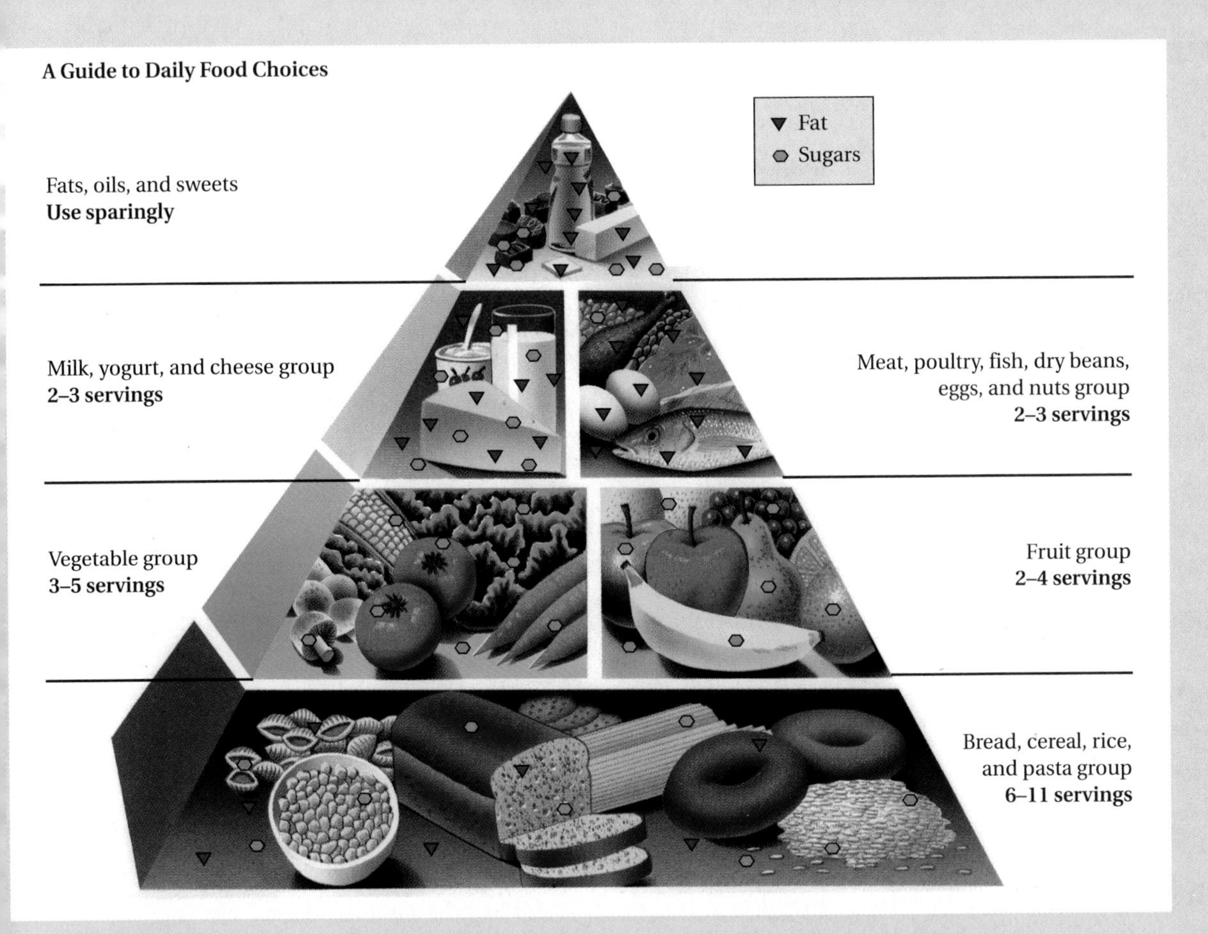


**Figure 5.2** ***Food Guide Pyramid*** These guidelines can help you plan a healthy diet. Each food group provides some but not all of the nutrients you need, so it's important to select from all groups. Emphasize the foods at the base of the pyramid and go easy on the fats, oils, and sweets at the top. Source: USDA Human Nutrition Information Service.

**Close-up**
Women and nutrition
**T0524**
Getting more information
**T0525**

amount of fat and sugars, supplies about 1,600 calories a day. Table 5.11 shows the amount of food in each of the major food groups that corresponds to a single serving. Table 5.12 shows some sample diets for selected calorie levels.

**TABLE 5.11**

**What Is a Serving?**[71]

| Food Group | A Serving Equals |
|---|---|
| Bread, cereal, rice, and pasta | 1 slice of bread<br>bun, bagel, or English muffin<br>1 small roll, biscuit, or muffin<br>3–4 small or 2 large crackers<br>1 ounce of dry ready-to-eat cereal<br>1 cup of cooked cereal, rice, or pasta |
| Vegetable | 1 cup of raw leafy green vegetables<br>1 cup of other kinds of cooked or chopped raw vegetables<br>$\frac{3}{4}$ cup of vegetable juice |
| Fruit | 1 medium apple, banana, or orange<br>$\frac{1}{2}$ grapefruit; a melon wedge; 1 cup of small or diced fruit; $\frac{3}{4}$ cup of fruit juice; 1 cup of chopped, cooked, or canned fruit; 1 cup of berries |
| Milk, cheese, and yogurt | 1 cup of milk or yogurt<br>1 ounce of natural cheese<br>2 ounces of processed cheese |
| Meat, poultry, fish, dry beans, eggs, and nuts | 2–3 ounces of cooked lean meat, poultry, or fish<br>Note that 1 cup cooked dry beans, 1 egg, or 2 tablespoons of peanut butter count as 1 ounce of lean meat |

Note: For mixed foods, estimate as best you can the number of servings of each of the ingredients. A serving of pizza, for instance, would include ingredients from the bread group (the crust), the milk group (cheese), and the vegetable group (tomato).

## Variety—The Keynote of Good Nutrition

Since the kinds and amounts of nutrients vary among foods, you need to eat a variety of foods to maintain good nutrition. How does your daily diet stack up in terms of variety? Here are some suggestions for adding variety to your daily diet, along with some tips for making healthful food choices:[73]

1. *Eat six or more servings of bread, cereals, rice, crackers, pasta, or other foods made from grains.* Note that servings are small, for example, one slice of bread. Include several servings of whole-grain products. Limit baked goods such as cakes, cookies, croissants, and pastries because of their high fat and sugar content. Use spreads such as butter sparingly. Use half the butter or margarine called for when preparing pasta, stuffing, and sauces from packaged mixes. Also substitute low-fat milk when milk or cream is called for.
2. *Eat at least three different kinds of vegetables a day.* Sample from dark-green leafy vegetables (spinach, romaine lettuce, broccoli), deep yellow vegetables (carrots, sweet potatoes), starchy vegetables (potatoes, corn, peas), legumes (navy,

TABLE 5.12

**Sample Daily Diets for Three Calorie Levels[72]**

| | Calorie Level | | |
|---|---|---|---|
| | Lower (about 1,600) | Moderate (about 2,200) | Higher (about 2,800) |
| *Bread Group Servings* | 6 | 9 | 11 |
| *Vegetable Group Servings* | 3 | 4 | 5 |
| *Fruit Group Servings* | 2 | 3 | 4 |
| *Milk Group Servings* | 2–3[a] | 2–3[a] | 2–3[a] |
| *Meat Group[b] (ounces)* | 5 | 6 | 7 |
| *Total Fat[c] (grams)* | 53 | 73 | 93 |
| *Total Added Sugars[d] (teaspoons)* | 6 | 12 | 18 |

[a]Women who are pregnant or breast-feeding, teenagers, and young adults to age 24 need 3 servings.
[b]Meat group amounts are in total ounces.
[c]Use a guide listing the grams of fat for foods in your diet.
[d]Use the guide showing added sugars in Appendix C.

pinto, and kidney beans, chickpeas), and other vegetables (lettuce, tomatoes, onions, green beans). Include all types regularly and eat dark-green leafy vegetables and legumes at least several times a week. Use fats as toppings sparingly, such as butter, mayonnaise, and salad dressing. Use low-fat salad dressing instead.

3. *Eat at least two different kinds of fruit or fruit juice.* Choose fresh fruits, fruit juices, and frozen, canned, or dried fruit rather than canned or frozen fruit in heavy syrup and sweetened fruit juices or juice drinks. Eat whole fruits often, especially fruits high in vitamin C, such as citrus fruits, melons, and berries.
4. *Vary your sources of meat, poultry, fish, or alternatives, such as eggs, dry beans, or nuts.* Limit fat by choosing lean meat and poultry without skin. Choose fish and dry beans and peas often. Limit fat when preparing meats by trimming all visible fat and by broiling, roasting, or boiling meat dishes instead of frying. Limit intake of egg yolks by using only one yolk per person in egg dishes; add extra egg whites in egg dishes to increase portion size. Moderate your intake of nuts and seeds, which are high in fat.

**Video**
The art of healthy eating
V0501

## Vegetarianism—Is It Healthier?

No doubt about it, vegetarianism is on the rise. Estimates indicate that about 10 million people in the U.S. are vegetarians, about 2 million more than there were a decade ago.[74] Vegetarianism has even become chic of late, with celebrities such as Madonna, Candice Bergen, and Phylicia Rashad revealing that they are vegetarians. Even the U.S. government's dietary guidelines recognize the healthfulness of a vegetarian diet. Some people adopt a vegetarian diet because they believe that killing animals for food is wrong. Others view vegetarianism as a healthier alternative to the typical high-fat meat-based American diet.

There are many different kinds of vegetarian diets. Some vegetarians practice a limited form of vegetarianism that includes dairy products, such as eggs and milk, but not fish or meat. Others, generally those who are motivated more by health concerns than moral beliefs, eat fish or perhaps chicken, but hold the line at red meat or pork. Since protein is generally less plentiful in vegetables than in animal foods, vegetarians must be especially careful to follow a diet providing a rich enough supply of protein and other essential nutrients from vegetable sources.

**Close-up**
More on vegetarianism
T0526

There is growing evidence that people who eat a diet rich in fruits and vegetables have a lower risk of developing some diseases, such as certain cancers, than do those whose diets are low in plant foods and high in meat and other animal sources of fat, such as cheese.[75] Cancers of the colon and prostate, for example, are more common among people who follow a high-fat, low-fiber diet than among vegetarians. Fruits and vegetables contain health-promoting nutrients that may lower the risk of certain cancers. Vegetarians also have lower levels of cholesterol and blood lipids (fats) than do comparable groups of meat eaters, which may lower their risk of cardiovascular disease. Vegetarians also tend to be thinner and have lower blood pressures than nonvegetarians. Vegetarianism per se may not explain these differences, since vegetarians may differ from nonvegetarians in other ways than diet. Still, evidence points to possible disease-preventive benefits from a vegetarian diet.

Yet strict vegetarianism may not be any healthier than alternative low-fat diets in which meat consumption is pared down but not eliminated. Nonvegetarians too may benefit from the healthful nutrients found in fruits and vegetables by eating ample portions of these foods. They may also decrease their health risks by eating less fat. Whatever the relative benefits of strict vegetarianism versus a low-fat nonvegetarian diet may be, the country has a long way to go toward meeting the federal government's health goals of having us consume at least five servings of fruits and vegetables daily. In 1991, the government reported that only 9% of Americans met this dietary goal.

## Making Fast Food a Healthier Choice

Our nation is obsessed with fast food. You probably live or work no more than a few miles from a fast-food restaurant—a McDonald's, Burger King, KFC, Taco Bell, or perhaps a Pizza Hut. We all know the rap against fast food: It's high in calories and fat and low in nutrition. But can fast food be good for you, not just good tasting? The answer is a surprising yes—but only if you watch what you order.

**What to Order** Among the choices that are lowest in calories and fat are the basic hamburgers from any of the large chains. Though the meat isn't lean, the average hamburger contains only about 2 ounces of beef, which keeps down the fat and calorie content. Not so for the Big Mac (500 calories; 26 grams of fat) and its major competitors, such as the Burger King Whopper (640 calories; 39 grams of fat). (They don't call it the "Whopper" for nothing.) Some people order fish or chicken in the belief that they are lower in fat and calories than hamburgers. However, chicken or fish that is breaded or fried or chicken with skin is typically loaded with fat and calories. Still, grilled chicken sandwiches (without sauce) are among the healthiest choices.

Consumer organizations and leading health magazines have rated the best and the worst in fast-food fare.[76] Among the best choices are grilled chicken sandwiches at McDonald's and Wendy's (hold the sauce), the BBQ chicken sandwich at KFC, Arby's Junior Roast Beef and Roy Rogers' Roast Beef sandwiches, and Taco Bell's Border Lights™ Taco Supreme and Border Lights™ Chicken Burrito Supreme. Because fast-food restaurants frequently change their menu selections, some of these selections may no longer be available. Salads are also good choices as long as you avoid adding cheese or eggs and use dressing sparingly. Among the worst selections are Boston Chicken Chunky Chicken Salad Sandwich and Burger King Chicken Sandwich, each of which contains more than 700 calories and 40 grams of fat.

You should also watch the sodium content along with the fat and calories, especially if you need to follow a low-sodium diet. Avoid using any added table salt and watch out for hidden sodium in other menu selections. For example, Burger King's BK Big Fish™ has a staggering 980 mg of sodium!

**Figure 5.3** ***Pizza—A Health Food?*** Not such a farfetched idea when you consider that the basic ingredients in pizza—bread, tomato sauce, and cheese—can fit within a healthy diet, so long as the cheese, high in saturated fat, is not used too generously as a topping. According to Pizza Hut, an average 4.4-ounce slice of their pizza is estimated to contain about 250 calories and 9 grams of fat; Godfather's claims that an average 4-ounce slice of their pizza has about 270 calories and 8 grams of fat. Pizza is a rich source of the complex carbohydrates that health experts encourage us to eat, as well as other nutrients, such as calcium and protein. All bets are off, though, if you add high-fat toppings like pepperoni, sausage, or extra cheese, which can easily double the amount of fat and quadruple the sodium in each serving, not to mention the extra calories. Try green peppers or mushrooms instead.

To learn more about the nutritional contents of the menu selections at some of the more popular fast-food restaurants, consult the table found in the Appendix C. You can also ask for a copy of the restaurant's latest nutritional guide before you order.

## Tips for Healthier Fast-Food Eating

1. *Hold the mayo and "special sauce."* "Special" is often a euphemism for "high-fat." As a rule of thumb, avoid using any gooey sauce. Ask for a plain sandwich with no sauce. Or use ketchup or a low-fat sauce. Avoid dipping sauces; many are loaded with fat and calories.
2. *Order food grilled, not fried.* Fried or breaded food adds calories and fat. People sometimes order a chicken cutlet or fish filet sandwich (breaded and fried) thinking these are healthier choices than a plain hamburger. Wrong.
3. *Order healthy salads.* Some salad selections are healthy choices, but others contain heaping helpings of salad dressing, cheese, sour cream, and meat that add calories, fat, and sodium. The Taco Bell Taco Salad, for example, contains about 80% of the recommended daily limit for fat intake.
4. *Skip the cheese and bacon.* Skipping the cheese, mayo, and bacon saves many grams of fat and calories.
5. *Substitute baked potatoes for french fries.* A plain baked potato has about 220 calories and 0 grams of fat, compared with more than 400 calories and 20 grams of fat for a large order of McDonald's french fries. A standard order of french fries typically has more fat and calories than a small hamburger. But don't add sour cream, cheese, or butter to the baked potato, or the low-fat advantage is lost.
6. *Order skinless chicken.* Ordering skinless chicken will cut the calories by about a third and the fat by one-half to three-quarters compared with roasted chicken with the skin. If chicken comes with skin, remove it.
7. *Skip the desserts and fruit pies.* When it comes to fast-food restaurants, dessert is just another word for fat.

Is it possible to eat *healthy* fast food? The answer is yes, so long as you eat modest portions (avoid those "supersize" portions), avoid high-calorie ("regular") soft drinks and shakes, and make sensible choices by ordering items that are lower in fat, calories, and sodium.

## Become a Health-Wise Consumer

Keep good nutrition in mind when choosing food at your local supermarket. Whenever we enter a supermarket we are bombarded with artfully constructed displays arranged with one purpose in mind: to get us to buy. Not buy healthy or smart. Just buy. Here are some guidelines to help you look beyond displays and make more healthful selections when shopping at the supermarket:

1. *Shop from a list.* Prepare a shopping list in advance that provides variety and nutritional balance and stick to it.
2. *Don't shop before meals or when you're hungry.* When you're hungry you're more likely to be tempted by high-fat foods.
3. *Become a label reader.* Consider the nutritional content of foods before you buy them.
4. *Avoid buying "fresh" packaged meats that are marinated with sauces.* Marinades and sauces are sometimes used to camouflage meats that have remained in the display case too long.
5. *Don't be misled by manufacturers' claims on food packages.* Claims like "new" or "improved" may simply mean that small, inconsequential changes have been made to the product.
6. *Don't assume that products claiming to be "lean" are necessarily low in calories or that "low-fat" foods are also low in cholesterol.* Note too that "fat free" does not mean "low calorie." Some "no-fat" or "low-fat" products actually pack a lot of calories (like some yogurt products). Check the food labels for both fat and calories.

**Decipher Food Claims** *Light! Lean! Low Fat! Reduced!* What does it all mean? For years, food manufacturers were casual with food claims like "light" and "low fat." Consumers were bewildered by these claims, some of which were outright distortions. Now, however, the federal government requires manufacturers to adhere to strict definitions for food claims. Table 5.13 provides the federally mandated definitions for some of the more common food claims.[77]

**TABLE 5.13 Food Claims and What They Mean**

| Food Claim | Definition |
|---|---|
| *Fat free* | Produce contains no or only negligible amounts of fat, saturated fat, cholesterol, sodium, sugar, and/or calories. |
| *Low fat* | No more than 3 grams of fat per serving. |
| *Low sodium* | Less than 140 milligrams per serving. |
| *Low cholesterol* | Less than 20 milligrams per serving. |
| *Low calorie* | No more than 40 calories per serving. |
| *Lean* | Less than 10 grams of fat, less than 4 grams of saturated fat, and less than 95 milligrams of cholesterol per serving. |
| *Extra lean* | Less than 5 grams of fat, less than 2 grams of saturated fat, and less than 95 milligrams of cholesterol per serving. |
| *Reduced* | Contains 25% less of a nutrient (such as fat) or of calories than the regular product. |
| *Light or Lite* | Contains at least a third fewer calories than the regular product or a reduction in fat content by 50% or more. (In foods containing 50% or more of their calories from fat, it's the fat that must be reduced for the product to earn the light claim.) Light may also apply to low-fat, low-calorie foods that have reduced sodium content by 50% or more. |

**Read Food Labels** The FDA began requiring a new food label format in 1994. The kind of information required by the new label is shown in Figure 5.4. Among other things, the new labels require that serving sizes be standardized and based on amounts that people normally eat (not the minuscule amounts food manufacturers often claim). For the first time, too, labels provide information about not only the total number of grams of fat but also the number of fat grams composed of saturated fat.

**Close-up**
Using the new food label
T0527
More on food labels
T0528

**Learn More about Nutrition** Health-wise consumers seek to become better informed about nutrition. Reading this chapter is a good start. Other sources of information are available from private and government organizations, and often the price is very right—free.

**Smart Quiz**
Q0507

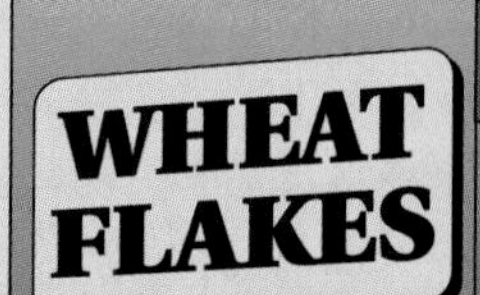
WHEAT
FLAKES
HEALTHY
The serving size is set by the Food and Drug Administration and reflects the amount most people typically eat.
The calories from fat. To get the percentage of fat, divide the fat calories by the total calories.
These percentages suggest how this food fits into daily food intake.
Vitamin A, vitamin C, calcium, and iron are listed. These are the vitamins and minerals for which it is especially important to avoid deficiencies.
Nutrition Facts
Serving Size: 3/4 cup (164g)
Servings Per Container: 12
Amount Per Serving
Calories 190
Calories from fat 60
%Daily Value*
Total Fat 7g 10%
Saturated Fat 3g 15%
Cholesterol 30mg 10%
Sodium 330mg 14%
Total Carbohydrate 33g 11%
Sugars 5g
Dietary Fiber 2g 8%
Protein 8g
Vitamin A 4% • Vitamin C 1% • Calcium 15% • Iron 4%
*Percents (%) of Daily Value are based on a 2,000 Calorie diet. Your Daily Values may vary higher or lower depending on your Calorie needs.

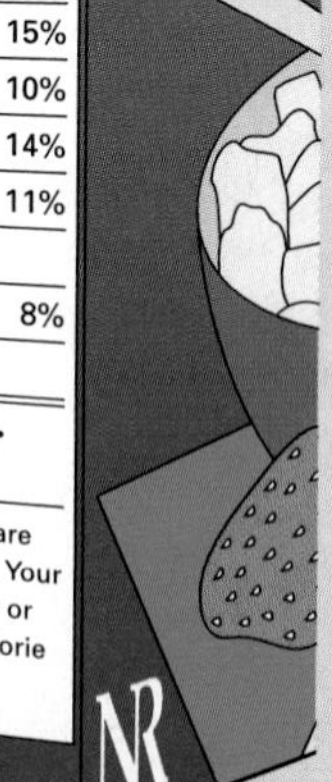

**Figure 5.4** ***Anatomy of a Food Label*** The information on food labels can help you to plan on getting adequate amounts of required nutrients—and to avoid consuming excessive amounts of fat, sodium, and cholesterol.

# SUMMING
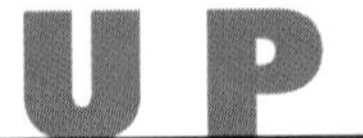

## Questions and Answers

### PROTEINS

**1. What are proteins?** Proteins are made up of amino acids that build muscle, bone, hair, blood, and other tissues. Nine amino acids must be obtained from the diet. People obtain most of their protein from animal sources.

**2. What are the health benefits of proteins?** Proteins are essential to growth and health. But excess protein is converted into body fat.

### CARBOHYDRATES

**3. What are carbohydrates?** Simple carbohydrates are sugars. Complex carbohydrates are starches and fiber. Starchy vegetables are abundant sources of energy.

**4. What are the health benefits of carbohydrates?** Starches provide a continual flow of energy. They are also low in fat and calories. Starches are also rich sources of vitamins and minerals. Some starches are also good sources of dietary fiber. Fiber provides bulk to the stool. Dietary fiber helps prevent gastrointestinal problems and may lower the risk of cardiovascular disease and colon cancer.

### FATS

**5. What are fats?** Fat consists of fatty acids: saturated, monounsaturated, and polyunsaturated.

**6. What are the relationships between health and consuming fats?** Fats, especially saturated fats, raise blood cholesterol levels, heightening the risk of heart disease and cancer.

### VITAMINS

**7. What are vitamins?** Vitamins are organic compounds that are needed, usually in small amounts, to maintain normal physiological functioning. Vitamins help regulate the chemical reactions that are involved in metabolism.

**8. What are the health benefits of vitamins?** Vitamins avert vitamin deficiency syndromes, such as scurvy. They may also afford some protection against heart disease and cancer. Antioxidants (vitamins C and E and beta-carotene) scavenge metabolic by-products called free radicals, which may help prevent them from damaging cells.

### MINERALS

**9. What are minerals?** Minerals are inorganic elements, like calcium, potassium, sodium, and magnesium, that are essential to health.

**10. What are the health benefits of minerals?** Minerals are involved in the formation of bones and teeth, the transmission of nerve signals, and the manufacture of hemoglobin.

### WATER AND ELECTROLYTES

**11. What about water and electrolytes?** Water helps transport nutrients and remove wastes through the blood system, and regulates body temperature. Electrolytes help conduct electrical currents in the body. Sodium is an essential electrolyte. Excess sodium may contribute to an increased risk of hypertension in susceptible people.

## References and Suggested Readings

### SMART REFERENCES FROM SCIENTIFIC AMERICAN

**Mirsky, S. Science and the Citizen: Chewing the Fat.** *Scientific American*, 276(1) (January 1997), 31. **R0501**

**Zorpette, G. Materials Science: Better Red than Dead?** *Scientific American*, 276(3) (March 1997), 36. **R0502**

### SUGGESTED READINGS

**Brody, J.** *Jane Brody's Nutrition Book.* New York: Bantam Books, 1987 (Updated and revised). A guide to better, more nutritious eating and weight control by the respected science writer and personal health columnist of *The New York Times.*

**Gershoff, S., and others.** *The Tufts University Guide to Total Nutrition.* New York: HarperCollins, 1996. Written by the dean emeritus of one of the nation's premier schools of nutrition, along with members of the editorial advisory board of the prestigious *Tufts University Diet & Nutrition Letter,* it presents the latest information on relationships between health and nutrition.

**Margen, S., and the Editors of the University of California at Berkeley** *Wellness Letter. The Wellness Encyclopedia of Food and Nutrition.* Berkeley, CA: University of California at Berkeley Press, 1995. A nutritional directory that provides hundreds of food facts and other tips for healthy eating.

*Tufts University Diet & Nutrition Letter.* A leading nutrition newsletter, it covers scientific developments concerning health and nutrition and separates facts from hype.

*Nutrition Action Healthletter.* Published by the Center for Science in the Public Interest, the *Nutrition Action Healthletter* debunks unsupported product claims and gives you the nutritional facts about what you bring home from the supermarket or eat in your neighborhood restaurants. To obtain a subscription, you can write to The Center for Science in the Public Interest, 1501 16th St. NW, Washington, DC 20036.

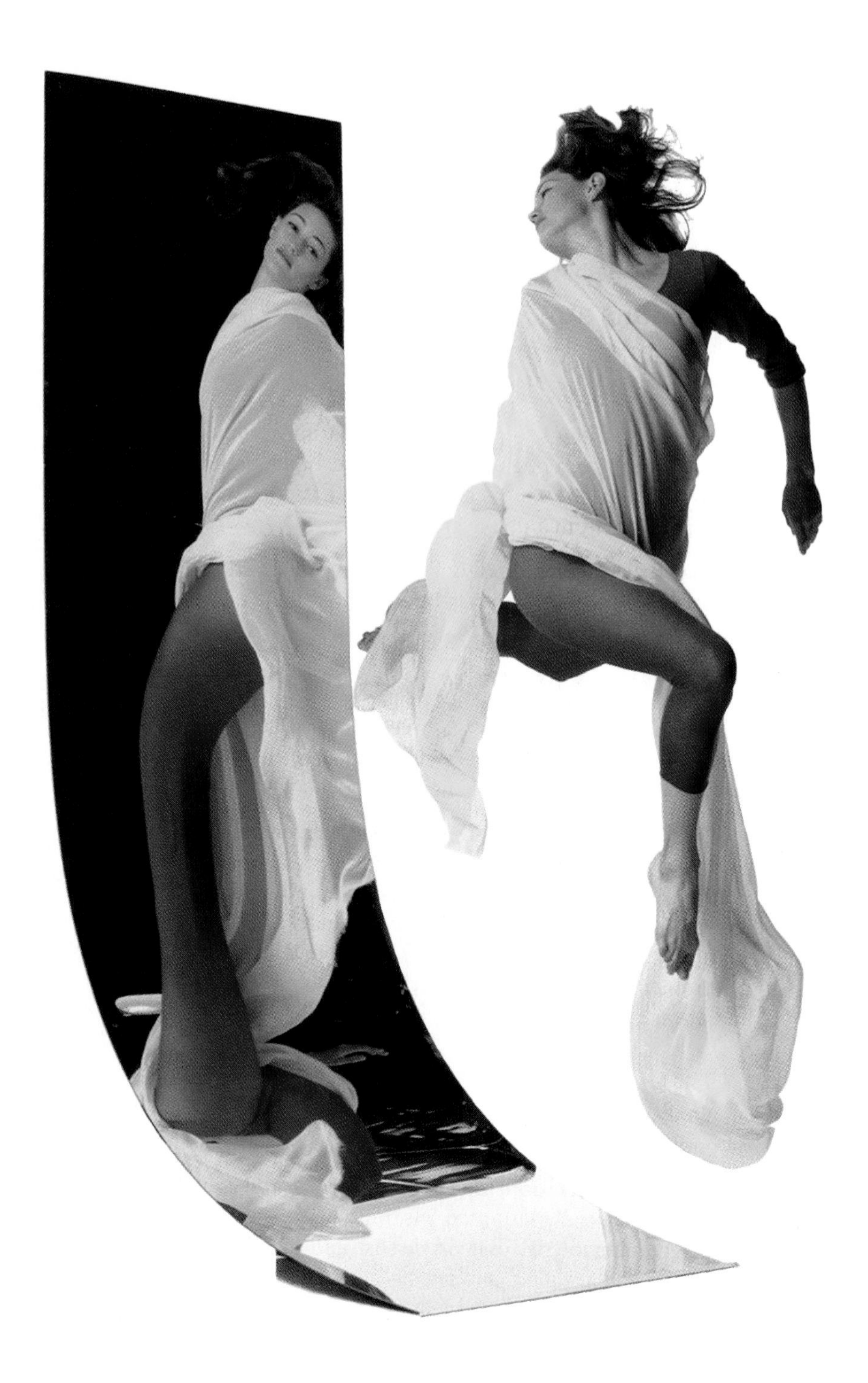

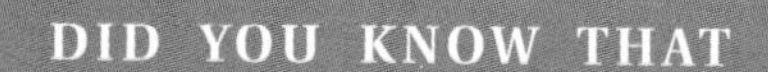

## DID YOU KNOW THAT

- The number of Americans who die from causes linked to obesity is equivalent to two jumbo jets crashing every day, with all passengers lost? p.144
- Dieting has become the normal way of eating for women in the United States? p.144
- You can be obese even if you are not overweight? p.148
- People who were adopted are typically closer in weight to their biological parents than to their adoptive parents? p.150
- Japanese-American men in California and Hawaii are more likely to be obese than Japanese men living in Japan? p.153
- Orange juice contains more calories than Coca-Cola? p.155
- You *can* be too rich or too thin? (At least you can be too thin.) p.156
- Most dieters eventually gain back the weight they lose? (And then some.) p.160
- Some obese people have their jaws wired to restrict them to low-calorie liquid diets? p.163

# 6



# Managing Your Weight

*We have some good news and some bad news. First, the good news. The United States has such an agricultural abundance that Americans take in 200 billion calories a day more than their bodies need. How much is 200 billion calories? Enough to feed the nation of Germany—80 million people. Now, the bad news. Unfortunately these excess calories are expanding our collective waistlines. More than one in three adults in the United States, more than 40 million people, are obese.[1]*

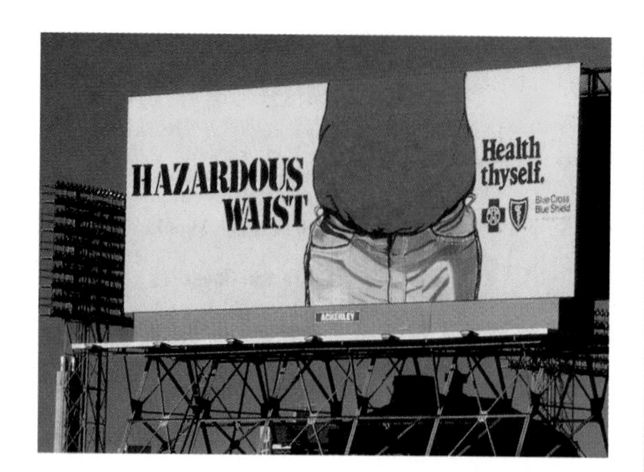


***Fat in America*** More than one in three Americans are obese. What health risks are associated with obesity?

**TABLE 6.1**

**Some Facts on Dieting in the U.S.**

- About one American in five—50 million people—is on a diet as you read this page.[5]
- In the United States, 40% of the men and 75% of the women have tried to lose weight; 10 to 20% have sought professional help.[6]
- About one in three Americans (35%) reports wanting to lose at least 15 pounds.[7]
- About 20% of young women attempt to lose weight even though they don't need to.
- Sixty-five million people in the United States diet each year, making use of nearly 30,000 different approaches.[8]
- More than 9 out of 10 dieters fail to keep off the weight they lose;[9] 2 out of 3 who lose weight on a diet will regain every pound that they lost within a few years—and then some.

So, as a nation we eat too much and weigh too much. Does it matter? Quite a bit as far as our health is concerned. **Obesity** is a risk factor in cardiovascular disorders, respiratory illnesses, diabetes, gall bladder disease, gout, and certain kinds of cancer. All in all, obesity contributes to about 300,000 deaths in the United States each year.[2] That's the equivalent of two jumbo jets crashing every day.

**Close-up** Obesity U.S.A. **T0601**

Losing weight has clear health benefits for obese people. Even a modest loss of 10 to 15% of body weight can reduce the health risks associated with obesity.[3] Concerns about weight are not limited to the obese. We can all benefit from learning skills to maintain a healthy weight and prevent obesity.

Our aim is to help readers attain and maintain a *healthy weight,* not to conform to an idealized image of thinness. The contemporary ideal is lean. Lean and, for many of us, mean. How mean? So mean that the pressures to meet an unrealistic standard of slenderness have led many of us to become obsessed with weight and dissatisfied with our bodies. About twice as many Americans consider themselves obese as actually meet clinical standards of obesity.[4]

We have become a nation of dieters. The pressure to be thin falls most heavily on women. It is so prevalent that dieting has become the normal eating pattern for American women. Four out of five young women in the United States have gone on a diet by the time they reach their eighteenth birthdays. Some facts about dieting are shown in Table 6.1.

**Obesity** A condition of excess body fat.

We are flooded with images of slender, sometimes emaciated models. Glamour magazines and TV commercials idealize them as standards of health and beauty. The cultural emphasis on thinness affects our self-perceptions. Most American women believe that they are heavier than men prefer, and heavier still than the feminine ideal.[10] This plump self-concept is found in girls as young

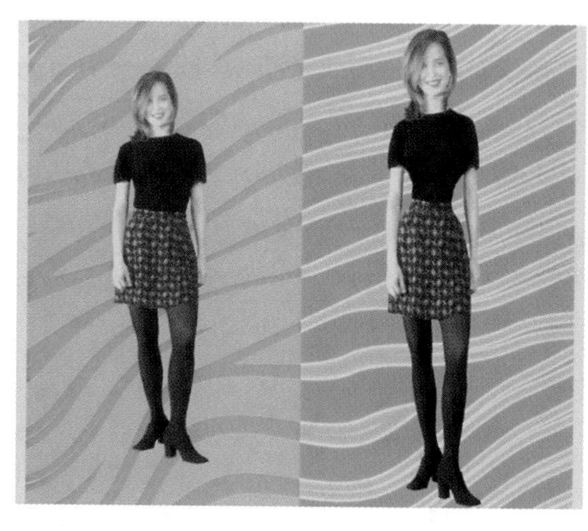

***Wanting to Be Barbie*** The Barbie doll has long epitomized the buxom but svelte female figure. However, if women were to be proportioned like Barbie dolls, they would look like the woman in the photograph on the right. To achieve these proportions, the typical woman on the left would have to grow nearly a foot in height, reduce her waist by 5 inches, and gain 4 inches in her bustline. How might exposure to such impossible standards of thinness affect the self-esteem and eating habits of young women?

as 10 to 15 years of age.[11] In contrast, college men are generally more satisfied with their bodies. Boys 10 to 15 years old generally believe that the ideal male physique is heavier than their own. However, boys naturally gain muscle mass and become heavier as they mature. Thus the gap between their own shape and their ideal shape is likely to narrow. Girls, on the other hand, encounter a greater discrepancy between their own body shapes and the cultural ideal of thinness as they mature and their figures fill out. Girls feel pressured to be thin even before they enter adolescence. Sadly, this pressure contributes to the development of eating disorders such as anorexia nervosa and bulimia nervosa and to a negative self-image.

Both men and women are somewhat off base in their estimates of the physiques preferred by the other sex.[12] College men actually prefer women somewhat heavier than women estimate. Ironically, women prefer men to be thinner than men imagine. Though women are more likely to perceive themselves to be overweight and are more likely to diet, the gender gap in obesity is actually quite narrow—27% of women versus 24% of men (see Figure 6.1).[13] Moreover, gender differences in obesity don't develop until midlife.

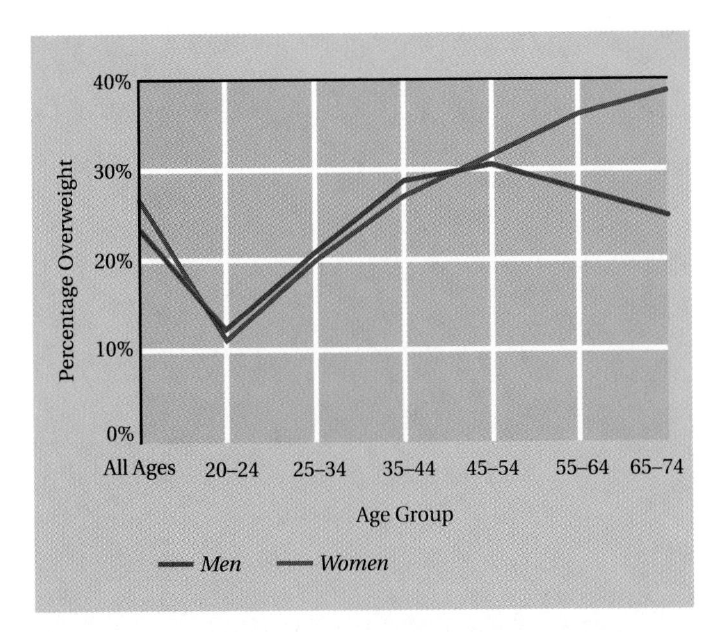


**Figure 6.1** ***Prevalence of Overweight by Gender and Age*** The percentages of men and women who are overweight are virtually the same until later life. Yet pressures to lose weight fall disproportionately on women. Why? Notice too that nearly one in three Americans in the 35 to 54 age range is overweight. Source: U.S. Department of Health and Human Services, Public Health Service, National Institutes of Health, National Heart, Lung, and Blood Institute (1993).

## CALORIES AND WEIGHT—A BALANCING ACT

Marathon runners can eat heaping portions of food day after day and never gain an ounce. Other people seem to gain weight if they have an extra helping at Sunday dinner. Gaining weight is not simply a matter of what we eat, or how much. It also depends on the food energy we expend in keeping our bodies running. We expend energy in maintaining normal bodily functions, such as breathing, heartbeat, circulation, and formation of new tissue. We expend energy in physical labor and exercise, and even in digesting and metabolizing food. We gain weight when we take in more food energy in the form of calories than we expend.

When food is metabolized, it releases energy, which is measured in units called calories. A **calorie** is the amount of energy required to raise the temperature of 1 gram of water 1 degree Celsius. Calories—food energy—maintain normal bodily processes and fuel physical activity.

### Metabolic Rates

The **basal metabolic rate (BMR)** is the minimum amount of energy needed to maintain bodily functions, apart from digestion. The **resting metabolic rate (RMR)** is the minimum energy that the body requires to maintain bodily functions, including digestion.

How many calories a day does your body need? The answer depends on many factors, including your age, weight, and level of activity. Younger adults need more calories than older adults. Active people need more than sedentary people.

Men generally require more calories than women, even if they are of the same weight and equally active. Why? Muscle tissue burns more calories than fat does, and a higher percentage of women's body weight is composed of fat. Men therefore tend to have a higher metabolic rate than women.

Consider the average woman 25 to 50 years of age. She's 5′4″ tall and weighs 138 pounds. She engages in light to moderate physical activity during her day. She needs about 2,200 calories a day to

**Calorie** A measure of food energy, which is equivalent to the amount of energy required to raise the temperature of 1 gram of water by 1 degree Celsius.

**Basal metabolic rate (BMR)** The minimum amount of energy needed to maintain bodily functions, apart from digestion.

**Resting metabolic rate (RMR)** The minimum energy that the body requires to maintain bodily functions including digestion.

maintain her weight. The average man of the same age is 5′10″ tall and weighs 174 pounds. If he also engages in light to moderate physical activity, he needs about 2,900 calories daily to maintain his weight. If more calories are consumed than expended, the excess calories are converted into body fat, extra weight, and added inches to waists and other parts.

Nutrients in our diet—proteins, fats, and carbohydrates—supply calories in varying amounts. All proteins and carbohydrates supply 4 calories per gram. All fats supply 9 calories per gram. Ounce for ounce, fats provide more than twice as many calories as proteins or carbohydrates. That is why fat-laden desserts are so, well, fattening. Since all fats have the same calorie content, switching from saturated to unsaturated fats may be good for your cholesterol levels (see Chapter 5), but it won't change your weight.

People who regularly engage in rigorous physical activity, like marathon runners, burn more energy than less active people. Physical activity in the form of regular exercise not only burns calories but also increases the basal metabolic rate by building muscle. (Again, muscular body tissue burns more calories, even at rest, than fatty body tissue.)

Calories not burned off through physical activity are converted into fat. The reverse is also true: Taking in fewer calories than you need causes your body to convert stored fat into energy. Maintaining weight is a matter of balance between energy in (calories consumed) and energy out (in the form of calories expended in bodily processes and activity, see Figure 6.2).

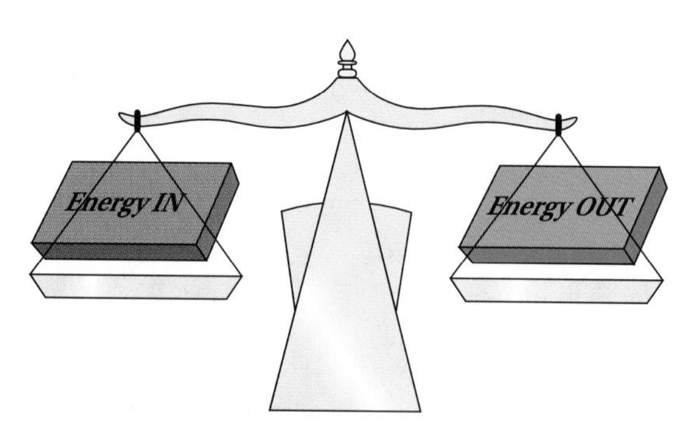


**Figure 6.2** ***Weight Management*** Maintaining your weight is a function of balancing energy input in the form of calories consumed and energy output in the form of calories expended.

## How Much Should You Weigh?

There are several ways for determining whether you weigh more or less than you should. The two most common methods involve the use of weight tables and calculation of the body mass index.

**Weight and Height Measurements** One yardstick for evaluating your weight is to compare it with the recommended healthy weights determined by the National Research Council of the National Academy of Sciences (Table 6.2).[14] The term *healthy weight* represents a change from earlier versions of the weight tables. They were based on the concept of *desirable weight*. What's the difference? The tables now focus on the health aspects of weight—not on appearance. For the first time, the tables now combine the recommended weight ranges for men and women.

**TABLE 6.2**

**Recommended Weights[17]**

| Heights[a] | Weight (in pounds)[b] | |
|---|---|---|
| | 19 to 34 years | 35 years and over |
| 5′0″ | 97–128[c] | 108–138 |
| 5′1″ | 101–132 | 111–143 |
| 5′2″ | 104–137 | 115–148 |
| 5′3″ | 107–141 | 119–152 |
| 5′4″ | 111–146 | 122–157 |
| 5′5″ | 114–150 | 126–162 |
| 5′6″ | 118–155 | 130–167 |
| 5′7″ | 121–160 | 134–172 |
| 5′8″ | 125–164 | 138–178 |
| 5′9″ | 129–169 | 142–183 |
| 5′10″ | 132–174 | 146–188 |
| 5′11″ | 136–179 | 151–194 |
| 6′0″ | 140–184 | 155–199 |
| 6′1″ | 144–189 | 159–205 |
| 6′2″ | 148–195 | 164–210 |
| 6′3″ | 152–200 | 168–216 |
| 6′4″ | 156–205 | 173–222 |
| 6′5″ | 160–211 | 177–228 |
| 6′6″ | 164–216 | 182–234 |

[a]Without shoes.
[b]Without clothes.
[c]The higher weights in the ranges generally apply to men, who have more muscle and bone. The lower weights more often apply to women, who have less muscle and bone.

Why does age matter? People normally put on weight as they age. Overweight is most common among those who are middle-aged and older. Two factors may explain these weight gains.[15] People tend to become less physically active as they age, and partly as a result, they also lose muscle mass. Modest weight gains are thus expected as people age. However, *major* weight gains or obesity are not the natural or inevitable consequences of aging.[16] The key factors are diet and exercise. Weight problems usually begin during a person's twenties or thirties. The people most at risk of major weight gains in midlife are those who were overweight in childhood or early adulthood. It's never too early to develop the healthful dietary and exercise habits that may prevent obesity later on.

What should you weigh? See Table 6.2. Find the range for your height and age range. Then narrow the weight range by adjusting for your gender and physique. Generally speaking, the higher weights in each range are intended for people with a greater proportion of muscle to fat—usually men. Recommended weights for men thus typically fall in the high end of each range and those for women in the low end. Very muscular women, however, may also use the weights in the upper range as a standard.

Figure 6.3 shows the recommended weight levels for young adults in graphical form together with two ranges of overweight.

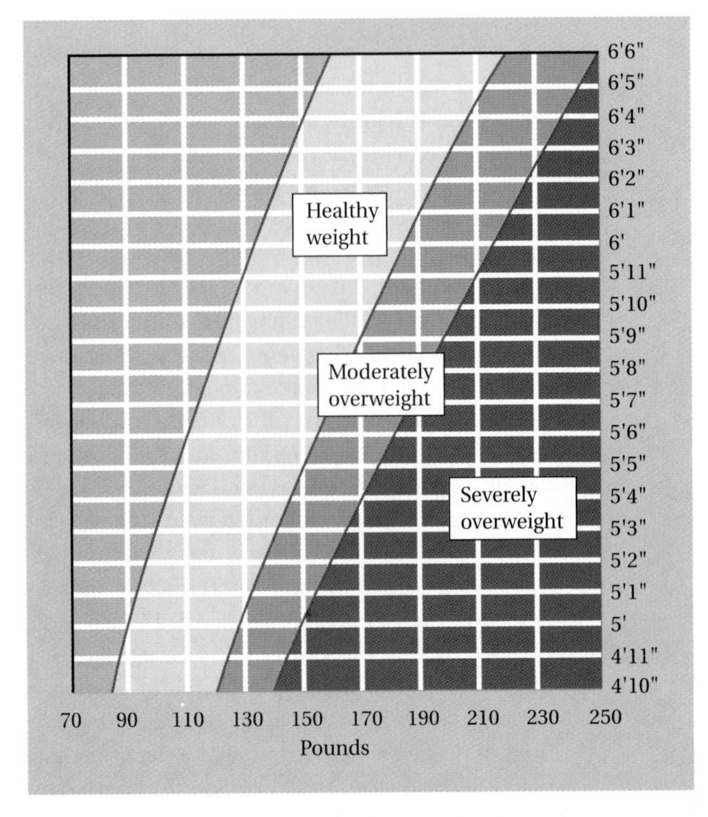


**Figure 6.3** ***How Much Should You Weigh?*** Are you overweight? This chart shows you the healthy weight range for persons of your height. Source: U.S. Government. Reprinted from UC Berkeley *Wellness Letter,* March 1996, p. 5.

**Body Mass Index** Another yardstick for evaluating one's weight is the **body mass index (BMI)**. The BMI takes into account your height in determining whether your weight falls in a healthy or obese range. The BMI formula is:

$$\text{BMI} = \text{kg}/\text{m}^2$$

It is computed by dividing one's body weight (in kilograms) by the square of one's height (in meters). BMIs of 25 or less are considered desirable.[18]

The National Center for Health Statistics defines obesity as a BMI equal to or greater than 27.8 in men and 27.3 in women.[19] These values correspond to body weights approximately 20% above desirable levels. People with BMIs above 40 are considered morbidly obese.[20] People with BMIs between 25 and 30 stand a somewhat larger than average risk of developing health problems associated with obesity. These include high blood pressure, elevated blood cholesterol, heart disease, and Type II (adult-onset) diabetes. The risks of these and other diseases increase sharply among people with BMIs of 30 or greater.

To calculate your own BMI, first multiply your weight in pounds (without clothes or shoes) by 700. Divide this amount by your height in inches. Then divide it again by your height. Your BMI equals ________ .

For example, if you weigh 130 pounds and are 5′6″, the following calculations yield your BMI:

130 × 700 = 91,000
91,000 divided by 66 inches = 1379
1379 divided by 66 = 21
Your BMI = 21

Health professionals agree that people with BMIs greater than 30 should reduce their weight. It has not been shown that otherwise healthy people with BMIs of 25 to 30 reduce their health risks by losing weight.

**Body mass index (BMI)** A measure of obesity that takes into account both weight and height. It is calculated by dividing body weight (in kilograms) by the square of the person's height (in meters).

## Are You Obese?

The answer is not a matter of how many pounds register on the scale. You also need to take into account such factors as your height and body composition. Though excess body weight is associated with obesity, obesity is actually a condition of excess body fat, or "overfat." The term **overweight** refers to those who weigh 20% or more than their healthy weight. In some unusual cases, people may be obese because they have too much body fat in relation to muscle mass, not because they are overweight. However, height/weight measurements and the BMI are usually reliable indications of obesity.

We can more precisely determine obesity by measuring body composition. That is, we compare the ratio of *lean body mass (lbm)*, such as muscle and bone, to body fat. A range of 8 to 15% body fat is generally considered healthful for men. A range of 15 to 22% is considered healthful for women.[21] Women normally carry a higher percentage of body fat because they have more fat deposits than men in their breasts and hips. One common standard of obesity is body fat in excess of 24% for men and 33% for women. There are several methods for assessing body fat, including skinfold measurements, underwater weighing, and bioelectrical impedance.

**Skinfold Measurements—How Many Inches Can You Pinch?** One widely used index of body fat is the thickness of skinfolds. **Skinfold thickness** is measured in places like the waist, underarms, and back. Skinfold calipers pinch the skin (painlessly) to measure skinfold thickness. The measurements are used to estimate the percentage of body fat.

A convenient but crude measure of skinfold thickness is the *pinch test.* Want to pinch yourself? Hold one arm out to the side. Pinch the skin with your other hand at various points along the underside of the outstretched arm. (Pinch only the fat lying under the skin, not the adjoining muscle tissue.) Can you pinch more than an inch? If so, you have more body fat than is desirable.

**Overweight** A body weight exceeding desirable weight for a person of a given age, height, and body frame, usually based on the criterion of 20% above desirable weight.

**Skinfold thickness** The thickness of the folds of skin, usually of the underarms, waist, or back, that is used to estimate the percentage of body fat.

**Hydrostatic weighing** A method of measuring body weight by weighing a person both underwater and out of water and comparing the results.

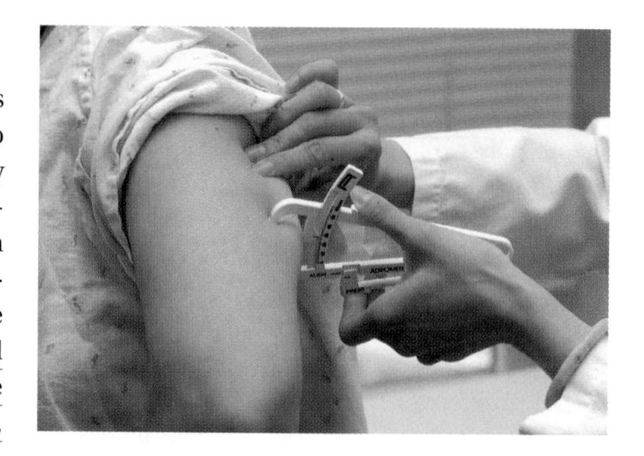

***Can You Pinch an Inch?*** Skin calipers are one way to measure the amount of fat in an individual. How much fat is too much fat?

**Hydrostatic Weighing** A more precise measure of body fat is provided by **hydrostatic weighing.** In this procedure, a person is weighed twice: once in the normal way and then submerged in water. Body fat is lighter than water; muscle and bone are heavier. The body's weight under water largely reflects the density of body mass. The more people weigh submerged, relative to dry weight, the less body fat they carry. This method is not flawless. It requires expensive equipment and a skilled technician. Measurements may also be thrown off by fluid retention and other factors.

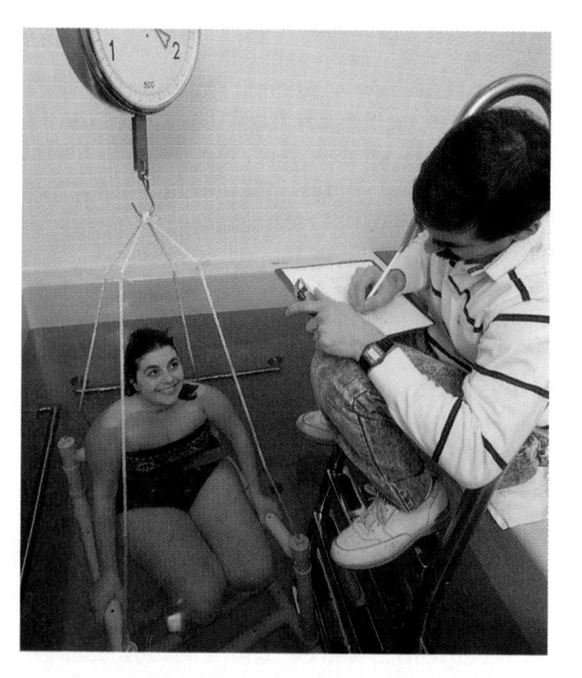

***Hydrostatic Weighing*** Hydrostatic weighing is another method for assessing the amount of fat in the body.

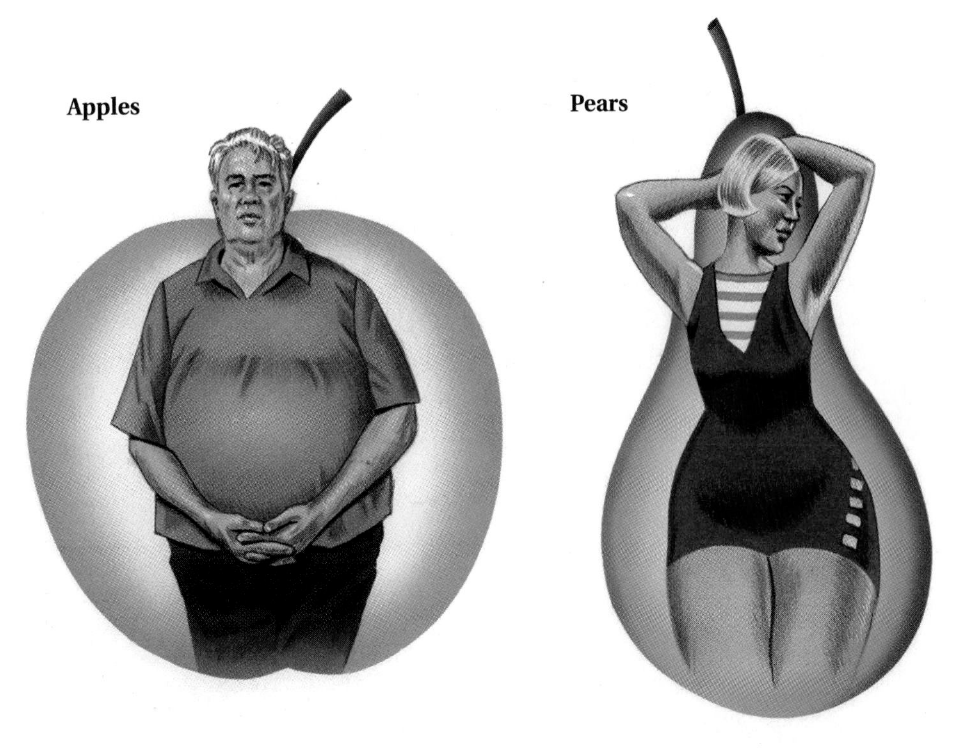


**Figure 6.4** ***Apples vs. Pears*** Apple-shaped people carry much of their excess weight around their middles, while pear-shaped people carry excess weight on their buttocks, thighs, and hips. Though both patterns of obesity are unhealthy, carrying fat around the waist is linked to a greater risk of serious chronic diseases, including heart disease, hypertension, and diabetes.

**Bioelectrical Impedance Analysis** Water conducts electricity; fat does not. **Bioelectrical impedance analysis** uses these facts to measure body fat. A harmless electric current is passed through the body. A technician analyzes the shifts in electrical conductance (impedance) to calculate the total amount of body water. The amount of body water is then used to compute percentages of lean and fat body weights. The results of this method may be affected by electrolyte balance or fluid retention.

Talking Glossary
Bioelectrical impedance analysis
G0601

**Body Fat Distribution and Health** Body shape, like body composition, is an index of health. Two people may weigh the same amount and even have the same amount of body fat. Yet different distributions of fat may affect their relative health risks. Some people are "pears"; they carry excess fat in their hips, buttocks, and thighs. Others are "apples"; they carry excess fat around their midsections (waists). (See Figure 6.4.) Though both kinds of obesity are associated with poor health, excess fat around the midsection appears to be a greater risk factor. Pears stand less of a risk of chronic diseases such as coronary heart disease, hypertension, and diabetes than apples. For example, a five-year study of 41,000 women aged 50 to 69 found that the higher the waist-to-hip ratio (the more "apple-shaped"), the greater the risk of death.[22]

Why are apples at greater risk than pears? A possible reason is that abdominal fat, which accumulates around the pelvis, is connected with higher blood levels of HDL. (HDL is the so-called good cholesterol that sweeps away artery-clogging deposits.) Fat in the waist is linked to lower levels of HDL. Men are more likely to be apples than women, so it is not surprising that they stand a greater risk of coronary heart disease (at least until about age 65, when the rates between men and women even out—see Chapter 17).

Just what is a desirable waist-to-hip ratio? For women, the desirable waist-to-hip ratio is less than 0.8.[23] That is,

**Bioelectrical impedance analysis**
A method of measuring body fat by analyzing the changes in electrical conductance (impedance) as a mild electric current is passed through the body.

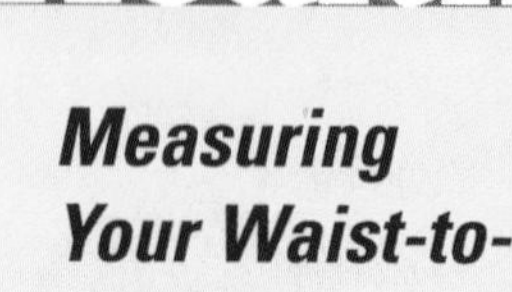

# Health*Check*

## *Measuring Your Waist-to-Hip Ratio*

Does your waist-to-hip ratio exceed the recommended level? To find out, follow this simple procedure.

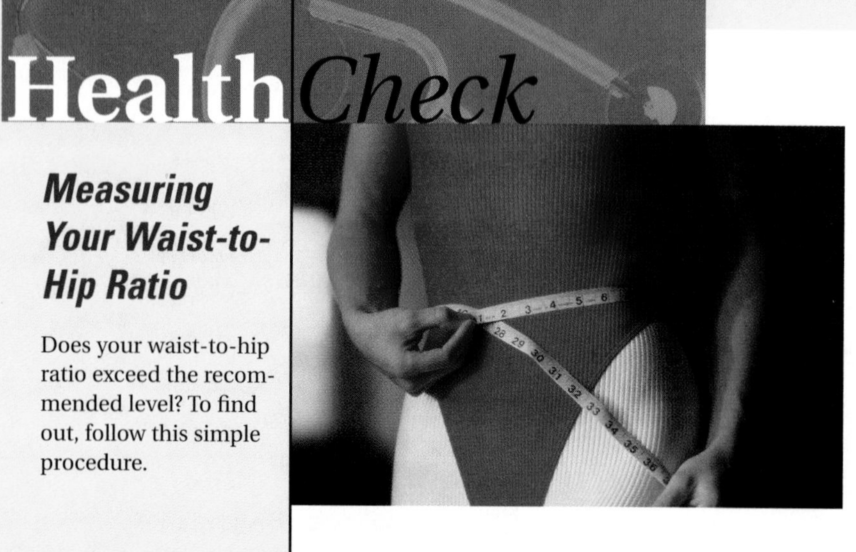

While standing relaxed, measure your waist around your navel. (Don't pull in your stomach while you do so. You will only be fooling yourself.)

Waist: ________ inches

Now measure your hips at their largest point, around your buttocks.

Hips: ________ inches

Now divide your waist measurement by your hip measurement to calculate your waist-to-hip ratio.

Waist/hip ratio ________

*Recommended waist-to-hip ratios are below 0.8 for women and 0.95 for men.*

the size of the waist should be less than 80% the size of the hips. (According to this recommendation, a woman with 35-inch hips should have a waist of 28 inches or less.) For men, the waist-to-hip ratio should be less than 0.95, meaning a waist less than 95% the size of the hips.

Smart Quiz
Q0601

### *think about it!*

- What is the connection between calories and weight?
- Why do men usually have more rapid metabolic rates than women do?
- How much should you weigh? Has your answer to this question changed as a result of reading this chapter?
- Do you believe you have too much body fat? How do you know?

## WHY DO PEOPLE BECOME OBESE?

People do not become obese because they lack willpower. Obesity is a complex problem that involves many factors, including heredity, body metabolism, and inactivity, to name a few.

### Heredity

Obesity runs in families. People whose parents are obese stand a better than average chance of becoming obese themselves. Why does obesity run in families? In part, obese parents may set poor examples for their children by consuming large amounts of fattening foods. Children acquire food preferences and eating habits in the home at early ages.

Evidence also points to a significant role of genetics in determining body weight. Studies of adopted children, for instance, have found that as adults, people who were adopted as children are closer in weight to their biological parents than to their adoptive parents.[24] Identical twins (who have the same genetic makeup) are also closer in weight in adulthood than fraternal twins are. Fraternal twins share only 50% of their genetic makeup. Whether they were reared apart or together, identical twins in one study weighed virtually the same amount in adulthood.

Close-up
Understanding obesity
T0602

We are beginning to identify the genetic factors in obesity. Scientists recently discovered a gene, dubbed the *ob gene,* linked to obesity in mice.[25] The gene regulates the production of *leptin,* a hormone believed to signal the brain that the body has had enough to eat. Mice with the defective gene have voracious appetites, become obese, and have low levels of leptin. When they are given leptin, however, their weight returns to normal. We don't yet know whether a defective ob gene plays a

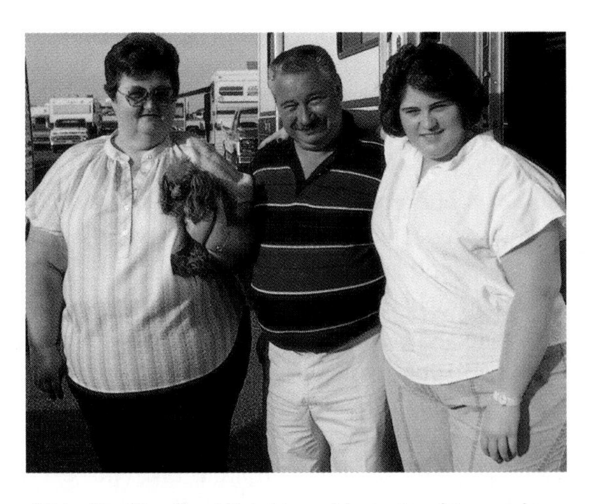

***All in the Family*** Weight problems tend to run in families. Both heredity and modeling of poor dietary habits appear to contribute to familial transmission of obesity.

role in human obesity. Many scientists believe that the ob gene may be one of many genes involved in regulating body weight in humans.

Even if our genes don't allow us to meet the cultural ideal of slim perfection, we can adopt healthy eating and exercise habits to achieve and maintain a healthy weight.[26]

## Metabolic Factors

Heredity may also influence body metabolism—the rate at which a body burns calories to maintain itself. Some people may have a faster metabolic rate than others. (Your authors were not so fortunate.) According to **set point theory,** regulatory mechanisms in the brain keep a person's body weight within a genetically predetermined range. When weight falls below the set point, say, a range of 150 to 160 pounds, regulatory mechanisms in the brain slow down metabolism. Further losses would thus be prevented. This may explain why dieters may find it harder and harder to continue to lose weight or even maintain the weight they've lost.

Dieters may not consume enough calories to satisfy their set points. Recent evidence shows that when people lose body weight by dieting, their metabolic rates decline.[27] The body reacts as if it were starving. By slowing down the metabolic rate, it preserves its fat reserves. However, as fewer calories are burned, the harder it becomes to lose weight, even on a diet. On the other hand, when people gain weight, researchers find that their metabolism speeds up.[28] Unfortunately, this mechanism may not compensate completely for weight gains. (Would that it were so!)

The ability of the body to slow its metabolic rate when calorie consumption decreases may be hard on dieters, but it may have helped humans survive through times of famine. You may be able to accelerate your weight loss for a while by further chopping your calorie intake. However, your body will eventually decrease your metabolic rate, further slowing your weight loss.

Then, too, when you lose weight, your body requires fewer calories than it did before. Generally speaking, a loss of 10% of body weight in a healthy person translates into 10% fewer calories the body needs just to maintain itself. Consider a 200-pound man who eats less and sheds 20 pounds, or 10%, of his body weight. At 180 pounds, his body requires about 10% fewer calories to maintain his new weight.

Are we doomed to regain the weight we lose? Not necessarily. Reducing gradually and exercising regularly may prevent a slowdown of metabolism. Exercise also maintains (or builds) muscle during weight loss, and muscle tissue burns more calories than fatty tissue.

## Fat Cells

**Fat cells** are cells that store fat. Fat cells are composed of **adipose tissue** (fatty tissue). Feelings of hunger are related to the number of fat cells in the body. As time passes since we have eaten, our blood sugar level drops. Low blood sugar leads to a release of fat from fat cells to fuel and nourish us. Depletion of fat in these cells is detected by the **hypothalamus,** a small structure in the midbrain. The hypothalamus triggers hunger, which motivates us to eat. Eating replenishes fat cells and restores the blood sugar level.

Obese people typically have more fat cells than other people.[29] People who are not obese have 25 or 30 billion fat cells. Severely obese people have 200 billion or more. So what does it matter how many fat cells you have? People with more fatty tissue in their bodies, and hence more fat cells,

**Talking Glossary**

Adipose tissue **G0602**

Hypothalamus **G0603**

**Set point theory** The theory that an individual's body weight is genetically set at a given weight range, or set point, that the body works to maintain.

**Fat cells** Body cells that store fat.

**Adipose tissue** The body tissue in which fat is stored.

**Hypothalamus** A midbrain structure involved in regulating body temperature, emotional states, and motivational states such as hunger and thirst.

feel hungry sooner than people with less fatty tissue, even when they weigh the same amount. Thus they may eat more often or feel hungry more of the time than people with less fatty tissue.

Heredity affects the number of fat cells in our bodies. But early dietary habits, such as excessive childhood eating, may also add fatty tissue. Unfortunately we do not shed fat cells when we lose weight. Rather, fat cells shrink but continue to signal the hypothalamus that they need to be replenished. Thus, dieters may experience relentless hunger. Nagging hunger can make it difficult for dieters to keep those extra pounds off. Some scientists believe that the human body is designed as a fat-storing machine, retaining its fat cells to provide reserves of energy in lean times. This may explain why you cannot shed fat cells once you have acquired them.

## Fat, Muscle, and Gender

Fatty tissue metabolizes or "burns" food more slowly than muscle tissue. Two people may weigh the same and consume the same amount of food. Yet they will metabolize food at different rates according to the proportions of fat and muscle in their bodies. People with higher fat-to-muscle ratios are more likely to put on extra pounds.

There is a gender difference in the fat-to-muscle ratio. Men's bodies average 40% muscle and 15% fat. Women's bodies average 23% muscle and 25% fat. Thus, men typically burn off excess calories more quickly than women of the same weight. Unfair as it may be, it is typically easier for men to keep off excess pounds.

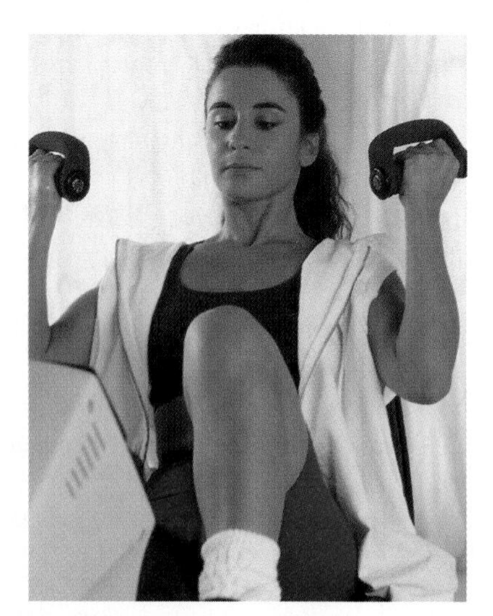

***Building Muscle***
Exercise helps control weight by burning calories in its own right and by building muscle. Muscle tissue burns more calories than an equal amount of fatty tissue.

## Inactivity

Obese people tend to be less active than other people.[30] A recent survey by the Centers for Disease Control showed that 33% of overweight men and 41% of overweight women are inactive. Inactivity was greater among the more severely overweight people.[31]

But which comes first, inactivity or obesity? Inactivity and obesity *interact*.[32] Inactivity contributes to obesity, and people tend to become less active as they gain weight. A program of regular exercise—like those described in Chapter 7—can help prevent weight gain and take off extra pounds.

**Close-up**
Get moving
**T0603**

Metabolic rates also fluctuate according to our activity levels. Watching TV, for example, may actually curb our metabolic rate.[33] One study reported an average decline of 12% in the metabolic rates of 7- to 11-year-old girls while they watched a TV program. Metabolic rates among overweight girls dropped even more, 16% on the average. Time spent in front of the tube is also time *not* spent walking, running, swimming, or engaging in other calorie-burning activities. Yet even couch potatoes can increase their activity levels by walking around during commercial breaks or exercising in place. And avoid snacking while watching the tube.

## Eating Habits

Problem eating habits also contribute to unwanted weight. Wolfing down one's food does not allow the brain the 15 minutes or so it takes to register sensations of satiety—feelings of fullness. You can consume a lot of excess food in the time it takes your brain to catch up to your stomach. People who seek to lose weight should control not only what they eat and how much they eat, but also how quickly they eat.

**Out of Sight, Out of Mouth?** Imagine a world in which there are no blinking neon signs advertising fried chicken or pizza. There are no TV commercials with images of melted cheese, drippy sauce, and scrumptious desserts. There are no magazines filled with pictures of cakes and pies. In such a world, people might eat only in response to their internal cues of hunger. Modern civilization, however, bombards us with external food cues—ads for tempting foods, aromas that permeate the air as we walk by the local bakery, and so on. Such cues can trigger food cravings even when we're not hungry.

## Socioeconomic, Sociocultural, and Ethnic Factors in Obesity

WORLD OF *diversity*

Rates of obesity vary from one racial or ethnic group in our society to another. Obesity is more prevalent among people of color, especially African Americans, Hispanic Americans, and Native Americans, than it is among non-Hispanic white Americans. Racial and ethnic differences are most pronounced among women (see Figure 6.5). The question is, why?

### Socioeconomic Factors

Socioeconomic factors play an important role in obesity. Obesity is more prevalent among poorer people.[34] People of color are typically of lower socioeconomic status than white Americans, so it is not surprising that rates of obesity tend to be higher among blacks and Hispanics, at least among women.[35]

Why are poorer people at greater risk of obesity? For one thing, more affluent people have greater access to information about nutrition and health. They are more likely to take health education courses. They have greater access to health care providers. The affluent also exercise more regularly than poorer people. They have the time and income to participate in organized fitness programs. Further, many poor people turn to food as a way of coping with the stresses of poverty, discrimination, crowding, and crime.

Results from a study in San Antonio, Texas, provide clear evidence of the link between socioeconomic status and obesity.[36] Obesity is less prevalent among both Mexican Americans and non-Hispanic white Americans living in higher-income neighborhoods than among those living in poorer neighborhoods. In other words, the link between socioeconomic level and obesity holds across ethnic groups.

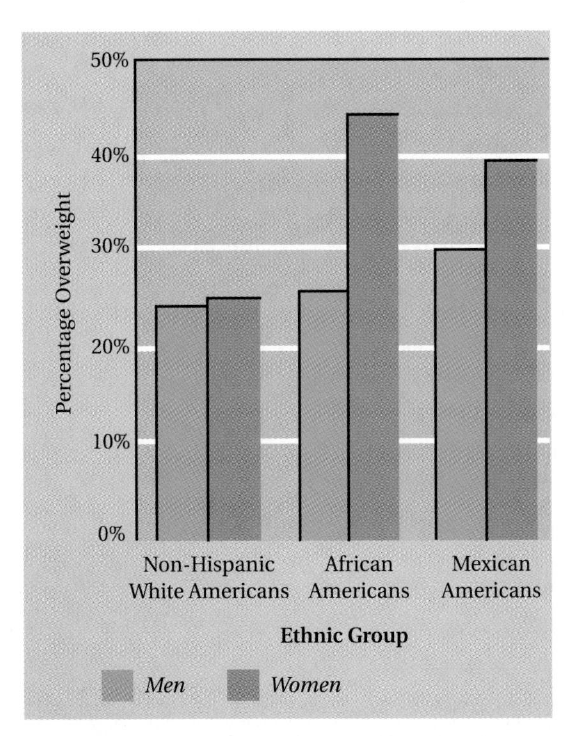


**Figure 6.5** ***Prevalence of Overweight People among Blacks, Whites, and Mexican Americans, by Gender*** Obesity varies with both gender and ethnicity. What factors might account for ethnic group differences in obesity?

### Dietary Patterns

Cultural differences in dietary customs may also contribute to excess body weight. African Americans, for example, are more likely than white Americans to consume high-fat, high-cholesterol foods. Whatever the underlying reasons for racial and ethnic differences, evidence shows that these differences may be narrowing. Though rates of obesity rose for men and women in all racial and ethnic groups during the 1980s, they rose most sharply among whites.[37]

### Acculturation

Acculturation is the process by which immigrant or native groups adopt the cultural values, attitudes, and behaviors of the host or dominant society. Acculturation may help immigrant people adapt more successfully to their new culture, but it can become a double-edged sword in terms of health if it involves adoption of unhealthful dietary practices from the host culture. Consider that Japanese-American men living in California and Hawaii eat a higher-fat diet than Japanese men do. Not surprisingly, the prevalence of obesity is two to three times higher among Japanese-American men than among men living in Japan.[38]

Acculturation may also contribute to high rates of obesity among Native Americans, who are more likely than white Americans to have diseases linked to obesity, such as cardiovascular disease and diabetes.[39] A study of several hundred Cree and Ojibwa Indians in Canada found that nearly 90 percent of the women in the 45 to 54 age group were obese. Moreover, the women were most likely to carry their extra pounds in the midsection. (They were "apples.") The adoption of a high-fat Western-style diet, the destruction of physically demanding native industries, and chronic unemployment combined with low levels of physical activity are factors contributing to obesity among Native Americans.

Preventing obesity calls for strategies that apply regardless of ethnicity or income level, such as cutting back on fat and sugar consumption and exercising regularly. But certain health initiatives need to be specifically aimed at meeting the needs of socially and economically disadvantaged groups, including the following:[40]

- Increased access to health education,
- Required health education curricula in all public schools,
- Guaranteed universal access to treatment of obesity,
- Increased access to healthful foods and recreational opportunities.

Some of us are more responsive to external cues than others. "External eaters" eat more in response to external cues than internal states of hunger. "Internal eaters" are not tempted to eat unless they are hungry. External eaters need to be especially aware of the effects that TV commercials and other cues have on them. That is why most weight-loss programs teach participants to limit their exposure to external cues. They recommend avoiding food-oriented magazines and keeping tempting treats out of sight (and preferably, out of the house). To paraphrase the familiar expression, "out of sight, out of mouth."

## Psychological Factors

We need to eat to survive, but food means more than survival. Psychologists have long recognized connections between eating and emotional states such as love, anger, fear, and depression. The giving and receiving of food is among the first interchanges between parent and child. It is intimately connected with the emotional warmth of the parent-child relationship. Food becomes a symbol of parental love. Parents may feel hurt or unloved if Junior fails to clean his plate or does not appreciate the nutritious meals they have prepared.

We celebrate achievements, family reunions, and holidays with food. Offering food to guests is a sign of hospitality. Refusing an offer (even a second or third helping) can be perceived as a rejection of hospitality.

Considering the emotional meanings of food, it is not surprising that people may turn to food when their emotional needs are not being met. Food may become a substitute for love; it may become a kind of natural tranquilizer, mood elevator, or sedative. When we eat, the parasympathetic nervous system activates digestive processes and lowers bodily arousal, which can calm feelings of anxiety or tension, or induce sleep. Some of us even eat in anger, as though we were biting the enemy. Eating because of negative emotions can compound emotional problems. It can lead to feelings of guilt and a negative body image if excess eating turns into unwanted body weight.

Negative emotions can also prompt binges. A binge is the consumption of a huge amount of food in a short period of time. Have you ever dreaded an approaching test and downed a carton of ice cream to quell your anxiety? We may attempt to drown disturbing emotions like anxiety, fear, and depression in chocolate cake. Frequent binge eating can lead to obesity.

In sum, many factors contribute to obesity: biological factors, inactivity, eating habits, and psychological factors. This chapter's ***Take Charge*** section suggests ways to achieve or maintain a healthy body weight by developing sensible eating and exercise habits.

## PREVENTION

### *Preventing Obesity*

Effective weight management means balancing the food energy (calories) you consume with the energy you expend. Here are some tips for managing your weight:

**Follow a Nutritionally Balanced Diet** You needn't become a calorie counter to control your weight.

- *Follow the nutritionally balanced diet outlined in the Food Pyramid (see Chapter 5, p. 137).* It will provide the calories to keep your weight at a healthful level. You will consume five or more servings of fruits and vegetables a day and take in ample minerals and vitamins.
- *Don't skip breakfast.* Weight watchers often try to save calories by skipping breakfast, but this deprives your body of the nutrition it needs to get started on the day. It may also lead to overeating later in the day as your body seeks to make up for the missed meal. Eat three balanced meals a day. Avoid unplanned snacks.
- *Keep healthful, low-fat foods handy for times you may be tempted to snack.* Make smart choices. Choose fat-free popcorn (the air-popped variety) over potato chips. Choose fat-free pretzels (read the labels). Switch from high-fat ice cream to low-fat or fat-free ice cream or frozen yogurt. Substitute fruits and vegetables for high-calorie snack foods. Fresh fruits make nutritious, low-calorie snacks. An average peach has 35 calories; an orange, 30 calories. Most fruits and vegetables are also rich sources of vitamins and fiber.
- *Reach for an extra helping of vegetables or bread, not an extra entree.*
- *Cut fat from your diet.* Substitute leaner cuts of meat. Don't eat red meat daily. Remove the skin from chicken. Switch from whole milk to low-fat or skim milk. Use butter sparingly, if at all. Use low-fat or fat-free salad dressings.

**Become Food Smart** You've heard of "book smarts" and "street smarts." Develop table smarts.

- *Become aware of the calorie and nutritional values of common foods.* Pocket-size calorie guides are available in bookstores and supermarkets. They will show you that:

    An 8-ounce serving of regular fruit-flavored yogurt has 230 calories.

Orange juice has more calories per ounce than Pepsi or Coke. Grapefruit juice has about as many calories as orange juice, and pineapple juice has even more (tomato juice has much less—see Table 6.3). Consider eating an orange or a grapefruit instead. (But don't rationalize drinking regular cola drinks as a substitute. They are not only loaded with calories; they have no nutritional value).

Nuts may be more fattening than candy (1 ounce of roasted peanuts contains 165 calories).

The point here is not to count calories, but to become more aware of the calorie and nutritional contents, including fat content, of the foods you typically consume. Arming yourself with this knowledge can help you make more sensible dietary choices.

- *Check out menu descriptions of meals.* Foods that are broiled, steamed, or cooked in their own juices are usually lower in fat and calories than foods that are fried, sauteed, or described as rich or crispy.
- *Beware of hidden calories.* What does it matter if your frozen waffles have no fat if you pour on gobs of butter and syrup? Food add-ons—sauces, butter, syrups, gravies, and dressings—are major sources of calories. A cup of fresh unsweetened peaches contains about 72 calories. Yet when it is packed in heavy syrup, it has 190 calories. And if you eat your fruit in cream, you are truly pouring on the fat and calories. A baked potato with skin contains about 220 calories and a trace of fat. One tablespoon of butter adds 11 grams of fat and 100 calories. Covering a meat dish with a cup of canned beef gravy adds some 125 calories. Chicken gravy adds 190 calories; mushroom gravy, 120 calories. Table 6.3 lists common foods that we don't usually think of as packing a lot of calories.

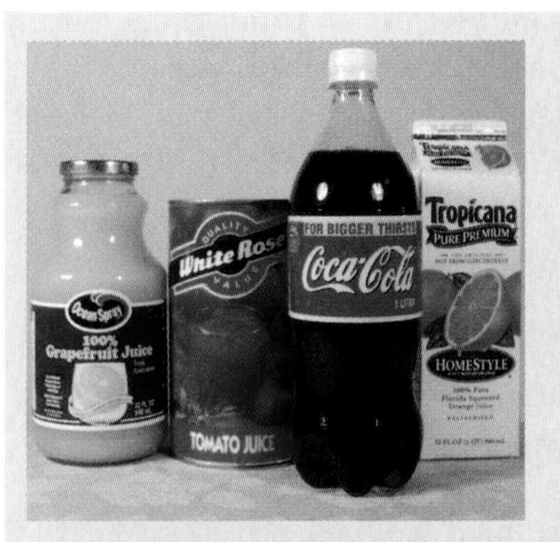


***Where Are the Calories?*** Calorie counters may be surprised to learn that Coca-Cola is lower in calories, ounce for ounce, than orange juice. However, orange juice is a rich source of vitamin C and other nutrients. Tomato juice is lowest in calories and also contains vitamins and other nutrients.

**TABLE 6.3**

**Sources of Hidden Calories[41]**

| Food | Calories | Fat (grams) |
|---|---|---|
| Plain yogurt (8 oz.) | 145 | 4 |
| Fruit-flavored yogurt (8 oz. container) | 230 | 2 |
| Beer (regular, 12 oz.) | 150 | 0 |
| Beer (light, 12 oz.) | 95 | 0 |
| Cola (regular, 12 fl. oz.) | 160 | 0 |
| Grapefruit juice (unsweetened, 12 fl. oz.) | 150 | Trace |
| Orange juice (unsweetened, 12 fl. oz.) | 180 | Trace |
| Tomato juice (unsweetened, 12 oz.) | 70 | Trace |
| Pineapple juice (unsweetened, 12 oz.) | 210 | Trace |
| Margarine (regular, tablespoon, $\frac{1}{8}$ stick) | 75 | Trace |
| Cashew nuts (dry roasted, 1 oz.) | 165 | 13 |
| Peanuts (roasted in oil, salted, 1 oz.) | 165 | 14 |
| Sunflower seeds (dry, 1 oz.) | 160 | 14 |
| Wine, dry table, red (12 fl. oz.) | 264 | 0 |
| Wine, dry table, white (12 fl. oz.) | 276 | 0 |
| Liquor (gin, rum, vodka, and whiskey—86 proof, 1 jigger) | 105 | 0 |

**Get into the Swing of Things—Follow a Regular Exercise Program** Exercise helps you maintain a healthful weight in two ways. It burns calories and increases your body's metabolic rate. Table 6.4 shows the numbers of calories expended in one hour for various activities. Which calorie-burners can you include in your regular routine?

**Close-up** Sisters together T0604

You needn't become an Olympic decathlete to include exercise as part of your weight-management effort. A half-hour swim at a typical pace burns about 240 calories for an average 125-pound person. This compares with less than 40 calories expended by sitting quietly for the same amount of time. Over the course of a year, substituting three 30-minute swims a week for time spent quietly sitting will burn off about 9 pounds without any changes in diet.

**TABLE 6.4**

**Calories Expended in One Hour According to Activity and Body Weight**

| | Body Weight (in pounds) | | | | |
|---|---|---|---|---|---|
| Activity | 100 | 125 | 150 | 175 | 200 |
| Sleeping | 40 | 50 | 60 | 70 | 80 |
| Sitting quietly | 60 | 75 | 90 | 105 | 120 |
| Standing quietly | 70 | 88 | 105 | 123 | 140 |
| Eating | 80 | 100 | 120 | 140 | 160 |
| Driving, housework | 95 | 119 | 143 | 166 | 190 |
| Desk work | 100 | 125 | 150 | 175 | 200 |
| Walking slowly | 133 | 167 | 200 | 233 | 267 |
| Walking rapidly | 200 | 250 | 300 | 350 | 400 |
| Swimming | 320 | 400 | 480 | 560 | 640 |
| Running | 400 | 500 | 600 | 700 | 800 |

**Focus on What You Eat, Not What You Weigh** Focus on what and how you eat, not on what you weigh. Body weight normally fluctuates from day to day due to water retention and other factors that can make weighing yourself daily a frustrating experience and discourage continued weight-control efforts. Weigh yourself at most once a week, without clothes and always at the same time of day. An alternative to weighing yourself is to keep tabs on your measurements. Measure your waistline, thighs, or hips, or the ratio between your hips and your waist, every month or so. A less formal but generally accurate measure of weight reduction is the closet test. See if you can fit into those clothes hanging in the back of your closet that you promised yourself you would wear once you lost weight. But be kind to yourself. Remember that people normally gain a moderate amount of weight, and some increased girth, as they age. (Your authors need to remind themselves of this fact from time to time.)

Smart Reference
Gaining on fat
R0601

**Take Corrective Action Early** Adjust your diet and activity level whenever your weight begins creeping upward or your clothes begin to feel tight. Don't go on a crash diet. Cut back gradually on the number or sizes of portions. Switch from high-calorie foods to low-calorie substitutes. You needn't go overboard increasing your exercise level either. Do it gradually. Don't risk injury. The "trick" is to take corrective action early to keep your weight within a stable range.

Smart Quiz
Q0602

## think about it!

- **What happens to body metabolism when people restrict calorie intake?**
- **Are you aware of the amount and the sources of calories in your diet? If not, should you be?**
- **Do you have unhealthy eating habits? What are you going to do about them?**

**critical thinking** **Agree or disagree and support your answer: Obese people simply eat too much.**

**critical thinking** **Do you believe that your own "set point" works for you or against you in maintaining a healthy weight? Explain.**

# EATING DISORDERS

You've probably heard the saying that you can't be too rich or too thin. Your authors can't say what it's like to be "too rich," although we wish we could. But being too thin can be hazardous to your health. In a nation of plenty, some people literally starve themselves—sometimes to death. They are obsessed with their weight and desire to achieve an exaggerated image of thinness. Others engage in cycles of binge eating and purging (as by vomiting) to control their weight. People with these problems have diagnosable psychological disorders called eating disorders. The two major types of eating disorders are anorexia nervosa and bulimia nervosa.

## Anorexia Nervosa

*Karen was the 22-year-old daughter of a renowned English professor. She had begun her college career full of promise at the age of 17, but two years ago, after "social problems" occurred, she had returned to live at home and taken progressively lighter course loads at a local college. Karen had never been overweight, but about a year ago her mother noticed that she seemed to be gradually "turning into a skeleton."*

*Karen spent literally hours every day shopping at the supermarket, butcher, and bakeries, and in conjuring up gourmet treats for her parents and younger siblings. Arguments over her lifestyle and eating habits had divided the family into two camps. The camp led by her father called for patience. That headed by her mother demanded confrontation. Her mother feared that Karen's father would "protect her right into her grave." She wanted Karen placed in residential treatment "for her own good." The parents finally compromised on an outpatient evaluation.*

*At an even 5 feet, Karen looked like a prepubescent 11-year-old. Her nose and cheekbones protruded crisply. Her lips were full, but the redness of the lipstick was unnatural, as if too much paint had been dabbed on a corpse for the funeral. Karen weighed only 78 pounds, but she had dressed in a stylish silk blouse, scarf, and baggy pants so that not one inch of her body was revealed.*

*Karen vehemently denied that she had a problem. Her figure was "just about where I want it to be." She engaged in aerobic exercise daily. A deal was struck in which outpatient treatment would be tried as long as Karen lost no more weight and showed steady gains back to at least 90 pounds. Treatment included a day hospital with group therapy and two meals a*

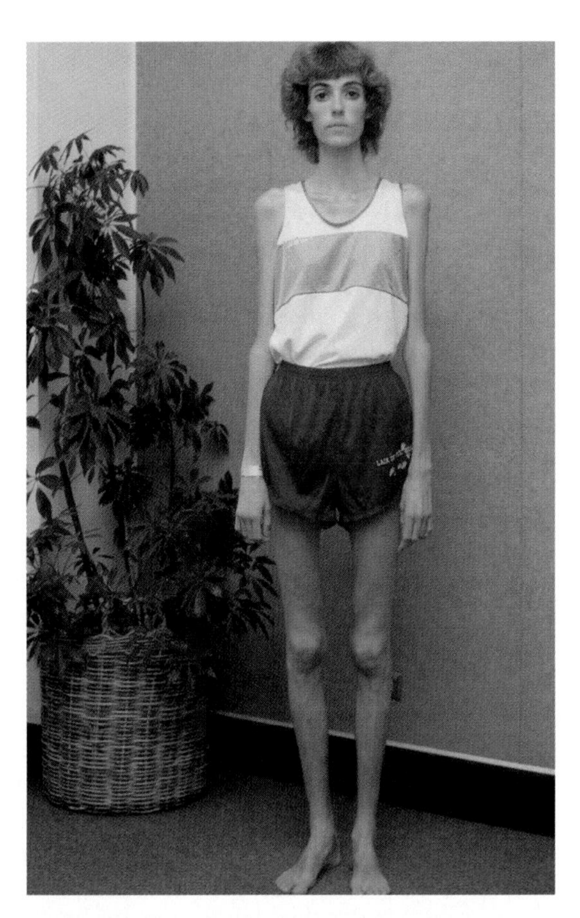

***Thin May Be "In," but What Are the Limits?*** Social pressure to be thin has contributed to serious eating disorders, such as anorexia nervosa (experienced by the woman in this photograph) and bulimia nervosa. Anorexia is a life-threatening eating disorder, characterized by a distorted body image and refusal to maintain a healthful body weight.

*day. But word came back that Karen was artfully toying with her food—cutting it up, sort of licking it, and moving it about her plate. She was not eating it. After 3 weeks Karen had lost another pound. At that point, her parents were able to persuade her to enter a residential treatment program, where her eating behavior could be more carefully monitored.*[42]

Karen has **anorexia nervosa.** The word *anorexia* derives from the Greek roots *an,* meaning "without," and *orexis,* meaning "a desire for." Anorexia typically develops during adolescence. It affects females more often than males by a ratio of about 20 to 1.[43] It is characterized by a body weight at least 15% below normal, intense fear of gaining weight or becoming fat, and a distorted body image. Anorexic people are convinced they are fat, despite the fact that others perceive them to be dangerously thin. Females with anorexia also experience **amenorrhea:** Their periods stop.

**Talking Glossary**
Amenorrhea
G0604

Anorexic people may literally starve themselves to death. Their mortality rate is believed to be about 4%.[44] Most fatalities are due to malnutrition. Other health consequences include:

- dermatological problems such as dry, cracking skin,
- fine, downy hair,
- yellowish coloration of the skin, which may continue for years after weight is regained,
- cardiovascular problems such as irregular heartbeat and low blood pressure,
- gastrointestinal problems such as chronic constipation, abdominal pain, and obstruction or paralysis of the bowels or intestines,
- muscular weakness,
- abnormal bone growth that may result in loss of height and osteoporosis.

Anorexia has become increasingly common, perhaps because of greater pressures on young women to adhere to unrealistic standards of thinness. Estimates are that about 1 to 2% of female adolescents have a history of anorexia.[45]

The typical person with anorexia is a young white female from a middle-class or upper-middle-class background. It is uncommon if not rare among men. In the typical case, a young woman begins to notice some added weight in adolescence. She becomes overly concerned about getting fat. She resorts to extreme dieting and in some cases excessive exercise to reduce her weight to a prepubescent level. She denies that she is too thin or losing too much weight, despite the concerns of others. In her mind's eye she views herself as heavier than she is.

## Bulimia Nervosa

*Nicole has only opened her eyes, but already she wishes it was time for bed. She dreads going through the day, which threatens to turn out like so many other days of her recent past. Each morning she wonders, is this the day that she will be able to get by without being obsessed by thoughts of food? Or*

**Anorexia nervosa** An eating disorder characterized by the maintenance of an unhealthily low body weight, an intense fear of gaining weight, a distorted body image, and, in females, an absence of menstruation.

**Amenorrhea** Absence of menstruation.

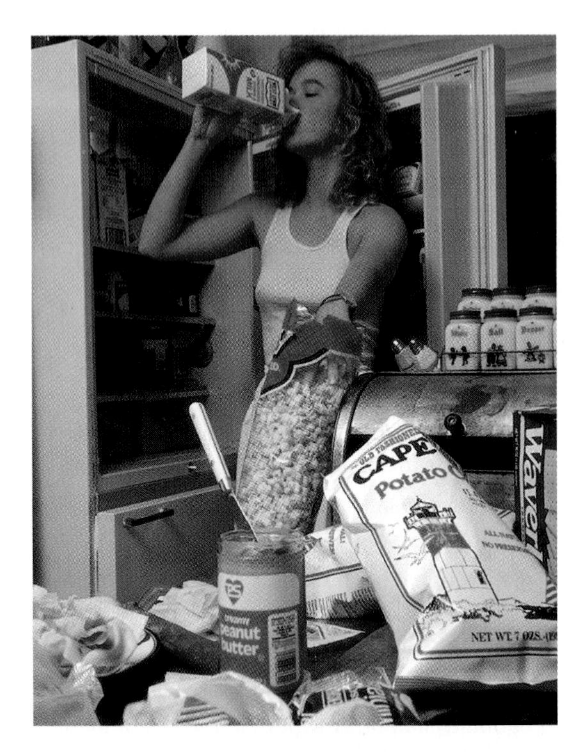


***On a Binge*** This woman with bulimia nervosa will binge-eat several thousand calories in one sitting. She will then purge by forcing herself to vomit.

> *will she "blow it again" and spend the day gorging herself? Today is the day she will get off to a new start, she promises herself. Today she will begin to live like a normal person. Yet she is not convinced that it is really up to her.*
>
> *Nicole starts the day with eggs and toast. Then she goes to work on cookies; doughnuts; bagels smothered with butter, cream cheese, and jelly; granola; candy bars; and bowls of cereal and milk—all within 45 minutes. Then she cannot take in any more food and turns her attention to purging what she has eaten. She goes to the bathroom, ties back her hair, turns on the shower to mask any noise she will make, drinks a glass of water, and makes herself vomit. Afterward she vows, "Starting tomorrow, I'm going to change." But she suspects that tomorrow may be just another chapter of the same story.*[46]

Nicole has **bulimia nervosa.** The word *bulimia* derives from the Greek roots *bous,* meaning "ox" or "cow," and *limos,* meaning "hunger," thus an image of continual eating like a cow chewing its cud. Bulimia is an eating disorder characterized by repeated episodes of binge eating followed by purging through such means as self-induced vomiting or excessive use of laxatives. Some people with bulimia purge regularly. Others purge only after a binge. Some engage in excessive, even compulsive exercise regimens to try to control their weight. Like those with anorexia, people with bulimia are obsessed with their weight. Unlike those with anorexia, bulimics typically maintain a relatively normal weight. Also, their perception of an ideal weight is similar to that held by other people.[47]

**Bulimia nervosa** An eating disorder characterized by repeated episodes of binge eating followed by purging and by persistent fears of gaining weight..

Bulimia usually begins in late adolescence, following a period of rigid dieting. As with anorexia, an estimated 1 to 2% of adolescent females develop the disorder.[48] Most bulimics are female, and most are from middle or upper socioeconomic classes. Some people have repeated binge-eating episodes but do not purge their food. They have another type of disorder classified as *binge-eating disorder.*

People with bulimia alternate food binges with strict dieting. The binge usually occurs in secret. It involves consumption of enormous amounts of usually forbidden fattening foods with little regard for taste or texture. One person with bulimia finished everything in her refrigerator, including scooping out margarine with her finger. As much as 5,000 to 10,000 calories may be consumed at a sitting. The binge may continue until the person is exhausted, in pain, or out of food. Upsetting events may trigger binges, or they may occur for no apparent reason. Purging follows immediately, out of fear of gaining weight or to punish oneself for violating one's diet. Afterward, the bulimic may feel exhausted, ashamed, and depressed.

Bulimia can cause a host of medical complications. Vomiting brings stomach acid to the mouth, where it can irritate the skin, block salivary ducts, and decay tooth enamel. Excessive use of laxatives can lead to bloody diarrhea and the development of laxative dependency. In some cases of laxative overuse, the bowel loses it ability to respond reflexively to pressure from waste material. Repeated vomiting can also induce potassium deficiencies. Lack of potassium upsets the electrolyte balance in the body and can cause irregular heart rhythms and even sudden death. People who use diuretics (drugs that increase the output of urine) to purge are at greatest risk. Females with bulimia, like those with anorexia, may experience amenorrhea.

**Close-up**
More on eating disorders
**T0605**

## Causes of Eating Disorders

The causes of eating disorders are the subject of much scientific inquiry and speculation. Psychoanalysts speculate that adolescents with anorexia unconsciously wish to remain little girls. They fear sexual maturity, which can bring pregnancy, separation from their families, and adult responsibilities. As they lose body fat, their breasts and hips flatten. Menstruation stops. They can maintain a distorted self-image of themselves as sexually undeveloped little girls. Evidence is sketchy, but some researchers find that girls with anorexia and bulimia do have problems with autonomy and independence.[49] Others suggest that adolescents may use refusal to eat as a weapon against their parents, a way of expressing resentment and rage. Some psychologists view anorexia as a type of weight phobia (excessive fear of gaining weight) that stems from the cultural idealization of the slender female form. Bulimic purging may be reinforced by a lessening of the fear of weight gain that accompanies a binge.

**HealthCheck**
Fear of fat scale
**H0601**

**All in the Family?** Biological factors also appear to be involved in eating disorders. Females with bulimia are often depressed and may respond well to treatment with antidepressant drugs. These drugs affect the appetite as well as the mood. Females with bulimia are also more likely than other women to have family members with mood disorders.[50] It is possible that bulimia and mood disorders share genetic roots. Perhaps both problems involve imbalances in key neurotransmitters in the brain.

## Treatment of Eating Disorders

Anorexics who become dangerously thin or malnourished are often hospitalized and force-fed if necessary. Drugs that stimulate appetite by curbing the actions of serotonin (a neurotransmitter that induces feelings of satiation) can lead to weight gains in people with anorexia.[51] Antidepressant drugs have the opposite effect: They increase the serotonin available in the brain, which suppresses appetite. Antidepressants can help people with bulimia by reducing their cravings for food and tendencies to binge.[52]

Psychological approaches also play important roles. With hospitalized anorexic patients, behavior therapists make reinforcements or rewards, such as increased ward privileges, contingent on eating or gaining weight. With bulimics, they may use a technique called *response prevention*. Bulimics are instructed to eat modest amounts of "forbidden" foods while the therapist stands by to prevent vomiting until the urge to purge has passed. In this way, bulimics learn to tolerate deviations from their rigid dieting rules without resorting to purging.

Psychodynamic treatment explores the psychological roots of the problem. Family therapy helps resolve family conflicts that contribute to or worsen the disorder. Cognitive-behavioral psychologists help people with eating disorders replace distorted beliefs about their bodies, food, and dieting with more rational beliefs. They encourage people with eating disorders not to define their self-worth in terms of their body weight. Although promising results of psychological and drug therapies are reported, many adolescents with eating disorders experience recurrent episodes into adulthood.

### think about it!

**critical thinking** Why do you think that females are more likely than males to have the eating disorders of anorexia nervosa and bulimia nervosa?

**critical thinking** Do you know anyone with an eating disorder? What do you think may be the cause? What, if anything, is being done to help the person?

**Smart Quiz**
**Q0603**

# Taking It Off and Keeping It Off

## Take Charge

*Super Diet! So Easy, They Call It a Miracle Diet! Lose Weight Fast, Effortlessly! Take Off Excess Weight Permanently . . . in Your Sleep! Hollywood Stars Reveal Their Diet Secrets!*

These are but a few of the magazine headlines that promise quick, easy, permanent weight loss. There are literally thousands of approaches to helping people lose weight. Despite the promises, taking it off and keeping it off is a constant struggle for most dieters. More than 90 percent of people who lose weight on a diet eventually gain it back, and then some.[53] These discouraging results have led many health professionals to conclude that dieting is ineffective.

Why don't quickie or crash diets work? In a nutshell, they fail to help people make lasting changes in eating and exercise habits. To be successful, diet programs need to set realistic, attainable goals and help people develop healthful eating and exercise habits that can become a part of their lifestyles.[54] Weight management is a lifelong challenge.

1. *Talk to a health professional.* Before making major dietary changes or starting an exercise program, talk things over with a health professional. You may have health concerns that may need to be taken into account when making these changes.
2. *Set realistic goals.* Establish a reasonable weight goal for yourself. You can use the height/weight table on p. 146 as a guide. Consider your body shape, family history, and age. Don't expect to fit into your high school prom suit or dress at the age of 40. Set a goal that is reasonable and attainable.
3. *Plan to lose weight gradually.* Plan to lose about a half a pound to a pound a week. The slower you take it off, the more likely you are to keep it off.[55] Remember: "Gradually on, gradually off."
4. *Plan a diet you can live with.* Plan a diet that meets your nutritional needs and cuts calories where you can best afford them. For example, reduce the size of servings, cut down on sweets and snacks, switch from high- to low-calorie foods, and use fats and oils sparingly. Plan to chop about 250 calories a day from your calorie intake to lose half a pound per week. Chop 500 calories a day to lose about 1 pound per week. (3,500 calories = 1 pound of body weight. Trimming 500 calories a day for 7 days amounts to a loss of 1 pound.) Make sensible *permanent* choices: Increase your intake of fruits and vegetables. Cut high-fat foods. Beware of fad diets and gimmicks that make claims that seem too good to be true.
5. *Shrink and switch.* Eat smaller portions. Substitute low-calorie foods for high-calorie foods. If you regularly eat two 6-ounce portions of meat a day, you can trim hundreds of calories a day by cutting back to two 4-ounce portions. Substitute a 4-ounce portion of skinless chicken or turkey for a portion of meat. Drink tomato juice rather than orange juice (at least part of the time).
6. *Track your eating habits.* Keep an eating diary for a week or two to track what you eat and to identify problem eating habits. Record everything you eat, jotting down in a diary what you ate, where you ate it, and what your feeling state (e.g., anxious, bored, angry, lonely, happy, or excited) and activity (e.g., watching TV, reading, talking on the telephone, or having a meal) were at the time.

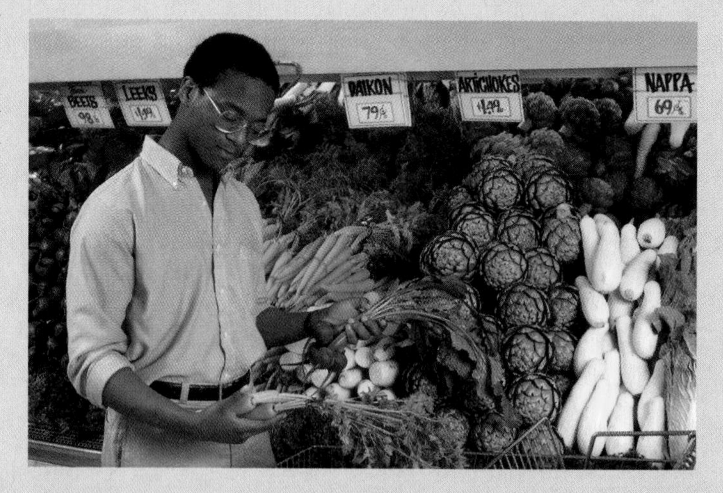


***Plan a Diet You Can Live With*** Eating vegetables and fruits is filling and helps control weight. Moreover, these foods are high in the kinds of vitamins, minerals, and fiber that help prevent chronic diseases such as cancer and cardiovascular disorders.

7. *Identify trouble spots.* Examine your eating diary to identify trouble spots, such as situations associated with unplanned or excessive snacking. Do you gobble down hundreds of calories in afternoon snacks or while watching late-night TV? If so, plan other activities at these times. Exercise or plan a low-calorie snack.
8. *Change self-defeating ideas about weight control.* Chronic dieters judge themselves harshly. They see themselves as "good" when they rigidly stick to their diets, or "bad" when they stray, even a little. They see themselves as total failures for breaking a minor dieting rule, such as using a spoonful of sugar in coffee if they run out of a sugar substitute. It's all-or-nothing thinking. Seeing themselves as failures may prompt them to binge ("What the heck—I'm off my diet, anyway").

   Changing irrational ideas can be as important as changing behavior. Replace irrational ideas with rational alternatives. Here are some adaptive thoughts you can substitute the next time you have a momentary lapse:
   - "No one is perfect. Everyone overeats now and then. Now let me get back to my regular diet."
   - "It's not the end of the world if I slip up. (Now let me . . . )"
   - "I am not a good or bad person because of what I eat. I am a complete person, not just an eating machine. (Now let me . . . )"
9. *Break the connections between food and bad feelings.* Do you use food to cope with negative emotions like anxiety, depression, and anger? If so, find other ways of handling your feelings. Write about them in a diary. Talk them over with a friend. Discuss what's on your mind with a counselor or a therapist. Don't try to solve your problems with food.
10. *Develop a regular exercise program and stick to it.* Combining a regular exercise program with a sensible calorie-reduction diet will help you lose weight more rapidly and keep the weight off. Unfortunately, many or most people who start exercise programs drop out within a few months. To boost your odds of sticking with an exercise plan, select one that's right for you, one that is conveniently located and fits your schedule. If possible, don't go it alone. Enroll with a friend or a spouse.

## The ABC's of Sensible Eating

How you eat can be as important as what you eat. Use **behavior modification** to replace unhealthy eating habits with healthy eating. Behavior modification focuses on the "ABC's" of eating and dieting. The *A*'s are the *antecedents* (stimuli or cues) that trigger eating. These include *external* or environmental cues, such as the sight and aroma of food. Antecedents for eating include the sight of other people eating in a cafeteria or the aromas emanating from a bakery. Emotional states, such as anger or boredom, are *internal* cues that also trigger the urge to eat. Hunger itself is an internal cue for eating. People who shop before dinner, when they are hungry, are more likely to buy fattening foods than people who shop after dinner. The more you are subjected to cues for eating, the more likely you are to overeat.

The *B*'s are the *behaviors* connected with eating and dieting. Behaviors such as taking large bites and swallowing without chewing thoroughly may not allow your brain the time it needs to feel satiated. You eat more—much more!—than your body requires to be satisfied.

The *C*'s are the *consequences* of eating and dieting. Food is a natural reinforcer. It provides immediate sensory pleasure and reduces feelings of hunger. These immediate rewards can outweigh the long-term problems connected with overeating, such as obesity and the health risks of obesity. Behavior modification changes the C's of eating by making the immediate consequences of sensible eating more rewarding and making the negative consequences of overeating more immediate.

Table 6.5 lists various behavior modification techniques based on the ABC's of effective dieting. These techniques are best combined with a sensible calorie reduction and exercise program. Behavior modification focuses on changing problem eating behaviors to keep lost weight off. People who participate in organized behavior modification programs typically lose between 1 and 2 pounds per week, or an average of about 21 pounds through the course of a 16-week program.[56] On average, participants keep off 60 to 70% of the weight they lost at a one-year follow-up. However, longer-term follow-ups are not as encouraging, as 90% or more of people who lose weight either by dieting alone or by behavior modification return to their baseline weights within five years.[57] Unfortunately, many people eventually return to unhealthy eating and exercise patterns and begin putting the weight back on. The lesson here is that losing weight and keeping it off requires a lifelong commitment to a healthy diet and regular exercise program.

How many of the ABC's listed in Table 6.5 can you use to make permanent changes in your eating habits?

## Other Methods

Many people find the social support and guidance of organized weight-loss programs helpful. But beware. Many of these programs don't make the grade. According to a *Consumer Reports* survey, users of Weight Watchers were more satisfied than users of competitors such as Jenny Craig, Physician's Weight Loss, Diet Center, Nutri/System, and liquid-fast programs.[59] Organized weight-loss programs are also offered by institutions such as hos-

**Take Charge**
Choosing for losing
C0601

**Behavior modification** Psychological interventions that apply learning principles to help people change their behavior.

TABLE 6.5

## Behavioral Techniques of Modifying the ABC's of Eating to Foster Weight Loss[58]

**Changing the A's of Overeating**

*Changing the Environmental A's*

- Avoid settings that trigger overeating.
- Don't leave tempting treats around the house.
- Serve food on smaller plates.
- Serve preplanned portions, and don't leave seconds on the table.
- Freeze leftovers, and don't keep them warm on the stove.
- Disconnect eating from other stimuli, such as watching TV, talking on the telephone, or reading.
- Establish food-free zones in your home. Place a mental barrier before the entrance to your bedroom: No food allowed!
- Shop quickly from a list. Don't browse through the supermarket.
- Treat the supermarket like enemy territory. Avoid the aisles of junk food and snacks. If you must walk down them, wear mental blinders.
- Never shop when hungry. Shop after dinner, not before dinner.

*Changing the Inner A's*

- Don't bury disturbing feelings in a box of cookies or a carton of ice cream.
- Relabel feelings of hunger as signals that you're burning calories.
- Don't let yourself get too hungry, however. Eat preplanned low-calorie snacks so that you are not tempted to binge.

**Changing the B's of Overeating**

*Slowing Down*

- Eat more slowly.
- Put utensils down between bites.
- Take smaller bites.
- Chew thoroughly.
- Savor each bite. Don't wolf bites down to make room for the next.
- Take a break during the meal. Put down your fork and converse with your family or friends for a few minutes. (Give your blood sugar level a chance to rise and signal your brain.)
- When you resume eating, ask yourself whether you need to finish every bite. Leave something over.

*Do Something Other than Eat*

- Substitute activities for food. When tempted to overeat, leave the house, take a bath, walk the dog, call a friend, walk around the block.
- Substitute low-calorie foods for high-calorie foods. Keep lettuce, celery, carrots, or fruit in the front of the refrigerator so that they are available for snacking.
- Fill spare time with activities unrelated to food. Volunteer at the local hospital, play golf or tennis, join exercise groups, read in the library (not the kitchen), take long walks.

**Changing the C's of Overeating**

- Reward yourself for meeting calorie-intake goals. To lose 1 pound per week, you need to cut 3,500 calories per week. Track what you eat and reward yourself for meeting weekly calorie goals. Reward yourself with gifts that you would not otherwise buy, like a new CD or tickets to a show. Repeat the reward program from week to week. If during some weeks you miss your calorie goals, don't give up. Get back on track next week.
- Use self-punishment. Charge yourself for deviating from your diet. Send one dollar to a political candidate you despise, or to a hated cause, each time the chocolate cake wins.

pitals, clinics, and YWCAs. These programs may be more affordable. (Y not give the Y a call?)

**Psychotherapy** Psychotherapy can help compulsive overeaters gain a better understanding of the psychological problems that may underlie their eating habits. For example, a person who feels chronically unloved or rejected may be using food as a substitute for love. Self-insight is not enough. It must be coupled with behavior change strategies to be successful.

**Very Low Calorie Diet Programs** A **very low calorie diet (VLCD)** program replaces a person's usual foods with a liquid protein mixture that provides 450 to 800 calories a day. The person typically stays on the VLCD for 12 weeks. Then she or he is gradually reintroduced to regular foods.

VLCD programs seem to be safe when properly supervised by a physician.[60] The protein mixtures are derived from nutritionally balanced dairy sources. They provide vital amino acids and other nutrients. Yet VLCD programs are not for everyone. Participants should be at least moderately obese. (If you want to lose five or ten pounds, this is not for you.) Participants are screened for medical conditions, such as heart problems, that could make a VLCD dangerous. The diet is often supplemented with behavior modification to help participants keep weight off.

VLCD typically leads to rapid and substantial weight losses (often 40 or 50 pounds over a 12-week period) in people who stick to it. VLCD programs have high dropout rates, however. Most people who complete a VLCD program also fail to keep off the weight when they return to regular food.[61] VLCD programs do not appear to offer any substantial long-term benefits over more conservative approaches like behavior modification.[62]

**Diet Drugs** Many people use over-the-counter appetite suppressants like Dexatrim and Accutrim. Diet pills work on the appetite control centers in the brain and may temporarily stave off hunger. Despite their popularity, however, these drugs yield only modest and temporary benefits.[63] Most people who lose weight with them put the pounds back on when they stop taking them.[64] Half the respondents to the *Consumer Reports* survey who had tried over-the-counter diet pills were very or completely dissatisfied with the results.[65] Fewer than 5% were very or completely satisfied with them. The drugs also have unpleasant side effects, such as dizziness and nausea. Many users report always feeling hungry, even though the drugs are supposed to suppress their appetites. The long-term safety of these drugs is also unknown.

**Video**
Use and abuse of diet drugs
**V0601**

Some people take prescription drugs to curb their appetite. One example is Redux, which was approved in 1996 for treating obesity. Unlike earlier prescription diet drugs that were amphetamine-based and made people jittery, Redux increases levels of the neurotransmitter serotonin in the brain, which makes people feel satiated. It literally fools the brain into thinking the body is full. However, users of Redux and of a similar drug, flenfluramine (Pondimin), have a much higher risk of a rare but potentially fatal lung disease, primary pulmonary hypertension.[66] Redux was intended only for people who are severely overweight.[67] In 1997, Redux and a similar drug, *fenfluramine* (the "fen" in the popular diet drug combination fen-phen), were linked to serious heart valve problems and were taken off the market.

Diet pills do not teach people more adaptive eating habits. Therefore, it is not surprising that when users discontinue the drug, their weight rebounds. Though diet drugs may have short-term benefits, they are not a substitute for developing sensible eating and exercise habits.

**Surgery** Surgery has revolutionized the treatment of morbidly obese people—that is, people whose weight exceeds *twice* the recommended level. Surgery may be indicated because of the serious health risks posed by morbid obesity. Then, too, other forms of treatment are often ineffective for people with extreme obesity.

One surgical method is *vertical-banded gastroplasty.* In this method, much of the stomach is stapled off, leaving but a small pouch for food. As people eat, the pouch quickly fills, leading to feelings of fullness.

Another procedure is gastric stomach bypass. A section of the small intestine is surgically connected to a pouch in the stomach so that food is rerouted directly from the stomach to the bowels for elimination. It bypasses the large intestine, where much of it would otherwise be digested. Bypass surgery has helped many morbidly obese people who could not lose weight through more conservative weight-loss treatments. However, about 10% of them develop complications.[68] Patients typically lose about 100 pounds within a two-year period after the surgery, but then start to regain weight slowly.

Other surgical treatments include jaw wiring, which restricts eating to low-calorie liquid diets, intestinal bypass (a shortening of the intestine to allow food to pass through more quickly), and insertion of a stomach balloon (to create a greater sense of fullness following eating). The outcomes of these techniques remain uncertain. A more common operation, which is not restricted to the morbidly obese, is *liposuction.* Liposuction is cosmetic surgery in which the surgeon removes fatty tissue from areas such as the hips or buttocks.

The safety and effectiveness of surgical treatments of obesity remain under scrutiny. Noting that 85% of the people who undergo surgical treatments for obesity are women, Sally E. Smith of the National Association to Advance Fat Acceptance argues, "Most women who get surgery do so more for psychosocial reasons such as getting a better self-image. These women are risking surgery because of the way society treats fat people."[69] Still, many severely obese people, men as well as women, have benefited from surgery.

**Very low calorie diet (VLCD)** A protein-sparing, low-calorie diet typically consisting of 800 calories or less.

**Keeping It Off** As if losing weight were not enough of a struggle, weight reducers face an even greater challenge in keeping it off. Most people who struggle to lose weight lose the battle of the bulge and eventually regain what they lose.

Smart Quiz Q0604

A regular exercise program appears to be the key to keeping weight off. In one study, men lost weight by following a calorie-reduction diet for a year. Men who then increased the time they spent exercising (as by walking or jogging) kept off more weight than those who continued to count calories or who tried to further reduce their calorie intake.[70] In fact, the men who increased their level of exercise consumed an average of 335 more calories daily than their calorie-counting counterparts. Yet they wound up regaining less than 2 pounds during the year follow-up period, compared with seven pounds gained back by the calorie counters. Exercise not only helps shed pounds; it helps keep them off.

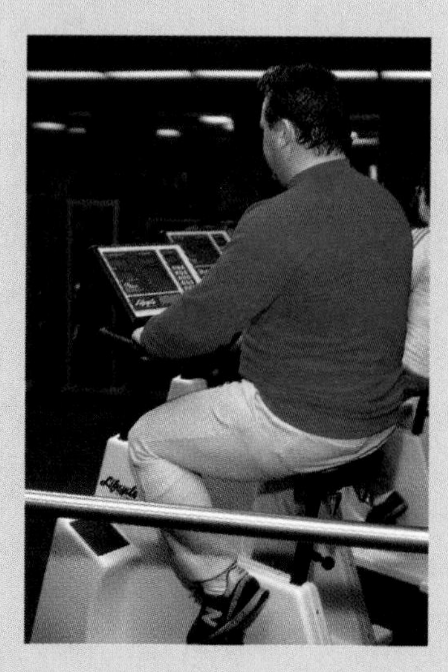

***Taking It Off and Keeping It Off*** Fitting regular exercise into your schedule helps shed extra pounds and keep them off.

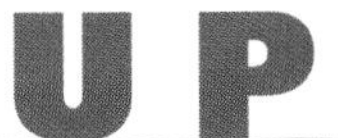

# SUMMING UP

## Questions and Answers

### CALORIES AND WEIGHT—A BALANCING ACT

1. **What health problems are connected with obesity?** These include cardiovascular disorders, respiratory illnesses, diabetes, gall bladder disease, gout, and certain kinds of cancer.

2. **What is the connection between calories and weight?** A calorie is the amount of energy required to raise the temperature of 1 gram of water 1 degree Celsius. The metabolic rate is the rate at which we burn calories. If we consume more calories than we metabolize ("burn"), we may gain weight. Muscle tissue burns calories more rapidly than fatty tissue. Therefore, men, who tend to have a higher muscle-to-fat ratio than women do, tend to burn calories faster than women of the same weight.

3. **How do you know if you weigh too much or have developed obesity?** One may consult weight charts, assess one's body mass index, take skinfold measurements, or measure one's hip-to-waist ratio.

### WHY DO PEOPLE BECOME OBESE?

4. **Why do people become obese?** Diet plays a role in obesity, but genetic factors are also involved. People find it difficult to lose weight because their metabolism slows down when they eat less. Inactivity and negative emotions, such as depression and anxiety, also play roles in obesity.

5. **What are fat cells?** These are adipose tissue that shrivels when people diet, triggering signals of hunger. Because of fat cells, people who *were* obese may be hungry nearly all the time when they try to *keep* weight off.

6. **What are the connections among socioeconomic, sociocultural, and ethnic factors and obesity?** Despite the fact that food costs money, poor people are more likely than affluent people to be obese. Cultural differences in diets, acculturation, and use of food in response to stress may also be involved in accounting for higher rates of obesity in some groups. For instance, Japanese Americans are heavier than Japanese nationals, at least among men, apparently because they eat higher-fat diets.

### EATING DISORDERS

7. **What is anorexia nervosa?** This is an eating disorder in which people starve themselves because of exaggerated concerns about weight gain. Anorexia is more common among women than men, largely because of the demanding cultural ideal of the slender female. Anorexic women have distorted body images, seeing themselves as fat when others see them as dangerously thin.

8. **What is bulimia nervosa?** This is an eating disorder characterized by cycles of binge eating and purging, as by vomiting or excessive use of laxatives.

### TAKING IT OFF AND KEEPING IT OFF

9. **How can people lose weight successfully?** People can lose weight and keep it off by changing their eating and exercise habits. They can eat lower-fat diets, consume fewer calories, and increase their metabolic rates through regular exercise. Diets high in vegetables, fruits, and grains not only help people lose weight but also help prevent cardiovascular disease and certain kinds of cancer.

## References and Suggested Readings

### SMART REFERENCES FROM SCIENTIFIC AMERICAN

**Gibbs, W.** Trends in Medicine: Gaining on Fat. *Scientific American,* 275(2) (August 1996), 88–94. **R0601**

### SUGGESTED READINGS

**Bellerson, K. J.** *The Complete & Up-to-Date Fat Book.* Garden City, NY: Avery Publishing Group, 1993. A comprehensive listing of the fat and calorie contents of over 25,000 food entries, including many brand-name food items. An essential resource if you are tracking the nutritional values of the foods you eat.

**Rodin, J.** *Body Traps.* New York: Quill, 1992. Avoiding diet traps and unrealistic expectations concerning body weight and shape, from a leading psychologist and obesity researcher.

**Brownell, K. D., and Wadden, T. A.** Etiology and treatment of obesity: Understanding a serious, prevalent, and refractory disorder. *Journal of Consulting and Clinical Psychology,* Vol. 60 (1992), pp. 505–517. A scholarly review of the causes and treatment of obesity.

**Nash, J. D.** *Maximize Your Body Potential.* Palo Alto, CA: Bull Publishing, 1986. This award-winning book focuses on the goal of lifetime weight management and contains information concerning good nutrition, healthful exercise, and eating habits.

**U.S. Department of Agriculture (USDA).** *Calories and Weight: The USDA Pocket Guide.* Washington, DC: U.S. Government Printing Office. This handy guide to the calorie values of common foods is available free of charge from the USDA.

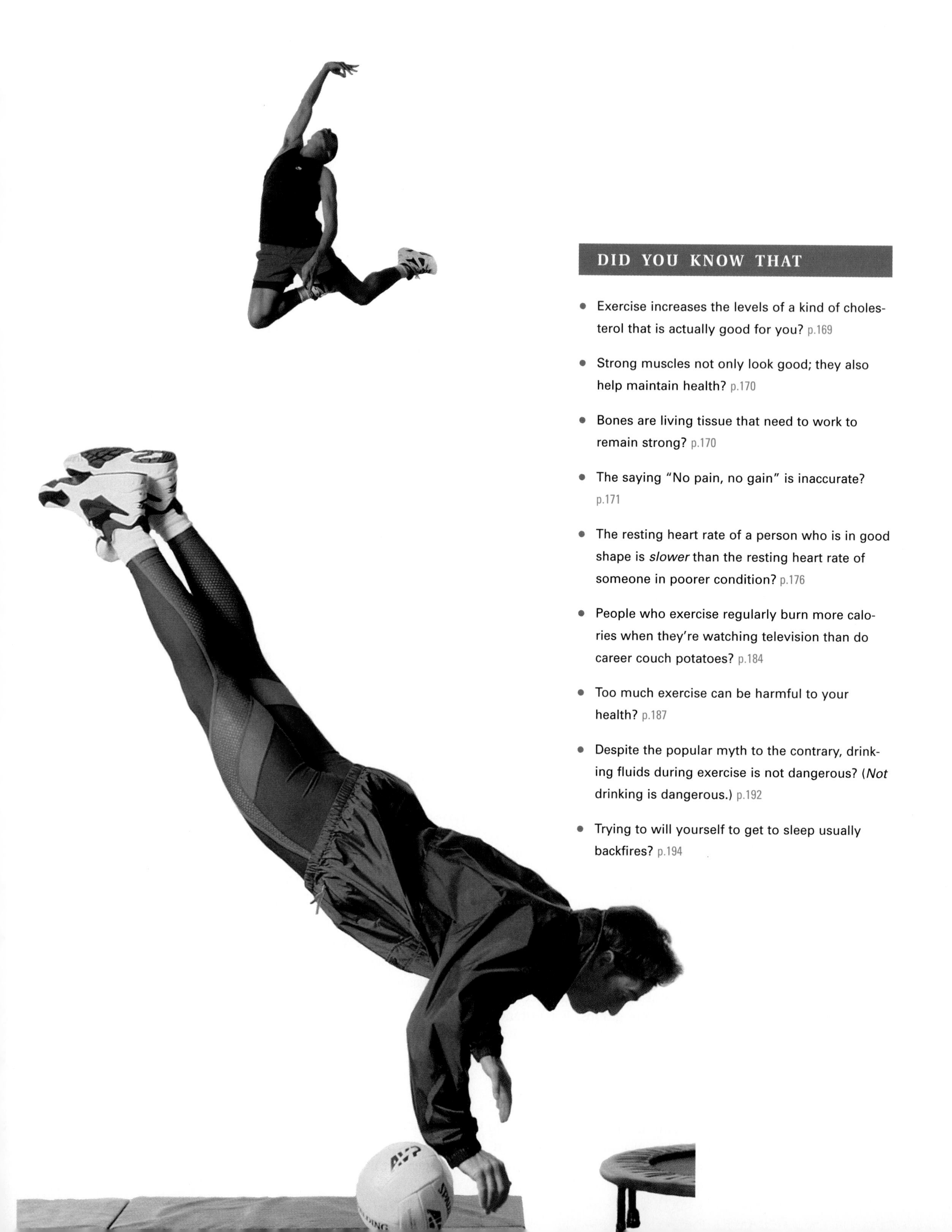

## DID YOU KNOW THAT

- Exercise increases the levels of a kind of cholesterol that is actually good for you? p.169
- Strong muscles not only look good; they also help maintain health? p.170
- Bones are living tissue that need to work to remain strong? p.170
- The saying "No pain, no gain" is inaccurate? p.171
- The resting heart rate of a person who is in good shape is *slower* than the resting heart rate of someone in poorer condition? p.176
- People who exercise regularly burn more calories when they're watching television than do career couch potatoes? p.184
- Too much exercise can be harmful to your health? p.187
- Despite the popular myth to the contrary, drinking fluids during exercise is not dangerous? (*Not* drinking is dangerous.) p.192
- Trying to will yourself to get to sleep usually backfires? p.194

# Fitness for Life

7



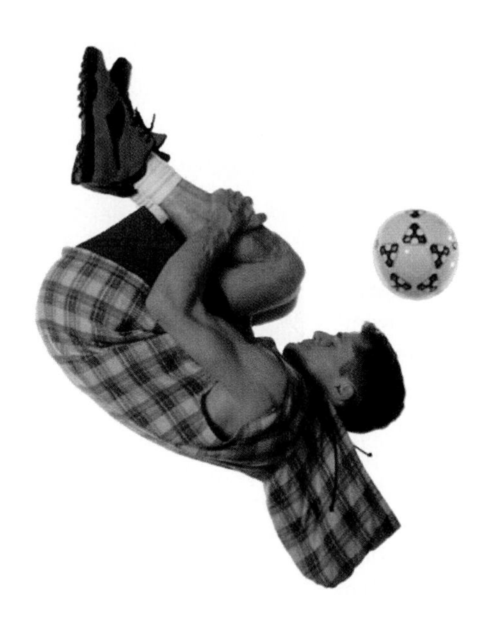

*Exercise builds and helps maintain health and vitality. It helps tone and build muscles, increases stamina and flexibility, strengthens the heart and improves lung capacity, combats stress and helps relieve depression and anxiety, sheds excess pounds, and reduces the risk of health problems such as coronary heart disease (CHD), adult-onset diabetes, and some forms of cancer. Exercise also gives you energy and a sense of well-being. It may even extend life. Whatever goals you set for yourself, from improving your physical appearance and mental outlook to lowering your risk of heart disease, exercise can help you achieve them.*

More than 40 centuries ago, the Chinese recognized that people who exercised regularly were sick less often than inactive people. The ancient Greeks believed that rigorous physical development was the key to self-betterment. Until the 1970s in the United States, exercise was largely confined to schools and professional sports. Then reports documenting the health benefits of exercise began to reach the public. A fitness boom began that is still going strong. New forms of exercise such as aerobic dance classes and in-line skating (rollerblading) caught on. Our roads became peopled by runners of all ages and descriptions. Bicycle riding became popular again. Health clubs and gyms sprang up everywhere. Today, millions of Americans stay in shape through **aerobic exercise.** Aerobic exercise includes running, lap swimming, brisk walking, aerobic dance classes, and other sustained, vigorous activities that elevate your heart rate and make you break into a sweat.

**Talking Glossary**
Aerobic exercise
G0701

To put the growing interest in exercise in perspective, consider this: In 1970, there were about 100 entrants to the first New York City Marathon. A marathon is a 26.2-mile race that sets the standard for endurance racing. By the 1990s, more than 40,000 marathoners were clamoring to enter the New York City Marathon. Among them were nearly 100 wheelchair racers.

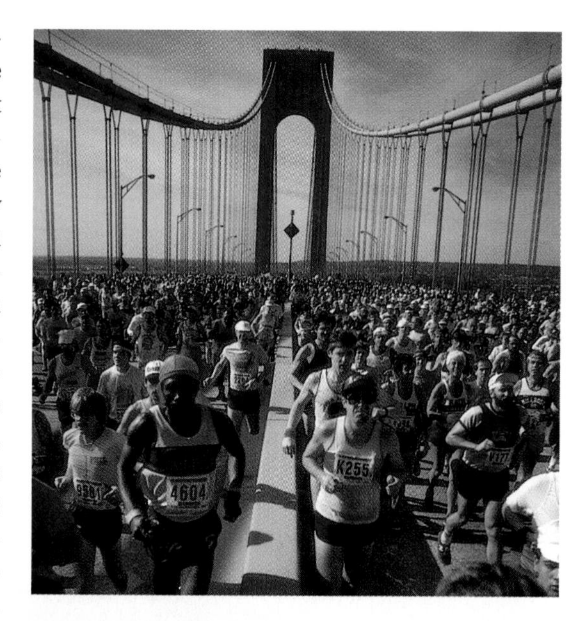


***The New York City Marathon*** Thousands of Americans have taken to long-distance running as a way of keeping fit. But you needn't become a marathon runner to reap health benefits of exercise. Many kinds of regular physical activity can improve fitness and health.

Participation has also grown in other types of exercise, such as walking, weight training, and the use of exercise machines such as stair-climbing and rowing machines. About 70 million Americans walk for fitness. More than 66 million swim.[1]

While many Americans participate in some form of exercise, the overall picture is less encouraging. One-quarter of all Americans are complete couch potatoes. They engage in no exercise routine whatsoever. Fewer than one in ten exercises vigorously or frequently enough to strengthen the heart and lungs.[2] People with lower incomes, children, and older women exercise least.[3] Nor is the average college student the model of fitness. Overall, the average level of cardiorespiratory fitness of entering freshmen in the 1990s was *lower* than that of freshmen who entered college a decade earlier.[4] Given that high rates of heart disease, obesity, and other health problems are linked to a sedentary lifestyle, many Americans are dangerously unfit.

A sedentary lifestyle is a key risk factor for coronary heart disease (CHD). It is comparable in importance to high blood cholesterol levels, hypertension, and smoking. A sedentary lifestyle can set the stage for obesity, adult-onset diabetes, osteoporosis, even some forms of cancer. Inactivity also leads to a general lack of energy, breathlessness during physical exercise, poor cardiac efficiency, and an increased risk of straining and spraining underused joints and limbs. All in all, inactivity represents a major risk factor for disease and reduced longevity.

**Aerobic exercise** Physical activity requiring sustained elevation in oxygen utilization.

# EXERCISE AND HEALTH

Regular exercise benefits our physical and psychological health in many ways.

## Physical Benefits of Exercise

**Reduced Risk of Cardiovascular Disease** Inactivity or sedentary living is a major risk factor for cardiovascular disease (heart and artery disease).[5] Cardiovascular disease is responsible for more deaths in the U.S. than any other cause, most often from heart attacks and strokes. Inactive people have about double the risk of developing heart disease as their most active peers. Fortunately, regular exercise reduces this risk. Even moderate activity, like gardening and physically demanding housework, can reduce the risk of cardiovascular disease if it is done daily, for at least 30 minutes a day. But to condition your heart and lungs, you need to engage in 20 minutes or more of vigorous activity at least three to four times a week. These activities include aerobic dancing, bicycling, cross-country skiing, hiking uphill, running, rowing, stair climbing, and fast walking.[6]

**Close-up**
Surgeon General's Report
T0701

Exercise has many healthful effects on the cardiovascular system. If done regularly, aerobic exercise widens blood vessels, allowing blood to circulate freely. This can help reduce high blood pressure (hypertension), a major risk factor for heart disease. Regular exercisers are between 30 and 50% less likely to develop hypertension than nonexercisers.[7] Even moderate exercise when done regularly can lower blood pressure in people with hypertension and reduce the amount of medication needed to control severe hypertension.[8]

**Healthcheck**
Fitness and Heart Disease IQ Test
H0701

Regular exercise also boosts levels of high-density lipoproteins (HDL cholesterol), dubbed "good" cholesterol because it sweeps away cholesterol deposits from artery walls. High levels of HDL are associated with a lowered risk of heart disease. Regular exercise also produces a more favorable ratio of HDL to total blood cholesterol.[9] A study of 7,000 male runners showed that the more miles the men ran, the higher their HDL levels.[10] Even men who logged only seven miles per week showed significantly higher HDL levels than people who do not exercise. Regular exercise also helps lower blood levels of **triglycerides,** a type of dietary fat that increases the risk of CHD, especially in people with low levels of HDL.[11]

Regular exercise helps people maintain a healthy body weight and avoid obesity, another risk factor for cardiovascular disease. Exercise helps people take off excess weight by burning calories, by increasing the ratio of muscle to fat, and by increasing body metabolism, the rate at which the body burns calories.

Exercise helps maintain a good supply of oxygen to the heart, which is vital to health. Exercise strengthens the heart muscle by increasing the size of the walls of the heart muscle. Because of this, people who regularly exercise may be better able to survive heart attacks. Exercise also lowers the resting heart rate. Thus the heart may pump with less wear and tear.

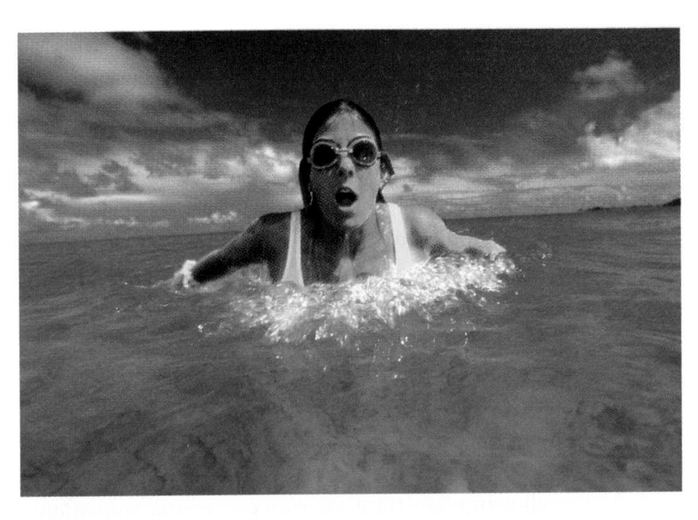

***Benefits of Exercise*** Regular exercise has many health benefits, including weight control, cardiovascular fitness, and even protection against certain kinds of cancer.

**Improved Immune System Functioning** Regular exercise may boost the **immune system,** the body's line of defense against disease-causing pathogens such as bacteria and viruses. The immune system is composed of specialized **white blood cells** (also called *leukocytes*) that identify, envelop, and eradicate microbes that invade the body. Some white blood cells produce specialized proteins called *antibodies* that attach to foreign bodies, inactivate them, and mark them for destruction. People who regularly exercise show higher levels of **natural killer (NK) cells** in their blood system, a type of white blood cell that destroys invading pathogens. In one study, previously inactive women who walked for 45 minutes a day five days a week showed greater NK cell activity when tested six weeks later.[12] Fifteen weeks into the program, the exercisers showed a higher level of virus-fighting antibodies than they did before the exercise program began. No changes were found for people in the study who did not exercise.

**Reduced Cancer Risk** Exercise helps reduce the risk of colon cancer.[13] It may also offer some protective benefit against other cancers, such as breast cancer and prostate cancer. Researchers from the National Can-

**Triglycerides** A type of lipid or fatty substance found in the blood.

**Immune system** The body's system of defense for identifying and eradicating invading bacteria and viruses, as well as diseased, mutated, and worn-out cells.

**White blood cells** *(leukocytes)* Blood cells that function in specialized roles as part of the body's immune system.

**Natural killer (NK) cells** A type of white blood cell that kills viruses.

cer Institute found that moderately active men had a 39% lower risk of cancer than inactive men. Among women, the moderately active had a 23% lower cancer risk.[14] Regular exercise is also associated with a reduction of as much as 60% in the risk of breast cancer in young women.[15] The sharpest reductions were found in women who regularly exercised for about four hours a week in vigorous activities such as running, swimming, or tennis. Even women who exercised two or three hours a week showed some reduction in risk.

What accounts for the cancer-preventive role of exercise? In the case of colon cancer, exercise helps speed waste material through the colon, allowing less time for cancer-causing substances to affect the lining of the colon. In the case of breast cancer, exercise may help by reducing levels of the female sex hormone estrogen. (Breast cancer is linked to length of exposure to estrogen.) Exercise also appears to boost the immune system, which rids the body of cancerous cells before they turn into malignant growths.

**Increased Energy** Regular exercise helps boost energy levels. People often report feeling energized and more alert after a brisk walk, swim, or workout. Moderate exercise seems to work best as an energy booster. Too much exercise can be exhausting. Regular exercise may also enhance feelings of energy and alertness. Why? We're not certain. Exercise may boost energy by inducing changes in brain chemicals or in the brain's electrical output. Exercise also increases the body's utilization of oxygen, which improves stamina and circulation.

**Other Physical Benefits** Regular exercise, especially vigorous exercise, can increase lung capacity, or the amount or volume of air the lungs can hold. Increased lung capacity is associated with greater longevity.

Regular exercise can also increase insulin sensitivity—the body's ability to utilize **insulin.** Insulin is a hormone produced by the pancreas that stimulates cells to absorb blood sugar (glucose) and other nutrients from the bloodstream. Insulin is essential to regulating the metabolism of glucose and in maintaining blood sugar at a proper level. In diabetes, a condition which afflicts about 16 million Americans, either the pancreas produces too little insulin, or cells in the body fail to utilize insulin efficiently (see Chapter 18). The body becomes less capable of using insulin efficiently as we age, which increases the risk of the most common form of the disorder, adult-onset diabetes. By increasing insulin sensitivity, regular exercise helps the body regulate blood sugar levels, which may reduce the risk of adult-onset diabetes or help manage it if it should develop.

**Insulin** A hormone produced by the pancreas that plays an essential role in the metabolism and regulation of blood sugar (glucose).

**Osteoarthritis** A chronic, degenerative disease of the joints that produces pain and restricted movement. More commonly called *arthritis.*

**Bones** Living tissues that support and move the body; consist of a matrix of the protein collagen and the mineral calcium.

**Osteoporosis** A degenerative condition characterized by the loss of bone density, which makes bones more brittle and prone to break.

**Benefits of Muscle-Strengthening Exercise** Maintaining strong muscles improves mobility, reduces the likelihood of injury, and helps prevent lower back problems. Muscle-strengthening exercise offers other important physical benefits, including reduced risks of osteoarthritis and osteoporosis. **Osteoarthritis** (also called *arthritis*) is a chronic, degenerative disease of the joints (see Chapter 19). It is linked to wear and tear on the joints and can result in painful and restricted movement. Muscle strengthening and stretching help keep joints and tendons flexible.

**Talking Glossary**
Osteoarthritis
G0702

Exercise is also important to healthy bones. **Bones** are living tissue. They consist of a lacelike matrix of the protein collagen and the mineral calcium. Bones grow in length until about age 21 but continue to change in density or thickness throughout life. Unless bones are worked, they become thinner and more brittle. Density gives bones their strength. Stronger bones are less vulnerable to fractures or breaks. When bones are not stressed through repeated use, they begin to lose density (become "demineralized") as the result of loss of calcium. Loss of density can lead to **osteoporosis,** which makes bones more vulnerable to fractures. Osteoporosis most often affects older women and is believed to account for more than 5 million fractures of the hip, spine, and wrists in women over the age of 45.[16]

*Resistance training* helps maintain bone density. Resistance training involves working against a weight or force, such as in lifting weights. On average, the bone mass (a measure of the density or strength of bones) of those who exercise regularly is 6 to 8% greater than it is in those who don't exercise.[17] Some types of exercise appear better than others for building bone mass and reducing the risk of fractures. Athletes in sports requiring greater muscular strength, such as weight lifting and gymnastics, typically have denser bones than distance runners, who require more endurance than strength.[18] Like aerobic exercise, strength training also raises HDL levels and lowers triglyceride levels, but apparently the effect is significant only in males.[19]

## Psychological Benefits of Exercise

People who exercise regularly report positive changes in their moods. They may feel less tense, anxious, and depressed during and after workouts. They are generally more relaxed and self-confident than inactive people. They're also more likely to engage in healthful behaviors and avoid harmful substances. The connection between improved mood and exercise is so strong that health professionals often encourage depressed people to exercise.

Exercise also provides a break from the strains of everyday life, which can help combat stress. Aerobic exercise helps normalize levels of neurotransmitters that are believed to play a role in depression. Exercise can also be enjoyable, which is another reason that it may help combat depression. Exercise can give us a sense of mastery and accomplishment, which boosts our self-image and self-confidence and may help us overcome the feelings of helplessness that are often associated with depression.

Some runners report feelings of euphoria known as the "runner's high." This phenomenon has been linked to the release of *endorphins*. Endorphins are the body's natural painkillers. They function in a similar way to the narcotic morphine.

## How Much Exercise Do You Need?

You don't need to become a marathon runner or sculpt your body like Arnold Schwarzenegger to reap the healthful benefits of exercise. You can gain the benefits of exercise without pain. The key is to make physical activity a regular part of your daily routine. A panel of fitness experts brought together by the Federal Centers for Disease Control and Prevention and the American College of Sports Medicine has encouraged Americans to engage in 30 minutes a day of moderate physical activity.[20] Moderate physical activity is equivalent to a level of effort required by brisk walking at a 3- to 4-mile-per-hour pace. Even such daily activities as walking briskly from your parking space to your office building, or climbing the stairs to your office, will help you meet your goals. Moderate physical activity may not make you aerobically fit, but it can reduce your risk of health problems such as CHD, hypertension, diabetes, colon cancer, depression, and anxiety.

**Close-up**
Physical activity and health
**T0702**

Note the use of the term *physical activity* rather than *exercise*. Virtually any form of physical activity of at least moderate intensity will fill the bill, including:

climbing stairs,
raking leaves,
taking a brisk walk,
playing actively with your children,
doing odd jobs around the house.

Many moderately vigorous activities can fit your daily routine (see Table 7.1, next page). You needn't accumulate your 30 minutes a day all at once or from the same activity. You can combine short bouts of activity throughout the day. Not just any activity counts, however. Walking around the house or the office doesn't measure up. Nor does most housework, unless it is physically demanding, like cleaning out your closet or washing the windows. In short, any physical activity that is equivalent in strenuousness to taking a brisk walk is beneficial, so long as you clock up 30 minutes a day. Table 7.1 lists different types of physical activities by their level of intensity: light, moderate, and vigorous. Activities that meet or exceed the recommended guidelines for moderate physical activities are found in the second and third columns.

**Why the Emphasis on Moderate Physical Activity?** For a long time health officials and fitness experts touted the benefits of regular aerobic exercise, the type of vigorous exercise (such as those in column 3 of Table 7.1) that gets your heart pumping and sweat dripping down your forehead. Though aerobic exercise has not gone out of favor, health officials are now touting the benefits of moderate exercise. Why?

One important reason is that moderate physical activity has health benefits.[22] In one study, researchers found that letter carriers have a lower risk of CHD than that of sedentary people and not very different from that of long-distance runners.[23] The letter carriers walked an average of 7 miles a

TABLE 7.1

**Examples of Physical Activities for Healthy U.S. Adults by Intensity of Effort[21]**

| Light Activity | Moderate Activity | Vigorous Activity |
|---|---|---|
| Walking slowly (strolling at 1–2 mph) | Walking briskly (3–4 mph) | Walking briskly uphill or with a load |
| Slow cycling, stationary | Cycling for pleasure or transportation (≤ 10 mph) | Cycling fast or racing (> 10 mph) |
| Swimming, slow treading | Swimming, moderate effort | Swimming, fast treading or crawl |
| Conditioning exercise, light stretching | Conditioning exercise, general calisthenics | Conditioning exercise, stair climber, ski machine |
| | Racket sports, table tennis | Racket sports, singles tennis, racquetball |
| Golf, power cart | Golf, pulling cart or carrying clubs | |
| Bowling | | |
| Fishing, sitting | Fishing, standing/casting | Fishing in stream |
| Boating, power | Canoeing, leisurely (2–4 mph) | Canoeing, rapidly (≧ 4 mph) |
| Home care, carpet sweeping | Home care, general cleaning | Moving furniture |
| Mowing lawn, riding mower | Mowing lawn, power mower | Mowing lawn, hand mower |
| Home repair, carpentry | Home repair, painting | |

day on their jobs but did not engage in vigorous activity.

Another reason for recommending moderate exercise is that most Americans do not exercise regularly. A national survey found that only a third or less of American adults exercise regularly.[24] About four of five Americans get little or no exercise.[25] Moderate physical activity may thus represent a more achievable goal for most Americans than strenuous aerobic exercise.[26]

Video
Getting fit?
V0701

### If Some Exercise Is Good, Is More Better?

Moderate physical activity certainly can have healthful effects, such as reducing the risk of cardiovascular diseases and adult-onset diabetes. Though moderate activity is certainly good for you, evidence indicates that more vigorous activity in the form of aerobic exercise helps even more.

Evidence from a long-term study of more than 17,000 male alumni of Harvard University suggests that only vigorous exercise increases longevity.[27] Vigorous exercise was defined in the study as a level of physical activity equivalent to three hours a week of activities like swimming laps briskly, running at a 6- to 7-mile-per-hour pace, playing singles tennis, or walking uphill or while carrying a load at 4 to 5 miles per hour. Men who engaged in this level of vigorous activity (equivalent to burning about 1,500 calories a week) had up to a 25% lower mortality rate than men who burned fewer than 150 calories in such activities.[28] This difference in relative risk of death was equivalent to that between smokers and nonsmokers and between overweight men and men of a healthful weight.

Investigators aren't quite sure why vigorous exercise is associated with longer life. One possibility is that vigorous exercise helps strengthen cardiorespiratory fitness. Another is that it reduces the risk of dying by lowering unhealthful LDL cholesterol or by raising healthful HDL cholesterol. In sum, when it comes to exercise, it appears that some exercise is preferable to none and more may be preferable to some.

Does the apparent life-extending effect of vigorous exercise mean that sedentary or moderately active people should begin to push themselves to the max? One point on which all authorities agree is the need for people to take it slowly when beginning an exercise program. Too much exercise too soon can jeopardize health, especially if it puts too much stress on the cardiovascular system. Most healthy adults may be able to begin an exercise program of moderate intensity without consulting their physicians. However, men over the age of 40 and women over the age of 50 should first see their physicians.[29] So too should people with health problems, risk factors for health problems, or physical limitations, so that safe and effective programs can be designed for them. Nonetheless, the problem for most of us is not exercising too much or too hard, but too little.

Exercise has many healthful benefits to our physical and psychological well-being. Making regular exercise a part of our lifestyle can help us achieve another important health and wellness goal: fitness.

Smart Quiz Q0701

**think about it!**

- **Could you use any of the physical benefits of exercise? Which ones?**
- **Could you use any of the psychological benefits of exercise? Which ones?**

**critical thinking** **How much exercise would make a difference in your life? Why?**

# FITNESS

**Fitness** is not a matter of how strong you are or whether you can run an eight-minute mile. Fitness involves the ability of an organism to withstand stress and pressure. Physical fitness is the ability to perform moderate to vigorous levels of physical activity without undue fatigue and the capability of maintaining such ability throughout life. If you can't climb the stairs to your office or walk uphill without losing your breath or exhausting yourself, consider yourself unfit. The good news is that you are not destined to remain unfit. You can improve your fitness by making exercise a regular part of your lifestyle.

## Components of Fitness

Fitness has two general components, performance-related fitness and health-related fitness.

**Performance-Related Fitness** This is the capacity to meet the demands that work or sports make on your body. We can measure performance-related fitness in terms of ability to compete on the playing field or in performance tests of occupational work (such as ability to carry fire hoses, if you work as a firefighter). Performance-related fitness depends on such factors as motor skills and coordination, muscular strength, endurance, cardiorespiratory power and capacity, motivation, and nutritional status. Though accomplished athletes are generally healthier than the average person, there is only a limited relationship between performance-related fitness and health.[30]

**Health-Related Fitness** Health-related fitness fosters good health and helps prevent disease. Health-related fitness includes:

1. *Cardiorespiratory endurance.* **Cardiorespiratory endurance** (also called *aerobic fitness* or *aerobic endurance*) refers to the ability of the **cardiorespiratory system**—the heart, lungs, and blood vessels—to deliver oxygen to working muscles and other body tissues at a rate sufficient to sustain vigorous activity. People with cardiorespiratory endurance can sustain vigorous, whole-body activity for extended periods of time without becoming breathless and exhausted. Their hearts and lungs can deliver the necessary fuel (mainly oxygen) for their muscles to work efficiently.

   People with good cardiorespiratory fitness are eight times less likely to die of cardiovascular disease than are unfit people.[31] Cardiovascular fitness creates favorable changes in the body's ability to use fat as an energy source. Like a car with a sick engine and transmission, a person whose heart and lungs are in poor condition can't go very far without stalling—or worse. The uniquely protective benefits of cardiorespiratory fitness make this the most important component of health-related fitness.

2. *Muscle strength and endurance. Muscle strength* refers to the amount of force a muscle can apply in a given contraction. *Muscle endurance* is the ability of a muscle or muscle group to repeatedly contract or to maintain force against a fixed object (such as holding a weight above the head). We need a certain degree of muscle strength to meet the demands of daily life, such as carrying a bag of groceries or opening a door. The stronger our muscles, the greater the number of tasks we can carry out, including those that are exercise- and sports-related, and the less prone we are to muscle strains and sprains. Muscle endurance enables us to use our muscles to perform repetitive tasks, such as running, repeated lifting, and so on.

   Muscle strength and endurance are

**Fitness** The ability to perform moderate to vigorous levels of physical activity without undue fatigue.

**Cardiorespiratory endurance** The ability of the cardiorespiratory system to deliver oxygen to working muscles at a rate sufficient to sustain vigorous activity over an extended period.

**Cardiorespiratory system** The system of heart, lungs, arteries, capillaries, and veins that circulates blood through the body and delivers oxygen to all body tissue, including muscle.

**Talking Glossary**
Musculoskeletal system
G0703

vital to overall fitness. Together with flexibility, they promote the health of the **musculoskeletal system**—the system of bones, muscles, and connective tissue (such as tendons, ligaments, and cartilage) that links the two. Muscle fitness helps minimize injuries, avoid degenerative bone diseases such as osteoporosis and osteoarthritis, and prevent lower back problems. Back pain is the second leading cause of missed work in the United States. Many cases are the result of weak stomach muscles and poor flexibility in the low back/hamstring region.

3. *Flexibility.* **Flexibility** refers to the ability of the joints to move through their entire range of motion without undue stress. The longer and more elastic the tissues are that surround the joints, the more fluidly the joints can move and the more flexible the body can become. Flexibility helps prevent strains and tears to muscles and their supporting tissues. It reduces the risk of injury during exercise and the risk of repetitive stress injuries (see Figure 7.1); improves posture; helps prevent lower back, shoulder, and neck problems; and allows for the range of motion needed for many forms of physical activity and exercise.
4. *Body composition.* Body composition refers to the makeup of the body in terms of the proportion of lean body mass (LBM) to fat tissue in the body. The lower the ratio, the higher the fat composition of the body and the less fit we are. People who are obese have an excess amount of fat on their bodies. The more obese we are, the less capable our bodies are of meeting physical demands. Obesity is linked to many health problems, including hypertension, high blood cholesterol, heart disease, strokes, respiratory illness, diabetes, gall bladder disease, gout, and certain kinds of cancer (see Chapter 6). Inactivity is a major culprit in obesity.[32]

Thin people can also have excess amounts of body fat, while some "husky" people may possess a more favorable ratio of LBM to fat tissue. To maintain a favorable body composition, we need to exercise regularly as well as watch our diets.

**Musculoskeletal system** The system of bones, muscles, and linking connective tissue, such as tendons, ligaments, and cartilage.

**Flexibility** The ability of the joints to move through their entire range of motion without undue stress. Flexibility is measured by the length and amount of stretch in the tissues surrounding the joints.

Fitness is closely linked to good health and prevention of disease. To become fit, you need to condition or "train" your body. Getting fit is one thing. *Remaining* fit requires that a fitness regimen become a regular part of your lifestyle.

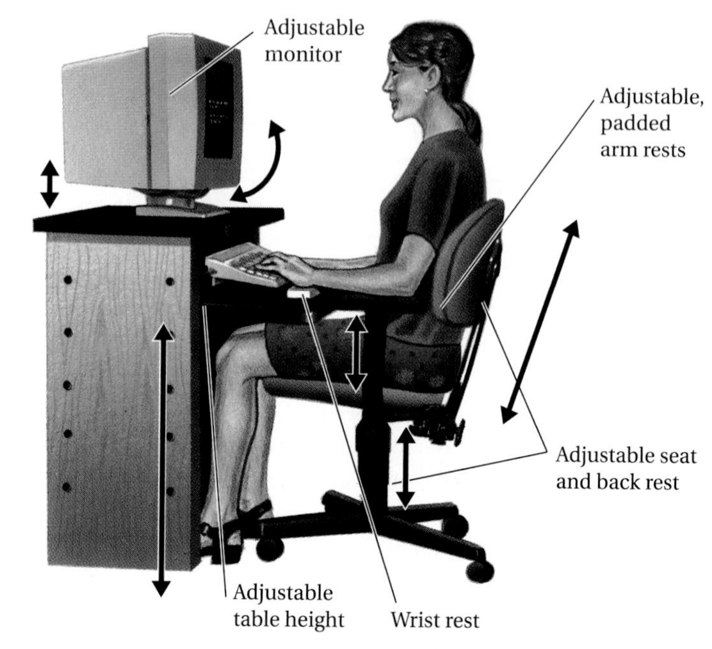


**Figure 7.1** ***Preventing Repetitive Stress Injury*** Repetitive motion injuries, such as those suffered by keyboard operators and meatpacking workers, are the fastest-growing type of occupational injuries. These injuries result in some $20 billion dollars annually in compensation claims. Use of ergonomically designed equipment and regular exercise programs can help avert many of these injuries.

One common type of repetitive motion injury is *carpal tunnel syndrome*; tissue that covers nerves in the wrist becomes inflamed, presses on nerves, and causes pain and impaired functioning. Use of ergonomically designed keyboards can help relieve stress on the wrist and hand, reducing the risk of this type of debilitating injury.

Other suggestions for preventing computer-related injuries include:

- Adjust the height of the keyboard so that your forearms remain parallel to the floor.
- Adjust the height of your chair so that your thighs are also parallel to the floor.
- Keep your wrists parallel to the floor—don't rest them on the desk.
- Use your arms to move your fingers around the keyboard. Don't let your fingers do all the stretching.
- Sit straight up in your chair and avoid leaning toward the keyboard.
- Take frequent breaks to stretch and move about the room or office.

## Getting Fit

The key to getting fit is working your body through a program of regular physical exercise. Exercise increases fitness in several ways:

- Vigorous exercise strengthens the heart and increases lung capacity, which can improve cardiorespiratory fitness (the ability to sustain strenuous effort) and reduce the risk of developing cardiovascular disease, the nation's #1 killer.
- Weight-bearing exercise, such as walking with weights, builds muscle strength and endurance (some exercises are better at building strength; others, endurance).
- Stretching and muscle-strengthening exercises increase joint mobility, making it easier for joints and muscles to work together with the full range of motion that daily activities require.
- Regular exercise increases body metabolism, promotes the loss of fat tissue, and improves the muscle-to-fat ratio.

The message is clear: To get fit, we need regular vigorous physical activity or exercise.

**Physical Activity versus Exercise** Perhaps you have a job waiting tables or baby-sitting. Given the exertion demanded of you, you may think that you're active enough and don't need to spend time working out. Or perhaps you get to the gym occasionally. Perhaps you ski several times in the winter and play softball every Sunday in the spring and summer. People who engage in even limited physical activity are better protected against heart disease than those who do nothing at all.[33] Thus you are better off than your sedentary friends. Without regular exercise, however, you're unlikely to be truly fit. Let's see why.

**Physical activity** is any demand made on muscles beyond their resting state. Activity can range from routine movements, such as walking from one place to another or throwing a ball, to exertions such as running long distances or moving a heavy object. **Exercise** incorporates physical activity into a structured sequence of movements that are performed consistently over a period of time sufficient to contribute to fitness.

Waiting tables can be physically demanding and may improve certain aspects of fitness, such as muscle strength in certain areas, especially the arms and wrists (those trays are heavy) and calves.

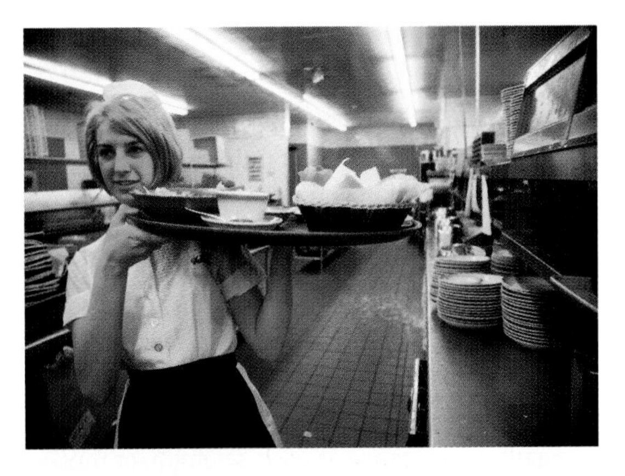

***Bursts of Activity*** Sustained exercise has greater health benefits than brief bursts of activity. Nevertheless, people whose jobs require physical activity appear to be more fit than people with sedentary jobs.

However, because the work is done in fits and starts, it is unlikely to improve cardiorespiratory fitness. A baby-sitter may expend energy chasing toddlers around the house, but this activity is usually not sustained. Even though you may be tired after a day of classes and an evening on the job, to ensure a healthful balance of endurance, strength, and flexibility, you'll want to find a way to incorporate regular exercise into your schedule.

## Training for Fitness

The body thrives on motion. It deteriorates and becomes vulnerable to disease when sedentary. While we benefit in many ways from labor-saving devices and other technological advances, to become fit and help safeguard our health we must compensate for lowered daily activity levels by challenging the body in programs of exercise.

**Training** (also called *conditioning*) refers to the gradual adjustment the body makes to increasingly demanding repetitive movements. Training is the key to overall fitness. Yet training is *specific.* The amount and type of exercise necessary to train for fitness varies according to the specific energy requirements and muscle groups required for a given activity. Certain kinds of training build aerobic endurance; others, strength; and still others, flexibility. The path to building fitness lies in progressively training the body to adapt to new demands.

**Smart Reference**

Training the Olympic athlete

R0701

**Physical activity** Any demand made on muscles beyond the resting state.

**Exercise** A structured sequence of movements performed consistently over a period of time that contribute to fitness.

**Training** (also called *conditioning*) The body's gradual adjustment to increasingly demanding levels of repetitive and progressive movements.

**General Principles of Training** Keep several general principles of training in mind:

1. *Specificity.* To improve fitness or endurance in a given activity, you must train specifically toward that end. If you want to strengthen your upper body, running won't be of much help. Each form of activity calls on different energy systems and muscle groups. To target a particular area for improvement, select an exercise that focuses on that area.
2. *Overload.* To improve any aspect of fitness, whether endurance, muscle strength, or muscle endurance, the parts of the body involved must be stressed or *overloaded* beyond their normal activity levels. **Overloading** refers to increasing the burden placed on the body—for example, by increasing the numbers of miles you jog or your running speed, or the amount of resistance you encounter in weight training. Overloading leads to both improved fitness and performance. The benefits achieved from overloading are referred to as a **training effect.**

   To build strong muscles, you must overload them by working them harder than you normally do. To increase aerobic endurance, you need to overload the demands placed on the heart and lungs by working them harder than usual.
3. *Progression.* Also called *progressive overload or progressive resistance,* the term *progression* refers to a process of gradually increasing the demands that challenge, or overload, your body. If you gradually demand more of your body, it can adapt to heavier workloads without becoming overtaxed or stressed beyond its ability to cope. Exercise too hard or too long and you risk injury; conversely, do too little and you won't see results.
4. *Warm-up and cool-down.* **Warm-up** and **cool-down** are advised for any vigorous exercise. Before strenuous exercise, warm up by engaging in mild exercise and stretching for 5 to 10 minutes. The warm-up period prepares your body for vigorous exercise by raising body temperature, increasing respiration and heart rate, and warming up muscles. The warm-up phase helps minimize injuries such as muscle strains and sprains. As you near the end of each exercise session, cool down for 5 to 10 minutes by slowing the rate of exertion. For instance, walk for 5 minutes after jogging. Follow this by 5 or 10 minutes of gentle stretching. Abruptly stopping in the midst of vigorous activity can cause dizziness, cramps, and muscle soreness, and may even lead to an irregular heartbeat.

**Overloading** The gradual increasing of the burden placed on the body to achieve a training effect.

**Training effect** The benefits to the heart, lungs, muscles, and bones produced by overloading.

**Warm-up** Mild exercise and stretching performed for 10 to 15 minutes prior to vigorous exercise.

**Cool-down** Reduced pace of activity, such as stretching, performed for 5 to 10 minutes before the end of exercise sessions.

**Cardiac output** The amount of blood the heart pumps per minute.

**Resting heart rate** The number of times per minute the heart beats at rest.

## Building Cardiorespiratory (Aerobic) Endurance

The word "aerobic" means "with oxygen." Aerobic exercise involves vigorous physical activity that requires a sustained elevation in the body's utilization of oxygen. Aerobic exercise builds cardiorespiratory endurance, also called aerobic fitness. In people with good cardiorespiratory endurance, the heart is able to pump and circulate oxygen-rich blood to muscles and other bodily tissues to meet the increased demands of strenuous activity. Cardiorespiratory endurance involves whole-body activities, especially those that use the legs and buttocks in rhythmic fashion, such as walking, running, and swimming. People who can swim, jog, or walk briskly for at least 20 minutes without becoming breathless are at least moderately aerobically fit.

During vigorous activity, muscles require more than ten times the amount of oxygen that they do when they are at rest. While you are sitting quietly, your heart is pumping about 5 quarts of blood throughout your body a minute. When you run around the track, however, your heart will pump at least four times as much blood, at least 20 quarts per minute. **Cardiac output**—the amount of blood the heart pumps per minute—can rise as high as 30 quarts or more per minute for those in excellent aerobic condition, for example, highly trained athletes.

A well-conditioned person's **resting heart rate** (the number of times per minute the heart beats at rest) is lower than that of an out-of-shape person's. This is because the trained heart is able to fill with a larger amount of blood and contract more forcefully, and thus move the same amount of blood with fewer beats. Because it is working at a much lower percent of its total capacity than that of an untrained heart, it is better prepared to meet strenuous demands and will suffer less wear and tear over the long run.

**Aerobic Exercise** Aerobic exercise—the type of exercise you get when you run, walk briskly, swim laps, work out in an aerobics class, or cycle quickly—uses large muscle groups in repetitive movements. In aerobic exercise, the heart is forced to pump at a rate above its resting state to supply the muscles with the increased oxygen they need. Table 7.2 describes several types of aerobic and anaerobic exercises.

***Aerobics*** Many visit their health clubs several times a week to maintain the benefits of aerobic exercise. (These classes are also good places to meet people!)

Aerobic exercise is performed at a low enough intensity to allow the body to provide a sufficient supply of oxygen to the exercising muscles. Many exercise physiologists believe that at least 20 minutes of continued effort is required to obtain the training effect of aerobic exercise—that is, to promote cardiorespiratory fitness.

**Anaerobic Exercise** **Anaerobic** (literally "without oxygen") **exercise** involves short bursts of intense muscle activity. Examples of anaerobic (or "nonaerobic") exercises are sprinting, some forms of weight training, calisthenics such as push-ups and sit-ups (which usually allow rest periods between repetitions), and periodic bursts of strenuous activity in baseball and some other sports (such as running to first base after hitting the ball). The intensity or all-out effort required by anaerobic activities can only be sustained for perhaps two or three minutes before muscle fatigue sets in.

Talking Glossary
Anaerobic
G0704

The intensity of anaerobic exercise exceeds the cardiorespiratory system's ability to supply working muscles with oxygen. In contrast, less intense aerobic activity continually feeds muscle fibers with the oxygen needed to fuel repetitive muscle contractions. We need to engage in aerobic rather than anaerobic exercise to build aerobic endurance. (Although anaerobic exercise alone does not improve aerobic fitness, it does build muscle strength and speed.)

**TABLE 7.2**

**Benefits of Selected Aerobic and Anaerobic Exercises**

| Exercise | Type | Benefits |
|---|---|---|
| *Aerobic dancing* | Aerobic | Cardiorespiratory system; whole-body muscle tone |
| *Jogging and running* | Aerobic | Cardiorespiratory system; leg muscle strength; endurance |
| *Bicycling* | Aerobic | Cardiorespiratory system; thigh muscle strength; endurance |
| *Swimming* | Aerobic | Cardiorespiratory system; whole-body muscle tone |
| *Sprinting* | Anaerobic | Leg muscle strength; endurance |
| *Weight training* | Lifting heavier loads for fewer repetitions is generally anaerobic; lifting lighter loads for more repetitions can be aerobic if done long enough within the target heart rate range | Muscle strength; endurance |
| *Push-ups* | Anaerobic | Arm and chest muscle strength; endurance |
| *Sit-ups* | Anaerobic | Abdomen and lower back muscle strength; endurance |

***Weight Training*** Weight training is one path to building muscle strength, but aerobic exercise—that is, sustained, vigorous physical activity—is superior for building cardiovascular fitness.

**Measuring Aerobic Endurance** Aerobic fitness can be measured by **maximal oxygen consumption,** commonly referred to as $VO_2$ max. Maximal oxygen consumption is the maximum amount of oxygen our body is able

**Anaerobic exercise** Short bursts of intense muscle activity not requiring sustained elevation in oxygen utilization.

**Maximal oxygen consumption** ($VO_2$ max) The maximum amount of oxygen the body is able to take in and consume.

to use during physical activity or exercise. The greater the intensity of the activity, the more oxygen will be consumed. Each person's maximum oxygen consumption level is genetically determined. Nevertheless, regular aerobic exercise boosts the body's ability to consume oxygen within this inherited range.[34] An aerobically fit person's $VO_2$ max should be within 50 to 85% of his or her maximum oxygen consumption.

$VO_2$ max can only be measured directly in the laboratory, with subjects breathing into a mouthpiece as they exercise. A more practical method of determining how aerobically fit we are involves monitoring the heart rate, or the number of heartbeats per minute, before, during, and after a workout. Raising the heart rate to between 60 and 85% or perhaps 90% of maximum level puts us in the **target heart rate range**—the range intense enough to overload the heart and muscles to improve fitness but not so intense that the exercise becomes anaerobic. Once an exercise becomes anaerobic, muscles burn carbohydrates in the form of glucose stored in muscle rather than fatty tissue. In other words, sustained anaerobic exercise not only exhausts us but actually depletes muscle rather than fat! In contrast, sustained aerobic exercise mostly uses stored body fat as fuel. So in addition to the cardiorespiratory benefits of aerobic exercise, it also fosters fat loss. To improve aerobic fitness, your heart rate should be elevated over a sustained period of time until its beat is within the target heart rate range. The accompanying ***HealthCheck*** offers some guidelines on determining your target heart rate range.

**Achieving Aerobic Fitness** To build aerobic endurance, the American Academy of Sports Medicine (AASM) recommends that you should exercise at least three times weekly, intensely enough to give your heart and lungs a good workout, for at least 20 minutes per session. Physical activities that increase aerobic endurance are those that increase the strength and efficiency of the heart, such as running, fast cycling, brisk walking, or swimming laps.

People who meet these guidelines should be rewarded with a 15 to 30% improvement in aerobic endurance.[35] Those who are *least fit* make the most gains—a nice motivating factor for couch potatoes who want to change their ways. People who exercise aerobically less than three days a week do not show much change in aerobic fitness. People who exercise more than five days a week do not show any greater improvement in fitness than those who stick to a three- to five-day program.

**Target heart rate range** The range of heartbeats per minute during vigorous exercise that is sufficient to overload the heart but not so intense as to be anaerobic. Range is between 60 and 85% of the person's maximum heart rate.

**Muscles** Cells grouped in long, slender bundles called muscle fibers that contract to move an organ or part of the body.

**Skeletal muscles** The muscles attached to the bones of the skeleton.

**Getting Started with Aerobic Exercise** As with any form of exercise, beginners should start slowly. Whether you opt for jogging, bicycling, or an aerobic dance class, remain at the lower end of your target heart range for several weeks. Do as much as you can without becoming breathless. Here are some additional suggestions for getting started:

- Pick an exercise you enjoy, and exercise continuously during your workout to achieve the aerobic effect.
- Remember that all training is specific. While any form of aerobic exercise benefits the heart and lungs, swimmers will not automatically be able to run around the track for 20 minutes, nor will runners find their first aerobic dance class to be a breeze. Each activity uses different muscle fibers, which in turn affects how the cardiorespiratory system responds.
- Apply the principles of overload and progression. Gradually challenge (overload) yourself to do more—jog another mile, swim another lap, or briskly walk another 10 minutes. After at least several weeks of exercising at the lower end of your target heart rate range—between 60 and 70%—for at least 20 minutes, try exercising for 30 minutes in the same range. After several more weeks, try working out for 20 minutes at 75% of your target heart rate range by increasing the intensity of your routine. Take your time to give your body time to adjust. *You can make gains without pain.*

## Building Muscle Strength and Endurance

Bones need muscles to move them. **Muscles** are cells grouped in long, slender bundles called muscle fibers. Muscles contract or shorten to move internal body organs or body parts such as the arms and legs. The muscles attached to the bones of the skeleton are called **skeletal muscles.** Most of the muscles in our bodies are skeletal muscles. They make up about half of our body weight.

## Health*Check*

### Determining Your Target Heart Rate Range

**Heart rate** (also called *pulse rate*) can be taken by applying the index and middle fingers to the carotid artery in the neck (located just under the jawbone and next to the Adam's apple) or the radial artery in the wrist (put your fingers on the thumb side). Press lightly while counting your pulse rate. The number of beats to count, as well as the figure used to multiply the beats, varies depending on whether you're measuring your resting or target heart rate. (Figure 7.2 illustrates this process.)

**Step 1.**
Before determining your target heart range, you should find out what your resting heart rate is. By doing so, you'll know how efficiently your heart is working at rest. The best time to measure resting heart rate is when you wake up in the morning or after you've been sitting for a while. Count your resting pulse for 20 seconds, then multiply by three. If you're out of shape, you should find your resting heart rate comes down after several months of regular aerobic exercise.

The average untrained resting heart rate for adult males is about 72 beats per minute; in adult females, about 80 beats per minute. With regular exercise, resting heart rate declines. Highly trained athletes may have resting heart rates as low as 35 to 40 beats per minute.

**Step 2.**
Next, you need to determine your recommended **maximum heart rate.** This is the fastest that your heart should be beating. You don't need to take a pulse to determine your maximum heart rate. Instead, subtract your age from the number 220 (if you are male) or 224 (if you are female), as follows:

| Males | | Females | |
|---|---|---|---|
| 220 | | 224 | |
| − ____ | (your age) | − ____ | (your age) |
| = ____ | (your maximum heart rate) | = ____ | (your maximum heart rate) |

Maximum recommended heart rates generally decline with age, but slowly, at the rate of one beat per year. The recommended target heart rate for sustained exercise is from 60 to 85% of your maximum heart rate. To compute your target heart rate, multiply your maximum heart rate by 0.60, and write the result here:

____ = the low end of your target heart rate range

Next, multiply your maximum heart rate by 0.85. Write the result here:

____ = the high end of your target heart range

Consider an example. A 30-year-old man's maximum heart rate is 220 minus 30 (his age in years), or 190. His target heart rate ranges from 114 beats per minute (that is, 190 × 0.60) to 161 beats per minute

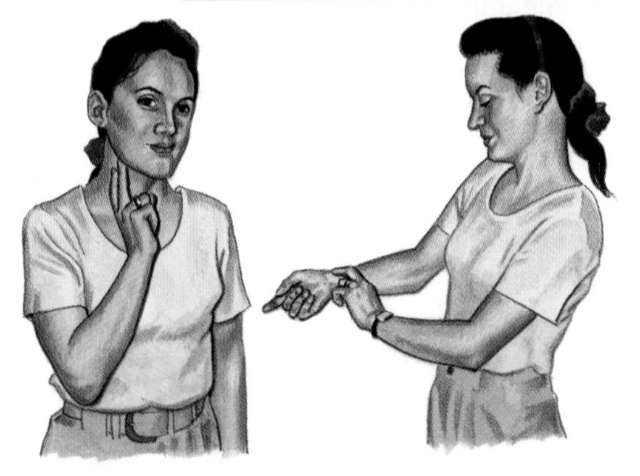

**Figure 7.2** ***Measuring Your Heart (Pulse) Rate***

(190 × 0.85). The 30-year-old, that is, can obtain the cardiorespiratory benefits of sustained activity by exercising intensely enough that his heart beats from 114 to 161 times per minute.

A 30-year old woman's maximum heart rate is 224 minus 30, or 194. Her target heart rate ranges from 116 beats per minute (that is, 194 × 0.60) to 165 beats per minute (194 × 0.85); figures are rounded off. Many people gauge whether they are exercising within their target heart rate range by taking their pulse 10 minutes into an exercise session. To measure your heart rate, count your pulse for 10 seconds and then multiply by six.

If you are just beginning an exercise program, you'll want to remain near the lower end of the target heart rate range—in the 60% range. When you are in good condition, you will be able to sustain heart rates in the higher part of your range during prolonged workouts. It should be emphasized, however, that studies have shown that the formula for determining maximum heart rate does not apply to everyone. Many people's hearts naturally beat faster than average. Others beat more slowly. If, after several months of regular exercise, these formulas leave you wide of the mark, you can use a simple technique to gauge whether you are in the target heart rate range. It's called the "talk test." If you can talk a little without gasping, and at the same time continue to exercise vigorously for a full 20 minutes without becoming exhausted, you can safely assume you are in your target heart rate range.

Skeletal muscles need **muscle tone,** or some firmness, to perform. We ordinarily maintain some degree of muscle tone by holding our heads up, standing upright, and moving around. Without more vigorous use, however, all but the most minimal muscle tone disappears—a condition called **muscle atrophy.** An example of muscle atrophy occurs after

**Heart rate** The number of heartbeats per minute.

**Maximum heart rate** The fastest rate that the heart should beat during exercise.

**Muscle tone** The degree of firmness in a muscle. A certain amount of muscle tone is needed for a muscle to perform.

**Muscle atrophy** A deterioration or loss of muscle tone.

you break a bone and it is immobilized in a cast. The muscles surrounding the bone atrophy through lack of use. To a lesser but significant extent, muscles can atrophy if we become sedentary.

**Muscle strength** is measured in the amount of force, or power, we can apply in a single contraction. **Muscle endurance** is our ability to contract muscles repeatedly. Building both muscle strength and endurance requires some form of resistance training. In **resistance training,** muscle force is repeatedly applied against an opposing force or weight for a certain number of *repetitions* (called "reps" or "sets"). This opposing force may be in the form of free weights (barbells), resistance machines such as Nautilus equipment, or your own body (as in push-ups and pull-ups). A **repetition maximum (RM)** is the maximum amount of force you are able to exert in one repetition.

Resistance training relies on the principles of specificity, overload, and progression: improvements are specific to the muscle groups worked, which are repeatedly and progressively (gradually) overloaded. When you overload a muscle through resistance training, the muscle cells adapt to the strain by increasing in size—a process called *muscle hypertrophy* (the opposite of atrophy)—which gives them the pumped-up look of body building. To keep growing, they need to work against greater amounts of resistance.

People who do *only* resistance training for strength may become "pumped up" but won't improve their aerobic endurance. Dedicated bodybuilders who run a three-mile race may end up panting after a half mile unless they have incorporated running into their exercise program. Runners who try to lift heavy barbells may discover that they are unable to do so unless they have incorporated strength training of the upper body into their exercise programs.

Resistance training that emphasizes *muscle strength* primarily builds muscle size or "mass." Resistance training geared toward *muscle endurance* increases the muscles' aerobic capacity, which in turn improves general aerobic endurance.

**Muscle strength** The amount of force, or power, that one or more muscles can apply in a single contraction.

**Muscle endurance** The ability to contract muscles repeatedly over time.

**Resistance training** Muscle training involving repeated movement or lifting against an opposing force or weight.

**Repetition maximum (RM)** The maximum amount of force a person is able to exert in one repetition.

**Isometric exercise** Contraction of a muscle which is not accompanied by any joint movement and in which the muscle remains the same length (does not shorten) even as tension increases.

**Isotonic exercise** Exercise in which muscles are repeatedly contracted under constant resistance throughout the full range of motion of the joint.

According to a recent fitness profile of 258 entering college freshmen, both male and female subjects had excellent levels of muscle strength but only average levels of muscle endurance and poor levels of aerobic endurance. The researchers concluded that college students may concentrate on strength while ignoring endurance.[36] It is advisable to enhance fitness in each area.

**Exercises for Building Muscle Strength and Endurance** Two general rules apply in building muscle strength and endurance: Use heavier weights and fewer repetitions ("high resistance, low repetitions"), and you'll see the greatest gains in muscle strength. Use lighter weights and more repetitions ("low resistance, high repetitions"), and you'll get the greatest gains in muscle endurance. If your initial goal is to increase muscle strength, use heavier weights for fewer repetitions. Once you are satisfied with the amount of strength you've achieved, switch to lighter weights for more repetitions to build endurance.

Three types of exercise—*isometric, isotonic,* or *isokinetic*—can be used to train for strength and endurance. These terms also refer to the different types of muscle contractions. Figure 7.3 illustrates each type of exercise.

**Isometric exercise** forces a "static" contraction of a muscle, which is a contraction occurring without joint movement. Isometric exercises involve placing pressure against an immovable object, such as pushing against a wall or placing your palms together and pushing. Rather than shortening as it normally does when it contracts, the muscle stays the same length even as the tension increases. Isometric exercise increases strength, but only at the single joint angle where the contraction occurs.

In performing isometric exercise, exert as much force as possible for six seconds, pause, and then repeat for a total of 5 to 10 repetitions. Because isometric exercise can raise blood pressure, though only briefly, it can prove dangerous for people with heart problems. Health professionals therefore advise people who have, or may be at risk for, cardiovascular problems not to do isometric exercises.

**Isotonic exercise** involves repetitive actions in which a muscle is contracted under constant resistance throughout the full range of motion. Examples include lifting dumbbells or barbells or using weight-training equipment, such as Nautilus or Universal equipment, which requires you to move or lift against constant resistance. Lifting a barbell

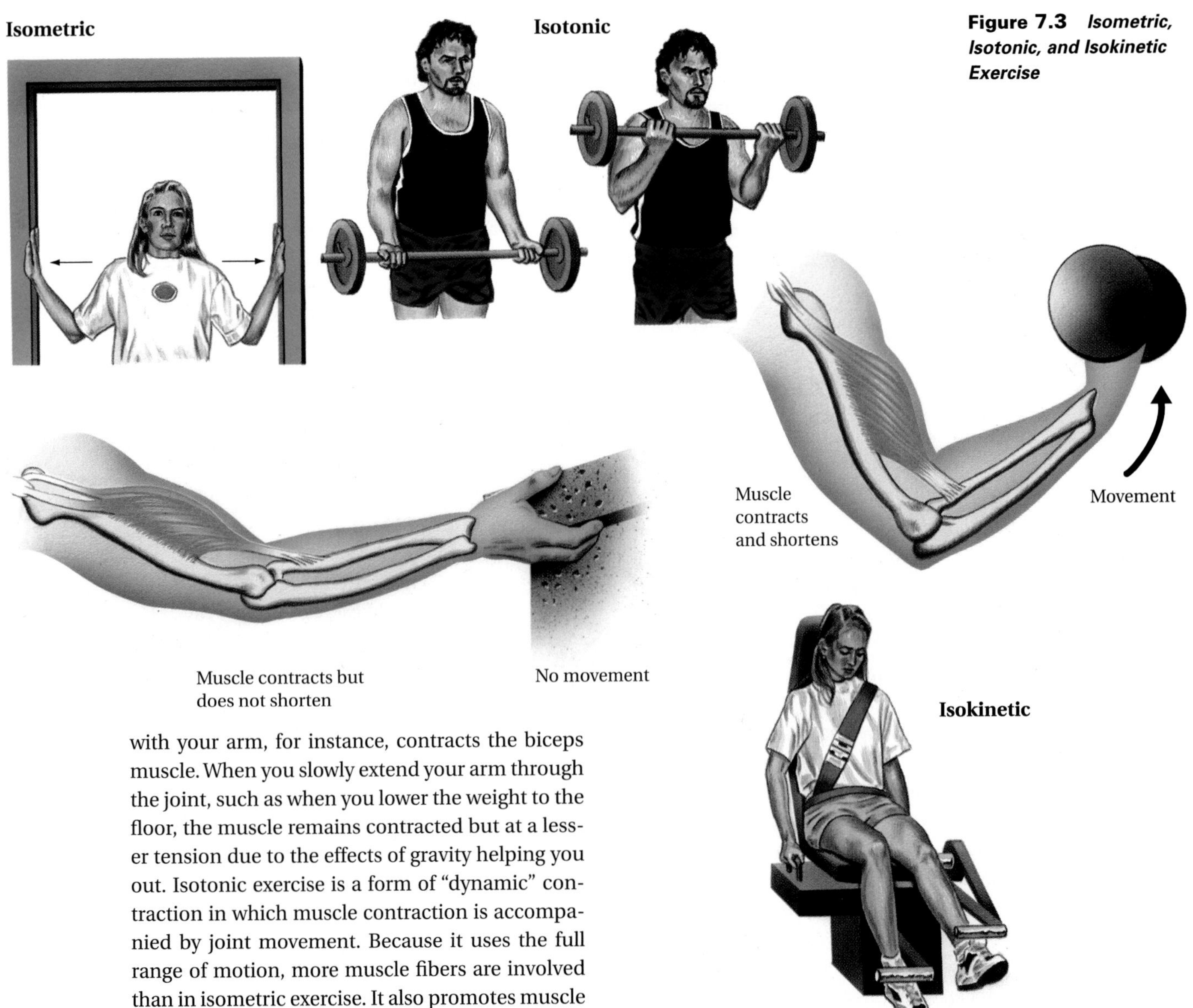


**Figure 7.3** ***Isometric, Isotonic, and Isokinetic Exercise***

with your arm, for instance, contracts the biceps muscle. When you slowly extend your arm through the joint, such as when you lower the weight to the floor, the muscle remains contracted but at a lesser tension due to the effects of gravity helping you out. Isotonic exercise is a form of "dynamic" contraction in which muscle contraction is accompanied by joint movement. Because it uses the full range of motion, more muscle fibers are involved than in isometric exercise. It also promotes muscle circulation and endurance. Sets of isotonic exercises involving high resistance (e.g., use of heavier weights) with a low number of repetitions are best for building muscle strength and mass. Low resistance, high repetition sets are most effective for building muscle endurance and flexibility.

**Isokinetic exercise** involves contractions of a muscle against resistance that varies with the exertion applied by the user throughout the full range of motion. Unlike isotonic exercises, isokinetic exercises require the use of an exercise machine (including models made by Cybex, Orthotron, and Mini-Gym) that provides variable resistance. Isokinetic exercise is believed to provide the most effective way of overloading muscles to strengthen them. As in isotonic exercise, you can vary the number and intensity of repetitions in isokinetic exercise. To build strength, set the machine on a heavier weight and do fewer repetitions; to build endurance, set the machine on a lighter weight and gradually increase the number of repetitions.

**Getting Started** For maximal health and fitness, you should strive to improve muscle strength and endurance throughout your body by exercising all your major muscle groups. This includes the muscle groups in the lower back (*latissimus dorsi*), chest (*pectorals*), upper and middle back (*trapezius*), shoulders (*deltoids*), arms (*biceps* and *triceps*), stomach (*abdominals*), buttocks (*gluteal muscles*), thighs (*quadriceps* and *hamstrings*), and lower legs or calves (*gastrocnemius*).

In addition, the following guidelines will help you exercise safely and more efficiently:

**Isokinetic exercise** Exercise in which muscles contract against a selected resistance through the full range of motion; requires use of an exercise machine.

- *Learn proper technique for lifting weights and using weight-training equipment.* Seek an instructor's guidance. Give yourself time to learn how to do the exercises, with proper body alignment and breathing.
- *Start easily.* Begin exercising muscle groups with low resistance *and* low repetitions for one set of 8 to 12 reps. Rest for 30 seconds to 3 minutes and then move on to another muscle group and repeat.
- *Allow muscles time to recuperate between sets and between exercise sessions.* This will enable them to repair themselves and adapt to the new demands. As a general rule, do not exercise the same muscle groups two days in a row. Allow 2 to 3 minutes between sets involving the same muscle groups.
- *When initially moving against resistance, try to complete the motion as quickly and smoothly as possible.* When returning to the starting position, slow the motion down. Don't allow gravity to take over and do the work for you.
- *Inhale when exerting force (for instance, while you lift) and exhale when relaxing the contraction.* Breathe evenly and avoid holding your breath. Try to breathe from your abdomen rather than your chest.
- *Pair your exercises so that opposing muscle groups are worked equally.* Each muscle group has an opposing, or antagonist, muscle group. Prime mover muscles are those that directly perform a movement. For instance, when you curl a weight toward your chest with your arm, your biceps muscles are acting as the prime movers. The triceps muscles in the back of the arm are used to extend the arm, so in this case they're the antagonist muscle group. After a set of biceps curls, follow with a set of exercises that target the triceps. Similarly, work both the quadriceps (muscles in the front of the thigh) and the hamstrings (muscles in the back of the thigh), and so forth. Consult an instructor to learn which exercises work prime mover and antagonist muscles.
- *To build strength, gradually increase the amount of resistance you can perform through a full range of motion for one to three sets of 8 to 12 reps each.* When you are able to accomplish three sets with relative ease, increase the amount of resistance.
- *To build endurance, use lower resistance for more repetitions—perhaps as many as 30, or until you can't push yourself further.* Do between three and five sets.
- *Resistance training guidelines.* To build muscle strength, the AASM recommends some form of resistance training for a minimum of two days per week and a maximum of three days. Resistance training should exercise each of the major muscle groups to the point of fatigue. Sessions should last between 20 and 60 minutes and include at least two sets of 8 to 12 repetitions "to near fatigue" for each major muscle group.[37]

## Improving Flexibility

The upper limits on flexibility are determined by factors such as heredity, body composition, and air temperature. Some people are born with more supple joints. The more fat that accumulates around the joints, the less they are able to move. Joints also tend to be more flexible on warm days. Whatever the upper limits, how-

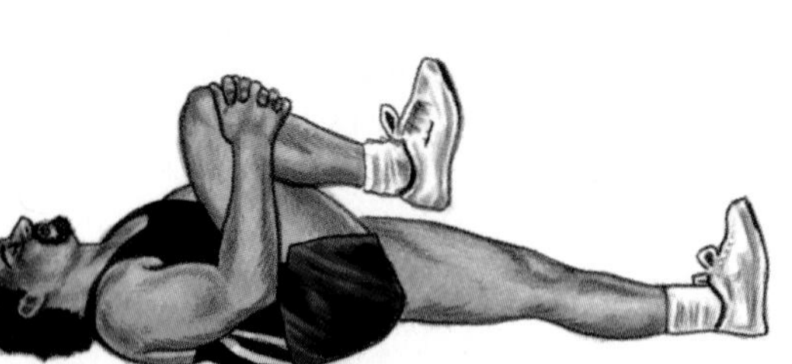

Pull each leg toward chest. Try to keep back of head on floor and lower back flat.

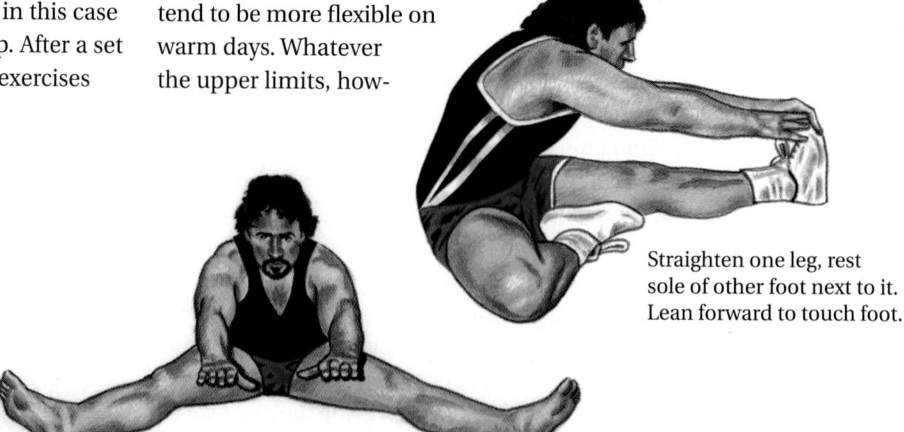

Straighten one leg, rest sole of other foot next to it. Lean forward to touch foot.

Sit on the floor and spread legs as far as possible. Now reach forward as far as possible, keeping back straight.

**Ballistic stretching** Stretching that involves repetitive bouncing motions.

**Static stretching** Stretching in which muscles are fully extended and then gradually stretched to the limit of the joint movement.

ever, you can improve the flexibility of your joints by means of regular stretching exercises.

There are two general types of stretching. **Ballistic stretching** involves repetitive bouncing motions, as when you repeatedly touch your toes from a standing position. We do not recommend this type of stretching, because jerking movements can lead to injuries such as tears in tendons, ligaments, and muscles.

Proper stretching should proceed slowly. The best way to accomplish this is through static stretching. In **static stretching,** muscles are fully extended and then slowly and gradually stretched to the limit of the joint movement. The extended position is then held for a while. Examples of static stretches are illustrated in Figure 7.4.

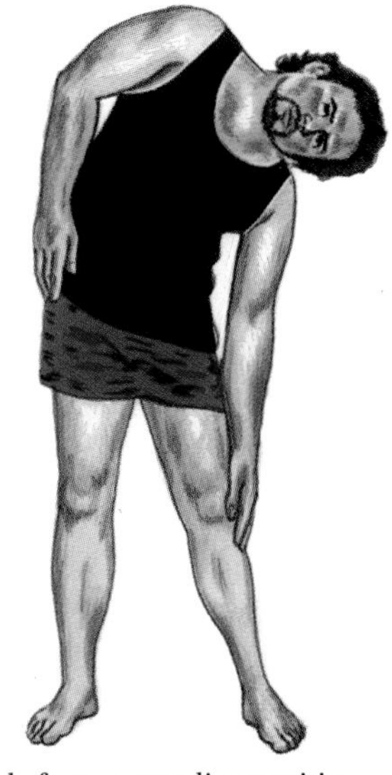

Bend to the side from a standing position. Touch leg as far down as possible. Repeat on the other side. Do six repetitions on each side.

**Figure 7.4** ***Examples of Stretching Exercises***
Stretching can improve flexibility and help prevent exercise-related injuries when practiced during the warm-up and cool-down phases of exercise routines. For each stretch, gently extend the muscle group into the stretch until you feel mild tension or tightness in the muscle. Don't stretch so hard that you feel pain. Hold the stretch for 10 to 30 seconds and complete 6 repetitions. If you have any questions about proper technique, consult a coach, trainer, or physical therapist.

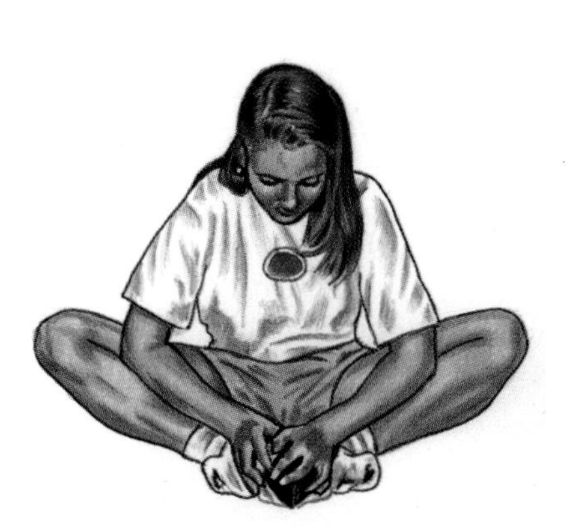

With arms exerting light resistance, slowly push down on knees.

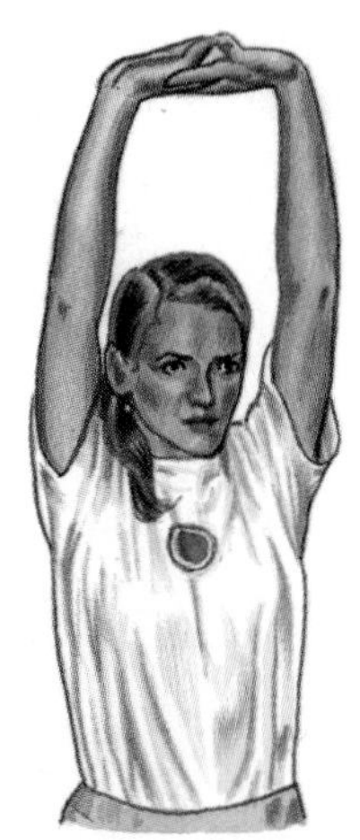

Standing or sitting, interlace fingers and push arms slightly back and up.

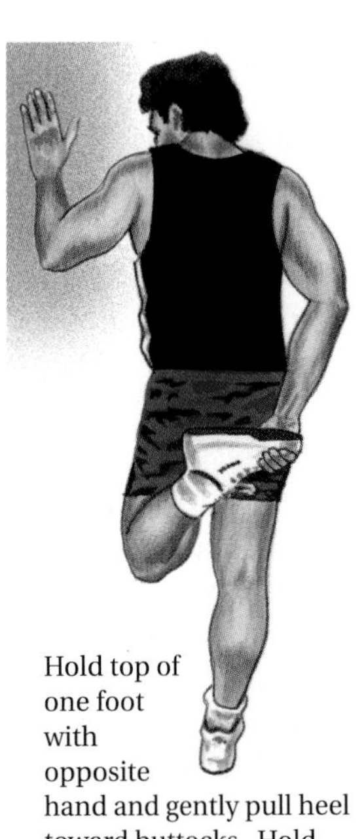

Hold top of one foot with opposite hand and gently pull heel toward buttocks. Hold 30 seconds.

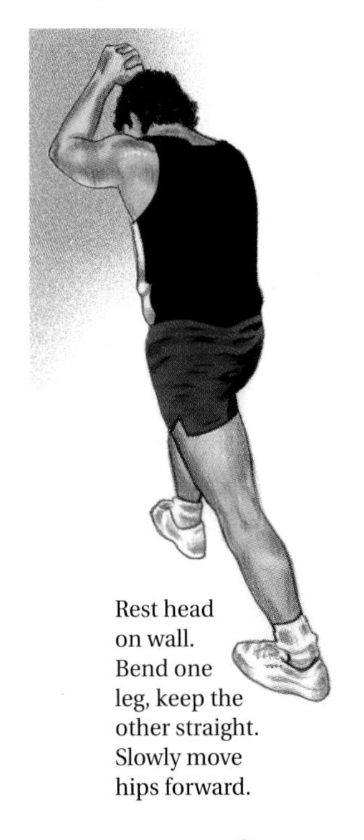

Rest head on wall. Bend one leg, keep the other straight. Slowly move hips forward.

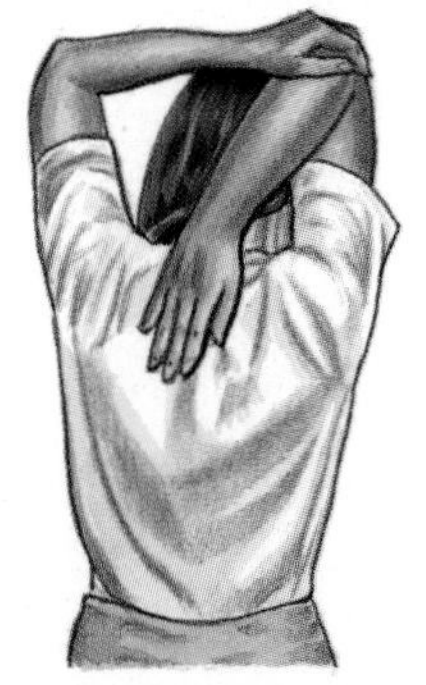

Hold elbow of each arm with other hand and slowly, gently pull behind arm.

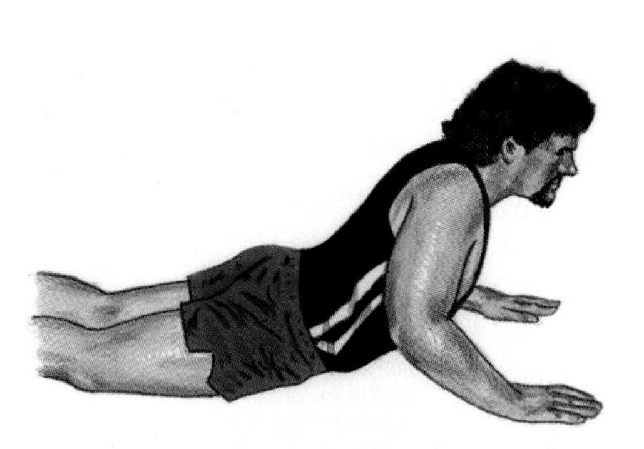

Lie face-down on the floor. Keeping hips flat against the ground, lift upper torso by pressing down with hands.

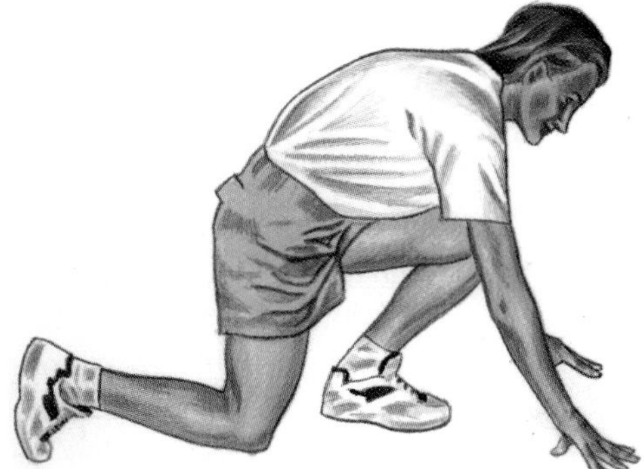

Put one leg forward, rest other knee on floor. Lower front of hip.

**Getting Started** Stretching exercises can be performed separately or incorporated into the warm-up and cool-down phases of other exercise routines. Here are some suggestions for proper stretching:

- *Warm up before vigorous stretching with light exercise, such as skipping rope or jogging slowly in place, until you've worked up a light sweat.* Warmed-up tissue is less prone to injury.
- *Apply the principles of specificity, overload, and progression to your stretching routine.* Select the muscle group you want to stretch and gradually stretch it until you feel a mild tension or tightness in the muscle. Don't overstretch until you feel pain. Some initial soreness is normal for beginners, but sharp or consistent pain can indicate an injury that should be evaluated medically. Begin with easy stretches and progress to more difficult ones. Stretch a bit further and hold the stretch a bit longer each time.
- *Breathe slowly while stretching.*
- *General guidelines.* Stretch at least three or four days per week. Many people like to stretch daily. Hold each stretch for 10 to 30 seconds. Repeat each stretch three or four times.

## Improving Body Composition

Exercise sheds fat while maintaining or building lean tissue such as muscle. Sustained aerobic exercise burns more calories than other forms of exercise. During aerobic exercise, muscles burn calories up to 50 times faster than when the body is in a resting state. Table 7.3 shows how many calories are burned by different types of activities.

Strength training burns far fewer calories per minute than aerobic exercise. However, strength training builds muscle, and muscles burn more calories than the equivalent weight of fat tissue—whether we're exercising or resting. At rest, 1 pound of muscle burns approximately 75 calories per hour, compared with a mere 2 calories burned per hour by a pound of fat. To get maximum results in reducing body fat, exercise specialists recommend a combination of aerobic exercise and muscle training.[39] Aerobic exercise also has another fat-burning advantage: It raises the rate at which fat is metabolized by the body. This is called the **afterburner effect.** People who exercise aerobically burn more calories than those who don't, even when they're watching television. Need we say more?

**Afterburner effect** Increased rate of metabolization of fat after exercise stops.

Exercise also has health benefits even for people who are overweight. A study at the Cooper Institute for Aerobics Research in Dallas tested more than 25,000 men. The men were assessed for cardiorespiratory endurance and proportion of body fat. The results showed that obese men who were either moderately or very fit had a 70% lower mortality risk than obese men who were unfit, even when such factors as age, smoking, cholesterol level, and general health were held equal.[40] Certainly it is healthier for obese people to lose weight than to remain obese. But it is also better for them to be fit than unfit.

**Guidelines for Getting Trim** To improve body composition by increasing the ratio of lean-to-fat tissue, the AASM recommends you engage in vigorous physical activity (the type of activity that causes you to break into a sweat) at a moderate pace at least three times weekly for a minimum of 30 minutes. Combine with muscle training to get the maximum results.

TABLE 7.3

**Calories Expended for Various Activities[38]**

| Activity | Calories Burned/Hour (approx.) |
|---|---|
| Bicycling, 6 mph | 240 |
| Bicycling, 12 mph | 410 |
| Cross-country skiing | 700 |
| Jogging, $5\frac{1}{2}$ mph | 740 |
| Jogging, 7 mph | 920 |
| Jumping rope | 750 |
| Running in place | 650 |
| Running, 10 mph | 1280 |
| Swimming, 25 yds./min. | 275 |
| Swimming, 50 yds./min. | 500 |
| Tennis—singles | 400 |
| Walking, 2 mph | 240 |
| Walking, 3 mph | 320 |
| Walking, $4\frac{1}{2}$ mph | 440 |

*Note:* Calories burned depend on the person's body weight. The calculations above are based on a body weight of 150 pounds. A 100-pound person burns about a third fewer calories, so you would multiply the above numbers by 0.7. A 200-pound person should multiply by 1.3. Note too that exercising more vigorously will only slightly increase the number of calories burned. To burn the maximum number of calories, it is better to increase the time spent exercising rather than the intensity.

WORLD OF *diversity*

## Fitness Is for Everyone—Exercise and the Physically Challenged

Janet Reed's videotape workout is similar in many ways to other exercise videos. Like other exercise tapes, Reed's has warm-up stretches, activities that foster relaxation and range of motion, and exercises that enhance flexibility, strength, balance, and coordination. But Reed's workout differs in a very important way: It is aimed at participants who are temporary or permanent users of wheelchairs.

Reed was thrown from a horse and suffered spinal cord injuries that paralyzed her from the waist down. She had difficulty accepting these new limitations for many years. One year, however, a friend asked her to dance during a fund-raiser, and her outlook began to change. The friend manipulated her wheelchair while she moved her upper body in time with the music. It was the most fun she had had since her accident and eventually led to the idea that she could help other physically challenged people profit from physical activity. She put together her "Wheelchair Workout" with the assistance of a physical therapist and found that creating the program helped her take charge of her life. Working out regularly "strengthens the body, relaxes the mind, and toughens the spirit," she says. "It can prove to you that you have what it takes to do what is necessary."[41]

When people are confined to wheelchairs or to generally sedentary lives, their cardiovascular functioning suffers, their muscles atrophy, and their joints stiffen. People in wheelchairs can also develop pressure sores. Exercise, of course, does not cure paralysis. However, it helps people with spinal cord injuries improve their upper body strength and flexibility, their cardiovascular condition, the functioning of other body systems—such as the nervous and urogenital systems—and their overall outlook on life and their self-esteem. Exercise may actually be more crucial to the well-being of physically challenged people than other people.

The benefits of exercise for the physically challenged have been known for some time. Physical activities, including tournaments, were organized as therapy for wounded war veterans after World War II. Wheelchair athletic organizations today encourage wheelchair users to participate in archery, basketball, bowling, Ping-Pong, racquetball, softball, swimming, track and field events, even weight lifting. The Special Olympics aims to foster independence and a sense of achievement among people with mental disabilities such as mental retardation. It provides training and competition in 22 sports to some 750,000 participants, many of whom are also physically challenged. A ranking system—a sort of literal "handicap" ranking—gives everyone a more or less equal chance to win.

Even group marathon "wheel chairing" is available to the physically challenged. At the Boston Marathon, wheelchair participants leave the starting gate a half-hour ahead of runners. The runners do not catch up to them until they hit the area of "Heartbreak Hill" on Commonwealth Avenue in Newton some 20 miles into the race.

Rehabilitation specialists suggest isometric exercises to enhance muscle strength in wheelchair users, such as pressing the palms together and making a fist. Isotonic exercises can help increase range of motion and stamina. One example is the "wheelchair sit-up." This is accomplished by locking the chair wheels, grasping the arms of the chair, and straightening the elbows, which lifts the person off of the seat.

Swimming is an ideal exercise for the physically challenged. It fosters flexibility, strength, and cardiovascular conditioning. The water helps support the body and swimming provides opportunities for social interaction.

At Philadelphia's Moss Rehabilitation Hospital, people in wheelchairs receive upper-body versions of martial

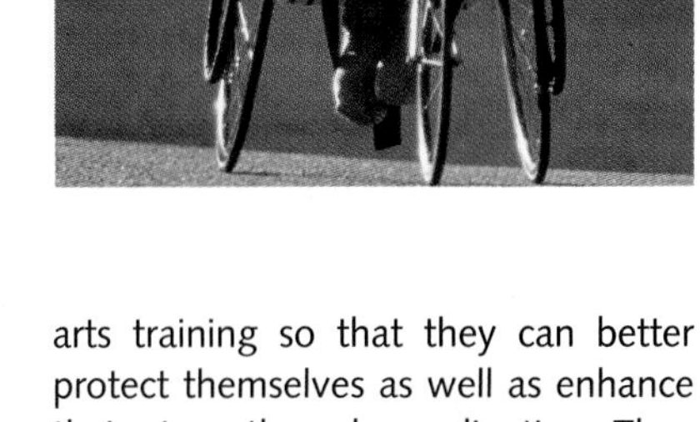

arts training so that they can better protect themselves as well as enhance their strength and coordination. They learn to jolt or fend off assailants with their fists, fingers, and arms.

In addition to more standard fare, the Handicapped Sports Program at Denver's Children's Hospital has programs in golf, horseback riding, river rafting, and skiing. One 15-year-old boy without a left leg and with a small right leg learned to ski with a brace on his one leg, one ski, and special ski "poles" with ski tips. In addition to enhancing his coordination and strength, skiing got him onto the slopes where he made friends and gained self-confidence.

Although exercise offers many benefits to people with disabilities, there are also some special hazards. For example, wheelchair-using athletes may overuse their upper bodies so that they incur injuries to muscles and joints in their hands, arms, shoulders, and necks. Wheelchair-using athletes are also apparently more susceptible to dangerous changes in body temperature. Drinking plenty of fluids helps avert a dangerous rise of body temperature (hyperthermia). Getting out of sweaty clothes at the end of a session and getting wrapped in a blanket can help prevent a dangerous drop of body temperature (hypothermia). Like other athletes, physically challenged people are encouraged to consult with health professionals before undertaking exercise regimens.

Smart Quiz Q0702

## think about it!

- Are you fit? In what way or ways?
- If you are not fit, what can you do to get fit?
- How can you enhance your strength or endurance? How can you maintain (or gain) flexibility?
- What is your target heart rate range? How can you get started with aerobic exercise?

# EXERCISE-RELATED INJURIES

Exercise has many health benefits, but it can be dangerous if it is carried out unsafely. Vigorous exercise and weight-bearing exercise exert tremendous forces on muscle, bone, and connective tissue such as tendons and ligaments. When stressed correctly, muscles generally adapt by becoming stronger. Most exercise-related injuries to muscles, bones, and connective tissue result from either overuse (exercising parts or all of the body too hard and too often) or improper technique.

## Muscle Soreness

When we begin an exercise program, we should expect some muscle soreness. This is especially so if our routine uses underused muscles. As muscles adapt to their workloads, the soreness should diminish, although it may not disappear. When soreness persists beyond a week and gets worse rather than better, it requires medical attention.

Muscles may also feel sore *during* exercise. Called *acute-onset muscle soreness,* this type of soreness is caused by inadequate circulation of blood to working muscles. Once you stop exercising, the soreness disappears. Soreness during exercise is a signal to stop and allow your muscles to relax before resuming.

Another form of muscle soreness, called *delayed muscle soreness,* usually appears a day or two after a workout and lasts from two to seven days, although it usually disappears in about three days. Delayed muscle soreness results from microscopic tears in muscle fibers, which irritate nerve endings. As the tears repair themselves, the muscle gets stronger. Delayed muscle soreness may be prevented by more gradually increasing the demands placed on muscles.

Muscle *cramps* are painful muscle spasms. Muscle cramps occurring during exercise often result from a depletion of fluids and/or an imbalance of **electrolytes** such as potassium and sodium. Cramps are usually alleviated through rest, fluid replacement, and massage.

Exercise-related injuries fall into two broad categories. *Sudden injuries* occur in a single, abrupt incident. Strains and sprains are sudden injuries, as are bone fractures or breaks, torn cartilage, and ruptured tendons. *Overuse injuries* develop more gradually as bone, muscle, or connective tissue are repeatedly stressed beyond their capacity to recover and adapt. Tendinitis, stress fractures, and shin splints are among the most common forms of overuse injuries. Sometimes a neglected overuse injury results in a sudden injury. For instance, untreated tendinitis may eventually lead to a ruptured tendon. Other exercise-related injuries include certain types of muscle soreness and weather-related injuries.

## Sudden Injuries

People who are sedentary most of the time and then try to compensate by going at it all at once—the so-called weekend athletes—are especially vulnerable to strains, sprains, and other types of sudden injuries.

**Muscle Strains** **Strains** ("muscle pulls") occur when a muscle is overstretched, which tears the muscle fibers or surrounding tissue. You may strain a muscle when you try to use it in an unusual way, as during vigorous exercise. Strains can occur in muscles in almost any part of the body, including the shoulders, back, hips, thighs, and lower legs. Virtually all of us experience occasional muscle strains. Recovery is usually quick and complete, typically within three to six weeks. Recovery is aided by the use of ice packs to reduce swelling and pain, avoiding use of the muscle for several days, and perhaps bandaging or strapping it for additional support. You should also avoid exercis-

**Electrolytes** A substance that when placed in solution conducts electricity; the body requires electrolytes, such as salts of sodium and potassium, to function.

**Strains** Stretches ("muscle pulls") or actual tears in muscle fibers or surrounding tissue.

## Health Check

### Overtraining—Are You Doing Too Much of a Good Thing?

You get involved in an exercise program and before long lose a few inches from your waist. You're basking in the pride of accomplishing something worthwhile that makes you feel firm and fit. And you want to do more. After all, if a half-hour on the treadmill is good, wouldn't an hour be better? You may find it more difficult to resist heading for the gym whenever time allows. Nothing wrong with this, right? Actually, it depends. You could be overtraining.

Exercise is a good thing as far as your health is concerned, but too much of a good thing can be dangerous. Unlike *overloading*, which gradually challenges the body to adapt to greater demands and is the path to fitness, *overtraining* means doing more than your body can handle. Workouts that are too frequent, intense, or lengthy can have unfortunate consequences.

Overtraining is a leading cause of exercise-related injuries as well as other health problems. Muscles and other tissue need time to recover to repair and renew themselves. If too little time is left for recovery, energy is depleted rather than renewed. Feelings of boredom and staleness may replace the more positive emotions usually connected with getting in shape.

Exercise to the point of exhaustion can weaken the immune system, increasing the risk of disease. When you exercise too strenuously, your body reacts as it does to other intense stressors, by pumping out stress hormones. Prolonged exposure to stress hormones can weaken the immune system's response to microbial invaders. We also know that grueling exercise reduces natural killer (NK) cell activity in both trained athletes and other people.[42] Even among a group of marathoners, researchers found, those who ran more than 60 miles a week in training experienced twice as many colds as those who ran less than 20 miles a week.[43]

How much exercise is too much? Use your body as a guide. Your body may be telling you something. Don't push yourself to the point of exhaustion. Overtraining usually takes place gradually, but sometimes even one too-intense workout can leave us feeling so weak that we're forced to rest for several days. Overtraining is the leading cause of overuse injuries. To prevent overuse injuries, be aware of the following signs of overtraining and use these cues to cut back:

- Elevated resting heart rate
- General fatigue or exhaustion
- Disturbed sleeping patterns
- A feeling of "staleness" rather than rejuvenation following exercise
- Decreased interest in exercise
- Loss of appetite
- Sudden weight loss
- Poor digestion
- Swollen lymph glands
- Increased frequency of colds or other illnesses
- Muscle pain
- Unsteadiness on your feet
- Excessive sweating
- Feeling faint
- Difficulty catching your breath

If these warning signs occur, cut back on your exercise routine. Then build gradually to a level that does not cause pain or distress. If pain or discomfort persists, see a health professional. The best way to avoid overtraining is to stick to the recommended training guidelines for each fitness component. Don't dramatically increase the intensity or length of time you exercise from one week to the next. Some experts recommend only a 5% weekly increase.[44] Follow the *hard/easy formula:* Alternate hard workouts with easier ones. If you suspect you're overtraining, an easy way to check is to take your resting heart rate in the morning. If your heart rate is 10% higher than usual, you may be overtraining.

Does this mean you should forget about lifting heavier loads or running more miles? Not at all. But if you experience any of the symptoms described here, you may need to modify the pace at which you pursue your fitness goals.

ing the muscle until it is healed (substitute another exercise in the meantime). If the muscle is ruptured or torn completely, it may require surgery.[45]

**Sprains** **Sprains** result from sudden joint twists that tear **ligaments,** the tough fibrous tissues that connect bones. The ankles, knees, fingers, and shoulders are most vulnerable to sprains. Depending on how severely the ligament is torn, sprains can be minor, with some tenderness and pain, or major, with significant swelling, pain, and loss of function. Pain that lasts for more than a few days should be brought to the attention of a health professional. In some cases, a cast or surgery may be necessary.

**Other Sudden Injuries** Other sudden injuries include bone **fractures** (broken bones), torn cartilage, and ruptured tendons. A broken bone results

**Sprains** Sudden joint twists that stretch or tear ligaments, the tough fibrous tissue connecting bone to bone.

**Ligaments** Tough fibrous tissue that connects bone to bone.

**Fracture** A broken bone.

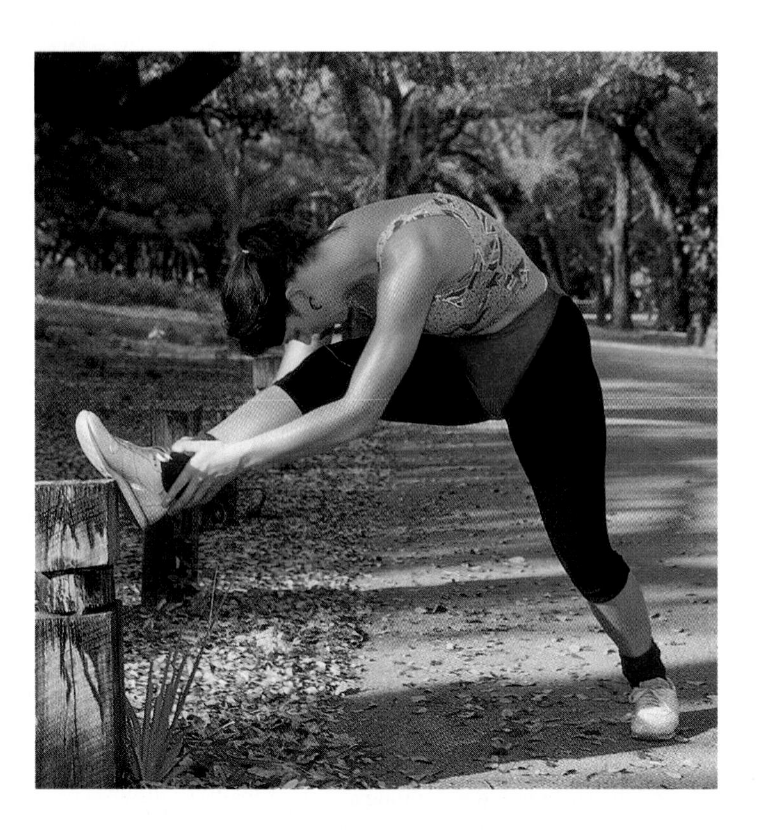

***Quite a Stretch?*** Warming up by stretching can help prevent muscle injuries.

from too much pressure or stress being placed on a bone. Broken bones are uncommon in physical activities like swimming, which have little impact on bones. They occur more often in contact sports, such as football, ice hockey, basketball, and boxing, especially fractures involving bones in the hands and nose. Fractures of bones in the feet are also common in runners, especially those who run on hard pavement.

**Cartilage** is tissue that acts as padding between the surfaces of a joint. The knee is the usual site of sports-related injuries involving damage to cartilage. Torn cartilage results from a sudden twisting of the knee joint, which may occur from taking a misstep or making an abrupt change in direction. These injuries, which typically require surgery, are common in running, tennis, football, and basketball.

**Tendons** are bands of tough fibrous tissue anchoring muscle to bone. They allow your muscles to move bones in various parts of your body, such as your fingers, hands, arms, legs, and feet. A ruptured tendon is a severe, sudden injury in which the tendon is torn away from the bone or actually snaps in half. If you sever a tendon, you will lose all or some movement of the bone to which it is connected. Ruptured tendons often produce searing pain (unless nerve damage is present) and demand immediate medical attention.

**Cartilage** A flexible, tough type of connective tissue that often covers the end of bones and acts as a "lining" for the joints.

**Tendons** Fibrous connective tissue that connects muscles to bones and other body parts.

**Tendinitis** Inflammation of tendons.

## Overuse Injuries

Overuse injuries such as tendinitis and stress fractures result when the body part affected is pushed past its ability to absorb the force of the exercise effectively. *Overtraining,* or exercising too much, is the usual cause.

**Tendinitis** When muscles contract, tendons pull on bones to make them work, bearing the brunt of the force that muscles exert. The most common form of tendon injury is **tendinitis,** or inflammation of tendons. Tendinitis results from doing too much of a repetitive motion. Through overuse, microscopic tears develop in the tendons, causing pain, redness, warmth, and swelling.

Tendinitis often occurs around the joints. The most common site is in the Achilles tendon *(Achilles tendinitis),* the large tendon in the back of the leg connecting calf muscles to the heel bone.

*Tennis elbow* is another common form of tendinitis. In tennis players, it results from repeated swinging of the racket placing undue stress on the affected tendons. Anyone who overstresses the tendons around the elbow joint, including gardeners, rowers, and even businesspeople who routinely lug a heavy briefcase, can develop "tennis elbow." Untreated tendinitis can lead to a rupture of the tendon.

**Stress Fractures** **Stress fractures** are microscopic breaks in bones (such as those in the foot, shin, and thigh) caused by repeated and excessive pressure or pounding. They result from more stress being placed on bone than it can withstand. At first, a stress fracture may cause a persistent, dull ache in the fracture area. If ignored, it may become extremely painful. Rest and ice applications may be all that's needed; if pain persists, however, the affected area should be X-rayed. More severe fractures require medical attention to realign and immobilize the broken bone pieces so that they heal correctly.

**Shin Splints** **Shin splints** feel somewhat like stress fractures but involve tears in muscle fibers rather than breaks in bone. Shin splints occur from slight tears in the muscles serving the **tibia,** the inner and larger of the two bones in the leg between the knee and the ankle. They cause tenderness and pain that may be severe if the affected area is directly squeezed with the fingers. A common injury in runners and beginning exercisers, shin splints may result from an imbalance between strong muscles in the back of the leg and weaker ones in front. Most cases resolve on their own once the muscles become accustomed to the exercise, but it's important to switch to a low-impact form of exercise until the condition improves (usually in about two weeks). Shoes should also supply ample arch support and overall cushioning.

## Weather-Related Injuries

You've made the decision. Tired of driving by all those healthy-looking joggers, you've resolved to join them. You begin by walking for several weeks, then proceed to a slow jog, and so on. All is going well until the weather changes. Suddenly it's 90 degrees in the shade, and the same 20-minute jog you breezed through yesterday leaves you weak and dizzy after just 10 minutes.

**Dangers of Heat Stress** Exercising in high temperatures can lead to **heat stress,** a condition in which body temperature rises, sometimes to dangerous levels. Heat stress may result in heat cramps, heat exhaustion, hyperthermia, and heat stroke.

Vigorous exercise produces 15 to 20 times the amount of body heat that is produced during rest.[46] As body temperature rises, the hypothalamus (a small structure located in the midbrain) signals the blood vessels to dilate, or open wider to allow more blood to flow to skin surfaces. This stimulates sweating, which in turn cools the skin through evaporation. Problems arise when the body produces more heat than it can remove through sweating. Heat then remains trapped in the body, raising temperatures to potentially dangerous levels.

**Heat cramps** are caused by an excess loss of body salt through sweating. Fluid replacement, rest, and massage will relieve a heat cramp. When rising body temperatures produce fatigue, **heat exhaustion** sets in. Symptoms include dizziness, cold skin, and a weak pulse. With both heat cramps and heat exhaustion, it is essential to move the person to a cool place, allow rest, and provide fluid replacement. Untreated heat exhaustion quickly leads to **hyperthermia,** or a rapid rise in body temperature. Unless checked immediately, hyperthermia leads to **heat stroke,** the most dangerous heat-related condition of all. In heat stroke, body temperature rises above 106 degrees Fahrenheit, all sweating stops, and the skin becomes very hot and dry. Heat stroke is a life-threatening condition demanding immediate medical attention. If left untreated, it can result in death.

**Cold-Weather Hazards** Just as too much heat can become trapped in the body in hot weather, too much heat can escape from the body in cold weath-

**Stress fractures** Microscopic breaks in bones caused by repeated and excessive pressure or pounding.

**Shin splints** Injuries that involve tears in muscle fibers.

**Tibia** The inner and larger of the two bones in the leg, extending from the knee to the ankle.

**Heat stress** A condition in which body temperature rises, sometimes to dangerous levels; may result in heat cramps, heat exhaustion, hyperthermia, and heat stroke.

**Heat cramps** Painful muscle spasms resulting from hard work in hot temperatures without an adequate supply of fluids and salt.

**Heat exhaustion** An acute reaction to excessive heat, characterized by dizziness, cold skin, weak pulse, nausea, weakness, and headache, leading to collapse.

**Hyperthermia** A bodily state characterized by unusually high fever.

**Heat stroke** A dangerous, potentially life-threatening reaction to excessive heat characterized by extremely high fever.

Talking Glossary
Hypothermia G0705

er. Extreme heat loss is called **hypothermia.** Blood vessels constrict, impeding circulation to all parts of the body. Prolonged exposure to extremely cold air or plunging into cold water may result in hypothermia. If untreated, hypothermia can lead to death.

**Frostbite** is skin damage produced by prolonged exposure to freezing temperatures. Any exposed area, including fingers, toes, earlobes, and nose, is vulnerable to frostbite. Frostbitten skin turns pale or white. Once circulation is restored, it becomes red and swollen. Though frostbite may affect any part of the body, the hands, toes, fingers, nose, and ears are most at risk. Skin that is severely frostbitten may turn darker red, purple, or black when warm. Severe frostbite requires immediate medical attention.

PREVENTION

### Preventing Exercise-Related Injuries

Since exercise-related accidents and injuries can happen to anyone, safety concerns should be an integral part of any exercise program or sports activity. While some injuries may be unavoidable, most can be prevented by taking a few precautionary steps:

- *Increase the intensity or duration of exercise gradually.*
- *Learn proper exercise techniques.* Check the proper use of an exercise machine or workout routine with a trainer.
- *Know when to stop.* Any point beyond mild discomfort, or any sign of dizziness or faintness, should be a cue to stop.
- *Warm up and cool down.* Warm up before vigorous exercise by performing some light exercise and stretching routines. Warming up helps prevent muscle sprains and strains because these injuries are more common when muscles are cold. Cool down by slowing down the pace of your exercise routine before stopping completely. Then do some stretching. Take an exercise class to learn specific techniques for warming up and cooling down. Warming up before each workout and cooling down afterward can sharply reduce the risk of injury.
- *Use proper equipment, especially appropriate athletic footwear and protective gear including helmets and pads.*
- *To minimize injuries to the feet and legs, avoid exercising on concrete surfaces.* Jog or run on grass or dirt. Run on flat terrain. A divot can cause a misstep and twist an ankle or a knee. Concrete floors raise the risk of injury in aerobic dance exercise. The wooden floors found in most gyms are safer.
- *Walk or run against traffic; if you bicycle, move with traffic.* Better yet, avoid running, bicycling, or walking in traffic.
- *Select an exercise that's right for your body.* If you have knee problems, select a low-impact activity (one that puts less stress on joints, especially those in the lower limbs). Don't just neglect your knees, however. Slowly and carefully develop a program to strengthen them.
- *Never exercise under the influence of alcohol or other drugs.*
- *Follow a balanced diet.* Drink plenty of fluids, especially if you lose body fluids through profuse perspiration during heavy exercise.
- *Make sure to get enough sleep.* Your muscles may be more resilient when they are rested.

**Hypothermia** Extreme loss of heat in the body characterized by an unusually low body temperature.

**Frostbite** Skin damage produced by prolonged exposure to cold air.

**Stress test** A method of evaluating cardiorespiratory fitness by measuring oxygen consumption and heart functioning in response to increasingly stressful physical demands during exercise, usually on a treadmill or stationary bicycle.

## Become Heart Smart

Now and then (but fortunately rarely) athletes die suddenly from heart attacks or other cardiovascular problems while exercising or in competition. Some runners have suffered heart attacks on the course. Nearly all exercise-related cardiac fatalities result from preexisting cardiovascular problems, such as narrowing of the arteries or heart defects. In people under age 35, sudden death during exercise is typically related to other cardiac abnormalities, such as irregular heart rhythms.

Cardiovascular risks can usually be detected by means of a stress test. In a **stress test,** heart function and blood pressure are monitored by medical personnel while the person engages in vigorous exercise, usually on a treadmill or bicycle. It's a good idea to get a medical evaluation before you embark on an exercise regimen, especially if you're in doubt about your general health or you are over 40 and sedentary. Medical evaluations are especially recommended for people who smoke, are overweight, or have family histories of cardiovascular disorders. However, it is much riskier not to exercise than to exercise, especially for people who are at risk of coronary heart disease. Safety concerns should not be an excuse for not exercising, but rather a reason to learn to exercise safely. Build up your intensity level gradually to allow your body to get accustomed to increased stress.

Also be aware of signs of heart problems when exercising—signs such as:

- Pain or pressure in the left or mid-chest area, left neck, shoulder, or arm during or just after exercising. (However, vigorous exercise may produce a side stitch, a pain below your bottom ribs, which is not a sign of a heart problem.)
- Sudden light-headedness, cold sweat, pallor, or fainting.[47]

Should you experience any of these signs, stop exercising and call your doctor for an evaluation.

## Gear Up—Use the Right Equipment

In one recent year alone, fitness and sports enthusiasts shelled out over 30 *billion* dollars on sports equipment, clothing, and athletic footwear.[48] Consumers face a dizzying array of choices in exercise gear, from countless kinds of stationary machines to a seemingly endless variety of athletic footwear. But while you can spend hours outfitting yourself in the latest activewear fashions, pay attention to a few key purchases to ensure that you are using the right equipment. These include proper footwear, comfortable sports clothing, and protective head and eye gear.

Properly fitting, well-cushioned, and supportive athletic shoes are a must for most forms of exercise. Feet absorb up to three times total body weight each time they land on the ground. Shoes that are well-cushioned help absorb much of this force, avoiding many kinds of painful injuries to knees, legs, and heels. Shoes should also be comfortable and leave the foot free of blisters or calluses.

Finding the right shoe depends on the type of exercise for which it is needed. *Jogging* and *running shoes* (see Figure 7.5) provide extra cushioning in the heel of the shoe, but this extra cushioning may not be much use, and may actually be harmful, in an aerobic dance class. *Aerobics shoes* provide more lateral support to help prevent excessive side-to-side movement, the kind of movement that can lead to stress injuries. When it comes to *walking shoes*, look for models that come with low heels and strong arch supports. These provide extra stability.[49]

Fitness magazines routinely provide evaluations of the pros and cons of the latest models in footwear. If you're confused about which brand to

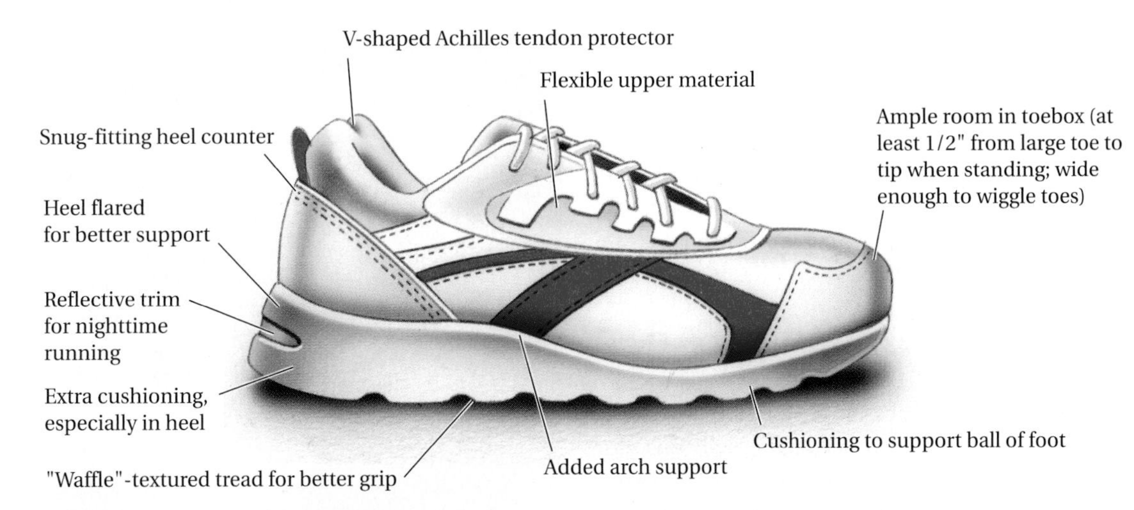


**Figure 7.5** ***Features of a Good Running Shoe*** When buying a running shoe, *Consumer Reports* suggests shopping late in the day, when your feet are their largest. Bring along an old pair of running shoes, so a skilled salesperson can examine the wear pattern to analyze your running motion. Make sure the shoes are flexible enough to bend easily at their widest point. Wear the socks you normally use when running and bring along any orthotics or other inserts you might regularly use. Jog around in the store to test out the comfort and feel.

buy, check out magazines at your library or newsstand that review competing models. Or tell the salesperson what you intend to use the shoe for. Walk around the store wearing the shoes for at least ten minutes to determine whether they are comfortable. Many stores today have liberal return policies; if you develop blisters or calluses, ask if you can exchange the shoes for another pair.

In general, sports clothing should be loose-fitting and made of material that easily absorbs moisture and permits sweat to evaporate. To avoid chafing and muscle tears, women should invest in a sports bra; men should purchase athletic supporters.

Match clothing to the exercise. Don't wear clothes that will catch in gears or wheels or that will cause you to trip. Pay particular attention to protecting the head and eyes. If you bicycle or engage in other sports that expose the head to possible trauma, *wear a helmet.* Head injuries are the leading cause of death in bicycle crashes; those who don't wear helmets are six times more likely to suffer a head injury than helmeted bicyclists.[50] Select a bicycle helmet that is certified by the Snell Memorial Foundation as meeting safety standards (look for the Snell sticker inside the helmet).

For in-line skating, wear protective wrist guards, elbow pads, and knee pads in addition to a safety helmet. Only 7% of in-line skaters outfit themselves with all of this protective gear and nearly half wear no safety equipment at all.[51] About 100,000 in-line skaters injure themselves so badly each year that they require emergency medical treatment. Moreover, hundreds of thousands of exercisers suffer sports-related eye injuries, yet only a small number wear protective eye guards. To avoid joining the ranks of the injured, use eye guards during any activity involving a flying object (such as squash and racquetball) and when swimming. Eye guards are also helpful in basketball.

## Weather the Weather

To avoid heat stress, drink plenty of fluids before, during, and after exercise. Lighten up on your usual exercise routine for a week or so until your body adjusts to the warmer temperature. Also, refrain from exercising in extreme heat unless you have accustomed yourself to these conditions over a lengthy period. Even then, frequent rest periods and constant fluid replacement are necessary. Watch out for any signs of heat stroke, such as feeling dizzy, weak, excessively tired, or light-headed, or a dangerous increase in body temperature or failure to perspire.

The keys to avoiding cold-weather injuries are wearing warm clothing, staying dry, and resting whenever necessary. Also important is warming up. Your body requires a longer warm-up on cold days. Pay particular attention to protecting extremities—ears, head, face, hands, and feet—from the cold. Wearing multiple layers of clothing is the secret to staying both warm and dry while exercising.[52] And wear a hat—most of your body's heat is lost through your head and neck. But don't overdress; sweat-soaked clothing can increase your risk of hypothermia.[53] Basically, wear one layer less than you normally would to stay warm if you were outside. And keep moving: Sustained exercise helps maintain body heat in the cold.

## Replenish Your Body's Needs for Food and Drink

Fitness magazines bulge with ads for "ergogenic" aids—supplements designed to boost performance and build stronger muscles. Save your money. Instead, by following a balanced diet and consuming plenty of fluids, you will ensure that you have all the nutrients you need to satisfy the energy requirements of exercise.

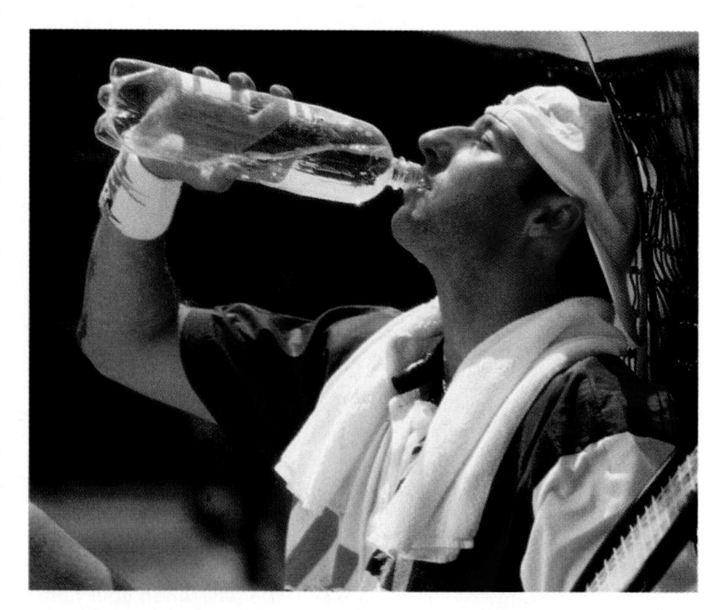

***Drink, Drink, Drink*** Drink liquids before, during, and after exercising. Your body needs to replenish fluid levels when you engage in sustained physical activity.

The components of a balanced diet are provided in Chapter 5. Most of our calories should come from complex carbohydrates, from starches like potatoes, rice, and pasta. In endurance training, it's even more important that the bulk of your diet (60 to 70%) derive from these high-octane sources.

Fluid replacement is essential. Lack of fluids can produce symptoms ranging from nausea and fatigue to heat stress. Don't just drink when you're thirsty: Many people don't feel thirsty until well after their bodies require fluids. And don't ignore your need for fluids on cold days. The cold may reduce your thirst, but not your body's need for fluids. To ensure that you get enough fluids:

- Drink several glasses of water before exercising.
- Drink 4 to 6 ounces every 15 minutes during exercise.
- Drink several more glasses after exercise to replace fluids lost in sweat.[54]

Another key element to healthful exercising is ensuring you get enough sleep (see "Getting Your Z's").

## Treating Injuries

Any injury that produces sharp pain or persistent swelling should be brought immediately to the attention of a health professional. Any serious injury, such as a fracture or ruptured tendon, also requires prompt attention. Severe weather-related injuries, such as heat stroke or frostbite, also require attention. Even a relatively minor strain or sprain or a persistently sore muscle should be medically evaluated to ensure that you are treating it correctly and not risking further damage. In many cases, a program of *rest, ice, compression, and elevation* (the **RICE principle**) may be sufficient to alleviate the problem. However, don't self-diagnose. Consult a health professional first.

The RICE principle involves four steps:

1. *Rest the injured area.* Avoid activities that stress the affected area until pain, swelling, and inflammation subside. You don't necessarily have to stop working out entirely, however. It may be possible to practice other forms of exercise that don't affect the injured area. Heading for the couch may perpetuate a vicious cycle: By getting out of shape, you're more likely to suffer another injury when you start to exercise again.
2. *Periodically apply ice to the parts that are swollen and inflamed.* Apply an ice pack to the injured area for 15 minutes, four times daily, for 48 hours after the injury. If symptoms persist, see the doctor.
3. *Compress: Wrap the injured area in a bandage.* Compression reduces the flow of blood to the site that is hurt, thereby reducing swelling and inflammation. If the injury is wrapped too tightly, however, the flow of blood will be cut off. You may wish to consult a physician or athletic trainer to determine how the injury should be wrapped and how long it should remain wrapped.
4. *Elevate the injured area whenever possible.* Keeping the injured area above heart level lets oxygen-poor blood drain away from the area while helping oxygen-rich blood flow back to the affected region.

When pain or swelling persists, don't take it for granted that the injury will eventually heal on its own. Check it out with a health professional.

PREVENTION

### *Getting Your Z's*

Adequate sleep is a key to fitness. When we get too little sleep, we may feel fatigued and lethargic and lack mental alertness. Our muscles may be less resilient, which can increase the risk of an injury during exercise.

Most people need between 6 and 8 hours of sleep nightly to feel refreshed. Yet many of us get too little sleep. We may go to bed later than we should or get up earlier than we'd like because of a need to get an early start on the day. In families with young children, a full night's rest is a wistful memory for many parents. Many people too are troubled by **insomnia,** a type of sleep disorder characterized by persistent or recurring problems falling asleep or remaining asleep, or achieving restorative sleep, the type of sleep that leaves you feeling refreshed and alert in the morning.

**Smart Reference**
Waking up
R0702

#### Insomnia—What It Is and What You Can Do About It

Occasional difficulty falling asleep or remaining asleep, especially during

**RICE principle** A program of rest, ice, compression, and elevation used in the treatment of exercise-related injuries.

**Insomnia** Difficulty falling asleep, remaining asleep, or achieving restorative sleep.

**Close-up**
Sleep apnea
**T0703**
More on insomnia
**T0704**

times of stress, is not abnormal. However, many of us, about one in three in a given year, are troubled by persistent problems with insomnia that last for a month or more.[55] In many cases, the sleep problem is actually a sign of an underlying physical cause, such as problems relating to drug or alcohol abuse, or a psychological disorder, such as depression. If the underlying problem is successfully resolved, chances are good that normal sleep patterns can be restored. In other cases, the insomnia itself is considered the primary problem.

The risk of primary insomnia increases with age and is greater among women than men. For younger people, insomnia usually takes the form of difficulty falling asleep, while older people are typically bothered by frequent awakenings during the night or awakening too early in the morning and having difficulty getting back to sleep.

Insomnia may have biological causes (such as changes as we age in the brain mechanisms that control sleep and wake cycles), but psychological problems are often involved. People with chronic insomnia tend to bring their worries to bed with them, which raises their anxiety and the accompanying bodily arousal to a level that prevents natural sleep. They may then worry about not getting enough sleep, which raises their arousal level even more. They may try to concentrate on falling asleep, which usually backfires by creating even more pressure and tension, making sleep even less likely.

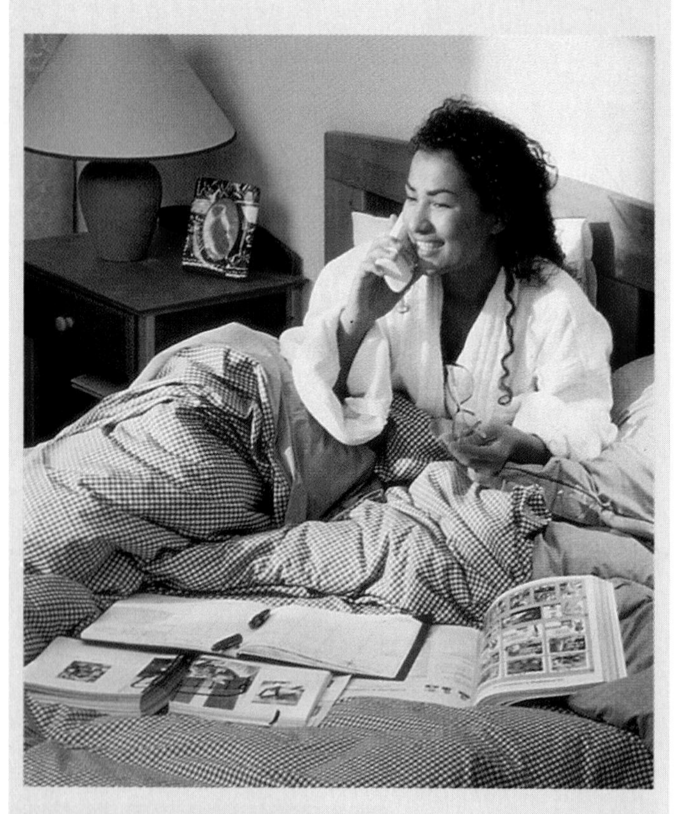

***Your Bed Is Not Your Office*** Using your bed as your office (or study hall) may make it more difficult for you to get to sleep at night. Let your bed become a cue for winding down, not gearing up.

Here are some suggestions that are useful in helping people overcome insomnia:

- *Recognize that sleep cannot be forced.* Sleep cannot be willed by conscious effort. You can only set the stage for sleep by relaxing and letting nature take its course.
- *Go to bed only when you are sleepy.* Don't try to sleep if you are wide-eyed and full of energy. Let your mind and body wind down before hitting the pillow.
- *Develop a regular sleep routine.* Establish a bedtime routine that allows your mind and body to get into a sleep mode before retiring. Read, watch TV, practice a relaxation exercise, or engage in some other relaxing activity for an hour or so before bed. Go to bed about the same time every night and rise about the same time each morning. You can sleep in on weekends, but be aware that sleeping till noon can throw off your body clock.
- *Make the bed a cue for sleeping.* Limit as much as possible other activities in bed, such as eating, talking on the phone, or watching TV.
- *Get up if you can't sleep.* If you don't fall asleep within 10 to 20 minutes, get out of bed and go to another room. Restore a state of relaxation by reading, meditating, or listening to calming music. Then go back to bed when you are feeling relaxed. Repeat this process until you fall asleep.
- *Avoid daytime naps.* Many people try to make up for nighttime sleeplessness by napping during the day. Napping can throw off your natural body clock, making it more difficult to fall asleep the following night.
- *Don't take your problems to bed.* Bedtime is not the time to try to solve your problems or organize your life. Remind yourself that you'll think about tomorrow, tomorrow.
- *Take a mind trip.* Mental fantasy is an excellent means of letting your thoughts slip away from consciousness, leading to sleep. Take a nightly mental excursion into a fantasy—travel, adventure, the past—wherever your mind takes you. Or you might try some pleasant mental imagery, such as lying on sun-drenched sand at the beach or walking through a lush, green meadow on a clear spring day. Let your mind wander.
- *Exercise regularly, but not before sleep.* Regular exercise can help relieve daily stress and reduce muscle tension, which can help you relax when you retire at night. But don't exercise directly before bedtime, as it temporarily increases your body's level of arousal.

- *Limit caffeinated beverages to the morning.* Caffeine is the stimulant found in coffee and tea (and in chocolate in lesser amounts). It can remain active in the body for 6 to 10 hours. You should also avoid smoking, not only because of its harmful effects to your health, but because it too contains a stimulant—nicotine.
- *Practice coping thoughts.* Thoughts that induce anxiety can keep you up long into the night. Replace anxious thoughts with calming alternatives. Instead of thinking, "I must get to sleep right now or I won't be able to concentrate tomorrow on the exam (conference, meeting, etc.)," substitute a thought like, "I might not be as sharp as usual, but I'm not going to fall apart. I've gotten by on little sleep before and I can do so again."

**Should You Take Sleeping Pills?** Sleep medications called **hypnotics** are the most common form of treatment of sleep disorders in the United States. Though these drugs can be helpful in the short-term treatment of insomnia, long-term use can lead to serious problems.

The most widely used hypnotics are those that belong to a family of minor tranquilizers called *benzodiazepines,* which include Valium, Librium, Dalmane, Xanax, and Halcion. These drugs help promote sleep by reducing the body's arousal state and inducing feelings of calmness. However, they tend to suppress rapid-eye-movement or **REM sleep,** the stage of sleep that was so named because the eyes can be seen darting rapidly under the lids. REM sleep is the sleep stage associated with dreaming. Lack of REM sleep can interfere with the natural restorative functions of sleep. Hypnotics can also produce "hangover" effects the following day and can lead to *rebound insomnia* when they are discontinued after a long period of use—meaning that they can lead to worse insomnia. Tapering off rather than withdrawing "cold-turkey" may reduce the likelihood of rebound insomnia.

Another problem is **tolerance.** That is, these drugs typically lose their effectiveness after a period of regular use, and larger doses are needed to achieve the same effect. Regular use, especially with increasing doses, can lead to the development of a physiological dependence (addiction) on these drugs. Moreover, high doses can be dangerous, especially if they are combined with other drugs. Regular users can also become *psychologically* dependent on sleep medications. They reach for a pill rather than learn more effective ways of coping with the stress in their lives. Because of the problems associated with regular use of sleep medications, especially the risk of dependence, they should be used only for a limited period of time (usually a few days at a time) and only under a physician's direction. At best they provide a temporary respite from sleeplessness in times of stress. If you are troubled by persistent insomnia, try using the techniques listed above. If the problem persists, consult a health professional for a more complete evaluation.

You should also avoid using alcohol to combat insomnia. Alcohol is a depressant drug that slows down your central nervous system, which may make you feel sleepy. However, alcohol use, especially if heavy, interferes with normal sleep patterns and can leave you feeling less refreshed on awakening.

## think about it!

- **Have you experienced an exercise-related injury? How did it happen? How was it treated, if at all?**
- **How can you tell if an exercise injury requires medical attention?**
- **How can you prevent exercise-related injuries?**
- **Do you get enough sleep? If not, what can you do about it?**

Smart Quiz
Q0703

**Hypnotics** Types of drugs that have sleep-inducing effects.

**REM sleep** The stage of sleep characterized by rapid eye movements under the sleeper's closed eyelids; associated with dreaming.

**Tolerance** The need for increasing amounts of a substance to achieve the same effects.

# Making Exercise a Part of Your Lifestyle

## Take Charge

What type of exercise activity is best for you? The choice depends on making a personal appraisal of your goals, needs, and interests. Here are some questions to get you started in this self-evaluation:

- What are my goals? What do I want to achieve by exercising?
- Do I have any physical conditions that limit the types of exercise I can do?
- What kinds of physical activities do I enjoy?
- Which kinds of activities am I most likely to stick with?
- What activities can I afford?
- Do I prefer competitive sports or individual effort?
- How can I fit working out or exercising into my schedule?
- Do I prefer to set aside specific time for exercise or incorporate more physical activity into my usual routine?

### Determine Your Goals

What are your exercise goals—strength training, cardiorespiratory fitness, weight loss, general health, or some combination? Identifying your goals can help you decide what type of exercise makes sense for you. Table 7.4 offers some suggestions.

**Healthcheck**
Choosing your sport
**H0702**

### Choose an Exercise Activity—What's Right for You?

Do you like to exercise alone or with others? Do you prefer indoor activities or outdoor activities? Would you prefer exercising at a health club or at home? What can you afford in the way of exercise equipment, classes, or club memberships?

**Treadmill, Stair-Stepper, or Cross-Country Skier: Which Is Best for You?** Though a vigorous workout on any exercise machine can have an aerobic effect, a recent study showed that working on a treadmill machine uses more energy (more calories burned) than other types of indoor exercise machines.[57] The stair-stepper came in second. Why is the treadmill such an energy user? One possible reason is that walking is something that almost all of us do regularly, so in the course of our daily routine we condition our large leg muscles to work vigorously with less stress and strain. Other activities—such as climbing stairs or skiing—use muscles that are not conditioned regularly. Does this mean that you should go out and buy a treadmill? Not necessarily. For one thing, a good treadmill is expensive, with motorized models running into the thousands

**TABLE 7.4**

**Physical Activities to Help You Achieve Your Fitness Goals**

| Goal | What's Involved | How Much Is Needed | Types of Physical Activities |
|---|---|---|---|
| Strength training | Building and toning muscles | Varies with the particular muscle group | Working with free weights or weight-bearing equipment, especially those that offer resistance when both contracting and releasing muscle tension |
| Cardio-respiratory (aerobic) endurance | Strengthening the heart and lungs; improving stamina and cardiovascular endurance | 20–30 minutes of vigorous exercise at least three times weekly | Any vigorous exercise that makes you break into a sweat and begin panting, such as running, rowing, bicycling at speeds greater than 10 mph or 90 rpm; aerobics classes; hiking uphill; cross-country skiing; or working out on a treadmill, stair-climber, or mechanical skier |
| Weight loss | Shedding excess pounds | To lose about a pound a week, increase physical activity to a level that burns an additional 3,500 calories per week | The more vigorous the activity, the more calories expended. See Table 7.3 for a listing of the calories expended for selected activities |
| General health | Making regular moderate exercise a part of your life-style | At least 30 minutes of moderate-intensity physical activity per day, nearly every day | Brisk walking; bicycling; swimming laps; heavy housework; walking up stairs; working out |

of dollars. For another, you can get the same benefit by running or walking briskly outdoors. You may also be able to reap the same benefit from stationary bicycles and cross-country skiers if you train well enough to build the muscle strength required to burn as much energy with the same amount of effort as on the treadmill.

## Stick with It

Motivation is the key factor determining whether you are likely to begin an exercise program and stick with it long enough to reap the benefits. The bicycle that remains in the garage or the indoor skier that is collecting dust is not going to help you achieve your fitness goals. Nearly half of the people who start an exercise program drop out within six months.[58] Why? Among the more common reasons for dropping out are scheduling difficulties, competing demands on time, lack of affordable or accessible programs, and a lack of confidence in one's ability to keep pace.

To maintain motivation, we must not only believe that we *need* to exercise, but we must also have a *desire* to exercise. Desire comes from an exercise routine that you enjoy. One study found that dedicated exercisers:[59]

- Believe they are responsible for their fitness and health, and that exercise is necessary for both.
- Select activities they enjoy.
- Exercise at a "comfortably hard" intensity (about 75% of the target heart rate range).
- Engage in activities that free their minds to think about other things while they're exercising—for instance, family, work, or nothing at all.

By contrast, exercise dropouts:

- Don't like the exercise they've selected.
- Exercise at a very hard intensity (at the upper limits of the target heart rate range or above).
- Push the limits when they feel tired or in pain.
- Punish themselves with thoughts like "C'mon, don't stop, wimp."
- Feel fatigued after a workout.

Steer clear of the pitfalls common to exercise dropouts. Rather than push yourself at all costs, exercise at a "comfortably hard" level of intensity (at the midpoint of your target heart rate range). Select an exercise routine that you enjoy. Avoid thinking that you must compete with others at the gym. Use a professional trainer or fitness expert to learn how to exercise correctly, but don't get wrapped up in evaluating the quality of your performance. Instead, use the time spent exercising to unwind mentally. Using these guidelines, you're very likely to design a workout that you will stay with.

Some additional tips for staying the course:[60]

- *Bring a buddy.* Set a regular time and place for the two of you to work out. Make it a social as well as a fitness occasion.
- *Reward yourself.* Pat yourself on the back for sticking with it. Do something pleasurable after completing each exercise routine—but not gorging on food.
- *Make exercise more enjoyable.* You may make exercise more enjoyable by listening to music on a personal stereo as you work out. Many people like to watch TV while they exercise.
- *Choose an activity you can stick with for a lifetime.* Tennis is more likely than football or ice hockey to be an activity you can continue to enjoy throughout your life. Swimming, fast walking, and racquetball are other such activities.
- *Don't overdo it.* If you overdo it, you increase the risk of injury and fatigue and may not want to return the next time.
- *Prepare for your next session.* Keep your exercise gear handy, so that you don't have to start rearranging your closets to get yourself ready each time you exercise. If you work out in a health club, keep your equipment at the club or in the trunk of the car.
- *Set realistic goals.* Set realistic and *attainable* short-term goals. Unrealistic goals may discourage you so that you drop out.

## Walk for Fitness

Walking is America's favorite fitness activity. And why not? You don't need special equipment (other than a good pair of walking shoes). Even people who can't swim, ski, or return a tennis ball can walk. And perhaps best of all, walking is free (after the initial outlay for athletic shoes), and you only need to go as far as the front door to get started. Like any fitness activity, it is important to work up to a fitness walk gradually.

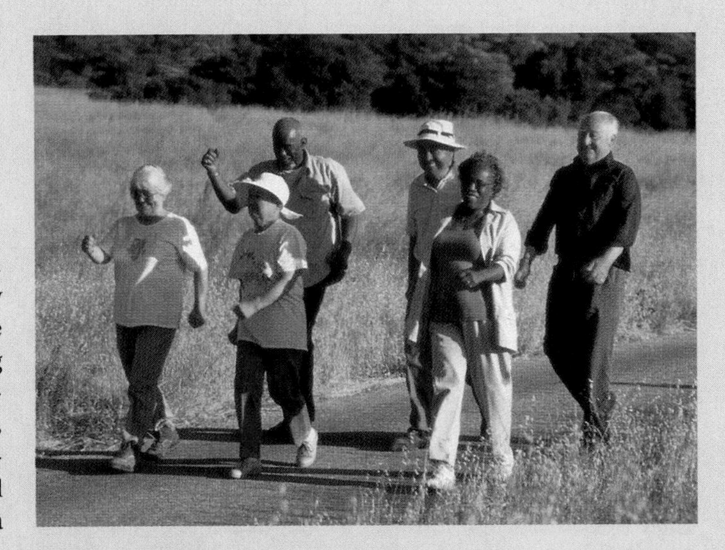

***Walking Is Excellent Exercise*** Brisk walking firms the muscles, builds cardiovascular fitness, and is "low-impact." For these reasons, it is a wonderful exercise choice for many of us, especially older people and people with sports injuries.

TABLE 7.5

**Types of Walking[62]**

| Type of Walking | What It Is | Advantages |
|---|---|---|
| *Strolling* | Walking at a leisurely pace. | Helps clear your mind, but probably too slow a pace to have any significant health benefits. Will burn some calories (about 100 calories per half-hour). This add up to about 1 pound lost per month, or 12 pounds per year. Not bad for enjoying a leisurely daily stroll. |
| *Fitness walking* | Walking at a brisk pace of about 3 to 4 miles per hour. | Meets the basic requirements for moderate exercise, if you can make it part of your daily routine. Experts believe that a program of regular brisk walking can lower risk of cardiovascular disease, adult-onset diabetes, and hypertension, and reduce excess weight. |
| *Race walking* | Fast walking in heel-toe fashion. Looks funny to observers, but speeds approach a running pace of 5+ miles per hour. | Lowers the risk of cardiovascular disease, adult-onset diabetes, and hypertension, and reduces excess weight. May increase longevity if practiced regularly at least three times weekly for 30 minutes. Burns calories with much less impact and risk of injuries than running. Swinging the arms with each step can also help tone chest and upper back muscles. |
| *Rugged walking* | Walking in rugged or hilly terrain at a brisk pace. Find a trail or make your own, but make sure to outfit yourself with athletic hiking shoes with good traction. | Depending on how vigorous the hike, it can have all the benefits of an aerobic workout with all that wonderful scenery to boot. But be careful jumping over those fallen logs and other natural obstacles. Because of the climbing involved, it also helps tone the thighs, hips, and butt. Keep those arms swinging to tone your chest and upper back muscles as well. |

There are different styles of walking and resulting health benefits (see Table 7.5). A fitness walk can be at either a moderate-exercise pace (3 to 4 mph) or an aerobics pace (4+ mph, especially on an incline). To reap the general health benefits of moderate exercise, you should plan to walk a half-hour a day, just about every day, at a 3- to 4-mile-per-hour pace. A more vigorous pace will help even more to improve your cardiorespiratory fitness and take off excess weight. Not sure how fast you're walking? Find the nearest quarter-mile track, perhaps at a nearby high school. Or take the car and mark off a quarter mile on the odometer. Then time yourself walking this distance. Divide 60 by your time in minutes, then divide again by 4. This gives your walking speed in miles per hour. At 4 miles per hour, you'll cover the quarter-mile course in 3.75 minutes. A rule of thumb is that you'll know you're walking at the aerobic threshold of 4 miles per hour if it becomes hard to walk and hold a conversation or you begin panting slightly.

Pump your arms as you walk, with your elbows bent at almost a 90 degree angle.[61] Pumping will increase your pace, burn more calories, and give your upper body a workout. Stretch before and after your walk.

## Make Exercise Part of Your Lifestyle

Regular exercisers fall into two groups: *Schedulizers* set aside specific times for exercise. They make exercise a regular part of their weekly schedules, usually before or after their workday. They place a high priority on exercise and juggle other responsibilities around exercise. *Routinizers* make exercise part of their everyday routine. There are many ways of making physical activity a regular part of your routine:

- *Walk to work.* Or if your workplace is too far to walk, take the car but park far enough away so that you must walk for at least 15 minutes at a brisk pace to get from your car to your job and back again.
- *Take the stairs rather than the elevator.*
- *Develop an outdoor interest, such as gardening, that requires sustained physical effort.*
- *Use a hand mower, not a power mower, to cut the grass.*
- *Walk from place to place to do your errands.* Don't move the car a few blocks when going from store to store. Look for a parking spot a few blocks away from your destination.
- *When playing with children, get on the floor and participate.* Don't just give directions from the couch or chair.
- *Take up dancing and step lively.* Slow ballroom dancing may be romantic, but it's not very physically demanding.

The recommended guidelines for daily moderate exercise do not require that the 30 minutes of exercise each day be completed all at once. Adding 15 minutes each way in walking between your car and your office will suffice, if you walk at a brisk pace.

Some people are both schedulizers and routinizers. Whichever pattern of physical activity you prefer, schedulizing or routinizing (or both), the most important factor in achieving the health benefits of regular exercise is to make it a part of your lifestyle.

Smart Quiz Q0704

# SUMMING UP

## Questions and Answers

### EXERCISE AND HEALTH

1. **What are the physical benefits of exercise?** Exercise helps people maintain a healthy weight by burning calories and increasing the metabolic rate. It reduces the risk of cardiovascular disease, increases levels of "good cholesterol" (HDL), enhances the functioning of the immune system, reduces the risks of certain kinds of cancer and other diseases, and increases one's energy level.

2. **What are the psychological benefits of exercise?** People who exercise regularly report feeling less tense, anxious, and depressed during and after workouts. They are generally more relaxed and self-confident than inactive people.

3. **How much exercise do you need?** Many of the health benefits of exercise can be reaped from 30 minutes a day of moderate physical activity. Virtually any form of physical activity will do, including climbing stairs, brisk walking, raking leaves, or pushing a stroller.

### FITNESS

4. **What is fitness?** Fitness has two main components, performance-related fitness and health-related fitness. We measure performance-related fitness in terms of ability to compete on the playing field or in performance tests. Health-related fitness refers to strength and endurance, flexibility, and a healthful muscle-to-fat ratio.

5. **What is fitness training?** Training, or *conditioning,* refers to the gradual adjustment the body makes to increasingly higher demands from repetitive movements. The movements can involve aerobic or nonaerobic exercise. Training requires overloading one's current capacity for activity. The recommended target heart rate for aerobic exercise is from 60 to 90% of your maximum heart rate. Flexibility is enhanced by stretching.

### EXERCISE-RELATED INJURIES

6. **What kinds of exercise-related injuries are there?** Most exercise-related injuries result from overuse (as in overtraining) or poor technique. Some muscle soreness is normal. Sudden injuries include sprains, strains, and fractures. There are also hot-weather (e.g., heat stroke) and cold-weather (e.g., frostbite) hazards.

7. **How can we prevent exercise-related injuries?** Injuries can be prevented by increasing the intensity and duration of exercise gradually, using proper techniques (including warming up and cooling down), knowing when to stop, following safety precautions (e.g., when bicycling in traffic), drinking liquids, and getting enough sleep.

8. **How do we cope with insomnia?** First, we should not *try* to get to sleep. We can only set the stage for sleep by relaxing when we are tired and allowing sleep to happen. In addition, we can get up at a regular time (tired or not), avoid napping during the day, challenge irrational ideas about sleep that keep us awake, allow our minds to wander into fantasy, and avoid excess caffeine. Sleeping pills can lead to tolerance and addiction.

## References and Suggested Readings

### SMART REFERENCES FROM SCIENTIFIC AMERICAN

**Kearney, J. Training the Olympic Athlete.** *Scientific American,* 274(6) (June 1996), 52–63. **R0701**

**Beardsley, T. In Focus: Waking Up.** *Scientific American,* 275(1) (July 1996), 14. **R0702**

### SUGGESTED READINGS

**Bricklin, M., and Spilner, M.** *Prevention's Practical Encyclopedia of Walking for Health.* Emmaus, PA: Rodale Press. 1992. By editors of *Prevention* magazine, this is a practical and comprehensive guide to walking for health and weight loss.

**Schlosberg, S., and Neporent, L.** *Fitness for Dummies.* Foster City, CA: IDG Books, 1996. Billed as a "reference for the rest of us!"™ this is a comprehensive, clear, and concise guide to fitness that offers easy-to-understand suggestions with a touch of humor.

**Cooper, K. H.** *Kid Fitness.* New York: Bantam Books, 1991. The "father" of aerobics, Dr. Kenneth Cooper, offers advice to parents about getting their children involved in fitness programs.

**Noakes, T.** *Love of Running.* (3rd ed.). Champaign, IL: Human Kinetics Press, 1991. A complete guide to running for the novice or the seasoned runner, with special attention to running-related injuries—what they are, how to avoid them, and how to treat them.

# Healthy Relationships

## DID YOU KNOW THAT

- Early self-disclosure of intimate information may destroy, rather than deepen, a budding relationship? p.204
- Small talk is an excellent way to begin a relationship? p.204
- Opposites usually do *not* attract? p.206
- The proportion of people remaining single into their late 20s and early 30s has more than doubled since 1970? p.211
- People who cohabit before getting married are *more* likely, not *less* likely, to get divorced later on? p.213
- College students today are more conservative in their attitudes toward casual sex than the preceding generation? p.214
- The divorce rate, having doubled from 1960 to 1990, has leveled off in the 1990s? p.215
- Conflict is inevitable in relationships—even in healthy relationships? p.218

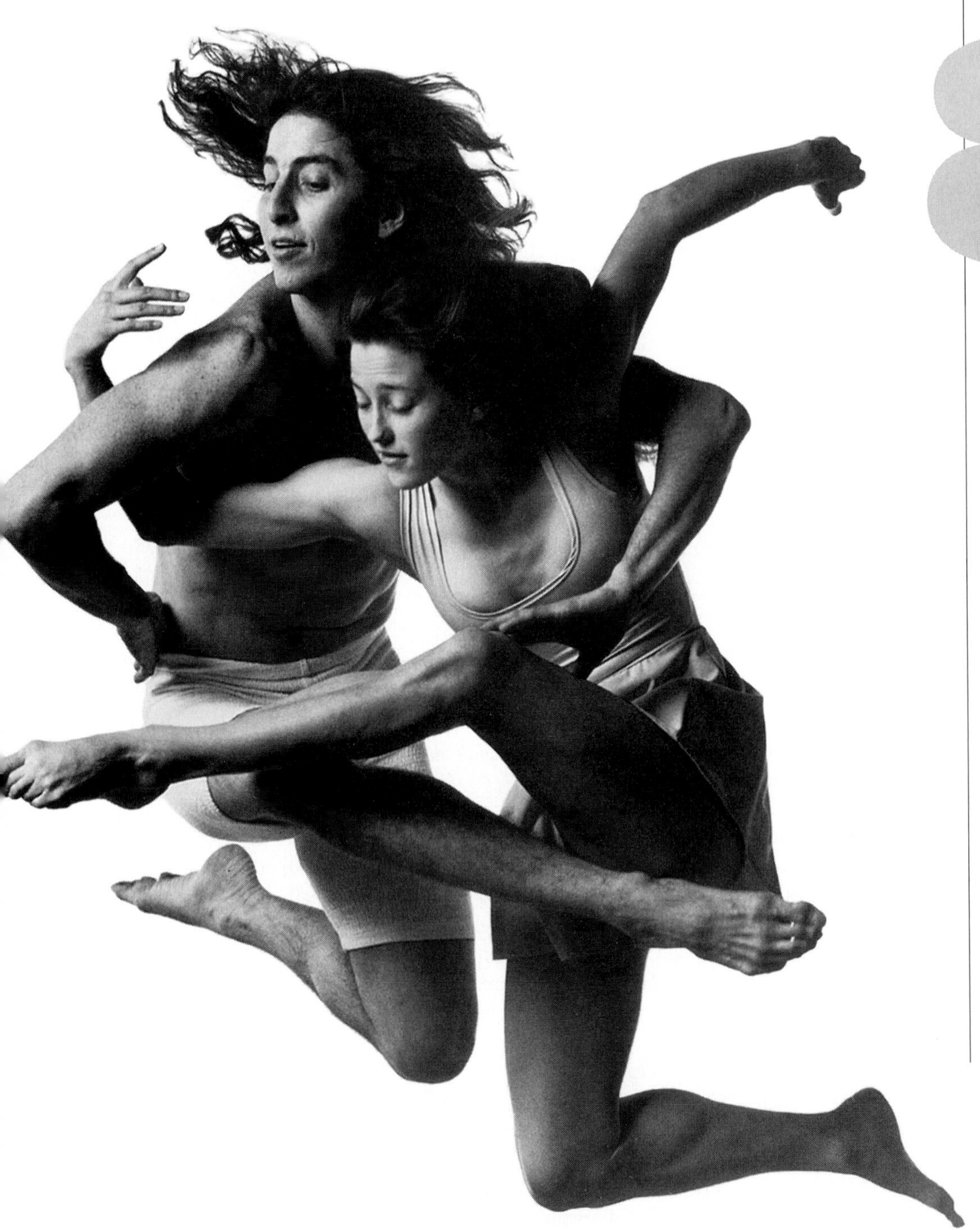

# 8 THE ABC(DE)'S OF RELATIONSHIPS



*We are all social creatures. Social relationships are important to our psychological well-being. Psychological problems are often characterized by social withdrawal or by difficulties in relating to others. Social relationships also affect our physical health. For example, people often suffer health problems when they undergo the stress of divorce or separation. Moreover, married people—men, anyhow—tend to be healthier and live longer than those who are single.*

# THE ABC(DE)'S OF RELATIONSHIPS

You have relationships of many sorts—with your parents, kids, friends, neighbors, and even with the shopkeepers in your neighborhood. We focus here on the development of an intimate, romantic relationship with a partner or lover. Healthy relationships, like healthy people, undergo stages of development. During each stage, positive factors or rewards encourage partners to maintain and enhance their relationship. Negative factors or costs lead to deterioration. George Levinger applied an **ABCDE model** to describe the stages of relationships: (1) *A*ttraction, (2) *B*uilding, (3) *C*ontinuation, (4) *D*eterioration, and (5) *E*nding.[1]

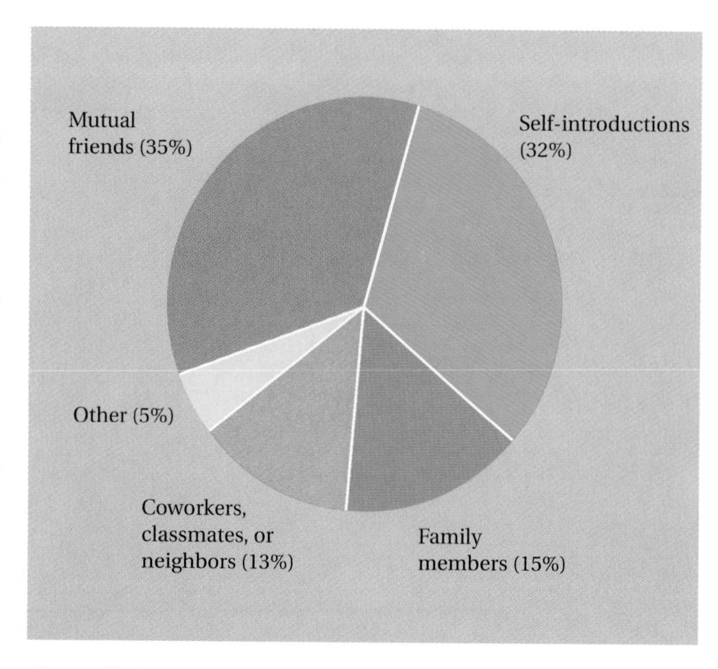


**Figure 8.1** ***How We Meet*** Spouses are most likely to have met through mutual friends or self-introductions.

## The A's—Attraction

Attraction occurs when two people become aware of each other and find each other appealing or enticing. We may find ourselves attracted to an enchanting person "across a crowded room" or in a nearby office. We may meet others through blind dates, introductions by friends, computer matchups, or by "accident." Initial feelings of attraction are largely based on visual impressions, though we may also be intrigued by a conversation or by what others say.

Married and unmarried couples are most likely to have met through mutual friends (35%) or by self-introductions (32%)[2] (Figure 8.1). Other sources of introductions are family members (15%) and coworkers, classmates, or neighbors (13%).

**Physical Attractiveness—How Important Is Looking Good?** We might like to think that we are attracted to people because of what they are like on the inside, not because of how they look on the outside. We might like to believe that sensitivity, warmth, and intelligence are more important to us. However, psychologists find that physical appearance is the key factor in determining attraction. It's not that sensitivity and other qualities aren't important. Rather, we may never learn about other people's personalities if we are not physically attracted to them.

What is it that we find physically attractive? Both genders find slenderness attractive, especially for females. College undergraduates—both male and female—rate women of average weight with a waist-to-hip ratio of 0.7 to 0.8 as most appealing. Women consider taller men to be more attractive. College women like their dates to be about six inches taller than they are. College men generally prefer women who are a few inches shorter.

**ABCDE model** Levinger's view describes five stages of romantic relationships: attraction, building, continuation, deterioration, and ending.

**What Do You Look for in a Long-Term, Meaningful Relationship?** Looks aren't everything, at least when it comes to making judgments about potential mates or partners in long-term relationships. Traits of warmth, fidelity, honesty, and sensitivity were rated by a sample of college students, both men and women, as more important than physical attractiveness when considering potential partners for meaningful, long-term relationships.[3] Still, men do place greater emphasis on the physical characteristics of their partners than do women. Women place more value on qualities such as warmth, assertiveness, wit, and an achievement orientation. The single most highly desired quality students wanted in long-term partners was honesty. Honestly.

When it comes to selecting mates, women in our culture place greater emphasis than men do on traits like vocational status, earning potential, expressiveness, kindness, dependability, and fondness for children. Men give relatively more consideration to youth, physical attractiveness,

## Gender Differences in Mate Preferences across 37 Cultures

WORLD OF *diversity*

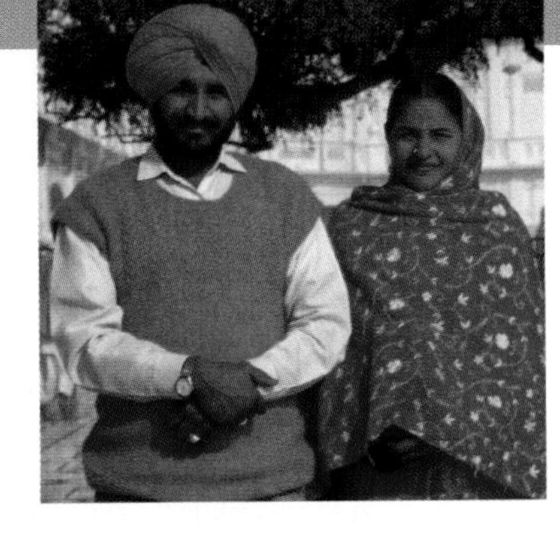

What do men in Nigeria, Japan, Brazil, Canada, and the United States have in common? For one thing, men in these countries report that they prefer mates who are younger than themselves. Psychologist David Buss reviewed evidence on the preferred age difference between oneself and one's mate in 37 cultures (representing 33 countries) in Europe, Africa, Asia, Australia and New Zealand, and North and South America.[4] In every culture men preferred younger mates (the range was from 0.38 year to 6.45 years). Women, however, preferred older mates (the range was from 1.82 years to 5.1 years).

Gender differences in the preferred age of mates paralleled actual differences in age of men and women at the time of marriage. Men were between 2 and 5 years older on average than their brides at the time of marriage. The smallest age difference at marriage, 2.10 years, was found in Poland. The largest difference, 4.92 years, was found in Greece. Men in the United States and Canada are about 2.5 to 2.7 years older than women at the time of marriage.

Buss finds that in all 37 cultures, men placed greater value on a prospective partner's "good looks" than did women. On the other hand, women in 36 of 37 cultures placed greater value on "good earning capacity" of prospective mates.

The sampling techniques in these surveys varied widely, and the samples may not be truly representative of the larger cultures in these countries. The consistency of findings nevertheless lends credence to the general notion that there are gender differences in preferences with respect to age, physical characteristics, and financial status of prospective mates. Generally speaking, men across cultures place greater value on the physical attractiveness and relative youth of prospective mates, whereas women place relatively greater value on the earning capacity of prospective mates. Buss interprets women's preference for relatively older mates as additional evidence that women appraise future mates on the basis of their ability to provide for a wife and family, since age and income tend to be linked among men.

Despite these gender differences in preferences for mates, Buss finds that both men and women placed greater weight on personal qualities than on looks or income potential of prospective mates. In *all* 37 cultures, the characteristics "kind—understanding" and "intelligent" were rated higher than earning power or physical attractiveness.

**Close-up**
More on culture
T0801

thrift, and cooking ability. The ***World of Diversity*** feature shows that these differences are not unique to our culture and are, in fact, quite similar across cultures.

Table 8.1 shows the results of a U.S. national sample of more than 13,000 English- or Spanish-speaking people, aged 19 or above. The pollsters asked respondents how willing they would be to marry someone who was older, younger, of a different religion, unlikely to hold a steady job, not good-looking, and so forth. Each item was followed by a 7-point scale in which 1 meant "not at all" and 7 meant "very willing." As the table shows, women were more willing than men to marry someone who was not good-looking. On the other hand, women were less willing to marry someone unlikely to hold a steady job.

**TABLE 8.1**

**Gender Differences in Mate Preferences[5]**

| How willing would you be to marry someone who | Men | Women |
|---|---|---|
| Was not "good-looking"? | 3.41 | 4.42* |
| Was older than you by 5 or more years? | 4.15 | 5.29* |
| Was younger than you by 5 or more years? | 4.54 | 2.80* |
| Was not likely to hold a steady job? | 2.73 | 1.62* |
| Would earn much less than you? | 4.60 | 3.76* |
| Would earn much more than you? | 5.19 | 5.93* |
| Had more education than you? | 5.22 | 5.82* |
| Had less education than you? | 4.67 | 4.08* |
| Had been married before? | 3.35 | 3.44 |
| Already had children? | 2.84 | 3.11* |
| Was of a different religion? | 4.24 | 4.31 |
| Was of a different race? | 3.08 | 2.84* |

*Difference statistically significant at the .01 level of confidence or better.

**The Matching Hypothesis—Who Is "Right" for You?** Most of us mere mortals, less than exquisite in appearance, are saved from permanent singlehood by virtue of the **matching hypothesis**. People tend to develop romantic relationships with people who are similar to themselves in physical attractiveness rather than with the neighborhood Denzel Washington or Cindy Crawford look-alikes. The central motive for seeking "matches" seems to be fear of rejection by more attractive people.

There are exceptions to the matching hypothesis. Now and then we find a beautiful woman married to a plain or unattractive man (or vice versa). How do we explain it? What, after all, would *she* see in *him?* In such cases, we tend to seek a factor that will balance the physical attractiveness of one partner, such as wealth or social status. For some mismatched couples, similarities in attitudes and personalities may balance differences in physical attractiveness.

**Close-up**
"Ideal men"
T0802

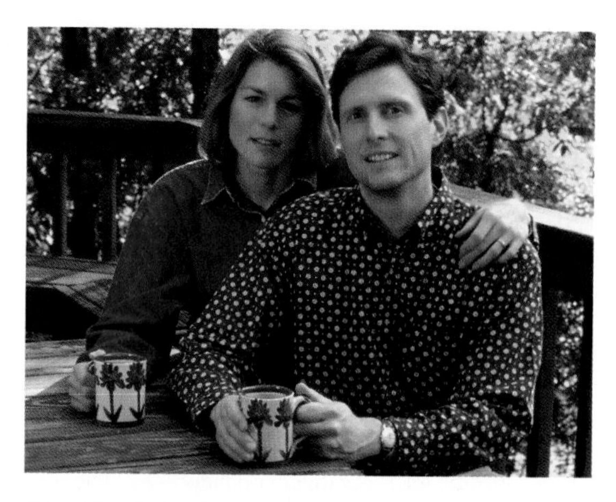

***Matching Hypothesis*** People tend to develop romantic relationships with people who have similar physical features and who share similar likes and dislikes. The choice of identical coffee mugs may not be crucial, however.

## The B's—Building

The stage of building a relationship follows initial attraction. Factors that motivate us to try to build relationships include similarity in the level of physical attractiveness, similarity in attitudes, and mutual liking.

**Seeking Common Ground through Not-So-Small Talk** We often decide whether to develop a relationship with someone on the basis of **small talk**. Small talk allows an exchange of basic information. It stresses breadth of topic coverage rather than in-depth discussion. Small talk may seem "phony." Yet early self-disclosure of intimate information may turn off the other person. Small talk is a trial balloon for friendship. Successful small talk encourages people to probe beneath the surface. At a cocktail party, people often flit from person to person exchanging small talk. Now and then a couple finds common ground and pairs off. In the early stages of a relationship, the partners tend to make **surface contact**: They continue to probe for common ground, for shared attitudes and interests. They check out each other as potential partners.

**Matching hypothesis** The concept that people tend to develop romantic relationships with people who are similar to themselves in attractiveness.

**Small talk** A superficial kind of conversation that stresses breadth of topic coverage rather than in-depth discussion.

**Surface contact** A probing phase of building a relationship in which people seek common ground and check out feelings of attraction.

**The "Opening Line"—How Do You Get Things Started?** One kind of small talk is the greeting, or opening line. We usually precede greetings with eye contact. We decide to talk if eye contact is reciprocated. Avoidance of eye contact may mean that the other person is shy, but it could also mean lack of interest. If you want to progress from attraction to surface contact, try a smile and eye contact. If the eye contact is reciprocated, choose an opening line (see Table 8.2 for some samples, but feel free to invent your own). A simple "Hi" or "Hello" is very useful. A friendly glance followed by a cheerful hello ought to give you some idea of whether your feelings of attraction are reciprocated. If the hello is returned with a friendly smile and inviting eye contact, follow it up with another opening line. Refer to your surroundings; offer your name. The other person will probably reciprocate. Self-introductions are a great ice-breaker.

Early exchanges include names, occupations, marital status, and place of residence. This has been likened to exchanging "name, rank, and serial number." Each person seeks a sociological profile of the other. Discovery of common ground may provide a basis for pursuing the conversation. An unspoken rule seems to be at work: "If I provide you with some information about myself, you will reciprocate by giving me an equal amount of information about yourself." Not everyone will respond, of course. The following section offers some general suggestions to help you improve date-seeking skills.

**TABLE 8.2**

**How to Pick Up . . . a Relationship—Opening Lines**

*Verbal salutes,* such as "Good morning."

*Personal inquiries,* such as "How are you doing?"

*Compliments,* such as "I like your outfit."

*References to your surroundings,* such as "What do you think of that painting?" or "Do you like what they did with this place?"

*References to people or events outside the immediate setting,* such as "How do you like this weather we've been having?"

*References to the other person's behavior,* such as "I couldn't help noticing you were sitting alone," or "I see you out on this track every Saturday morning."

*References to your own behavior, or to yourself,* such as "Hi, my name is Darren Jiminez."

**Improving Date-Seeking Skills** You have seen someone interesting. What do you do now? How do you go about making a date?

The following steps may help you sharpen your own date-seeking skills:[6]

1. *Easy Practice Level* Select a person with whom you are friendly, but one whom you have no desire to date. Practice making small talk about the weather, about new films that have come into town, television shows, concerts, museum shows, political events, and personal hobbies.

   Select a person you might have some interest in dating. Smile when you pass this person at work, school, or elsewhere, and say "Hi." Practice saying hello to other people as well, not just potential dates, to help increase your skills at greeting others.
2. *Medium Practice Level* Sit down next to the person you want to date and engage him or her in small talk. If you are in a classroom, talk about an assignment, the seating arrangement, or the instructor (be kind). If you are at work, talk about the building or some recent interesting event in the neighborhood. Ask your intended date how he or she feels about the situation. If you are at a group function, tell the other person that you are there for the first time and ask for advice on how to relate to the group.

   Engage in small talk about the weather and local events. Channel the conversation into an exchange of personal information. Give your "name, rank, and serial number"—who you are, your major in college or your occupation, where you're from, why or how you came to be where you are.

   Rehearse asking the person out. You may wish to ask the person out for "a cup of coffee." Or you may rehearse asking the person to accompany you to a cultural event, such as an exhibition at a museum or a concert—it's "sort of" a date, but also less anxiety-inducing.
3. *Target Behavior Level* Ask the person out on a date, using the skills you rehearsed. If the person can't make it because of a previous commitment, you may wish to say something like, "That's too bad" or "I'm sorry you can't make it," and add something like, "Perhaps another time." You should be able to get a feeling for whether the person you asked out was just seeking an excuse or has a genuine interest in you and, as claimed, could not in fact accept the specific invitation.

   Before asking the person out again, pay attention to his or her apparent comfort level when you return to small talk on a couple of occasions. If there is still a chance, the person should smile and return eye contact. The other person may also offer you an invitation. In any event, if you are turned down twice, do not ask a third time. And don't make a catastrophe out of the refusal. Look up. Note that the roof hasn't fallen in. The birds are still chirping in the trees. You are still paying taxes. Then give someone else a chance to appreciate your finer qualities.

**More than Beauty** Serious relationships and marriages are made in the neighborhood, not in heaven. That is, we tend to choose people who are like us in race, ethnic background, age, level of education, and religion. They are generally people from the same neighborhood, or nearby. Certainly there are exceptions, but findings from a national survey illustrate these patterns, as seen in Table 8.3 (next page).

**Similarity in Attitudes—Do Opposites Attract?** Why do most of us have partners from our own backgrounds? For one thing, we tend to live among people who are similar to us in background and thus to come into contact with them. Similarity in attitudes and tastes is also a key contributor to attraction, friendships, and love relationships.[8] People with similar backgrounds are more likely to have similar attitudes. The popular

TABLE 8.3

**Snapshot, USA—Who Are Our Lovers and Spouses?[7]**

According to a recent national survey of partners in heterosexual relationships:

- The sexual partners of nearly 94% of unmarried white men are white women. About 2% of single white men have Hispanic-American women as partners, 2% have Asian-American women, and fewer than 1% have African-American women.
- The sexual partners of nearly 82% of African-American men are African-American women. Nearly 8% of African-American men have white women as partners. Fewer than 5% have Hispanic-American women as partners.
- About four of five of the women and men in this survey report choosing partners within 5 years of their own age and of the same or a similar religion.
- All (100%) of the women with a graduate college degree had a partner who had finished high school.
- Relatively few men with college degrees have sexual relationships with women with either much more or much less education than they have.

belief that opposites attract does not bear up under scrutiny. To paraphrase Woody Allen, the lamb may lie down with the lion, but will not get very much sleep.

Let us note a gender difference. Women place greater weight on attitude similarity as a factor determining their attraction to prospective partners than do men. Men place more value on physical attractiveness.[9]

**Reciprocity—If You Like Me, You Must Have Excellent Judgment** Has anyone told you that you are good-looking, brilliant, and emotionally mature to boot? That your taste is elegant? Ah, what superb judgment! When we receive a compliment or hear someone tell us that he or she cares for us, we are likely to reciprocate in kind. **Reciprocity** is a major building block of healthy relationships. Reciprocating positive words and actions can deepen feelings of attraction and help a relationship move toward greater intimacy.

**Reciprocity** Mutual exchange.

**Intimacy** Feelings of closeness and connectedness characterized by sharing of inmost thoughts and feelings.

**Self-disclosure** The revelation of personal, perhaps intimate, information.

**Intimacy** **Intimacy** involves feelings of emotional closeness and connectedness with another person and the desire to share each other's inmost thoughts and feelings. Intimate relationships are also characterized by attitudes of mutual trust, caring, and acceptance.

Friends, lovers, and family members become emotionally intimate when they care deeply for each other and share their private feelings and experiences. It is not necessary for people to be *sexually* intimate to have an emotionally intimate relationship. Nor does sexual intimacy automatically produce emotional intimacy. People who are sexually involved may still fail to touch one another's lives in emotionally intimate ways. Even couples who fall in love may not be able to forge an intimate relationship because they are unwilling or unable to exchange inmost thoughts and feelings. Sometimes husbands or wives share greater emotional intimacy with friends than with their spouses.

Consider some of the factors that help to build intimacy:

- *Knowing and liking yourself* When you know and value yourself, you are able to identify your inmost feelings and needs and have the security to share them.
- *Self-disclosure: You tell me and I'll tell you . . . carefully* Opening up, or **self-disclosure,** is central to building intimate relationships. Yet

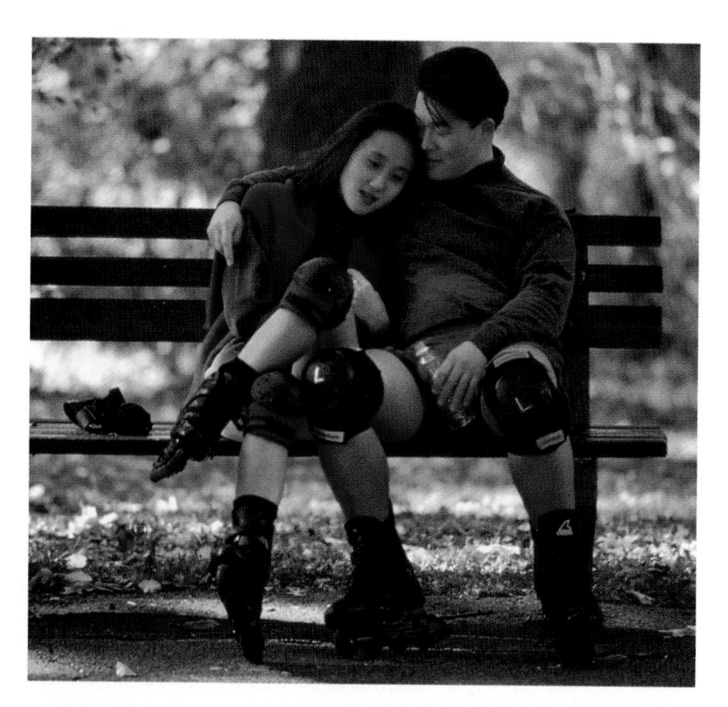

***Sharing Intimacy*** Intimate couples share their inmost thoughts and feelings. Intimacy also involves attitudes of mutual trust, caring, and acceptance.

those who disclose too much too soon are perceived to be less mature, secure, well-adjusted, and genuine than other people.

If surface contact provided by small talk and initial self-disclosure has been mutually rewarding, partners in a relationship may develop deeper feelings of liking for each other. Self-disclosure may continue to build gradually through the course of a relationship as partners come to trust each other enough to share confidences and more intimate feelings.

Women commonly report that the men in their lives are loath to disclose information about themselves or to express their feelings. Men may adhere to the traditional "strong and silent" male stereotype. Though men today may not be as bound by these traditional gender roles, this cultural tradition can interfere with the building of intimate relationships.

- *Trust and caring* Two key ingredients of intimate relationships are trust and caring. When trust exists in a relationship, partners feel secure that disclosing intimate feelings will not lead to ridicule, rejection, or other kinds of harm. Trust usually builds gradually, as partners learn whether it is safe to share confidences. Caring is an emotional bond that allows intimacy to develop. In caring relationships, partners seek to gratify each other's needs and interests.

  Tenderness can be expressed by a caring arm around a partner's shoulder or by verbalizations of love, caring, and appreciation. In romantic relationships, tenderness also takes the form of kissing, hugging, cuddling, and holding hands.

- *Honesty* Since intimacy involves the sharing of one's inmost thoughts and feelings, honesty is a core feature of intimacy. Without honesty, partners see only one another's facades. A person need not be an "open book" to develop and maintain intimacy, however. Some aspects of experience are kept even from one's most intimate partners, for they may be too embarrassing or threatening to reveal. For example, we would not expect partners to disclose every passing sexual fantasy.

  Total honesty could devastate a relationship. It would not be reasonable, for example, to expect intimate partners to divulge the details of past sexual experiences. Nor is intimacy established by brutal criticism, even if it is honest.

- *A sense of commitment* People sometimes open up to strangers on airplanes or trains yet find it hard to be open with people they care about most. An intimate relationship involves more than an isolated baring of the soul. It is a commitment to work to overcome problems rather than run for the exit at the first sign of trouble. When we open up to strangers on a plane, we know it is unlikely that we will have to face them again.

**Video**
What do you look for in a mate?
**V0801**

**Love, Sweet Love** The vast majority of people in the United States believe that romantic love is a prerequisite for marriage. More than half believe that falling out of love is an adequate reason for divorce.[10] So what is love? Until recently, scientists left the study of love to the poets, philosophers, and theologians. Recently, scientific attention has turned to studying this "funny thing called love." One leading model, proposed by psychologist Robert Sternberg,[11] describes love as having three distinct components:

1. *Intimacy* Feelings of closeness with the other person. Sharing one's innermost feelings.
2. *Passion* Intense romantic or sexual desire.
3. *Decision/commitment* The decision that one is in love. The commitment to maintain the relationship through good times and bad.

Sternberg conceptualizes love as a triangle. Each vertex represents one of these basic elements of love (see Figure 8.2, next page). The balance of the components can be represented by the shape of the triangle. For example, a love in which all three components are equally balanced is represented by an equilateral triangle, as in Figure 8.3. Couples are well matched on these dimensions of love if each partner possesses corresponding levels of passion, intimacy, and commitment. Relationships may become troubled when partners are mismatched. A relationship may fizzle rather than sizzle when one partner experiences more passion than the other. Or it may end when one wants a long-term commitment but the other's idea of commitment is to stay the night.

According to the Sternberg model, various combinations of the elements of love characterize different love relationships (see Figure 8.2 and Table 8.4, page 209). For example, *infatuation* (passionate love) is typified by strong sexual desire but not by intimacy and commitment. Infatuation may be a passing fancy or it may lead to deeper feelings of intimacy and commitment.

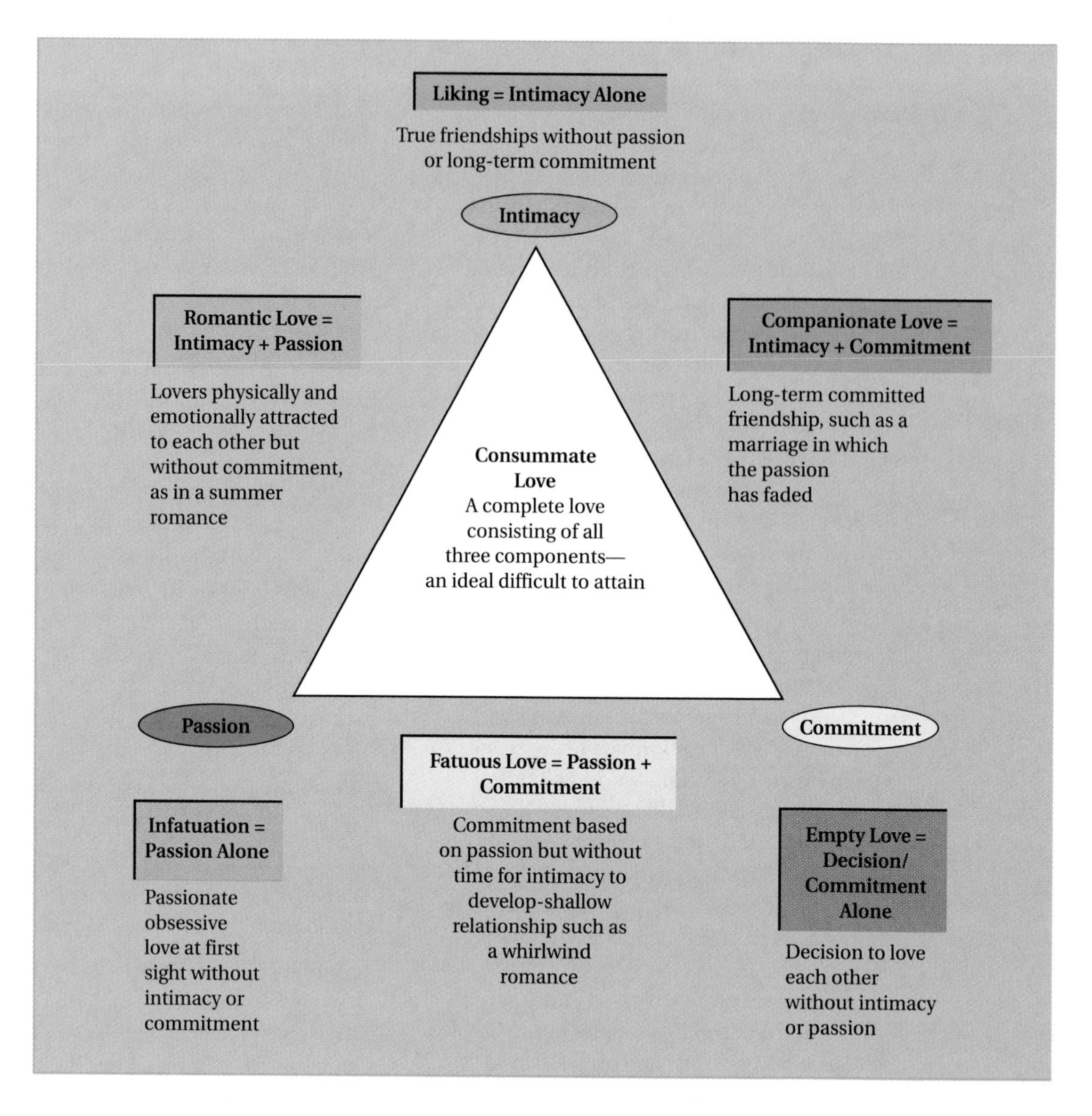
Liking = Intimacy Alone
True friendships without passion or long-term commitment
Intimacy
Romantic Love = Intimacy + Passion
Lovers physically and emotionally attracted to each other but without commitment, as in a summer romance
Companionate Love = Intimacy + Commitment
Long-term committed friendship, such as a marriage in which the passion has faded
Consummate Love
A complete love consisting of all three components—an ideal difficult to attain
Passion
Commitment
Fatuous Love = Passion + Commitment
Commitment based on passion but without time for intimacy to develop-shallow relationship such as a whirlwind romance
Infatuation = Passion Alone
Passionate obsessive love at first sight without intimacy or commitment
Empty Love = Decision/ Commitment Alone
Decision to love each other without intimacy or passion

**Figure 8.2** ***Love Triangle*** Psychologist Robert Sternberg conceptualizes love as a triangle. Each vertex represents one of these basic elements of love.

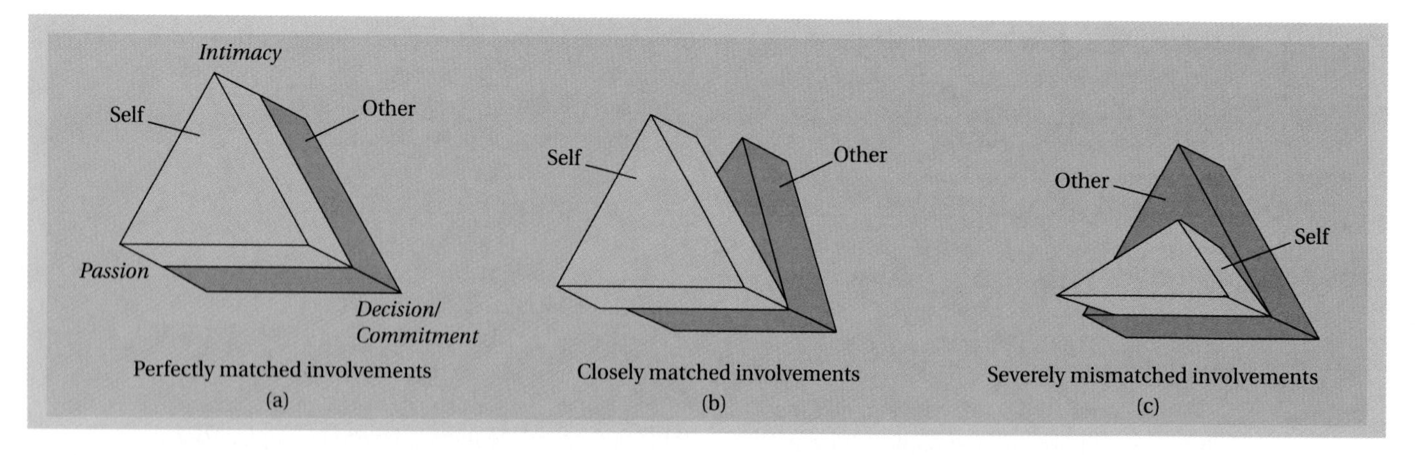
Intimacy
Self
Other
Passion
Decision/ Commitment
Perfectly matched involvements
(a)
Self
Other
Closely matched involvements
(b)
Other
Self
Severely mismatched involvements
(c)

**Figure 8.3** ***Are Your Love Triangles Compatible?*** Couples match if they possess corresponding levels of passion, intimacy, and commitment. (a) A perfect match. The triangles are congruent. (b) A good match. The partners are similar in the three dimensions. (c) A mismatch. Major differences exist between the partners on all three components.

TABLE 8.4

**Types of Love in the Sternberg Model**[12]

| | |
|---|---|
| 1. *Nonlove* | A relationship in which all three components of love are absent. Most of our personal relationships are of this type—casual interactions or acquaintanceships that do not involve any elements of love. |
| 2. *Liking* | A loving experience with another person or an intimate friendship in which intimacy is present but passion and commitment are lacking. |
| 3. *Infatuation* | A kind of "love at first sight" in which one experiences passionate desire for another person in the absence of both the intimacy and decision/commitment components of love. |
| 4. *Empty love* | A kind of love characterized by the decision (to love) and the commitment (to maintain the relationship) in the absence of either passion or intimacy. Stagnant relationships that no longer involve the emotional intimacy or physical attraction that once characterized them are of this type. |
| 5. *Romantic love* | A loving experience characterized by the combination of passion and intimacy, but without the decision/commitment components of love. |
| 6. *Companionate love* | A kind of love that derives from the combination of the intimacy and decision/commitment components of love. This kind of love often occurs in marriages in which passionate attraction between the partners has died down and has been replaced by a committed friendship. |
| 7. *Fatuous love* | The type of false love associated with whirlwind romances and "quicky marriages" in which the passion and decision/commitment components of love are present, but intimacy is not. |
| 8. *Consummate love* | The full or complete measure of love involving the combination of passion, intimacy, and decision/commitment. Many of us strive to attain this type of complete love in our romantic relationships. Maintaining it is often harder than achieving it. |

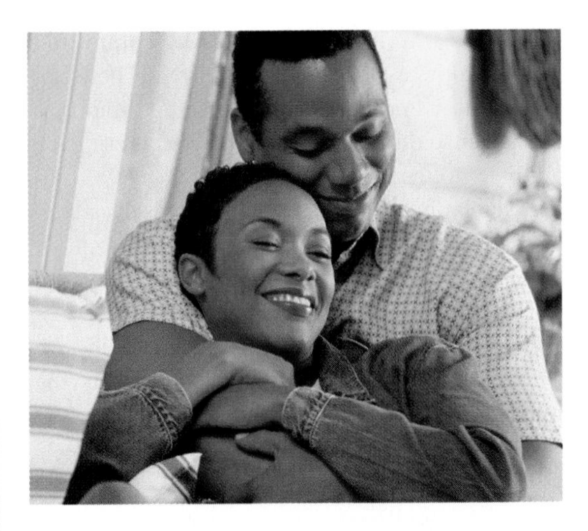

***Consummate Love*** In consummate love, sexual desire is accompanied by deep intimacy and commitment. Many people strive to achieve the ideal of consummate love.

*Liking* is very much like friendship. It consists of feelings of closeness and emotional warmth without passion or decision/commitment. This form of love is reserved for people to whom one feels close enough to share inmost feelings and thoughts. Liking may develop into a passionate love, however.

*Romantic love* has both passion and intimacy but lacks commitment. Romantic love may burn brightly, then flicker out. Or it may develop into a more complete love, called *consummate love,* in which all three components flower. The flames of passion can be stoked across the years, even if they do not burn quite as brightly as once they did. Consummate love is most special, and for many people an ideal toward which they strive.

**HealthCheck**
Are you in love?
**H0801**

In *companionate love,* intimacy and commitment are strong, but passion is lacking. This form of love typifies long-term (so-called Platonic) friendships and marriages in which passion has ebbed but a deep and abiding friendship remains.

**Mutuality—When the "We," Not the "I's," Have It** Many couples build a relationship to the point that they think of themselves as "we"—not two "I's" who happen to be in the same place at the same time. The sense of "we" is what Levinger terms a state of **mutuality.** The development of mutuality favors the continuation and further deepening of the relationship.

**Mutuality** A phase in building a relationship in which a couple come to regard themselves as "we."

**Maintaining Individuality** In committed relationships, a delicate balance exists between individuality and mutuality. In healthy unions, a strong sense of togetherness does not erase each partner's individuality. Partners in healthy committed relationships are free to be themselves. Neither seeks to dominate or submerge himself or herself in the personality of the other. Each partner maintains individual interests, likes and dislikes, needs and goals. Troubled relationships, on the other hand, are often characterized by the squelching of one partner's individuality by the other.

## The C's—Continuation

Factors that encourage continuation of a relationship include seeking ways to introduce variety and maintain interest (such as trying out new sexual practices and social activities) and showing continued evidence of caring and positive evaluation (such as remembering to send birthday or Valentine's Day cards). A relationship is also more likely to continue if the partners feel satisfied with the relationship and perceive a sense of fairness in it.

Factors that can throw the relationship into a downward spiral include boredom, bickering, forgetting or ignoring anniversaries and other important dates, dissatisfaction or perceived unfairness in the relationship, and jealousy.

### Jealousy

*O! beware, my lord, of jealousy;*
*It is the green-ey'd monster . . .*

From Shakespeare's *Othello*

Thus Othello, the Moor of Venice, was warned of jealousy in the play that bears his name. Yet Othello could not control his feelings and murdered his wife Desdemona. The English poet John Dryden labeled jealousy a "tyrant of the mind." Jealousy appears to be more common and intense among cultures with a *machismo* tradition in which men are expected to display their virility.

Jealousy is aroused when an intimate relationship is threatened by a rival. Jealousy can hurt a relationship by producing feelings of mistrust. Feelings of possessiveness, which are related to jealousy, also place stress on relationships.

What causes jealousy? In some cases, people become mistrustful of their present partners because their former partners had cheated. Jealousy can also derive from low self-esteem or lack of self-confidence. People with low self-esteem may fear that they will not be able to find someone else if their partner leaves. Some people play jealousy games. They let their partners know that they are attracted to other people. They flirt openly. Some even manufacture tales to make their partners pay more attention to them, to test the relationship, to inflict pain, or to take revenge for a partner's disloyalty. Such acts can damage, and even destroy, relationships.

## The D's—Deterioration

Deterioration, the fourth stage of a relationship, is not inevitable. A relationship begins to deteriorate when partners find it less enticing or rewarding than it had been. Couples who work to maintain and enhance relationships may make them stronger and more meaningful. Deterioration that proceeds unchecked can lead to the end of a relationship.

**PREVENTION**

### *Preventing a Relationship from Deteriorating*

When relationships deteriorate, couples can respond in active or passive ways. Active responses involve taking steps to enhance the relationship, such as improving communication, negotiating differences, or seeking outside help. Passive responses include waiting for the relationship to improve on its own or to end. Relationships usually don't improve on their own. Maintaining a good relationship requires time and effort. Here are some concrete suggestions for preventing a relationship from deteriorating:

- *Enhance communication skills.* (See pages 218–220 in this chapter.)
- *Spend focused time together.* Try new things together to develop common interests.
- *Tolerate differences.* (No two people are perfectly matched.) Allow your partner to express some personal interests that do not interest you.
- *Be flexible in carrying out chores and in making important decisions.*
- *Be helpful.* Offer your partner a helping hand. Offer to spend more time with the children or to take care of household chores.
- *Share power in the relationship.* Ask your partner for his or her opinions. Listen to them.
- *Talk privately and intimately.* Set aside time for the two of you to have heart-to-heart talks, with the TV turned off and after the kids are in bed.

- *Take time for physical intimacy.* Hug. Hold hands. Give your partner a backrub or a massage. Set aside time for physical intimacy.
- *Work together to solve problems.* Be open-minded. Brainstorm. Select a potential solution. Try it out. Evaluate the results.
- *Be sensitive about financial issues.* Listen to your partner's fears. Compromise about money. Check with your partner before making a sizable purchase.
- *Compromise about rearing children.* Explain *why* you make recommendations. Listen to your partner. (Listen to your *children.*)

### The E's—Ending

Ending is the fifth and final stage of a relationship. Ending, like deterioration, need not be inevitable. Some couples prevent a deteriorating relationship from ending by investing in it. They invest when they are committed to maintaining the relationship or when they believe they will be able to overcome their problems.

Relationships end when the partners gain little satisfaction from them. They end when the barriers to breaking up are low—that is, when the social, religious, and financial constraints are manageable. Troubled relationships tumble down especially when alternate partners are available.

The end of a relationship can be a healthful outcome. When people are incompatible, when efforts to preserve the relationship have faltered, ending it can offer partners a chance for happiness with someone else. On the other hand, troubled relationships can often be salvaged, sometimes by the couple themselves working on their differences, sometimes with the help of a professional counselor.

Smart Quiz
Q0801

**think about it!**

- **Are you in a relationship now? What stage? What do you anticipate will happen to the relationship?**
- **Are you or have you been in love? How do you know? What kind(s) of love, according to Sternberg's model?**

**critical thinking** **What attracts you to others? Are your reasons for being attracted typical for your gender? Why or why not?**

## TYPES OF LIFESTYLES

People entering adulthood today face a wider range of relationship choices and lifestyles than did those in earlier generations. The sexual revolution of the 1960s loosened traditional constraints on sexual choices, especially for women. Couples today experiment with lifestyles that would have been unthinkable in earlier generations. An increasing number of young people choose to remain single as a way of life, not merely as a way station preceding marriage.

A similar variety of lifestyles exists within the gay community. Though the legal status of gay marriages continues to be debated, many gay couples consider themselves to be married even if their unions are not recognized as marriages by the state.

In this section, we discuss several different forms of relationships in society today, including singlehood, cohabitation, and marriage.

### Singlehood

Recent years have seen a sharp increase in the numbers of single young people in the United States. The proportion of people who remain single into their late 20s and early 30s has more than doubled since 1970. "Singlehood," not marriage, is the most common lifestyle among people in their early 20s. Marriages may be made in heaven, but many of us are saying that heaven can wait. In the United States of the mid-1990s, one in four people 18 years of age and older had never married, compared with about one in six in 1970 and one in five in 1980.

Several factors contribute to the increased proportion of singles. For one thing, more people are postponing marriage to pursue educational and career goals. Many young people are deciding to "live together" (cohabit), at least for a while, rather than get married. The increased prevalence of divorce also swells the ranks of single adults.

Many single people do not choose to be single. Some remain single because they have not yet met someone they want to marry. Yet many young people see singlehood as an alternative, open-ended way of life. As career options have expanded for women, they are not as financially dependent on men as were their mothers and grandmothers. Some young women, like some young men, choose to remain single (at least for a while) to focus their energies on their careers.

Singlehood is not without its problems. Many single people complain of loneliness. Some express concern about a lack of a steady, meaningful relationship. Others are fearful, understandably so, about the risk of sexually transmitted diseases. Others, usually women, worry about their physical safety. Some singles find it difficult to satisfy their needs for intimacy, companionship, and sex. Despite these concerns, most singles are well-adjusted and content.

**Take Charge**
Coping with loneliness
C0801

There is no one "singles scene." Single people differ in their sexual interests and lifestyles. Many achieve security through intimate relationships with friends. Most are sexually active. Many practice **serial monogamy.** That is, they become involved in one exclusive relationship after another. They do not have multiple sexual relationships at the same time. Other singles have a primary sexual relationship with one steady partner but occasional brief relationships with others. A few, even in this age of AIDS, are "swinging singles" pursuing casual sexual encounters, or "one-night stands."

Some singles remain celibate, either by choice or for lack of opportunity. People choose **celibacy** for a number of reasons. Nuns and priests do so for religious reasons. Others believe that celibacy allows them to focus their energies and attention on work or to commit themselves to an important cause. Others remain celibate because they view sex outside of marriage as immoral. Others do so out of fear of sexually transmitted diseases.

## Cohabitation—Darling, Would You Be My POSSLQ?

*Marriage is a great institution, but I'm not ready for an institution yet.*

Mae West

*POSSLQ?* This unromantic abbreviation was introduced by the Census Bureau. It stands for People of Opposite Sex Sharing Living Quarters and applies to unmarried couples who live together. The rest of us refer to it as **cohabitation** or simply "living together."

Some social scientists believe that cohabitation has become fully accepted into the social mainstream. Whether or not this is so, society in general has become more tolerant of it. We seldom see cohabitation referred to as "living in sin" as we once did.

The number of households consisting of unmarried adults of opposite sexes living together in the United States grew from about $1\frac{1}{2}$ million couples in 1980 to nearly 3 million couples in 1990 and is still growing.

Much attention has been focused on college students who live together. Yet cohabitation is more prevalent among the less educated and less affluent classes. The cohabitation rate is about twice as high among African-American couples as white couples. Children live with about one cohabiting couple in three.

About one cohabitor in three is divorced. Divorced people are more likely than people who have never married to cohabit. Apparently, the experience of divorce makes some people less willing to take the plunge into marriage. Perhaps, too, they may be more willing to share their lives than their bank accounts—the second or third time around.

Willingness to cohabit is related to liberal attitudes toward sexual behavior, untraditional views of marriage, and untraditional views of gender roles. People who cohabit are less likely than married people to attend church regularly.

**Why Do People Cohabit?** Cohabitation, like marriage, can be an alternative to the loneliness of living alone. Lovers may have deep feelings for each other but not be ready to get married. Some couples prefer cohabitation because of its relative lack of legal and economic entanglements.

Many cohabitors feel less committed to their relationships than married people do. Ruth, 84 years old, has been living with her partner, aged 85, for four years. "I'm a free spirit," she says. "I need my space. Sometimes we think of marriage, but then I think that I don't want to be tied down."[13] Being a "free spirit" knows no age boundaries.

Ruth's comments are of interest because they counter stereotypes of women and older people. However, it is more often the man who is unwilling to make a marital commitment, as in the case of Mark. Mark, a 44-year-old computer consultant, lives with Nancy and Janet, their 7-year-old daughter. Mark says, "We feel we are not primarily a couple but rather primarily individuals who happen to be in a couple. It allows me to be a little more at arm's length. Men don't like committing, so maybe this is just some sort of excuse."[14]

**Serial monogamy** A pattern of involvement in one exclusive relationship after another, as opposed to engaging in multiple sexual relationships at the same time.

**Celibacy** Complete sexual abstinence.

**Cohabitation** Living together as though married but without legal sanction.

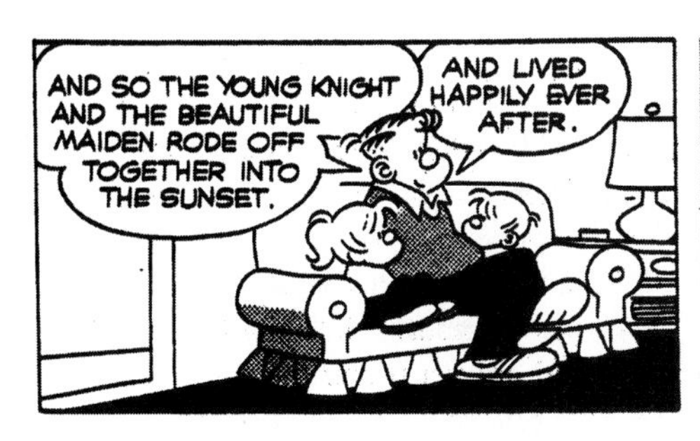
AND SO THE YOUNG KNIGHT AND THE BEAUTIFUL MAIDEN RODE OFF TOGETHER INTO THE SUNSET.
AND LIVED HAPPILY EVER AFTER.

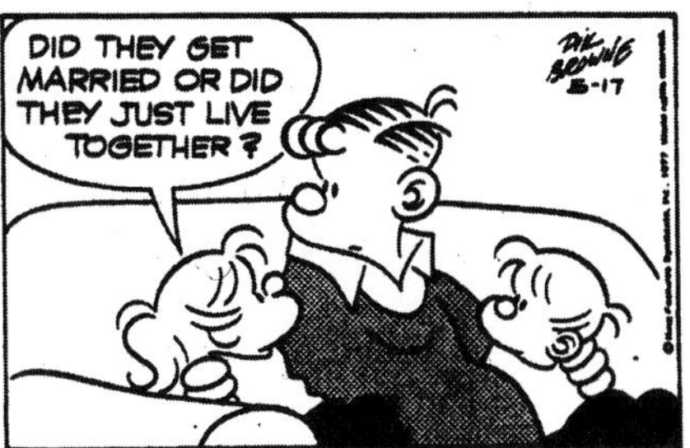
DID THEY GET MARRIED OR DID THEY JUST LIVE TOGETHER ?

Economic factors come into play as well. Couples who are committed to each other may cohabit because of the economic advantages of sharing household expenses. Cohabiting individuals who receive public assistance (Social Security or welfare checks) risk losing support if they get married. Some older people live together rather than marry because of resistance from adult children. Some children fear that a parent might be victimized by a predatory partner. Others may not want their inheritances to come into question. Younger couples may cohabit secretly to maintain parental support that would be lost if they were to get married or reveal their living arrangements.

**Does Cohabitation Affect the Success of Marriage?** Cohabiting couples may believe that cohabitation will strengthen eventual marriage by helping them iron out the kinks in their relationship. Yet cohabitors who later marry actually have a greater risk of divorce than noncohabitors.[15] We must be cautious about drawing causal conclusions, however. People who cohabit before marriage tend to be less committed to traditional values associated with the institution of marriage. Lack of commitment, and not cohabitation itself, may account for the higher rates of divorce among people who had cohabited.

About 40% of cohabiting couples eventually get married.[16] The majority of other cohabiting couples break up within three years.

## Marriage

Marriage is our most common lifestyle. According to the U.S. Census Bureau, about 65% of the adult men and 60% of the adult women in the U.S. are married and living with their spouses. The average age of first marriage has risen from the early twenties in 1975 to the midtwenties in the 1990s. Men marry about 2 years later than women do, on average.

Since ancient times, Western society has largely been characterized by forms of **patriarchy** (from the Greek *pater* meaning "father," and *archein,* meaning "to rule") or male dominance. Among the ancient Hebrews, for example, men had the right to choose wives for their sons and could take concubines or additional wives for themselves. Men alone could initiate divorce. Failure to bear children was grounds for divorce. A wife was considered a man's property. In classical Greece and Rome, women were also the property of men. Their central purposes were to care for the household and to bear children. Women were in effect given by their fathers to their husbands, usually for political or economic gain. The Christian tradition also has a strong patriarchal foundation.

**Talking Glossary**
Patriarchy
G0801

Over time, patriarchal traditions in Western culture weakened. Women came to be viewed as loving companions rather than mere property—**chattels** (from an old French word meaning "cattle"). They gradually gained more household responsibilities and were recognized as being capable of profiting from education. The notion that a married woman might seek personal fulfillment through a career of her own is a recent development, however. The perception that married women have a right to sexual fulfillment is also new. As late as the nineteenth century, sex for a married woman was largely seen as a means for bearing children and satisfying the husband's sexual needs. Women were assumed to be motivated sexually only by the desire for children.

**Talking Glossary**
Chattels
G0802

Marital roles in modern society have changed, and they are changing still. Some couples still adhere to traditional gender roles. They still believe in breadwinning responsibilities for the husband and child care and homemaking roles for the wife. Today, however, American couples are more likely to share or even reverse marital roles. Table 8.5 lists some of the features of traditional and contemporary marriages. The nearby ***HealthCheck*** will provide you with insight into your own attitudes toward marital roles.

**Patriarchy** A form of social organization in which the father or eldest male runs the group or family. More broadly, government, rule, or domination by men.

**Chattel** A movable piece of personal property, such as furniture or livestock.

TABLE 8.5

**A Comparison of Traditional and Contemporary Marriages[18]**

| Traditional Marriage | Contemporary Marriage |
|---|---|
| The emphasis is on ritual and traditional roles. | The emphasis is on companionship. |
| Couples do not live together before marriage. | Couples may live together before marriage. |
| The wife takes the husband's last name. | The wife may choose to keep her maiden name. |
| The husband is dominant; the wife is submissive. | Neither spouse is dominant or submissive. |
| The roles for the husband and the wife are specific and rigid. | Both spouses have flexible roles. |
| There is one income (the husband's). | There may be two incomes; that is, the couple may share the breadwinning role. In some cases, the woman is the breadwinner. |
| The husband initiates sexual activity; the wife complies. | Either spouse may initiate (or refuse) sex. |
| The wife cares for the children. | The parents share child-rearing chores. |
| Education is considered important for the husband, not for the wife. | Education is considered important for both spouses. |
| The husband's career decides the location of the family residence. | The career of either spouse may determine the location of the family residence. |

**Why Do People Marry?** Marriage meets personal and cultural needs. It legitimizes sexual relations, establishes a home life, and provides an institution for rearing children and socializing them to adopt the norms of the family and the culture at large. Marriage also permits the orderly transmission of wealth from one family to another and from one generation to another. As late as the seventeenth and eighteenth centuries, most European marriages were arranged by parents as a means of enhancing the financial stability of the families.

Notions like romantic love, equality between spouses, and the concept that men as well as women would do well to aspire to the ideal of faithfulness are very recent additions to the institution of marriage. Not until the nineteenth century did the notion of love as a basis for marriage become widespread in Western culture.

Today, most young people endorse the idea that people in love may engage in sexual activity whether or not they are married. It's not that young people today generally approve of casual sex. College students today are actually more conservative than the preceding generation of the 1970s. A 1996 survey reported that only 41% of college freshmen today approve of casual sex, down from 50% of the students polled in 1975.[19] Still, sex has become a less significant motive for entering into marriage. Other goals have become more important. Marriage provides a sense of security and offers opportunities to form a special attachment to another person that allows for intimacy and companionship. Even in these more liberated times, most young people endorse the traditional ideal that marriage is a lifetime commitment.

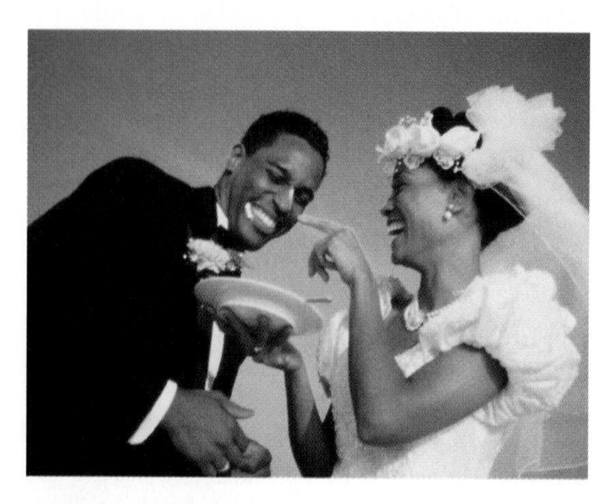

*To Wed* Despite increases in the proportion of single adults, marriage remains our most common lifestyle.

**Whom Do We Marry?** Parents today seldom arrange marriages. (Even so, they may still encourage their child to date that wonderful son or daughter of the solid churchgoing couple who live down the street.) Because we are free to marry whom we choose, we tend to marry those who attract us and who are similar to us in physical attractiveness and attitudes. Storybook Cinderella-like marriages are the exception to the rule.

# Health Check

## Do You Endorse a Traditional or a Liberal Marital Role?

What do you believe? Should the woman cook and clean, or should housework be shared? Should the man be the breadwinner, or should each couple define its own roles? Are you traditional or nontraditional in your views on marital roles for men and women?

The items reveal the degree to which you endorse traditional roles for men and women in marriage.[17] Answer each one by circling the letters (AS, AM, DM, or DS), according to the code given below. Then turn to the scoring key in Appendix B at the back of the book to interpret your scores. (Ignore the numbers beneath the codes for the time being.) You may also be interested in seeing whether the responses of your date or partner agree with your own.

AS = Agree strongly
AM = Agree mildly
DM = Disagree mildly
DS = Disagree strongly

1. A wife should respond to her husband's sexual overtures even when she is not interested.

   AS AM DM DS
   1 2 3 4

2. In general, the father should have greater authority than the mother in the bringing up of children.

   AS AM DM DS
   1 2 3 4

3. Only when the wife works should the husband help with housework.

   AS AM DM DS
   1 2 3 4

4. Husbands and wives should be equal partners in planning the family budget.

   AS AM DM DS
   4 3 2 1

5. In marriage, the husband should make the major decisions.

   AS AM DM DS
   1 2 3 4

6. If both husband and wife agree that sexual fidelity isn't important, there's no reason why both shouldn't have extramarital affairs if they want to.

   AS AM DM DS
   4 3 2 1

7. If a child gets sick and his wife works, the husband should be just as willing as she to stay home from work and take care of that child.

   AS AM DM DS
   4 3 2 1

8. In general, men should leave the housework to women.

   AS AM DM DS
   1 2 3 4

9. Married women should keep their money and spend it as they please.

   AS AM DM DS
   4 3 2 1

10. In the family, both of the spouses ought to have as much say on important matters.

    AS AM DM DS
    4 3 2 1

**Talking Glossary**
Homogamy
**G0803**

The concept of "like marrying like" is termed **homogamy** (from the Greek *homos,* meaning "same," and *gamos,* meaning "marriage"). We usually marry people of the same racial and ethnic background, educational level, and religion. Interracial marriages account for less than 1% of marriages. More than 90% of marriages are between people of the same religion. Marriages between individuals who are alike may stand a better chance of survival, since the partners are more likely to share values and attitudes. Dissimilar couples, however, can work to overcome the barriers that divide them. They can develop common interests and mutual respect for their differences.

## Divorce

*Whenever I date a guy, I think, is this the man I want my children to spend their weekends with?*

Rita Rudner

Nearly half of the marriages in the United States end in divorce. The divorce rate doubled from 1960 to 1990 but has remained stable during the 1990s.[20]

The relaxation of legal restrictions on divorce has made divorces easier to obtain. Until the mid-1960s, adultery

**Homogamy** The practice of marrying people who are similar in social background and standing.

was the only legal grounds for divorce in New York State. Other states were equally strict. But now no-fault divorce laws have been enacted in nearly every state. These laws allow divorce without a finding of marital misconduct. The increased economic independence of women has also contributed to the rising divorce rate. More women today can afford to break away from troubled marriages. Today, more people consider marriage an alterable condition than in prior generations.

Ironically, people today hold higher expectations of marriage than did their parents or grandparents. They expect marriage to be personally fulfilling as well as an institution for rearing children. Many demand the right to be happy in marriage. The most common reasons given for divorce today are problems in communication and lack of understanding. Years ago it was more likely to be lack of financial support.

Divorce is often associated with financial and emotional problems. When a household splits, the resources often cannot maintain the earlier standard of living for each partner. A woman who has not pursued a career may struggle to compete with younger, more experienced workers. Divorced mothers often face the combined stress of the sole responsibility for rearing their children (women receive custody in most divorce cases) and the need to increase their incomes to make ends meet. Not surprisingly, single mothers (including divorced and never-married mothers) are more likely to feel depressed and dissatisfied with life than single fathers or married parents are. Divorced fathers may also find it difficult to pay alimony and child support while attempting to establish a new lifestyle.

Divorce may also prompt feelings of failure as a spouse and parent, loneliness and uncertainty about the future, and depression. Married people appear to be better able to cope with the stresses and strains of life, perhaps because they can rely on each other for emotional support. Those who are divorced or separated have higher rates of physical and mental illness and suicide than those who are married. On the other hand, divorce may be a time of personal growth and renewal. It can provide an opportunity for people to take stock of themselves and establish a new and more rewarding life for themselves.

Children can suffer in a divorce. They can also suffer in troubled marriages. Marital problems before and after divorce can spill over into parent-child relations. Boys tend to show greater problems adjusting to marital conflict or divorce, such as conduct problems at school and increased anxiety and dependence. Some children of divorce show a "sleeper effect." That is, they appear to be well-adjusted throughout childhood, but problems emerge later on. For example, they may not trust that their partners in intimate relationships will make lasting commitments. Researchers attribute children's problems not only to the divorce itself, but also to a decline in the quality of parenting following divorce. Children's adjustment is enhanced when parents set aside their differences long enough to agree on child-rearing practices, encourage each other to continue to play important roles in their children's lives, and avoid saying negative things about each other in front of the children.

Most divorced people eventually bounce back. The majority remarry. Among older people, divorced men are more likely than divorced women to remarry. Why? For one thing, men usually die earlier than women do. Thus, fewer prospective husbands are available for older women. Another reason is that older men tend to remarry younger women.

**Stepfamilies** By the beginning of the next century, the stepfamily may be the most common family unit in the United States. Yet most stepfamilies eventually disband. A prime reason is the weight of the financial and emotional pressures of coping with the demands of a reconstituted family. However, people whose remarriages survive are as happy as people in their first marriages. They are much happier than divorced people who remain single.

### *think about it!*

- **What is your marital status? Why? What do you anticipate for yourself in the future? Why?**
- **What does marriage mean to you? Why would you get married? Under what circumstances—if any—would you get divorced?**
- **Do you know people who have gotten divorced? What have been the effects of divorce on them? On their children?**

**critical thinking** **Agree or disagree and support your answer: Couples should live together before marriage to iron out the kinks in their relationship.**

Smart Quiz
Q0802

# Health*Check*

## *Are You a Tiger or a Doormat? The Rathus Assertiveness Schedule*

Evaluating your tendency to be assertive will expand your perspective on resolving conflicts in relationships, the subject of the next ***Take Charge.***

Being assertive is not simply speaking up, it includes:

- expressing your true feelings—positive as well as negative
- standing up for your legitimate rights, and refusing unreasonable requests
- withstanding improper social pressures (for example, refusing to participate in repulsive hazing activities)
- disobeying authority figures you believe are making immoral demands
- refusing to conform to group standards that run counter to your own beliefs (for example, refusing to use drugs even if it seems that "everyone's doing it")
- expressing positive feelings like love and admiration
- initiating new relationships—friendships and romances.

How assertive are you? Do you demand your rights, or do you permit others to walk all over you? Do you say what's on your mind or what you think others want to hear? Do you launch relationships with attractive people, or do you shy away from them?

You can gain insight into how assertive you are by completing the following questionnaire.[21] Turn to the scoring key in Appendix B at the end of the book to see how to compute and interpret your score. (The asterisks are explained there.)

*Indicate how well each item describes you by using this code:*

3 = very much like me
2 = rather like me
1 = slightly like me
−1 = slightly unlike me
−2 = rather unlike me
−3 = very unlike me

____ **1.** Most people seem to be more aggressive and assertive than I am.*
____ **2.** I have hesitated to make or accept dates because of shyness.*
____ **3.** When the food served at a restaurant is not done to my satisfaction, I complain about it to the waiter or waitress.
____ **4.** I am careful to avoid hurting other people's feelings, even when I feel that I have been injured.*
____ **5.** If a salesperson has gone to considerable trouble to show me merchandise that is not quite suitable, I have a difficult time saying "No."*
____ **6.** When I am asked to do something, I insist upon knowing why.
____ **7.** There are times when I look for a good, vigorous argument.
____ **8.** I strive to get ahead as well as most people in my position.
____ **9.** To be honest, people often take advantage of me.*
____ **10.** I enjoy starting conversations with new acquaintances and strangers.
____ **11.** I often don't know what to say to attractive persons of the opposite sex.*
____ **12.** I hesitate to make phone calls to business establishments and institutions.*
____ **13.** I would rather apply for a job or for admission to a college by writing letters than by going through with personal interviews.*
____ **14.** I find it embarrassing to return merchandise.*
____ **15.** If a close and respected relative were annoying me, I would smother my feelings rather than express my annoyance.*
____ **16.** I have avoided asking questions for fear of sounding stupid.*
____ **17.** During an argument I am sometimes afraid that I will get so upset that I will shake all over.*
____ **18.** If a famed and respected lecturer makes a comment that I think is incorrect, I have the audience hear my point of view as well.
____ **19.** I avoid arguing over prices with clerks and salespeople.*
____ **20.** When I have done something important or worthwhile, I manage to let others know about it.
____ **21.** I am open and frank about my feelings.
____ **22.** If someone has been spreading false and bad stories about me, I see him or her as soon as possible and have a talk about it.
____ **23.** I often have a hard time saying "No."*
____ **24.** I tend to bottle up my emotions rather than make a scene.*
____ **25.** I complain about poor service in a restaurant and elsewhere.
____ **26.** When I am given a compliment, I sometimes just don't know what to say.*
____ **27.** If a couple near me in a theater or at a lecture were conversing rather loudly, I would ask them to be quiet or to take their conversation elsewhere.
____ **28.** Anyone attempting to push ahead of me in a line is in for a good battle.
____ **29.** I am quick to express an opinion.
____ **30.** There are times when I just can't say anything.*

# Resolving Conflicts in Relationships

## Take Charge

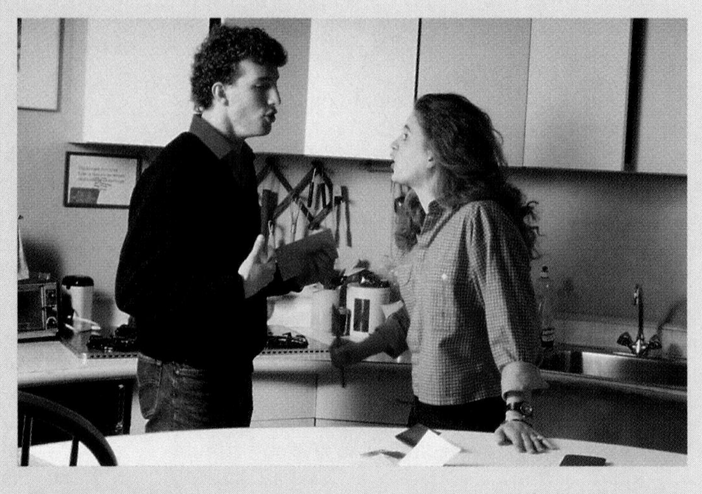

*Handling Conflicts* Conflicts are inevitable, even in healthy relationships. People need to resolve conflicts with their partners in constructive ways that do not tear down their relationships, or each other.

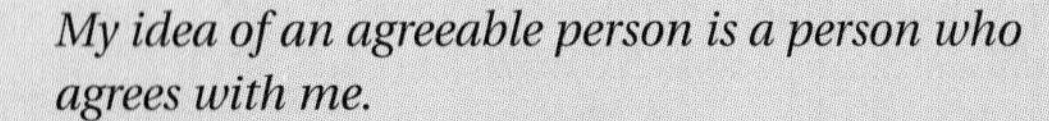

*My idea of an agreeable person is a person who agrees with me.*

Benjamin Disraeli

Conflict is inevitable in relationships—even in healthy relationships. No two people agree on everything, except the authors of your text of course. Unless you are a doormat, you will encounter occasional conflicts. Lack of skill in handling conflicts can transform social interactions into unhealthy burdens.

Conflicts in relationships arise over things like money—for example, how much should be spent for food and whether or not to leave the lights on when no one is home. Conflicts arise from:

- difficulties in communication (for example, not discussing problems until an explosion occurs),
- personal interests (one partner wants to spend money on a collection of sports memorabilia, the other partner wants to save for a house)
- sex (what kind? how much?)
- in-laws (is any example needed?),
- friends (for example, going out drinking with "the boys" or with "the girls"), and
- children (how many, when to have them, how to rear them).

When couples take up housekeeping, they need to decide who does what. Even among "liberated" partners, responsibilities are often delegated according to feminine and masculine stereotypes. Women often get stuck with the cooking and cleaning. Men may be more likely to make repairs and take care of the car, or take out the garbage. When men take an apartment on their own, they usually have the bathrooms cleaned every few weeks or months, whether they need to be cleaned or not.

When conflicts arise, the following measures may help in ironing them out.

### Challenge Unreasonable Ideas and Expectations

We accept disagreements with friends as normal, but when it comes to lovers, we may expect perfection and believe (erroneously) that well-matched couples do not disagree. Challenge the following unhealthy misconceptions:

| Unhealthy misconception: | Challenge with: |
|---|---|
| Conflicts about sex, distribution of chores, or a partner's family indicate that the relationship is on the rocks. | If there are two or more people, there will be disagreements from time to time. Finding good solutions can be a positive, creative experience. |
| My partner should know what's bothering me without my needing to mention it explicitly. | No one is a mind reader. I need to find a positive way to state my problem and engage my partner in helping to solve it. |
| I must accept the fact that my partner just won't or can't change. So we're stuck with the problem. | Everyone can make changes—if the change is reasonable and there is motivation to do so. |

### Make a Deal—Exchange New Behavior

One method for resolving conflicts is to make a contract to exchange behaviors. We all do some things that irk others. Partners can list the behavior that disturbs them. They then offer to modify their own objectionable behavior if their partners will modify theirs, for example:

I agree to keep the stereo off after 8:00 P.M. every weekday evening if you agree not to allow your friends to smoke in the apartment.

I agree to replace the toilet paper when we run out if you clean your hair out of the bathroom sink.

Another key way to resolve conflicts is to enhance communication skills.

## Communicate!

Do you take communication for granted? After all, people communicate often with other students, instructors, friends, and families. But do you communicate in a way that helps you learn about other people's needs? Do you express your own needs well? How do you criticize someone you love? How do you disagree with others without hurting feelings or jeopardizing the relationship? Can you accept criticism and keep your self-respect? What do you do when a discussion reaches an impasse?

The following guidelines should help you to communicate more effectively.

**Get Started** How do you get started on tough topics? Here are a couple of possibilities.

- *Talk about talking.* Open the discussion by mentioning that it is hard for you to talk about problems and conflicts. This encourages the other person to invite you to proceed.
- *Request permission to raise a topic.* Say, "There's something on my mind. Do you have a few minutes? Is now a good time to tell you about it?" Or, "There's something that we need to talk about, but I'm not sure how. Can you help me with it?"

**Listen to the Other Side** Hearing the other person out is an essential aspect of conflict resolution. Listening gives you information and shows the other person how she or he can better listen to you.

- *Listen actively.* Show you are listening actively by maintaining eye contact. Show you understand the other person's feelings by nodding your head when appropriate. Ask helpful questions, such as, "Would you please give me an example?"
- *Paraphrase.* Recast or restate what the other person is saying. This helps to convey and confirm your understanding. If your partner says, "You hardly ever say anything positive to me. You don't need to tell me you love me all the time, but sometimes I wonder how you feel about me." You can paraphrase it by saying something like this: "So it's hard to tell if I care for you."
- *Reinforce the other person for communicating.* Even when you disagree, maintain a good relationship and keep channels of communication open by saying things like, "Thanks for spending this much time with me," "I hope you'll think it's OK if I continue to see things differently," or "I'm glad we had a chance to talk about it."
- *Use unconditional positive regard.* Unconditional positive regard refers to enduring feelings of warmth and acceptance that are not contingent on what another person does from minute to minute. When one disagrees with a partner, one can say, "I care for you very much, but it annoys me when you . . ."
- *Learn about the other person's needs.* Listening is basic to learning about another person's needs, but it can help to go further. Ask questions to draw the other person out.
- *Use self-disclosure.* Communicate your own feelings and ideas to invite reciprocation. If you want to find out if your partner is concerned about your relationship with a friend, you can try something like, "You know, I have to confess that sometimes I worry that you feel much closer to your friends than to me. I get the feeling that I play a role in your life, but that there are some things that you would only do with them . . ."
- *Grant permission for the other person to be honest.* Ask your partner to level with you about an irksome issue. Say that you will try your best to listen carefully and not get upset.

**Ask for What You Want (You Just Might Get It)** Ask people to change their behavior—to do something differently or to stop doing something that annoys you.

- *Take responsibility.* The first step in making requests lies with you. Take responsibility for what happens to you. If you want others to change, you must be willing to ask them to change.
- *Be specific.* It is more useful to say, "I am concerned about your harsh tone of voice with me in front of our friends" than to say, "Be nicer to me." The other person may not realize that her or his behavior is *not* nice and may not understand your request.
- *Use "I-talk."* Use the words *I, me,* and *my* in your speech. Saying "I would appreciate it if you would put your shoes away rather than leave them lying on the floor," is likely to attain better results than accusing the other person of sloppiness or laziness.

**Deliver Criticism Tactfully** Delivering criticism is a skill. It requires focusing other people's attention on the problem and changing their behavior without inducing resentment or guilt or fear.

- *Be tactful.* Is it your primary intention to punish the other person or to gain cooperation? If your goal is conflict resolution, be tactful.
- *Pick the right time and place.* Deliver criticism privately—not in front of other people.
- *Be specific.* Be specific about the *behavior* that disturbs you. When your partner forgets to jot down a telephone message, it is more productive to explain that missing your messages may lose a job opportunity than to accuse your partner of being completely irresponsible.
- *Express displeasure in terms of your own feelings.* It is less threatening to express displeasure in terms of your own feelings than to attack the other person. Say, "You know, it's really bad news for me when an important message doesn't get through." Don't say, "You're so self-absorbed that you never think about anyone else."

- *Keep the focus on present complaints.* Avoid bringing up old grievances.
- *Express criticism positively.* Express criticism positively and combine it with a concrete request. Tell your partner, "You know, you're really a much better cook than I am. I'd really enjoy it if you cooked a meal for us," rather than, "You don't do any of the cooking, and I'm sick of it."

Making requests and delivering criticism are examples of assertive behavior. Why not complete the nearby questionnaire to see how assertive you are in comparison with other college students?

### Deal with Criticism Productively

> *Honest criticism is hard to take, particularly from a relative, a friend, an acquaintance, or a stranger.*
>
> Franklin P. Jones

Criticizing someone can be tricky, especially when you want to inspire cooperation. Receiving criticism can be even trickier. The following suggestions offer some help.

- *Ask clarifying questions.* When you are delivering criticism, it helps to be specific. Similarly, when you receive criticism, encourage the other person to be specific. If your partner indicates irritation with your behavior, ask for particulars.
- *Acknowledge the criticism if you are at fault.* Admitting mistakes can improve communication. It shows your partner that you are listening to what he or she has to say and that you are fair and open-minded. Admitting mistakes defuses anger and helps you move from arguing to searching cooperatively for solutions.
- *Reject the criticism if you are not at fault.* You don't have to accept unfair or abusive criticism.

**Handle Impasses Positively** Even when communication skills are excellent, partners now and then reach an impasse. Here are some ideas for handling impasses.

- *Look at the situation from the other person's perspective.* It may be possible to resolve some of the conflict by saying something like, "I still disagree with you, but I can see where you're coming from. I can understand why you think as you do."
- *Seek information.* If you do not understand the other person's concerns, you can say something like, "Believe me, I'm trying to see this from your point of view, but I can't. Would you try to help me understand your point of view?"
- *Take a break.* Count to ten, or twenty. When you reach a stalemate, stand back for a while. Perhaps a resolution will dawn on one of you later.
- *Tolerate differences.* Remember that no two people are exactly alike. Let your relationship be a broadening experience.
- *Agree to disagree.* When all else fails, people can agree to disagree on specific matters. You can handle an impasse by focusing on things that you and other people have in common, such as mutual respect and caring.

With relationships, as with other aspects of life, don't sit back and hope for the best. Make good things happen. Be honest with yourself, be fair, and be assertive. Achieving and maintaining good health involves taking charge of your life. This is as true for your relationships as it is for your physical health.

Smart Quiz
Q0803

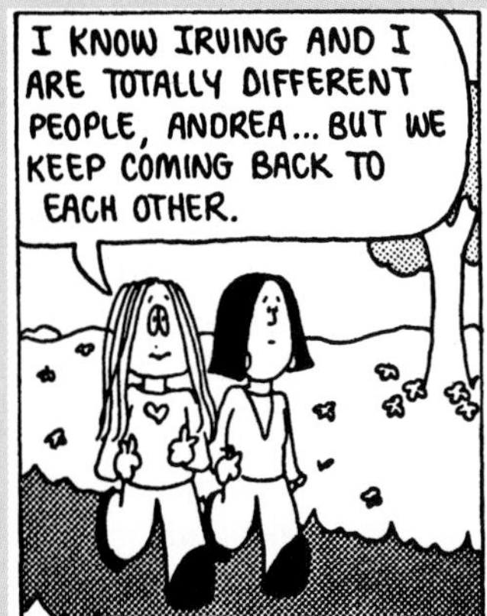
I KNOW IRVING AND I ARE TOTALLY DIFFERENT PEOPLE, ANDREA... BUT WE KEEP COMING BACK TO EACH OTHER.

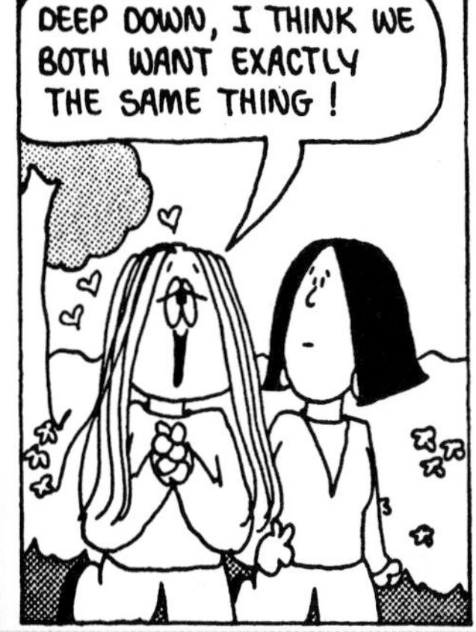
DEEP DOWN, I THINK WE BOTH WANT EXACTLY THE SAME THING!

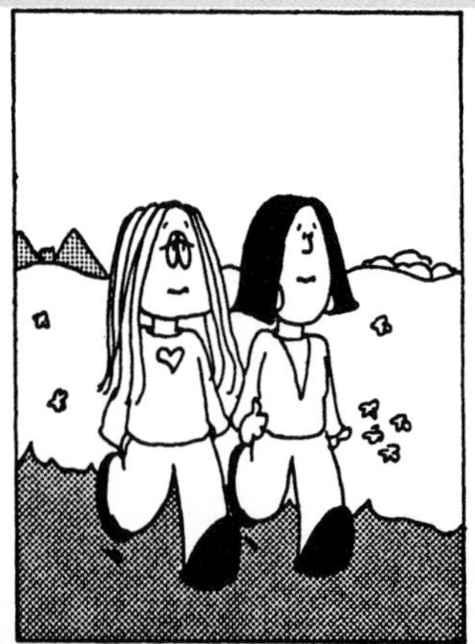

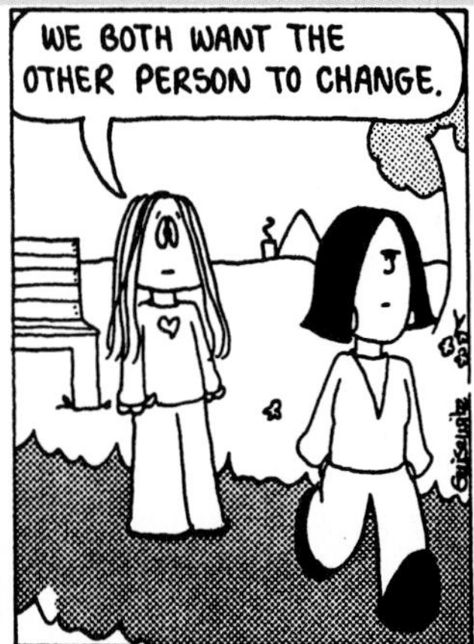
WE BOTH WANT THE OTHER PERSON TO CHANGE.

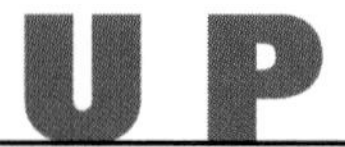

# SUMMING UP

## Questions and Answers

### THE ABC(DE)'S OF RELATIONSHIPS

**1. What are the five stages of relationships, according to Levinger?** Remember the ABC(DE)'s: These stages are termed *a*ttraction, *b*uilding, *c*ontinuation, *d*eterioration, and *e*nding.

**2. What factors contribute to interpersonal attraction?** These include physical appearance; traits such as warmth, fidelity, honesty, and sensitivity; matching of attitudes; and reciprocity.

**3. What gender differences are there in attraction?** Generally speaking, women pay relatively more attention to vocational status and men pay relatively more attention to appearances.

**4. What factors are involved in building intimacy with another person?** These include knowing and liking yourself, self-disclosure, trust and caring, honesty, and commitment.

**5. What are the components of love, according to Sternberg?** These are intimacy, passion, and decision/commitment.

**6. How does jealousy affect relationships?** Jealousy can hurt a relationship by producing feelings of mistrust and possessiveness.

**7. When do relationships come to an end?** Factors that bring relationships to an end include loss of satisfaction, low barriers to ending the relationship, and the availability of alternate partners.

### TYPES OF LIFESTYLES

**8. Why are more people remaining single these days?** Factors that contribute to increased "singlehood" include pursuit of educational and career goals and increased rates of cohabitation.

**9. What are the trends in cohabitation?** The numbers of cohabiting couples are on the rise, partly because there is less stigma attached to it, partly because of unwillingness to make a permanent commitment to another person, partly for financial reasons.

**10. Why do people get married?** People marry these days because of love, to share a home life, and to create an environment for rearing children.

**11. Why do so many people get divorced?** About half of the marriages in the United States end in divorce. Reasons include relaxation of restrictions on divorce and the widespread belief that falling *out* of love is sufficient reason to get divorced.

## Suggested Readings

**Rubin, L. B.** *Intimate Strangers: Men and Women Together.* New York: Harper & Row, 1983. A sensitive and probing study of the struggle to establish and maintain intimate relationships.

**Tannen, D.** *You Just Don't Understand: Women and Men in Conversation.* New York: Morrow, 1990. Written by a linguistics professor, this down-to-earth, best-selling book examines how gender-based differences in conversational styles lead to misunderstandings in relationships between men and women.

**Tennov, D.** *Love and Limerence: The Experience of Being in Love.* New York: Stein & Day, 1979. A clearly written book describing the experience of love.

**Lerner, H. G.** *The Dance of Anger.* New York: Harper & Row, 1985. Examines how couples can constructively handle anger in their relationships.

**Brehm, S.** *Intimate Relationships.* New York: McGraw-Hill, 1992. A leading text explores theory and research on marriage and relationships.

# Gender and Sexuality

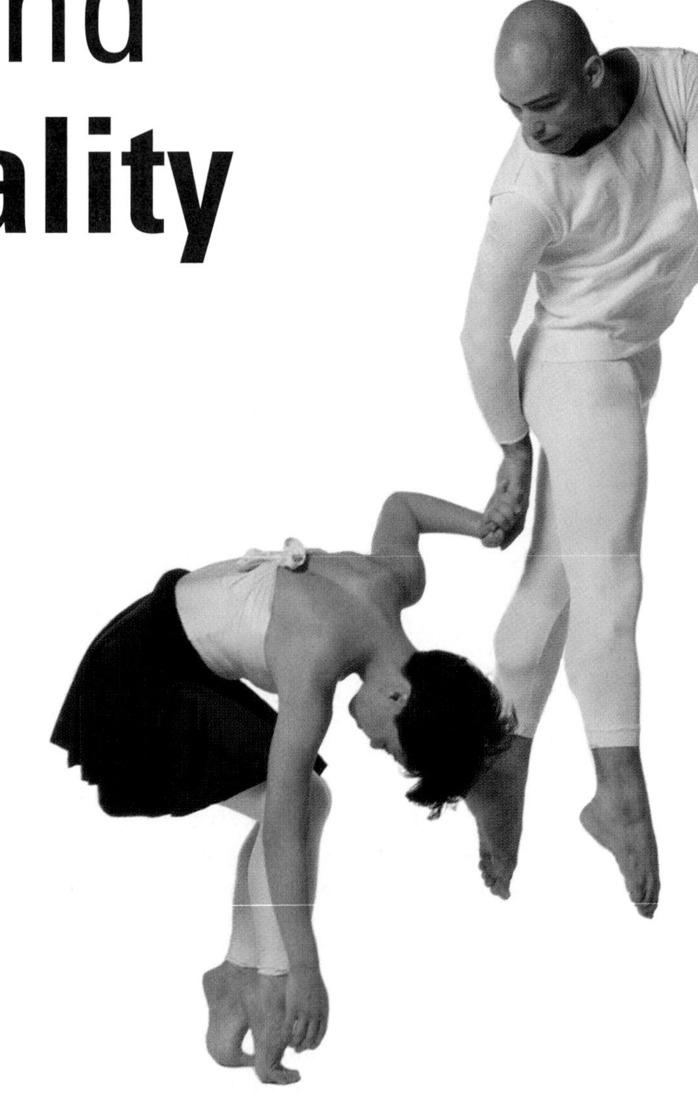

## DID YOU KNOW THAT

- We would all develop female sexual organs if male sex hormones were not present during prenatal development? p.224
- Women, but not men, have a sex organ whose only known function is sexual pleasure? p.228
- Women are born with all the egg cells they will ever have? p.231
- The size of a woman's breasts does not determine how much milk she can produce while nursing? p.232
- The penis contains neither bone nor muscle? p.238
- It is common for married people to masturbate? p.245
- Oral sex has become the norm among today's young married couples? p.246
- Gay men and lesbians are not any more psychologically disturbed than heterosexual men and women? p.249
- Sexual dysfunctions are actually quite common? p.249
- Both men and women produce testosterone? p.250

# 9

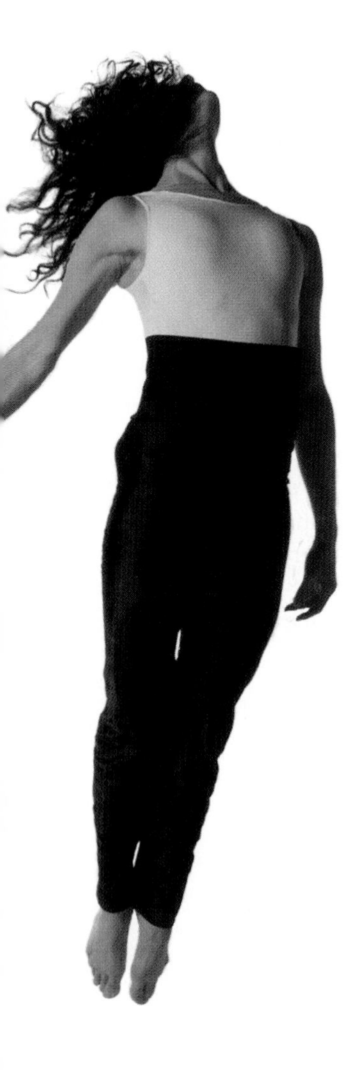



*What does it mean to be male? To be female? Our awareness of ourselves as females or males is part of our sexuality, as is our capacity for erotic experiences and responses. Our sexuality is an essential part of ourselves, whether or not we ever engage in sexual fantasy or sexual intercourse, or even if we lose sensation in our genitals because of injury. Sexuality is also an important part of a healthy lifestyle. It is the wellspring of intimate relationships and serves as a major source of pleasure and gratification as well as a means of reproduction. Although sexuality is a natural function, it is strewn with misunderstanding, myth, prejudice, and confusion. In this chapter we examine and, we hope, clarify many aspects of our sexuality. We begin by considering the most fundamental aspect of our identity, our sense of ourselves as male or female.*

# GENDER IDENTITY AND GENDER TYPING

**Gender** is the state of being male or female. Gender is so important to people that parents usually ask "Is it a boy or a girl?" before they begin counting fingers and toes. Our **gender identity** is our psychological sense of being male or female. How do we acquire gender identity? The answer may seem obvious enough. For the great majority of us, our gender identity conforms to our anatomic sex. For **transsexuals**, however, gender identity and anatomic sex are mismatched. Transsexuals have the gender identity of one gender but possess the sexual anatomy of the other. They report feeling trapped in the body of the wrong sex. Many undergo **gender reassignment surgery** to correct what they see as nature's mistake.

If anatomical sex does not dictate gender identity, what determines it? And what leads some people to feel alien in their own bodies? As it turns out, gender identity is a complex process involving both biological and psychological factors.

## Biological Influences

According to the Bible, Adam was created first, and Eve was created from one of his ribs. From the standpoint of biology, however, it would be more accurate to say that "Adams" develop from "Eves." Let us trace the development of **sexual differentiation.**

When a sperm cell fertilizes an egg cell or ovum, 23 **chromosomes** from the male parent normally combine with 23 chromosomes from the female parent. They form 23 pairs. The twenty-third pair are the sex chromosomes. An ovum always carries an X sex chromosome. A sperm may carry either an X or a Y sex chromosome. If a sperm with an X sex chromosome fertilizes the ovum, the newly conceived person will normally develop as a female, with an XX sex chromosomal structure. If the sperm carries a Y sex chromosome, the child will normally develop as a male (XY).

**Gender** The state of being male or female.

**Gender identity** The psychological sense of being male or female.

**Transsexual** A person who has a gender-identity disorder and who feels trapped in the body of the wrong gender.

**Gender reassignment surgery** Surgery that modifies a person's genitalia into a likeness of the genitalia of the opposite sex.

**Sexual differentiation** The process by which males and females develop distinct reproductive anatomy.

**Chromosomes** Rodlike structures found in the nuclei of every living cell that carry the genetic code in the form of genes.

**Embryo** The stage of prenatal development that begins with the implantation of a fertilized ovum in the uterus and concludes with the development of the major organ systems at about two months after conception.

**Testes** The male gonads, which produce sperm and the male sex hormone testosterone.

At about 5 to 6 weeks, the **embryo** is only $\frac{1}{4}$- to $\frac{1}{2}$-inch long. The embryonic structures of both genders develop along similar lines. Both look female at this time. The basic blueprint of the embryo is female. At this point, the Y sex chromosomes cause it to deviate from the female course. "Adams" develop from embryos that would otherwise become "Eves."

At about the seventh week after conception, the chromosomal code (XX or XY) begins to assert itself. Changes occur. The Y sex chromosome causes the **testes** to differentiate. If the Y chromosome is absent, ovaries begin to form at 11 or 12 weeks.

**The Role of Sex Hormones in Sexual Differentiation** Once the testes develop in the embryo, they begin to produce **androgens**—male sex hormones. These hormones, including **testosterone,** further spur development of male reproductive organs.

Small amounts of androgens are produced in female fetuses, too, but normally not enough to cause male sexual differentiation. Female sex hormones **estrogen** and **progesterone** are not involved in prenatal sexual differentiation. They do become important following puberty in regulating the menstrual cycle and reproductive functions. If a fetus with an XY sex chromosomal structure failed to produce testosterone, it would develop female reproductive organs. Thus we would all develop female sexual organs if male sex hormones were not present during critical stages of prenatal development.

**Talking Glossary**
Estrogen, Progesterone
G0901

**Prenatal Sexual Differentiation of the Brain** The brain, like the sex organs, undergoes prenatal sexual differentiation. Testosterone in the blood causes cells in the male fetal brain to become insensitive to the female sex hormone estrogen. In the absence of testosterone, as in female fetuses, the brain becomes sensitive to estrogen. Sensitivity of the brain to estrogen is important in the later regulation of the menstrual cycle.

Prenatal sculpting of the brain may also be involved in the development of gender identity. A disturbance in the prenatal sexual differentiation of the brain may underlie the development of gen-

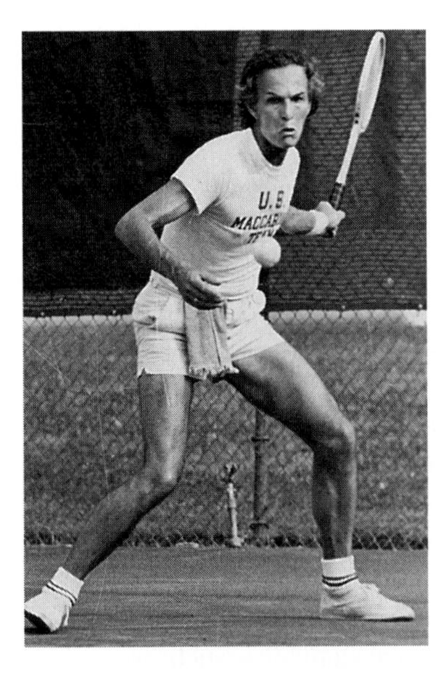

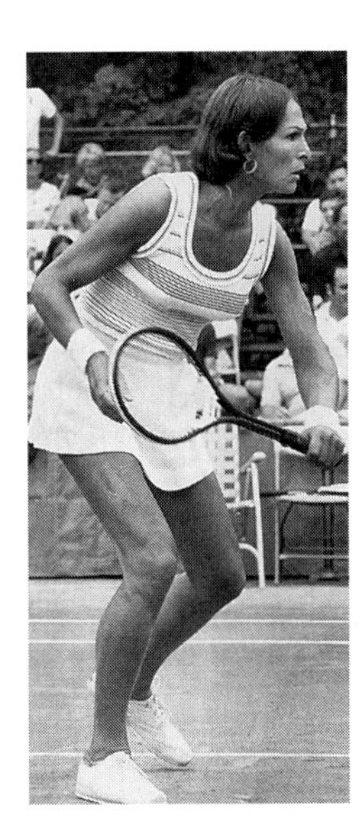

***Renée Richards (née Richard Raskin)*** Physician Richard Raskin (left), who became Renée Richards (right) after gender reassignment surgery. Renée Richards played professional tennis on the women's circuit.

der identity problems such as transsexualism. Perhaps the developing brains of transsexuals differentiate in one direction while their sexual organs differentiate in the other. We say "perhaps" because no one has yet been able to trace the origins of transsexuality. Yet it is conceivable that genetic, hormonal, and possible environmental factors to which the fetus was exposed may alter the architecture of the brain in this way.

## Psychological Influences

Our gender identity is interwoven with our **gender typing.** At birth we are assigned a gender and reared accordingly. For nearly all of us, our assigned gender is consistent with our anatomic sex. But some rare individuals are born with ambiguous-looking external sex organs that may not be consistent with their internal reproductive organs and chromosomal sex. Their gender identity may be shaped to a certain extent by whether they are reared as boys or girls. In other words, gender identity may not be fixed at birth. Experience may contribute to gender identity. In any event, most children become aware of their anatomic sex by about 18 months. By age 3, most children have achieved a firm gender identity as male or female.

## Gender Roles and Stereotypes

The complex clusters of ways in which males and females are expected to behave in a given culture are called **gender roles.** Fixed, conventional views of "masculine" and "feminine" behavior are called **gender-role stereotypes.** In our culture the stereotypical female is perceived as gentle, dependent, kind, helpful, patient, and submissive. The masculine gender-role stereotype is tough, gentlemanly, and protective. Females are generally seen as warm and emotional. Males are seen as independent, assertive, and competitive.

Children become aware of gender roles and stereotypes by about the age of 3. By that age, they have learned to distinguish behaviors and toys deemed acceptable for their gender from those deemed acceptable for the other gender. Boys and girls begin to recognize that boys build things and play with transportation toys, such as cars and fire trucks, while girls enjoy playing with dolls. By the time they are 3, most children also become aware of stereotypical differences in adult dress and jobs.

Biological differences may play a role in explaining some forms of gender-typed behavior. Perhaps men tend to be more aggressive than women because of the prenatal influence of the male sex hormone testosterone on their brains. Whatever the role of underlying biological factors, cultural learning has an important, perhaps crucial, effect on gender-typed behavior. Once children discover that they are girls or boys, they seek to learn about traits that society deems appropriate for their gender and to live up to them. Jack will retaliate when provoked, if boys in his culture are expected to do so. Jill will be "sugary and sweet," if such is expected. Children's self-esteem is linked to how they measure up to gender-role stereotypes.

**Socialization** also plays a role in gender typing. Babies are treated according to their anatomic sex.

**Androgens** Male sex hormones.

**Testosterone** The male sex hormone that fosters the development of male sex characteristics and is connected with the sex drive.

**Estrogen** A generic term for female sex hormones that promote the development of female secondary sex characteristics and regulate the menstrual cycle.

**Progesterone** A steroid hormone involved in regulation of the menstrual cycle.

**Gender typing** The process by which children acquire behavior that is deemed appropriate to their gender.

**Gender roles** Complex clusters of ways in which males and females are expected to behave in a given culture.

**Gender-role stereotypes** Fixed, conventional ideas about the roles performed by men and women.

**Socialization** The process of guiding people into socially acceptable behavior patterns by means of information, rewards, and punishments.

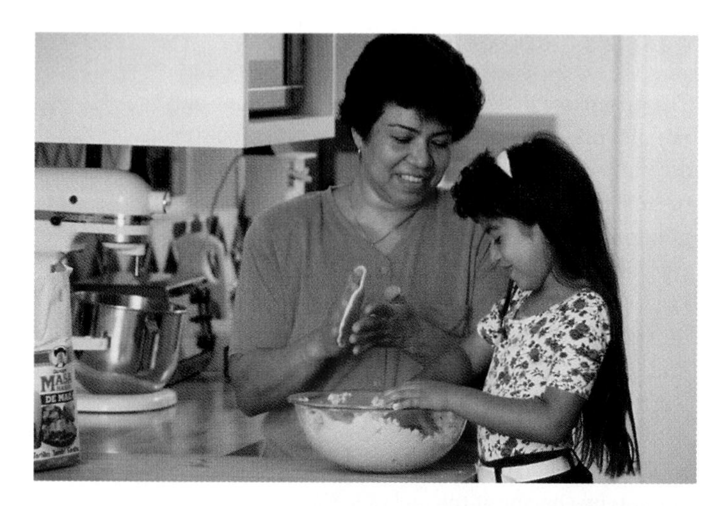

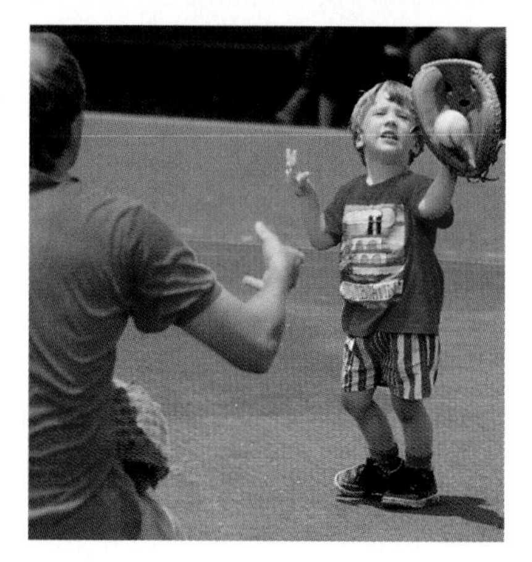

***Gender Typing and Socialization*** How we are socialized by our parents and others has an important bearing on our adoption of behaviors deemed appropriate for our gender. Gender expectations are changing, however. What influence did your upbringing have on your adoption of gender-typed behavior?

The popular media—books, magazines, radio, film, television—also convey gender stereotypes. The media usually portray men and women in traditional roles. One observer notes, "Women are often still depicted on television as half-clad and half-witted, and needing to be rescued by quick-thinking, fully clothed men."[1] Ageism buttresses sexism. Women of age 40 and above are only rarely depicted in roles other than mothers and grandmothers.

Parental roles in gender typing have been changing. Today more mothers are working outside the home. Daughters are thus exposed to more career-minded role models than they were in earlier generations. More parents today encourage their daughters to become career-minded and to engage in strenuous physical activities, such as organized sports. Many boys today are exposed to fathers who take a larger role than men used to in child care and household responsibilities. Perhaps changes in gender typing will improve everyone's psychological health. Perhaps people will feel freer to express their genuine feelings and pursue life paths that appeal to them—regardless of their gender.

Parents tend to talk more to baby girls. Fathers engage in more roughhousing with boys. Parents reward children for behavior they consider gender-appropriate. Parents punish or ignore them for behavior they consider inappropriate. Girls are encouraged to practice caretaking behaviors that prepare them for traditional feminine roles. Boys are handed erector sets or doctor sets to prepare them for traditional masculine roles.

Fathers generally encourage their sons to develop assertive behavior. They encourage sons to get things done, to accomplish things. They encourage daughters to become nurturant and cooperative. Fathers are likely to cuddle their daughters gently. They are likely to carry their sons like footballs or toss them into the air. Being a nontraditionalist, your second author made sure to toss his young daughters into the air. This behavior raised objections from relatives who chastised him for being too rough. Disapproval led him to modify his behavior. He tossed his daughters into the air when the relatives weren't around.

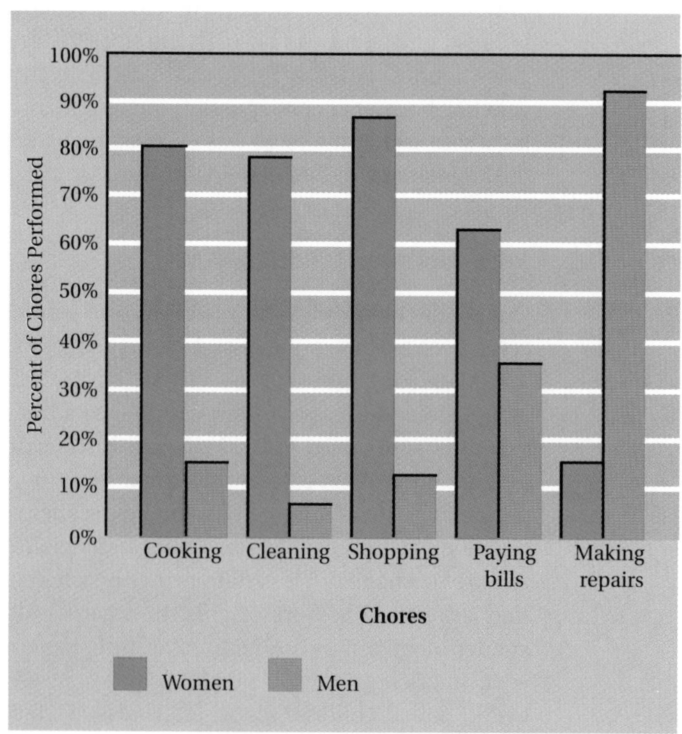


**Figure 9.1** ***When Mommy's Got a Job*** Women who work often put in a second shift when they return home. Except for making repairs, most of the household and child care chores are left to women.

Even though women, as well as men, now bring home the bacon, women are still more often expected to fry it in the pan and clean up afterward. In addition to doing most household chores, women also still bear the primary responsibility for child rearing (Figure 9.1). This is not universal, however; in some cultures women are reared to be the hunters and food gatherers while men stay close to home and tend the children.

### Gender Differences—Vive La Différence or Vive La Similarité?

The genders are anatomically different. (No argument.) How do the genders differ in mental abilities and personality?

**Mental Abilities** In our culture, girls are generally more advanced in verbal abilities. Boys tend to show greater mathematical problem-solving ability, beginning in adolescence. Three factors should caution us not to attach too much importance to these gender differences, however:

1. In most cases, they are small, and getting smaller.[2]
2. These gender differences are *group* differences. Despite differences between groups of boys and girls, millions of boys exceed the average girl in writing and spelling. Likewise, millions of girls outperform the average boy in problem-solving and spatial tasks. Men have produced their Shakespeares. Women have produced their Madame Curies.
3. Small differences in abilities may reflect environmental influences and cultural expectations, not inborn differences.

The point is that men who are interested in writing should be encouraged to write. Women who are interested in math, engineering, and science should be encouraged to enter these fields.

**Personality** There are also some gender differences in personality. Research shows that females are generally higher in such traits as extroversion, anxiety, trust, and nurturance.[3] Males tend to be more aggressive, assertive, and tough-minded, and to have higher self-esteem. Women are generally more ready to disclose their feelings and personal experiences. Whether such differences reflect biological or psychosocial factors, or a combination of both, remains open to debate. But consider two psychosocial factors that may largely account for females' relatively lower self-esteem:

- Most parents prefer to have boys.
- Society has created an unlevel playing field for girls and women. Females have to perform better than males to be seen as doing equally well.

**think about it!**

- **Do you consider yourself a stereotypical male or female? Why or why not?**

**critical thinking Do you believe that gender differences in aggression and nurturance are inborn or the result of cultural influences? Why?**

Smart Quiz
Q0901

## SEXUAL ANATOMY AND PHYSIOLOGY

Our sexual anatomy includes external and internal organs and structures that bring us sensual pleasure and provide for reproduction. (If reproduction were a painful or unpleasant process, none of us might be here to tell the story.)

### Female Sexual Anatomy—Outside

Taken collectively, the external reproductive structures of the female are termed the pudendum or the **vulva.** *Vulva* is a Latin word that means "wrapper" or "covering." The vulva consists of the *mons veneris,* the *labia majora* and *minora* (major and minor lips), the *clitoris,* and the vaginal opening (see Figure 9.2, next page).

Talking Glossary
Mons veneris
G0902

**The Mons** The **mons veneris** (from the Latin phrase, "mount of Venus") consists of fatty tissue that covers the joint of the pubic bones in front of the body, below the abdomen and above the clitoris. At puberty the mons becomes covered with pubic hair. The mons cushions a woman's body during sexual intercourse.

**The Labia** The **labia majora** (Latin for "large lips" or "major lips") are large folds of skin that

**Vulva** The external sexual structures of the female.

**Mons veneris** A mound of fatty tissue that covers the joint of the pubic bones, below the abdomen and above the clitoris.

**Labia majora** Large folds of skin that run downward from the mons along the sides of the vulva.

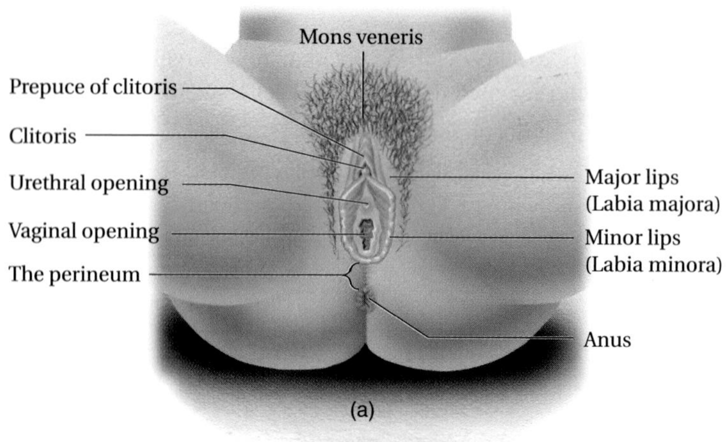


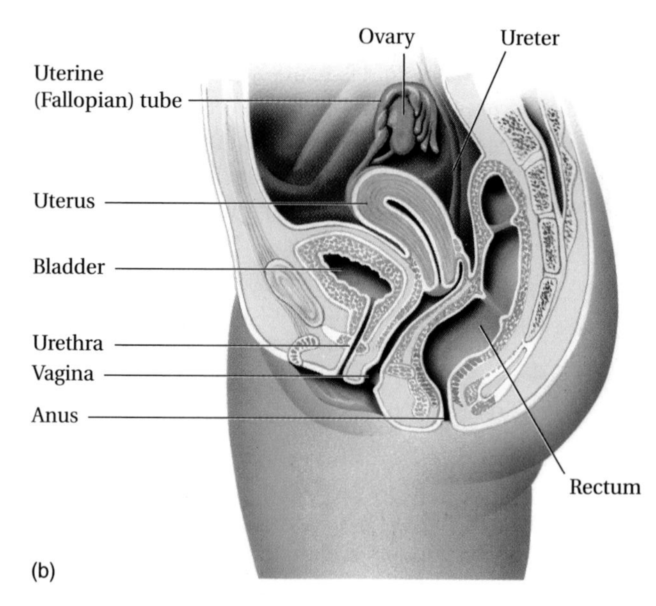


**Figure 9.2** ***External Female Sexual Organs and the Reproductive System*** (a) This illustration shows the vulva with the labia opened to reveal the urethral and vaginal openings. (b) This cross section locates many of the internal sexual organs that compose the female reproductive system.

run downward from the mons along the sides of the vulva. The **labia minora** ("minor lips") are hairless, light-colored membranes located between the major lips. They surround the urethral and vaginal openings.

**Talking Glossary**
Labia majora, Labia minora G0903
Clitoris G0904

**The Clitoris** The body of the **clitoris,** termed the clitoral shaft, contains spongy masses that fill with blood and become erect in response to sexual stimulation. The **prepuce** or hood covers the clitoral shaft. The clitoral glans is a smooth, round knob or lump of tissue. It is highly sensitive to touch.

In some respects, the clitoris is the female counterpart of the penis. Both organs receive and transmit sexual sensations, but the penis is directly involved in reproduction and excretion. The penis serves as a conduit for sperm and for urine. The clitoris is a unique sex organ. It serves no known purpose other than sexual pleasure.

**Labia minora** Hairless, light-colored membranes located between the labia majora.

**Clitoris** A female sex organ consisting of a shaft and glans located above the urethral opening. It is extremely sensitive to sexual sensations.

**Prepuce** The fold of skin covering the glans of the clitoris (or penis).

**Urethral opening** The opening through which urine passes from the female's body.

**Cystitis** An inflammation of the urinary bladder.

**Gynecologist** A physician who treats women's diseases, especially of the reproductive tract.

**Clitoridectomy** Surgical removal of the clitoris.

**The Urethral Opening** Urine passes from the female's body through the **urethral opening,** which is connected by a short tube called the urethra to the bladder, where urine collects (Figure 9.2). The urethral opening, urethra, and bladder are unrelated to the reproductive system. Many males believe erroneously that women urinate and engage in sexual activity through the same opening. The confusion may arise from the fact that urine and semen both pass through the penis, or that the urethral opening lies near the vaginal opening.

**PREVENTION**

## *Preventing Cystitis*

The proximity of the urethral opening to the external reproductive organs may pose some hygienic problems for sexually active women. The urinary tract, which includes the urethra, bladder, and kidneys, may become infected from bacteria that are transmitted from the vagina or rectum. Pathogens may also pass from the male's sex organs to the female's urethral opening during sexual intercourse. Manual stimulation of the vulva with dirty hands may transmit bacteria through the urethral opening to the bladder. Anal intercourse followed by vaginal intercourse may transfer pathogens from the rectum to the bladder. For similar reasons, women should first wipe the vulva, then the anus, when using the bathroom. In this way, they can prevent organisms that normally dwell in the rectum or intestines from infecting the urinary or reproductive tracts.

**Talking Glossary**
Cystitis G0905

**Cystitis,** or bladder inflammation, can stem from any of these sources. Its primary symptoms are burning and frequent urination (also called *urinary urgency*). Pus or a bloody discharge are common. There may be an ache just above the pubic bone. These symptoms may disappear after several days. Yet consultation with a **gynecologist** (from

WORLD OF *diversity*

## Female Circumcision—Health Measure or Mutilation?

**Talking Glossary**
Clitoridectomies
G0906

Like male circumcision, female circumcision is rooted in religious and cultural tradition. Yet, unlike male circumcision, which involves the removal of the penile foreskin, female circumcision as practiced in some African and Middle Eastern Islamic cultures involves removal of the entire clitoris, not just the clitoral hood. In some practices, even more of the female external genitalia are removed. Also, while male circumcision is generally performed shortly after birth, female circumcision is generally performed at puberty as a rite of initiation into womanhood. Female circumcision, which many observers see as ritualized genital mutilation, is usually performed under unsanitary conditions without benefit of anesthesia. Medical complications are common, including infections, bleeding, scarring, painful menstruation, and obstructed labor.

There is no hygienic or health basis for female circumcision. Why, then, is it performed? The clitoris gives rise to feelings of sexual pleasure in women. Its removal or mutilation is believed to be rooted in an ancient attempt to destroy women's ability to take pleasure in sex and thus ensure female chastity.[4] However, for some groups in rural Egypt and in the northern Sudan, **clitoridectomies** continue to be performed as a long-standing social custom, not ostensibly as a means of controlling female sexuality. Some people perceive it as part of their faith in Islam. However, neither Islam nor any other religion requires it.[5] Ironically, many young women do not perceive themselves as victims. They assume that clitoridectomy is a natural part of becoming a woman.

An even more radical form of clitoridectomy, Pharaonic circumcision, is practiced widely in the Sudan. Pharaonic circumcision involves removal of the clitoris, the labia minora, and the inner layers of the labia majora. Medical complications are common, including menstrual and urinary problems, and even death. Mutilation of the labia is now illegal in the Sudan, although the law continues to allow removal of the clitoris. Some African countries have outlawed clitoridectomies, although such laws are rarely enforced.

Nearly 100 million women in Africa and the Middle East have undergone removal of the clitoris and the labia minora.[6] Clitoridectomies remain common, even universal, in nearly 30 countries in Africa, many countries in the Middle East, and parts of Malaysia, Yemen, Oman, Indonesia, and the Indian subcontinent.[7]

Do not confuse male circumcision with the maiming inflicted on girls in the name of circumcision. Former member of Congress Patricia Schroeder depicts the male equivalent of female genital mutilation as cutting off the penis and its surrounding tissue. The Pulitzer Prize–winning African-American novelist Alice Walker has drawn attention to female genital mutilation in her novel *Possessing the Secret of Joy*. She has called for its abolition in her book and movie *Warrior Marks*.

Calls from Westerners to ban female circumcision in parts of Africa and the Middle East have sparked controversy on the grounds of "cultural condescension." Critics complain that Westerners have no right to dictate the cultural traditions of other peoples. A leader of an influential women's rights organization in Kenya put the issue thus: "Let indigenous people fight it [female circumcision] according to their own traditions. . . . It will die faster than if others tell us what to do." Yet for Alice Walker, "torture is not culture." As the debate continues, 2 million African girls are mutilated each year.

Greek *gyne*, meaning "woman") is recommended, because untreated cystitis can lead to serious kidney infections.

So-called honeymoon cystitis is caused by the tugging on the bladder and urethral wall that occurs during sexual intercourse. It may occur when a woman first becomes sexually active (not necessarily on her honeymoon) or when she resumes sexual activity after lengthy abstinence. Figure 9.2 shows the close proximity of the urethra and vagina.

A few precautions may help women prevent inflammation of the bladder:

- Drinking two quarts of water a day to flush the bladder.
- Drinking cranberry juice to maintain an acid environment that discourages growth of infectious organisms.
- Decreasing use of alcohol and caffeine (from coffee, tea, or cola drinks) that may irritate the bladder.
- Washing hands before masturbation or self-examination.
- Washing both partners' genitals before and after intercourse.
- Preventing objects that have touched the anus (fingers, penis, toilet tissue) from subsequently coming into contact with the vulva.
- Urinating after intercourse to help wash away bacteria.

The **hymen** (Greek for "membrane") is a fold of tissue across the vaginal opening. It may remain partly intact until a woman becomes sexually active. For this reason the hymen has been called the "maidenhead." Its presence has been taken as proof of virginity; its absence, as evidence of sexual activity. However, some women are born with incomplete hymens. Other women's hymens are torn accidentally, as through exercising. Some people believe incorrectly that virgins cannot insert tampons into their vaginas, but most hymens will readily accommodate them. Most women experience little pain or distress when they become sexually active, despite old horror stories.

## Female Sexual Anatomy—Inside

The internal reproductive organs of the female include the innermost parts of the vagina, the cervix, the uterus, ovaries, and Fallopian tubes (Figure 9.2). These structures make up the woman's internal reproductive system.

**The Vagina** The **vagina** (Latin for "sheath") extends back and upward from the vaginal opening. It is usually 3 to 5 inches long at rest. Menstrual flow and babies during birth pass out of the body from the uterus through the vagina. The penis is contained within the vagina during sexual intercourse. When at rest, the walls of the vagina touch like a deflated balloon. The vagina expands during sexual arousal. The vagina also expands to accommodate a baby's head and shoulders during childbirth.

The vaginal walls secrete substances that help maintain the vagina's normal acidity (pH 4.0 to 5.0). Douching or spraying may alter the natural chemical balance of the vagina, which can increase the risk of infection. Feminine deodorant sprays can irritate the vagina and cause allergic reactions. The normal, healthy vagina cleanses itself through regular chemical secretions that are evidenced by a slight white or yellowish discharge.

**Hymen** A fold of tissue across the vaginal opening that is usually present at birth and remains at least partly intact until a woman engages in coitus.

**Vagina** The tubular female sex organ that contains the penis during sexual intercourse and through which a baby is born.

**Vaginitis** Vaginal inflammation.

**Cervix** The lower end of the uterus.

**Uterus** The hollow, muscular, pear-shaped organ in which a fertilized ovum implants and develops until birth.

PREVENTION

### *Preventing Vaginitis*

**Vaginitis** refers to any vaginal inflammation, whether it is caused by an infection, an allergic reaction, or chemical irritation. Vaginitis may also stem from use of birth-control pills or antibiotics that alter the natural body chemistry, or from other factors, such as lowered resistance (from fatigue or poor diet). Changes in the natural body chemistry or lowered resistance permit microscopic organisms normally found in the vagina to multiply to infectious levels. Vaginitis may be recognized by abnormal discharge, itching, burning of the vulva, and sometimes urinary urgency. Women with vaginitis are advised to seek medical attention, but let us note some suggestions that may help prevent vaginitis:[8]

1. *Wash your vulva and anus regularly with mild soap.* Pat dry (taking care not to touch the vulva after the anus).
2. *Wear cotton panties.* Nylon underwear retains heat and moisture that cause harmful bacteria to flourish.
3. *Avoid pants that are tight in the crotch.*
4. *Be certain that sex partners are clean.* Condoms may also reduce spread of infections from one's sex partner.
5. *Use a sterile, water-soluble jelly like K-Y jelly if artificial lubrication is needed for intercourse.* Do *not* use Vaseline. Birth-control jellies can also be used for lubrication.
6. *Avoid intercourse that is painful or abrasive.*
7. *Avoid diets high in sugar and refined carbohydrates since they alter the normal acidity of the vagina.*
8. *Women who are prone to vaginal infections may find it helpful to douche occasionally with plain water, a solution of 1 or 2 tablespoons of vinegar in a quart of warm water, or a solution of baking soda and water.* Douches consisting of unpasteurized plain (unflavored) yogurt may help replenish the "good" bacteria that are normally found in the vagina and may be destroyed by use of antibiotics. Do not douche if you are pregnant or suspect you may be pregnant. Consult your physician before douching or applying preparations to the vagina.
9. *Watch your general health.* Eating poorly or getting insufficient rest will reduce your resistance to infection.

**The Cervix** The **cervix** is the lower end of the uterus. Sperm pass from the vagina to the uterus through the cervical canal. Babies pass from the uterus to the vagina during childbirth.

**The Uterus** The **uterus,** or womb, is the pear-shaped organ in which a fertilized ovum implants and develops until birth. The inner layer of the uterus is called the **endometrium.** Endometrial tissue is discharged through the cervix and vagina at menstruation. In some women endometrial tissue may also grow in the abdominal cavity or elsewhere in the reproductive system. This condition is called **endometriosis.** The most common symptom is abdominal pain, usually around the time of the menstrual period. Treatments are available for endometriosis, but it sometimes leads to infertility.

Talking Glossary
Endometriosis
G0907

One woman in three in the United States has a **hysterectomy** by the age of 60. Most hysterectomy patients are between the ages of 35 and 45. The hysterectomy is now the second most commonly performed operation on women in this country. (Caesarean sections are the most common.) A hysterectomy may be performed when a woman develops cancer of the uterus, ovaries, or cervix, or another disease that causes pain or excessive bleeding. A hysterectomy may be partial or complete. A complete hysterectomy is the surgical removal of the ovaries, Fallopian tubes, cervix, and uterus. It is usually performed to reduce the risk of cancer spreading throughout the reproductive system. A partial hysterectomy removes the uterus but spares the ovaries and Fallopian tubes. Sparing the ovaries allows the woman to continue to ovulate and produce adequate amounts of female sex hormones.

The hysterectomy has become a controversial procedure. In many cases it may be possible to use less radical medical interventions to treat the underlying problem. Women whose physicians recommend a hysterectomy are advised to seek a second opinion before proceeding.

Talking Glossary
Fallopian tubes
G0908

**The Fallopian Tubes** The two **Fallopian tubes** extend from the upper end of the uterus toward the ovaries (Figure 9.2). Ova (egg cells) pass through the Fallopian tubes to the uterus. *Tubal ligation* is a form of sterilization that ties off the Fallopian tubes. Thus ova cannot pass through them or become fertilized.

**The Ovaries** Two almond-shaped **ovaries** lie on either side of the uterus. The ovaries produce ova and the female sex hormones estrogen and progesterone. Estrogen promotes the changes of puberty and regulates the menstrual cycle. Estrogen also helps older women maintain mental functioning and feelings of well-being.

The human female is born with all the ova she will ever have (about 2 million), but they are immature. Of these, about 400,000 survive into puberty. Each is contained in the ovary within a capsule, or **follicle.** During a woman's reproductive years, from puberty to menopause, about one ovum per month will be released by its follicle for possible fertilization.

## PREVENTION

### *The Pelvic Examination—What to Expect*

Women should have an internal (pelvic) examination at least once a year by the time they reach their late teens, or earlier if they become sexually active. The physician (usually a gynecologist) first examines the patient externally for irritations, swellings, abnormal vaginal discharges, and clitoral adhesions. The physician normally inserts a **speculum** to help inspect the cervix and vaginal walls for discharges (which can be signs of infection), discoloration, lesions, or growths. This examination is typically followed by a **Pap smear** (named after the originator of the technique, Dr. Papanicolaou) to detect cervical cancer. A sample of vaginal discharge may also be taken to test for the sexually transmitted disease gonorrhea.

Talking Glossary
Speculum
G0909

To take a Pap smear, the physician will hold open the vaginal walls with a plastic or metal speculum so that a sample of cells (a "smear") may be scraped from the cervix with a wooden spatula. Women should not douche before a Pap smear or schedule one during menstruation. (Douches and blood confound analysis of the smear.)

The speculum exam is normally followed by a bimanual (two-handed) vaginal exam. The index and middle fingers of one hand are inserted into the vagina while the lower part of the abdomen is palpated (touched) by the other hand from the outside. The physician uses this technique to examine the location, shape, size, and movability of the internal reproductive organs, searching for abnormal growths and other problems. Palpation may be uncomfortable, but severe pain means that something is wrong. A woman

**Endometrium** The innermost layer of the uterus.

**Endometriosis** A condition caused by the growth of endometrial tissue in the abdominal cavity or elsewhere outside the uterus.

**Hysterectomy** Surgical removal of the uterus.

**Fallopian tubes** Tubes that extend from the upper uterus toward the ovaries and conduct ova to the uterus.

**Ovaries** Organs that produce ova and the hormones estrogen and progesterone.

**Follicle** A capsule within an ovary that contains an ovum.

**Speculum** A medical instrument used to enlarge openings of body canals or cavities to allow inspection of the inner areas.

**Pap smear** A sample of cervical cells that is examined to screen for cervical cancer and other abnormalities.

should not try to be "brave" and deny pain. She may be masking a symptom (that is, depriving the physician of useful information). Physical discomfort is usually mild, however. Psychological discomfort is often relieved by discussing feelings with the examiner.

**Close-up**
More on the Pap smear
T0901

Finally, the physician should do a recto-vaginal examination in which one finger is inserted into the rectum while the other is inserted into the vagina. This procedure yields information about the health of the internal reproductive organs and the rectum.

It is normal for a woman to be anxious about her first pelvic exam, or her first exam with a new doctor. The doctor should be reassuring if the woman expresses concern. If the doctor is not, the woman should feel free to consult another doctor. She should not forgo the pelvic examination itself, however. It is essential for early detection of health problems.

## The Breasts

*The degree of attention which breasts receive, combined with the confusion about what the breast fetishists actually want, makes women unduly anxious about them. They can never be just right; they must always be too small, too big, the wrong shape, too flabby. The characteristics of the mammary stereotype are impossible to emulate because they are falsely simulated, but they must be faked somehow or another. Reality is either gross or scrawny.*

Germaine Greer, *The Female Eunuch*

College women recall:[9]

*I was very excited about my breast development. It was a big competition to see who was wearing a bra in elementary school. When I began wearing one, I also liked wearing see-through blouses so everyone would know. . . .*

*My breasts were very late in developing. This brought me a lot of grief from my male peers. I just dreaded situations like going to the beach or showering in the locker room. . . .*

In some cultures the breasts are a means for feeding infants, period. In our culture, however, breasts have also achieved erotic significance. In fact, a woman's self-esteem may become linked to her feelings about her bustline.

The breasts contain milk-producing **mammary glands.** Each gland opens at the nipple through its own duct. The mammary glands are separated by soft, fatty tissue. The amount of fatty tissue, not the amount of glandular tissue, determines the size of the breasts. There is not much variation among women in the amount of glandular tissue. Thus breast size does not determine the quantity of milk that can be produced.

The nipple contains smooth muscle fibers that cause the nipple to become erect when they contract. Milk ducts conduct milk from the mammary glands through the nipples. Nipples are richly endowed with nerve endings. Stimulation of the nipples can be sexually arousing. The **areola,** or area surrounding the nipple, darkens during pregnancy and remains darker after delivery. Oil-producing glands in the areola help lubricate the nipples during breast-feeding.

**Talking Glossary**
Areola
G0910

## The Menstrual Cycle

**Menstruation** is the cyclical bleeding that results from the shedding of the uterine lining (endometrium). Menstruation takes place when an ovum is not fertilized. The word *menstruation* derives from the Latin *mensis,* meaning "month." The menstrual cycle averages 28 days in length.

The menstrual cycle involves finely tuned relationships among the **hypothalamus,** the **pituitary gland,** the ovaries, and the uterus. All these structures are parts of the endocrine system. That is, they secrete hormones directly into the bloodstream. (The ovaries and uterus are also reproductive organs.) Other bodily secretions, such as milk, saliva, sweat, and tears, arrive at their destinations through narrow tubes called ducts.

The menstrual cycle is divided into four phases (see Figure 9.3). The first, or **proliferative phase,** begins with the end of menstruation and lasts about 9 or 10 days in a 28-day cycle. Low levels of estrogen and progesterone are circulating in the blood as menstruation draws to an end. When the hypothalamus senses a low level of estrogen in the blood, it triggers the pituitary gland to release **follicle-stimulating hormone (FSH).** When FSH reaches the ovaries, it stimulates some follicles to

**Mammary glands** Milk-secreting glands.

**Areola** The dark ring on the breast that encircles the nipple.

**Menstruation** The cyclical bleeding that stems from the shedding of the uterine lining (endometrium).

**Hypothalamus** A brain structure below the thalamus involved in regulating body temperature, motivation, and emotion.

**Pituitary gland** The so-called master gland that secretes hormones involved in growth, regulation of the menstrual cycle, and childbirth.

**Proliferative phase** The first phase of the menstrual cycle during which the endometrium proliferates.

**Follicle-stimulating hormone (FSH)** A pituitary hormone that stimulates development of follicles in the ovaries.

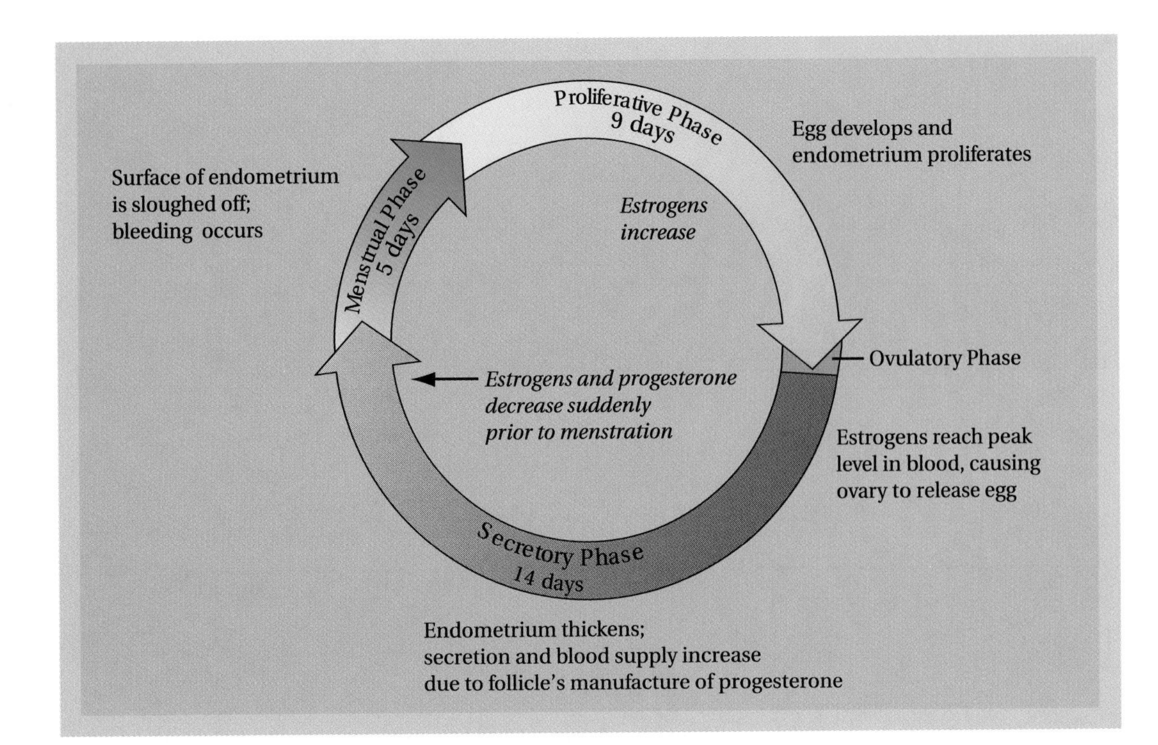


**Figure 9.3** ***The Four Phases of the Menstrual Cycle*** The menstrual cycle has proliferative, ovulatory, secretory (luteal), and menstrual phases.

mature. As the follicles ripen, they begin producing estrogen. Estrogen further ripens ova (egg cells) within their follicles. During this phase the endometrium develops, or "proliferates."

The second phase is the **ovulatory phase. Ovulation,** the release of the ovum, is triggered by peak estrogen levels. The hypothalamus detects these estrogen levels and triggers the pituitary to release FSH and **luteinizing hormone (LH).** The surge of LH triggers ovulation, which usually begins 12 to 24 hours after the peaking of LH (Figure 9.4, next page). A mature ovum is released *near* a Fallopian tube—not *into* a Fallopian tube. If two ova are released during ovulation, and both are fertilized, fraternal (nonidentical) twins will develop. Identical twins develop when one fertilized ovum divides into two separate embryos.

**Talking Glossary**
Luteinizing hormone
G0911

A woman's *basal body temperature (BBT),* taken by oral or rectal thermometer, dips slightly at ovulation (Figure 9.4) and rises by about 1 degree Fahrenheit on the day after. Many women use their BBT to help them know when to engage in intercourse (if they wish to conceive) or avoid intercourse (if they wish to avoid pregnancy). Unfortunately the BBT method is not highly reliable. Some women have discomfort or cramping during ovulation, termed *mittelschmerz* ("pain in the middle" in German).

The third phase of the cycle is called the *secretory,* or *luteal,* phase. The **luteal phase** begins right after ovulation and continues through the beginning of the next cycle. The term *luteal phase* is derived from the follicle that releases the ovum, which is called the **corpus luteum.** LH signals the corpus luteum to produce large amounts of progesterone and estrogen. Progesterone causes the endometrium to thicken to support an embryo. Levels of these hormones peak around the 20th or 21st day of the cycle.

**Talking Glossary**
Corpus luteum
G0912

If the ovum goes unfertilized, the hypothalamus responds to the high levels of progesterone. It signals the pituitary to stop producing LH and FSH. This feedback process is similar to that of a thermostat in a house, which reacts to rising temperatures by shutting down the furnace. The levels of LH and FSH decline rapidly, causing the corpus luteum to decompose. After the corpus luteum breaks down, estrogen and progesterone levels plummet. The falloffs trigger the fourth, or menstrual, phase, which leads to the beginning of a new cycle. The **menstrual phase** is the sloughing off of the endometrium. The low estrogen levels of the menstrual phase

**Ovulatory phase** The second stage of the menstrual cycle during which a follicle ruptures and releases a mature ovum.

**Ovulation** The release of an ovum from an ovary.

**Luteinizing hormone (LH)** A hormone that helps regulate the menstrual cycle by triggering ovulation.

**Luteal phase** The third phase of the menstrual cycle, named after the corpus luteum, which begins to secrete large amounts of progesterone and estrogen following ovulation.

**Corpus luteum** The follicle that has released an ovum and then produces copious amounts of progesterone and estrogen during the luteal phase of a woman's cycle.

**Menstrual phase** The fourth phase of the menstrual cycle, during which the endometrium is sloughed off in the menstrual flow.

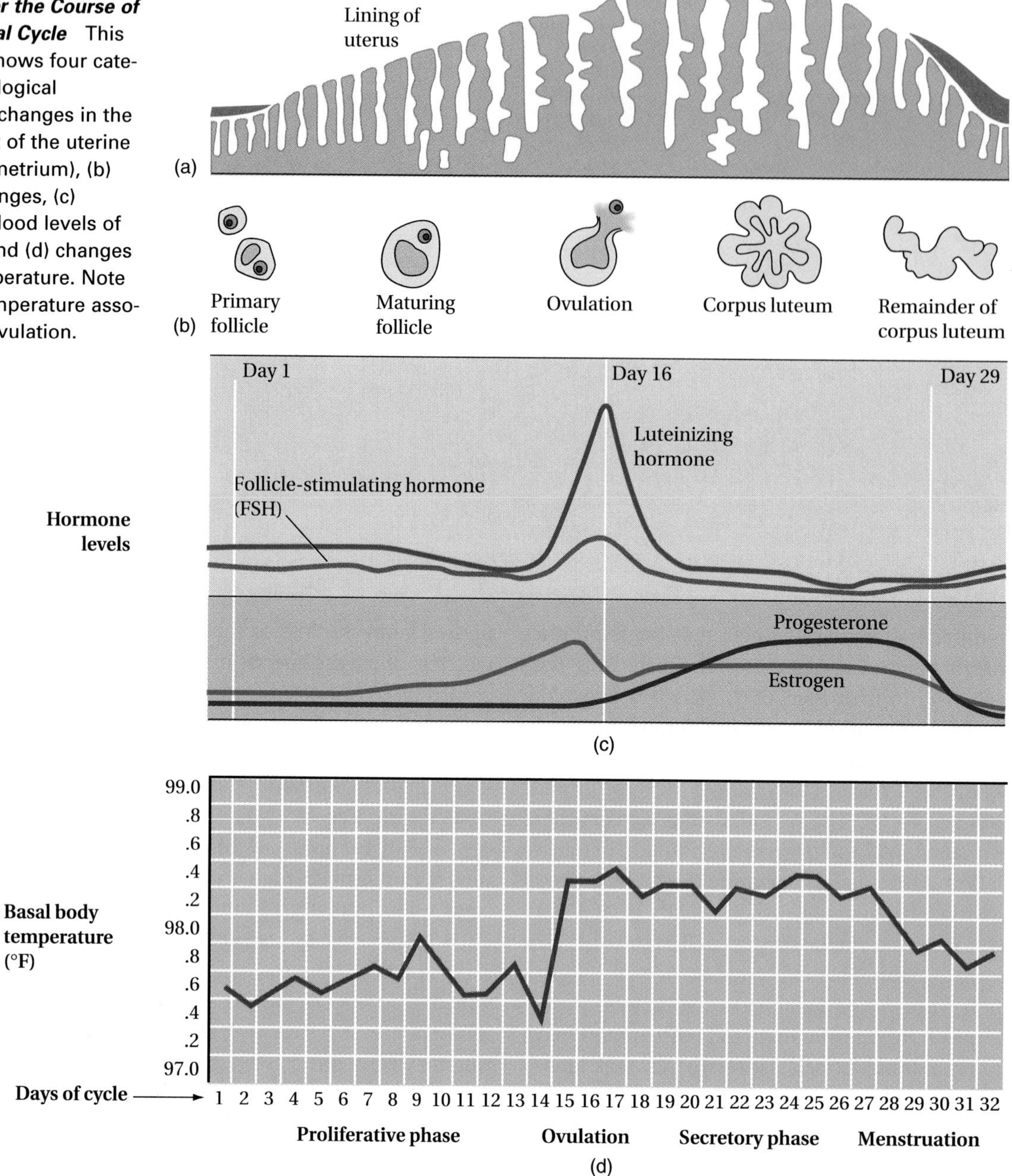


**Figure 9.4** ***Physiological Changes over the Course of the Menstrual Cycle*** This illustration shows four categories of biological changes: (a) changes in the development of the uterine lining (endometrium), (b) follicular changes, (c) changes in blood levels of hormones, and (d) changes in basal temperature. Note the dip in temperature associated with ovulation.

signal the hypothalamus to stimulate the pituitary to secrete FSH. FSH, in turn, prompts ovarian secretion of estrogen and the onset of another proliferative phase. A new cycle begins. The menstrual phase is a beginning as well as an end.

Although the menstrual flow can persist for 5 days or more, most women lose only 2 or 3 ounces of blood (4 to 6 tablespoonfuls). A typical blood donor, by contrast, donates 16 ounces of blood at a sitting. Most American women use external sanitary napkins or pads, or internal tampons, to absorb the menstrual flow. Tampons enable women to swim without concern while menstruating, wear more revealing or comfortable apparel, and feel less burdened.

## Menstrual Discomfort

Although menstruation is a natural biological process, most women experience some discomfort before or during menstruation (see Table 9.1).

TABLE 9.1

**Common Symptoms of Menstrual Problems**

| Physical Symptoms | Psychological Symptoms |
| --- | --- |
| Breast swelling or tenderness | Depressed mood, sudden tearfulness |
| Bloating | Loss of interest in usual social or recreational activities |
| Weight gain | Anxiety, tension (feeling "on edge" or "keyed up") |
| Food cravings | Anger |
| Abdominal discomfort | Irritability |
| Cramps | Changes in body image |
| Lack of energy | Concern over skipping routine activities at school or work |
| Sleep disturbance, fatigue | A sense of loss of control or ability to cope |
| Migraine headache | |
| Pains in muscles and joints | |
| Aggravation of chronic disorders like asthma and allergies | |

Talking Glossary
Dysmenorrhea
G0913

**Dysmenorrhea** Pain or discomfort during menstruation—**dysmenorrhea**—is the most common menstrual problem. Most women have mild menstrual discomfort at least occasionally. Pelvic cramps are the most common complaint. Cramps may be accompanied by headache, backache, nausea, or bloated feelings. Dysmenorrhea may be caused by problems such as endometriosis, pelvic inflammatory disease, and ovarian cysts. Some discomfort is connected with hormonal changes themselves.

Cramps are the feelings associated with uterine spasms. Spasms can result from the secretion of hormones called **prostaglandins.** Prostaglandins cause muscle fibers in the uterine wall to contract, and powerful, persistent contractions are painful. They may also deprive the uterus of oxygen, another source of discomfort. Prostaglandin-inhibiting drugs, such as ibuprofen and aspirin, often help. Menstrual cramps sometimes decrease after childbirth, as a result of the hormonal changes of pregnancy. Pelvic pressure and bloating may be traced to pelvic swelling—congestion in the pelvic region.

Headaches frequently accompany menstrual discomfort. Most headaches stem from muscle tension in the shoulders, back of the neck, and scalp. Pelvic discomfort may cause general muscle tension, contributing to headaches.

**Amenorrhea** The absence of menstruation is termed **amenorrhea.** It is a primary sign of infertility. Amenorrhea has various causes, including structural or hormonal abnormalities, growths such as cysts and tumors, and psychological problems, such as stress. Amenorrhea is normal during pregnancy and following menopause. Amenorrhea is also a symptom of anorexia nervosa. Hormonal changes that accompany emaciation in anorexic women are believed responsible for the cessation of menstruation. Amenorrhea may also occur in women who exercise strenuously, such as competitive runners. It is unclear whether the cessation of menstruation in athletes is due to exercise itself or to related physical factors such as low body fat and the stress of training, or a combination of factors.

**Premenstrual Syndrome (PMS)** **PMS** describes symptoms some women experience during the 4 to 6 days before menstruation starts. These include anxiety, depression, irritability, fluid retention, and abdominal discomfort. PMS

**Dysmenorrhea** Pain or discomfort during menstruation.

**Prostaglandins** Hormones that cause muscle fibers in the uterine wall to contract, as during labor.

**Amenorrhea** The absence of menstruation.

**Premenstrual syndrome (PMS)** Physical and psychological symptoms that afflict many women during the days before their menstrual period.

also appears to be linked with imbalances in serotonin—one of the chemical messengers or neurotransmitters of the nervous system. Serotonin imbalances are also linked to changes in appetite.

Though PMS is quite common, the great majority of cases involve mild to moderate discomfort. Only 10% of women report menstrual symptoms severe enough to impair their social, academic, or occupational functioning. In fact, fewer than 1% of the employed women in one study reported missing work because of PMS.[10]

The causes of PMS are unclear. Hormonal factors and chemical changes in the brain are suspected, though scientists have not yet pinpointed the underlying mechanism. Researchers have yet to find differences in levels of estrogen or progesterone between women with severe PMS and those with mild symptoms or no symptoms.[11] Perhaps it is not hormone levels themselves but the sensitivity of the brain to these hormones that predisposes some women to PMS.

Treatments for PMS range from exercise and dietary control (for example, limiting salt and sugar), to use of vitamin supplements, to hormone treatments (usually progesterone), to drugs that increase the amount of serotonin in the nervous system.

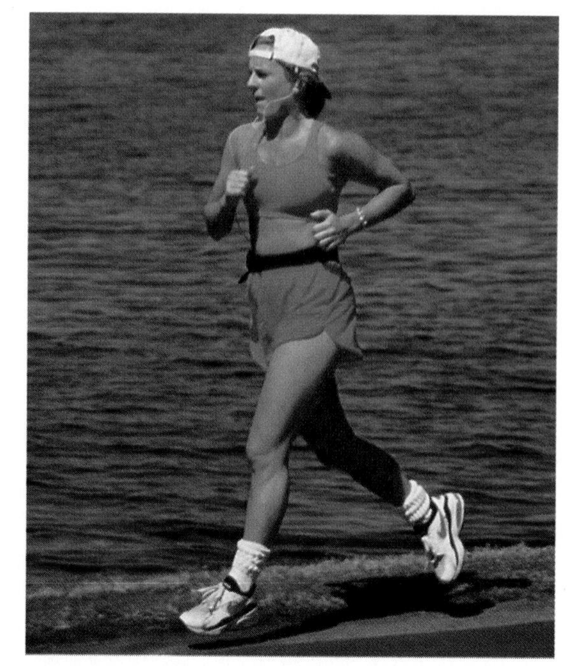

***Managing Menstrual Discomfort*** Some women find that vigorous exercise helps relieve premenstrual and menstrual discomfort.

### How to Handle Menstrual Discomfort

Most women experience some degree of menstrual discomfort. Women with persistent menstrual distress may profit from the suggestions listed below. Researchers are exploring the effectiveness of these techniques in scientific studies. For now, women may wish to try these techniques to see whether they are helpful.

1. *Don't blame yourself!* Menstrual problems were once erroneously attributed to women's "hysterical" nature. This is nonsense. Menstrual problems appear to largely reflect hormonal variations or chemical fluctuations in the brain during the menstrual cycle. Menstrual discomfort is very real.
2. *Keep a menstrual calendar.* It will allow you to track your symptoms and identify patterns. Knowledge of how and when you feel discomfort can help you form strategies to deal with it.
3. *Develop strategies for dealing with your worst days.* Plan activities to enhance your pleasure and minimize your stress on those days. Distract yourself. Go to a movie or read a novel.
4. *Ask yourself whether you harbor any self-defeating attitudes toward menstruation.* Might such attitudes be compounding your distress? For example, do relatives or friends see menstruation as an illness, as a "female problem" or even a "dirty" thing? Have you adopted any of these attitudes?
5. *See a doctor about your concerns, especially if you have severe symptoms.* Severe symptoms can be caused by disorders like endometriosis and **pelvic inflammatory disease (PID).** If so, you can be helped.
6. *Develop nutritious eating habits.* Consider limiting intake of alcohol, caffeine, fats, salt, and sweets, especially during the days preceding menstruation.
7. *Try exercise.* Some women find that jogging, swimming, bicycling, fast walking, dancing, skating, or even jumping rope helps relieve premenstrual and menstrual discomfort.
8. *Check out vitamins.* Ask your doctor whether vitamin and mineral supplements (such as calcium and magnesium) may help. Vitamin $B_6$ appears to have helped some women.

**Pelvic inflammatory disease (PID)** An infection of the female internal reproductive organs that can lead to infertility.

**Menopause** The cessation of menstruation.

9. *Consider medication.* Ibuprofen (brand names Advil, Medipren, Motrin, etc.) and other medicines available over the counter may be helpful for cramping. Prescription drugs such as fluoxetine (Prozac) may also be useful. Ask your doctor for a recommendation.
10. *Remind yourself that menstrual problems are time-limited.* Unlike getting through life or a career, you just need to get through the next couple of days.

## Menopause

As women age, their menstrual cycles shorten and become irregular. **Menopause,** or the "change of life," involves the cessation of menstruation. Menopause most commonly occurs between the ages of 45 and 55. In menopause, the ovaries no longer ripen egg cells or secrete estrogen and progesterone. Low estrogen levels may cause unpleasant physical sensations. There may be night sweats, hot flashes (suddenly feeling hot), and hot flushes (suddenly looking reddened). Hot flashes and flushes may alternate with cold sweats, in which a woman feels suddenly cold and clammy. Hot flashes and flushes stem largely from "waves" of dilation of blood vessels across the face and upper body. These sensations occur when body mechanisms that normally dilate or constrict the blood vessels to maintain an even body temperature are disrupted. Other signs of estrogen deficiency include dizziness, headaches, joint pains, tingling in the hands or feet, burning or itchy skin, and heart palpitations. The skin becomes drier. There is some loss of breast tissue, and vaginal lubrication decreases. Women may also awaken more frequently at night and have difficulty returning to sleep.

# HealthCheck

## How Much Do You Know about Menopause?

Menopause is a major life change for most women. Menopause can symbolize many midlife issues, including changes in appearance, sexuality, and health. Yet exactly what changes do we find? Many of us harbor misleading ideas about menopause—ideas that can be harmful to women. Complete this ***HealthCheck*** to see how much you know about menopause.

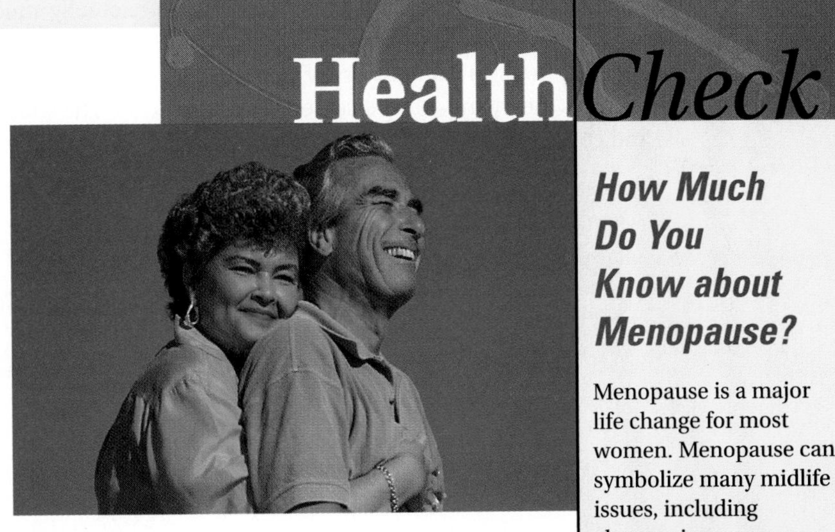

***Menopause and Sexuality***
Menopause does not mark the end of a woman's sexual life. Many postmenopausal women, in fact, feel more sexually liberated because of the freedom from concerns about unwanted pregnancies.

Mark each item as true or false. Then check the key in Appendix B at the end of the book to see what is truth and what is fiction.

| True | False | |
|---|---|---|
| ___ | ___ | 1. Menopause is abnormal. |
| ___ | ___ | 2. The medical establishment considers menopause a disease. |
| ___ | ___ | 3. After menopause, women need complete replacement of estrogen. |
| ___ | ___ | 4. Menopause is accompanied by depression and anxiety. |
| ___ | ___ | 5. At menopause, women suffer debilitating hot flashes. |
| ___ | ___ | 6. A woman who has had a hysterectomy will not undergo menopause. |
| ___ | ___ | 7. Menopause signals an end to a woman's sexual appetite. |
| ___ | ___ | 8. Menopause ends a woman's childbearing years. |
| ___ | ___ | 9. A woman's general level of activity is lower after menopause. |
| ___ | ___ | 10. Men are not affected by their wives' experience of menopause. |

Long-term estrogen deficiency can lead to **osteoporosis,** a condition involving loss of bone density that leaves bones more brittle and subject to fractures. Some women develop a bent posture called "dowager's hump." The risk of serious fractures increases, especially of the hip. Many older women never recover fully from these fractures.

Estrogen deficiency also has psychological effects. It can impair mental functioning and feelings of well-being.

**Hormone-Replacement Therapy** Some women with severe physical symptoms have been helped by **hormone-replacement therapy (HRT).** HRT typically consists of synthetic estrogen and progesterone. The hormones offset the losses of their natural counterparts. HRT may help reduce hot flushes and other symptoms of menopause. It may also prevent osteoporosis, although other treatments are available for this condition.[12] Other drugs are also available to help women with menopausal problems such as hot flashes.

HRT is controversial. Although HRT has been helpful with symptoms of menopause, some studies link the use of estrogen to an increased risk of cancers of the breast and uterus.[13] (HRT is not recommended for women with a family history of breast cancer.) On the other hand, estrogen replacement lowers a woman's risk of cardiovascular disorders (heart and artery disease), osteoporosis, and colon cancer. HRT may reduce the risk of cardiovascular disease by lowering the levels of cholesterol in the bloodstream. A study of 49,000 postmenopausal nurses found that HRT was connected with 44% fewer heart attacks and a reduced risk of death from heart disease of 39%.[14] Combination pills that contain progestin (synthetic progesterone) along with estrogen eliminate the added risk of uterine cancer and appear to provide just as much protection against heart disease as estrogen alone.[15]

**Close-up** HRT and cancer T0902

## Male Sexual Anatomy—Outside

The external male reproductive organs include the penis and the scrotum (see Figure 9.5).

**The Penis** The **penis,** like the vagina, is the sex organ used in sexual intercourse. Unlike the vagina, however, urine also passes through the penis. Semen and urine pass out of the penis through the urethral opening at the tip of the penis.

In many mammals, bones stiffen the penis to enable copulation. Despite the slang term "boner," the human penis contains no bones. Nor, despite another slang term, "muscle," does the penis contain muscle tissue. The penis is not a muscle; it is actually more like a sponge. It contains spongy material that fills with blood and stiffens, resulting in erection.

The **glans** (tip) of the penis, like the clitoral glans, is extremely sensitive to sexual stimulation.

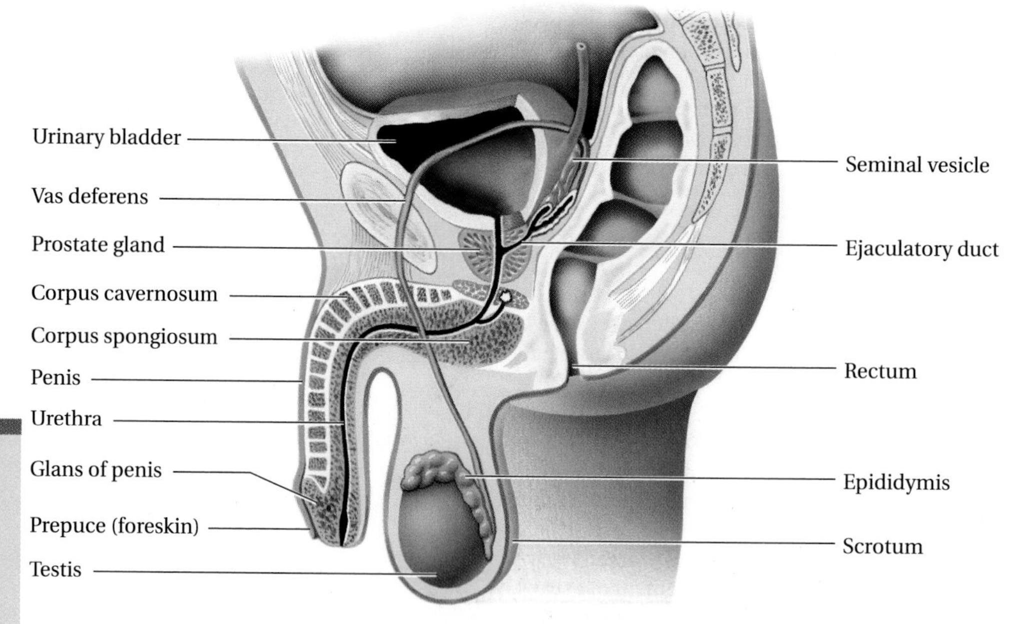


**Figure 9.5** ***The Male Reproductive System*** The external male sex organs include the penis and the scrotum.

**Osteoporosis** A condition characterized by a decline in bone density, such that bones become porous and brittle.

**Hormone-replacement therapy (HRT)** The use of artificial female sex hormones in postmenopausal women.

**Penis** The male organ that becomes erect during sexual arousal and through which sperm and urine pass.

**Glans** The head of the penis or clitoris.

So is the **corona,** or coronal ridge, that separates the glans from the body of the penis. The body of the penis is called the penile *shaft.* When sexual excitement engorges the penis with blood, the result—erection—is obvious.

Some skin of the penis, like the labia minora in the female, folds over to partially cover the glans. This covering is the prepuce, or **foreskin.** It covers part or all of the penile glans just as the clitoral prepuce (hood) covers the clitoral shaft. In the male, as in the female, a cheeselike secretion called **smegma** may accumulate below the prepuce, causing the foreskin to adhere to the glans.

The urethra is the tube through which urine passes from the bladder through the penis. Men, like women, are subject to bladder and urethral inflammations. These are generally referred to as **urethritis.** The symptoms include frequent urination (urinary frequency), a strong need to urinate (urinary urgency), burning urination, and a discharge from the penis. The urethra also may become constricted when it is inflamed, slowing or halting urination. Preventive measures for urethritis parallel those suggested for cystitis (bladder infection): drinking more water, drinking cranberry juice (four ounces, two or three times a day), and lowering intake of alcohol and caffeine. Cranberry juice is highly acidic, and its acid may help destroy the bacteria that cause urethritis.

**Circumcision** Surgical removal of the foreskin is termed **circumcision** (from Latin *circumcidere,* "to cut around"). Male circumcision has a long history as a religious rite. Jews traditionally carry out male circumcision shortly after a baby is born. Circumcision is performed as a sign of the covenant between God and the people of Abraham. Muslems also practice circumcision for religious reasons.

Circumcision is also performed by people of different faiths for hygienic reasons, although the health benefits of the practice continue to be debated. Circumcision eliminates a site where smegma might accumulate and bacteria might grow. However, regular washing can eliminate these problems. Urinary tract infections appear to be more common among uncircumcised male infants. Such infections respond to treatment, however, if they should develop. Uncircumcised men may also be at greater risk of becoming infected by HIV, the virus that causes AIDS. Cells in the foreskin may be especially susceptible to HIV infection.[16]

**The Scrotum** The **scrotum** is a pouch of loose skin that consists of two compartments that hold the testes. Sperm production is optimal at a temperature that is slightly cooler than the 98.6 degrees Fahrenheit that is desirable for most of the body. Typical scrotal temperature is several degrees lower than body temperature. The scrotum thus permits the testes to escape the higher body heat, especially in warm weather.

## Male Sexual Anatomy—Inside

The internal male reproductive organs consist of the testes, tubes, and ducts that conduct sperm through the male reproductive system, and organs that nourish and activate sperm.

**The Testes** The testes (testicles) are analogous to the ovaries. They secrete sex hormones and produce **germ cells** (from the Latin *germen,* meaning "bud"). In the case of the testes, the sex hormones are androgens (from the Greek *andros,* meaning "man," and *gene,* meaning "born") and the germ cells are **sperm.** The most important androgen is testosterone. Testosterone stimulates prenatal differentiation of male sex organs, sperm production, and development of secondary sex characteristics.

In contrast to the dramatic changes in hormone levels in women during the phases of the menstrual cycle, the hypothalamus, pituitary gland, and testes keep blood testosterone levels at a more or less even level. The same pituitary hormones that regulate the ovaries—FSH and LH—also regulate the testes. FSH induces the testes to produce sperm. LH stimulates the testes to release testosterone. Low testosterone levels in the blood signal the hypothalamus to secrete a releasing hormone. Like dominoes falling in line, the releasing hormone causes the pituitary gland to secrete LH, which in turn stimulates the testes to secrete testosterone (see Figure 9.6).

When the level of testosterone in the blood is adequate, the hypothalamus stops

**Corona** The ridge that separates the glans from the body of the penis.

**Foreskin** The loose skin that covers the penile glans.

**Smegma** A secretion that accumulates under the foreskin or around the clitoris.

**Urethritis** An inflammation of the bladder or urethra.

**Circumcision** Surgical removal of the foreskin of the penis.

**Scrotum** The pouch of loose skin that contains the testes.

**Germ cell** A cell from which a new organism develops.

**Sperm** The male germ cell.

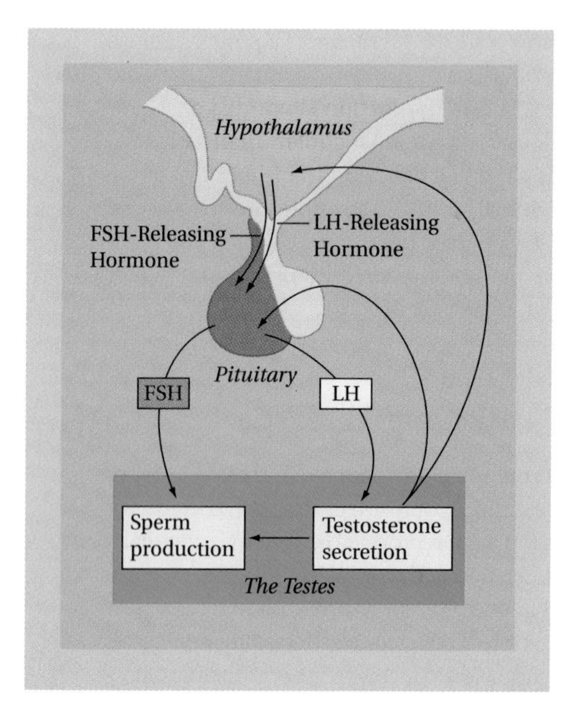


**Figure 9.6** ***Hormonal Control of the Testes*** Several endocrine glands—the hypothalamus, the pituitary gland, and testes—keep blood testosterone levels at a more or less constant level. Low testosterone levels signal the hypothalamus to secrete LH-releasing hormone. Like dominoes falling in line, LH-RH causes the pituitary gland to secrete LH, which in turn stimulates the testes to release testosterone into the blood system. Follicle-stimulating-hormone releasing hormone from the hypothalamus causes the pituitary to secrete FSH which, in turn, causes the testes to produce sperm cells.

the pituitary gland from secreting LH. This system for circling information among endocrine glands is called a *feedback loop.* This particular feedback loop is *negative.* That is, increases in hormone levels in one part of the system trigger another part to shut down, and vice versa.

The forerunners of sperm cells contain 46 chromosomes, including one X and one Y sex chromosome. Each of these divides into two mature sperm cells, with 23 chromosomes. Half have X sex chromosomes. The other half have Y sex chromosomes. Whereas ova are nearly visible, sperm cells are about $\frac{1}{5,000}$ of an inch long, one of the smallest cells in the body. The testes churn out about 1,000 sperm per second, or some 30 billion—yes, *billion*—per year. Sperm proceed within the testis (testicle) through a maze of ducts that converge in a single tube called the **epididymis.** The epididymis lies against the back wall of the testicle and serves as a storage facility. Sperm continue to mature in the epididymis.

**Epididymis** A tube that lies against the back wall of each testicle and serves as a storage facility for sperm.

**Vas deferens** A tube that conducts sperm from the testicle to the ejaculatory duct of the penis.

**Vasectomy** A sterilization procedure in which both vas deferens are severed, preventing sperm from reaching the ejaculatory duct.

**Seminal vesicles** Small glands that lie behind the bladder and secrete fluids that combine with sperm in the ejaculatory ducts.

**Ejaculatory ducts** Ducts through which sperm pass through the prostate gland and into the urethra.

**The Vas Deferens** Each epididymis empties into a **vas deferens.** The vas is a thin tube about 16 inches long. A **vasectomy** is an operation in which the right and left vas deferens are severed, rendering the man infertile since sperm have no way of getting through and out of the penis. They are simply, harmlessly, absorbed into the body. The vas leaves the scrotum, follows a path up into the abdominal cavity, then loops back along the surface of the bladder (see Figure 9.7).

**Talking Glossary**
Vas deferens
G0914

**The Seminal Vesicles** The two **seminal vesicles** are small glands that lie behind the bladder. They open into the **ejaculatory ducts,** where the

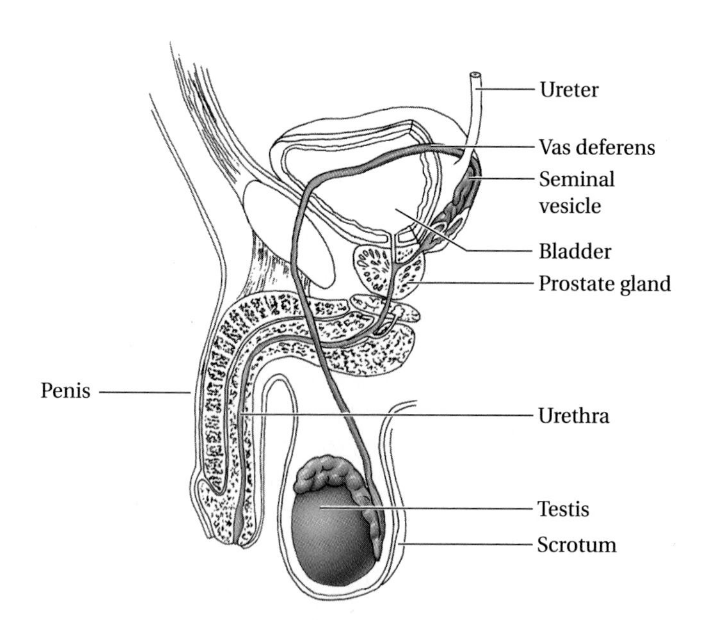


**Figure 9.7** ***Passage of Spermatozoa*** Throughout the course of a lifetime, hundreds of billions of sperm are produced and stored by threadlike tubules within the testes. During ejaculation, sperm cells travel through the vas deferens, up and over the bladder, into the ejaculatory duct, and then through the urethra. Secretions from the seminal vesicles, the prostate, and other glands join with sperm to compose semen.

fluids they secrete combine with sperm. Fluid produced by the seminal vesicles is rich in fructose, a sugar that nourishes sperm and helps them become active, or motile. Sperm motility is a major factor in male fertility. Once sperm become motile, they propel themselves by whipping their tails.

At the base of the bladder, each vas deferens joins a seminal vesicle to form a short ejaculatory duct that runs through the prostate gland. In the prostate the ejaculatory duct opens into the urethra, which leads to the tip of the penis. The urethra carries sperm and urine out through the penis, but not at the same time.

**The Prostate Gland** The **prostate gland** lies beneath the bladder and is chestnut-like in shape and size. The prostate gland secretes a milky and alkaline fluid that makes up part of the **semen,** or seminal fluid. Sperm and the fluids contributed by the seminal vesicles and other glands are also found in the semen (ejaculate), the whitish fluid expelled during ejaculation.

A vasectomy prevents sperm from reaching the urethra but does not cut off fluids from the seminal vesicles or prostate gland. A man who has had a vasectomy thus emits an ejaculate that appears normal but contains no sperm.

Many infectious agents can inflame the prostate, causing **prostatitis.** The chief symptoms are an ache or pain between the scrotum and anal opening and painful ejaculation. Prostatitis is usually treated with antibiotics. Other conditions affecting the prostate include prostate enlargement (a common occurrence in men as they age) and prostate cancer, both of which are discussed in Chapter 18.

## Manopause (*Man*opause)?

Men cannot undergo menopause; they have never menstruated. Yet one now and then hears of a "male menopause," or "*man*opause." Some older men are loosely referred to as menopausal. Sadly, this description is usually meant to convey the negative, harmful stereotype of the aging person as crotchety and irritable. Such stereotypes are not consistent with the biology or psychology of aging.

The scientific jury is still out on the existence of a male menopause. Women encounter a relatively sudden age-related decline in sex hormones and fertility during menopause. Men experience a gradual decline in testosterone levels as they age. There is nothing comparable to the sharp plunge in estrogen levels that women experience during menopause. Testosterone levels begin to fall in the forties. They may decline to one-third or one-half of their peak levels by age 80.

The drop in testosterone levels among older men may be connected with age-related symptoms such as reduced muscle mass and strength, accumulation of body fat, reduced energy levels, lowered fertility, and reduced erectile ability. However, despite a decline in testosterone levels, most men can attain erections throughout their lives.

Testosterone replacement may help avert erectile problems, bone loss, and frailty in much the same way that estrogen replacement benefits postmenopausal women.[17] But some health professionals worry that excessive use of testosterone may increase the risks of prostate cancer and cardiovascular disease.

Men experience a gradual decline in the number and motility of sperm as they age, which reduces their fertility. However, some viable sperm continue to be produced even in late adulthood. It is not surprising, biologically speaking, to find a man in his seventies or older fathering a child. Men can remain sexually active and father children at advanced ages. For both genders, marital satisfaction and attitudes toward aging can affect sexual behavior and self-esteem as profoundly as physical changes.

### think about it!

- **What kinds of health problems may affect your reproductive organs? What are you doing to prevent these problems?**
- **What were your beliefs about menstrual problems and menopause? Does the information in this section contradict any of your beliefs?**

**critical thinking** **Had you heard of "manopause"? Is there evidence for the existence of manopause?**

Smart Quiz
Q0902

**Prostate gland** The gland that lies beneath the bladder and secretes prostatic fluid, which gives semen its characteristic odor and texture.

**Semen** The whitish fluid that constitutes the ejaculate, consisting of sperm and glandular secretions.

**Prostatitis** Inflammation of the prostate gland.

# SEXUAL RESPONSE AND PRACTICES

What happens to our bodies when we are sexually aroused? How are men and women alike in their sexual response? How do they differ? What are the varieties of sexual experience people seek to find sexual gratification?

## The Sexual Response Cycle

The physical changes that take place as people become aroused are referred to as the **sexual response cycle.** Famed sex researchers William Masters and Virginia Johnson[18] divided the cycle into four phases: *excitement, plateau, orgasm,* and *resolution.*

Men and women both respond early in the sexual response cycle with vasocongestion and myotonia. **Vasocongestion** is the swelling of the genital tissues with blood. It causes erection of the penis and engorgement of the area surrounding the vaginal opening. The testes, nipples, even the earlobes become engorged as blood vessels in these areas dilate. Figures 9.8 and 9.9 show the physiological changes that occur during the phases of the sexual response cycle in men and women.

**Talking Glossary**
Vasocongestion
G0915

**Myotonia** is muscle tension. Myotonia causes facial grimaces, spasms in the hands and feet, and eventually, the spasms of orgasm. Let us follow the changes that make up the sexual response cycle.

**Excitement** Vasocongestion during the **excitement phase** produces erection in men. The testes increase in size. The testes and scrotum become elevated.

In women, vaginal lubrication may start 10 to 30 seconds after stimulation begins. Vasocongestion swells the clitoris, flattens and spreads the labia majora, and expands the labia minora. The inner two-thirds of the vagina expand. The vaginal walls thicken. Because of the inflow of blood, they turn from their normal pink to a deeper hue. The uterus becomes engorged and elevated. The breasts enlarge.

The nipples may become erect in both genders, especially in response to direct stim-

**Sexual response cycle** The four-phase model of sexual response.

**Vasocongestion** The swelling of the genital tissues with blood, which causes erection of the penis and engorgement of the area surrounding the vaginal opening.

**Myotonia** Muscle tension.

**Excitement phase** The first phase of the sexual response cycle, characterized by erection in the male, vaginal lubrication in the female, and muscle tension and heart rate increases in males and females.

**Figure 9.8** *The Male Genitals During the Phases of the Sexual Response Cycle*

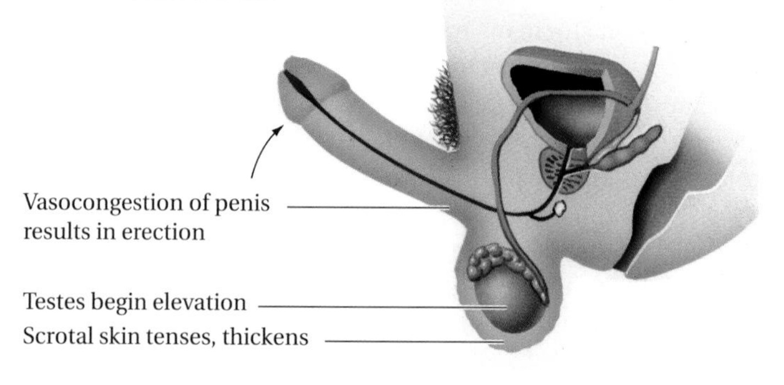
1. EXCITEMENT PHASE
Vasocongestion of penis results in erection
Testes begin elevation
Scrotal skin tenses, thickens

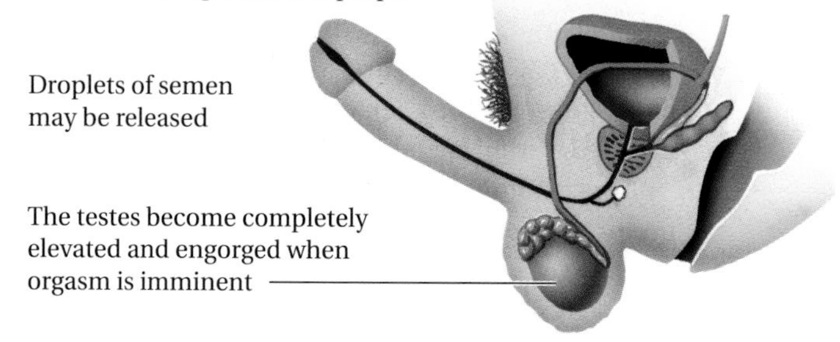
2. PLATEAU PHASE
The coronal ridge of the glans increases in diameter and turns a deeper reddish purple
Droplets of semen may be released
The testes become completely elevated and engorged when orgasm is imminent

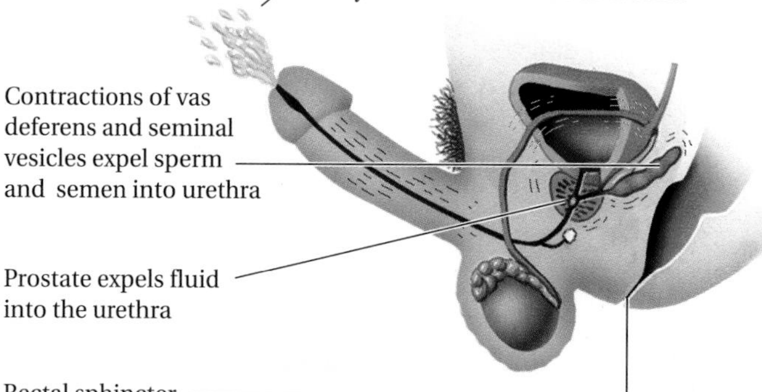
3. ORGASM PHASE
Sperm and semen expelled by rhythmic contractions of urethra
Contractions of vas deferens and seminal vesicles expel sperm and semen into urethra
Prostate expels fluid into the urethra
Rectal sphincter contracts

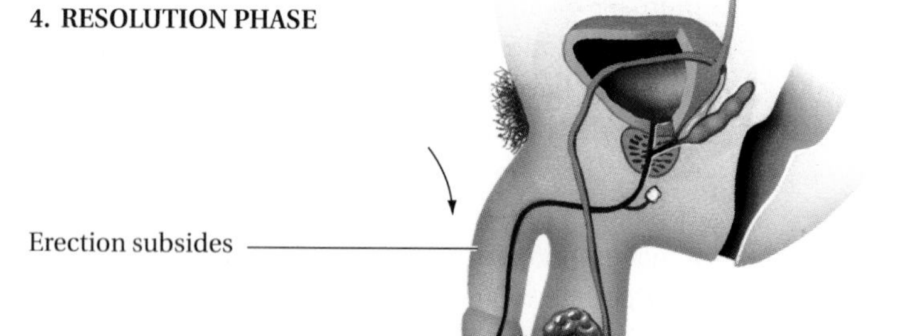
4. RESOLUTION PHASE
Erection subsides
Testes descend
Scrotum thins, folds return

**Figure 9.9** ***The Female Genitals During the Phases of the Sexual Response Cycle***

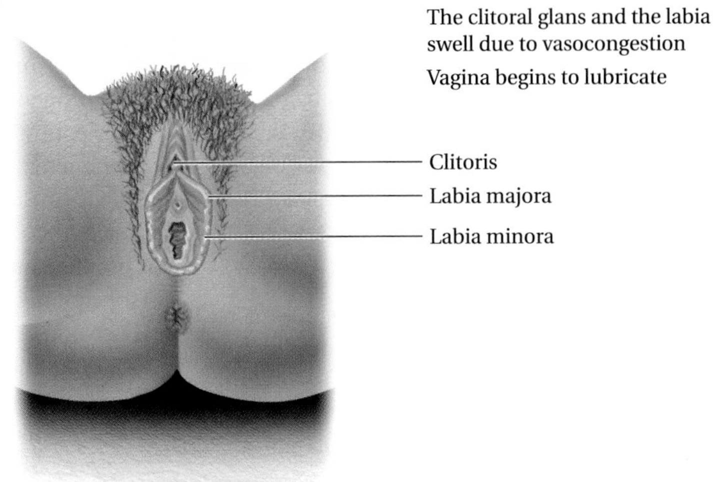
The clitoral glans and the labia swell due to vasocongestion
Vagina begins to lubricate
Clitoris
Labia majora
Labia minora
1. EXCITEMENT PHASE

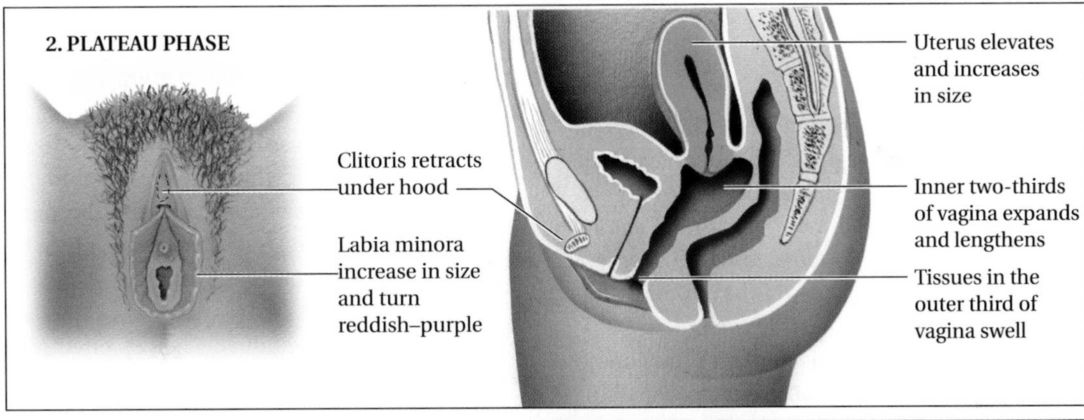
2. PLATEAU PHASE
Clitoris retracts under hood
Labia minora increase in size and turn reddish–purple
Uterus elevates and increases in size
Inner two-thirds of vagina expands and lengthens
Tissues in the outer third of vagina swell

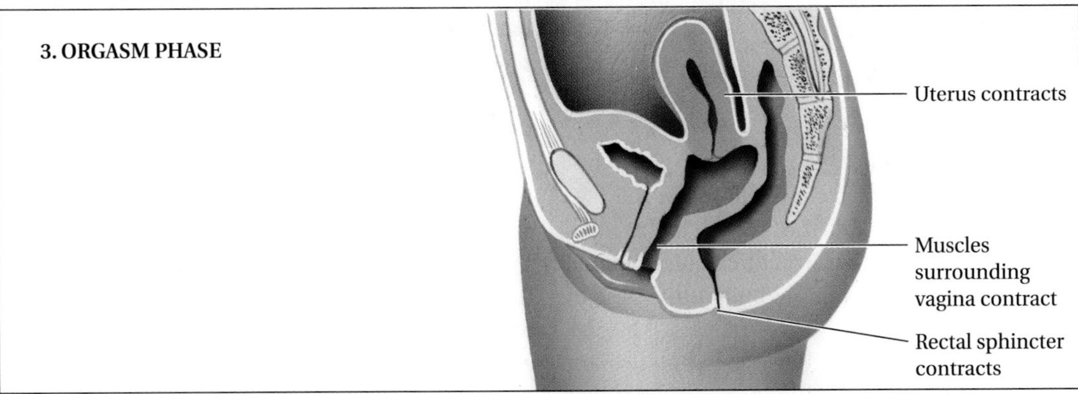
3. ORGASM PHASE
Uterus contracts
Muscles surrounding vagina contract
Rectal sphincter contracts

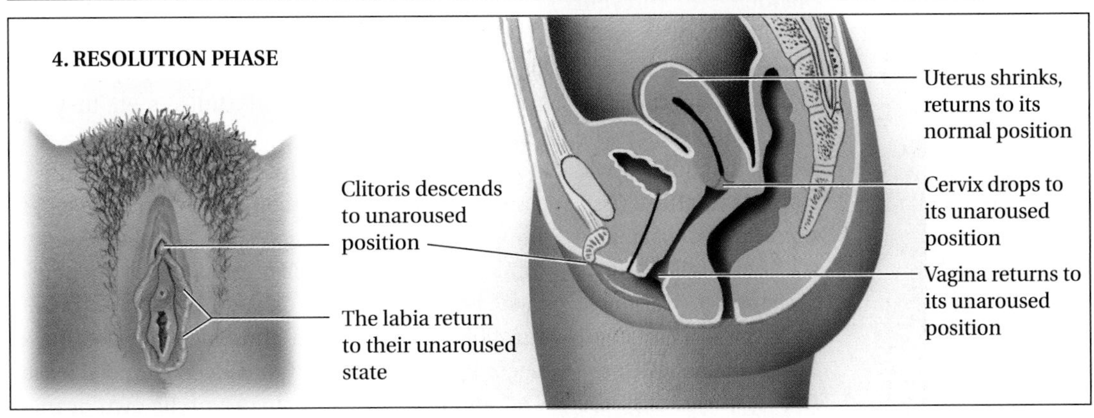
4. RESOLUTION PHASE
Clitoris descends to unaroused position
The labia return to their unaroused state
Uterus shrinks, returns to its normal position
Cervix drops to its unaroused position
Vagina returns to its unaroused position

ulation. Men and women show some increase in myotonia, heart rate, and blood pressure.

Erection and vaginal lubrication are reflexes. People set the stage for these reflexes by participating in sexual activity or engaging in sexual fantasy. (The brain is really the primary sex organ.) But erection and lubrication are involuntary. They cannot be forced or willed.

**Plateau** The level of sexual arousal remains somewhat constant during the **plateau phase** of sexual response, the phase that precedes orgasm. The tip of the penis turns a purplish hue, a sign of vasocongestion. The testes are elevated further into position for ejaculation. Droplets of sperm-carrying seminal fluid are secreted and found at the tip of the penis. This is why women can become pregnant even if the man doesn't ejaculate.

In women, vasocongestion swells the tissues of the outer third of the vagina. The inner part of the vagina expands fully. The uterus becomes fully elevated. The clitoris withdraws beneath the clitoral hood and shortens. The labia minora become a deep wine color in women who have borne children, bright red in women who have not.

Myotonia may cause spasmodic contractions in the hands and feet and facial grimaces. Breathing becomes rapid, like panting. The heart rate may increase to between 100 and 160 beats a minute. Blood pressure continues to rise.

**Orgasm** In the male, the **orgasmic phase** has two stages of muscular contractions. In the first stage, contractions of the vas deferens, the prostate gland, and other structures cause seminal fluid to collect in the urethral bulb at the base of the penis. Muscles close off the urinary bladder to prevent urine from mixing with semen. The collection of semen in the urethral bulb produces the feeling that nothing will stop ejaculation. This sensation of ejaculatory inevitability lasts perhaps 2 to 3 seconds.

In the second stage, contractions of muscles surrounding the urethra and urethral bulb and the base of the penis propel the ejaculate through the urethra and out of the body. Sensations of pleasure tend to be related to the strength of the contractions and the amount of semen. The first few contractions are most intense.

In the female, orgasm involves contractions of the pelvic muscles that surround the vagina. As in the male, the contractions release sexual tension and produce intense feelings of pleasure.

Orgasm, like erection and lubrication, is a reflex. We can set the stage for orgasm through erotic stimulation, but orgasm cannot be forced or willed. In both genders, orgasm is accompanied by muscle spasms throughout the body. Blood pressure and heart rate reach their peaks. The heart beats up to 180 times a minute. The sensations of orgasm have challenged the descriptive powers of poets. Words like "rush," "warmth," "explosion," and "release" do not adequately capture them.

**Resolution** The **resolution phase** follows orgasm. In this phase, the body returns to its prearoused state. Following ejaculation, the man loses his erection. The testes and scrotum return to normal size. The scrotum regains its wrinkled appearance.

In women, blood gradually leaves engorged areas. The swelling of the areolas decreases. The nipples return to normal size. The clitoris, vagina, uterus, and labia gradually shrink to their prearoused sizes. The labia minora turn lighter.

Most muscle tension (myotonia) dissipates within 5 minutes after orgasm in both men and women. Blood pressure, heart rate, and respiration return to normal within a few minutes. Both men and women may feel relaxed and satisfied.

There is an important gender difference during the resolution phase. Unlike women, men enter a **refractory period.** In this period, they cannot experience another orgasm or ejaculation. The refractory period of adolescent males may last only minutes. That of men age 50 and above may last from several minutes to a day. Women do not undergo a refractory period. Unlike men, they are capable of becoming quickly rearoused to the point of repeated (multiple) orgasms.

Myotonia and vasocongestion may take an hour or more to dissipate in people who are aroused but do not reach orgasm. Persistent pelvic vasocongestion may cause unpleasant pelvic throbbing in both men and women if they have become highly aroused and do not find release. The unpleasantness dissipates on its own or may be relieved through masturbation.

**Plateau phase** The second phase of the sexual response cycle, characterized by increases in vasocongestion, muscle tension, heart rate, and blood pressure in preparation for orgasm.

**Orgasmic phase** The third phase of the sexual response cycle, characterized by the rhythmic contractions of orgasm.

**Resolution phase** The fourth phase of the sexual response cycle, during which the body gradually returns to its prearoused state.

**Refractory period** A period of time following a response (e.g., orgasm) during which an individual is no longer responsive to stimulation (e.g., sexual stimulation).

## Varieties of Sexual Experience

**Take Charge**
Talking to your kids about sex
**C0901**

There is great variety in human sexual expression. Some of us practice few, if any, of the techniques in this chapter. Some of us practice most or all of them. Some of us practice some of them some of the time. Our aim is to describe the diversity of sexual expression and to note some behavior patterns that are unhealthful.

The human body is sensitive to many forms of sexual stimulation. Yet biology is not destiny. A biological capacity does not impose a behavioral requirement. Cultural expectations, personal values, knowledge of health, and individual experience—not only our biological capacities—determine our sexual behavior. What is right for you may not necessarily be right for your neighbor.

### Masturbation

The word *masturbation* derives from the Latin *masturbari,* from the roots for "hand" and "to defile." The derivation provides clues to cultural attitudes toward the practice. **Masturbation** may be practiced by manual (hand) stimulation of the genitals, perhaps with the aid of artificial stimulation, such as a vibrator. Even before we conceive of sexual experiences with others, we may learn early in childhood that touching our genitals can produce pleasure.

According to the findings of the National Health and Social Life Survey (NHSLS), conducted by researchers at the University of Chicago, there are numerous reasons people masturbate, ranging from lack of a partner to help in getting to sleep to fear of AIDS.[19]

Until recent years masturbation was thought to be physically and mentally harmful, as well as morally degrading. Many eighteenth-century physicians, including Benjamin Rush (a signer of the Declaration of Independence), believed that masturbation caused tuberculosis, "nervous diseases," poor eyesight, memory loss, and epilepsy.

In the nineteenth-century United States, medical advice was largely disseminated to the general public through pamphlets and guides written by leading medical authorities. One of the more influential writers was the superintendent of the Battle Creek Sanatorium in Michigan, Dr. J. H. Kellogg (1852–1943). He is better known to you as the creator of the modern breakfast cereal. Kellogg identified 39 signs of masturbation, including acne, paleness, heart palpitations, rounded shoulders, weak backs, and convulsions. Kellogg believed that sexual desires could be controlled by a diet of simple foods, especially grains, including the corn flakes that have since borne his name.

Despite this history, there is no scientific evidence that masturbation is harmful to health. Masturbation does not cause insanity, grow hair on the hands, or cause warts or any of the other ills once ascribed to it. Masturbation is physically harmless, save for rare injuries to the genitals due to rough stimulation. Nor is masturbation in itself psychologically harmful. Masturbation *may* be a sign of an adjustment problem if people use it as an exclusive sexual outlet when opportunities for sexual relationships are available.

Of course, people who consider masturbation wrong, harmful, or sinful may experience anxiety or guilt if they masturbate or think about masturbating. These negative emotions are linked to their attitudes toward masturbation, not to masturbation per se.

Despite the widespread condemnation of masturbation in our society, surveys indicate that most adults masturbate at some time. The incidence of masturbation is generally greater among men than women.[20] Despite the loosening of traditional sexual restraints a generation or two ago during the so-called sexual revolution, engaging in sexual activity only for pleasure may still be more of a taboo for women than for men.[21]

Married people are less likely to have masturbated during the past 12 months than never-married and formerly married people. Nevertheless, only 43% of the married men and 63% of the married women sampled said that they did not masturbate at all during the past year.

**Kissing** Kissing is a nearly universal form of foreplay. **Foreplay** refers to sexual activities that are intended to arouse partners so that they can engage in sexual intercourse. Other forms of foreplay include cuddling, touching, petting, even oral sex. Women usually prefer longer periods of foreplay (and "afterplay") than men do. Kissing, genital touching, and oral sex may also be experienced as ends in themselves, not as preludes to intercourse.

Kissing may also be an affectionate gesture without erotic significance, as in kissing someone good night. Some people kiss relatives and close friends affectionately on the lips. Others limit kissing relatives to the cheek. Sustained

**Masturbation** Sexual self-stimulation.

**Foreplay** Physical interactions that are sexually stimulating and set the stage for intercourse.

kissing on the lips and tongue kissing are almost always erotic gestures.

**Oral Sex** Oral stimulation of the male genitals is called **fellatio.** Oral stimulation of the female genitals is called **cunnilingus.** Oral sex has entered the mainstream of sexual practices among contemporary couples. According to the recent national survey, about three of four men (77%) and two of three women (68%) have taken the active role in oral sex.[22] Nearly four men in five (79%) and three women in four (73%) report having been on the receiving end of oral sex at some point during their lifetimes. Oral sex has become the norm among today's married couples; 80% of the men and 71% of the women report engaging in oral sex with their partners.

Talking Glossary
Fellatio, Cunnilingus
G0916

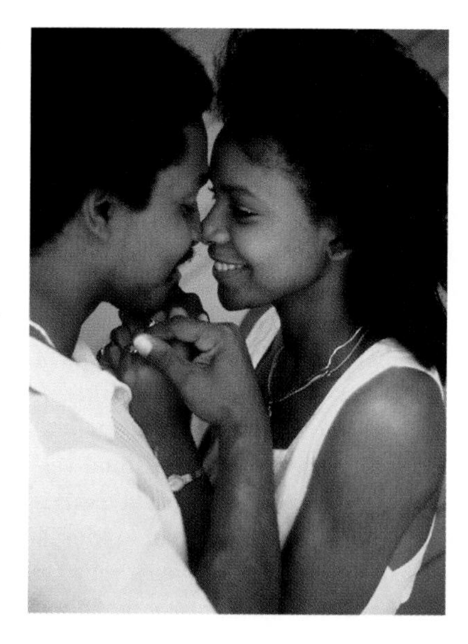

***A Touching Experience*** Touching is not only a form of sexual foreplay but also a means of expressing tenderness, caring, and love.

**Sexual Intercourse** The number of positions for sexual intercourse (also called **coitus**) is virtually endless. We will focus on four of the most commonly used positions: the male-superior (man-on-top) position, the female-superior (woman-on-top) position, the lateral-entry (side-entry) position, and the rear-entry position.

In the male-superior position ("superiority" is used purely in relation to body position, but it has sometimes been taken as a symbol of male domination), the partners face each other. The man lies above the woman. (He should support himself on his hands and knees rather than applying his full weight against his partner.) Movement is easier for the man than for the woman, which may suggest that he is in charge.

It may be preferable for the woman rather than the man to guide the penis into the vagina. The woman can feel the location of the vaginal opening and determine the angle of entry. Entry is thus more likely to be comfortable for her. The male-superior position is not advisable during the late stages of pregnancy, when the man's body would place pressure against the woman's abdomen.

In the female-superior position, the couple face each other with the woman on top. The woman straddles the man. She controls the angle of entry and the depth of thrusting. Some women maintain a sitting position; others lie on top of their partners. Many women vary their position. In the female-superior position, the woman is psychologically, and to some degree physically, in charge. She can move as rapidly or as slowly as she wishes. She can adjust the angle and depth of penetration. Many women find it easier to achieve orgasm in this position. Men may also experience better control over ejaculation in this position.

In the lateral-entry position, the man and woman face one another, side by side. This position allows each partner relatively free movement. They can easily kiss each other and stroke one another's bodies. The position is not taxing, because both partners are supported by the bedding. Thus it is an excellent position for prolonging intercourse or for couples who are tired.

In the rear-entry position, the man faces the woman's rear. The woman usually supports herself on her hands and knees. The man supports himself on his knees, entering her from behind. The rear-entry position may be highly stimulating for both partners.

Some people object to the rear-entry position because it is the mating position used by most other mammals. The position is also impersonal in the sense that the partners do not face one another, which may create a sense of emotional distance. Since the man is at the woman's back, the couple may feel that he is very much in charge. He can see her, but she cannot readily see him. Physically, the penis may not provide enough direct stimulation of the clitoris. He (or she) may reach underneath to provide direct clitoral stimulation by use of the hand. Many couples alternate positions during intercourse to heighten their sensations.

**Fellatio** Oral stimulation of the male genitals.

**Cunnilingus** Oral stimulation of the female genitals.

**Coitus** Sexual intercourse.

**Anal Sex** **Anal intercourse** can be practiced by male-female couples and male-male couples. It involves insertion of the penis into the rectum. The rectum is highly sensitive to sexual stimulation. Both women and men may reach orgasm through anal sex. Rectal tissues are more sensitive than vaginal tissues to penetration, so couples need to use ample lubrication and avoid thrusting too vigorously.

Anal intercourse is also referred to as "Greek culture," or sex in the "Greek style," because of bisexuality in ancient Greece among males. It is also the major act that comes under the legal definition of *sodomy.* Many couples are repulsed by the idea of anal sex. They view it as unnatural, immoral, or risky. Others find anal sex to be an enjoyable sexual variation, though perhaps not a regular activity.

The recent national survey, the NHSLS, found that one man in four (26%) and one woman in five (20%) reported engaging in anal sex at some time during their lives.[23] Yet only about one person in ten (10% of the men and 9% of the women) had engaged in anal sex during the past year.

Some couples kiss or lick the anus in their foreplay. This practice is called **anilingus.** Oral–anal sex carries a serious health risk, however. Microorganisms causing intestinal diseases and many sexually transmitted diseases can be spread through oral–anal contact.

Talking Glossary
Anilingus
G0917

Many couples avoid anal sex because of the fear of AIDS and other sexually transmitted diseases (STDs). Many STDs can be spread by anal intercourse, because small tears in the rectal tissues may allow the microbes to enter the recipient's bloodstream. Women also incur a greater risk of contracting HIV, the virus that causes AIDS, from anal intercourse than from vaginal intercourse—just as receptive anal intercourse in gay men carries a high risk of infection.[24] However, monogamous partners who are both infection-free are at no risk of contracting HIV or other STD-causing organisms through any sexual act. HIV and other STD-causing organisms can be transmitted only by people who are infected with them. But people who are uncertain whether their partners are infected would be prudent to avoid anal sex, or at least to use a latex condom and a spermicide that can kill the AIDS virus. Further guidelines for reducing the risk of STDs, including AIDS, are provided in Chapter 16.

In sum, our bodies can respond to many forms of sexual stimulation. Whether we engage in some, many, or all of the techniques described here, or whether we remain **celibate,** reflects many factors, especially our personal needs, desires, and values.

### think about it!

- **Are you surprised to learn that erection, vaginal lubrication, and orgasm are reflexes? Why?**
- **What were your beliefs about masturbation before reading this section? Has the information presented altered your views? How?**
- **How does your choice of sexual practices reflect your personal values?**

Smart Quiz
Q0903

## SEXUAL ORIENTATION

**Sexual orientation** refers to the direction of one's erotic interests. **Heterosexuals** are sexually attracted to, and interested in forming romantic relationships with, people of the other gender. **Gay males** and **lesbians** are sexually attracted to, and interested in forming romantic relationships with, people of their own gender. **Bisexuals** are sexually attracted to, and interested in forming romantic relationships with, both women and men. Research in the United States, Britain, France, and Denmark finds that about 3% of men surveyed identify themselves as gay.[25] About 2% of the U.S. women surveyed consider themselves lesbians.

The concept of *sexual orientation* is not to be confused with *sexual activity.* Sexual orientation is not a matter of choice; one does not choose to be homosexual any more than one chooses to be heterosexual. However, one *does* choose whether to engage in sexual activity, whether with a same-sex partner or an opposite-sex partner. Nor does sexual activity

**Anal intercourse** A sexual practice involving insertion of the penis into the rectum of either a male or female partner.

**Anilingus** Oral–anal sexual stimulation.

**Celibacy** Abstinence from sexual activity.

**Sexual orientation** The direction of one's sexual interests—toward members of the same gender, the opposite gender, or both genders.

**Heterosexuals** People who are erotically attracted to, and who prefer to have romantic relationships with, members of the opposite gender.

**Gay males** Male homosexuals.

**Lesbians** Female homosexuals.

**Bisexuals** People who are erotically attracted to, and have interest in developing romantic relationships with, both men and women.

with members of one's own gender necessarily mean that one has a gay male or lesbian sexual orientation. Male–male sexual behavior may reflect limited sexual opportunities or even ritualistic cultural practices, as in the case of the Sambians, a tribe in New Guinea. American adolescent males may manually stimulate one another while fantasizing about girls. Men in prisons may similarly turn to each other as sexual outlets. Sambian male youths engage in sexual practices with older males exclusively, since it is believed that they must drink "men's milk" to achieve the fierce manhood of their tribe. Their sexual activities are limited to female partners once they reach marrying age, however.

## Origins of Sexual Orientation

The origins of sexual orientation remain obscure. The originator of psychoanalysis, Sigmund Freud, believed that a heterosexual orientation arises from a "normal" process of identification with the parent of the same sex, whereas homosexuality derives from an overidentification with the parent of the other sex. In men, this is believed to stem from a "classic pattern" of child rearing in which there is a "close binding" mother and a "detached hostile" father. Boys reared in such a home environment would be expected to identify more strongly with their mothers than their fathers. Within this view, gay men would be expected to be effeminate and disdain traditional masculine interests. Though the backgrounds of some gay men (as well as some heterosexual men) conform to the "classic" pattern, many do not. Moreover, there is much variation in gender-role patterns of gay men and women. Only a minority conform to the stereotypes that Freud expected.

Learning theorists believe that early reinforcement of sexual behavior (as by orgasm achieved through interaction with members of one's own gender) can influence one's sexual orientation. Though we cannot discount the potential role of learning experiences in shaping one's developing sexual orientation, we should recognize that many gay males and lesbians were aware of their sexual orientation before they had any sexual experience with other people.[26]

Biological models, which focus on an interplay of genetic and hormonal factors, have gained more favor in recent years. Heredity may have something to do with sexual orientation. Researchers find that identical (MZ) twins have a higher agreement rate for a gay male sexual orientation (52%) than do fraternal (DZ) twins (22%).[27] Since MZ twins share 100% of their genes, compared with a 50% overlap among fraternal twins, the higher concordance rate among MZ twins supports the belief that genes play a role.

We also know that prenatal sex hormones can masculinize or feminize the brains of laboratory animals in ways that direct the development of brain structures. Perhaps prenatal sex hormones in humans affect sexual orientation before birth by affecting the differentiation of the developing brain. Drugs (such as androgens) and maternal stress could also be involved. Why maternal stress? Stress causes the release of hormones such as adrenaline. Since stress hormones can interact with testosterone and affect the prenatal development of the brain, it's possible that hormonal effects may have prenatally feminized the brains of some gay males and masculinized the brains of some lesbians.[28] These views are intriguing but remain speculative in the absence of direct evidence that prenatal hormones are involved in determining sexual orientation.

Some evidence does point to structural differences between the brains of heterosexual and gay men. Researchers who conducted autopsies on the brains of men believed to be homosexual and heterosexual, all of whom had died of AIDS, found that a segment of the hypothalamus in the brains of the gay men was less than half the size of the same segment in the heterosexual men.[29] The same brain segment was larger in the brain tissues of heterosexual men than in those of a comparison group of six apparently heterosexual women. No meaningful differences in size were found between brain tissues of the women and the homosexual men, however. Might these structural differences in the brains of gay men and heterosexual men upon autopsy date back to prenatal development, perhaps reflecting the influence of prenatal sex hormones sculpting the brain in one direction or the other? It is too early to say. We should also note that the fact that AIDS was involved might have been a confounding factor.

The determinants of sexual orientation remain mysterious and complex. Research suggests that they may involve prenatal hormone levels—which can be affected by factors such as heredity, drugs, and maternal stress—and possible early learning experiences. However, the precise interaction of these influences remains obscure.

**Close-up**
Sexual orientation
**T0903**

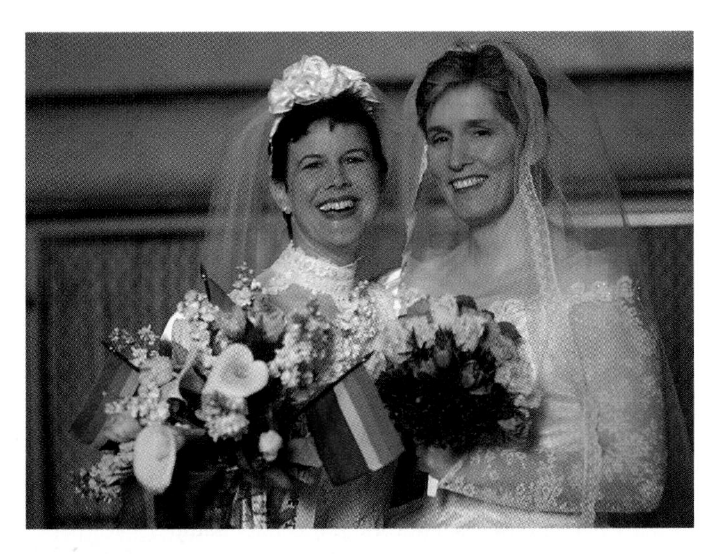

***A Sign of the Times*** The legal basis of gay marriages continues to be debated. Whatever the legal outcome, gay couples who exchange marital vows consider themselves to be just as committed to each other as do heterosexual couples.

### Adjustment of Gay Males and Lesbians

**Close-up** Homosexuality: A mental disorder? T0904

Gay men and lesbians are not more emotionally unstable or subject to more psychological disorders (like anxiety and depression) than other people.[30] Having a gay or bisexual sexual identity is not considered a psychological disorder, any more than having an exclusively heterosexual orientation.

Gay men, lesbians, and bisexuals occupy all socioeconomic and vocational levels. Gay people who live with partners in stable, intimate relationships are about as well adjusted as married heterosexuals. Older gay people who live alone and have few sexual contacts tend to be less well adjusted. So, too, are many heterosexual people with similar lifestyles. All in all, differences in adjustment are more likely to reflect one's lifestyle than one's sexual orientation.

**Smart Quiz** Q0904

**think about it!**

- **Does it surprise you that gay males and lesbians are as well adjusted (or poorly adjusted) as heterosexuals? Why or why not?**

**critical thinking** **Do you believe that you chose your sexual orientation at some point in your life? Why or why not?**

## SEXUAL DYSFUNCTIONS

Sexual dysfunctions involve problems with sexual interest, arousal, or response. Many of us are troubled by sexual problems from time to time. Men occasionally have problems achieving an erection or ejaculate sooner than they or their partners would like. Most women occasionally have problems lubricating or reaching orgasm. When such problems become persistent and distressing, they are classified as **sexual dysfunctions.**

The NHSLS, a recent national survey, found that many types of sexual dysfunctions are quite common (see Table 9.2). Women overall were more likely to report lack of interest in sex, painful sex, lack of sexual pleasure, and inability to reach orgasm. Men were more likely to report reaching climax too early and being anxious about their performance. The NHSLS figures represent *persistent current* problems. Many more people have occasional problems. Or they had these problems at some point during their lives but not presently.

**TABLE 9.2**

**Current Sexual Problems**[31]

| | Percentage of respondents reporting the problem within the past year | |
|---|---|---|
| | **Men** | **Women** |
| Pain during sex | 3 | 14 |
| Sex not pleasurable | 8 | 21 |
| Unable to reach orgasm | 8 | 24 |
| Lack of interest in sex | 16 | 33 |
| Anxiety about performance* | 17 | 12 |
| Reaching climax too early | 29 | 10 |
| Unable to keep an erection | 10 | — |
| Having trouble lubricating | — | 19 |

*Anxiety about performance is not itself a sexual dysfunction. However, it figures prominently in sexual dysfunctions.

### Types of Sexual Dysfunctions

Health professionals group sexual dysfunctions into four categories:[32]

1. *Sexual desire disorders.* These are defined by lack of sexual desire or aversion to sex. Lack of sexual desire is about twice as common in women as in men. Nevertheless, the belief that all men are always eager and willing is a myth.

**Sexual dysfunctions** Persistent difficulties with sexual interest, arousal, or response.

2. *Sexual arousal disorders.* In men, sexual arousal disorders involve problems in achieving or maintaining erections. In women, these disorders involve problems in becoming sexually aroused or adequately lubricated. Disorders in sexual arousal were once labeled *impotence* in the male and *frigidity* in the female. Because these terms carry pejorative connotations, professionals prefer using more descriptive labels for these disorders: **male erectile disorder** and **female sexual arousal disorder.**
3. *Orgasm disorders.* Men or women may have problems reaching orgasm. Or they may reach orgasm sooner than they or their partners would like. In **female orgasmic disorder** or **male orgasmic disorder,** people have problems reaching orgasm or cannot reach it at all. A person who reaches orgasm through masturbation or oral sex may not necessarily be able to reach orgasm with a partner. Women are more likely to experience these kinds of problems. Another type of orgasm disorder in males, **premature ejaculation,** was the most common male sexual dysfunction reported in the NHSLS study. Nearly 3 men in 10 experience this disorder (see Table 9.2).
4. *Sexual pain disorders.* Sexual pain disorders include dyspareunia and vaginismus. Both men and women, but more commonly women, may suffer from **dyspareunia** (painful intercourse). Women may experience vaginismus. Dyspareunia is a common complaint of women seeking gynecological services and often stems from gynecological infections. **Vaginismus** involves an involuntary contraction of the muscles surrounding the vagina during attempts at penetration, making intercourse painful or preventing it altogether. Vaginismus is a psychological problem that often stems from a history of sexual trauma, such as rape or child sexual abuse.

**Male erectile disorder** Persistent difficulty achieving or maintaining an erection sufficient to allow the man to engage in or complete sexual intercourse.

**Female sexual arousal disorder** Persistent difficulty in becoming sexually aroused, denoted by a lack of vaginal lubrication in response to sexual stimulation.

**Female orgasmic disorder** Inability or persistent difficulty achieving orgasm.

**Male orgasmic disorder** Inability or persistent difficulty achieving orgasm.

**Premature ejaculation** A sexual dysfunction in which ejaculation occurs too rapidly or with minimal sexual stimulation.

**Dyspareunia** Painful intercourse.

**Vaginismus** A sexual dysfunction characterized by involuntary contraction of the muscles surrounding the vagina, preventing penile penetration or rendering penetration painful.

## Causes of Sexual Dysfunctions

Some sexual dysfunctions stem completely or mostly from biological causes. Others are caused mainly by psychosocial factors such as sexual anxieties and marital dissatisfaction. Still others involve a combination of biological and psychosocial factors.

**Biological Causes** Sexual desire is stoked by testosterone, which is produced by men in the testes and by both genders in the adrenal glands. Yes, women produce small amounts of testosterone. The testes in men also produce small amounts of the female sex hormones estrogen and progesterone. Low testosterone levels may dampen sexual desire and reduce sexual responsiveness. This may occur among women after menopause if their adrenal glands are removed surgically.

**Talking Glossary**
Dyspareunia, Vaginismus
G0918

A gradual decline in sexual desire, at least among men, may be explained in part by the reduction in testosterone levels that occurs in middle and later life. Abrupt losses of sexual desire are more often explained by psychosocial factors, for example, depression, stress, or relationship problems.

Fatigue is connected with reduced sexual responsiveness in both men and women. Painful sex is a sign that something is wrong, often an underlying infection. For women, pain during sex may also result from inadequate lubrication. In such cases, additional foreplay or artificial lubrication may help.

Health problems can prevent both genders from becoming sexually aroused or reaching orgasm. Diabetes mellitus, multiple sclerosis, spinal cord injuries, epilepsy, complications from surgery (such as prostate surgery in men[33]), and hormonal problems are but a few of the medical conditions that can impair sexual performance or responsiveness. Prescription drugs, alcohol, and illicit drugs can reduce sexual desire and impair sexual arousal and orgasm. Regular use of cocaine reduces sexual responsiveness in both genders. People with sexual dysfunctions are advised to have physical examinations to learn whether their problems may be biologically based.

**Psychosocial Causes** Children reared in sexually repressive cultures or households may learn to respond to sexual stimulation with feelings of anxiety and shame rather than sexual arousal and pleasure. Women are more likely than men to be taught to repress their sexual desires. Self-control and vigilance—not sexual awareness and acceptance—are sometimes considered feminine virtues. Women reared with repressive attitudes are less likely to explore their sexual potential and to assert their sexual wishes with their partners.

With some couples, sex becomes a routine. Perhaps only one partner takes the lead, leaving the other partner feeling unsatisfied. Couples who fail to communicate their preferences or to experiment may find themselves losing interest in sex.

Problems in a couple's relationship are not easily left at the bedroom door. Couples usually find that their sexual relationship is no better than other facets of their relationship. Couples who harbor resentments toward one another may make sex an arena of combat. Problems in communication may play a role. Troubled relationships are usually characterized by poor communication. Partners who have difficulty communicating about other matters may also be unlikely to communicate their sexual desires.

Victims of rape or other sexual trauma may harbor feelings of disgust and revulsion toward sex. A deep-seated fear of sex may make it difficult for them to respond sexually, even with a loving partner. These factors may inhibit lubrication or cause vaginismus, making sexual relations painful or impossible. Other emotional factors, especially depression, can lessen sexual response.

Anxiety—especially **performance anxiety**—plays an important role in sexual dysfunctions. Performance anxiety occurs when a person becomes overly concerned with how well he or she is doing something. Performance anxiety can stifle sexual responsiveness, leading a woman to fail to become adequately lubricated or a man to fail to achieve or maintain an erection. Failure to perform adequately may lead the person to attend more to self-doubts and fears of repeated failure than to erotic sensations. The person thinks, "Will I be able to do it this time? Will this be another failure?" Performance anxiety can set the stage for a vicious cycle in which a sexual failure increases anxiety. Anxiety then leads to repeated failure, and so on.

## Sex Therapy

Sex therapy involves the direct treatment of sexual dysfunctions. When dysfunctions have psychosocial causes, some sex therapists help clients learn about these causes through counseling and psychotherapy. Sex therapy aims to:

- *Reduce performance anxiety.* Sex therapists break the vicious cycle of performance anxiety and failure by removing the need to perform. The couple may be told to practice touching each other in nongenital areas but not to attempt to engage in intercourse. Sex becomes pleasurable once more, not anxiety-provoking.
- *Foster sexual skills or competencies.* Clients are taught about their sexual anatomy and sexual response. They learn how to obtain adequate sexual stimulation and how to stimulate their partners sexually. They learn how to relax so that the natural reflexes of erection, lubrication, and orgasm can take place.

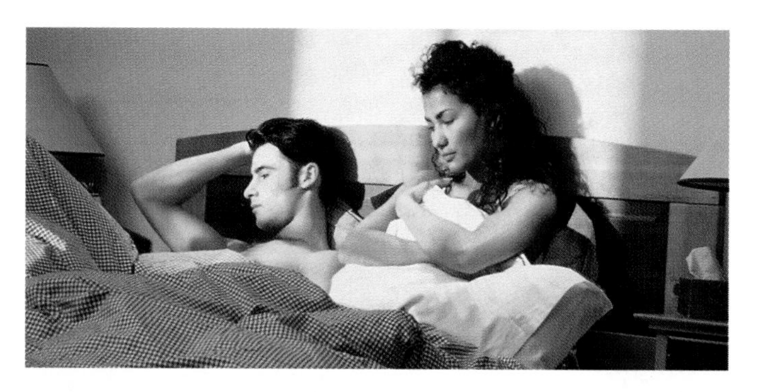

***Communication Problems*** Problems in communication can lead to sexual difficulties or prevent couples from resolving them. Sexual problems may arise when partners fail to communicate their sexual needs or desires. Problems may persist when they fail to work together to find solutions.

Readers who wish to learn more about sex therapy are advised to consult a human sexuality textbook,* contact their state's psychological association, or ask their professor or college counseling centers for a referral.

*Here's a randomly selected sexuality textbook: Rathus, S.A., Nevid, J.S., and Fichner-Rathus, L. *Human Sexuality in a World of Diversity* (3rd ed.). Boston: Allyn & Bacon, 1997.

### think about it!

- **Can you think of any examples in your own life in which you have been hampered by performance anxiety of one kind or another?**
- **What kinds of health problems are associated with sexual dysfunctions?**

**critical thinking** **When does a sexual problem become a sexual dysfunction?**

Smart Quiz
Q0905

**Performance anxiety** Anxiety stemming from an overconcern with the quality of one's performance.

# Making Breast Self-Exams and Testicular Self-Exams a Monthly Habit

## Take Charge

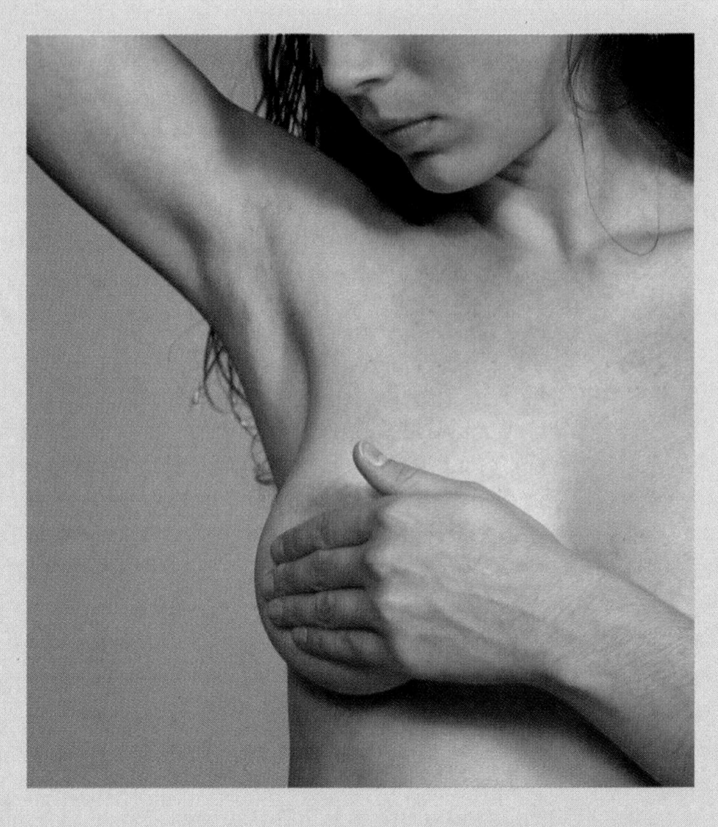

Breast cancer is the second leading cancer killer of women, after lung cancer, claiming the lives of some 44,000 women in the U.S. annually. Cancer of the testicles (testicular cancer) is a relatively rare form of cancer, accounting for about 6,000 new cases annually, or about 1% of all new cancers in men. However, it accounts for nearly 10% of all cancer deaths among men in the 20 to 34 age group.[34]

Early detection and treatment is the key to increasing your chances of surviving these and other forms of cancer. You can help protect yourself by practicing monthly self-examinations and obtaining regular medical checkups.

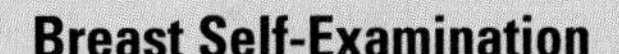

### Breast Self-Examination

Regular breast self-examination, combined with regular visits to a physician, is the best protection against breast cancer, since it can lead to early detection and treatment (see Figure 9.10). One study estimated that regular breast self-examination may reduce breast cancer mortality by nearly 20%.[35] A woman may wish to undertake an initial breast self-examination with a physician in order to determine the degree of "lumpiness" that seems normal for her. Then she should conduct a breast self-examination at least once a month, preferably about a week after her period ends (when the breasts are least influenced by hormones), and report any changes promptly to a physician.

The following instructions for breast self-examination are based on American Cancer Society guidelines. Additional material on breast self-examination may be obtained from the American Cancer Society.

1. *In the shower.* Examine your breasts during bath or shower; hands glide more easily over wet skin. Keep your fingers flat and move gently over every part of each breast. Use the right hand to examine the left breast and the left hand for the right breast. Check for any lump, hard knot, or thickening.
2. *Before a mirror.* Inspect your breasts with your arms at your sides. Next, raise your arms high overhead. Look for any changes in the contour of each breast, a swelling, dimpling of skin, or changes in the nipple. Then rest your palms on your hips and press down firmly to flex your chest muscles. Your left and right breasts will not exactly match—few women's breasts do. Regular inspection shows what is normal for you and will give you confidence in your examination.
3. *Lying down.* To examine your right breast, put a pillow or folded towel under your right shoulder. Place your right arm behind your head—this distributes breast tissue more evenly on the chest. With your left hand, fingers flat, press gently with the finger pads (the top thirds of the fingers) of the three middle fingers in small circular motions around an imaginary clock face. Begin at the outermost top of your right breast for 12 o'clock, then move to 1 o'clock, and so on around the circle back to 12. A ridge of firm tissue in the lower curve of each breast is normal. Then move in an inch, toward the nipple. Keep circling to examine *every part of your*

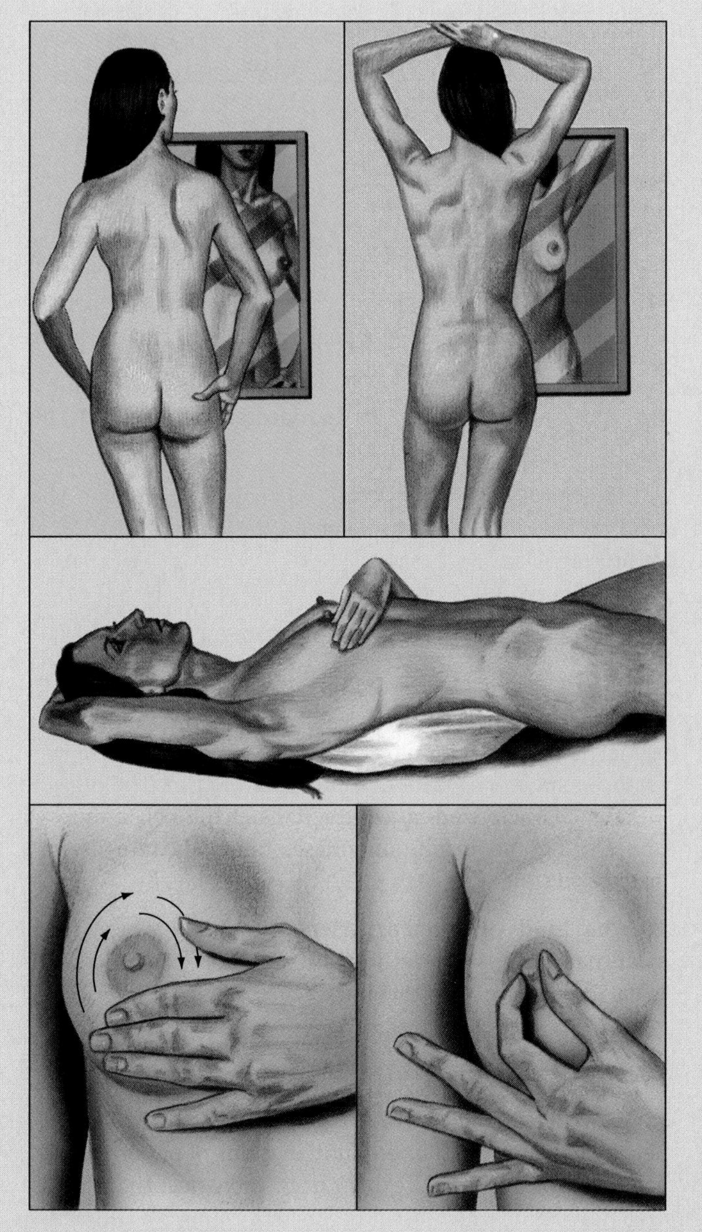

Figure 9.10 *Woman Examining Her Breasts for Lumps*

## Testicular Self-Examination

Self-examination (see Figure 9.11) is best performed shortly after a warm shower or bath, when the skin of the scrotum is most relaxed. The man should examine the scrotum for evidence of pea-sized lumps. Each testicle can be rolled gently between the thumb and the fingers. Lumps are generally found on the side or front of the testicle. The presence of a lump is not necessarily a sign of cancer, but it should be promptly reported to a physician for further evaluation. The American Cancer Society lists these warning signals:[36]

Smart Quiz
Q0906

1. A slight enlargement of one of the testicles.
2. A change in the consistency of a testicle.
3. A dull ache in the lower abdomen or groin. (Pain may be absent in cancer of the testes, however.)
4. A sensation of dragging and heaviness in a testicle.

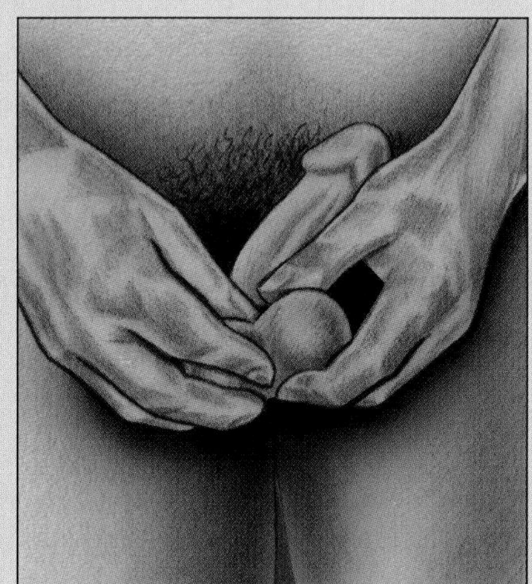

Figure 9.11 *Testicular Self-Examination*

*breast,* including the nipple. This requires at least three more circles. Now slowly repeat the procedure on your left breast. Place the pillow beneath your left shoulder, your left arm behind your head, and use the finger pads on your right hand.

After you examine your left breast fully, squeeze the nipple of each breast gently between your thumb and index finger. Any discharge, clear or bloody, should be reported to your doctor immediately.

# SUMMING UP

## Questions and Answers

### GENDER IDENTITY AND GENDER TYPING

**1. What are gender roles?** Gender roles are complex clusters of behavior expected of males and females within a given culture.

**2. What is sexual differentiation?** This is the process by which embryos differentiate into males and females. All embryos would develop female sexual structures in the absence of male sex hormones. Females have an XX sex chromosomal structure; males have an XY sex chromosomal structure. Testosterone induces the male fetal brain to become insensitive to estrogen.

**3. What is gender typing?** Gender typing is the process by which children develop to behave in accord with the stereotypical image of their biological sex. Sex hormones may account in part for gender differences in verbal skills, math, and aggressiveness, but cultural influences also play a role. Parents, peers, and the mass media socialize boys into acting like stereotypical males and girls into acting like stereotypical females.

### SEXUAL ANATOMY AND PHYSIOLOGY

**4. What are the external female reproductive organs?** They are collectively called the *pudendum* or *vulva.* They consist of the mons, labia, clitoris, and urethral opening.

**5. What are the internal female reproductive organs?** They consist of the inner vagina, the cervix, the uterus, ovaries, and Fallopian tubes. Ova pass through the Fallopian tubes on their way to the uterus and are normally fertilized within them. The ovaries lie on either side of the uterus and produce ova and the sex hormones estrogen and progesterone.

**6. What are the parts of the breasts?** The breasts consist of mammary glands, nipples, and areolas.

**7. What are the phases of the menstrual cycle?** The menstrual cycle has four stages or phases: proliferative, ovulatory, secretory, and menstrual. During the first phase, ova ripen and endometrial tissue proliferates. During the second phase, ovulation occurs. During the third phase, progesterone and estrogen cause the endometrium to thicken. If the ovum goes unfertilized, a plunge in estrogen and progesterone levels triggers the fourth, or menstrual, phase.

**8. How common are menstrual problems?** Most women experience some menstrual problems, such as dysmenorrhea, amenorrhea, or premenstrual syndrome (PMS).

**9. What is menopause?** Menopause is the cessation of menstruation. Estrogen deficiency in menopause may give rise to night sweats, hot flashes, hot flushes, cold sweats, dry skin, loss of breast tissue, decreased vaginal lubrication, and osteoporosis.

**10. What are the external male reproductive organs?** These include the penis and the scrotum.

**11. What are the internal male reproductive organs?** These consist of the testes, the vas deferens, the seminal vesicles, and the prostate gland.

### SEXUAL RESPONSE AND PRACTICES

**12. What are the phases of the sexual response cycle?** The excitement phase is characterized by erection in the male and vaginal lubrication in the female. The plateau phase is an advanced state of arousal that precedes orgasm. The orgasmic phase is characterized by contractions of the pelvic musculature. During the resolution phase, the body returns to its prearoused state.

**13. What kinds of sexual experience are there?** These include masturbation, kissing and touching another person, oral sex, sexual intercourse, and anal intercourse.

### SEXUAL ORIENTATION

**14. What are the origins of sexual orientation?** Psychological theories explain sexual orientation in terms of patterns of child rearing and early sexual experiences. Biological theories note possible roles for genetics and prenatal sex hormones.

**15. How well adjusted are gay males and lesbians?** Actually, they are as well adjusted as heterosexuals. The lifestyle of the individual more than sexual orientation seems connected with adjustment.

### SEXUAL DYSFUNCTIONS

**16. What are sexual dysfunctions?** These are persistent and distressing problems in sexual interest, arousal, or response. They include sexual desire disorders, sexual arousal disorders, orgasm disorders, and sexual pain disorders.

**17. What are the causes of sexual dysfunctions?** Sexual dysfunctions can have biological causes, such as declining hormone levels and health problems, and psychosocial causes, such as negative attitudes toward sex, communication problems, sexually traumatic experiences, and performance anxiety.

## Suggested Readings

**Barrett, M. B.** *Invisible Lives: The Truth About Millions of Women-loving Women.* New York: Morrow, 1990. Based on interviews with 125 lesbians, this book reveals what it is like to be a lesbian in contemporary America and seeks to develop understanding between lesbians and parents, children, and friends.

**Boston Women's Health Book Collective.** *The New Our Bodies, Ourselves.* New York: Simon & Schuster, 1984. A highly popular repository of information about women's health care, sexuality, and reproductive health.

**Stewart, F. H., and others.** *Understanding Your Body.* New York: Bantam, 1992. A comprehensive guide to women's reproductive health, gynecological problems, and contraceptive techniques.

**Reinisch, J.** *The Kinsey Institute New Report on Sex: What You Must Know to Be Sexually Literate.* New York: St. Martin's Press, 1990. The findings of a national survey of sexual knowledge, along with a comprehensive and well-researched compendium of information on contraception, sexually transmitted diseases, sexual development, sexual health, and problems with sexual functioning.

**Calderone, M. S., and Ramey, J.** *Talking with Your Child About Sex.* New York: Random House, 1982. A practical guide to parents in raising sexually healthy children. Provides parents with answers to questions that children frequently ask about sex.

**Griffin, C., Wirth, M., and Wirth, A.** *Beyond Acceptance.* Englewood Cliffs, NJ: Prentice-Hall, 1986. Written by parents of gay and lesbian children for parents of gay and lesbian children, this book sensitively discusses issues and conflicts that arise in the context of discovering that one's child is homosexual.

**Spark, R. F.** *Male Sexual Health: A Couple's Guide.* Mount Vernon, NY: Consumer Reports Books, 1991. A concise up-to-date guide to male sexual problems ranging from infertility to erectile dysfunction.

**Zilbergeld, B.** *The New Male Sexuality: A Guide to Sexual Fulfillment.* New York: Bantam, 1992. A thorough updating of this informative guide to male sexuality.

**McWhirter, D. P., Sanders, S. A., and Reinisch, J. M. (Eds.).** *Homosexuality/Heterosexuality: Concepts of Sexual Orientation.* The Kinsey Institute Series, Volume II. New York: Oxford University Press, 1990. A compendium of scholarly articles on the classification and understanding of sexual orientation.

**Michael, R. T., and others.** *Sex in America: A Definitive Survey.* Boston: Little Brown, 1994. A popularized version of a major national survey on sexual practices in the United States.

**Rathus, S. A., Nevid, J. S., and Fichner-Rathus, L.** *Human Sexuality in a World of Diversity* (3rd ed.). Boston: Allyn & Bacon, 1997. A comprehensive textbook on human sexuality, from two of the authors of this text.

DID YOU KNOW THAT

- Prolonged athletic activity may decrease fertility in the male? p.260
- A so-called test-tube baby does not develop in a test tube? p.261
- The ancient Egyptians used crocodile dung as a contraceptive? p.262
- Many contraceptives are useless in the prevention of sexually transmitted diseases? p.263
- Many birth-control pills fool the brain into acting as though the woman is already pregnant? p.263
- Besides contraception, birth-control pills have other healthful benefits? p.265
- There is an oral contraceptive that can be taken the morning after intercourse? p.265
- Many spermicides kill not only sperm but also STD-causing agents, including HIV? p.268
- Sterilization is not always permanent? p.274
- Testosterone may have a role as a male contraceptive device? p.275
- Abortions were legal in the United States before the Civil War? p.276

# Conception,

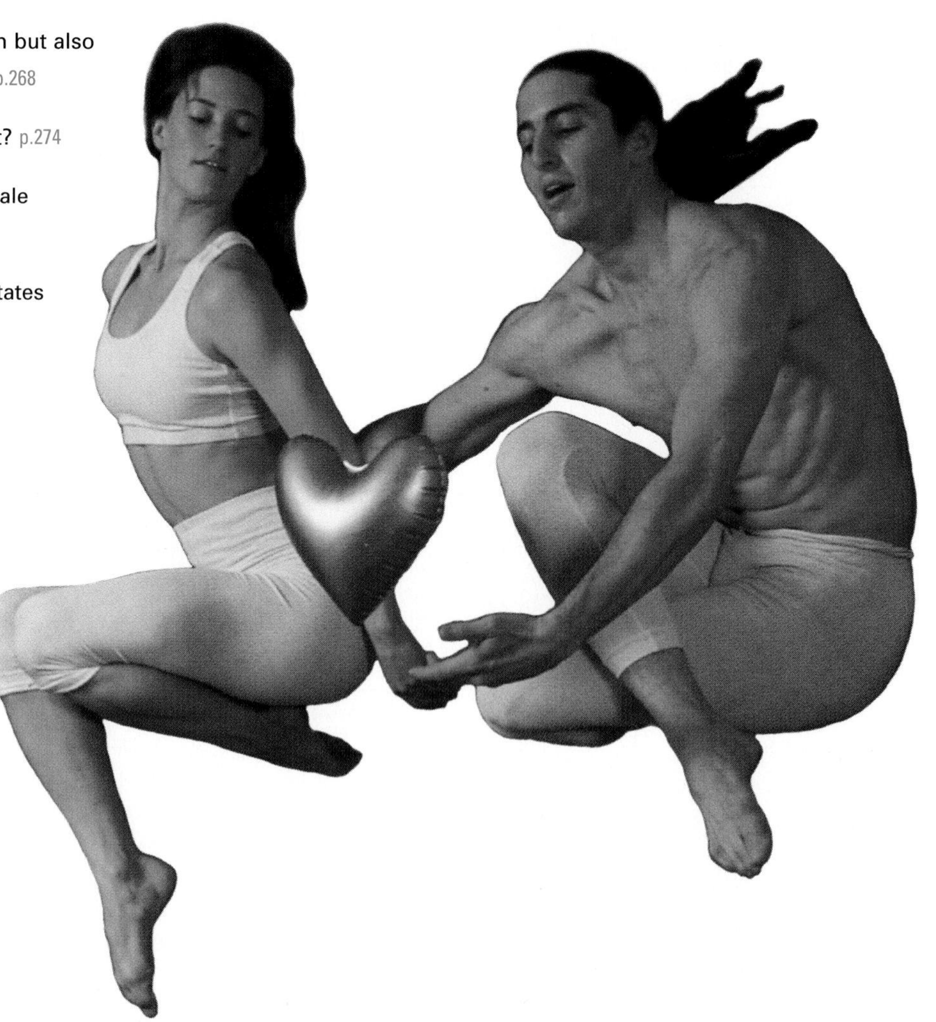

# 10

# Contraception, and Abortion



*On a balmy day in October, Anna and her husband Hector rush to catch the train to their jobs in the city. Anna's work day is outwardly much the same as any other. Within her body, however, a drama is unfolding. Yesterday, a follicle in her ovary ruptured, releasing its egg cell or ovum.*

*Anna had used an ovulation-timing kit the previous morning. It detected a surge in luteinizing hormone (LH), which meant that Anna was about to ovulate. So later that night, Anna and Hector had made love, hoping that Anna would become pregnant. They had been trying to conceive for five months and were becoming worried. Anna and Hector are ready for their child. Their home life is stable and they have thought things through.*

*Dennis and Elaine also made love the night before. Their home life is stable and they also thought things through. They decided that they are not ready for children, and so they used a method of contraception to avoid pregnancy. They chose the rhythm method because of their religious beliefs and the lack of side effects.*

Many couples want children and seek to conceive them. Many others are sexually active but do not want children. Thus they use methods of *contra*ception—methods designed to prevent an unwanted pregnancy. Some sexually active couples fail to use contraception, or the contraception they use fails, resulting in conception. Some of them decide to terminate their pregnancies through abortion.

This chapter focuses on conception, contraception, and abortion. We first look at the process of conception. We examine what couples can do to optimize their chances of conceiving and overcome infertility. We then consider how people can protect themselves from unwanted pregnancies through the use of contraception. Finally, we turn our attention to the practice of abortion, arguably the most divisive issue our nation faces today.

## CONCEPTION—AGAINST ALL ODDS

When Hector ejaculated, hundreds of millions of sperm were deposited within Anna's vagina. Only a few thousand survived the journey through the cervix and uterus to the Fallopian tube that contained the ovum. Of these, a few hundred remained to bombard the ovum. This month one succeeded in penetrating the ovum's covering, resulting in conception. From a single cell formed by the union of sperm and ovum, a new life begins to form.

Anna is 37. Like many other women today, she had delayed marriage and childbearing for the sake of her education and career. Four months into her pregnancy, Anna will undergo **amniocentesis** to check for the presence of chromosomal abnormalities in the fetus, such as **Down syndrome,** which results in mental retardation. Down syndrome is more common among children born to women in their late thirties and older. Amniocentesis will also indicate the gender of the fetus. Many parents want to know their baby's gender before it is born. Anna and Hector ask their doctor *not* to tell them, however. "Why ruin the surprise?" Hector explains to his friends. Anna and Hector are thus left to debate both boys' names and girls' names for the next few months.

**Talking Glossary**
Amniocentesis
G1001

**Conception** is the union of a sperm cell and an ovum, or egg. It is the beginning of a new human life and also the end of a fantastic voyage. At journey's end, one of the several hundred ova that will ripen during a woman's lifetime unites with one of the 200 to 400 million sperm produced by the man in the average ejaculate. This number of sperm may seem excessive. After all, only one can fertilize an egg. Only 1 in 1,000 will ever arrive in the egg's vicinity, however. Millions flow out of the woman's body because of gravity, unless she remains lying down for quite some time. Vaginal acidity kills many more. Surviving sperm battle the current of fluid coming from the cervix and reach the uterus. Some sperm may reach the Fallopian tubes 60 to 90 minutes after ejaculation. About half the sperm end up in the wrong tube—that is, the one not containing the egg. Perhaps some 2,000 sperm find their way into the right tube. Fewer still manage to swim the final two inches against the current in the tube.

**Fertilization** normally occurs in a Fallopian tube. Ova contain chromosomes, proteins, fats, and nutritious fluid. They are surrounded by a gelatinous layer that must be penetrated if fertilization is to occur. Sperm that have completed their journey secrete an enzyme that briefly thins this layer, enabling one sperm to penetrate. Once a sperm has entered, the layer thickens, locking

**Amniocentesis** A procedure for drawing off and examining fetal cells in the amniotic fluid to check for fetal disorders.

**Down syndrome** A chromosomal abnormality that leads to mental retardation, caused by an extra chromosome on the twenty-first pair.

**Conception** The inception of pregnancy that results from the fertilization of an ovum.

**Fertilization** In humans, the union of an ovum and a sperm cell, resulting in the formation of a zygote.

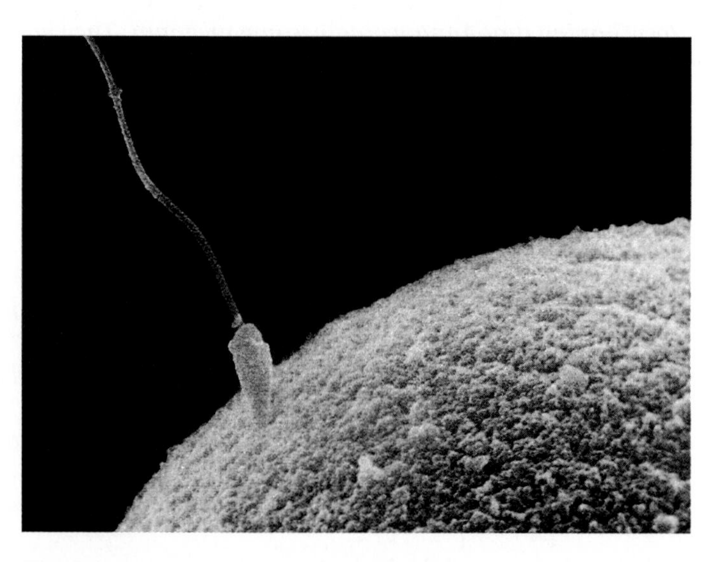

***The Dance of Life*** A sperm and ovum unite.

other sperm out. Corresponding chromosomes in the sperm and ovum line up opposite each other in a dance of creation. Conception occurs as the chromosomes from the sperm and ovum combine to form 23 new pairs, which carry a unique set of genetic instructions.

Hector's sex chromosome was a Y. Thus Anna and Hector conceived a boy.

## Optimizing the Chances of Conception

Some couples wish to optimize their chances of conceiving at a particular time. Others have difficulty conceiving and wish to maximize their chances for a few months before consulting a fertility specialist. Some fairly simple procedures increase the chances that couples will conceive.

The ovum can be fertilized for about one day after ovulation. Sperm are most active within 48 hours after ejaculation. One way of enhancing the chances of conception is to engage in sexual relations within a few hours of ovulation, as Anna and Hector did. There are a number of ways to predict ovulation.

### Using the Basal Body Temperature Chart

Few women have perfectly regular cycles. They can only guess when they are ovulating. A basal body temperature (BBT) chart helps provide a more reliable estimate. See Figure 9.4, page 234. As shown in the figure, body temperature is fairly even before ovulation. Early morning body temperature is generally below 98.6° Fahrenheit. Just before ovulation, BBT dips slightly. On the day after ovulation, the temperature tends to rise by about 0.4 to 0.8 degrees above the level before ovulation. It remains higher until menstruation. A woman may be able to detect these changes by tracking her BBT upon awakening each morning before rising from bed. Thermometers that provide finely graded readings, such as electronic digital thermometers, are best suited for the purpose. The couple record the woman's temperature and the day of the cycle (as well as the day of the month) and indicate whether they have engaged in sexual relations. If a woman's cycles are fairly regular, six months of charting may help her learn to predict ovulation.

**Tracking Vaginal Mucus** Women can track the thickness of their vaginal mucus during the phases of the menstrual cycle by rolling it between their fingers and noting changes in texture. The mucus is thick, white, and cloudy during most phases of the cycle. It becomes thin, slippery, and clear for a few days before ovulation. A day or so after ovulation the mucus again thickens and becomes opaque. Unfortunately, these changes may not be apparent enough to use reliably as a basis for planning conception.

### Analyzing Urine for Luteinizing Hormone

The most reliable method for predicting ovulation involves the use of ovulation-timing kits. These kits, which are available over the counter, predict ovulation by analyzing the woman's urine for the surge in luteinizing hormone (LH) that precedes ovulation. The couple then engages in intercourse following this LH surge.

**Additional Considerations** Sex with the man on top allows sperm to be deposited deeper in the vagina. It minimizes leakage of sperm out of the vagina due to gravity. Women may improve their chances of conceiving by lying on their backs and drawing their knees close to their breasts following ejaculation. This position, perhaps with a pillow beneath the buttocks, causes gravity to work for rather than against conception. Women may also lie as still as possible for 30 to 60 minutes following ejaculation.

The man should penetrate the woman as deeply as possible just prior to ejaculation, hold still during ejaculation, then withdraw slowly in a straight line to avoid dispersing the pool of semen.

## Infertility and Ways of Becoming Parents

For couples who want children, few problems are more frustrating than inability to conceive. Health professionals often recommend that couples try to conceive on their own for six months before seeking assistance. The term **infertility** is usually not applied until the problem has persisted for more than a year.

Infertility affects millions of Americans. Because the incidence of infertility increases with age, it is partially the result of a rise in couples who postpone childbearing until their thirties and forties. All in all, about one American couple in six has fertility problems. About half of them eventually succeed in conceiving a child. Many treatment options are available, ranging from drugs to stimulate ovulation to newer reproductive technologies, such as in vitro fertilization.

**Infertility** Inability to conceive a child.

**Male Fertility Problems** Although most concerns about fertility have traditionally centered on women, fertility problems are found in men in about 30% of cases of infertility.[1] In about 20% of cases, problems are found in both partners.

Fertility problems in the male reflect abnormalities such as:

1. low sperm count
2. irregularly shaped sperm (for example, malformed heads or tails)
3. low sperm **motility**
4. chronic diseases like diabetes, as well as infectious diseases like sexually transmitted diseases
5. injury to the testes
6. an **autoimmune response** in which antibodies produced by the man deactivate his own sperm
7. hormonal problems (for example, a pituitary imbalance or thyroid disease).

Problems in producing normal, abundant sperm may also be caused by genetic factors, advanced age, varicose veins in the scrotum, drugs (alcohol, narcotics, marijuana, tobacco), antihypertensive medications, environmental toxins, excess heat, and stress. Sperm production gradually declines with age, but normal aging does not produce infertility. Men in late adulthood may father children, even though conception may require more attempts.

Low sperm count (or absence of sperm) is the most common problem. Sperm counts of 40 to 150 million sperm per milliliter of semen are considered normal. A count of fewer than 20 million is generally regarded as low. Sperm production may be low among men with undescended testes that were not surgically corrected before puberty. Frequent ejaculation can reduce sperm counts. Sperm production may also be impaired in men whose testicles are consistently 1 or 2 degrees above the typical scrotal temperature of 94 to 95 degrees Fahrenheit. Some men may encounter fertility problems from prolonged athletic activity, use of electric blankets, or even long, hot baths. In such cases the problem can be readily corrected. Male runners with fertility problems are often counseled to take a few weeks off to increase their sperm counts.

Sometimes the sperm count is adequate, but prostate, hormonal, or other factors sap sperm of motility or deform them. Motility can also be hampered by scar tissue from infections, which may prevent sperm from passing through parts of the male reproductive system. Sperm counts have been increased by surgical repair of varicose veins in the scrotum. Microsurgery can open blocked passageways that prevent the flow of sperm. Researchers are also investigating the effects on sperm production of special cooling undergarments.

**Motility** Self-propulsion. A measure of the viability of sperm cells.

**Autoimmune response** The production of antibodies that attack naturally occurring substances in the body that are (incorrectly) recognized as being foreign or harmful.

**Artificial insemination** Introduction of sperm into a woman's reproductive tract through means other than sexual intercourse.

***Artificial Insemination*** The sperm of men with low sperm counts can be collected and quick-frozen. Sperm from multiple ejaculations can be injected into a woman's uterus at the time of ovulation. This is one kind of **artificial insemination.** The sperm of men with low sperm motility can also be injected into their partners' uteruses, so that the sperm start their journey closer to the Fallopian tubes. Sperm from a donor can be used to artificially inseminate a woman whose partner is completely infertile or has an extremely low sperm count. The child then bears the genes of one of the parents, the mother. A donor can be chosen who resembles the man in physical traits and ethnic background.

A variation of artificial insemination has been used with some men with either very low (or zero) sperm counts in the semen, immature sperm, or immotile sperm. Immature sperm can be removed from a testicle by a thin needle and then directly injected into an egg in a laboratory dish. The method has even been successful with a few men who have only tail-less immature sperm.

**Female Fertility Problems** Major causes of infertility in women include:

1. irregular ovulation, including failure to ovulate
2. obstructions or malfunctions of the reproductive tract, which are often caused by infections or disease
3. endometriosis
4. declining hormone levels of estrogen and progesterone that occur with aging. (They may prevent the ovum from becoming fertilized or remaining implanted in the uterus.)

About 10% to 15% of female infertility problems stem from failure to ovulate. Many factors can play a role in failure to ovulate, including hormonal irregularities, malnutrition, genetic factors, stress, and chronic disease. Extreme dieting can prevent ovulation, as in the case of the eating disorder anorexia nervosa. But even women who are only 10 to 15% below their normal body weights may fail to ovulate.

Ovulation may be induced by fertility drugs such as clomiphene (Clomid). Clomiphene stimulates the pituitary gland to secrete FSH and LH (see pp. 232–233). LH, in turn, stimulates maturation of ova. Clomiphene leads to conception in most cases of infertility that are due *solely* to irregular or absent ovulation. But infertility can have multiple causes. Therefore, only about half the women who use clomiphene become pregnant. Another fertility drug, Pergonal, contains a high concentration of FSH, which directly stimulates maturation of ovarian follicles. Like clomiphene, Pergonal has high success rates with women whose infertility is due to lack of ovulation. Clomiphene and Pergonal have been linked to multiple births, including quadruplets and quintuplets. However, fewer than 10% of such pregnancies result in multiple births.

Other causes of female infertility include cervical mucus that impedes the passage of sperm, antibodies produced by the woman that destroy sperm, infections that leave scars that block the passage of ova and sperm through the Fallopian tubes, and endometriosis.

In endometriosis, cells break away from the uterine lining (the endometrium) and become implanted and grow elsewhere. When they develop on the surface of the ovaries or Fallopian tubes, they may block the passage of ova or impair conception for other reasons. About one case in six of female sterility may be due to endometriosis. Hormone treatments and surgery sometimes reduce the blockage to the point that women can conceive.

Several new methods help many couples with problems such as blocked Fallopian tubes bear children.

***In Vitro Fertilization*** When Louise Brown was born in England in 1978 after being conceived by the method of **in vitro fertilization (IVF),** the event made headlines around the world. Louise was dubbed the world's first "test-tube baby." However, her conception took place in a laboratory dish (not a test tube). The fetus was then implanted in the mother's uterus, where it developed to term. In in vitro fertilization, fertility drugs are first used to stimulate ripening of ova. Ripe ova are then surgically removed from an ovary and placed in a laboratory dish along with the father's sperm. Fertilized ova are then injected into the mother's uterus in the hope they will become implanted in the uterine wall. They do not grow in a test tube or laboratory dish.

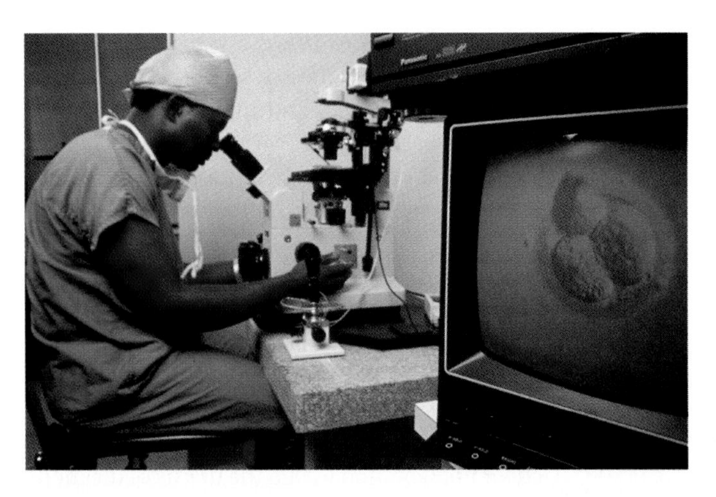

***In Vitro Fertilization*** In in vitro fertilization, a mother's egg cell is surgically removed and fertilized with a sperm cell from the father. The fertilized ovum, as seen here on the monitor, is then injected into the mother's uterus.

**Video**
In vitro fertilization
**V1001**
How old is too old?
**V1002**

**Talking Glossary**
Gamete intrafallopian transfer
**G1002**

***GIFT*** In **gamete intrafallopian transfer,** or **GIFT,** sperm and ova are inserted together into a Fallopian tube for fertilization. Unlike in vitro fertilization, conception occurs in a Fallopian tube rather than a laboratory dish.

***ZIFT*** **Zygote intrafallopian transfer (ZIFT)** combines IVF and GIFT. Sperm and ova are combined in a laboratory dish. The fertilized ovum (called a **zygote**) is placed in the mother's Fallopian tube, from which it journeys to the uterus. Unlike GIFT, ZIFT allows fertility specialists to determine that fertilization has occurred before insertion.

**In vitro fertilization (IVF)** A method of conception in which mature ova are surgically removed from an ovary and placed in a laboratory dish along with sperm.

**Gamete intrafallopian transfer (GIFT)** A method of conception in which sperm and ova are inserted into a Fallopian tube to encourage conception.

**Zygote intrafallopian transfer (ZIFT)** A method of conception in which an ovum is fertilized in a laboratory dish and then placed in a Fallopian tube.

**Zygote** A fertilized ovum.

***Donor IVF*** **Donor IVF** is a variation of the IVF procedure in which the ovum is taken from another woman, fertilized, and then injected into the uterus or Fallopian tube of the intended mother. The procedure is used in cases in which the intended mother does not produce ova.

***Embryonic Transfer*** A similar method for women who do not produce ova of their own is **embryonic transfer.** In this method a woman volunteer is artificially inseminated by the male partner of the infertile woman. Five days later the embryo is removed from the volunteer and inserted for implantation within the uterus of the mother-to-be.

Talking Glossary
Intracytoplasmic injection
G1003

***Intracytoplasmic Injection*** **Intracytoplasmic injection** has been used when the man has too few sperm for IVF, or when IVF fails. In this method, sperm is injected directly into an ovum.

In vitro and transfer methods are costly and successful in only a minority of cases. Frustration and lack of hope lead many couples to drop out of infertility programs. Coping with infertility can also place strain on the marriage.

***Surrogate Motherhood*** A **surrogate mother** is artificially inseminated by the husband of the infertile woman and carries the baby to term. The surrogate agrees to turn the baby over to the infertile couple. Such contracts have been invalidated in some states, however. Surrogate mothers in these states cannot be compelled to hand over their babies.

**Adoption** Adoption is yet another way for people to obtain children. We often hear of conflicts in which adoptive parents are pitted against biological parents who change their minds about giving up their children. These cases are the exception, however. Most adoptions result in the formation of loving new families. Many people in the United States find it easier to adopt infants from other countries, infants with special needs, or older children.

**Donor IVF** A variation of in vitro fertilization in which the ovum is taken from one woman, fertilized, and then injected into the uterus or Fallopian tube of another woman.

**Embryonic transfer** A method of conception in which a woman volunteer is artificially inseminated by the male partner of the intended mother. The embryo is later transferred to the uterus of the intended mother.

**Intracytoplasmic injection** A method of conception involving the injection of sperm directly into an ovum.

**Surrogate mother** A woman who is impregnated through artificial insemination with the sperm of a prospective father, carries the baby to term, and then gives it to the prospective parents.

**Contraception** Methods or devices that prevent conception.

**Abortion** Termination of a pregnancy before the fetus achieves viability outside the womb.

**Coitus interruptus** A method of contraception in which the penis is withdrawn from the vagina before ejaculation.

**Condom** A sheath made of animal membrane or latex that covers the penis during coitus and serves as a barrier to sperm following ejaculation.

Smart Quiz
Q1001

### think about it!

- **What are the factors that optimize the chances of conception?**
- **If you wished to optimize the chances of conception, how could you do it?**

**critical thinking What are the various ways that people with problems with infertility can attempt to become parents? Which ways would appeal to you if you faced this situation? Why?**

## CONTRACEPTION

Methods of birth control include contraception and abortion. **Contraception** refers to techniques that prevent conception. **Abortion** is the termination of a pregnancy before the fetus can survive outside the womb.

People have been devising means of contraception since they became aware of the relationship between sexual intercourse and conception. The Bible contains many references to contraceptive techniques, including use of contraceptive concoctions applied to the vagina and **coitus interruptus,** or withdrawal. Of course, the safest and most effective method of contraception is also the least popular: abstinence.

Talking Glossary
Coitus interruptus
G1004

HealthCheck
What about abstinence?
H1001

Ancient Egyptian methods of birth control included douching after coitus with wine and garlic, and soaking crocodile dung in sour milk and stuffing the mixture deep within the vagina. The dung blocked the passage of many—if not all—sperm through the cervix and also soaked up sperm. The dung may also have done its job by discouraging all but the most ardent suitors.

Greek and Roman women placed absorbent materials within the vagina to absorb semen. The use of coverings for the penis can be traced to ancient Egypt (1350 B.C.). The term **condom** was not used to describe sheaths until the eighteenth century. At that time, sheaths made of animal intestines became popular as means of preventing sexually transmitted diseases and unwanted pregnancies. Condoms made of rubber (hence the slang "rubbers") were introduced shortly after Charles Goodyear's invention of the vulcanization of rubber in 1843. Many other forms of contraception were also used widely in the nineteenth century, though not necessarily effectively, including withdrawal, vaginal sponges, and douching.

There are many methods of contraception, including oral contraceptives (the pill), Norplant, intrauterine devices (IUDs), diaphragms, cervical caps, spermicides, condoms, douching, withdrawal (coitus interruptus), timing of ovulation (rhythm), and some devices under development. Some contraceptive techniques also provide protection against sexually transmitted diseases (STDs). Many do not. Table 10.1 (next page) shows the failure rates, continuation rates, reversibility, and degree of protection against STDs associated with various contraceptive methods.

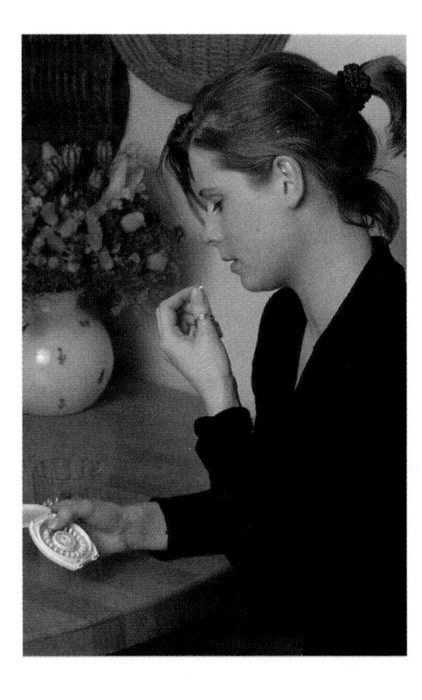

***The Pill*** Oral contraceptives are a highly effective method of birth control.

## Oral Contraceptives ("the Pill")

**Oral contraceptives** are commonly referred to as birth-control pills, or simply "the pill." However, there are many kinds of birth-control pills. They vary in the type and dosages of hormones they contain. Birth-control pills fall into two major categories: combination pills and minipills.

**Combination pills,** such as Ortho-Novum, Ovcon, and Loestrin, contain synthetic forms of estrogen and progesterone (progestin). Most combination pills provide a steady dose of these hormones. Other combination pills, called *multiphasic* pills, vary the dosage of these hormones across the menstrual cycle. They reduce the overall doses to which the woman is exposed. The **minipill** contains progestin only.

Oral contraceptives are available only by prescription. Birth-control pills are the most popular form of contraception among single women. About one in two never-married women who use contraception takes oral contraceptives.[2]

Women cannot conceive when they are already pregnant because their bodies suppress the maturation of egg follicles and ovulation. The combination pill fools the brain into acting as though the woman is already pregnant. Thus no additional ova mature or are released. If ovulation does not take place, a woman cannot become pregnant. The woman continues to have menstrual periods, but no ovum is sloughed off in the menstrual flow.

The progestin in the combination pill also increases the thickness and acidity of the cervical mucus. The mucus thus becomes a more resistant barrier to sperm and inhibits development of the endometrium. Therefore, even if an egg were somehow to mature and be released into a Fallopian tube, sperm would not be likely to survive the passage through the cervix. Even if sperm were to fertilize an egg, the undeveloped endometrium would not permit implantation of the fertilized ovum in the uterus. Progestin would also impede the progress of an ovum through the Fallopian tube.

Minipills contain progestin only. They act like the progestin in combination pills. They thicken the cervical mucus to impede the passage of sperm and render the inner lining of the uterus less receptive to a fertilized egg. Since the minipill contains no estrogen, it does not usually prevent ovulation. The combination pill, by contrast, prevents ovulation. Since ovulation and fertilization may occur in women who use the minipill, some people see use of the minipill as an early abortion method. Others reserve the term "abortion" for methods of terminating pregnancy following implantation.

**Oral contraceptive** A contraceptive consisting of sex hormones that is taken by mouth.

**Combination pill** A birth-control pill that contains synthetic estrogen and progesterone.

**Minipill** A birth-control pill that contains synthetic progesterone but no estrogen.

TABLE 10.1

## Approximate Failure Rates of Various Methods of Birth Control

| Method | Percentage of Women Experiencing an Accidental Pregnancy within the First Year of Use | | Percentage of Women Continuing Use at One Year[3] | Reversibility | Protection against Sexually Transmitted Diseases (STDs) |
|---|---|---|---|---|---|
| | Typical Use[1] | Perfect Use[2] | | | |
| *Chance*[4] | 85 | 85 | | yes (unless fertility has been impaired by exposure to an STD) | no |
| *Spermicides*[5] | 21 | 6 | 43 | yes | some |
| *Periodic Abstinence* | 20 | | 67 | yes | no |
| *Calendar* | | 9 | | | |
| *Ovulation method* | | 3 | | | |
| *Sympto-thermal*[6] | | 2 | | | |
| *Post-ovulation* | | 1 | | | |
| *Withdrawal* | 19 | 4 | | yes | no |
| *Cervical Cap*[7] | | | | | |
| *Parous women** | 36 | 26 | 45 | yes | some[8] |
| *Nulliparous women*** | 18 | 9 | 58 | yes | some[8] |
| *Diaphragm*[7] | 18 | 6 | 58 | yes | some[8] |
| *Condom Alone* | | | | | |
| *Female ("Reality")* | 21 | 5 | 56 | yes | yes[8] |
| *Male* | 12 | 3 | 63 | yes | yes[8] |
| *Pill* | 3 | | 72 | yes | no, but may reduce the risk of PID[9] |
| *Progestin only* | | 0.5 | | | |
| *Combined* | | 0.1 | | | |
| *IUD* | | | | | |
| *Progesterone T* | 2.0 | 1.5 | 81 | yes, except if fertility is impaired | no, and may increase the risk of PID |
| *Copper T 380A* | 0.8 | 0.6 | 78 | | |
| *LNg 20* | 0.1 | 0.1 | 81 | | |
| *Depo-Provera* | 0.3 | 0.3 | 70 | yes | no |
| *Norplant (6 capsules)* | 0.09 | 0.09 | 85 | yes | no |
| *Female Sterilization* | 0.4 | 0.4 | 100 | not usually | no |
| *Male Sterilization* | 0.15 | 0.10 | 100 | not usually | no |

[1] Among typical couples who initiate use of a method (not necessarily for the first time), the percentage who experience an accidental pregnancy during the first year if they do not stop use for any other reason.
[2] Among couples who initiate use of a method (not necessarily for the first time) and who use it perfectly (both consistently and correctly), the percentage who experience an accidental pregnancy during the first year if they do not stop use for any other reason.
[3] Among couples attempting to avoid pregnancy, the percentage who continue to use a method for one year.
[4] The percentages failing in columns (2) and (3) are based on data from populations where contraception is not used and from women who cease using contraception in order to become pregnant. Among such populations, about 89% become pregnant within one year. This estimate was lowered slightly (to 85%) to represent the percentage who would become pregnant within one year among women now relying on reversible methods of contraception if they abandoned contraception altogether.
[5] Foams, creams, gels, vaginal suppositories, and vaginal film.
[6] Cervical mucus (ovulation) method supplemented by use of a menstrual calendar in the pre-ovulatory period and basal body temperature in the post-ovulatory period.
[7] With spermicidal cream or jelly.
[8] These methods provide better protection against STDs if a spermicide such as nonoxynol-9 is used simultaneously.
[9] Pelvic inflammatory disease.
* Women who have borne children.
** Women who have not borne children.

*Sources:* For failure rates and percentages of women discontinuing use, adapted from Hatcher, R. A., et al. *Contraceptive Technology 1992–1994* (16th rev. ed.). New York: Irvington Publishers, 1994.
For reversibility and protection against sexually transmitted diseases, adapted from Reinisch (1990).

When the pill is taken properly, the failure rate is negligible (see Table 10.1). Failures occur when women do not take the pill regularly, do not use backup methods when they first go on the pill, or switch brands.

Use of oral contraceptives may temporarily reduce fertility after they are discontinued. They do not lead to permanent infertility. The great majority of women ovulate regularly within a few months after they discontinue the pill. When a woman does not ovulate after coming off the pill, a fertility drug like clomiphene may help her ovulate.

The great advantage of the pill is its effectiveness. The pill also does not interfere with sexual spontaneity or lessen sexual sensations. The pill does have some disadvantages, however. It confers no protection against STDs and may reduce the effectiveness of antibiotics used to treat them. Going on the pill requires medical consultation. Women must be on the pill several weeks before becoming sexually active.

The main drawbacks of the pill are its side effects and possible health risks. The estrogen in combination pills may produce such side effects as nausea and vomiting, fluid retention (feeling "bloated"), weight gain, increased vaginal discharge, headaches, tenderness in the breasts, and dizziness. Many of these side effects are temporary. When they persist, women may switch from one pill to another. Pregnant women produce high estrogen levels in the corpus luteum and placenta. Because the combination pill raises estrogen levels, side effects can mimic the early signs of pregnancy, such as weight gain and nausea ("morning sickness"). Estrogen causes fluid retention, leading to weight gain. Progestin increases appetite and develops muscle tissue. In the past, the pill was also linked to high blood pressure and blood clots. But lower doses of hormones are used today, making these problems less likely.

Some, but not all, evidence links oral contraceptives to a small increased risk of breast cancer in younger women.[3] This evidence cautions women who have a family history of breast cancer or other risk factors for breast cancer to carefully consider their choice of contraception in consultation with their primary health care providers.

Women with the following health problems are usually advised not to use the pill: circulatory problems or blood clots, histories of cardiovascular disease or cancers of the breast or uterus, undiagnosed genital bleeding, liver tumors, or sickle-cell anemia. The combination pill is usually not prescribed for heavy smokers over the age of 35 because of their increased risk of cardiovascular problems. Healthy nonsmokers aged 35 to 44 can apparently use the pill safely.[4] Nursing mothers should not use the pill because the hormones are passed to the baby in the mother's milk.

On the other hand, birth-control pills have some healthful benefits. They appear to reduce the risk of rheumatoid arthritis, ovarian cysts, pelvic inflammatory disease (PID), and fibrocystic (benign) breast growths. The pill helps regularize the menstrual cycle in women with irregular periods. It also reduces menstrual cramping and premenstrual discomfort. The pill may also be helpful in the treatment of iron-deficiency anemia and facial acne. Long-term use of oral contraceptives appears to reduce the risk of some cancers, including endometrial (uterine) cancer and one of the deadliest forms of cancer affecting women, ovarian cancer (cancer of the ovary).[5] These preventive effects appear to continue even for years after the woman has stopped taking the pill.

The pill may also have psychological effects. Some users report depression or irritability. Switching brands or altering doses may help.

Progestin fosters the development of male secondary sex characteristics. Women who take the minipill may develop acne, facial hair, thinning of scalp hair, reduction in breast size, vaginal dryness, and missed or shorter periods. Irregular or "breakthrough" bleeding between menstrual periods is a common side effect of the minipill.

**Close-up**
More on the pill
T1001

**"Morning-After" Pills** "Morning-after" pills are contraceptives taken after intercourse. They contain high doses of estrogen and progestin. They do not prevent ovulation. Rather, they stop fertilization from taking place or prevent the fertilized egg from implanting in the uterus. Some people therefore consider them to be an early abortion technique. Morning-after pills are most effective when taken within 72 hours after ovulation. They are of no help to women who wait to see whether they have missed a period.

Morning-after pills have a higher hormone content than most birth-control pills. For this reasons, nausea is a common side effect. The morning-after pill is not intended to be a regular method of birth control, but rather an "emergency" backup if the couple's regular contraception should fail for some reason.

## Norplant

The contraceptive implant Norplant consists of six matchstick-sized silicone tubes that contain progestin. They are surgically embedded in a woman's upper arm under local anesthesia. The tubes release a small, steady dose of progestin into the bloodstream, providing birth-control protection for up to five years. The contraceptive effect begins within 24 hours of insertion. After five years the tubes are replaced. The alternative Norplant-2 consists of two hormone-releasing tubes that provide about three years of protection.

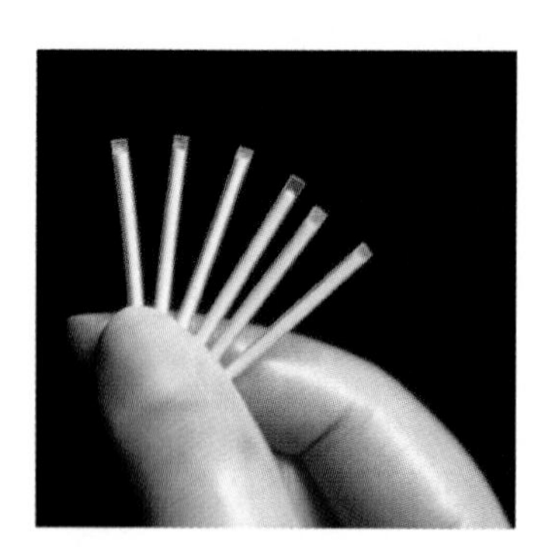

***Norplant*** Norplant consists of silicone rods that are surgically implanted in the woman's arm, which then gradually release progestin, the same female sex hormone found in the minipill.

Norplant, like the pill, has an extremely low failure rate. Moreover, it is fully reversible. Removing the tubes restores a normal likelihood of pregnancy. The key advantage of Norplant is convenience: The hormone is dispensed automatically. The most common side effect is abnormal menstrual bleeding.

**Close-up**
More on Norplant
**T1002**

## Intrauterine Devices

Camel drivers setting out on long desert journeys placed round stones in the uteruses of female camels to prevent them from becoming pregnant en route. The stones may have acted as primitive **intrauterine devices (IUDs).** IUDs are small objects inserted into the uterus by a health practitioner as a form of birth control. They are usually left in place for a year or more. Fine plastic threads or strings hanging down into the vagina enable the woman to check that the IUD remains in place.

The nearby photo shows the two currently available IUDs: the Progestasert T, which releases small quantities of progestin daily, and the Copper T 380A (ParaGard), a T-shaped, copper-based device. The Progestasert T is replaced annually. ParaGard can be used for up to 10 years, unless the woman is allergic to copper.

We do not know exactly how IUDs work. They may work by irritating the uterine lining, making it unreceptive to the implantation of the fertilized ovum. Irritation also causes mild inflammation and the production of antibodies that may be toxic to sperm or fertilized ova. Progestin released by the Progestasert T also has the effects of the minipill: It lessens the chances of fertilization and implantation. Since the contraceptive effects of the IUD may occur following fertilization, some people view it as a method of early abortion. Those opposed to early abortion in any form may also oppose use of the IUD.

**Intrauterine device (IUD)** A small object that is inserted into the uterus and left in place to prevent conception.

The failure rate of the Progestasert T is about 2%. Most failures occur because the device shifts position or is expelled. ParaGard is more effective, with a first-year failure rate under 1%.

The IUD may irritate the muscles in the uterine wall, causing contractions that may expel it. Expulsions occur in perhaps 2 to 10% of users within the first year.[6] IUDs can be easily removed by health professionals, and the effects are reversible. The great majority of former IUD users who seek to become pregnant are able to do so within a year.

The IUD has a number of advantages:

1. It is highly effective.
2. It does not diminish sexual spontaneity or sexual sensations.
3. The woman need not "do anything" to prevent pregnancy other than check that the IUD remains in place.
4. The IUD does not interfere with the woman's normal hormone production.

If IUDs are so effective and relatively "maintenance free," why are they not more popular? One reason is that insertion can be painful. Another reason is side effects. The most common side effects are menstrual cramping, irregular bleeding

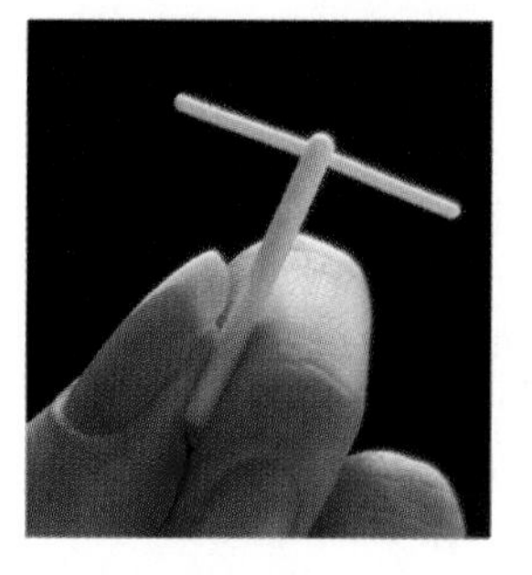

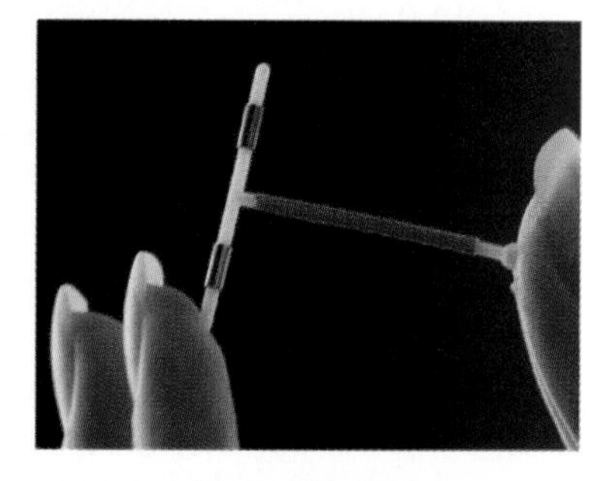

***IUDs*** Two IUDs, the Progestasert T (left) and the Copper T 380A (right). Though IUDs have a number of advantages, concerns about side effects and potential complications have limited their popularity.

(spotting) between periods, and heavy menstrual bleeding. The major health concern is a small increased risk of pelvic inflammatory disease (PID).[7] PID can produce scar tissue that blocks the Fallopian tubes, causing infertility. It is also dangerous in its own right. The risk of PID is mostly connected with insertion of the IUD introducing bacteria into the woman's reproductive system.

The IUD may also perforate (tear) the uterine or cervical walls. Perforation causes bleeding, pain, and adhesions, and it may become life-threatening. Perforations are usually caused by improper insertion of the IUD. IUD users are also at greater risk for ectopic pregnancies, both during and after usage, and for miscarriage. Despite the fact that the IUD irritates uterine tissues, there is no evidence that IUD users run a greater risk of cancer.

Close-up
More on the IUD
T1003

## The Diaphragm

The **diaphragm** is a shallow cup or dome made of thin latex rubber (Figure 10.1). The rim is a flexible metal ring covered with rubber. Diaphragms are available by prescription and must be fitted to the vagina by a health professional. Several sizes and types of diaphragms may be tried during a fitting. The diaphragm forms a barrier to sperm but should be used in conjunction with a spermicidal cream or jelly.

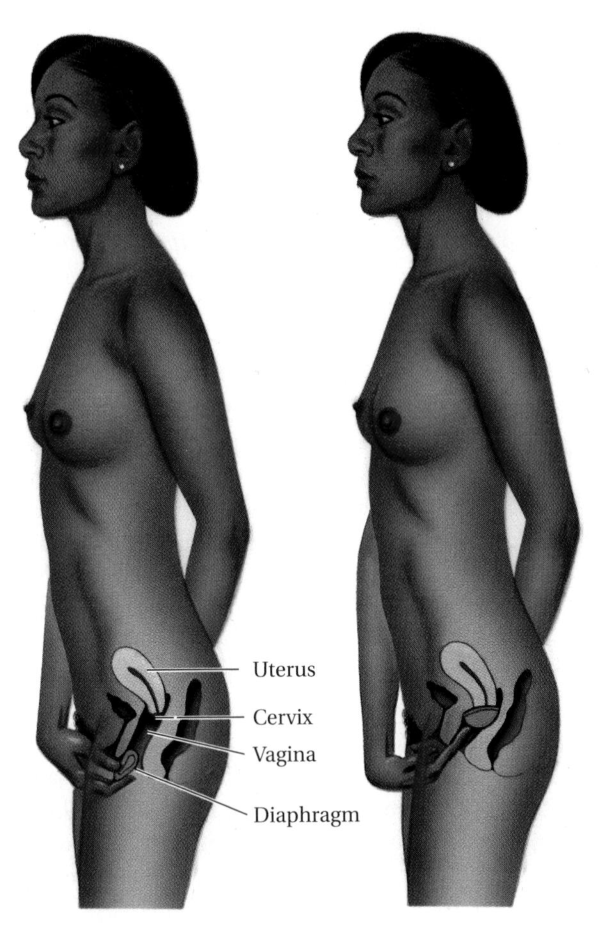


**Figure 10.2** ***Insertion and Checking of the Diaphragm*** Women are instructed in insertion of the diaphragm by a health professional. In practice, a woman and her partner may find insertion an erotic experience.

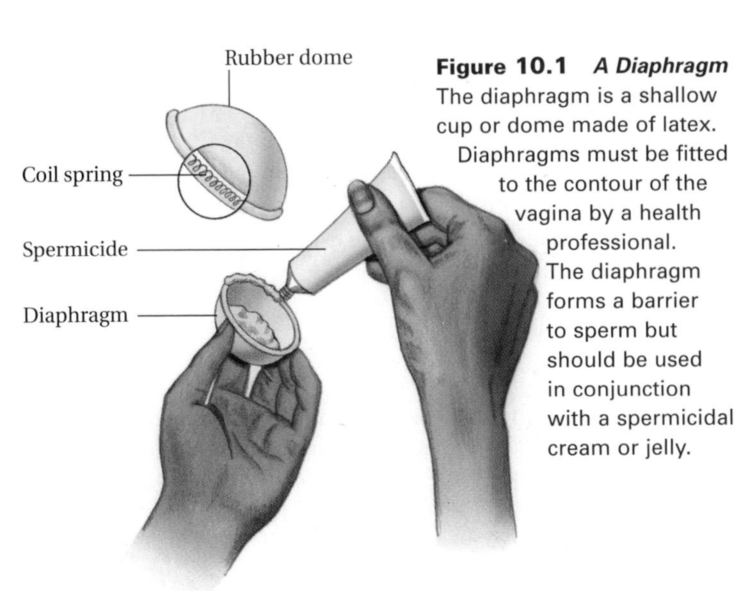


**Figure 10.1** ***A Diaphragm*** The diaphragm is a shallow cup or dome made of latex. Diaphragms must be fitted to the contour of the vagina by a health professional. The diaphragm forms a barrier to sperm but should be used in conjunction with a spermicidal cream or jelly.

The diaphragm is inserted and removed by the woman who uses it, much like a tampon. Like a condom, it forms a barrier against sperm when fitted over the cervical opening. A diaphragm is unreliable when used alone and so should be used with a spermicidal cream or jelly (see Figure 10.2).

After use, the diaphragm should be washed with mild soap and warm water and stored in a dry, cool place. When cared for properly, a diaphragm can last about two years. Women may need to be refitted after pregnancy or a change in weight of about ten pounds or more.

The diaphragm should be inserted no more than two hours before coitus, since the spermicides that are used may begin to lose effectiveness beyond this time. The woman or her partner places a tablespoonful of spermicidal cream or jelly on the inside of the cup and spreads it inside the rim. (Cream

**Diaphragm** A shallow rubber cup or dome, fitted to the contour of a woman's vagina, that is coated with a spermicide and inserted before coitus to prevent conception.

spread outside the rim might cause the diaphragm to slip.) The woman opens the inner lips of the vagina with one hand and folds the diaphragm with the other by squeezing the ring. She inserts the diaphragm against the cervix, with the inner side facing upward (see Figure 10.2). The diaphragm should be left in place *at least six hours* (but no longer than 24 hours) to allow the spermicide to kill any remaining sperm in the vagina.

If used consistently and correctly, the failure rate of the diaphragm is estimated to be 6% during the first year of use (see Table 10.1). In typical use, the failure rate is 18%. Some women become pregnant because they insert the diaphragm too early or do not leave it in long enough after sexual intercourse. For some, the diaphragm does not fit well, or it may slip. A diaphragm may also develop tiny holes or cracks. Diaphragm users are advised to inspect them for wear and tear and to consult their health professionals when in doubt. The effects of the diaphragm are fully reversible. To become pregnant, the woman simply stops using it.

**Close-up**
More on the diaphragm
T1004

When used correctly, the diaphragm is a safe and effective means of birth control. It does not alter the woman's hormone production or reproductive cycle. The diaphragm can be used as needed. By contrast, the pill must be used daily and the IUD remains in place whether or not the woman needs it. Side effects are virtually absent. Another advantage is that spermicides that contain the chemical nonoxynol-9 are toxic to many pathogens that cause STDs, including HIV.

The major disadvantage is the high failure rate connected with typical use. Moreover, the couple may find the need to insert the diaphragm before sex to be disruptive. The diaphragm and the spermicide may also cause some local irritation.

## Spermicides

Spermicides are chemical agents that kill sperm. They coat the cervical opening and block and kill sperm by chemical action. Spermicides come in different forms, including jellies and creams, suppositories, aerosol foam, and a contraceptive film. Spermicidal jellies, creams, foam, and suppositories should be applied no more than 60 minutes before sexual relations. They need to be left in place for several hours after sexual relations. Jellies and creams come in tubes with plastic applicators (see Figure 10.3). The foam is a fluffy white cream with the consistency of shaving cream. It is contained in a pressurized can and is introduced with a plastic applicator. Suppositories are inserted into the upper vagina, where they release spermicide as they dissolve. Spermicidal film dissolves into a gel and releases the spermicide. Unlike spermicidal jellies, creams, and foam, which become effective immediately, suppositories and films must be inserted several minutes before sex so that they have time to dissolve. Spermicides are most effective when they are combined with other forms of contraception, such as the diaphragm or condom.

Spermicides do not alter reproductive potential. Couples who wish to become pregnant simply stop using them. Spermicides also do not alter the woman's natural biological processes. Unlike a diaphragm, they do not require a prescription or a fitting. They can be bought in virtually any drugstore. Their cost is modest. Spermicides that contain nonoxynol-9 afford some protection against STD-causing organisms. The major disadvantage is the high failure rate. Spermicides are generally free of side effects, but they may cause local irritation in some people. Failure rates are estimated to be about 20% a year in typical use.

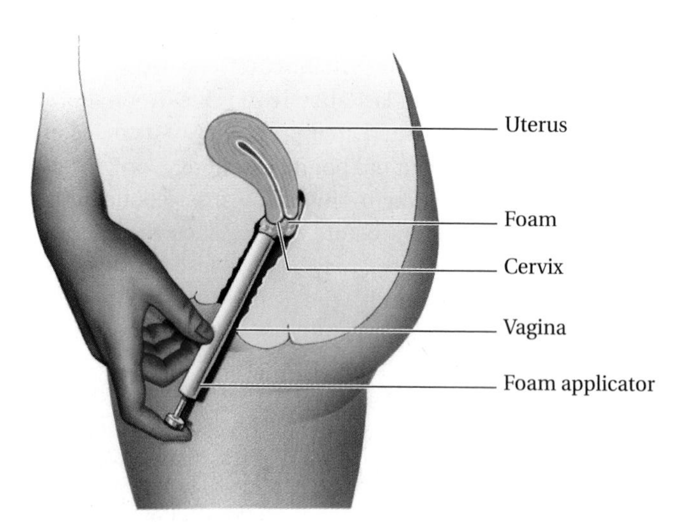


**Figure 10.3** ***The Application of Spermicidal Foam*** Spermicidal jellies and creams come in tubes with plastic applicators. Spermicidal foam comes in a pressurized can and is applied with a plastic applicator in much the same way as spermicidal jellies and creams.

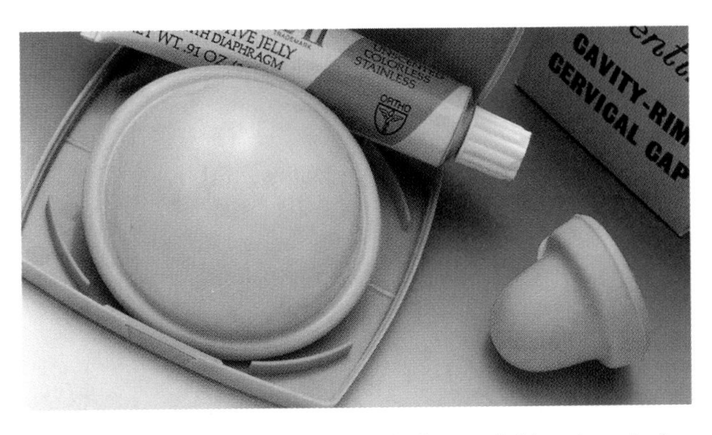


***Diaphragm and Cervical Cap*** The diaphragm (left) and cervical cap (right) must be used with spermicide to be maximally effective.

## The Cervical Cap

The cervical cap, like the diaphragm, is a dome-shaped rubber cup. It comes in different sizes and must be fitted by a health professional. It is smaller than the diaphragm, and fits snugly over the cervical opening.

The cap is intended to be used with a spermicide. The woman or her partner fills the cap about one-third full of spermicide. Then, squeezing the edges together, the woman presses the cap firmly against the cervix. It should be left in place for several hours after intercourse. The cap provides continuous protection for about 48 hours without the need for additional spermicide, no matter how many times intercourse occurs. The cap should not be left in place longer than 48 hours.

Unfortunately, the failure rate of the cap is high. One user in three to five will become pregnant within a year. Many failures can be attributed to the cap's becoming dislodged.

Like the diaphragm, the cap is a mechanical device that does not affect the woman's hormonal production or menstrual cycle. Some women find it uncomfortable. Reported side effects include urinary tract infections and allergic reactions.

## Condoms

Condoms are also called "rubbers," "safes," **prophylactics** (because latex condoms protect against STDs), and "skins" (referring to condoms made from lamb intestines). Condoms lost popularity with the advent of the pill and the IUD. They are less effective than the pill or IUD, may disrupt sexual spontaneity, and can decrease sexual sensations. Condoms have been making a comeback, however, because the latex condom can help prevent the spread of many STD-causing agents, including HIV.

**Talking Glossary**
Prophylactics
G1005

The renewed popularity of condoms has also been spurred by the increased assertiveness of contemporary women, who believe that contraception is as much the man's responsibility as the woman's. Condoms thus alter the psychology of sexual relations. Condoms are the only contraceptive device used by men. They are inexpensive and can be obtained without prescription from pharmacies, family-planning clinics, rest rooms, even from vending machines in some college dormitories.

A condom is a barrier. A latex (rubber) condom prevents the passage of sperm and pathogens from the man to his partner. It prevents infected vaginal fluids from entering the man's urethral opening or penetrating small cracks in the skin of the penis. Some condoms have plain ends. Others have nipples or reservoirs that catch semen and

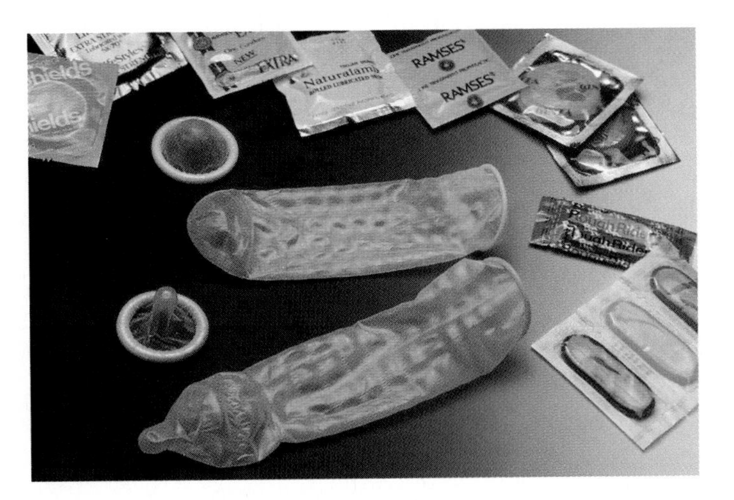


***Condoms*** There are many different types of condoms on the market today. Some are ribbed, like the two shown here. Some have nipple tips (bottom of photo) while others are plain tipped (middle of photo). Though both natural and latex condoms can prevent unwanted pregnancies, natural condoms provide less effective protection against STDs.

**Prophylactic** An agent that protects against disease.

may help prevent the condom from bursting during ejaculation.

**Close-up**
More on condoms and spermicides
**T1005**

Thinner, more expensive condoms ("skins") are made from the intestinal membranes of lambs. These allow greater sexual sensation but do not protect as well against STDs. Condoms made of animal intestines have pores large enough to permit the AIDS virus and other viruses to slip through. A few condoms are made from other materials, such as plastic (polyurethane). Questions remain about the effectiveness of polyurethane condoms.

Condoms can slip or break, allowing sperm and pathogens to leak through. To use a condom effectively and help prevent breakage or slippage, the following guidelines are recommended:[8]

- Use a condom each and every time you engage in sexual relations. Inexperienced users should practice applying a condom before they have occasion to use one with a partner.
- Handle the condom carefully to avoid damage with fingernails or other sharp objects.
- Place the condom on the erect penis before it touches the vulva.
- Uncircumcised men should pull back the foreskin before putting on the condom.
- If you use a spermicide, place some inside the tip of the condom before placing the condom on the penis. Many condoms are also coated with spermicides.
- Do not pull the condom tightly against the tip of the penis. Leave space at the end of a condom without a reservoir to catch semen. (Do not allow air to be trapped at the tip.) Some condoms come with reservoir (nipple) tips that hold semen. Unroll the condom all the way to the bottom of the penis (see Figure 10.4).
- If the condom breaks during intercourse, withdraw the penis immediately. The woman should apply a spermicide containing nonoxynol-9 to provide additional protection.
- After ejaculation, carefully withdraw the penis, while it remains erect, if possible. Hold the rim of the condom firmly against the base of the penis as the penis is withdrawn to prevent the condom from slipping off. Remove the condom carefully from the penis, ensuring that semen doesn't leak out.
- Check the removed condom for evidence of any tears or cracks. If any are found, the woman should use a spermicide containing nonoxynol-9.

About one woman in eight or ten whose partner uses a condom will become pregnant within a year. The failure rate is reduced if the condom is combined with use of a spermicide.

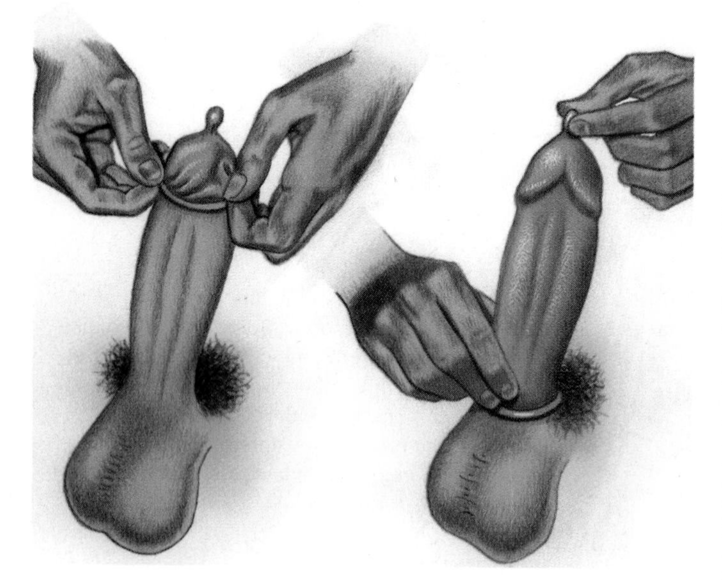

**Figure 10.4** ***Applying a Condom*** First the rolled-up condom is placed on the head of the penis, and then it is rolled down the shaft. If a condom without a reservoir tip is used, a one-half-inch space should be left at the tip for the ejaculate to accumulate.

**PREVENTION**

## *Avoiding Condom Failure—What Not to Do with Condoms*[9]

It should be no surprise that a condom works best when it is used correctly. Mistakes in using condoms can result in both STD transmission and unwanted pregnancies. Among the most common mistakes are the following:

- Rolling the condom on the flaccid (limp) penis.
- Not putting on the condom until after intercourse has begun.
- After ejaculation, allowing the penis to become fully limp before withdrawing it from the vagina.
- Failing to roll the condom all the way down the penis.
- Failing to leave a reservoir tip at the end of a plain-tipped condom.

And most commonly:

- Failing to use a condom at all or using it only occasionally.

These are some things you should *never* do with a condom:

- Never use teeth, scissors, or sharp nails to open a package of condoms. Open the condom package carefully to avoid tearing or puncturing the condom.
- Never test a condom by inflating it or stretching it.
- Never use an oil-based lubricant, such as petroleum jelly (like Vaseline), cold cream, baby oil or lotion, mineral oil, vegetable oil, Crisco, hand or body lotions, and most skin creams. These can erode the latex material. If a lubricant is desired, use a water-based lubricant such as contraceptive jelly or K-Y jelly. Do not use saliva as a lubricant because it may contain infectious organisms, such as viruses.
- Never use a damaged condom. Condoms that are sticky or brittle or otherwise appear damaged should not be used.
- Never use a condom after the expiration date (if any).
- Never use a condom if the sealed packet containing the condom is damaged, cracked, or brittle, as the condom itself may be damaged or defective.
- Do not open the sealed packet until you are ready to use the condom. A condom contained in a packet that has been opened can become dry and brittle within a few hours, causing it to tear more easily.
- Never use the same condom twice. Also, use a new condom if you switch the site of intercourse, such as from the vagina to the anus, or from the anus to the mouth, during a single sexual act.
- Do not store condoms where they could be exposed to extreme heat, such as the glove compartment of a car. Condoms should be stored in a cool, dry place, such as a medicine cabinet or dresser drawer.
- If you want to carry a condom with you, place it in a loose jacket pocket or purse, not in your pants pocket or in a wallet held in your pants pocket, where it might be exposed to body heat.
- Never buy condoms from vending machines that are exposed to extreme heat or placed in direct sunlight.

## Douching

Talking Glossary
Douches
G1006

Some couples believe that if a woman **douches** shortly after sex, she will not become pregnant. Unfortunately, douching is an ineffective birth-control technique. Large numbers of sperm are beyond the range of the douche seconds after ejaculation. In addition, squirting a liquid into the vagina may actually propel sperm *toward* the uterus. Regular douching may also alter the natural chemistry of the vagina, increasing the risk of vaginal infection. In short, douching is a "non-method" of contraception.

## Withdrawal (Coitus Interruptus)

Withdrawal means that the man removes his penis from the vagina before ejaculating. Withdrawal has a high failure rate. One in five to one in four women who use the method become pregnant within a year. There are several reasons for failure. The man may not withdraw in time. Even if he does, sperm may be present in the *pre*-ejaculatory secretions of seminal fluid.

## Fertility Awareness Methods (Rhythm Methods)

Fertility awareness, or *rhythm*, methods rely on awareness of the fertile segments of the woman's menstrual cycle. Terms such as *natural birth control* or *natural family planning* also refer to these methods. Sexual relations are avoided on days when conception is most likely. Since rhythm methods do not employ artificial devices, they may be morally acceptable to people whose religious teachings prohibit artificial contraception. Rhythm methods seek to predict ovulation so that the couple can abstain from sexual relations when the woman is likely to be fertile.

**The Calendar Method** The **calendar method** assumes that ovulation occurs 14 days before menstruation. The couple abstains from intercourse during the period that begins 3 days before day 13 (because sperm are unlikely to survive for more than 72 hours in the female reproductive tract) and ends 2 days after day 15 (because an unfertilized ovum is unlikely to remain receptive to fertilization for longer than 48 hours). The period of abstention thus covers days 10 to 17 of the woman's cycle.

Defining the period of abstention is easy enough for women with regular cycles. Women with irregular cycles are generally advised to chart their

**Douche** To rinse or wash the vaginal canal by inserting a liquid and allowing it to drain out.

**Calendar method** A fertility awareness (rhythm) method of contraception that relies on prediction of ovulation by tracking menstrual cycles.

cycles for 10 months to a year to determine their shortest and longest cycles. The first day of menstruation counts as day 1 of the cycle. The last day of the cycle is the day preceding the onset of menstruation.

One way of determining the period of abstention is to subtract 18 days from the woman's shortest cycle to determine the start of the "unsafe" period and 11 days from her longest cycle to determine the last "unsafe" day. Some women have such irregular cycles that the range of "unsafe" days cannot be predicted reliably even if baseline tracking is extended.

**The Basal Body Temperature (BBT) Method** Women who use the **basal body temperature (BBT) method** track their body temperature. A drawback to the BBT method is that it does not indicate the several *unsafe* pre-ovulatory days during which sperm deposited in the vagina may remain viable. Rather, it indicates when a woman *has* ovulated. Thus, many women use the calendar method to predict the number of "safe" days before ovulation. They turn to the BBT method to determine the number of "unsafe" days afterward. A woman would avoid sexual relations during the "unsafe" pre-ovulatory period (as determined by the calendar method). She would continue to avoid sexual relations for three days when her temperature rises and remains elevated, which indicates ovulation. Some women triple check themselves by also tracking their cervical mucus.

**The Cervical Mucus (Ovulation) Method** The **ovulation method** tracks changes in the **viscosity** of the cervical mucus. Following menstruation, the vagina feels rather dry. There is also little or no discharge from the cervix. These dry days are relatively safe. Then a mucous discharge appears in the vagina that is at first thick and sticky, and white or cloudy in color. Sexual relations are avoided at the first sign of any mucus. As the cycle progresses, the mucus discharge thins and clears, becoming slippery or stringy, like raw egg white. These are the **peak days.** This mucus discharge, called the *ovulatory mucus,* may be accompanied by a feeling of vaginal lubrication or wetness. Ovulation takes place about a day after the last peak day (about four days after this ovulatory mucus first appears). Then the mucus becomes cloudy and tacky once more. Intercourse may resume four days following the last peak day.

The method is not without problems. Some women have difficulty detecting changes in cervical mucus. Such changes may also result from infections, medications, or contraceptive creams, jellies, or foam. Sexual arousal may also induce changes in viscosity.

**Basal body temperature (BBT) method** A fertility awareness method of contraception that relies on prediction of ovulation by tracking a woman's temperature during the menstrual cycle.

**Ovulation method** A fertility awareness method of contraception that relies on prediction of ovulation by tracking the viscosity of the cervical mucus.

**Viscosity** Stickiness, consistency.

**Peak days** The days during the menstrual cycle during which a woman is most likely to be fertile.

**Sterilization** Surgical procedures that render people incapable of reproduction without affecting sexual response.

**Ovulation-Prediction Kits** Ovulation-prediction kits are more accurate than the BBT method. Some couples use them as a means of birth control to find out when to avoid sexual relations. However, ovulation kits are expensive. They also require that the woman test her urine each morning. Nor do they reveal the full range of the unsafe *pre*-ovulatory period during which sperm may remain viable in the vagina. A couple might thus choose to use the kits to determine the unsafe period following ovulation, and the calendar method to determine the unsafe period preceding ovulation.

Rhythm methods are most reliable when a combination of rhythm methods is used and when the woman's cycles are regular. Although failure rates in typical use are high, these rates can be greatly reduced if rhythm methods are supplemented with other methods of birth control, such as the condom or diaphragm.

Because they are a natural form of birth control, rhythm methods appeal to many people who, for religious or other reasons, prefer not to use artificial means. Since no devices or chemicals are used, there are no side effects or health complications. Nor do they cause any loss of sensation, as condoms do. Nor is there disruption of lovemaking, although lovemaking could be said to be quite "disrupted" during the period of abstinence. All rhythm methods are fully reversible. To conceive, the couple discontinue timing ovulation or engage in sexual relations at about the time of ovulation.

## Sterilization

Many people choose **sterilization** when they plan to have no children or no more children. With the exception of abstinence, sterilization is the most effective form of contraception. More than a mil-

**Figure 10.5** ***Vasectomy***
The male sterilization procedure is usually carried out in a doctor's office, using local anesthesia. Small incisions are made in the scrotum. Each vas deferens is cut and the ends are tied off or cauterized to prevent sperm from reaching the urethra. Sperm are harmlessly reabsorbed by the body after the operation.

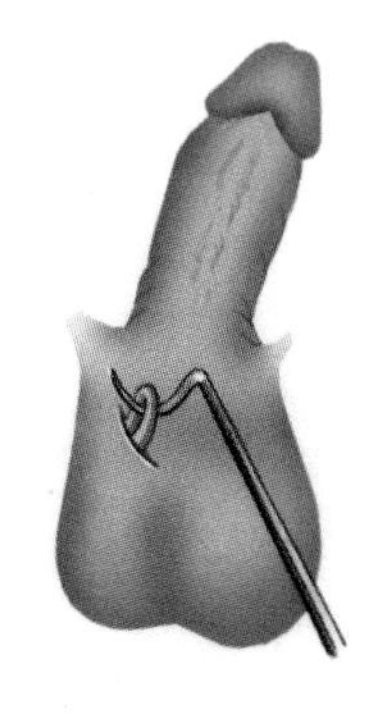

1. Isolation of vas from surrounding tissue

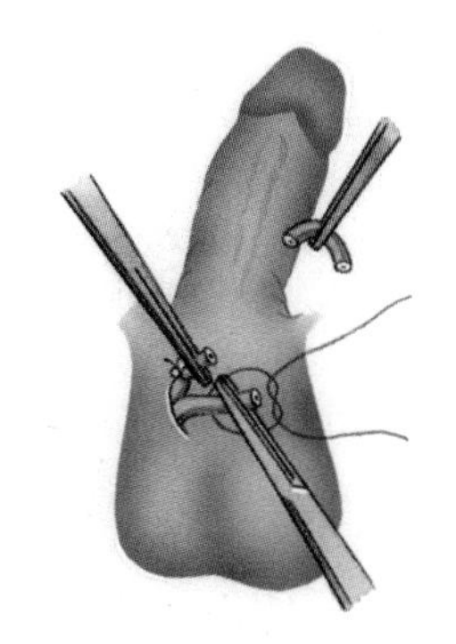

2. Removal of segment of vas; tying of ends

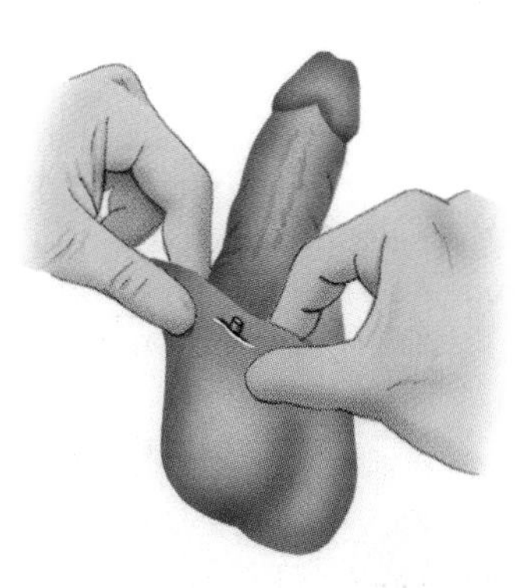

3. Return of vas to position; incision is closed and process is repeated on the other side

lion sterilizations are performed in the United States each year. It is the most widely used form of birth control among married couples age 30 and above. Married people are far more likely than single people to choose sterilization.

**Male Sterilization** The male sterilization procedure used today is the **vasectomy.** About 500,000 vasectomies are performed each year in the United States. More than 15% of men in the United States have had vasectomies.[10]

A vasectomy is usually carried out in a doctor's office, under local anesthesia. It takes 15 to 20 minutes. Small incisions are made in the scrotum. Each vas is cut. A small segment is removed. The ends are usually tied or closed off to prevent them from growing back together (Figure 10.5). Now sperm can no longer reach the urethra. Instead, they are harmlessly reabsorbed by the body.

Vasectomy does not affect the sex drive, erectile or ejaculatory ability, or sensations of ejaculation. Male sex hormones and sperm are still produced by the testes. Without a passageway to the urethra, however, sperm are no longer expelled with the ejaculate. Since sperm account for only about 1% of the ejaculate, the amount of ejaculate is not noticeably different.

Some vasectomies result in temporary local inflammation or swelling. Rarer still is a risk of infection of the epididymis. There are no confirmed long-term health risks of vasectomy. Nevertheless, two studies of more than 73,000 men who had vasectomies raise concerns that vasectomy may be connected with a slightly increased risk of prostate cancer.[11] The results of these studies conflict with earlier studies showing either no link between vasectomies and the risk of prostate cancer or a *lower* risk among vasectomized men. Health experts recommend more research to clarify the relationship between vasectomy and prostate cancer.[12]

Vasectomies should be considered permanent. In an operation to reverse a vasectomy, the ends of the vas deferens are sewn together, and, in a few days, grow together. Fertility is not guaranteed, however.

**Female Sterilization** The most common method of female sterilization is the **tubal ligation.** Nearly 650,000 tubal sterilizations are performed each year in the United States. Nearly 40% of married women under the age of 45 have been sterilized. Tubal sterilization prevents ova and sperm from passing through the Fallopian tubes.

The two major surgical techniques used for female sterilization are *minilaparotomy* and *laparoscopy.* In a **minilaparotomy,** the Fallopian tubes are reached through a small incision in the abdomen, just above the pubic

**Vasectomy** The surgical method of male sterilization in which each vas deferens is cut and closed off.

**Tubal ligation** The Fallopian tubes are surgically blocked to prevent the meeting of sperm and ova.

**Minilaparotomy** Tubal sterilization in which a small incision is made in the abdomen to provide access to the Fallopian tubes.

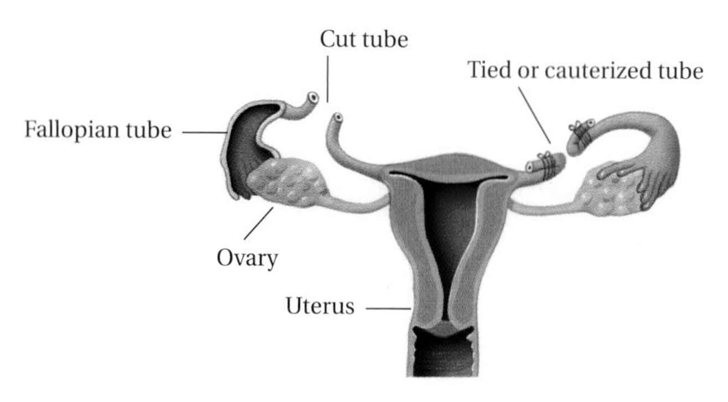


**Figure 10.6** ***Laparoscopy*** In this method of female sterilization, the surgeon approaches the Fallopian tubes through a small incision in the abdomen just below the navel. A narrow instrument called a laparoscope is inserted through the incision, and a small section of each Fallopian tube is cauterized, cut, or clamped to prevent ova from joining with sperm.

**Talking Glossary**
Laparoscopy
G1007

hairline. Each tube is cut and tied back or clamped with a clip. In a **laparoscopy** (Figure 10.6) (sometimes called "belly button surgery"), the Fallopian tubes are approached through a small incision just below the navel. The surgeon inserts a narrow, lighted viewing instrument called a *laparoscope.* A small section of each of the tubes is cauterized, cut, or clamped. The woman usually returns to her daily routine in a few days and can resume sexual relations when they become comfortable. The Fallopian tubes can also be approached through an incision in the back wall of the vagina.

Although many tubal ligations are successfully reversed, women should assume that they are permanent. Reversal is difficult and costly.

None of these methods disrupts sex drive or sexual response. Surgical sterilization does not affect production of sex hormones. The menstrual cycle is undisturbed. The unfertilized egg is reabsorbed by the body, rather than being sloughed off in the menstrual flow.

Some tubal ligations cause medical complications. Most common are abdominal infections, excessive bleeding, inadvertent punctures of nearby organs, and scarring. The use of general anesthesia (typical in laparoscopies and in some minilaparotomies) poses additional risks, as in any major operation.

**Laparoscopy** A method of sterilization in which a laparoscope is inserted through a small incision just below the navel and used to close off the Fallopian tubes.

**Vaginal ring** A contraceptive device shaped like a diaphragm that is worn in the vagina; slowly releases either a combination of estrogen and progestin or progestin only.

A hysterectomy also results in sterilization. However, hysterectomy is a major operation that is inappropriate as a method of sterilization.

Male or female sterilization affords no protection against STDs, of course. People who are sterilized may still need to use condoms and spermicides for protection against STDs.

## Other Devices

A number of other contraceptive devices have recently been introduced or are under development.

**Close-up**
More on the female condom
T1006

**The Female Condom** The female condom consists of a polyurethane (plastic) sheath that lines the vagina during intercourse. It is held in place at each end by a flexible plastic ring. The female condom provides a secure but flexible barrier against sperm. However, the female condom appears to be less effective than the male latex condom in preventing pregnancies and transmission of STDs. Many women complain that the female condom is bulky and difficult to insert.

**The Vaginal Ring** The **vaginal ring** can be worn in the vagina for three months before replacement. Shaped like a diaphragm, the ring contains either a combination of estrogen and progestin or progestin only. The hormones are slowly released and pass into the bloodstream through the mucosal lining of the vagina. Research on the effectiveness of the vaginal ring is under way.

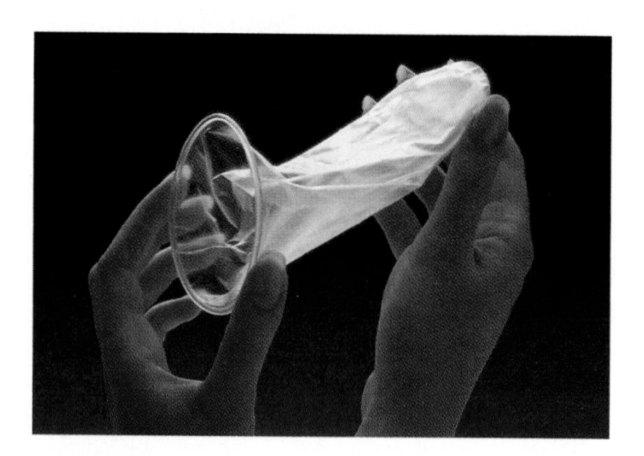

***Female Condom*** The female condom is inserted in the vagina to prevent sperm from reaching the woman's internal reproductive tract. The female condom does not appear to provide the same level of protection against pregnancies and STDs as the male latex condom.

Talking Glossary
Depo-Provera
G1008

**Depo-Provera** **Depo-Provera** is a long-acting, synthetic form of progesterone that works as a contraceptive by inhibiting ovulation. The progesterone signals the pituitary gland in the brain to stop producing hormones that would lead to the release of mature ova by the ovaries. Administered by injection once every three months, Depo-Provera is an effective form of contraception. A World Health Organization study of 12,000 women found no links between the drug and the risk of ovarian or cervical cancer.[13] Yet the drug may produce side effects such as weight gain, menstrual irregularity, and spotting between periods.

**Experimental Efforts** Other methods of contraception are in experimental stages, including sterilization techniques that promise greater reversibility. A "male pill"—that is, an oral contraceptive for men—is in the experimental stage. The male sex hormone testosterone has shown promise in reducing sperm production. The pituitary gland normally stimulates the testes to produce sperm. Testosterone suppresses the pituitary, in turn suppressing sperm production. Men who have received testosterone injections have shown declines in sperm production. Potential complications include concerns about an increased risk of prostate cancer and elevated cholesterol levels. In any event, a survey of college men found that only one in five expressed willingness to take a male pill.[14] The men believed that taking a male pill would be more of a bother than having one's partner take a female pill and more "contrary to nature"!

Close-up
Under development
T1007

Another approach was suggested when investigators in China found extremely low birth rates in communities in which cottonseed oil was used in cooking. They extracted a drug from the cotton plant, gossypol, which shows promise as a male contraceptive. Chinese studies reveal the drug to be nearly 100% effective in preventing pregnancies. The drug appears to nullify sperm production without affecting hormone levels or the sex drive. However, toxic effects of gossypol have limited its acceptability.

Some men are infertile because they produce antibodies that destroy their own sperm. Researchers suspect that it may be possible to develop ways to induce the body to produce such antibodies. Ideally this procedure would be reversible.

Applying ultrasound waves to the testes has been shown to produce reversible sterility in laboratory rats, dogs, and monkeys. As with the IUD, no one is quite certain how ultrasound works. Moreover, its safety with men has not been demonstrated.

The perfect contraceptive will be dispensed automatically, have no side effects, and be fully reversible. We are not there yet.

### think about it!

- **Have you discussed methods of contraception with your peers? If so, what factors account for their choices?**
- **Which methods of contraception also confer some protection against sexually transmitted diseases?**
- **Which methods of contraception are most and least disruptive of sexual spontaneity? Why?**

**critical thinking Are some or all of the methods of contraception morally and ethically unacceptable to you? Explain.**

Smart Quiz
Q1002

## ABORTION

An **induced abortion** (in contrast to a spontaneous abortion, or miscarriage) is the purposeful termination of a pregnancy before the embryo or fetus is capable of sustaining independent life. Perhaps more than any other contemporary social issue, induced abortion (hereafter referred to simply as abortion) has divided neighbors and family members into opposing camps.

Nearly 40 million abortions worldwide, including about 1.2 million in the U.S., are performed annually. Nearly 90% of abortions in the United States occur during the first trimester, when they are safest for women and least costly. Nearly four women in five who have abortions are unmarried. According to the latest available statistics, the annual abortion rate stands at 21 women of every 1,000 in the 15 to 44 age group.[15] The abortion rate in the U.S. has actually been declining in recent

**Depo-Provera** A synthetic form of progesterone that works as a contraceptive by inhibiting ovulation.

**Induced abortion** The purposeful termination of a pregnancy before the embryo or fetus is capable of sustaining independent life.

years and reached a 20-year low in 1994. The decline is attributed at least partly to better access to contraception, resulting in fewer unwanted pregnancies.

More than half (55%) of the women who have abortions are in their twenties. Women aged 15 to 19 account for about one in four (25%) abortions. Most of the remainder of women who have abortions are between 30 and 39 years of age.

The national debate over abortion has been played out in recent years against a backdrop of demonstrations, marches, and occasional acts of violence, such as firebombings of abortion clinics, even murder. The right-to-life (pro-life) movement asserts that human life begins at conception and thus views abortion as the murder of an unborn child. Some in the pro-life movement allow no exception to their opposition to abortion. Others would permit abortion to save the mother's life or when a pregnancy results from rape or incest. The pro-choice movement contends that abortion is a matter of personal choice and that the government has no right to interfere with a woman's right to terminate a pregnancy. Pro-choice advocates argue that women are free to control what happens within their bodies, including pregnancies.

## When Does Human Life Begin?

Moral concerns about abortion often turn on the question of when human life begins. For some Christians, the matter revolves around when they believe the fetus obtains a soul.

In his thesis on ensoulment, the thirteenth-century Christian theologian Thomas Aquinas wrote that a male fetus does not acquire a human soul until 40 days after conception. A female fetus does not acquire a soul until after 80 days. Scientists, too, have attempted to define when human life can be said to begin. The late astronomer Carl Sagan, for example, wrote that fetal brain activity can be considered a secular or scientific marker of human life.[16] He argued that brain activity is needed for thought, the quality that is considered most "human" by many. Brain wave patterns typical of children do not begin until about the thirtieth week of pregnancy. Before then, the human fetus lacks the brain architecture to begin thinking. Of course, this argument raises the question of whether fetal brain wave activity can be equated with thought. (What would a fetus "think" about?) Moreover, some argue that a newly fertilized ovum carries the *potential* for human thought in the same way that the embryonic or fetal brain does. It could even be argued that sperm cells and ova are living things in that they carry out the biological processes characteristic of cellular life. All in all, the question of when *human* life begins is a matter of definition that is apparently unanswerable by science.

## Historical and Legal Perspectives on Abortion

Societal attitudes toward abortion have varied across cultures and times in history. Abortion was permitted in ancient Greece and Rome, but women in ancient Assyria were impaled on stakes for attempting abortion. For much of its history, the Roman Catholic Church held to Thomas Aquinas's belief that ensoulment of the fetus did not occur for at least 40 days after conception. In 1869, Pope Pius IX declared that human life begins at conception. Thus an abortion at any stage of pregnancy became murder in the eyes of the church.

In colonial times and through the mid-nineteenth century, women in the United States were permitted to terminate a pregnancy until such time as they felt fetal movement. More restrictive abortion laws emerged after the Civil War. By 1900 virtually all the states had enacted legislation banning abortion except to save the woman's life.

Abortion laws remained essentially unchanged until the late 1960s, when some states liberalized their abortion laws under mounting public pressure. Then, in 1973, the United States Supreme Court in effect legalized abortion nationwide in the *Roe* v. *Wade* decision. *Roe* v. *Wade* held that a woman's right to an abortion was protected under the right to privacy guaranteed by the Constitution. The decision legalized abortion for any reason during the first trimester. In its ruling, the Court noted that a fetus is not considered a person and is thus not entitled to constitutional protection. The Court ruled that states may regulate a woman's right to have an abortion during the second trimester to protect her health, as in requiring her to obtain an abortion in a hospital rather than a doctor's office. The Court also held that when a fetus becomes viable, its rights override the mother's right to privacy. Because the fetus may become viable early in the third trimester, states may prohibit third-trimester abortions, except when an abortion is necessary to protect a woman's health or life.

# HealthCheck

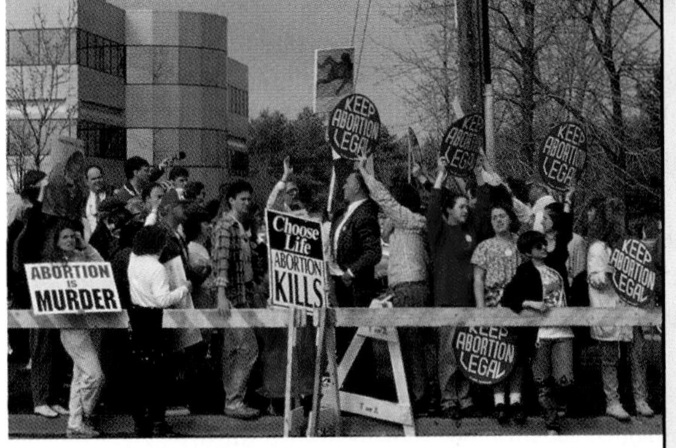
KEEP ABORTION LEGAL
ABORTION IS MURDER
Choose Life
ABORTION KILLS

## Pro-Choice or Pro-Life? Where Do You Stand?

What does it mean to be "pro-life" on the abortion issue? What does it mean to be "pro-choice"? Which position is closer to your own views?

The *Reasoning about Abortion Questionnaire (RAQ)*[17] assesses agreement with pro-life or pro-choice reasoning about abortion. To find out which position is closer to your own, indicate your level of agreement or disagreement with each of these items by circling the number that best represents your feelings. Refer to the answer key in Appendix B at the end of the book to interpret your score.

1 = Strongly disagree
2 = Disagree
3 = Mixed feelings
4 = Agree
5 = Strongly agree

| | | | | | | |
|---|---|---|---|---|---|---|
| **1.** | Abortion is a matter of personal choice. | 1 | 2 | 3 | 4 | 5 |
| **2.** | Abortion is a threat to our society. | 1 | 2 | 3 | 4 | 5 |
| **3.** | A woman should have control over what is happening to her own body by having the option to choose abortion. | 1 | 2 | 3 | 4 | 5 |
| **4.** | Only God, not people, can decide if a fetus should live. | 1 | 2 | 3 | 4 | 5 |
| **5.** | Even if one believes that there may be some exceptions, abortion is still basically wrong. | 1 | 2 | 3 | 4 | 5 |
| **6.** | Abortion violates an unborn person's fundamental right to life. | 1 | 2 | 3 | 4 | 5 |
| **7.** | A woman should be able to exercise her right to self-determination by choosing to have an abortion. | 1 | 2 | 3 | 4 | 5 |
| **8.** | Outlawing abortion could take away a woman's sense of self and personal autonomy. | 1 | 2 | 3 | 4 | 5 |
| **9.** | Outlawing abortion violates a woman's civil rights. | 1 | 2 | 3 | 4 | 5 |
| **10.** | Abortion is morally unacceptable and unjustified. | 1 | 2 | 3 | 4 | 5 |
| **11.** | In my reasoning, the notion that an unborn fetus may be a human life is not a deciding issue in considering abortion. | 1 | 2 | 3 | 4 | 5 |
| **12.** | Abortion can be described as taking a life unjustly. | 1 | 2 | 3 | 4 | 5 |
| **13.** | A woman should have the right to decide to have an abortion based on her own life circumstances. | 1 | 2 | 3 | 4 | 5 |
| **14.** | If a woman feels that having a child might ruin her life, she should consider an abortion. | 1 | 2 | 3 | 4 | 5 |
| **15.** | Abortion could destroy the sanctity of motherhood. | 1 | 2 | 3 | 4 | 5 |
| **16.** | An unborn fetus is a viable human being with rights. | 1 | 2 | 3 | 4 | 5 |
| **17.** | If a woman feels she can't care for a baby, she should be able to have an abortion. | 1 | 2 | 3 | 4 | 5 |
| **18.** | Abortion is the destruction of one life for the convenience of another. | 1 | 2 | 3 | 4 | 5 |
| **19.** | Abortion is the same as murder. | 1 | 2 | 3 | 4 | 5 |
| **20.** | Even if one believes that there are times when abortion is immoral, it is still basically the woman's own choice. | 1 | 2 | 3 | 4 | 5 |

Since *Roe* v. *Wade,* a majority of states have enacted laws requiring parental consent or notification before a minor child may have an abortion. Most adults in the United States believe that parental permission should be required for teenage girls to have abortions. Many pregnant teenage girls, however, especially those living in families with alcoholic or abusive parents, fear telling their parents that they are pregnant. In 1990, in rulings involving state laws in Ohio and Minnesota, the United States Supreme Court upheld the rights of states to require that a minor seeking an abortion notify at least one parent and wait 48 hours before an abortion can be performed. The Court provided an "escape clause," however: The minor girl may go before a judge instead. A 1993 U.S. Supreme Court ruling let stand a Mississippi law requiring minors to obtain approval from both parents or from a judge.

In 1989 a decision by the United States Supreme Court in a Missouri case, *Webster* v. *Reproductive Health Services,* considerably narrowed abortion rights granted previously under *Roe* v. *Wade.* By a five-to-four decision, the Supreme Court upheld Missouri state laws (1) restricting public employees from performing or assisting in abortions, except in cases in which an abortion is needed to save a woman's life; (2) prohibiting the use of public facilities for performing abortions; and (3) requiring doctors to perform medical tests to determine the viability of a fetus before granting a woman's request for an abortion if she is believed to be at least 20 weeks pregnant. The *Webster* decision made it more difficult (and expensive) for women to obtain late second-trimester abortions by allowing states to require medical testing for viability at 20 weeks.

Many people in the pro-choice movement argue that if abortions were to be made illegal again, thousands of women, especially poor women, would die or suffer serious physical consequences from botched or nonsterile abortions. People in the pro-life movement counter that women can allow unwanted children to be adopted and that no one is forced to have an illegal abortion. Pro-choice advocates argue that the debate should also address the quality of life of an unwanted child. They argue that minority and physically or mentally disabled children are often hard to place for adoption. These children often spend their childhoods shuffled from one foster home to another. Pro-life advocates counter that killing a fetus eliminates any potential that it might have, despite hardships, of living a fruitful and meaningful life. The debate about abortion continues. No consensus is in the offing.

**Vacuum aspiration** Removal of the uterine contents by suction. An abortion method used early in pregnancy.

## Methods of Abortion

Regardless of the moral, legal, and political issues that surround abortion, many abortion methods are in use today.

**Vacuum Aspiration** **Vacuum aspiration,** or suction curettage, is the safest and most common method of abortion. It accounts for more than 90% of abortions in the United States. It is relatively painless and inexpensive. It can be done with little or no anesthesia in a medical office or clinic, but only during the first trimester. Later, thinning of the uterine walls increases the risks of perforation and bleeding. In the procedure, the cervix is usually dilated first by progressively larger rods, or "dilators." Or the cervix is dilated more gently by a stick of seaweed called *Laminaria digitata. Laminaria* expands as it absorbs cervical moisture. Then a tube connected to an aspirator (suction machine) is inserted through the cervix into the uterus. The uterine contents are then evacuated (emptied) by suction (Figure 10.7). Possible complications include perforation of the uterus, infection, cervical lacerations, and hemorrhaging, but these are rare.

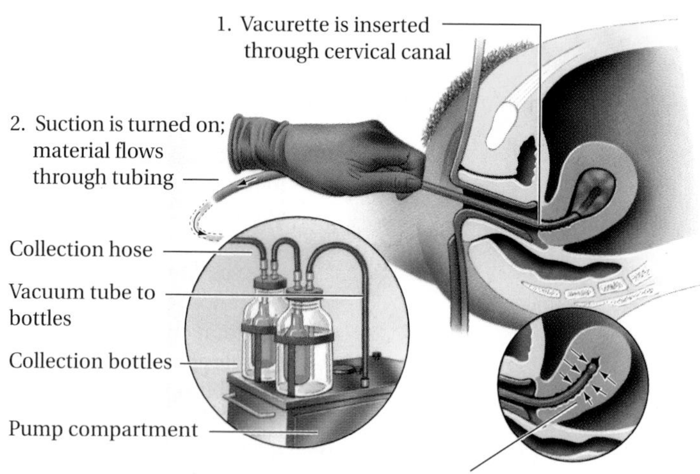
1. Vacurette is inserted through cervical canal
2. Suction is turned on; material flows through tubing
Collection hose
Vacuum tube to bottles
Collection bottles
Pump compartment
3. Empty uterus collapses

**Figure 10.7** ***Vacuum Aspiration*** This is the safest and most common method of abortion, but it can be performed only during the first trimester. An angled tube is inserted through the cervix into the uterus, and the uterine contents are then evacuated (emptied) by suction.

**Dilation and Curettage (D&C)** Dilation and curettage was once the customary method of performing abortions. It now accounts for only a small number of abortions in the United States. It is usually performed 8 to 20 weeks following the last menstrual period. Once the cervix has been dilated, the uterine contents are scraped from the uterine lining.

D&Cs are carried out in a hospital, usually under general anesthesia. The scraping increases the chances of hemorrhaging, infection, and perforation. Because of these risks, D&Cs have largely been replaced by vacuum aspiration. D&Cs are still used to treat various gynecological problems, however, such as abnormally heavy menstrual bleeding.

**Dilation and Evacuation (D&E)** Dilation and evacuation is used most commonly during the second trimester, when vacuum aspiration alone would be too risky. The D&E combines suction and the D&C. First the cervix is dilated. Then a suction tube is inserted to remove some of the contents of the uterus. But suction alone cannot safely remove all uterine contents. The remaining contents are removed with forceps. The uterine wall may be scraped to make sure that the lining has been fully removed. Like the D&C, the D&E is usually performed in the hospital under general anesthesia. Most women recover quickly and relatively painlessly. In rare instances, however, complications can arise. These include excessive bleeding, infection, and perforation of the uterine lining.

**Intra-amniotic Infusion** Second-trimester abortions are sometimes performed by chemically inducing premature labor and delivery. The procedure is performed in a hospital. It is called instillation, or **intra-amniotic infusion.** It is usually performed when fetal development has progressed beyond the point at which other methods are deemed safe. A saline (salt) solution or a solution of prostaglandins (hormones that stimulate uterine contractions during labor) is injected into the amniotic sac. Prostaglandins may also be administered by vaginal suppository. Uterine contractions (labor) begin within a few hours after infusion. The fetus and placenta are expelled from the uterus within the next 24 or 48 hours.

Talking Glossary
Intra-amniotic infusion
G1009

Intra-amniotic infusion accounts for only a small number of abortions. Medical complications, risks, and costs are greater with this procedure than with other methods of abortion. Overly rapid labor can tear the cervix, but previous dilation of the cervix with *Laminaria* lessens the risk. Perforation, infection, and hemorrhaging are rare if prostaglandins are used, but about half the recipients experience nausea and vomiting, diarrhea, or headaches. Saline infusion can cause shock and even death if the solution is carelessly introduced into the bloodstream.

**Hysterotomy** The **hysterotomy** is, in effect, a caesarean section. A hysterotomy is major surgery that must be carried out under general anesthesia in a hospital. Incisions are made in the abdomen and uterus, and the fetus and uterine contents are removed. Hysterotomy may be performed during the late second trimester. It is usually performed only when intra-amniotic infusion is not advised. Hysterotomy involves risks of complications from the anesthesia and the surgery itself.

Talking Glossary
Hysterotomy
G1010

**Abortion Drugs** Most early abortions are accomplished by vacuum aspiration, which is a surgical technique. Most women in the United States would prefer a drug-induced abortion if it were available.[18]

One drug-induced abortion method is available in France and many other parts of the world. It is the abortion pill, RU-486. The pill contains *mifepristone,* which induces early abortion by blocking the effects of progesterone. (Progesterone stimulates proliferation of the endometrium, allowing implantation of the fertilized ovum.) By the mid-1990s, 46% of the French women seeking abortion preferred RU-486 to surgical methods, including vacuum aspiration.

Supporters of RU-486 argue that it offers a safe, noninvasive substitute for more costly and unpleasant abortion procedures. RU-486 may make abortion physically easier, but not necessarily psychologically easier. The

**Dilation and curettage (D&C)** An operation in which the cervix is dilated and uterine contents gently scraped away.

**Dilation and evacuation (D&E)** An abortion method in which the cervix is dilated before vacuum aspiration.

**Intra-amniotic infusion** An abortion method in which a substance is injected into the amniotic sac to induce premature labor.

**Hysterotomy** An abortion method in which the fetus is removed by caesarean section.

## Japan's Abortion Agony—In a Country That Prohibits the Pill, Reality Collides with Religion[24]

WORLD OF *diversity*

Japan is perhaps the richest, most technologically advanced nation in the world, but it depends on an antiquated system of birth control that forces women to rely heavily on abortion in a society that at the same time disapproves of it.

Japan's abortion rate is one of the highest among the world's industrialized nations. One reason for this is the lack of birth-control alternatives. The government bans the use of the birth-control pill as a contraceptive, and doctors do not encourage sterilization, IUDs, or diaphragms. Nearly 75% of Japanese continue to rely on condoms and rhythm methods despite their high failure rate.

Over the years Japanese officials defended the ban against the pill by arguing that oral contraceptives are unsafe and would promote promiscuity. In 1992, a review by the Health and Welfare Ministry found birth-control pills to be safe but decided to uphold the ban because of concerns about AIDS. Though Japan has had relatively few AIDS cases by international standards, the health ministry feared that lifting the ban on the pill might discourage condom use and lead to an epidemic of AIDS. Some women in Japan are able to skirt the ban by consulting sympathetic physicians who are willing to prescribe the pill ostensibly to treat gynecological complaints.

In part because of limited contraceptive options, the Japanese use condoms more than any other people in the world. Condoms are widely available in drugstores, supermarkets, and vending machines; embarrassed housewives can buy them from door-to-door saleswomen. Abortion is the widely used backup for failed contraception. And yet, while abortions have now been legal and easily accessible in Japan for over 40 years, women who have them feel stigmatized because abortion is regarded by many Japanese, even those who accept it, as "killing a baby."

Most Japanese draw little distinction between a fetus and an infant. According to Samuel Coleman, the author of *Family Planning in Japanese Society,* the reasons lie at least partially in Shinto and Buddhism, Japan's two major religions. Although neither religion promotes active opposition to abortion, Buddhism is based on the ideal of overcoming one's sense of ego. In this context, a woman who aborts wrongly puts her ego before her fetus. Shinto, an ancient religion based on ancestor and nature worship, holds that an aborted fetus can place a curse on the woman who aborts.

### Offerings at the Temple

Hiroshi Hihara is a gynecologist in Tokyo. He makes his living from infertility treatment and abortions, many of them for married women whose method of contraception has failed. Although Hihara is a member of a Buddhist temple, he does not consider himself religious. But he says he is not comfortable with abortion. "Abortion is legal and approved of by the government, and if a patient wants it, I can't turn her down," he says. "She's entitled to it. But I am not happy to do it." And yet, he performs some 200 abortions a year and quietly admits, when asked, that his fees from abortion represent "a large portion of my income."

Caught in this moral and economic trap, he resolves his feelings in a uniquely Japanese way. First, he tells each abortion patient to make an offering after the operation at any of the Buddhist temples selling miniature stone statues, or mizuko-juko, which women can buy in memory of an aborted fetus. Thousands of such statues stand on display at temples these days, and although some are for miscarriages and stillborn children, the vast majority are for abortions. Many of the statues are decorated with crocheted hats, plastic bibs, and little pinwheels, all put there by women to keep the soul of the aborted fetus warm and amused.

Debate is going on in Japan over whether to legalize the pill and promote other forms of birth control such as the diaphragm. Whether Japanese women will use the pill if it is legalized is an open question. In a 1990 survey released by one of Japan's largest newspapers, results showed that fewer than 10% of Japanese women would use it even if it were available.

developer of RU-486, Dr. Étienne-Emile Baulieu, remarks, "It's insulting to women to say that abortion now will be as easy as taking aspirins. . . . It is always difficult, psychologically and physically, sometimes tragic."[19] Moreover, questions remain about the safety of the procedure. Commonly reported side effects include heavy menstrual bleeding and cramping. RU-486 has not yet been introduced in the United States, largely because of opposition by pro-life groups. Opponents argue that RU-486 makes abortions more accessible and difficult to regulate.

As the abortion debate continues, so does research into the use of other drugs. A combination of the cancer drug methotrexate and the ulcer drug misoprostol, for example, can be used to terminate early pregnancy. Methotrexate is toxic to the embryo, and misoprostol causes uterine contractions. In a pilot study, an injection of methotrexate followed by a vaginal suppository with misoprostol led to successful abortions in 171 of 178 women.[20] (The remaining seven subsequently underwent aspiration.) Moreover, it would appear that the combination of methotrexate and misoprostol has fewer side effects than RU-486. It seems likely that additional methods of chemical induction of abortion will become available as the years go on. None of them is likely to defuse the abortion debate, however.

**Close-up**
More on abortion drugs
T1008

## Psychological Consequences of Abortion

The woman who faces an unwanted pregnancy may experience a range of negative emotions, including fear ("What will I do now?"), self-anger ("How could I let this happen?"), guilt ("What would my parents think if they knew I was pregnant?"), ambivalence ("Will I be sorry if I have an abortion? Will I be sorry if I don't?"), and sometimes desperation ("Is suicide a way out?").[21] Whether to have an abortion is typically a painful decision—perhaps the most difficult decision a woman will ever make. Even women who apparently make the decision without hesitation may later have feelings of guilt, remorse, anger, and sadness. Although the woman's partner is often overlooked in the research on abortion, he may experience similar feelings.

Women's reactions depend on various factors, including the support they receive from others (or the lack thereof) and the strength of their relationships with their partners. Women with greater support from their male partners or parents tend to show a more positive emotional reaction following an abortion.[22] Generally speaking, the sooner the abortion occurs, the less stressful it is. Women who have a difficult time reaching an abortion decision, who blame the pregnancy on their character, who have lower coping ability, and who have less social support tend to experience more distress following abortion.[23]

### *think about it!*

- **Do you know anyone who has had an abortion? What motivated the abortion? How did she react to the abortion? How did you feel at the time?**

**critical thinking** **One of the issues concerning abortion is whether it is the taking of a human life. How do you define human life? When do you believe human life begins? At conception? When the embryo becomes implanted in the uterus? When the fetus begins to assume a human shape or develops human facial features? When the fetus is capable of sustaining independent life? Explain.**

**critical thinking** **What are your own views on abortion? Are some abortion methods more acceptable to you than others? Why, or why not?**

**Smart Quiz**
Q1003

# Preventing Unwanted Pregnancies

## Take Charge

What do you call sexually active couples who fail to use contraception? Parents. Taking charge of your reproductive health involves taking steps to protect yourself and your partner from unwanted pregnancies. Unfortunately, too many couples wait until it is too late and they are faced with an unwanted pregnancy. Where do you begin? With perhaps the most important four-letter word in the English language: Talk.

Close-up
Preventing teenage pregnancy
T1009

### Talking to Your Partner about Contraception

When is the right time to discuss contraception? Between the appetizer and main course on your first date? When you are invited to meet your partner's family? When you are lost in amorous embraces? Broaching the topic can be awkward. *Not* broaching the issue can be disastrous. Often a man responds to the news that his partner is pregnant by saying "But I thought you were using *something!*"

Technically speaking, the right time to discuss birth control is *any time* that allows your contraceptive to become effective before sexual relations occur. That can mean weeks or months before, if you decide to use a prescription contraceptive such as the birth-control pill, the IUD, the diaphragm, or the cervical cap. Or it can mean a few moments before, if you decide to use a condom and have one available. Despite the obvious advantage to deciding on contraception before sex, the issue is often broached, if at all, only *after* the partners become sexually intimate.

Practically speaking, it is awkward—and perhaps presumptuous!—to discuss contraception when you meet or are on a first date. But if penile-vaginal sexual contact is a possibility, the person should come prepared. The man or woman may bring along a condom. The woman may already be on the pill, have an IUD in place, or a diaphragm.

Talking about contraception can help build the relationship. In talking about birth control, partners demonstrate their willingness to share responsibility for their behavior. As a result, the woman is less likely to be resentful that the responsibility rests entirely on her. Yes, it can be awkward or difficult to raise the topic. Couples may not feel that their relationship is secure enough. They may take the view, "We'll cross that bridge when we come to it." Not planning ahead, however, prevents the effective use of contraceptives that require advance planning.

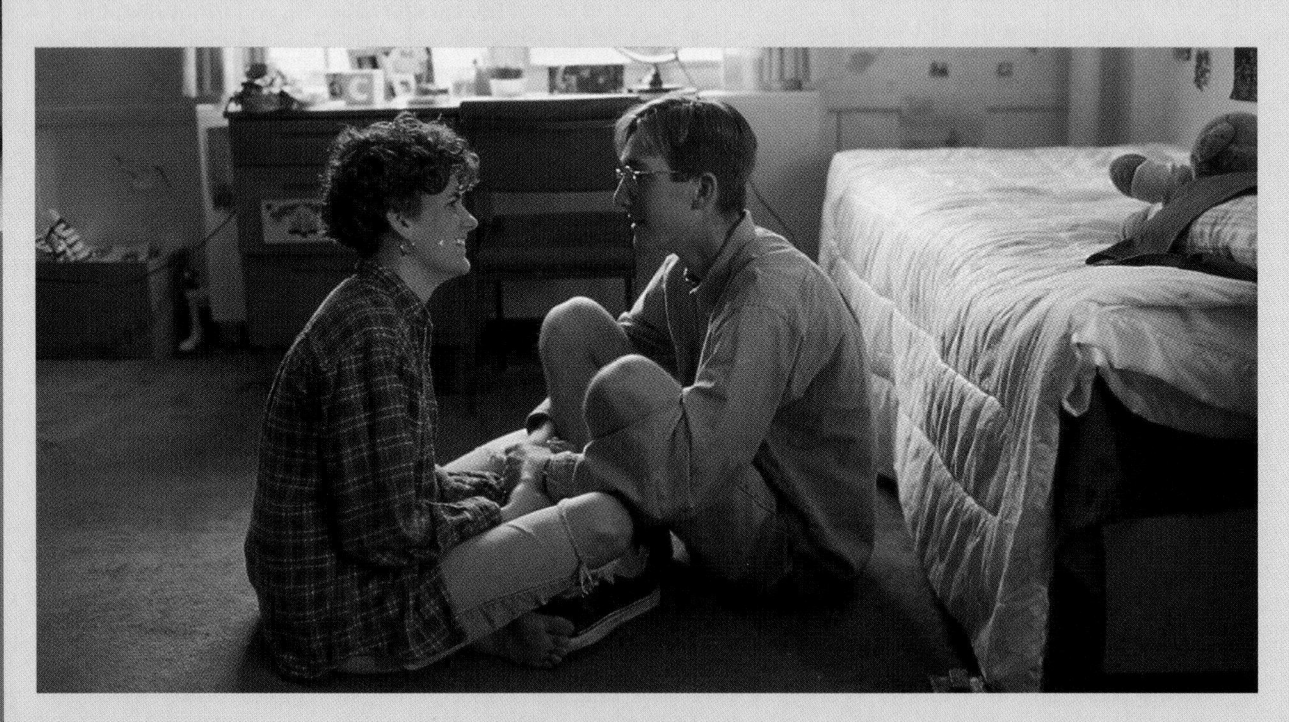

***Talking to Your Partner*** The time to discuss birth control with your partner is before sexual relations begin.

## Selecting a Method of Contraception

If you believe that you and your partner should use a method of contraception, how will you determine which one is right for you? There is no simple answer. What is right for your friends may be wrong for you. You and your partner will make your own selections, but there are some issues you may want to consider:

1. *Convenience.* Is the method convenient? The convenience of a method depends on a number of factors: Does it require a device that must be purchased in advance? If so, can it be purchased over the counter, or is a prescription required? Will the method work at a moment's notice, or, as with the birth-control pill, will it require time to reach maximum effectiveness? Couples may feel that few things dampen ardor and spontaneity more quickly than the need to apply a contraceptive device in the heat of passion. Use of contraceptives like the condom and the diaphragm need not interrupt sexual activity, however. Some couples find that applying a contraceptive device can become an erotic part of lovemaking.
2. *Moral acceptability.* A method that is morally acceptable to one person may be objectionable to another. For example, some oral contraceptives prevent fertilization. Others permit fertilization but prevent implantation of the fertilized ovum in the uterus. In the second case, the method may be considered a form of early abortion. It is thus likely to concern people who object to abortion, no matter how early. Yet the same people may have no moral objection to preventing conception.
3. *Cost.* Methods vary in cost. Some more costly methods involve devices (such as the diaphragm, the cervical cap, and the IUD) or hormones (pills or Norplant) that require medical visits in addition to the cost of the devices themselves. Other methods, such as rhythm methods, are essentially free.
4. *Sharing responsibility.* Most forms of birth control place the burden of responsibility largely on the woman. She must consult her doctor to obtain pills or other prescription devices, such as a diaphragm, a cervical cap, Norplant, or an IUD. She must remember to take birth-control pills reliably or check to see that her IUD remains in place. Some couples prefer methods that allow for greater sharing of responsibility, such as alternating use of the condom and diaphragm. A man can share the responsibility for the birth-control pill by accompanying his partner on her medical visits. He can share the expense. He can help her remember to take the pill.
5. *Safety.* How safe is the method? What are the side effects? Can your partner's health or comfort be affected by its use?
6. *Reversibility.* In most cases the effects of birth-control methods can be fully reversed by discontinuing their use. In other cases reversibility may not occur immediately, as with pills. Sterilization should be considered irreversible, although many attempts at reversal have been successful.
7. *Protection against sexually transmitted diseases (STDs).* Birth-control methods vary in the degree of protection they afford against STDs. *Most methods confer no protection against STDs.* Protection against STDs is especially important to people who are sexually active with partners who are *not known* to be free of them.
8. *Effectiveness.* Techniques and devices vary widely in effectiveness. Despite the widespread availability of contraceptives, about two of three pregnancies in the United States are unplanned. About half of these result from contraceptive failures.[25] Consult Table 10.1 earlier in the chapter to learn more about contraceptive effectiveness.

Even the best contraceptive methods are ineffective if they are practiced incorrectly or inconsistently. Or left at home in your dresser drawer. When it comes to your reproductive choices, the responsibility for avoiding unwanted pregnancies rests with you—not with your partner, your doctor, or, worse, blind luck.

Smart Quiz
Q1004

# SUMMING UP

## Questions and Answers

### CONCEPTION—AGAINST ALL ODDS

**1. What is conception?** Conception is the union of a sperm cell and an ovum. Fertilization normally occurs in a Fallopian tube.

**2. How can a couple optimize the chances of conception?** Optimizing the chances of conception means engaging in sexual relations at the time of ovulation. Ovulation can be predicted by calculating the woman's basal body temperature, analyzing the woman's urine for luteinizing hormone, or tracking the thickness of vaginal mucus.

**3. How can infertile couples become parents?** Many alternatives are available to help infertile couples become parents, including artificial insemination, in vitro fertilization, gamete intrafallopian transfer (GIFT), zygote intrafallopian transfer (ZIFT), donor IVF, embryonic transfer, intracytoplasmic injection, surrogate motherhood, and adoption.

### CONTRACEPTION

**4. What should couples consider when selecting a method of contraception?** Issues surrounding the choice of a method of contraception involve its convenience, moral acceptability, cost, sharing of responsibility between the partners, safety, reversibility, the protection it affords from STDs, and effectiveness.

**5. How do oral contraceptives work?** Birth-control pills include combination pills and minipills. Combination pills contain estrogen and progestin and fool the brain into acting as though the woman is already pregnant, so that no additional ova mature or are released. Minipills contain progestin, thicken the cervical mucus to impede the passage of sperm through the cervix, and render the inner lining of the uterus less receptive to a fertilized egg. "Morning-after" pills prevent implantation of a fertilized ovum in the uterus.

**6. What is Norplant?** Norplant consists of tubes containing progestin that are surgically embedded under the skin of the woman's upper arm. Norplant provides continuous contraceptive protection for as long as five years.

**7. What are intrauterine devices (IUDs)?** IUDs apparently irritate the uterine lining, causing inflammation and the production of antibodies that may be toxic to sperm or fertilized ova and/or may prevent fertilized eggs from becoming implanted. The IUD is highly effective, but there are possible troublesome side effects and the potential for serious health complications.

**8. What is the diaphragm?** The diaphragm is a device that covers the cervix and should be used with a spermicidal cream or jelly. It must be fitted by a health professional.

**9. What are spermicides?** Spermicides block the passage of sperm and kill sperm. Their failure rate is high, but spermicides that contain nonoxynol-9 may also provide some protection against organisms that cause STDs.

**10. What is the cervical cap?** Like the diaphragm, the cap covers the cervix and is most effective when used with a spermicide.

**11. What are condoms?** Latex condoms afford protection against STDs. Condoms are the only contraceptive device worn by men and the only readily reversible method of contraception that is available to men.

**12. What are the facts on douching and withdrawal?** Douching is ineffective as a contraceptive because large numbers of sperm may pass beyond the range of the douche within seconds after ejaculation. Withdrawal requires no special equipment but has a high failure rate.

**13. What are fertility awareness methods?** Fertility awareness (rhythm) methods rely on awareness of the fertile segments of the woman's menstrual cycle. Rhythm methods include the calendar method, the basal body temperature method, and the cervical mucus method. Their failure rate is high in typical use.

**14. What about sterilization?** Sterilization methods should be considered permanent, although they may be reversed in many cases. The vasectomy is usually carried out under local anesthesia in 15 to 20 minutes. Female sterilization methods prevent ova and sperm from passing through the Fallopian tubes.

### ABORTION

**15. What is abortion?** An induced abortion (in contrast to a spontaneous abortion, or miscarriage) is the purposeful termination of a pregnancy before the embryo or fetus is capable of sustaining independent life.

**16. What is the history of abortion?** In colonial times and through the mid-nineteenth century, women in the United States were permitted to terminate a pregnancy until fetal movements occurred. More restrictive abortion laws came into being after the Civil War. In 1973, the U.S. Supreme Court in effect legalized abortion nationwide in the landmark *Roe* v. *Wade* decision.

**17. What abortion methods are available?** Abortion methods in use today include vacuum aspiration, D&C, D&E, induction of labor by intra-amniotic infusion, and hysterotomy.

## Suggested Readings

**Asbell, B.** *The Pill: A Biography of the Drug That Changed the World.* New York: Random House, 1995. A fascinating account of the history of the birth-control pill and how oral contraceptives have affected sexual values and behavior.

**Hatcher, R. A., and others.** *Contraceptive Technology.* New York: Irvington. The authoritative guide to the most recent developments in contraception, revised every two years.

**Tribe, L.** *Abortion: The Clash of Absolutes.* New York: Norton, 1990. An illuminating discussion of the controversy over abortion.

# Pregnancy and

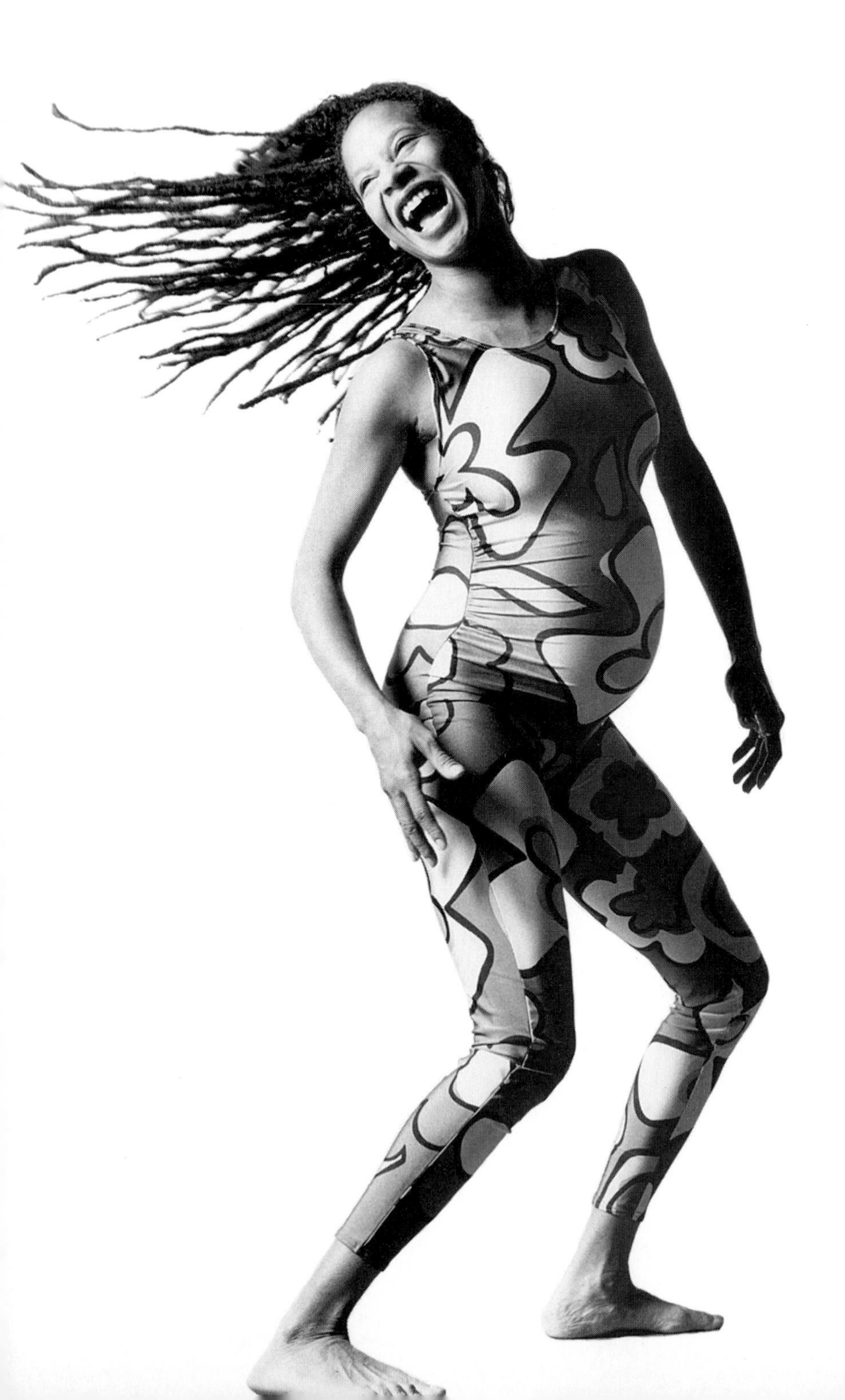

DID YOU KNOW THAT

- Physicians no longer use the "rabbit test" to determine that a woman is pregnant? p.288
- A fertilized egg cell is not attached to its mother's body for the first week or so following conception? p.291
- The fetus does somersaults in the womb? p.293
- The baby may signal its mother when it is ready to be born? p.296
- The proportion of C-sections more than doubled between the 1970s and 1990s? p.300
- Most new mothers experience some mood changes in the days or weeks following childbirth? p.301
- High doses of certain vitamins can lead to birth defects? p.305
- Most babies born to HIV-infected mothers do not become infected themselves? p.305
- Pregnant women cannot assume that it is safe to have even one or two alcoholic beverages a day? p.307

# Childbirth

*Pregnancy and childbirth are major milestones in parents' lives. They are also the beginnings of new lives. We have learned much in recent years about the health issues involved in these milestones. We are in a better position than we have ever been to ensure the health of mothers and children. Unfortunately, however, not all pregnant women have access to health care. For them, health-related knowledge and skills are not used often enough. For other women, some contemporary techniques, like caesarean section, may be used too often.*

*This chapter chronicles the key events of pregnancy and childbirth. The information here will help readers understand what they need to enhance their own health and that of their children.*

11

# PREGNANCY

People react to pregnancy in different ways. For those who are psychologically and economically prepared, pregnancy may be greeted with joyous celebration. Some women feel that pregnancy helps fulfill their sense of womanhood:

> *Being pregnant meant I was a woman. I was enthralled with my belly growing. I went out right away and got maternity clothes.*
>
> *It gave me a sense that I was actually a woman. I had never felt sexy before . . . I felt very voluptuous.*
>
> The New Our Bodies, Ourselves, *1992*

On the other hand, an unwanted pregnancy may evoke feelings of fear and hopelessness, as occurs with many teenagers.

In this section we examine biological and psychological aspects of pregnancy. The nearby ***HealthCheck*** invites you to consider whether you believe you should have a child.

## Early Signs of Pregnancy

For many women, the first sign of pregnancy is missing a period. Missing a period may be greeted with joy or despair, depending on whether the woman wants the pregnancy and is prepared for it. But since some women have irregular menstrual cycles or miss a period because of stress, missing a period is not a fully reliable indicator of pregnancy. Some women also experience cyclic bleeding or spotting during pregnancy, although the blood flow is usually lighter than normal. If a woman's basal body temperature remains high for about three weeks after ovulation, there is reason to suspect pregnancy—despite spotting.

## Pregnancy Tests

You may have heard your parents say that they learned your mother was pregnant by means of the "rabbit test." In that test, a urine sample was injected into a laboratory animal. This procedure, which was once commonly used to confirm pregnancy, relied on the fact that women produce **human chorionic gonadotropin (HCG)** shortly after conception. HCG causes rabbits, mice, or rats to ovulate.

**Talking Glossary**
Human chorionic gonadotropin (HCG)
G1101

Today, instead of the "rabbit test," pregnancy is confirmed in minutes by tests that detect HCG in the urine as early as the third week of pregnancy. A blood test—the *beta subunit HCG radioimmunoassay* (RIA)—can detect HCG in the woman's blood as early as the eighth day of pregnancy, about five days before her expected period.

Over-the-counter home pregnancy tests also test the woman's urine for HCG. They can be used as early as one day after a missed period. Home tests are somewhat less accurate than laboratory tests. Women are advised to consult their physicians if they suspect that they are pregnant or wish to confirm a home test result.

About a month after a woman misses her period, a health professional may confirm pregnancy by pelvic exam. Women who are pregnant usually show **Hegar's sign.** Hegar's sign is softness of a section of the uterus between the uterine body and the cervix. The area may be palpated (felt) by placing a hand on the abdomen and two fingers in the vagina.

## Early Effects of Pregnancy

A few days after conception, a woman may note that her breasts feel tender. Hormonal stimulation of the mammary glands may make the breasts more sensitive and cause sensations of tingling and fullness.

**Morning sickness,** which may actually come at any time of day, refers to the nausea, food aversion, and vomiting experienced during pregnancy. About half of all pregnant women experience morning sickness during the first few months of pregnancy. In some cases, morning sickness is so severe that the woman cannot eat regularly. Some women are then hospitalized to ensure adequate nutrition. Morning sickness usually subsides by about the twelfth week of pregnancy. Pregnant women may also experience fatigue during the early weeks. They tend to sleep longer and fall asleep more readily than usual. Women may also experience frequent urination. It is caused by pressure from the swelling uterus on the bladder.

**Human chorionic gonadotropin (HCG)** A hormone produced by women shortly after conception which stimulates the corpus luteum to continue to produce progesterone. The presence of HCG in a woman's urine indicates that she is pregnant.

**Hegar's sign** Softness of a section of the uterus between the uterine body and the cervix; indicates that a woman is pregnant.

**Morning sickness** A symptom of pregnancy; may include nausea, food aversions, and vomiting.

# Health Check

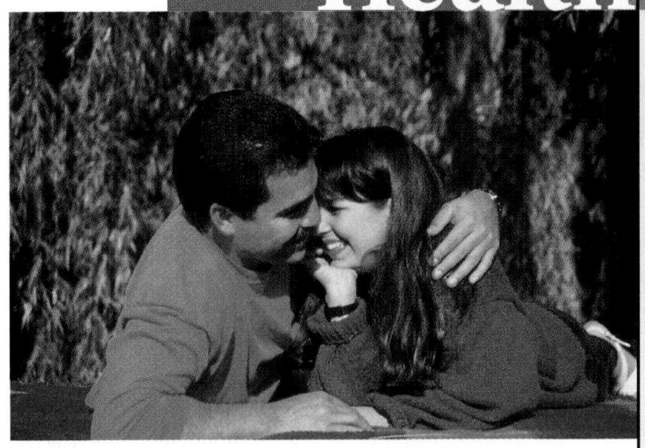

## Should You Have a Child?

Whether to have children is one of the most significant life decisions you will face. Children have a way of needing a generation (or a lifetime) of love and support. We have no simplistic way of arriving at a recommendation. Instead, we offer the following questionnaire to help you consider your own reasons for having or not having children. You can complete the questionnaire by checking the blank spaces of the pros and cons. The items are not intended to be equal in weight. Nor should your total score govern your decision. You be the judge. It's your life and your choice.

### Reasons to Have Children

*Couples offer reasons such as the following for having children. Check those that seem to apply to you:*

____ 1. *Personal experience.* Having children is a unique experience. To many people, no other experience compares with having the opportunity to love them, experience their love, help shape their lives, and watch them develop.

____ 2. *Personal pleasure.* There is fun and pleasure in playing with children, taking them to the zoo and the circus, and viewing the world through their fresh, innocent eyes.

____ 3. *Personal extension.* Children carry on our family heritage, and some of our own wishes and dreams, beyond the confines of our own mortality. We name them after ourselves or others in our families and see them as extensions of ourselves. We identify with their successes.

____ 4. *Loving relationship.* Parents have the opportunity to establish extremely close and cherished bonds with other human beings.

____ 5. *Personal status.* Within our culture, parents are afforded respect *just because* they are parents. Consider the commandment: "Honor thy father and thy mother."

____ 6. *Personal competence.* Parenthood is a challenge. Competence in the social role of mother or father is a source of gratification to many people.

____ 7. *Personal responsibility.* Parents have the opportunity to be responsible for the welfare and education of their children.

____ 8. *Companionship for the later years.* Many people expect their children to provide them with comfort, companionship, and perhaps crucial aid in their later years.

____ 9. *Moral worth.* Some people feel that having children provides the opportunity for a moral, selfless act in which they place the needs of others—their children—ahead of their own.

____10. *Religious beliefs.* The biblical injunction to "be fruitful and multiply" is followed by many people across a range of religious affiliations.

### Reasons *Not* to Have Children

*Many couples who decide not to have children cite reasons such as the following. Check those that you endorse:*

____ 1. *Strain on the earth's resources.* Because the world is overpopulated, it is wrong to place additional strain on limited resources. More children will only geometrically increase the problem of overpopulation.

____ 2. *Time together.* Child-free couples may be able to spend more time together as a couple and develop a more intimate relationship.

____ 3. *Freedom.* Children have a way of erasing leisure time. They may also make it more difficult to pursue educational and vocational advancement. Child-free couples may be more able to live spontaneously, to go where they please and do as they please.

____ 4. *Dual careers.* Child-free couples may both pursue careers without the demands of child rearing.

____ 5. *Financial drain.* Children are a financial burden, especially considering the costs of child care and education.

____ 6. *Difficulty.* Parenthood is demanding. It requires sacrifice of time, money, and energy, and not everyone makes a good parent.

____ 7. *Irrevocable decision.* Once you have children, the decision cannot be changed.

____ 8. *Failure.* Some people fear that they will not be good parents. People with poor relationships with their own parents may fear that they will repeat the same mistakes their parents made with them.

____ 9. *Other children.* People can enjoy children other than their own, such as nieces and nephews, or become "Big Brothers" or "Big Sisters," without assuming the full brunt of parental responsibility.

____10. *Sense of danger.* The world is perceived to be a dangerous place, with the threats, for example, of crime, environmental destruction, and nuclear war. People may feel that it is better not to bring children into such a world.

## Miscarriage (Spontaneous Abortion)

**Miscarriages** have many causes. Chromosomal defects in the fetus and abnormalities of the placenta and uterus are among them. Most miscarriages occur early, in the first trimester. (Some miscarriages occur so early that the woman is not aware that she was pregnant.) Following a miscarriage, a couple may feel a deep sense of loss, especially when the miscarriage occurs later in pregnancy. Emotional support from friends and family often helps the couple cope. In most cases women who miscarry carry later pregnancies to term.

## Sex during Pregnancy

Most health professionals concur that coitus (sexual intercourse) is safe throughout the course of pregnancy until the start of labor, provided that the pregnancy is developing normally and the woman has no history of miscarriages. But women who experience bleeding or cramps during pregnancy may be advised by their obstetrician not to engage in coitus.[1]

## Psychological Changes during Pregnancy

A woman's psychological response to pregnancy reflects her desire to be pregnant, her physical changes, and her attitudes toward these changes. Women with the financial, social, and psychological resources to meet the needs of pregnancy and child rearing may welcome pregnancy. Some describe it as the most wondrous experience of their lives. Other women may question their ability to handle their pregnancies, childbirth, and child rearing. Or they may fear that pregnancy will interfere with their careers or their relationships with their partners. In general, women who choose to become pregnant are better adjusted throughout their pregnancies.

The typical nine-month term of pregnancy can be divided into three trimesters of three months each. The first trimester may be difficult for women who are ambivalent about pregnancy. At this stage, symptoms like morning sickness are most pronounced. Women must come to terms with being pregnant. The second trimester is generally less tempestuous. Morning sickness and other symptoms may have dissipated if not vanished, and it is not yet difficult to move about. Delivery is still in the future. Women first note the fetal movements during the second trimester. For many, the experience is stirring:

> *I was lying on my stomach and felt—something, like someone lightly touching my deep insides. Then I just sat very still and . . . felt the hugeness of having something living growing in me. Then I said, No, it's not possible, it's too early yet, and then I started to cry. . . . That one moment was my first body awareness of another living thing inside me.*
>
> The New Our Bodies, Ourselves, *1992*

During the third trimester it is normal, especially for first-time mothers, to worry about the mechanics of delivery and whether the child will be normal. The woman becomes heavier and is literally "bent out of shape." It may become difficult to get out of a chair or a bed. Muscle tension from supporting the extra weight in her abdomen may cause backaches. She may feel impatient in the days and weeks just before delivery, wanting the pregnancy to be over—now!

Men, like women, respond to pregnancy according to the degree to which they want the child. They may feel pride and look forward to having the child. In such cases, pregnancy may bring parents closer together. Fathers who are financially or emotionally unprepared may consider the pregnancy a trap. Now and then an expectant father experiences symptoms that resemble signs of pregnancy, including morning sickness and vomiting. This reaction is termed a **sympathetic pregnancy.**

**Miscarriage** The sudden, involuntary expulsion of the embryo or fetus from the uterus before it is capable of independent life. Also called *spontaneous abortion.*

**Sympathetic pregnancy** The experiencing of signs of pregnancy by the father.

### think about it!

- **How did people in your life react on learning that they were pregnant? Why?**
- **Has anyone you know had a miscarriage? How did she react?**
- **How did the psychological state of people you know (or yourself) change during the course of a pregnancy?**

Smart Quiz
Q1101

# PRENATAL DEVELOPMENT

We can date pregnancy from the onset of the last menstrual cycle before conception. In this case, the normal gestation period is 280 days. We can also date pregnancy from the date at which fertilization was assumed to have occurred. This date normally corresponds to two weeks after the beginning of the woman's last menstrual cycle. In this case, the normal gestation period is 266 days.

Once pregnancy is confirmed, the delivery date may be calculated by *Nagele's rule:*

- Jot down the date of the first day of the last menstrual period.
- Add seven days.
- Subtract three months.
- Add one year.

Assume that the last period began on November 12, 2000. Add seven days. We arrive at November 19, 2000. Then we subtract three months and obtain the date August 19, 2000. Finally, we add one year. We thus have a "due date" of August 19, 2001. Few babies are born right on schedule.* The great majority are delivered during the ten-day period that spans the date.

Shortly after conception, the single cell that results from the union of sperm and egg begins to multiply. It becomes two cells, then four, then eight, and so on. During the weeks and months that follow, tissues, structures, and organs begin to form. The fetus gradually takes on the shape of a human being. By the time the fetus is born, it consists of hundreds of billions of cells—more cells than there are stars in the Milky Way galaxy.

We noted that prenatal development is often divided into three trimesters of three months each. In terms of many health issues, it is sometimes preferable to divide pregnancy into three unequal periods:

- the *germinal stage,* which corresponds to about the first two weeks;
- the *embryonic stage,* which coincides with the first two months; and
- the *fetal stage,* which is the balance of the pregnancy, some seven months long.

*The second author wishes to boast, however, that his daughters Allyn and Jordan were born precisely on their due dates. At least one of them has been just as compulsive ever since. The first author adds that he and his wife Judy had their son Michael and daughter Daniella within one day of their due dates. (Close but no cigar, notes the second author.) The third author wants to know why men must be competitive about everything.

## The Germinal Stage

The period from conception to implantation is termed the **germinal stage,** or the *period of the ovum.* Within 36 hours after conception, the *zygote* divides into two cells. It then divides repeatedly. It becomes 32 cells within another 36 hours. As division proceeds, the zygote journeys to the uterus. It takes the zygote perhaps three or four days to reach the uterus. The mass of dividing cells then wanders about the uterus for another three or four days before it begins to implant in the uterine wall. Implantation takes another week or so. Implantation may be accompanied by bleeding. Bleeding results from normal rupturing of small blood vessels that line the uterus. Bleeding can also be a sign of a miscarriage. However, most women who experience implantation bleeding have normal pregnancies and healthy babies.

## The Embryonic Stage

The period from implantation to about the eighth week of development is called the **embryonic stage.** The major organ systems of the body begin to differentiate during this stage.

The development of the embryo follows two trends—**cephalocaudal** (from Latin roots meaning "head" and "tail") and **proximodistal** (from Latin roots meaning "near" and "far"). The apparently oversized heads depicted in Figure 11.1 (following page) represent embryos and fetuses at various stages of prenatal development. Growth of the head (the cephalic region) takes precedence over the growth of the lower parts of the body. You can also think of the body as containing a central axis that coincides with the spinal cord. The growth of the organ systems that lie close to this axis (that is, *proximal* to the axis) takes precedence over those that lie further away toward the extremities (that is, *distal* to the axis). Relatively early maturation of the brain and organ systems that lie near the central axis allows these organs to facilitate further development of the embryo and fetus.

By about three weeks after conception, two ridges appear in the embryo. The

**Talking Glossary**
Cephalocaudal, Proximodistal
G1102

**Germinal stage** Prenatal development from conception through implantation in the uterus.

**Embryonic stage** The stage of prenatal development that lasts from implantation through the eighth week; the major organ systems differentiate.

**Cephalocaudal** From the head downward.

**Proximodistal** From the central axis of the body outward.

14 days

18 days

24 days

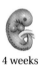


ridges fold together to form the **neural tube.** This tube develops into the nervous system.

During the third week of development, the head and blood vessels also begin to form. By the fourth week, a primitive heart begins to beat and pump blood in an embryo that is but a fifth of an inch long. The heart will normally continue to beat without rest for the better part of a century. By the end of the first month of development we see the beginnings of the arms and legs: "arm buds" and "leg buds." The mouth, eyes, ears, and nose begin to take shape. The brain and other parts of the nervous system begin to develop.

The arms and legs develop in accordance with the proximodistal principle. First the upper arms and legs develop. Then the forearms and lower legs. Then the hands and feet form, followed by webbed fingers and toes by about six to eight weeks into development. The webbing is gone by the end of the second month. By this time the head has become rounded and the limbs have elongated and separated. Facial features are visible. All this has occurred in an embryo that is about an inch long and weighs $\frac{1}{30}$ of an ounce. During the second month, nervous impulses also begin to travel through the developing nervous system.

**The Amniotic Sac** The embryo—and later, the fetus—develop within a protective environment in the mother's uterus called the **amniotic sac.** This sac is surrounded by a clear membrane called the **chorion.** The embryo and fetus are suspended within the sac in **amniotic fluid.** The fluid acts like a shock absorber. It cushions the embryo from damage that might otherwise result from the mother's movements. The fluid also helps maintain a steady temperature.

**The Placenta** Nutrients and waste products are exchanged between mother and embryo (and later, the fetus) through the **placenta.** The placenta is unique in origin. It develops from material supplied by both mother and embryo. Toward the end of the first trimester, it becomes a flattish, round organ about 7 inches in diameter and 1 inch thick—larger than the fetus itself. The fetus is connected to the placenta by the **umbilical cord.** The mother is connected to the placenta by the system of blood vessels in the uterine wall. The umbilical cord develops about five weeks after conception

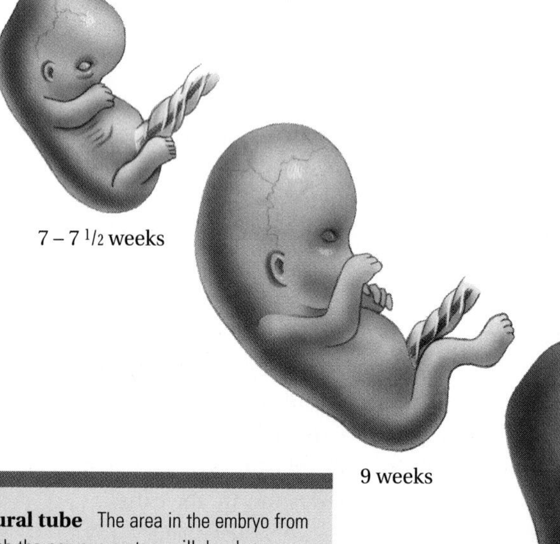


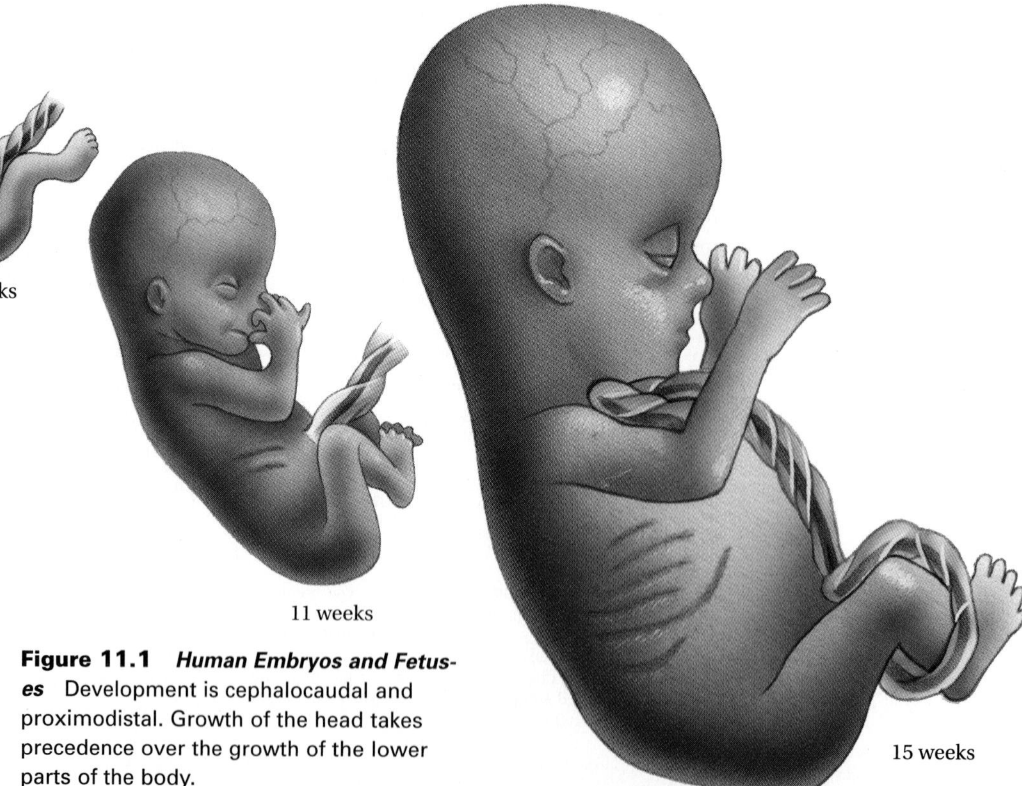


**Figure 11.1** ***Human Embryos and Fetuses*** Development is cephalocaudal and proximodistal. Growth of the head takes precedence over the growth of the lower parts of the body.

**Neural tube** The area in the embryo from which the nervous system will develop.

**Amniotic sac** The sac containing the fetus.

**Chorion** The membrane that envelops the amniotic sac and fetus.

**Amniotic fluid** Fluid within the amniotic sac that suspends and protects the fetus.

**Placenta** An organ connected to the fetus by the umbilical cord. The placenta serves as a relay station between mother and fetus, allowing the exchange of nutrients and wastes.

**Umbilical cord** A tube that connects the fetus to the placenta.

and reaches 20 inches in length. It contains two arteries through which maternal nutrients reach the embryo. A vein transports waste products back to the mother.

The bloodstreams of mother and embryo do not mix. A membrane in the placenta permits only certain substances to pass through. Oxygen passes from the mother to the fetus. So do nutrients; some microscopic disease-causing organisms; and some drugs, including aspirin, narcotics, alcohol, and tranquilizers. Carbon dioxide and other wastes pass from the embryo or fetus to the mother. They are eliminated by the mother's lungs and kidneys.

The placenta is also an endocrine gland. It secretes hormones that preserve the pregnancy, stimulate the uterine contractions that induce childbirth, and help prepare the breasts for breastfeeding. Some of these hormones may also cause the signs of pregnancy. HCG (human chorionic gonadotropin) stimulates the corpus luteum to continue to produce progesterone. The placenta itself secretes estrogen and progesterone. Ultimately, the placenta passes from the woman's body after delivery. For this reason it is also called the "afterbirth."

## The Fetal Stage

The fetal stage begins by the ninth week and continues until birth. By about the ninth or tenth week, the fetus begins to respond to the outside world by turning in the direction of external stimulation. By the end of the first trimester, the major organ systems, the fingers and toes, and the external genitals have been formed. The sex of the fetus can be determined visually. The eyes have become clearly distinguishable.

During the second trimester the fetus increases dramatically in size. Organ systems continue to mature. The brain now contributes to the regulation of basic body functions. The fetus increases in weight from 1 *ounce* to 2 *pounds* and grows from about 4 to 14 inches in length. Soft, downy hair grows above the eyes and on the scalp. The skin turns ruddy because of blood vessels that show through the surface. (During the third trimester, layers of fat beneath the skin will give the red a pinkish hue.)

The mother can usually feel the first fetal movements by the middle of the fourth month. By the end of the second trimester, the fetus moves its limbs so vigorously that the mother may complain of being kicked—often at 4 A.M. It opens and shuts its eyes, sucks its thumb, alternates between periods of wakefulness and sleep, and perceives lights and sounds. The fetus also does somersaults, which the mother will definitely feel. Fortunately, the umbilical cord will not break or strangle the fetus, no matter what acrobatic feats the fetus performs.

Near the end of the second trimester the fetus approaches the **age of viability.** Still, only a minority of babies born at the end of the second trimester who weigh under 2 pounds will survive—even with intense medical efforts.

During the third trimester, the organ systems continue to mature and enlarge. The heart and lungs become increasingly capable of maintaining independent life. Typically during the seventh month the fetus turns upside down in the uterus so that it will be head first, or in a **cephalic presentation,** for delivery. But some fetuses do not turn during this month. If such a fetus is born prematurely it can have either a **breech presentation** (bottom first) or a shoulder-first presentation. Either presentation can complicate problems of

***Prenatal Development*** Prenatal development progresses rapidly. Compare the embryo at approximately 6 to 7 weeks after conception (a) with a fetus at approximately 16 weeks (b). Notice how the fetus has taken on a human form by this point in prenatal development.

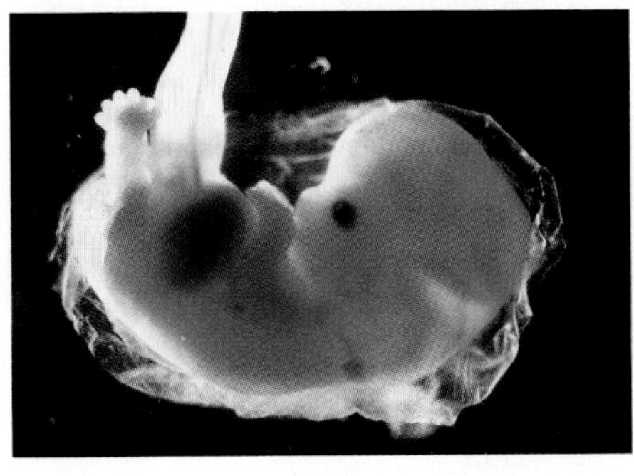

(a)

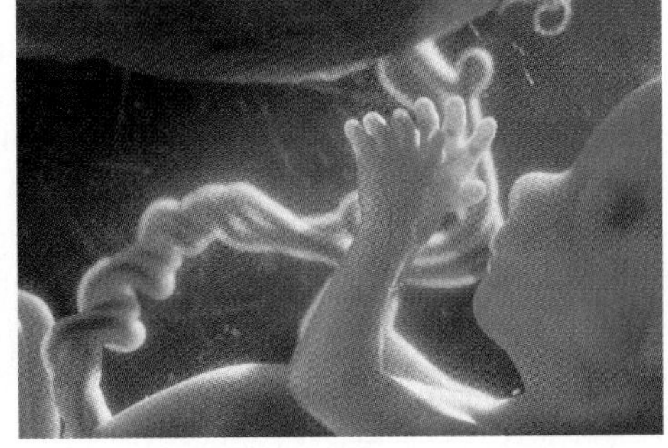

(b)

**Age of viability** The age at which a fetus can sustain independent life.

**Cephalic presentation** Emergence of the baby head first from the uterus.

**Breech presentation** Emergence of the baby feet first from the uterus.

prematurity. The closer to term (the full nine months) the baby is when born, the more likely it is that the presentation will be cephalic. If birth occurs at the end of the eighth month, the odds are overwhelmingly in favor of survival.

During the final months of pregnancy, the mother may become concerned that the fetus seems to be less active than before. Most of the time the change in activity level is normal. The fetus has grown so large that its movements are constrained.

## Toxemia

**Toxemia** during pregnancy is a potentially life-threatening condition characterized by high blood pressure. It may affect women late in the second or early in the third trimester of pregnancy. The first stage of toxemia is termed *preeclampsia,* which may be relatively mild. It is diagnosed by protein in the urine, swelling from fluid retention, and high blood pressure. As preeclampsia worsens, the mother may have headaches, visual problems, and abdominal pain. If untreated, the disease may progress to the final stage, *eclampsia.* Eclampsia can lead to maternal or fetal death. Babies born to women with toxemia are often undersized or premature. An obstetrician will be able to diagnose and treat toxemia—yet another reason for regular prenatal visits.

Toxemia appears to be linked to malnutrition, although the causes are unclear. Ironically, undernourished women may gain weight rapidly through fluid retention. However, their swollen appearance may discourage them from eating. Pregnant women who gain weight rapidly but have not increased their food intake should consult their obstetricians.

**TABLE 11.1**

**Some Chromosomal and Genetic Abnormalities**

| | |
|---|---|
| *Cystic Fibrosis* | A genetic disease in which the pancreas and lungs become clogged with mucus, which impairs the processes of respiration and digestion. |
| *Down Syndrome* | A condition characterized by a third chromosome on the twenty-first pair. The child with Down syndrome has a characteristic fold of skin over the eye and mental retardation. The risk that a child will have Down syndrome increases as parents age. |
| *Hemophilia* | A sex-linked disorder in which the blood fails to clot properly. |
| *Huntington's Disease* | A fatal neurological disorder; onset occurs in middle adulthood. |
| *Neural Tube Defects* | Disorders of the brain or spine, such as *anencephaly,* in which part of the brain is missing, and *spina bifida,* in which part of the spine is exposed or missing. Anencephaly is fatal shortly after birth, but some spina bifida victims survive for a number of years, albeit with severe handicaps. |
| *Phenylketonuria* | A disorder in which a child cannot metabolize dietary phenylalanine, which builds up in the form of phenylpyruvic acid and causes mental retardation. The disorder can be diagnosed at birth and controlled by diet. |
| *Retina Blastoma* | A form of blindness caused by a dominant gene. |
| *Sickle-Cell Anemia* | A blood disorder that afflicts mainly African Americans. Deformed blood cells obstruct small blood vessels, decreasing their capacity to carry oxygen and heightening the risk of occasionally fatal infections. |
| *Tay-Sachs Disease* | A fatal neurological disorder that primarily afflicts Jews of European origin. |

## Chromosomal and Genetic Abnormalities

Not all of us have the normal complement of chromosomes. Some of us have genes that threaten our health or our existence (see Table 11.1).

**Down Syndrome** The risk of a child's having **Down syndrome** increases with the mother's age (see Table 11.2). Down syndrome is usually caused by an extra chromosome on the twenty-first pair. In the great majority of cases, Down syndrome is transmitted by the mother. The inner corners of the eyes of people with the syndrome have a downward-sloping crease of skin that gives them a superficial likeness to Asians. This is why the syndrome was once called *mon-*

**TABLE 11.2**

**Risk of Giving Birth to an Infant with Down Syndrome**

| Age of Mother | Probability of Down Syndrome |
|---|---|
| 30 | 1/885 |
| 35* | 1/365 |
| 40 | 1/109 |
| 45 | 1/32 |
| 49 | 1/11 |

*Age at which amniocentesis is usually first recommended.

**Toxemia** A life-threatening condition during pregnancy that is characterized by high blood pressure.

**Down syndrome** A chromosomal abnormality that leads to mental retardation; caused by an extra chromosome on the twenty-first pair.

*golism,* a term that is now rejected because of racist overtones.

Children with Down syndrome have characteristic round faces; wide, flat noses; and protruding tongues. They often have respiratory problems and heart malformations, problems that tend to claim their lives by middle age. People with Down syndrome are also moderately mentally retarded, but they usually can learn to read and write. With help from family and social agencies, they may hold jobs and lead largely independent lives. Despite their intellectual limitations, they are as capable of feeling as the rest of us, and they usually have warm, loving relationships with their families.

**Sickle-Cell Anemia and Tay-Sachs Disease** Sickle-cell anemia and Tay-Sachs disease are genetic disorders that are most likely to afflict certain racial and ethnic groups. Sickle-cell anemia is most prevalent in the United States among African Americans. One of every 375 African Americans is affected by the disease. Eight percent are carriers of the sickle-cell trait.[2] In **sickle-cell anemia,** the red blood cells assume a sickle shape—hence the name. They form clumps that obstruct narrow blood vessels and lower the oxygen supply. As a result, people have problems ranging from swollen, painful joints to pneumonia and heart and kidney failure. Infections are a leading cause of death among those with the disease.

**Tay-Sachs disease** is a fatal neurological disease of young children. Overall, only one in 100,000 people in the United States is affected. Among Jews of Eastern European background, the figure jumps to one in 3,600.[3] The disease is characterized by degeneration of the central nervous system. It gives rise to retardation, loss of muscle control, paralysis, blindness, and deafness. The disease leads to death usually before the age of four.

**Sex-Linked Genetic Abnormalities** Some genetic disorders, like hemophilia, are sex-linked. They are carried only on the X sex chromosome. They are transmitted from generation to generation as **recessive traits.** Females each have two X sex chromosomes. They are less likely than males to have sex-linked disorders, because the genes that carry the disorder would have to be present on both of their sex chromosomes for it to be expressed. Sex-linked disorders are more likely to affect sons of female carriers. The sons have only one X sex chromosome, which they inherit from their mothers.

England's Queen Victoria in the nineteenth century was a carrier of hemophilia. She transmitted the condition to many of her children. They carried it into several ruling houses of Europe. For this reason, hemophilia has been dubbed the "royal disease."

PREVENTION

## *Preventing Chromosomal and Genetic Abnormalities*

In recent years, a health specialty called genetic counseling has developed. Genetic counselors take information about a couple's medical background and family history of genetic defects. They help couples appraise the risks of passing along genetic health problems to their children. Some couples who face a high risk of transmitting genetic defects to their children decide to adopt. Some couples decide on abortion if medical tests uncover a chromosomal or genetic abnormality in the fetus. Others facing the same situation decide to continue the pregnancy to term. Advances in medical procedures allow couples to detect various fetal abnormalities.

**Smart Reference**
Fetal check-up
R1101

**Amniocentesis** **Amniocentesis** is usually performed about four months into pregnancy. Fluid is drawn from the amniotic sac with a syringe. Fetal cells in the fluid are grown in a culture and examined under a microscope for the presence of biochemical and chromosomal abnormalities.

**Talking Glossary**
Chorionic villus sampling (CVS)
G1103

**Chorionic Villus Sampling** An alternative to amniocentesis, **chorionic villus sampling (CVS)** is performed several weeks earlier. A narrow tube is used to snip off material from the *chorion,* the membrane that contains the amniotic sac and fetus. The material is analyzed. CVS is somewhat riskier than amniocentesis, so most obstetricians prefer to use the latter. Both tests detect

**Sickle-cell anemia** An inherited form of anemia characterized by the appearance of sickle-shaped red blood cells.

**Tay-Sachs disease** An inherited, incurable neurological disease most common among Jews of Eastern European background.

**Recessive trait** A trait that is not expressed when the gene or genes involved have been paired with dominant genes.

**Amniocentesis** A procedure for drawing off and examining fetal cells in the amniotic fluid to determine the presence of various disorders in the fetus.

**Chorionic villus sampling (CVS)** A test for prenatal abnormalities involving analysis of material snipped from the chorion, the membrane containing the amniotic sac and fetus.

Down syndrome, sickle-cell anemia, Tay-Sachs disease, spina bifida, muscular dystrophy, Rh incompatibility, and other conditions. The tests also identify the sex of the fetus.

**Ultrasound** **Ultrasound** is also used to detect fetal abnormalities. In ultrasound, high-pitched sound waves are bounced off the fetus like radar. They reveal a picture of the fetus on a TV monitor. Obstetricians also use ultrasound to locate the fetus during amniocentesis to lower the probability of injuring it with the syringe.

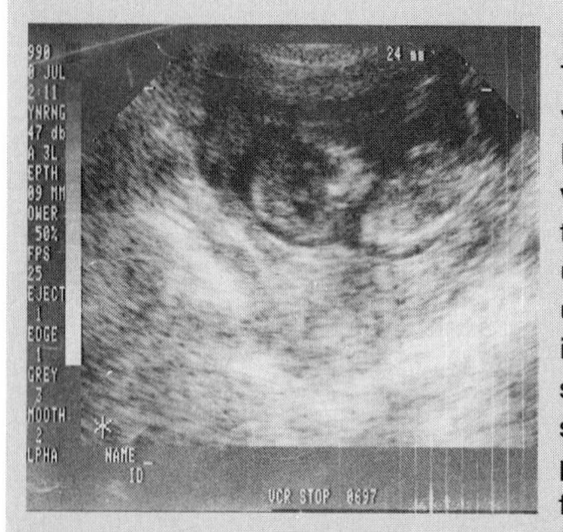

***Ultrasound Image*** This grainy image is of your first author's son Michael, taken at 12 weeks after conception. The head and upper torso (facing upward) can be seen in the upper middle section. He was handsome even then, his perfectly objective father points out.

**Blood Tests** Parental blood tests can suggest the presence of problems such as sickle-cell anemia, Tay-Sachs disease, and neural tube defects. Still other tests examine fetal DNA. They can indicate the presence of Huntington's disease, cystic fibrosis, and other disorders.

Smart Quiz Q1102

**think about it!**

- **Have you been with anyone during a pregnancy? How did she react when she first detected fetal movements?**
- **Do you know anyone who drank alcohol or smoked during pregnancy? What did she say about it?**

**critical thinking**

**Do you want to know if you or your partner is at risk of carrying a genetic abnormality? Why or why not? How would such knowledge affect your decisions about having children?**

**Ultrasound** The use of high-pitched sound waves bounced off the fetus to reveal its form.

**Braxton-Hicks contractions** So-called false labor contractions, these are relatively painless.

**Prostaglandins** Hormones that stimulate uterine contractions.

**Oxytocin** A pituitary hormone that stimulates uterine contractions.

# CHILDBIRTH

Early in the ninth month of pregnancy, the fetus's head settles in the pelvis. This shift is called "dropping" or "lightening." The woman may actually feel lighter. Pressure lessens on the diaphragm. About a day or so before the beginning of labor, the woman may notice blood in her vaginal secretions. (Fetal pressure on the pelvis may rupture superficial blood vessels in the birth canal.) Tissue that had plugged the cervix, possibly preventing entry of infectious agents from the vagina, becomes dislodged. This results in a discharge of bloody mucus, which is known as the "bloody show."

At about this time, one woman in ten also has a rush of warm "water" from the vagina. The "water" is amniotic fluid, and it means that the amniotic sac has burst. Labor usually begins within a day after rupture of the amniotic sac. For most women the amniotic sac does not burst until the end of the first stage of childbirth. Other signs of impending labor include indigestion, diarrhea, abdominal cramps, and an ache in the small of the back. Labor begins with the onset of regular uterine contractions.

The first uterine contractions are relatively painless. They are called **Braxton-Hicks contractions** or false labor contractions. They are "false" because they do not widen the cervix or advance the baby through the birth canal. They tend to increase in frequency but are less regular than labor contractions. Braxton-Hicks contractions may warm the muscles that will be used in delivery. "Real" contractions, by contrast, become more intense when the woman moves around or walks.

The initiation of labor may involve the secretion of hormones by the fetus that stimulate the placenta and mother's uterus to secrete **prostaglandins.** Prostaglandins stimulate the uterine musculature to contract. It would make sense for the fetus to have a mechanism for signaling to the mother that it is mature enough to sustain independent life. We should caution that the mechanisms that initiate and maintain labor are not fully understood, however. Later in labor, the pituitary gland releases the hormone **oxytocin.** Oxytocin stimulates contractions strong enough to expel the baby.

## The Stages of Childbirth

Childbirth begins with the onset of labor and progresses through three stages.

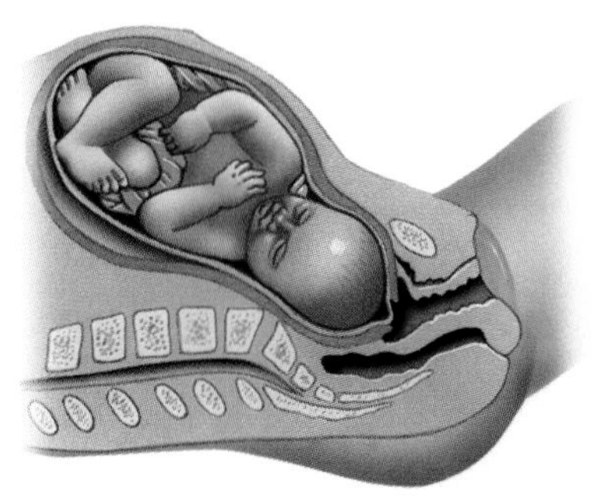
1. The second stage of labor begins

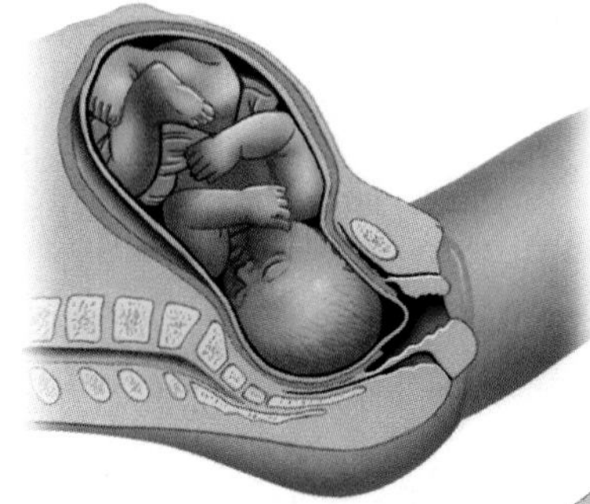
2. Further descent and rotation

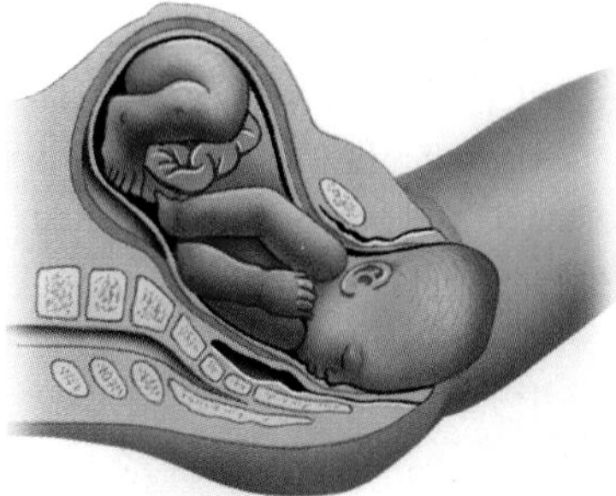
3. The crowning of the head

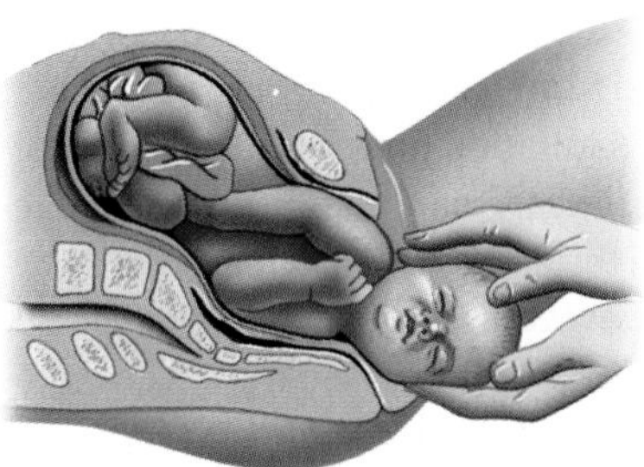
4. Anterior shoulder delivered

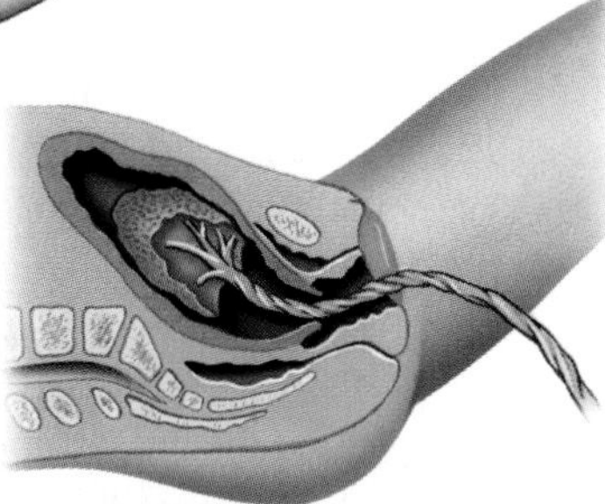
5. The third stage of labor begins with separation of the placenta from the uterine wall.

**Figure 11.2** ***The Stages of Childbirth*** In the first stage, uterine contractions efface and dilate the cervix to about 4 inches so that the baby may pass. The second stage begins with movement of the baby into the birth canal and ends with the birth of the baby. During the third stage the placenta separates from the uterine wall and is expelled through the birth canal.

**The First Stage** In the first stage, uterine contractions **efface** and **dilate** the cervix to about 4 inches (10 cm) in diameter, so that the baby may pass. Stretching of the cervix causes most of the pain of childbirth. A woman may experience little or no pain if her cervix dilates easily and quickly. The first stage may last from a couple of hours to more than a day. For a first pregnancy 12 to 24 hours of labor is considered about average. In later pregnancies labor typically takes about half this time.

The initial contractions are usually mild and spaced widely. They come at intervals of 10 to 20 minutes and may last 20 to 40 seconds. As time passes, contractions become more frequent, long, strong, and regular.

**Transition** occurs when the cervix becomes nearly fully dilated and the baby's head begins to move into the vagina, or birth canal. Contractions usually come quickly during transition. Transition usually lasts 30 minutes or less and is often accompanied by feelings of nausea, chills, and intense pain.

**The Second Stage** The second stage of childbirth follows transition. It begins when the cervix has become fully dilated. Then the baby begins to move into the vagina and first appears at the opening of the birth canal (Figure 11.2). The woman may be taken to a delivery room for the second stage of childbirth. The second stage is shorter than the first stage. It lasts from a few minutes to a few hours, and ends with birth of the baby.

Each contraction of the second stage propels the baby farther along the birth canal (vagina). When the baby's head becomes visible at the vaginal opening, it is said to have *crowned.* The baby typically emerges fully a few minutes after crowning.

**Talking Glossary**
Episiotomy
G1104

An **episiotomy** may be performed on the mother when the baby's head has crowned. Episiotomies are controversial, however. The incision can be painful in itself and can cause discomfort and itching as it heals. In some cases the discomfort interferes with sexual activity for months. Many obstetricians no longer perform episiotomies routinely. However, most health professionals concur that an episiotomy is preferable to random tearing if the tissues of the **perineum** become extremely effaced.

With or without an episiotomy, the baby's passageway to the ex-

**Efface** To become thin.

**Dilate** To open or widen.

**Transition** The process during which the cervix becomes nearly fully dilated and the head of the fetus begins to move into the birth canal.

**Episiotomy** A surgical incision in the perineum that widens the birth canal, preventing random tearing during childbirth.

**Perineum** The area between the vulva and the anus.

ternal world is a tight fit at best. As a result, the baby's facial features and the shape of its head may be temporarily distended. The baby may look as if it has been through a prizefight. Its head may be elongated, its nose flattened, and its ears bent. Parents may be concerned about whether the baby's features will assume a more typical shape. They almost always do. (Sigh of relief.)

**The Third Stage** The third, or placental, stage of childbirth may last a few minutes to an hour or more. During this stage, the placenta is expelled. Detachment of the placenta from the uterine wall may cause some bleeding. The uterus begins the process of contracting to a smaller size. The obstetrician sews the episiotomy or any tears in the perineum.

**In the New World** As the baby's head emerges, mucus is cleared from its mouth by means of suction aspiration. Aspiration prevents obstruction of the breathing passageway. Aspiration may be repeated when the baby is fully delivered. Now that suction aspiration is used, newly delivered babies are no longer routinely held upside down to help expel mucus. Nor, as in old films, is the baby slapped on the buttocks to stimulate breathing.

Once the baby is breathing adequately, the umbilical cord is clamped and severed about 3 inches from the baby's body. (After the birth of the second author's third child, he was invited by the obstetrician to cut the umbilical cord. His wife seized the scissors and cut the umbilical cord herself, squirting blood on the obstetrician's glasses in the process. "Who gave the obstetrician the right to determine who would cut the umbilical cord!" she wanted to know.) The stump of the umbilical cord dries and falls off in its own time, usually in seven to ten days.

While the mother is in the third stage of labor, the nurse may perform procedures on the baby, such as placing drops of silver nitrate or an antibiotic ointment into the eyes. This procedure is required by most states to prevent bacterial infections in the newborn's eyes. Typically the baby will now be footprinted. If the baby has been born in a hospital, she or he will be given an identification bracelet. The baby may also receive an injection of vitamin K, which is essential to the clotting of blood. (Newborns do not manufacture vitamin K on their own.)

**General anesthesia** The use of drugs to put people to sleep and eliminate pain, as during childbirth.

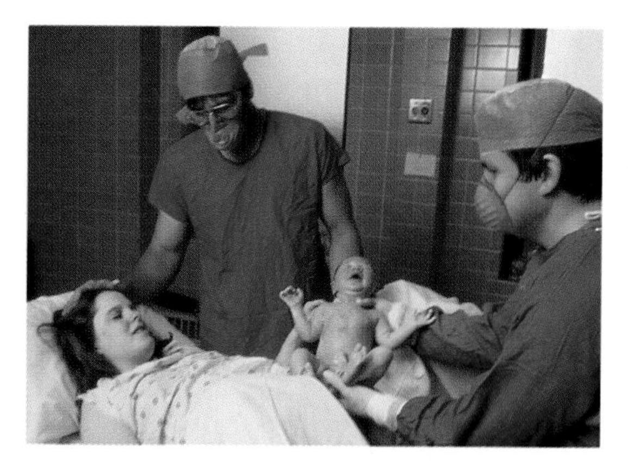

***Into the World*** Despite the sterile hospital environment, the birth of a child is for many parents the most wondrous experience of life.

## Methods of Childbirth

Until this century, childbirth was usually a family event. It happened at home and involved the mother, a midwife, family, and friends. Today, women in the United States and Canada typically give birth in hospitals. They are attended by obstetricians who use surgical instruments and anesthetics to protect mothers and children from infection, complications, and pain. Medical procedures save lives but also make childbearing more impersonal. Social critics argue that these procedures have "medicalized" a natural process. They have usurped control over women's bodies. Through the use of drugs, they have also denied many women part of the natural experience of giving birth.

### Anesthetized Childbirth

*In sorrow thou shalt bring forth children.*

Genesis 3:16

The Bible suggests that the ancients saw suffering as a woman's lot. But during the past two centuries, science and medicine have led to an expectation of less painful childbirth. Today some form of anesthesia is used in most U.S. deliveries.

**General anesthesia** first became popular in 1853. In that year, Queen Victoria of England delivered her eighth child under chloroform. General anesthesia, like the chloroform of old, induces unconsciousness. The drug sodium pentothal, a barbiturate, may be used to induce general anesthesia. Barbiturates (sedating drugs) may also be used to reduce anxiety while the woman remains awake. Women may also receive tranquilizers like Valium to help them relax or narcotics like Demerol to deaden pain.

Anesthetic drugs, as well as tranquilizers and narcotics, decrease the strength of uterine contractions during delivery. They may thus prolong cervical dilation and labor. They also weaken the woman's ability to push the baby through the birth canal. Because they cross the placental membrane, they also lower the newborn's overall responsiveness.

Regional or **local anesthesia** blocks pain in parts of the body without generally depressing the mother's alertness or putting her to sleep. In a *pudendal block,* the external genitals are numbed by local injection. In an *epidural block* and a *spinal block,* an anesthetic is injected into the spinal canal. It temporarily numbs the mother's body below the waist. To prevent injury, the needles used for these injections do not touch the spinal cord itself. Although local anesthesia decreases the responsiveness of the newborn baby, medicated childbirth is not associated with serious or long-term effects on children.

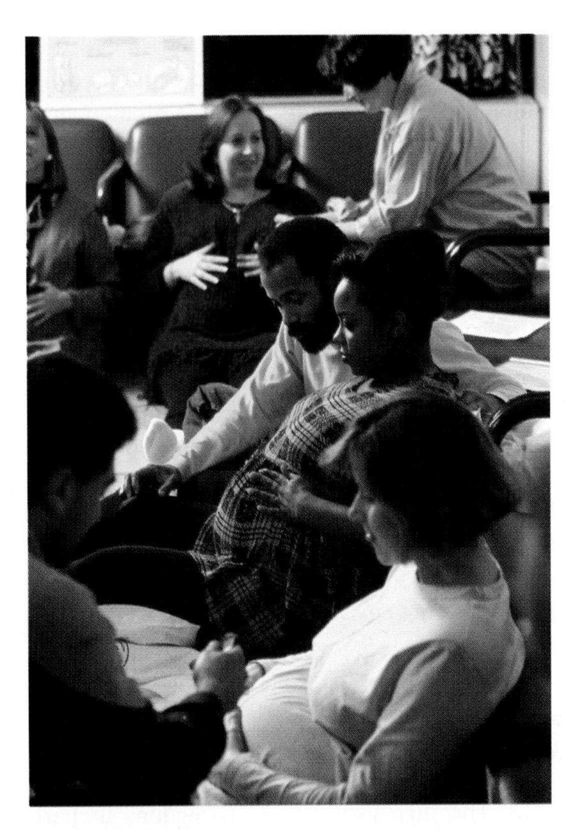

***Prepared Childbirth*** The Lamaze method helps expectant parents prepare for childbirth.

**Natural Childbirth** Partly as a reaction against the use of anesthetics, English obstetrician Grantly Dick-Read endorsed **natural childbirth** in his 1932 book *Childbirth without Fear.* Dick-Read argued that women's labor pains were heightened by their fear of the unknown and resulting muscle tensions. Dick-Read emphasized the value of informing women about the biological aspects of reproduction and childbirth, encouraging physical fitness in the mother, and teaching her relaxation and breathing exercises. Many of Dick-Read's contributions have become accepted practice in modern childbirth procedures.

**Prepared Childbirth—The Lamaze Method** The French obstetrician Fernand Lamaze visited the Soviet Union in 1951 and found that many Russian women bore babies without anesthetics or a great deal of pain. Lamaze returned to Western Europe with some of the techniques the women used. They are now usually termed the **Lamaze method,** or *prepared childbirth.* Lamaze argued that women can learn to conserve energy during childbirth and reduce the pain of uterine contractions by learning coping responses. For example, they can visualize pleasant mental images, such as beach scenes, or practice breathing and relaxation exercises.

A pregnant woman usually attends Lamaze classes with a "coach"—typically the father. The coach assists her in the delivery room by timing contractions, offering support, and coaching her in breathing and relaxation exercises. The woman and coach are also generally educated about childbirth. The father is fully integrated into the process. Many couples report that their marriages are strengthened as a result.

The Lamaze method is flexible about the use of anesthetics. The woman is the boss. She is free to use or not use anesthetics. This allows her to feel in control of the delivery.

**Caesarean Section** In a **caesarean section** (C-section), the baby is delivered through surgery rather than naturally through the vagina. The term "section" is derived from the Latin for "to cut." Julius Caesar is said to have been delivered in

**Local anesthesia** Anesthesia that eliminates pain in a specific area of the body, as during childbirth.

**Natural childbirth** A method of childbirth in which women use no anesthesia but are given other strategies for coping with discomfort.

**Lamaze method** A childbirth method in which women learn to relax and to breathe in patterns that conserve energy and lessen pain.

**Caesarean section** A method of childbirth in which the fetus is delivered through a surgical incision in the abdomen.

this way, but health professionals believe this unlikely. In a C-section, the woman is anesthetized and incisions are made in her abdomen and uterus, through which the baby is taken out. The incisions are sewn up and the mother can begin walking, often on the same day.

C-sections are most likely to be advised when normal delivery is difficult or threatening to the health of the mother or child. Vaginal deliveries can become difficult if the baby is large or the mother's pelvis is small or misshapen, or if the mother is tired or weakened. Viral agents that may be present in the birth canal of infected women, such as herpes viruses and HIV, can be bypassed by performing a C-section. C-sections are also likely to be performed if the baby presents for delivery in the breech position or the **transverse position** (lying crosswise), or if the baby is in distress.

Use of the C-section has mushroomed. In the 1990s, nearly one million births each year are by C-section. This works out to nearly one birth in four. Compare this figure to about one in ten births in 1975. The increased rate of C-sections in part reflects advances in health technology, such as fetal monitors that detect fetal distress.[4] Critics claim that many C-sections are unnecessary. They reflect overly aggressive medical practices. Even the Centers for Disease Control and Prevention (CDC) believe that as many as one in three C-sections are unnecessary.[5]

Health specialists once thought that after a woman had a C-section, subsequent deliveries also had to be C-sections. Otherwise, the uterine scar might rupture during labor. Today, however, many women who have had C-sections deliver subsequent children vaginally.

## Alternatives to the Hospital—Where Should a Child Be Born?

In the United States, most births occur in hospitals. Medical equipment and personnel are thus available to handle complications. But hospital deliveries have their disadvantages. Hospitals are often impersonal and very expensive, although the costs may be offset by medical insurance. Giving birth in a hospital also tends to instill the perception that pregnancy is an illness instead of a healthy, natural process. The hospital environment may also encourage mothers to assume a more passive role and surrender responsibility for their care to doctors and nurses. For various reasons, then, many pregnant women and their partners have sought alternatives to the hospital.

**Transverse position** A crosswise birth position.

**Birth Center** Birth centers seek to provide the atmosphere associated with home delivery, although they typically have some medical equipment available. They are frequently located within or adjacent to medical centers to permit immediate access to medical facilities if, for example, an emergency C-section is needed. Birth centers are intended for women who are at low risk for birth complications.

The birthing room itself is typically decorated and furnished cheerfully, like a bedroom. Family members, friends, and siblings of the baby may all be present. Women in labor can move about the room freely. They eat, drink, rest, or chat with friends and family as they wish. Following the birth, the family generally remains together in the room. They share what for most is a loving and joyous experience. Today, even maternity wards in hospitals are changing their decor and ambiance to resemble more the comforting environment of birthing centers.

**Home Births** Home birth provides familiar surroundings and the psychological sense that the woman and her family are in charge. Some advocates of home birth argue that it is safe enough for women who have been medically screened for complications and have a history of normal births.

Critics charge that it is not possible to screen women for every possible complication. They add that home delivery exposes the mother and child to unnecessary risks, especially if unexpected complications occur. Many physicians refuse to deliver babies in the mother's home.

### think about it!

- **Do you know anyone who has used the Lamaze method? What does she (or he) say about it?**
- **Do you know anyone who had a caesarean section? What was her experience like?**

**critical thinking** **Agree or disagree and support your answer: Children should be born in a hospital.**

Smart Quiz Q1103

## BIRTH PROBLEMS

Most deliveries are uncomplicated, or "unremarkable" in medical parlance. Of course, childbirth is the most remarkable experience of many parents' lives. Problems can and do occur, however. Some of the most common birth problems are anoxia and the birth of preterm and low birth weight babies.

Talking Glossary
Prenatal anoxia
G1105

### Anoxia

**Prenatal anoxia** can cause various problems in the neonate and affect later development. It leads to such complications as brain damage and mental retardation. Prolonged anoxia during delivery can also result in **cerebral palsy** and death.

The baby is supplied with oxygen through the umbilical cord, which is squeezed when the baby passes through the birth canal. Temporary squeezing, like holding one's breath for a moment, is unlikely to cause problems. (Slight oxygen deprivation at birth is not unusual. The transition from receiving oxygen through the umbilical cord to breathing on its own may not happen immediately after the baby emerges.) Anoxia can result if constriction of the cord is prolonged, however. Prolonged constriction is more likely to occur with a breech presentation. In that case, the baby's head presses the umbilical cord against the birth canal during delivery. Fetal monitoring can help detect anoxia early, before damage occurs. An immediate C-section can be performed if the fetus appears to be in distress.

### Preterm and Low Birth Weight Children

A **neonate** is considered to be premature, or **preterm,** if it is born before 37 weeks of gestation. The normal period of gestation is 40 weeks. The fetus normally makes dramatic gains in weight during the last weeks of pregnancy. Therefore, prematurity is linked with low birth weight. Regardless of the length of gestation, a newborn baby is considered to have a low birth weight if it weighs less than 5 pounds (about 2,500 grams). Preterm or low birth weight babies face a heightened risk of infant mortality. A birth weight of $3\frac{1}{4}$ pounds (1,500 grams) is considered to be the cutoff with respect to the likelihood of infant mortality.

Preterm babies are relatively thin; they have not yet formed the layer of fat that accounts for the round, robust appearance of most full-term babies. Their muscles are immature. Thus their sucking and breathing reflexes are weak. Also, in the last weeks of pregnancy fetuses secrete **surfactants** that line the airways to keep them from sticking together. Muscle weakness and incomplete lining of the airways contribute to **respiratory distress syndrome.** This syndrome is responsible for many neonatal deaths. Preterm babies may also suffer from underdeveloped immune systems, which leave them vulnerable to infections.

Preterm infants usually remain in the hospital for a time. There they can be monitored and placed in incubators. Incubators are temperature-controlled environments that provide some protection from disease. If necessary, preterm babies are also given oxygen.

**think about it!**

- **Do you know of anyone who has experienced birth problems? What problems? What was the outcome?**

**critical thinking** **Agree or disagree and support your answer: The government should spend more on health care for poor pregnant women.**

Smart Quiz
Q1104

## THE POSTPARTUM PERIOD

The weeks following delivery are called the **postpartum** period. The first few days postpartum are frequently happy ones. The long wait is over. So are the discomforts of childbirth. A sizable number of women experience feelings of depression, however, following childbirth.

### Maternal Depression

Mood changes following childbirth are experienced by many new mothers. During the days or weeks following

**Prenatal anoxia** Oxygen deprivation.

**Cerebral palsy** A muscular disorder characterized by spastic paralysis; caused by damage to the central nervous system usually occurring prior to or during birth.

**Neonate** A newborn child.

**Preterm** Born before 37 weeks of gestation.

**Surfactants** Substances that prevent the walls of the airways from sticking together.

**Respiratory distress syndrome** A cluster of breathing problems, including weak and irregular breathing, to which preterm babies are especially prone.

**Postpartum** Following birth.

WORLD OF *diversity*

## Ethnicity and Infant Mortality

The United States has some of the world's most sophisticated health technology. Back in 1950, there were more than 25 infant deaths per 1,000 live births in the United States. That number has been dropping sharply, to 8.5 in 1992 and 7.9 in 1994. Yet within the United States, rates of infant mortality differ dramatically across ethnicities. Infant mortality rates are lowest for Chinese Americans and Japanese Americans.[6] Hispanic Americans of Cuban, Mexican, or Central or South American descent have the next lowest infant mortality rates. Non-Hispanic white Americans follow. Then come African Americans. The infant mortality rate for African Americans is about twice that for non-Hispanic white Americans. In 1992, African Americans made up about 12% of the U.S. population. However, they accounted for about one-third of the infant deaths in the nation.[7]

Although the United States has sophisticated health care, not all Americans receive it. Much of the ethnic difference in infant mortality can be attributed to differences in prenatal health care. Table 11.3 shows 1990 infant health statistics obtained from public records in New York City. As you can see, residents of the affluent white Kips Bay–Yorkville area have healthier newborns than residents of the poorer East Harlem community or the middle-income and mainly white community of Astoria–Long Island City. East Harlem is a low-income neighborhood made up mostly of African Americans. East Harlem mothers, like other low-income mothers, are more likely than wealthier women to have babies with low birth weights and babies who die during infancy.[8] Maternal malnutrition and use of chemical substances such as alcohol and tobacco during pregnancy are all linked to low birth weight and increased mortality during the first year of life.[9]

The differences in infant health shown in the table are also connected with the prenatal care received by the mothers in the three neighborhoods. According to 1990 New York City Department of Health records, nearly 36% of East Harlem mothers receive either late prenatal care or none. This figure compares with about 6% in Kips Bay–Yorkville and about 10% in Astoria–Long Island City. Research has shown that comprehensive prenatal care is associated with higher birth weights.[10]

**TABLE 11.3**

**Infant Health Statistics for Three New York City Neighborhoods[11]**

| Infant Health Statistics | East Harlem | Astoria–Long Island City | Kips Bay–Yorkville |
|---|---|---|---|
| Infant deaths per 1,000 live births | 23.4 | 14.9 | 7.3 |
| Low birth weight babies per 100 live births (less than 5.5 pounds) | 18.5 | 6.1 | 6.0 |
| Very low birth weight babies per 100 live births (less than 3.3 pounds) | 3.8 | 0.98 | 0.87 |
| Live births per 100 in which mothers received late or no prenatal care | 35.8 | 10.4 | 6.1 |

delivery, most new mothers experience periods of sadness, tearfulness, and irritability. These periods are commonly called the "postpartum blues," the "maternity blues," or the "baby blues." This downswing in mood typically occurs about three days after delivery and lasts about 48 hours. It is generally believed to be a normal response to the hormonal and psychological changes that attend childbirth.

Some mothers experience more persistent and severe mood changes, called **postpartum depression (PPD).** PPD may last a year or even longer. PPD can involve extreme sadness or despair, apathy, changes in appetite and sleep patterns, low self-esteem, and difficulty concentrating. A study of some 1,000 married, middle-class, first-time mothers from the Pittsburgh area who had full-term, healthy infants found that nearly one in ten had experienced PPD.[12]

Like the "maternity blues," PPD may reflect a combination of physiological and psychological factors. Hormonal changes may play a role in PPD, but stress, a troubled marriage, or the need to

**Postpartum depression (PPD)** Persistent and severe mood changes during the postpartum period, involving feelings of despair and apathy and characterized by changes in appetite and sleep, low self-esteem, and difficulty concentrating.

adjust to an unwanted or sick baby may all contribute to PPD. Adjusting to a new baby imposes inevitable, and often stressful, changes on all parents. First-time mothers, single mothers, and mothers who lack social support from their partners or family members face the greatest risk of PPD.

**Close-up**
Reducing the risk of SIDS
T1101

New fathers may also have bouts of depression. New mothers are not the only ones who must adjust to the responsibilities of parenthood. Fathers too may feel overwhelmed or unable to cope. Perhaps more fathers might experience the "paternity blues," except for the fact that mothers generally shoulder most child-rearing chores.

## Breast-Feeding versus Bottle-Feeding

Only a minority of U.S. women breast-feed their children. One reason is that many women return to the workforce shortly after childbirth. Thus they are unavailable for regular feedings. Some choose to share feeding chores with the father. (The father is equally equipped to prepare and hold a bottle, but not to breast-feed.) Other women find breast-feeding inconvenient or unpleasant. Long-term comparisons of breast-fed and bottle-fed children show few, if any, meaningful differences. Breast-feeding does reduce the general risk of infections to the baby, however. The risk is lowered through transmission of the mother's antibodies to the baby. Breast-feeding also reduces the incidence of allergies in babies, particularly in allergy-prone infants.

**Close-up**
Breast-feeding: a best bet?
T1102

Uterine contractions that occur during breast-feeding help return the uterus to its typical size. Breast-feeding also delays resumption of normal menstrual cycles. Breast-feeding is not a perfectly reliable birth-control method, however. (Nursing women are advised not to use birth-control pills. The hormone content of the pills is passed to the infant through the milk.)

Should a woman breast-feed her baby? Although breast-feeding has benefits for both mother and infant, each woman must weigh these benefits against her personal feelings and the difficulties breast-feeding may impose on her. Difficulties include assuming the sole responsibility for nighttime feedings, the physical demands of producing and expelling milk, possible soreness in the breasts, and the inconvenience of being continually available to meet the infant's feeding needs. Women should breast-feed because they want to, not because they think they must.

## Resumption of Ovulation and Menstruation

For close to a month after delivery, women experience a reddish vaginal discharge called **lochia.** A nonnursing mother does not resume actual menstrual periods until two to three months postpartum. The first few cycles are likely to be irregular.

Many women incorrectly assume that they will first menstruate and then ovulate two weeks later. In most cases, the opposite is true. Ovulation precedes the first menstrual period after childbirth. Thus, a woman may become pregnant before the menstrual phase of her first postpartum cycle.

## Resumption of Sexual Activity

The resumption of sexual activity depends on a couple's level of sexual interest, the healing of episiotomies or other injuries, fatigue, the obstetrician's recommendations, and, of course, tradition. Obstetricians usually advise a six-week waiting period for safety and comfort. However, many sexual activities other than intercourse are safe and do not cause discomfort.

Women who breast-feed may find that they have less vaginal lubrication, which can cause discomfort during sexual activity. K-Y jelly or other lubricants may help in such cases.

The return of sexual interest and resumption of sexual activity take longer for some couples than for others. Sexual interest depends more on psychological than on physical factors. Many couples encounter declining sexual interest and activity in the first year following childbirth, because child care can sap energy and limit free time. One of the big challenges that new parents face is learning to incorporate sexual activity within their busy schedules.

### *think about it!*

- **Do you know of anyone who was depressed after delivering a baby? How serious was the depression? How was it resolved?**

**critical thinking** **Agree or disagree and support your answer: It is the mother's responsibility to breast-feed her child.**

**Smart Quiz**
Q1105

**Lochia** A reddish vaginal discharge that may persist for a month after delivery.

# Enhancing Prenatal Health

## Take Charge

Health professionals have not only made us more aware of the changes that take place during prenatal development; they have also heightened our awareness of prenatal health problems and how we can prevent them. Here we focus on what pregnant women can do to enhance their own health and that of the fetus.

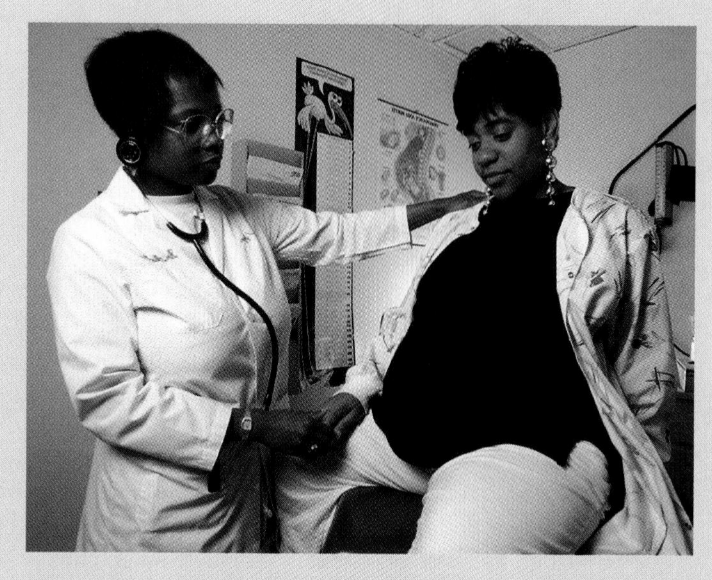

***Prenatal Care*** Obtaining regular prenatal care, following a sensible diet and exercise program, and avoiding exposure to teratogens are the most important steps pregnant women can take to ensure their own health and the health of the fetus.

### Obtain Regular Prenatal Care

A healthy pregnancy can make the difference between a joyous experience and a lifetime of regrets. One way to help ensure a healthy pregnancy is to obtain adequate prenatal health care. This means early and regular visits to an obstetrician, a medical specialist who provides care to pregnant women.

Many women learn about obstetricians from friends and relatives. Others, especially women in a new locale, rely on the phone book. In either case, there are things you will want to know about the obstetrician, questions that you will need to ask. Many of them concern the degree to which the obstetrician will allow you to be in control of your own childbirth. Here are some suggestions for selecting an obstetrician.

1. *As in consulting any helping professional, you should inquire about the obstetrician's academic credentials and experience.* Degrees, licenses, and certificates about residencies should be displayed. If they are not, you might want to ask why.
2. *Ask a lot of questions.* You're going to be bursting with questions over the next several months. If the obstetrician does not handle them well now, you may be in for problems. Here are some types of questions you may want to ask:
   - Ask what kinds of problems the obstetrician runs into most often: How does she or he handle them? This is an indirect way of inquiring about frequency of C-sections, for example. Then, too, you never know what "bombshells" will be dropped when you ask an open-ended question.
   - Ask follow-up questions, such as, "What percentage of your deliveries are caesareans?" or, "I've been reading that too many caesareans are done these days. What do you think?"
   - Ask questions about medication use during childbirth, such as, "What are your attitudes toward medication?" You'll quickly get a sense of whether the obstetrician is open-minded about medication and sensitive to your wishes and preferences.
   - Ask something like, "What do you see as the role of the father during childbirth?" You'll quickly learn whether the obstetrician's attitudes coincide with your own.
   - You may also want to ask questions about the obstetrician's beliefs concerning routine testing, weight gain, vitamin supplements, use of amniocentesis or ultrasound, and a whole range of issues. Each will provide you with specific information. They also give you the opportunity to determine how the obstetrician is relating to you as a person.
3. *See how the obstetrician handles you during the initial examination.* You should have the feeling that you are being handled gently, respectfully, and competently. If you're not sure, do some comparison shopping. It's your body and your child. You have the right to gather enough information so that you are confident you are making the right choice.

## Follow a Sensible Diet

It is a common misconception that the fetus will take what it needs from its mother. *Not so.* Maternal malnutrition can impair fetal health. Maternal malnutrition during the third trimester, when the fetus normally makes substantial weight gains, is linked to low birth weight and increased infant mortality. Pregnant women who are well nourished are more likely to deliver healthy babies at least average in size. Women should consult their obstetricians regarding any special dietary needs they may have.

**Vitamins** Many obstetricians prescribe multivitamins for pregnant women to maintain their own health and to promote fetal development. Prescribed doses of vitamins are healthful.[13] "Too much of a good thing" is risky, however. High doses of vitamins such as A, $B_6$, D, and K have been linked to birth defects. Vitamin A excesses have been linked with such problems as cleft palate and heart problems.[14] Excesses of vitamin D are linked to mental retardation. All pregnant women need to consume 400 mcg of folic acid daily to prevent neural tube defects, such as spina bifida (see Chapter 5).

## Follow a Healthy Exercise Program

Being pregnant is not an excuse for avoiding physical activity. Just the opposite is true: Exercise is healthy for mother and baby. Pregnancy certainly imposes some limitations, but a safe exercise program can be devised with an obstetrician's advice.

## Avoid Exposure to Teratogens

Talking Glossary
Teratogens
G1106

Environmental influences or agents that can harm the embryo or fetus are called **teratogens** (from the Greek *teras,* meaning "monster"). These include drugs taken by the mother and certain substances produced by the mother's body, such as Rh-positive antibodies. Other teratogens include the metals lead and mercury, radiation, and pathogens. Exposure to particular teratogens causes the greatest harm during **critical periods of vulnerability.** Critical periods correspond to the times at which the structures most affected are developing (see Figure 11.3, following page). The heart, for example, develops rapidly from the third to the fifth week following conception. It is most vulnerable to certain teratogens at this time. The arms and legs, which develop later, are most vulnerable from the fourth through the eighth week of development. The major organ systems differentiate during the embryonic stage. Therefore, the embryo is most vulnerable to the effects of teratogens.

Environmental contaminants such as lead and mercury are present in the air and soil in small amounts and do not pose much risk except under unusual circumstances, such as breathing high levels of lead dust released from deteriorated old paint during home renovations (see Chapter 22). Pathogens (disease-causing organisms) and drugs pose more serious risks.

**Infectious Diseases Affecting the Mother** Many pathogens cannot pass through the placenta to infect the embryo or fetus. However, some can, including potentially dangerous pathogens responsible for such infectious diseases as syphilis, measles, mumps, and chicken pox. Here we consider the risks posed by several infectious diseases that can be serious threats to the fetus and newborn.

***Rubella (German Measles)*** **Rubella** is a viral infection. Women who contract rubella during the embryonic stage, when rapid organ differentiation is taking place, may bear children who are deaf or develop mental retardation, heart disease, or cataracts. Most American women have rubella as children and acquire immunity to it. Women who are unsure whether they have had rubella may be tested for immunity. If they are not immune, they can be vaccinated *before pregnancy.* Inoculation during pregnancy is risky because it causes a mild case of the disease in the mother, which can affect the embryo or fetus.

***Syphilis*** Maternal **syphilis** may cause miscarriage or **stillbirth.** It can be passed along to the child in the form of congenital syphilis. Congenital syphilis can impair vision and hearing, damage the liver, or deform bones and teeth. Routine blood tests early in pregnancy can diagnose syphilis and other problems. The bacteria that cause syphilis do not readily cross the placenta during the first months of pregnancy. Thus the fetus will probably not contract syphilis if an infected mother is treated with antibiotics before the fourth month of pregnancy.

***Acquired Immunodeficiency Syndrome (AIDS)*** **AIDS** is caused by the human immunodeficiency virus (HIV). HIV is blood-borne and is sometimes transmitted through the placenta to infect the fetus. The rupturing of blood vessels in mother and baby during childbirth provides another opportunity for transmission of HIV. However, most babies born to mothers who are infected with HIV do not become infected themselves. HIV-infected women can greatly lessen the chances of viral transmission in utero by taking the antiviral drug AZT (see Chapter 16). HIV can also be transmitted to children by breast-feeding. Pregnant women (and those who suspect they may become pregnant) who fear that they may have HIV should consult with their obstetrician about the need to be tested for the virus.

**Teratogens** Environmental influences or agents that can damage an embryo or fetus.

**Critical period of vulnerability** A period of time during which an embryo or fetus is vulnerable to the effects of a teratogen.

**Rubella** A viral infection that can cause mental retardation and heart disease in an embryo. Also called *German measles.*

**Syphilis** A sexually transmitted disease caused by a bacterial infection.

**Stillbirth** The birth of a dead fetus.

**Acquired immunodeficiency syndrome (AIDS)** A sexually transmitted disease that destroys white blood cells in the immune system, leaving the body vulnerable to various "opportunistic" diseases.

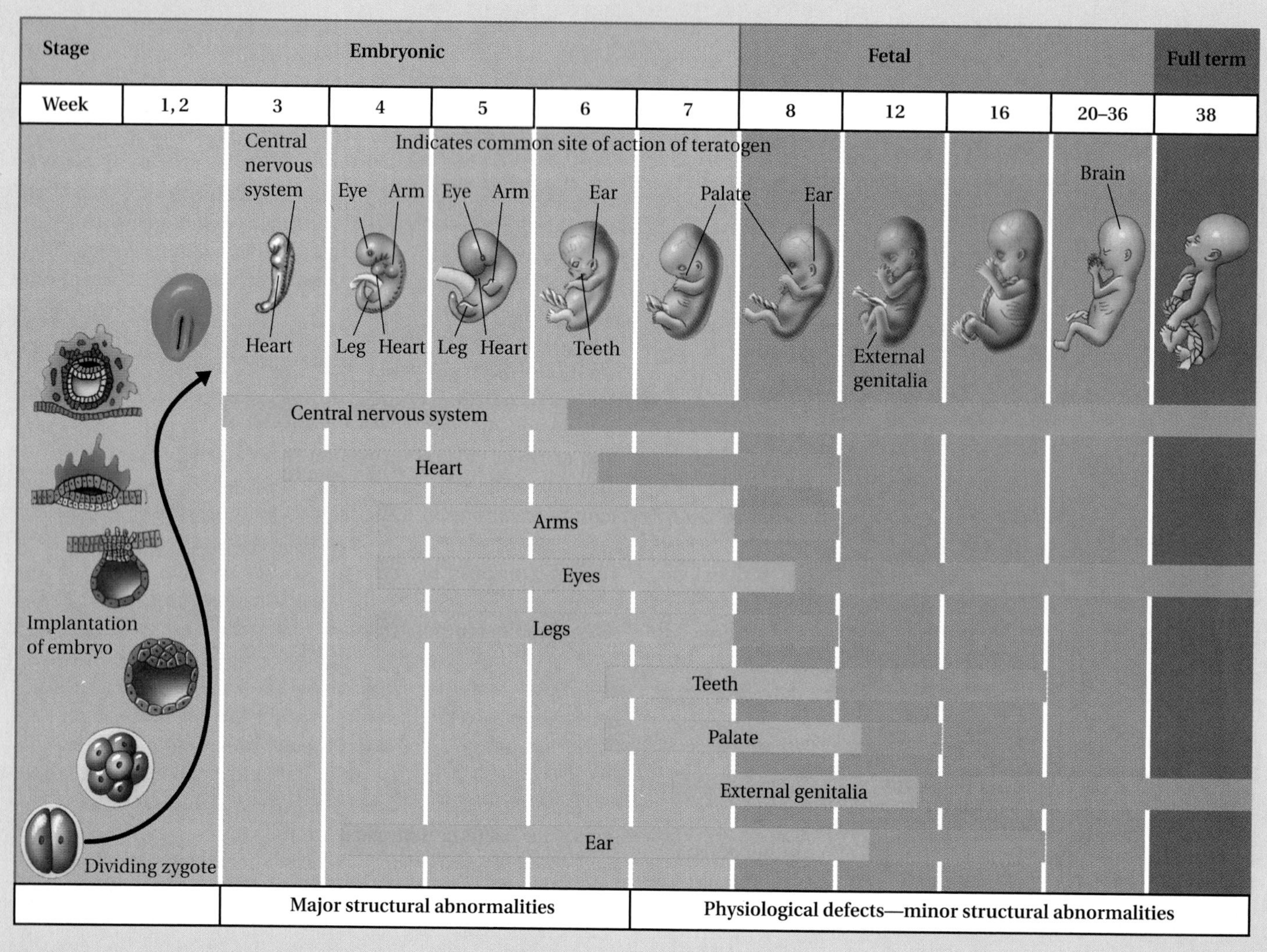


**Figure 11.3** ***Critical Periods in Prenatal Development*** The developing embryo is most vulnerable to teratogens when the organ systems are taking shape. The periods of greatest vulnerability of organ systems are shown in orange. Periods of lesser vulnerability are shown in blue.

**Rh Incompatibility** In **Rh incompatibility,** antibodies produced by the mother are transmitted to a fetus or newborn infant. *Rh* is a blood protein found in some people's red blood cells. Rh incompatibility occurs when a woman who does not have this blood factor, and thus is *Rh negative,* is carrying an *Rh-positive* fetus. (This can happen if the father is Rh-positive.) The negative-positive combination is found in about 10% of U.S. married couples. However, it becomes a problem only in a minority of such couples' pregnancies. In these cases the mother's antibodies attack the red blood cells of the fetus, which can cause fetal brain damage or death. Rh incompatibility does not usually adversely affect a first child because women will usually not yet have formed antibodies to the Rh factor. It is most likely that Rh-positive fetal red blood cells will enter the Rh-negative mother's body during childbirth. The mother will then produce antibodies to the baby's Rh-positive blood.

Blood typing of pregnant women significantly decreases the threat of Rh incompatibility. If an Rh-negative mother is injected with the vaccine Rhogan within 72 hours after delivery of an Rh-positive baby, she will not develop the harmful antibodies. She will thus not pass them to the fetus during a later pregnancy. A fetus or newborn child at risk may also receive a preventive blood transfusion to remove the mother's antibodies.

**Rh incompatibility** A condition in which antibodies produced by a pregnant woman are transmitted to the fetus and may cause brain damage or death.

**Drugs Taken by the Mother (and Father)** Expectant mothers should avoid taking any drugs during pregnancy unless they are directed to do so by a physician. There's good reason for this because many drugs can be harmful to the developing fetus, especially if they are taken during critical periods of fetal development. Even widely used over-the-counter drugs, like aspirin and antihistamines, can damage the fetus, as can several antibiotics. The antibiotic tetracycline, for example, may yellow the teeth and deform the bones. Other antibiotics have been implicated in deafness and jaundice. Some acne drugs have been shown to cause physical and mental abnormalities in children of women who used them during pregnancy. Maternal use of illicit drugs such as narcotics, cocaine, and marijuana also places the fetus at risk.

**Close-up**
More on drugs and pregnancy
T1103

***Narcotics*** Narcotics such as heroin and methadone readily pass from mother to fetus through the placenta. Narcotics are addictive. Fetuses of women who use them regularly can become addicted in utero. At birth, they may undergo drug withdrawal and show muscle tension and agitation. Women who use narcotics must inform their obstetricians or health care providers and receive appropriate drug treatment. The information will be kept confidential, and measures can be taken to help their babies.

***Tranquilizers and Sedatives*** The tranquilizers Librium and Valium cross the placental membrane and may cause birth defects such as harelip. Sedatives, such as the barbiturate phenobarbital, are suspected of decreasing testosterone production and causing reproductive problems in the sons of pregnant women who use them.

***Cocaine*** Maternal use of cocaine, a stimulant drug, can cause miscarriages and is associated with later developmental problems. Cocaine is usually consumed by snorting (in powder form) or smoking (in the hardened form called "crack")—see Chapter 12. Many babies born to crack-addicted mothers develop problems later in childhood, including behavior problems and difficulty concentrating.

***Hallucinogens and Marijuana*** Use of hallucinogenic drugs such as marijuana and LSD during pregnancy has been linked to chromosomal damage in fetuses. The active ingredient in marijuana, THC, readily crosses the placenta. So does LSD. Use of marijuana can lead to decreased androgen production in male fetuses, which can impede sexual differentiation.

It's not just illicit drugs that can cause fetal damage. The most widespread damage is caused by two legally available substances, alcohol and tobacco.

***Alcohol*** Mothers who drink heavily during pregnancy expose their fetuses to serious risk of birth defects, low birth weight, infant mortality, sensory and motor problems, and mental retardation. Nearly 40% of children whose mothers drink heavily during pregnancy develop **fetal alcohol syndrome (FAS).** FAS is a leading cause of mental retardation and is associated with the development of facial deformities such as an underdeveloped upper jaw, flattened nose, and widely spaced eyes.[15] The critical period for the development of these deformities is the first two months, when the head is taking shape.[16] FAS affects between 1 and 3 children of every 1,000 live births.[17]

Some research suggests that light drinking is unlikely to harm the fetus in most cases.[18] However, FAS has been found among children whose mothers drank only two ounces of alcohol a day during the first trimester.[19] It is not true that pregnant women can have one or two alcoholic beverages a day without harming their babies. No safe minimal amount of drinking for pregnant women has been clearly established. Therefore, pregnant women are advised to abstain from alcohol—period.

***Smoking*** About one pregnant woman in four smokes cigarettes. Cigarette smoke contains chemicals such as carbon monoxide and the stimulant nicotine. Both are transmitted to the fetus. Maternal smoking increases the risk of spontaneous abortion, stillbirth, premature birth, low birth weight, and infant mortality.[20] The health risks increase with the amount smoked.

Low birth weight is the most common risk factor for infant disease and mortality. Maternal smoking during pregnancy more than doubles the risk of low birth weight. The combination of smoking and drinking alcohol places the child at yet greater risk.[21] The earlier the pregnant smoker quits, the better for the baby (and herself!).

Maternal smoking also increases the risk of asthma and sudden infant death syndrome (SIDS). Passive exposure to second-hand smoke during infancy is also linked to increased risk of SIDS.[22] Evidence also points to more academic problems for children of smokers: reduced attention spans, hyperactivity, and lower IQs and achievement test scores.[23]

One in four smokes cigarettes. Many of them do not suspend drug use until they learn that they are pregnant. Unfortunately, they may not learn they are pregnant until several weeks into the pregnancy. Damage to the fetus may thus have already occurred. Even then, only about 20 percent of pregnant smokers quit.[24]

It may be easier for women to quit if they perceive quitting as limited to the terms of their pregnancies, not as permanent. If they should remain abstinent after the baby is born, so much the better.

It is best to consider any substance that passes a pregnant woman's lips, legal or not, prescription or over-the-counter, as a potential hazard to the fetus. Every pregnant woman—and every woman who suspects that she might be pregnant—should consult her obstetrician or health care provider before taking any medications or other drugs. She should definitely avoid tobacco, alcohol, and illicit drugs such as cocaine, marijuana, and narcotics.

***Paternal Drug Use*** Paternal use of certain drugs also may endanger the fetus. For example, some drugs may alter the genetic material in the father's sperm. The mother's inhalation of second-hand cigarette smoke from the father (or other people) can harm the fetus (see Chapter 14). Exposure to marijuana smoke may also harm the fetus. If the father smokes during his wife's pregnancy, he should not do so in her presence. Pregnant women should also avoid enclosed areas in which people are smoking.

**Other Agents** X-rays increase the risk of malformed organs in the fetus, especially within a month and a half following conception. (Ultrasound has *not* been shown to harm the embryo or fetus.) To enhance prenatal health, pregnant women are advised to consult their health care providers before undergoing any medical or dental procedure, including dental X-rays.

Smart Quiz
Q1106

**Fetal alcohol syndrome (FAS)** A cluster of symptoms caused by maternal drinking in which the child shows developmental lags and facial deformities.

# SUMMING UP

## Questions and Answers

### PREGNANCY

**1. What are the early signs of pregnancy?** Early signs include a missed period, presence of HCG in the blood or urine, and Hegar's sign.

**2. How do pregnancy tests work?** Pregnancy tests detect the presence of HCG—human chorionic gonadotropin—in the woman's urine or blood.

**3. What are the early effects of pregnancy?** Early effects include tenderness in the breasts and morning sickness.

**4. What are the causes of miscarriage?** Miscarriages have many causes, including chromosomal defects in the fetus and abnormalities of the placenta and uterus.

**5. What are the effects of sexual intercourse during pregnancy?** Most health professionals concur that coitus is normally safe until the start of labor.

**6. What psychological changes occur during pregnancy?** A woman's psychological response to pregnancy reflects her desire to be pregnant, her physical changes, and her attitudes toward these changes. Men, like women, respond to pregnancy according to the degree to which they want the child.

### PRENATAL DEVELOPMENT

**7. What are the stages of prenatal development?** The germinal stage is the period from conception through implantation. The embryonic stage begins with implantation and extends to about the eighth week of development and is characterized by differentiation of the major organ systems. The fetal stage begins by the ninth week and continues until the birth of the baby. The fetal stage is characterized by continued maturation of the fetus's organ systems and dramatic increases in size.

**8. What are some health problems involved with prenatal development?** These include toxemia, a potentially life-threatening condition characterized by high blood pressure, and chromosomal and genetic abnormalities. Environmental factors can also affect prenatal development, including the mother's diet, maternal diseases and disorders, and use of certain medications and drugs. Maternal malnutrition has been linked to low birth weight and infant mortality. Exposure to particular teratogens causes the greatest harm during critical periods of vulnerability.

**9. What are some effects of chromosomal and genetic abnormalities?** Chromosomal and genetic abnormalities can lead to cystic fibrosis, Down syndrome, hemophilia, Huntington's disease, neural tube defects, phenylketonuria, retina blastoma, sickle-cell anemia, and Tay-Sachs disease. Parental blood tests, amniocentesis, and ultrasound allow parents to learn whether a fetus or infant has or is at risk for many such disorders.

### CHILDBIRTH

**10. What are the stages of childbirth?** In the first stage uterine contractions efface and dilate the cervix so that the baby may pass. The first stage may last from a couple of hours to more than a day. The second stage lasts from a few minutes to a few hours and ends with the birth of the baby. During the third stage the placenta is expelled.

**11. What are some contemporary methods of childbirth?** Contemporary methods of childbirth include anesthetized childbirth, natural childbirth, the Lamaze method, and caesarean section.

**12. What are some places other than hospitals where children are born?** In the United States most births occur in hospitals. Some parents seeking more intimate arrangements, however, opt for a birth center or home delivery.

### BIRTH PROBLEMS

**13. What are some birth problems?** Prenatal anoxia can cause brain damage and mental retardation. Preterm and low birth weight babies have a heightened risk of infant mortality.

### THE POSTPARTUM PERIOD

**14. What is maternal depression?** Transient mood changes following childbirth are experienced by many new mothers. Women with postpartum depression experience lingering depression following childbirth.

**15. What are the effects of breast-feeding versus bottle-feeding?** Breast-feeding is connected with fewer infections and allergic reactions in the baby than bottle-feeding. Long-term studies show little difference between children whose parents used one or the other feeding method, however.

**16. When can sexual activity resume?** Obstetricians usually advise a six-week waiting period following childbirth before resuming coitus. Couples need not wait this long to enjoy other forms of sexual activity.

# References and Suggested Readings

## SMART REFERENCES FROM SCIENTIFIC AMERICAN

**Beardsley, T. Medical Diagnostics: Fetal Checkup.** *Scientific American,* 276(1) (January 1997), 38. **R1101**

## SUGGESTED READINGS

**Eisenberg, A., Murkoff, H., and Hathaway, S. E.** *What to Expect the First Year.* New York: Workman Publishing, 1989. A comprehensive guide to infant development during the first year of life.

**Greenburg, M.** *The Birth of a Father.* New York: Continuum, 1985. A first-hand account of the experience of fatherhood.

**Leach, P.** *Your Baby & Child: From Birth to Age Five.* (Rev. ed.). New York: Knopf, 1989. A comprehensive, clearly presented, and well-illustrated guide to child care.

**Nillsson, L., and Hamberger, L.** *A Child Is Born.* New York: Delacorte, 1990. Breathtaking pictures of fetal development with accompanying text.

**Samuels, M., and Samuels, N.** *The Well Pregnancy Book.* New York: Harper & Row, 1986. A comprehensive and sensitive guide to pregnancy and childbirth.

**Lamaze, F.** *Painless Childbirth.* New York: Simon & Schuster, 1970. This is the Fernand Lamaze classic that helped begin the Lamaze method of childbirth.

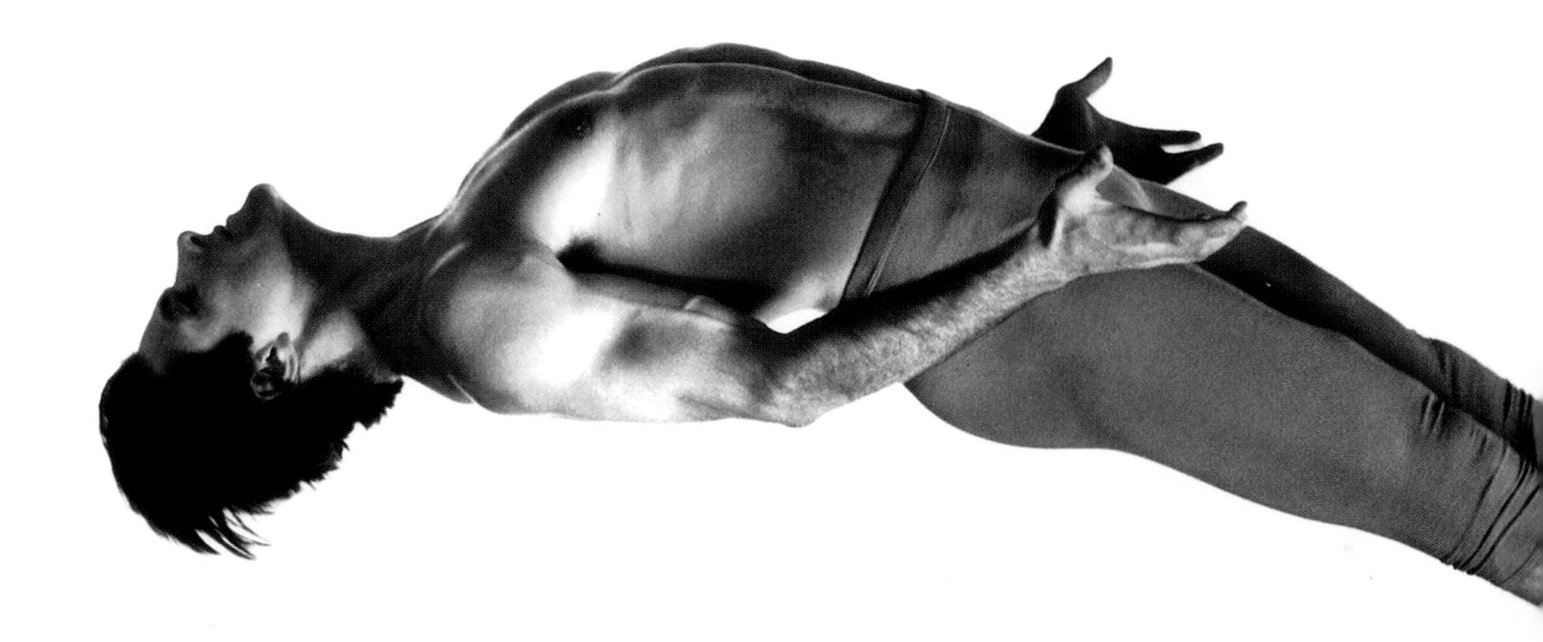

## DID YOU KNOW THAT

- Today's prescription drug may be tomorrow's over-the-counter drug? p.313
- Some of the most addictive and harmful drugs are perfectly legal? p.315
- The active ingredient in over-the-counter sleep aids like Nytol and Sominex is also used to dry up runny noses? p.316
- The brain has "docking stations" designed to receive narcotic drugs like morphine and heroin? p.328
- Heroin was originally touted as a nonaddictive substitute for morphine for use in deadening pain? p.328
- You may very well be hooked on a drug you have with breakfast every morning? p.330
- Coca-Cola once contained cocaine? p.331
- Some people who used LSD have flashbacks of their drug experiences years later? p.334
- One common way of treating heroin addiction is to substitute another addictive drug in its place? p.338

# Drug Use and Abuse

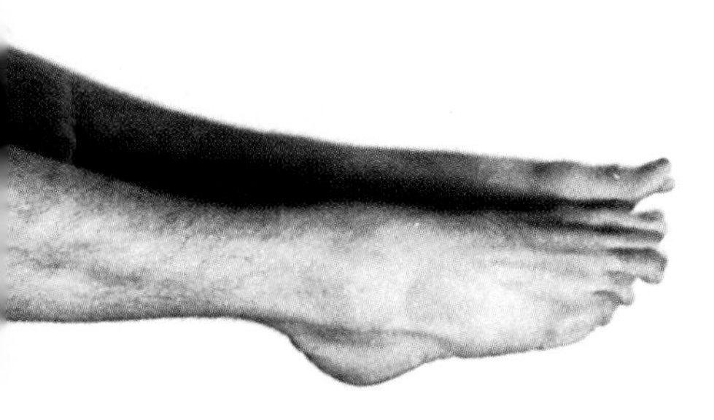

*Ask people to list the major problems facing our society, and drugs are surely one of the most often mentioned. About three of four people in the United States rank illegal drug use among the most serious problems facing the country today.*[1] *Only 2% consider it unimportant. For more than a generation, the government has been fighting a war on drugs. Images of that war—drug busts, seizures of cocaine and heroin, gun battles between drug dealers and the police, innocent people cut down in the crossfire in turf wars among drug dealers—are paraded before us on our television screens.*

12

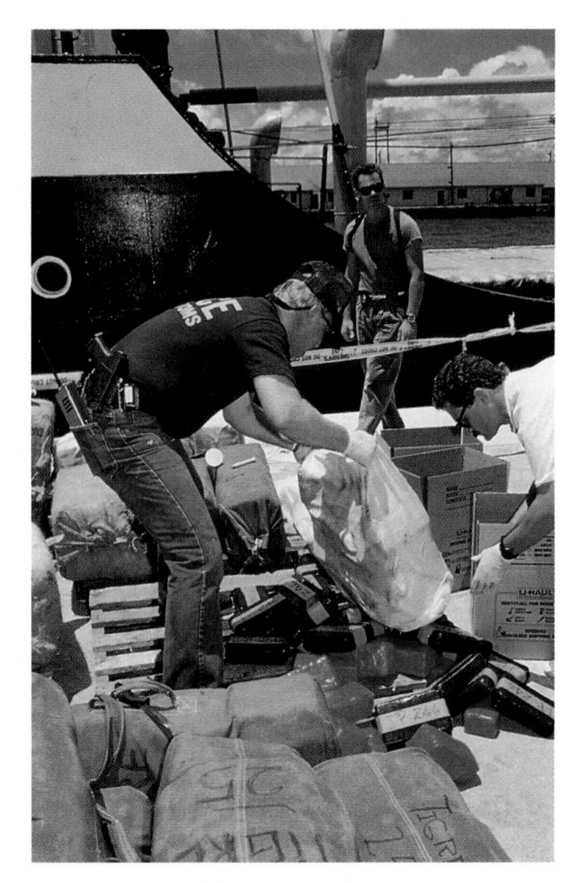

***America's War on Drugs*** About three of four Americans cite illegal drugs as one of the most serious problems facing the country today.

So what *are* drugs? **Drugs** are chemical substances that can affect your health, your feelings, and your behavior. Although the word *drugs* may suggest people shooting up a harmful substance in an alleyway, drugs can be healthful or harmful. Using the right drug at the right time can relieve a health problem or save a life. Using the wrong drug at the wrong time can create a health problem or take a life.

**Drug misuse** is the use of a drug for the wrong reason, in the wrong way, or by the wrong person. Using sleeping pills or tranquilizers prescribed for a friend is an example of drug misuse. The drugs might be harmful for you. Popping an antibiotic for a cough without consulting the doctor is also misuse. Antibiotics combat bacteria, but the drug would be useless against a cough caused by a virus. A prescription cough syrup containing the opiate drug codeine would be misused if you used it to get high rather than to relieve a cough or if you took higher than recommended doses.

**Drug** A chemical agent that affects biological function.

**Drug misuse** Use of a drug for the wrong reason.

**Drug abuse** Repeated use of a drug even when it is causing or aggravating personal, occupational, or health problems.

**Pharmacology** The study of drugs and their role in medicine.

**Pharmacy** The discipline relating to the preparation and dispensing of drugs.

**Over-the-counter (OTC) drugs** Drugs available for sale without a prescription.

The American Psychiatric Association defines **drug abuse** as repeated use of a drug even when it is causing or aggravating a personal, occupational, or health problem.[2] If you are missing school or work because you are drunk or "sleeping it off," you are abusing alcohol. It is not the amount of alcohol that matters, according to this definition. It is whether using alcohol interferes with your life. From a legal point of view, *any* use of illegal or illicit drugs such as marijuana, cocaine, or heroin is labeled drug abuse. Use of alcohol or nicotine by a minor is also drug abuse according to the legal standard.

The scientific study of drugs and their role in health is called **pharmacology. Pharmacy,** on the other hand, has to do with preparing and dispensing drugs. Pharma*cologists* work in laboratories and develop drugs. Pharma*cists* work in pharmacies (drugstores) and dispense them. Pharmacists may not have the research skills of pharmacologists, but they know about the effects and interactions of hundreds of drugs and can offer useful information on whether a drug is right for you.

# TYPES OF DRUGS

Some drugs, such as antibiotics and analgesics, are medicines used for treating or preventing disease or relieving physical discomfort. Other drugs are used or abused for their psychological effects, for relaxation, stimulation, pleasure, or to alter perceptions. First, let's distinguish between over-the-counter (OTC) drugs and prescription drugs. Then let's examine differences between psychoactive and nonpsychoactive drugs.

## Over-the-Counter versus Prescription Drugs

**Over-the-counter (OTC) drugs** are available without prescription. This means that you can decide whether to use these drugs on your own. If you have the idea that OTC drugs are harmless, however, you are quite wrong. For example, many vitamin pills can be bought OTC, but excessive use of

TABLE 12.1

**Over-the-Counter Pain Relievers**

| | Acetaminophen | Aspirin | Ibuprofen | Naproxen Sodium |
|---|---|---|---|---|
| *Brand Names* | Panadol, Tylenol | Anacin, Bayer, Bufferin, Ecotrin | Advil, Motrin, Nuprin | Aleve |
| *Useful for* | Aches and pains, fever | Aches and pains, inflammation, fever, arthritic pain | Aches and pains, inflammation, fever, arthritic pain, sports injuries | Aches and pains, menstrual cramps, arthritic pain |
| *Reduces Pain and Fever?* | Yes | Yes | Yes | Yes |
| *Reduces Inflammation?* | No | Yes | Yes | Yes |
| *Possible Side Effects* | Unlikely if used briefly as directed; overdoses are harmful to liver | Bleeding in digestive tract, stomach upset, ulceration | Bleeding in digestive tract, stomach upset, ulceration | Bleeding in digestive tract, stomach upset, ulceration |
| *Comments* | Especially useful when other analgesics are not tolerated | Ask pharmacist about coated versions that are less likely to upset the stomach | Should not be taken by people who are allergic to aspirin, or who have asthma or heart or kidney problems | Should not be taken by people who are allergic to aspirin, or who have asthma or heart or kidney problems |

vitamins can cause health problems such as jaundice and kidney stones. Aspirin can be bought OTC, and it is surely one of the wonder drugs of the day. Not only can aspirin relieve many aches and pains; it is also widely used to help reduce the risk of heart attacks.[3] Though aspirin can help relieve tension headaches, it has no effect on migraine headaches. Moreover, aspirin can upset the stomach and cause bleeding and ulcers in the digestive tract in high-risk individuals. Aspirin can also cause **Reye's syndrome** in children with chicken pox. (Reye's syndrome can be deadly; it involves kidney damage, brain swelling, and convulsions.) Is aspirin an over-the-counter drug? Yes. Is aspirin harmless? Not necessarily.

In some cases, yesterday's prescription drug has become today's OTC drug. Examples include the **analgesics** ibuprofen (Advil, Motrin, etc.) and naproxen sodium (Aleve) (see Table 12.1), and medicines that are taken for allergies and asthma (such as Benadryl and Bronkaid Mist), skin irritation (Cortaid), heartburn and ulcers (Pepcid, Axid, Zantac, etc.), lice (Nix, etc.), and yeast infections (Monistat 7, Gyne-Lotrimin). Many sleeping pills and diet pills are also sold over the counter.

When in doubt about an over-the-counter drug, ask your doctor or ask the pharmacist. Also keep in mind that OTC drugs are *misused* when they are used for the wrong condition. You should therefore be sure of your diagnosis before using an OTC medication. OTC medications are best used when recommended by a physician for treatment of recurrent or chronic conditions.

Prescription drugs are only available if prescribed by a physician, because their use needs to be monitored to be safe and effective. In later chapters we examine the use of the different kinds of prescription drugs in treating microbial infections and combating chronic diseases such as heart disease and cancer. Confused about the codes doctors use when writing prescriptions? Figure 12.1 helps you decipher their meaning.

Some antimicrobial drugs are available OTC. However, you should not attempt to diagnose or medicate yourself. For one thing, you might *mis*diagnose yourself and fail to identify a serious illness that requires medical attention. For another, you might medicate yourself with a drug that is ineffective against the particular disease-causing organism. Worse, using the wrong medication (or failing to complete treatment) can actually make disease-causing organisms hardier, leading to drug-resistant forms of disease. When it comes to an infection for anything but the common cold, it is essential that it be evaluated by a health professional to determine the appropriate diagnosis and treatment.

**Reye's syndrome** A potentially fatal brain disease that can follow a viral infection, most commonly in children.

**Analgesics** Drugs that relieve pain.

These are some of the abbreviations that doctors use when writing prescriptions.

| ABBREVIATION | MEANING |
|---|---|
| AA | OF EACH |
| AC | BEFORE MEALS |
| AM | MORNING |
| BID | TWICE A DAY |
| C | WITH |
| CAP | CAPSULE |
| CC | CUBIC CENTIMETER |
| D | DAYS |
| DISP | DISPENSE |
| GT | DROP |
| GTT | DROPS |
| H | HOUR |
| HS | AT BEDTIME |
| ML | MILLILITER |
| OD | RIGHT EYE |
| OS | LEFT EYE |
| PC | AFTER MEALS |
| PM | EVENING |
| PO | BY MOUTH |
| PRN | AS NEEDED |
| Q | EVERY |
| QD | ONCE A DAY. EVERY DAY |
| QID | FOUR TIMES A DAY |
| S̄ | WITHOUT |
| SIG | LABEL AS FOLLOWS |
| STAT | AT ONCE. FIRST DOSE |
| TAB | TABLET |
| TID | THREE TIMES A DAY |
| X | TIMES |

**Figure 12.1** ***How to Read a Prescription*** This prescription is for 30 pills of ampicillin in a strength of 250 mg (ampicillin 250 mg DISP = 30). One pill is to be taken by mouth three times a day for 10 days (1PO TID X 10D). Ampicillin is an antibiotic prescribed for such ailments as earaches, sinus infections, and other bacterial infections. *Source:* Reprinted from *Live Longer Live Better,* copyright © 1995 The Reader's Digest Association, Inc.

## PREVENTION

### *Using Medications Wisely*[4]

Prescription and OTC medications can cause serious problems if they are used inappropriately. You and your family should learn about the drugs you take and their possible side effects. Be very careful to take them exactly the way your doctor advises. To be safe, don't mix them together or with alcohol without first talking to your doctor. The following tips can help you avoid risks and get the best results from your medicines:

**Close-up**
Giving medicine to children
**T1201**

DO review your drug record with the doctor at every visit and whenever your doctor prescribes new medicine. Your doctor often gets new information about drugs that might be important to you.

DO always ask your doctor about the right way to take any medicine before you start to use it.

DO always tell your doctor about past problems you have had with drugs, such as rashes, indigestion, dizziness, or not feeling hungry.

DO make sure you can read and understand the drug name and the directions on the container.

DO take medicine in the exact amount and on the same schedule prescribed by your doctor.

DO call your doctor right away if you have any problems with your medicines.

DO keep a daily record of all the drugs you take. Include prescription and OTC drugs.

DO check the expiration dates on your medicine bottles. Throw the medicine away if it has passed this date.

There are also some things you should not do:

DO NOT stop taking a prescription drug unless your doctor says it's OK—even if you are feeling better. If you are worried that the drug might be doing more harm than good, talk with your doctor. He or she may be able to change your medicine to another one that will work just as well.

DO NOT take more or less than the prescribed amount of any drug.

DO NOT mix alcohol and medicine unless your doctor says it's OK. Some drugs may not work well or may make you sick if taken with alcohol.

DO NOT take drugs prescribed for another person or give yours to someone else.

Before leaving your doctor's office with a prescription, ask these questions:

What is the name of the drug and what will it do?

How often should I take it? How long should I take it?

When should I take it? As needed? Before, with, after, or between meals? At bedtime?

If I forget to take it, what should I do?

What side effects might I expect? Should I report them?

Is there any material about this drug that I can take with me?

If I don't take this drug, is there anything else that would work as well?

Smart Quiz Q1201

## think about it!

- **Which over-the-counter drugs do you and your family use? Do you read the labels and follow instructions?**
- **Are you certain that the over-the-counter drugs used by you and your family are the right ones? Why or why not?**
- **Do you always take prescription drugs as directed? (Give some examples.) Why or why not?**

### Psychoactive versus Nonpsychoactive Drugs

Drugs that act on the brain to affect one's mental state are called **psychoactive drugs.** They affect mood, thought processes, perceptions, and behavior. They may also affect one's judgment and ability to operate an automobile or perform other complex motor skills. Some psychoactive drugs have legitimate medical uses in the treatment of psychological disorders. Others are used or abused by people seeking to alter their mental states—to get "high" or to feel relaxed or more alert. Some of these drugs induce a rush of euphoric pleasure that washes away awareness of the struggles and stresses of daily living.

Most drugs are not psychoactive. Antibiotics, for example, may eradicate bacteria but do not directly alter our psychological states. Pain relievers may affect how we feel by relieving pain, but they do not alter our psychological states.

The remainder of the chapter focuses on the uses and misuses of psychoactive drugs. We discuss types of psychoactive drugs, their effects on health, and how you can avoid problems associated with drug misuse and abuse.

## PSYCHOACTIVE DRUGS

There are three major classes of psychoactive drugs: *depressants, stimulants,* and *hallucinogens.* Depressants, including alcohol, barbiturates, tranquilizers, and opiates such as heroin, lower the level of activity of the central nervous system to bring about feelings of calmness and drowsiness. Stimulants, such as nicotine, caffeine, cocaine, and amphetamines, increase the activity of the central nervous system. They increase arousal and alertness. Hallucinogens, such as LSD, psilocybin, mescaline, and marijuana, lead to sensory distortions and hallucinations. Psychoactive drugs vary in their intensity and specific effects. Caffeine and nicotine, for example, are mild stimulants. They do not produce the intense effects or euphoric highs of stronger stimulants like cocaine and methamphetamine ("ice"). Nor does alcohol, a depressant, produce the euphoric rush of another depressant, heroin.

Some drugs are addictive. Some are illegal. You might think that only addictive drugs are illegal, yet some of the most strongly addictive drugs—including nicotine and alcohol—are legal, although the sale of tobacco products (which contain nicotine) and alcohol to minors is prohibited. Nicotine, alcohol, and caffeine (yes, caffeine) are so widely used that many people don't realize that they are psychoactive drugs. Caffeine, the psychoactive ingredient in coffee and tea, is a mild stimulant. Nicotine, also a mild stimulant, is found in tobacco products such as cigarettes, pipe tobacco, and cigars. Alcoholic beverages contain the depressant drug *ethyl alcohol.*

Close-up
Straight facts about drugs and alcohol
T1202

Illegal (or *illicit*) drugs include opiates such as morphine, opium, and heroin; stimulants such as methamphetamine and cocaine; and hallucinogens such as LSD, mescaline, marijuana, and hashish. In some cases, illegal drugs have legitimate medical uses, but such use must be authorized by a physician.

Are legal drugs less harmful to one's health than illicit drugs? Not necessarily. Despite the attention focused on illicit drugs, two legally available drugs, alcohol and tobacco, account for more deaths, disease, and health costs than all other drugs combined. Because of their effects on health, we devote the following two chapters to them.

**Psychoactive drugs** Drugs that act on the brain to affect mental processes.

### Medical Uses of Psychoactive Drugs

Most people who use opiates are not drug addicts. Nor are they breaking the law. Opiates have legitimate medical uses as pain relievers, and most people who use them do so under a doctor's care. They are used most widely to deaden postsurgical pain or to treat severe pain arising from some medical conditions. The opiate codeine is often used as a cough suppressant. Because of opiates' high potential for abuse and addiction, their medical use is strictly regulated. (Opiates are *controlled substances;* that is, they are subject to strict regulation.) Yet many people use opiates illegally to "get high." They obtain them on the street from drug dealers.

Some psychoactive drugs, called psychotherapeutic drugs or *psychotropics,* are used to treat psychological disorders. They include antidepressants (like Elavil and Prozac), antianxiety agents (like Valium and Xanax), stimulants (like Ritalin), and antipsychotic drugs (like Thorazine and Haldol).

Other drugs with psychoactive properties are available over the counter. Sleep aids such as Nytol and Sominex contain **antihistamines** (e.g., pyrilamine maleate), which have sedating effects on the central nervous system. Antihistamines are also used in allergy and cold medications such as Contac and Nyquil, which is why many cold medications carry warnings that they may cause drowsiness. Antihistamines may also have adverse reactions when combined with alcohol. While OTC sleep medications may provide temporary relief from insomnia, they have drawbacks. Their effectiveness tends to diminish over time, and they may interfere with natural sleep cycles and make it difficult to achieve a truly deep, restful sleep. People may also become unable to sleep without them.

Other OTC drugs with psychoactive properties include decongestants and diet aids. Decongestants—Sudafed, for example—help relieve the nasal congestion that often accompanies colds or allergies. The active ingredient in these drugs, **pseudoephedrine,** has a mild stimulant effect. It should not be used by people with certain medical conditions, such as high blood pressure and heart disease, unless they are directed to do so by a physician.

Talking Glossary

**Antihistamine** A drug that blocks the actions of histamine, a substance released in the body during an allergic reaction.

**Pseudoephedrine** A sympathomimetic drug used as a nasal decongestant.

**Sympathomimetic** An agent that activates the sympathetic nervous system.

Diet aids such as Dexatrim suppress the appetite. The active ingredient in these drugs is phenylpropanolamine hydrochloride, a **sympathomimetic** or chemical agent that excites the sympathetic nervous system, causing such effects as dry mouth and a loss of appetite. Although they may help curb appetite, they have only modest and temporary benefits in helping people lose weight (see Chapter 6).

Talking Glossary
Sympathomimetic
G1202

**think about it!**

- **What are some medical uses of psychoactive drugs?**
- **What are the drawbacks to using sleeping pills?**

Smart Quiz
Q1202

## EFFECTS OF DRUGS

The effects of drugs vary with a number of factors, including the type of drug, how it is used, the person's biological responsiveness to the drug, the person's frame of mind, the presence of other drugs, and the social setting.

### Routes of Administration

Drugs can enter the body in different ways. Alcohol, barbiturates, and amphetamines are taken orally in liquid or pill form and pass into the bloodstream through the digestive system. Other drugs enter the body through the lungs, either by smoking or, as in the case of powder cocaine, inhaling or snorting. Inhalants are chemical fumes that are inhaled for their psychoactive effects, usually by drawing the fumes into the nose or mouth. They can have dangerous, even deadly, effects.

Smoking is the usual route of administration for cigarette and pipe tobacco and for such illegal drugs as marijuana, hashish, and crack cocaine. Chewing tobacco is typically placed between the cheek and gum, where it is chewed or sucked and the juices absorbed through the mucosal lining of the mouth. Snuff, a powder form of smokeless tobacco, may be inhaled through the nostrils or placed inside the cheek and sucked.

Some drugs are injected into the body. Drugs may be injected *intravenously* (into a vein), *intramuscularly* (into a muscle), or *intracutaneously* (into the subcutaneous layer of the skin). The term

**injecting drug user (IDU)** refers to a person who injects drugs in any of these ways. The term **intravenous drug user** (**IVDU** or IV drug user) is reserved for a person who injects a drug into a vein. Some drugs may be administered in two or more ways.

A drug's route of administration can influence its effects. Injection of a drug typically produces stronger reactions than swallowing. Heroin, for instance, is usually injected, which intensifies its effects, but it can also be snorted or smoked. Drugs that are injected into a vein enter the bloodstream directly and may travel to the brain relatively intact. Drugs that enter the body by way of the stomach may be partially broken down by digestion before they reach the bloodstream. Drugs that are injected, smoked, or snorted also have more immediate effects than those that are swallowed. The former drugs may reach the brain in a matter of seconds, whereas drugs that are swallowed may take 30 minutes or longer to move through the digestive system before they enter the bloodstream and reach the brain.

The site of injection also matters. Intravenous injection delivers more immediate effects than intramuscular or intracutaneous injections because the drug is deposited directly into the bloodstream. Drugs injected into muscle or skin tissue can take several minutes to seep into the blood. Although intravenous injection delivers the drug immediately to the bloodstream, it is not necessarily the fastest way of delivering a drug to the brain. The nicotine in tobacco smoke reaches the brain 7 to 10 seconds after a puff of a cigarette. This is a few seconds sooner than it takes heroin to reach the brain when it is injected into a vein.[5]

People who inject opiates like morphine or heroin intravenously typically experience an initial "rush" of pleasure followed by a second, longer phase of a tranquil, dreamlike state in which they feel emotionally disconnected from reality.[6] Injecting the drug under the skin, however, does not produce the early high concentration of the drug in the brain that causes the initial euphoric rush. The predominant effect is the tranquility associated with the second phase.

## Dosage Level

The effects of a drug depend in part on the dosage level, or amount of the drug consumed. The relationship between the dosage level of a drug and its effects is called the **dose-response relationship.** The dose-response relationship is not necessarily linear (a straight line). That is, the effects may not increase as much with each increase in dose. The difference in effect of your second and third alcoholic drinks, for instance, will be greater than that between your eighth and ninth drinks. For some drugs, such as LSD, the effects of the drug reach a plateau level with increasing dosage, so that even higher doses above a certain level do not further intensify the effect.

Dosage level is also an important determinant of the risk of overdose ("OD"). Some drugs have a greater overdose potential than others. Generally, the greater the dosage, the greater the overdose risk. The amount of a drug needed to induce an overdose, even a fatal overdose, also varies among individuals. Some people can OD on relatively low dosages of a drug. Others can tolerate much larger amounts. People with certain heart conditions can suffer cardiac irregularities that result in death from the ingestion of a small amount of cocaine, for example.

## Biological Responsivity

People vary in their responsiveness to particular drugs. The same amount of a given drug affects different people in different ways. The effects of a given dose may depend on the person's weight and sex, even a genetic predisposition or sensitivity to the effects of certain drugs. A heavier person may be less responsive to the effects of a given dosage of a drug, especially alcohol, than a person who weighs less. Women tend to become intoxicated at lower doses of certain drugs, such as alcohol, than men do. Regular use of a drug may also alter the person's responsiveness to it. With continued use of a drug, a state of physical habituation, or **tolerance,** may develop, such that higher dosages are needed to achieve the same effect.

## Frame of Mind

A person's reaction to a drug reflects not only the biological effects of the drug but also the user's frame of mind. A cheerful person may experience greater euphoria from amphetamines or heroin than a gloomy person. A person's expectations about the effects of a

**Injecting drug user (IDU)** A person who injects psychoactive drugs.

**Intravenous drug user (IVDU)** An injecting drug user (IDU) who injects drugs intravenously (into a vein).

**Dose-response relationship** The relationship between the dosage level of a drug and its effects on the user.

**Tolerance** A feature of drug dependence in which the user comes to need larger amounts of the drug to achieve the same effect.

drug also come into play. If you expect that a drug will make you feel high, you may feel high even if the drug turns out to be nothing more than a sugar pill. If you believe that alcohol is a sexual stimulant, you may feel sexually aroused when you are drinking, even though alcohol, like other depressants, actually dampens sexual responsiveness.

### Drug Interactions

Drugs can interact in ways that increase their **toxicity.** Therefore, mixing drugs can be a dangerous, even deadly, practice. Mixing alcohol and barbiturates, for example, can lead to a fatal overdose, as was reported to be the case in the deaths of entertainers Marilyn Monroe and Judy Garland. Mixing alcohol and cocaine was reported to be involved in the death of the actor River Phoenix.

Combining drugs can also intensify their effects. In some cases the psychoactive effects of combining drugs are *cumulative* or *additive,* meaning that the overall effect is equal to the sum of the effects of each drug. Other drug combinations (as with alcohol and barbiturates) have a **synergistic effect.** That is, the combined effects of the drugs can be many times greater than the additive effects of the individual drugs themselves. Combining alcohol and barbiturates creates effects four times as powerful as those caused by either drug used alone. A given drug may also **potentiate** the effects of another drug. That is, the second drug intensifies the effects of the first drug. Alcohol, for instance, can potentiate the effects of marijuana.

**Close-up**
Food and drug interactions
T1203

Some drugs can block the effects of other drugs. These drugs, called **antagonists,** have no effects of their own but are useful in the treatment of drug addictions since they can block the rewarding effects of addictive drugs. The drug naloxone, for instance, is an antagonist for opiates like heroin and morphine. So long as the opiate addict takes naloxone, the pleasurable effects of heroin or morphine are blocked.

**Toxicity** The quality or degree of being poisonous.

**Synergistic effect** As applied to drug interactions, the action of two or more drugs operating together to enhance the overall effect to a level greater than the sum of the effects of each drug operating by itself.

**Potentiate** Relating to drugs, to enhance a drug's effects or potency.

**Antagonists** Drugs that block or neutralize the actions of other drugs.

**Polyabusers** People with drug abuse problems involving two or more drugs.

**Physiological dependence** A state of bodily need for a drug, evidenced by the appearance of characteristic withdrawal symptoms upon abrupt cessation of use of the drug.

### Social Factors

The social setting in which drugs are used can affect people's response to them. Drinking a given amount of alcohol might make you mellow and drowsy if you are alone at home, but giddy and bubbly at a party or with friends. Marijuana use may induce paranoia if it is smoked in an abandoned building in a crime-ravaged inner-city neighborhood, but not when it is taken in a setting in which the user feels more secure.

**think about it!**

- **What drugs have you taken, orally, nasally, or by injection? What were the purposes and effects of the drugs?**
- **Have you ever taken too much of a drug? If so, what were the effects?**

**Smart Quiz**
Q1203

## DRUG ABUSE AND DEPENDENCE

Not everyone who uses drugs, even addictive drugs, becomes a drug abuser or addict. Some people experiment with a drug but do not become regular users. Only between 10 and 15% of people who try snorting cocaine become cocaine abusers.[7] Many of us end the day with a nightcap or a glass of wine but we do not become alcoholics.

What is the line between drug use and abuse? What are the warning signs of drug abuse? How would you know if you or someone else was hooked?

*Drug abuse* involves the repeated use of a drug even when its use is harmful to a person's health, impairs a person's ability to meet academic, occupational, or family responsibilities, or exposes the person or others to danger (as in driving while intoxicated). People who abuse more than one drug at a time are called **polyabusers.**

### Physiological Dependence

**Physiological dependence** (also called *chemical dependence*) is a condition in which a person's body chemistry has changed as the result of using a drug so that the body comes to depend on a steady supply of the drug. **Drug addiction** involves the development of physiological dependence accompanied by a pattern of compulsive or habitual use of the drug in which the person demonstrates impaired control over its use. Addicts may continue to use drugs even when they know that their drug use is ruining their lives.

In chemically dependent persons, stopping drug use abruptly (going "cold turkey") or cutting back sharply leads to an **abstinence syndrome** (also called a *withdrawal syndrome*), or cluster of unpleasant and possibly dangerous withdrawal symptoms. Resumption of drug use to relieve withdrawal symptoms is a major reason why a drug dependence is so difficult to break. Another feature of drug dependence is tolerance. Tolerance develops when a user's biological responsivity to a drug changes such that more is needed to achieve the same effect.

Psychoactive drugs that are clearly addictive include opiates, such as heroin and morphine; the stimulants nicotine and cocaine; and depressants, such as barbiturates, tranquilizers, and alcohol. The addictive properties of drugs such as marijuana and the hallucinogens (LSD, mescaline, psilocybin) remain questionable, since no clear abstinence pattern has been established for them.

## Psychological Dependence

**Psychological dependence** involves a pattern of compulsive or habitual use of a drug in the absence of physiological signs of dependence. People who are psychologically dependent on a drug come to depend on it to meet their psychological needs. They may repeatedly turn to the drug to counter unpleasant feelings or to cope with stress. The psychologically dependent person may feel compelled to use the drug despite knowledge of the harm it is causing. Psychological dependence may or may not be accompanied by physiological dependence. Some drugs, such as nicotine, alcohol, and heroin, can lead to both psychological and physiological dependence. Others, such as PCP and cannabis (marijuana), can produce psychological dependence but are not known to lead to physiological dependence or addiction.

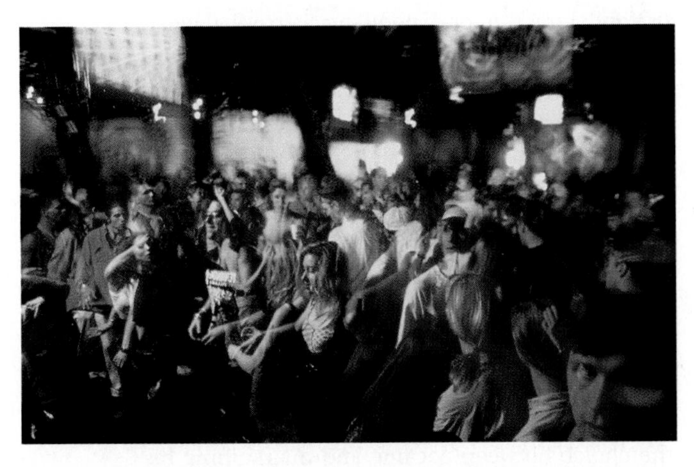

***Peer Pressure*** Many young people start using drugs because of social pressure from friends who use drugs or because it is perceived as cool within their peer group.

## Factors in Drug Abuse and Dependence

There are as many different reasons why people use drugs as there are drugs to use. Some people use drugs to help them relax, others to perk themselves up. Some use drugs to alter their experience of reality. Depressants or "downers" are used to induce sleep or calm nerves. Stimulants or "uppers" help maintain alertness, fend off sleep, or "jump-start" the morning. Others use drugs as a form of escape from troubling emotional states, such as anxiety and depression. Still others use drugs to counter boredom or loneliness or to blunt awareness of life's hardships. Some drugs, like cocaine and heroin, produce feelings of intense pleasure that are experienced as a euphoric rush or "high." Yet most people encounter feelings of boredom, anxiety, and emotional pain from time to time without becoming drug abusers or addicts. Why, then, do some people abuse drugs while others cope with life's ups and downs without turning to drugs? To understand the problems of drug abuse and dependence, we need to take into account environmental, psychological, and genetic factors.

**Environmental Factors** Peer pressure and exposure to family members and friends who abuse drugs can encourage young people to experiment with drugs. Continued use may be reinforced by the pleasurable effects of the drugs, their "rush" or "high," as well as by peer support from friends who also use drugs. Some young

**Drug addiction** A state of physiological dependence on a drug that is accompanied by a lack of control over its use.

**Abstinence syndrome** A cluster of withdrawal symptoms that is characteristic of abrupt cessation of use of a particular drug.

**Psychological dependence** A pattern of compulsive or habitual use of a drug indicating impaired control over the use of the drug but without physiological signs of dependence.

people who feel alienated from the mainstream culture come to identify with subcultures in which drug use is sanctioned or encouraged, such as the gang subculture.

Unemployment often figures into drug abuse. Unemployed young adults (18 to 34 years of age) are more than twice as likely as their peers who are working to abuse drugs.[8] The relationship seems to work both ways: Drug abuse may contribute to unemployment, and unemployment may contribute, in turn, to drug abuse.

**Psychological Factors** People use and abuse drugs for psychological reasons as well, including feelings of hopelessness, relief from troubling emotions, and needs for **sensation-seeking.** Young people whose hopes for a successful future are dashed at an early age may turn to drugs out of hopelessness and despair. If the future doesn't hold much promise, why not live for the pleasure of the moment that drugs can provide? People who feel unable to cope with negative emotions like anxiety, tension, and depression, and who see nowhere else to turn for help, may seek relief through alcohol and other drugs. People with high needs for sensation may come to rely on drugs to provide the stimulation they seek.[9] They get easily bored with the ordinary activities that fill most people's days. Though some sensation-seekers engage in stimulating activities, like riding motorcycles, in-line skating, bungee-jumping, or downhill skiing, some seek the rush of sensations caused by mind-altering drugs.

**Genetic Factors** Genetic factors may put people at greater risk of developing problems with alcohol and drugs. For one thing, evidence points to genetic factors making it more likely for some people to find the effects of drugs more rewarding or stimulating.[10] For another, people may also inherit greater tolerance of the negative effects (such as nausea) of alcohol, which can make it more difficult for them to learn when to say when.

## Pathways to Drug Dependence

People do not become drug addicts overnight. A progression of steps leads from occasional use to addiction. For some, the slide into addiction is rapid; for others, gradual. While the particular steps to addiction may vary among addicts and from one drug to another, there are some common pathways.[11]

**Sensation-seeking** The tendency to seek exciting or highly stimulating activities that heighten one's physical sensations.

**Stage 1. Experimentation** The first stage, experimentation, involves occasional use of a drug—perhaps on weekends, perhaps monthly. The drug produces pleasant, even euphoric, feelings. The user feels in control and capable of stopping at any time. Experimentation typically lasts a short time, weeks or months, before giving way to routine use.

**Stage 2. Routine Use** The user begins taking the drug more often, eventually daily. More time is spent obtaining and using drugs. Schedules get shifted around as the need to buy drugs becomes a priority. Users try to deny the effects of the drugs on their lives. Values change. Things that once were important—school, work, or a child's recital or baseball game—now pale in comparison with the need to find and use drugs.

Problems mount as routine drug use continues. Family possessions, even heirlooms, are pawned for a fraction of their worth. To cover their tracks, drug users are ingenious: A woman claims to have been robbed of her wedding ring at gunpoint. A man claims that a burglar made off with the large-screen TV. Lying and manipulation become everyday activities. Family relationships become strained to the breaking point. More and more days are lost from work and family finances become depleted. Mortgage and car payments are skipped. The drug abuser may even steal from family members or others to feed the habit.

**Stage 3. Addiction** The line between routine use and addiction or dependency is crossed when the user begins to feel powerless to resist cravings for the drug and when the physical signs of dependence—tolerance and withdrawal symptoms—appear. With heroin, the slide into addiction can be rapid: "One morning you awaken with what seems to be a cold—running nose, a slight feeling of chilliness. You mention it to a friend, who says: 'That's no cold. Try some heroin and see how fast it goes away. You're hooked!'"[12] Pursuit and use of the drug dominates virtually everything else in life, becoming more important than family relationships. For Eugene, a 41-year-old cocaine addict, the choice between cocaine and maintaining his marriage became no choice at all:[13]

*She had just caught me with cocaine again after I had managed to convince her that I hadn't used it in over a month. Of course I had been tooting [snorting] almost every day, but I had managed to cover my tracks a little better than usual. So she said to me that I was going to have to make a choice—either cocaine or her. Before she finished the sentence, I knew what was coming, so I told her to think carefully about what she was going to say. It was clear to me that there wasn't a choice. I love my wife, but I'm not going to choose* anything *over cocaine. It's sick, but that's what things have come to. Nothing and nobody comes before my coke.*

Denial plays a prominent role, even in the addiction stage.[14] A 48-year-old executive sought a psychiatric consultation at the urging of his wife. His once-successful business had been nearly ruined by his erratic and irresponsible behavior. His savings were being quickly exhausted, as he was spending $7,000 a month on his addiction. C is the clinician, E is the executive.

C: Have you missed many days at work recently?

E: Yes, but I can afford to, since I own the business. Nobody checks up on me.

C: It sounds like that's precisely the problem. When you don't go to work, the company stays open, but it doesn't do very well.

E: My employees are well trained. They can run the company without me.

C: But that's not happening.

E: Then there's something wrong with them. I'll have to look into it.

C: It sounds as if there's something wrong with you, but you don't want to look into it.

E: Now you're on my case. I don't know why you listen to everything my wife says.

C: How many days of work did you miss in the last two months?

E: A couple.

C: Are you saying that you missed only two days of work?

E: Maybe a few.

C: Only three or four days?

E: Maybe a little more.

C: Ten? Fifteen?

E: Fifteen.

C: All because of cocaine?

E: No.

C: How many were because of cocaine?

E: Less than fifteen.

C: Fourteen? Thirteen?

E: Maybe thirteen.

C: So you missed thirteen days of work in the last two months because of cocaine. That's almost two days a week.

E: That sounds like a lot but it's no big deal. Like I say, the company can run itself.

C: How long have you been using cocaine?

E: About three years.

C: Did you ever use drugs or alcohol before that in any kind of quantity?

E: No.

C: Then let's think back five years. Five years ago, if you had imagined yourself missing over a third of your workdays because of a drug, and if you had imagined yourself spending the equivalent of $84,000 a year on that same drug, and if you saw your once-successful business collapsing all around you, wouldn't you have thought that was indicative of a pretty serious problem?

E: Yes, I would have.

C: So what's different now?

E: I guess I just don't want to think about it.

## Codependence

A **codependent** is a person who, perhaps unintentionally, helps the drug-dependent person remain dependent on drugs. The codependent is an *enabler,* a person who remains silent about the drug abuser's behavior, makes excuses for the behavior, or lightens its impact—for example, by calling in sick for the drug abuser who is on a binge and telling the boss the person is out with the flu, by making excuses to a child for the drug-abusing parent's missing the child's birthday party, and so on. The process of recovery is hampered because abusers in codependent relationships never have to face the full consequences of their actions and the damage caused by their drug-using behavior. Codependents may not be aware of their enabling behavior, or if they are, they may minimize or rationalize it. They may realize that their loved one has a problem with drugs but mistakenly believe that the best way to deal with it is to shower the person with love and support and hope that the person will somehow get the message that he or she should stop using drugs. Codependents often choose drug-dependent people as mates and lovers because it serves their personal needs to have someone dependent on them.

**Codependent** A person involved in a close relationship with a drug-dependent person who plays a part in enabling or maintaining the other person's chemical dependency.

# Health Check

## Are You a Codependent?

Are you involved in a relationship with a drug-dependent person? If so, do you recognize any of the following signs of codependence in yourself?

- Have you looked the other way when a friend or lover showed signs of using drugs?
- Have you willingly accepted someone else's excuses for his or her unkempt appearance, missed appointments, and changes in behavior, without looking further to see if drugs were involved?
- Have you ever failed to confront a loved one whom you knew was high on drugs?
- Have you made excuses for a person's behavior to others (employers, teachers, friends) when you suspected that drugs were involved?
- If someone you know or love is using drugs, do you readily accept the person's promises that he or she will stop, no matter how often such promises have been broken in the past?
- Do you tell yourself and others that the drug-dependent person only needs time to deal with the problem and will eventually "come around"?
- Have you ever recorded phone numbers or passed along messages to the drug abuser from strangers whom you suspect might be drug contacts?
- Have you accompanied a drug-dependent person to buy drugs out of concern for the person's safety?
- Have you ever lent money to the person to buy drugs?

If you recognize any of these behaviors in yourself, think seriously about how your behavior may be helping to maintain the drug-dependent person's drug habits. Codependency does not displace responsibility from the drug-abusing person. The drug abuser is the one responsible for his or her own behavior. However, people in codependent relationships need to understand how their own behavior contributes to the problem and how they can change their behavior to promote rather than hinder recovery.

### Gateway Drugs

A **gateway drug** is a stepping-stone drug, one that a person uses in progressing to harder drugs. Many users of so-called hard drugs like cocaine and heroin, for example, began their illicit drug career with marijuana. Alcohol and tobacco are gateway drugs for harder-drug use among many adolescents.[15] Adolescents who drink heavily are more likely than other adolescents to progress to hard-drug use, except, it seems, for Asian Americans. Hard-drug use among Asian-American adolescents typically *precedes* rather than follows the use of alcohol. Asians are generally more sensitive to alcohol's effects. They are more likely to experience an unpleasant "flushing" response (sweating and reddening of the face) when drinking alcohol, which may discourage excess drinking. Perhaps for Asian-American adolescents, heavy drinking follows a prior commitment to harder-drug use.

**Gateway drug** A drug serving as a stepping-stone or gateway to use of other, usually harder, drugs.

Regular cigarette smoking among adolescents is also linked to hard-drug use.[16] One possible reason for this link is that smoking has come to be viewed, even by adolescents, as risky behavior. People who are prone to take risks with one drug may be more likely to take risks with others.[17]

**think about it!**

- **Are you (or have you been) addicted to any drug? How do you know?**
- **Are you or is someone you care about now addicted to any drug? If so, what will you do about it?**

**critical thinking** **Agree or disagree and support your answer: I have control over any drugs I am using.**

Smart Quiz Q1204

## Health Check

### Warning Signs of Drug Dependence

Have you become dependent on drugs? Are you in danger of becoming dependent?

Answer each of the following questions yes or no. While no exact number of yeses guarantees dependence, the more questions you answer yes, the more likely it is that you are dependent.

If you are becoming dependent on drugs, the time to act is now. Talk to someone who can evaluate your drug problem. If you don't know where to go for help, contact the referral sources listed later in the chapter. If you don't feel that you can make the call yourself, ask someone you trust for help.

**Yes No**

___ ___ 1. Do you use the drug regularly or daily?

___ ___ 2. Does your life seem to revolve around finding and using drugs?

___ ___ 3. Have you put yourself in dangerous situations to get drugs?

___ ___ 4. Have you had to sacrifice valuable possessions to secure drugs?

___ ___ 5. Have you borrowed money from others or stolen things to support your drug habit?

___ ___ 6. Has your physical or mental health been affected by your drug use?

___ ___ 7. Do you worry or become frantic if you begin to run out of the drug?

___ ___ 8. Do you feel a lack of control over your drug use?

___ ___ 9. Do you find yourself increasingly turning to drugs when you're feeling down or stressed out?

___ ___ 10. Have you missed appointments or days at work or school because of drugs?

___ ___ 11. Have your friends told you they are concerned about you?

___ ___ 12. Have you neglected your responsibilities to your loved ones?

___ ___ 13. Do you continue to use drugs despite negative consequences?

___ ___ 14. Have you tried to stop but were unable?

___ ___ 15. Do you feel more like yourself when you are using drugs than when you are not?

___ ___ 16. Has your drug use gotten you into trouble with the law? Your boss? Your teachers?

___ ___ 17. Have you been using drugs alone? To cope with emotional pain?

___ ___ 18. Do you use drugs to get going in the morning or wind down at night?

___ ___ 19. Do you need to take larger and larger amounts of the drug to achieve the same effect?

___ ___ 20. Are you using the drug more often than you used to?

___ ___ 21. Do you experience withdrawal symptoms if you stop taking the drug for a few days?

___ ___ 22. Do you shy away from people who don't use drugs?

___ ___ 23. Are you shying away from people in general?

___ ___ 24. Do you attempt to keep your drug habits a secret from others?

___ ___ 25. Is your drug use affecting your personal relationships?

___ ___ 26. Have you been lying to your loved ones about your drug habit?

___ ___ 27. Do you socialize with others because they can get you drugs, not because you like them?

## WHO USES ILLICIT DRUGS?

More than one in three people in the United States age 12 or older, more than 75 million people in total, report having used an illegal drug at least once in their lives. About 13% report having used an illegal drug during the past year and 6% report using one during the past month.[18] About half of high school students have used an illegal drug by the time they reach their senior year.[19] Despite the widespread use of illegal drugs, use of these drugs is dwarfed by the numbers of people who use alcohol and cigarettes (see Figure 12.2).

### Drug Use among Young People

The federal government regularly surveys drug use among young people. The survey taps high school seniors, college students, and young adults, who are asked whether they have ever used various drugs, and if so, how regularly they use them.

**Figure 12.2**
***Prevalences of Drug Use in the United States***

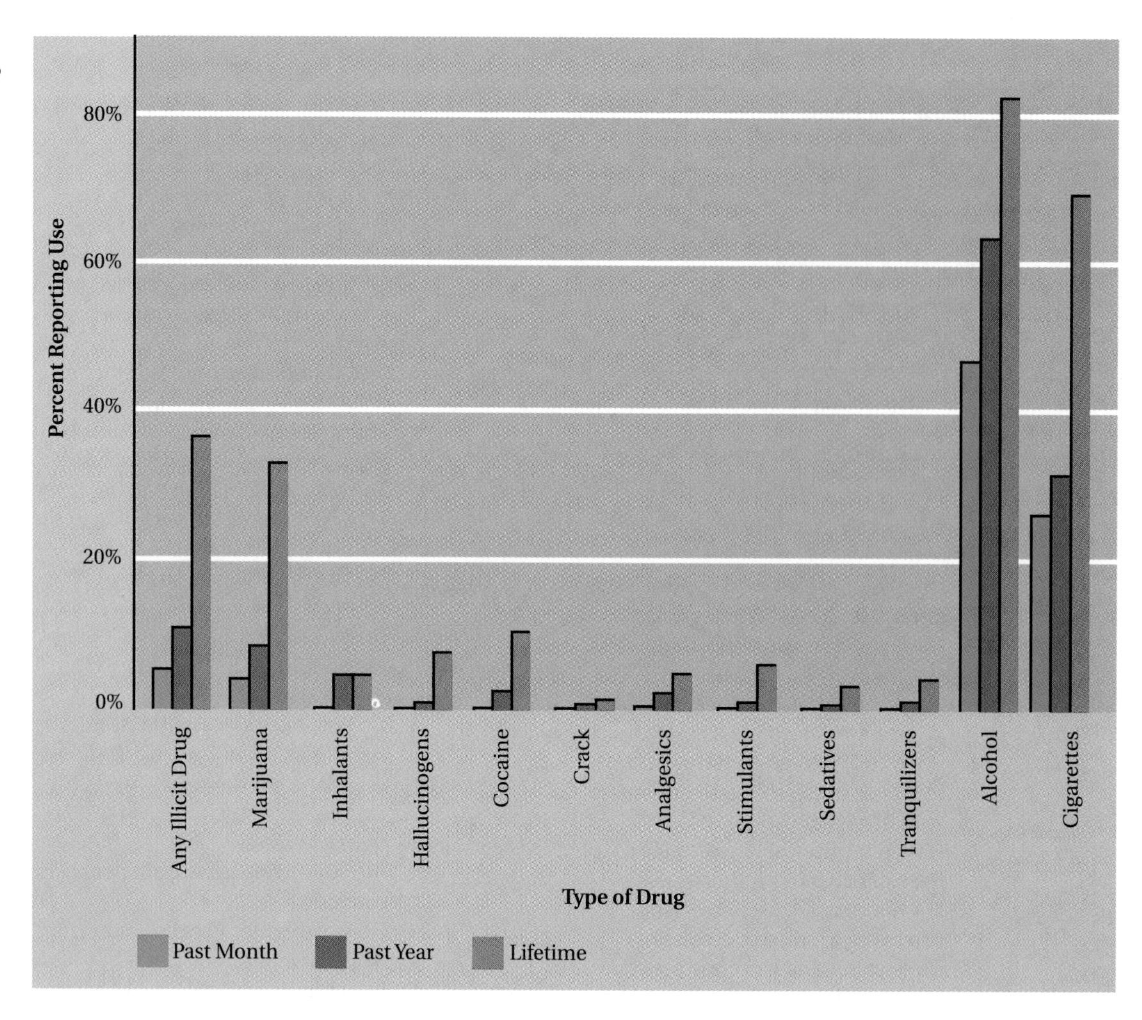


**Close-up**
Student drug use up
**T1204**

Though cocaine use among college students has fallen off in recent years, there has been a rise in use of many illicit drugs among high school students, especially marijuana, inhalants, hallucinogens, cocaine and other stimulants, and heroin.[20] Some wonder whether the school-age population is beginning to look like the generation of the 1960s. By 1995, two in five twelfth-graders and one in five eighth-graders had tried marijuana.[21] Use of illicit drugs among teenagers shot up 80% from 1991 to 1996. From 1995 to 1996 alone, use of illicit drugs was up by a staggering 33%.[22]

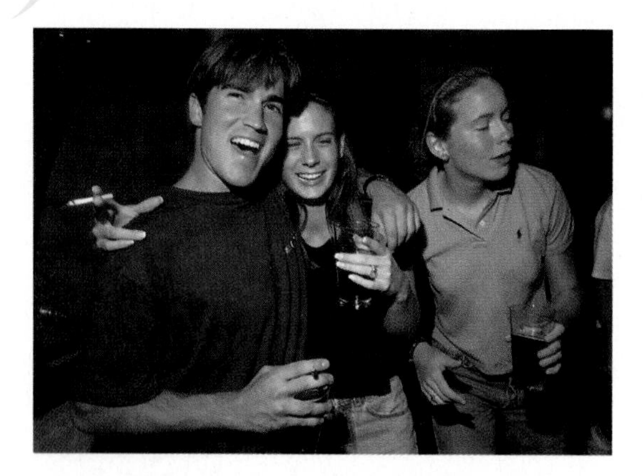

***Drugs on Campus*** Though use of marijuana among college students has increased in the 1990s, the major drugs on campus remain alcohol and tobacco (which contains nicotine, a stimulant).

Table 12.2 highlights findings for drug use among college students from 1980 through 1994. Note the marked decline in the use of cocaine and other stimulants. Current (past month) use of marijuana also declined steadily during the 1980s but began rising again in the 1990s. Heroin, cocaine, and MDMA are currently used by fewer than 1% of college students.

The mainstays of the drug scene on campus, alcohol and cigarettes, remain popular, although use of alcohol declined slowly but steadily through much of the 1980s and early 1990s. Not so for cigarettes, which have continued to be used regularly by one in four to one in five college students.

## Drugs in the Workplace

While illicit drug use is greater among the unemployed, seven of ten people who use illicit drugs are employed.[24] About 8% of workers overall (and about 24% of male workers aged 18 to 25) use drugs, most commonly marijuana and cocaine. Drug use by workers can impair job performance and reduce productivity, increase absenteeism and health care utilization, and contribute to accidents and injuries.

**Close-up** Drugs in the workplace T1205

## Costs of Drug Abuse

The effects of drug abuse are all too obvious. Babies are born addicted to crack cocaine because their mothers used it during pregnancy. Emergency rooms are crowded with people who overdose on drugs or commit crimes of aggression while high on drugs. Potentially useful lives are laid waste by drugs. Families are torn apart. Use of alcohol and other drugs is involved in more than half of fatalities resulting from automobile crashes and in about one in four heavy-truck accidents.[25]

The use of illicit drugs is also a major factor in social problems, including dropping out of school, unemployment, and crime.

Tax dollars are poured into the seemingly endless war on drugs. Health insurance premiums become more costly because of the health care needs of people with alcohol and drug problems. Whether we personally use illicit drugs or not, we all pay the costs of their use.

The costs of the drug epidemic are also reflected in increased rates of transmission of HIV, the virus that causes AIDS. Intravenous drug use is a leading cause of HIV infection. Sexually active teens are less likely to use condoms under the influence of drugs, thereby placing themselves and their partners at greater risk of contracting sexually transmitted diseases, including AIDS.

**Close-up** Drugs and AIDS T1206

Children often suffer the most. Parental drug abuse disrupts family life and contributes to child abuse and neglect. Many, perhaps most, cases of child abuse are linked to parental drug or alcohol abuse. About one in three children placed in foster care are children of drug abusers who were no longer able or willing to care for them.

TABLE 12.2

**Trends in Drug Use among College Students during Lifetime and during Last 30 Days (in Percent)[23]**

| Drug | Used . . . | 1980 | 1982 | 1984 | 1986 | 1988 | 1990 | 1992 | 1994 |
|---|---|---|---|---|---|---|---|---|---|
| Marijuana | Ever? | 65.0 | 60.5 | 59.0 | 57.9 | 51.3 | 49.1 | 44.1 | 42.2 |
| | Last 30 days? | 34.0 | 26.8 | 23.0 | 22.3 | 16.3 | 14.0 | 14.6 | 15.1 |
| Inhalants | Ever? | 10.2 | 10.6 | 10.4 | 11.0 | 12.6 | 13.9 | 14.2 | 12.0 |
| | Last 30 days? | 1.5 | 0.8 | 0.7 | 1.1 | 1.3 | 1.0 | 1.1 | 0.6 |
| Hallucinogens (includes LSD) | Ever | 15.0 | 15.0 | 12.9 | 11.2 | 10.2 | 11.2 | 12.0 | 10.0 |
| | Last 30 days? | 2.7 | 2.6 | 1.8 | 2.2 | 1.7 | 1.4 | 2.3 | 2.1 |
| Cocaine (includes crack) | Ever? | 22.0 | 22.4 | 21.7 | 23.3 | 15.8 | 11.4 | 7.9 | 5.0 |
| | Last 30 days? | 6.9 | 7.9 | 7.6 | 7.0 | 4.2 | 1.2 | 1.0 | 0.6 |
| MDMA ("ecstacy") | Ever? | NA | NA | NA | NA | NA | 3.9 | 2.9 | 2.1 |
| | Last 30 days? | NA | NA | NA | NA | NA | 0.6 | 0.4 | 0.2 |
| Heroin | Ever? | 0.9 | 0.5 | 0.5 | 0.4 | 0.3 | 0.3 | 0.5 | 0.1 |
| | Last 30 days? | 0.3 | 0.0 | 0.0 | 0.0 | 0.1 | 0.0 | 0.0 | 0.0 |
| Stimulants (other than cocaine) | Ever? | NA | 30.1 | 27.8 | 22.3 | 17.7 | 13.2 | 10.5 | 9.2 |
| | Last 30 days? | NA | 9.9 | 5.5 | 3.7 | 1.8 | 1.4 | 1.1 | 1.5 |
| Barbiturates | Ever? | 8.1 | 8.2 | 6.4 | 5.4 | 3.6 | 3.8 | 3.8 | 3.2 |
| | Last 30 days? | 0.9 | 1.0 | 0.7 | 0.6 | 0.5 | 0.2 | 0.7 | 0.4 |
| Alcohol | Ever? | 94.3 | 95.2 | 94.2 | 94.9 | 94.9 | 93.1 | 91.8 | 88.1 |
| | Last 30 days? | 81.8 | 82.8 | 79.1 | 79.7 | 77.0 | 74.5 | 71.4 | 67.5 |
| Cigarettes | Ever? | NA | NA | NA | NA | NA | NA | NA | NA |
| | Last 30 days? | 25.8 | 24.4 | 21.5 | 22.4 | 22.6 | 21.5 | 23.5 | 23.5 |

**Drug Abuse during Pregnancy** Many children are born addicted to drugs used by their mothers during pregnancy and experience withdrawal symptoms when they are born. Maternal drug use during pregnancy is associated with an increased risk of babies being born of low birth weight, which in turn increases the risk of infant mortality and developmental problems.[26]

One newborn in ten in the United States is exposed to drugs in the uterus, and of these, 75% are exposed to cocaine. The government estimates that by 2000, 60% of the student body in inner-city public schools may well consist of children who were exposed to drugs in utero. About half of them will require specialized educational and psychological services.[27]

**Economic Costs of Drug Abuse** The economic costs of drug abuse can be measured in terms of lost productivity, absenteeism, medical treatment for drug-related problems and treatment of drug-related accidents and injuries, costs slated for the interdiction of drugs, and the apprehension, trial, and incarceration of people engaged in the drug trade. A study by the United States Postal Service showed that the absenteeism rate among recently hired workers who tested positive for illicit drug use was 59% higher than among new hires who tested negative.[28] Prisons are populated by illicit drug users, many of whom were incarcerated for drug sales or crimes committed to obtain money to buy drugs. Seven of ten prisoners in state facilities have histories of illegal drug use. Half of the inmates in federal prisons are serving time for drug offenses. The costs of caring for children who are exposed to drugs in the womb is estimated to run as high as $750,000 per child through the age of 18.

The economic strain resulting from drug abuse burdens the health care system. Emergency rooms in inner cities are already filled to capacity with people with little or no health insurance who have nowhere else to turn for medical attention. They are further strained by people with drug overdoses and gunshot wounds resulting from drug-related violence. At Albert Einstein Medical Center in Philadelphia, 75% of all newly admitted trauma patients test positive for drugs.[29]

**Depressants** Drugs such as barbiturates, tranquilizers, opiates, and alcohol that lower the rate of nervous system activity.

**Barbiturates** A class of depressant drugs with sedating or calming effects.

**Methaqualone** A type of sedative drug with addictive properties; can induce coma when ingested in large doses.

**Sedative** A central nervous system depressant that has calming and relaxing effects.

**think about it!**

- **Have you ever used an illicit drug? What factors contributed to your use?**
- **How do you measure the costs of drug abuse?**

**critical thinking Agree or disagree and support your answer: The most dangerous drugs are legal and widely available.**

Smart Quiz Q1205

## TYPES OF PSYCHOACTIVE DRUGS

Let us now consider the effects of psychoactive drugs. Most of these are illegal, but some have legitimate medical uses. Nevertheless, they are abused when they are used improperly or illicitly.

### Depressants

**Depressants** dampen the activity of the central nervous system. They produce feelings of relaxation and provide relief from anxiety and tension. Tranquilizers are depressants that have widespread use in treating anxiety disorders. Alcohol is also a depressant. Alcohol has become the most widely used (and abused) over-the-counter tranquilizer (see Chapter 13). In high doses, depressants can kill by arresting vital body functions, such as breathing. Some depressants, notably opiates, produce a "rush" of pleasure in addition to relaxation.

**Barbiturates** **Barbiturates** are a class of depressant drugs that have sedating effects and help relieve anxiety. They are used medically to block pain during surgery, to regulate high blood pressure, and to prevent epileptic seizures. Formerly they were used to treat anxiety and insomnia. Some of the more commonly used barbiturates are amobarbital, pentobarbital, phenobarbital, and secobarbital. Barbiturates have a high addictive potential, which is why physicians no longer use them to treat anxiety or insomnia. **Methaqualone** (brand names Quaalude, or "ludes," and Sopor, or "sopors") is a **sedative** that is similar in effect to barbiturates. It also holds similar dangers and potential for dependence.

Talking Glossary Methaqualone G1203

Barbiturates and methaqualone have become popular street drugs. They induce mild euphoria

## WORLD OF *diversity*

### Ethnicity and Drug Use—Do Statistics Lie?

Statistics may not actually lie, but they can certainly mislead if we are not careful when interpreting them. Consider the following findings reported by the federal government:

The U.S. government regularly conducts representative surveys of households in the U.S. to measure the prevalence of use of various drugs. The results from recent years show that blacks and Hispanics are more likely than (non-Hispanic) whites to be current (past month) users of cocaine.[30] Blacks are also more likely to be currently using marijuana. The government does not report comparable statistics for Asian Americans or Native Americans. Figure 12.3 shows the current (past month) reported rates of use of cocaine, marijuana, and any illicit drug in relation to ethnicity. Can we thus conclude that ethnicity is a key factor in drug use? Are illicit drugs mainly a problem for blacks and Hispanics, or for society in general?

Statistics relating ethnicity to drug use can be misleading if they fail to account for socioeconomic and educational differences between groups. For example, blacks have disproportionately high rates of unemployment, and people who are unemployed more often abuse drugs. As a group, they are also more likely than white people to be poor and to live in socially distressed neighborhoods. People living under such conditions are more likely to use drugs than more affluent people who live in more secure neighborhoods. People who drop out of high school are also more likely to use drugs than those who complete school. Researchers find that African Americans who remain in high school through their senior year are actually less likely to use cocaine or marijuana than white seniors are.[31]

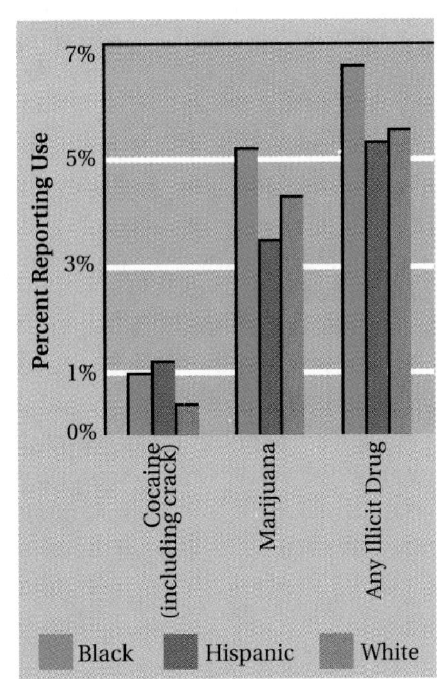


**Figure 12.3** ***Drug Use and Ethnicity***
Percent of individuals surveyed who reported use of illicit drugs. Use of heroin, stimulants, and hallucinogens during the month was less than 0.5% (1 in 200 people) for all groups.

Recently, researchers reanalyzed the data from the government's 1988 national household survey, which had reported higher prevalences of crack cocaine use among blacks and Hispanics than among whites. The reanalysis used a statistical technique to take into account the neighborhoods in which study participants lived.* The results showed that for people living in the same neighborhoods, blacks and Hispanics were no more likely than (non-Hispanic) whites to use crack.[32] Consider too that a nationally representative survey that controlled for income and educational differences showed that alcohol and drug dependence was actually less frequent among blacks than whites and was no more common among Hispanics than whites.[33]

Without taking factors such as education and socioeconomic background into account, statistics concerning drug-use prevalence may serve only to reinforce racial prejudices and divert public attention from the social conditions that may serve as better explanations of drug use than membership in a particular ethnic or racial group.[34]

*By accounting for the neighborhoods in which study participants lived, the researchers were able to hold constant those characteristics that people in the same neighborhood tend to share, such as drug availability, social conditions, and general income level.

and relaxation that can last for hours. They can also cause drowsiness, slurred speech, irritability, and impaired motor functioning and judgment. Overdoses can cause convulsions, coma, and death. Mixing barbiturates and methaqualone with alcohol is extremely dangerous. Barbiturate and methaqualone addicts should undergo withdrawal under medical supervision, as abrupt withdrawal can cause convulsions and death.

**Opiates** **Opiates** are narcotic drugs derived from the poppy plant, including crude opium, morphine, heroin, and codeine. **Narcotics** are addictive drugs that have pain-relieving and sleep-inducing properties. Synthetic opiates, such as Demerol, Per-

**Opiates** Narcotics derived from the opium poppy or synthesized to have opiatelike properties and effects.

**Narcotics** Drugs, primarily opiates, that have sleep-inducing and pain-relieving effects with a high potential for addiction.

codan, and Darvon, are drugs which are synthesized in the laboratory to be similar to natural opiates in chemical structure and effects.

Opiates are often given to postsurgical patients to deaden pain. They can have unpleasant side effects such as nausea and vomiting and cause people to drift between states of alertness and drowsiness. Because of their high potential for addiction, their medical use is regulated. Opiates also produce feelings of pleasure or a "rush" of pleasurable excitement, which is a primary reason for their popularity as street drugs. They also dampen awareness of problems, which is attractive to people who seek to escape the stresses of everyday life.

How do opiates work? As you'll recall, neurons (nerve cells) have receptor sites, or docking stations, for receiving chemical messengers called neurotransmitters. Neurotransmitters relay messages between neurons. Certain neurons in the brain have receptor sites that fit the chemical structure of opiates. Opiates fit into them like keys fit into locks. The brain is apparently configured to dock opiates because they are similar to chemical substances naturally produced by the body—called **endorphins**—that dock at these sites. The term *endorphin* means "endogenous morphine," or morphine from within. Endorphins are neurotransmitters that play a role in regulating states of pleasure and pain. Opiates mimic the actions of endorphins—our own "natural opiates"—and thereby stimulate brain centers involved in regulating pain.[35]

***Opium, Morphine, and Codeine*** **Opium** is a resinous substance extracted from the juice of the opium poppy. It can be smoked or sniffed in powder form and is highly addictive. Two commonly used narcotic drugs, morphine and codeine, are derived from opium.

**Endorphins** Chemical substances produced by the body that are similar in their effects to morphine.

**Opium** A narcotic drug derived from the opium poppy.

**Morphine** A narcotic drug, one of the most powerful derivatives of the opium poppy.

**Codeine** Another narcotic drug derived from the opium poppy that is used medically to deaden pain and to suppress coughing.

**Heroin** A naturally occurring opiate derived from morphine that has strong addictive properties.

**Morphine** derives its name from the Greek god of dreams, Morpheus. Morphine is among the most powerful derivatives of the opium poppy. Introduced around the time of the U.S. Civil War, morphine quickly became widely used to deaden pain in injured soldiers. In fact, morphine addiction became dubbed the "soldier's disease." Morphine continues to be used as an analgesic following surgery. **Codeine** is also used extensively in medicine to deaden pain and may be combined with other analgesics, such as acetaminophen. It is also used in some prescription cough syrups.

***Heroin*** **Heroin** was developed in 1875 in the belief that it would be a nonaddictive alternative to morphine. But heroin turned out to be highly addictive, even more addictive than morphine. Heroin is strongly addictive because it stimulates centers of the brain responsible for pleasure and for the development of physical dependence.

Heroin is a white crystalline powder that can be snorted, smoked, or, most commonly, injected. Heroin may be injected under the skin (skin popping) or directly into a vein (mainlining). Heroin ("horse," "junk," "smack") accounts for most cases of opiate addiction. Nearly 1 million people in the United States are addicted to heroin today.[36] Heroin use, unlike most other drug use, occurs more commonly among people over age 35 than among younger people.[37] About one-third of heroin users are women, and about a third of these are prostitutes. They are especially vulnerable to contracting HIV because of sexual activity with multiple partners and sharing needles in injecting heroin.

When injected into a vein, heroin produces a euphoric rush that can last from 5 to 15 minutes. It is so intense and pleasurable that some compare it to the pleasure of orgasm. A second phase of pro-

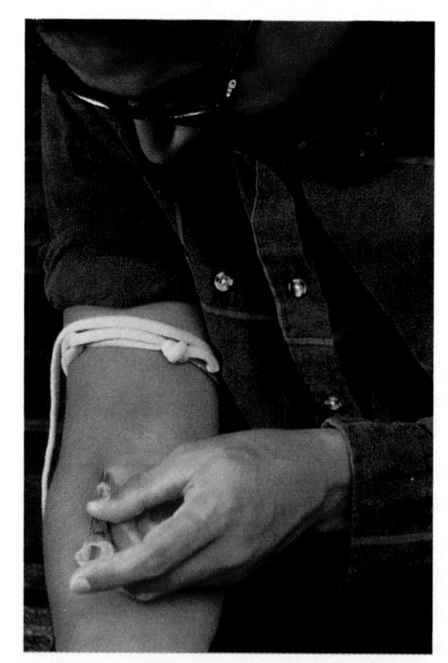

***Shooting Up*** Heroin is a highly addictive narcotic drug that can be snorted, smoked, or, most commonly, injected.

longed relaxation follows, with feelings of satisfaction, mild euphoria, drowsiness, and well-being. This period lasts from 3 to 5 hours. Under the influence of heroin, worries and cares evaporate. Drives for sex or food become blunted. Once this carefree state begins to wear off, users may seek their next fix to return to the drugged state. Heroin addicts begin to organize their lives around pursuit and use of the drug, often turning to crime or prostitution to support their habits.

Addicts develop tolerance (need for higher doses) and an unpleasant abstinence syndrome that can be likened to a very bad case of the flu.[38] Withdrawal symptoms include rapid pulse and respiration, increased blood pressure, profuse sweating, muscle cramps, tremors, watery eyes, runny nose, loss of appetite, nausea, hot and cold flashes, panic, vomiting, insomnia, diarrhea, and strong cravings. While these symptoms may be unpleasant, they can be managed under medical supervision and can often be relieved through prescribed drugs.

Injecting heroin can lead to the development of skin abscesses, inflammation of the veins, and the transmission of microscopic organisms causing such diseases as hepatitis and AIDS. A heroin overdose, characterized by such symptoms as shallow breathing, clammy skin, convulsions, and coma, can also be deadly. The risk of complications and overdose is accentuated when heroin is used in combination with other drugs such as alcohol or cocaine. Serious complications may also occur when agents used to cut the drug are contaminated by poisons. Chronic use of heroin may also depress the body's immune system. Babies whose mothers used heroin during pregnancy may be born addicted themselves and experience withdrawal effects.

The sharing of hypodermic needles among heroin addicts is a principal means of transmission of HIV, the virus that causes AIDS. Nearly one-third of new cases of AIDS are linked to injecting drugs, either from sharing contaminated needles or from sexual contact with people who became infected by needle sharing.[39] The issue of whether public health officials should distribute clean needles to addicts continues to be debated. Some heroin addicts inhale or smoke heroin to avoid the risks posed by contaminated needles.

## Stimulants

**Stimulants** are a class of drugs that heighten the activity of the central nervous system. They include amphetamines, cocaine, and the most widely used psychoactive drug of all, caffeine.

**Caffeine** Does it surprise you to learn that most drug-dependent people live perfectly normal lives and may never realize that they are hooked on a mind-altering drug? That drug is available in any supermarket and is probably sitting in your kitchen cabinet right now. It is **caffeine,** the mild stimulant found in coffee, tea, colas, and chocolate (see Table 12.3). Caffeine is our most widely used drug. More than 420 million cups of coffee

TABLE 12.3

**Sources of Caffeine[44]**

| | Milligrams of Caffeine |
|---|---|
| Coffee (5 fl.oz.) | |
| Brewed | |
| Drip | 110–150 |
| Percolated | 64–124 |
| Decaffeinated | 2–5 |
| Instant | |
| Regular | 40–108 |
| Decaffeinated | 2 |
| Tea | |
| Hot, steeped 3 minutes (6 fl. oz.) | 36 |
| Iced (1 tsp. instant powder in 8 fl. oz. water) | 31 |
| Soft drinks (12 fl. oz.) | |
| Cola (regular and diet) | 46 |
| Pepsi Cola (regular and diet) | 36–38 |
| Mountain Dew | 54 |
| Milk drinks | |
| Hot cocoa (heaping 3/4 tsp. powder in 6 fl. oz. water) | 4 |
| Chocolate milk (2 tbsp. chocolate syrup in 8 fl. oz. milk) | 6 |
| Foods with chocolate | |
| Cadbury milk chocolate (1 oz.) | 15 |
| Chocolate instant pudding (1/2 cup) | 4–12 |
| Unsweetened baking chocolate (1 oz.) | 25 |
| Drugs (standard dose) | |
| Excedrin | 130 |
| Anacin | 64 |
| Midol | 65 |
| No Doz tablets | 200 |

**Stimulants** Psychoactive drugs that increase the level of activity of the central nervous system.

**Caffeine** A mild stimulant found in coffee, tea, colas, and chocolate.

are consumed each day in the United States, or more than two cups for every adult.[40] If you regularly drink caffeinated beverages, you are probably hooked, as are your authors. Caffeine is the least harmful of addictive substances and actually has the benefit of enhancing wakefulness and mental alertness,[41] which is why many of us start the day with coffee or tea. Caffeine even improves performance on some mental and physical tasks.

How do you know if you're hooked? The question is whether you can skip caffeine for a day or two without withdrawal symptoms. If you feel on edge, depressed, fatigued, or anxious, have headaches or flulike symptoms, or experience strong cravings for caffeine, you're probably hooked. Regular use of just a cup or two of coffee or tea a day, or a few cans of caffeinated soft drinks, is enough to become addicted.[42]

The effects of caffeine are dose-related. At 100 milligrams (equivalent to the amount in an average cup of coffee), people tend to report feeling stimulated, energetic, and talkative. As the dosage rises from 200 to 600 milligrams, more negative effects are reported, such as feelings of jitteriness, nervousness, and shakiness.

Because caffeine crosses the placenta and enters the fetal bloodstream, questions have been raised about the safety of caffeine for pregnant women. No links have been found between low levels of caffeine (a cup or two of coffee or tea daily) and miscarriage or reduced growth in the fetus.[43] However, higher levels of caffeine (greater than 300 mg per day, or equivalent to three or more cups of coffee or tea daily) may lower birth weights in infants. Low birth weight increases the risk of infant mortality and some developmental problems. Pregnant women are advised to ask their doctors about caffeine.

**Close-up**
Decaf and cancer
T1207

Some people should avoid or limit caffeine because they are highly sensitive to it. Some people can down a strong cup of coffee at bedtime and still sleep like a baby, but others toss and turn for hours if they have had even one cup of coffee or tea after noon. For some people, coffee and tea cause side effects such as nervousness, headaches, trembling, even diarrhea.

If you decide to cut caffeine down or out, you need not go "cold turkey." While withdrawal symptoms usually taper off within 48 hours and are gone within a week or so, cutting down gradually reduces or eliminates withdrawal symptoms. You can gradually cut the number of cups of caffeinated coffee or tea per day, or brew mixtures of caffeinated and decaffeinated coffee. Gradually reduce the caffeinated proportion until you've reached your goal. Be aware of other sources of caffeine, such as cola drinks, that may more than make up for eliminating caffeine from your coffee.

**Amphetamines** A class of synthetic stimulants.

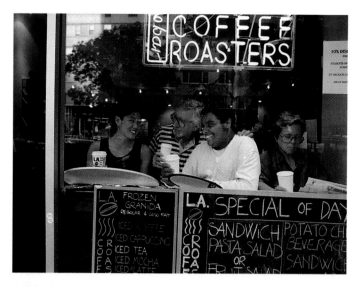


***Coffee Bar*** Is the recent popularity of coffee bars explained by a craving for caffeine or by the pleasures of socializing?

**Amphetamines** The most common **amphetamines** are amphetamine sulfate (trade name Benzedrine), methamphetamine (Methedrine), and dextroamphetamine (Dexedrine). Amphetamines are known on the street as "speed," "crank," or "meth" (for Methedrine), "uppers" or "bennies" (for Benzedrine), and "dexies" (for Dexedrine). They are synthetic compunds (manufactured in the laboratory—not found in nature). Related drugs include the stimulant methylphenidate (Ritalin), used in the treatment of childhood hyperactivity, pemoline (Cylert), and phenmetrazine (Preludin).

Amphetamines activate the sympathetic branch of the autonomic nervous system, thus increasing heart rate and respiration rates and raising blood pressure. Like cocaine, amphetamines stimulate the reward pathways in the brain that control feelings of pleasure. In low doses, they increase mental alertness and concentration and lessen fatigue. In high doses, they can produce a euphoric rush. Because they also suppress the appetite, they are used by some dieters.

Amphetamines stimulate the release of the neurotransmitters norepinephrine and dopamine. They also interfere with the reabsorption of these neurotransmitters (through a process called reuptake) by the transmitting neuron, thereby increasing the availability of these chemicals. As a result, neurons continue to fire, maintaining a state of high arousal.

Amphetamines can be taken in pill form or smoked in a relatively pure form of methamphetamine called "ice" or "crystal meth." "Ice" heightens alertness and excitability and can produce a euphoric high. Prolonged use of the drug can cause potentially fatal lung and kidney damage and cause psychological disorders. The most potent form of amphetamine, liquid methamphetamine, is injected into the veins, producing an intense rush. When highs come to an end, users may "crash"—fall into deep sleep or stupor, or experience deep, prolonged depression. Some people commit suicide on the way down from amphetamine highs. In 1994, 3.4% of high school seniors had used crystal methamphetamine at least once in their lifetimes, up from 2.7% in 1990.[45]

Amphetamines can quickly lead to psychological dependence, especially in people who use them to fight depression. Tolerance can also develop quickly. Some people overdose—fatally—as they take more and more to try to reach highs similar to those they achieved when they first started using amphetamines. At high doses, amphetamines can cause restlessness, irritability, loss of appetite, anxiety, insomnia, tremors, chest pain, heart irregularities, even cardiovascular collapse and death. Chronic amphetamine users may develop **amphetamine psychosis.** This is a psychotic state that resembles paranoid schizophrenia. Symptoms include hallucinations (seeing, hearing, or feeling things that are not there). Chronic use of methamphetamine can also cause permanent brain damage or death. It is unclear whether amphetamines are addictive.

**Close-up** More on "meth" T1208

**Cocaine** Coca-Cola was once advertised as "the real thing." While the sugar and caffeine that Coca-Cola contains are likely to give drinkers a boost, Coca-Cola hasn't actually been "the real thing" since 1906. In that year, **cocaine** ("coke") was removed from the brew. The name Coca-Cola reflects its original sources, the coca plant, from which a cocaine extract was derived and added to the original formula for the drink, and the cola nut, which was used for flavoring. Cocaine is a natural stimulant that is derived from the leaves of the coca plant.

Cocaine exerts such powerfully rewarding effects that users may not be able to predict or control their use of the drug. Occasional use can quickly lead to habitual use, even among people who want to stop.

Next to marijuana, cocaine is the most widely used illicit drug in the United States. From the mid-1970s to the mid-1980s, cocaine users were mainly middle class. The drug was primarily available in powder form and was snorted. By the mid-1980s, a new epidemic began: crack cocaine. **Crack** is readily smokable and was being sold in unit doses for $3 to $5. The affordability of crack led to a marked expansion of cocaine use among young people, especially in poorer, inner-city neighborhoods. Crack cocaine has been used by nearly 2% of the U.S. population aged 12 and older.[46]

Cocaine can also be injected in liquid form or ingested as a tea brewed from coca leaves. **Freebase cocaine** is derived from a chemical process that intensifies the effects of the drug. Cocaine is heated with ether, which frees the psychoactive base of the drug, and then smoked. Ether, however, is highly flammable, which makes its use very hazardous.

***Effects of Cocaine*** Like other stimulants, cocaine increases mental clarity and alertness and heightens arousal. Like amphetamines, cocaine stimulates reward pathways in the brain, producing a state of euphoria. Smoking crack transports the drug to the brain almost immediately, producing an intense and sudden high. The rush wears off in a few minutes, leaving the user wanting more. The high from snorting powder cocaine lasts perhaps 15 to 30 minutes; the high from smoking crack, only 5 to 10 minutes. Because of the immediacy and intensity of the high, combined with its short duration, crack is the most habit-forming street drug.[47] The user needs to take the drug at frequent intervals to maintain the crack high. Repetition can

**Amphetamine psychosis** An acute psychotic reaction induced by the ingestion of amphetamines that mimics acute episodes of paranoid schizophrenia.

**Cocaine** An addictive stimulant drug derived from coca leaves that increases mental alertness and induces a euphoric rush.

**Crack** A hardened form of cocaine that comes in the form of pebbles ("rocks") that can be smoked.

**Freebase cocaine** A form of cocaine in which the drug is first heated with ether to separate its more potent component (the "free base") and then smoked.

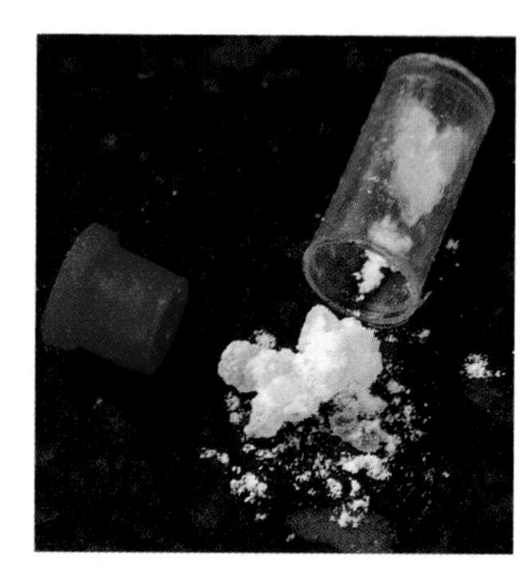

***Crack Pebbles*** Crack pebbles or "rocks" produce a powerful but short-lived rush when smoked. Small, ready-to-smoke doses are priced at relatively modest cost, making them affordable to adolescents, who can quickly become hard-core users.

lead to compulsive use as the user seeks to maintain highs and avoid the lows of withdrawal. Cocaine abusers typically fall into a cycle of binges lasting 12 to 36 hours followed by days of abstinence during which cravings increase sharply, prompting another binge.[48]

Prolonged use of cocaine can lead to psychological disturbances, including anxiety, irritability, and depression. Cocaine-induced depression is sometimes severe enough to prompt a suicide attempt. High doses or chronic use can trigger a break with reality—a **cocaine psychosis**—that is characterized by hallucinations and delusions of persecution.

Cocaine is highly addictive. The abstinence syndrome involves intense cravings for the drug, depression, and inability to experience pleasure.[49] Cocaine addicts often resume using the drug to relieve withdrawal symptoms. A tolerance effect, yet another sign of physiological dependence, develops quickly with repeated cocaine use. Severe psychological dependence may also occur. Cocaine becomes the focus of the addict's life.

High doses or prolonged use of the drug can damage the cardiovascular system, with deadly effects. Cocaine causes an abrupt rise in blood pressure, constricts blood vessels (which limits the supply of oxygen to the heart), and accelerates the heart rate. During cocaine binges, users attempt to maintain the high by taking more and more of the drug, which can lead to irregular heartbeats, heart stoppage, and strokes caused by spasms of blood vessels in the brain.[50] An overdose can also disrupt breathing, causing gasping and leading to respiratory arrest. Death often results, as in the case of the athletes Len Bias, Dave Croudip, and Don Rogers. Most cocaine deaths do not make the headlines, however.

**Close-up**
More on cocaine
**T1209**

Occasional snorting of cocaine can lead to nasal congestion and a chronic runny nose. Chronic heavy snorting can cause more damage to the nasal cavity, ulcerating the mucous membrane and causing the nasal septum to collapse. Habitual smoking of crack cocaine or freebase cocaine can damage the mouth, throat, and lungs, and lead to lung cancer. The health effects of cocaine are summarized in Table 12.4.

Pregnant women who use cocaine increase their risk of miscarriage, premature birth, and other complications. Because cocaine constricts the blood vessels leading to the womb, less oxygen reaches the fetus, retarding fetal development and growth. Cocaine use during pregnancy can cause hemorraghing, threatening the lives of mother and fetus.

**Cocaine psychosis** An acute psychotic reaction induced by the use of cocaine, often involving paranoid delusions.

**Psychedelics** Hallucinogenic drugs that have been used in religious ceremonies among Native American peoples and others for their mind-expanding and hallucinogenic effects.

**Hallucinogenic drugs** Psychoactive drugs that alter sensory processes and induce hallucinations.

**Lysergic acid diethylamide (LSD)** A hallucinogenic drug, more commonly known by its abbreviation.

**Psilocybin** A hallucinogenic drug derived from certain types of mushrooms.

**Mescaline** A hallucinogenic drug derived from the peyote cactus.

## Hallucinogens

Also known as **psychedelics** ("mind-revealing"), **hallucinogenic drugs** or *hallucinogens* alter sensory perceptions, distorting reality and producing hallucinations. Hallucinogens also produce feelings of relaxation or euphoria in some cases, and paranoia or panic in others.

About 1 to 2% of people in the United States report using hallucinogens during the past year.[52] Hallucinogen use is greatest among adolescents and young adults, and among males overall. Hallucinogens can produce strong psychological dependence, especially when people turn to them as a means of coping with problems or distracting themselves from stress. They are not known to be addictive, however. The hallucinogens include **lysergic acid diethylamide (LSD), psilocybin,** and **mescaline.**

**Talking Glossary**
Lysergic acid diethylamide, Psilocybin, Mescaline
**G1204**

**LSD** LSD ("acid") is a synthetic hallucinogenic drug that can produce vivid hallucinations and sensory distortions. LSD is among the most potent psychoactive drugs. The experience of taking the drug is called a "trip." LSD trips may last as long as

TABLE 12.4

**Health Effects of Cocaine[51]**

| **Physical Effects and Risks** | |
|---|---|
| *Effects* | *Risks* |
| 1. Increased heart rate | Accelerated heart rate may give rise to heart irregularities that can be fatal, such as ventricular tachycardia (extremely rapid contractions) or ventricular fibrillation (irregular, weakened contractions). |
| 2. Increased blood pressure | Rapid or large changes in blood pressure may place too much stress on a weak-walled blood vessel in the brain, which can cause it to burst, producing cerebral hemorrhage or stroke. |
| 3. Increased body temperature | Can be dangerous to some individuals. |
| 4. Possible grand mal seizures (epileptic convulsions) | Some grand mal seizures are fatal, particularly when they occur in rapid succession or while someone is driving a car. |
| 5. Respiratory effects | Overdoses can produce gasping or shallow irregular breathing that can lead to respiratory arrest. |
| 6. Dangerous effects in special populations | Special populations are at greater risk from cocaine use or overdose. People with coronary heart disease have died because their heart muscles were taxed beyond the capacity of their arteries to supply oxygen. |
| **Medical Complications of Cocaine Use** | |
| Nasal problems | When cocaine is administered intranasally (snorted), it constricts the blood vessels serving the nose, decreasing the supply of oxygen to these tissues, leading to irritation and inflammation of the mucous membranes, ulcers in the nostrils, frequent nosebleeds, and chronic sneezing and nasal congestion. Chronic use may lead to tissue death of the nasal septum, the part of the nose that separates the nostrils, requiring plastic surgery. |
| Lung problems | Freebase smoking may lead to serious lung problems within 3 months of initial use. |
| Malnutrition | Cocaine suppresses the appetite so that weight loss, malnutrition, and vitamin deficiencies may accompany regular use. |
| Seizures | Grand mal seizures, typical of epileptics, may occur due to irregularities in the electrical activity of the brain. Repeated use may lower the seizure threshold, described as a type of "kindling" effect. |
| Sexual problems | Despite the popular belief that cocaine is an aphrodisiac, frequent use can lead to sexual dysfunctions, such as impotence and failure to ejaculate among males, and decreased sexual interest in both sexes. Although some people report initial increased sexual pleasure with cocaine use, they may become dependent on cocaine for sexual arousal or lose the ability to enjoy sex for extended periods following long-term use. |
| Other effects | Cocaine use may increase the risk of miscarriage among pregnant women. Sharing of infected needles is associated with transmission of hepatitis, endocarditis (infection of the heart valve), and HIV. Repeated injections often lead to skin infections as bacteria are introduced into the deeper levels of the skin. |

12 hours before wearing off. In 1994, about 7% of Americans reported having used LSD at least once, up from 4.2% in 1985.[53] Fewer than 1% reported using LSD during the past year.

LSD causes dilation of the pupils; increased body temperature, heart rate, and blood pressure; sweating; loss of appetite; sleeplessness; dry mouth; and tremors.[54] The psychological effects of LSD are variable and unpredictable. They depend on the amount taken as well as the user's expectations, personality, mood, and surroundings.[55] Some users report vivid displays of colors and visual distortions and hallucinations, especially with larger doses. Emotions may merge or shift rapidly. There may be changes in the sense of time and of self. Sensations may cross over so that users feel that they hear colors or see sounds. Some users report that the drug expands their consciousness, helping them to discover a deeper reality or to acquire new insights. These discoveries are usually fleeting and do not lead to constructive life changes.

***LSD Trip*** LSD is a hallucinogenic drug that can produce vivid hallucinations and sensory distortions. Some users report "bad trips" that may involve feelings of fear or panic or even psychotic reactions. Some people are affected by flashbacks even years later.

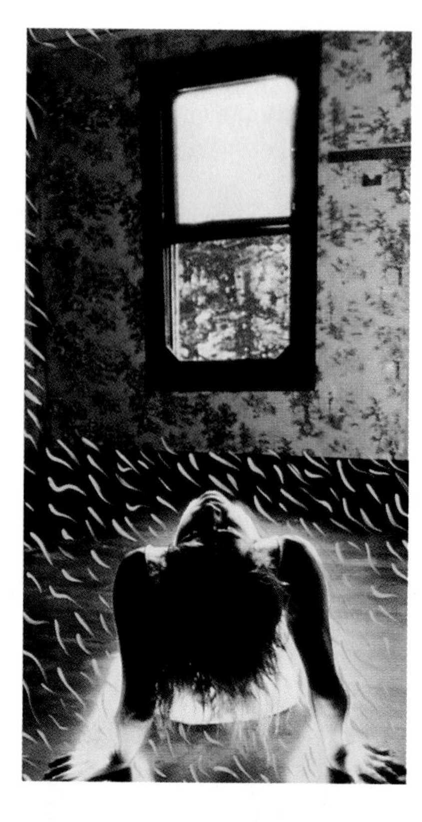

Some users have "bad trips." Feelings of intense fear or panic may occur. Users may fear death, or losing control or sanity. Fatal accidents have sometimes occurred during LSD trips.

Flashbacks, typically involving a recurrence of some of the perceptual distortions of the trip, may occur weeks or years afterward. Flashbacks tend to occur suddenly and without warning. Other disturbing complications from LSD may occur, including psychotic reactions.

**Mescaline** Used for centuries in religious rites by Native Americans in the southwestern U.S., Mexico, and Central America, mescaline ("mesc") is derived from the peyote cactus. Like LSD, it can produce hallucinations, vivid lights, and visual distortions that can last more than 12 hours.

**Psilocybin** Psilocybin is derived from certain mushrooms. These "magic mushrooms" have long been used in religious practices among Native Latin Americans. Although less potent than LSD, psilocybin can produce colorful images and hallucinations that last perhaps 4 to 6 hours. The hallucinations are often accompanied by feelings of elation and uncontrollable laughter.[56] However, the drug's effects are not predictable (psychedelic mushrooms vary in potency), and users may have negative experiences, with panic or frightening hallucinations. Flashbacks may occur days or weeks afterward.

**Phencyclidine** **Phencyclidine (PCP),** or "angel dust" as it is commonly called, achieved popularity as a street drug in the 1970s because it could be cheaply and quickly synthesized in basement or garage-type laboratories. By the mid-1980s, more than 20% of young people age 18 to 25 had used PCP.[57] Its popularity has since waned, in large part because of its unpredictable effects. Today, only about 2.5% of 18- to 25-year-olds have used PCP.[58]

PCP is a **deliriant.** That is, it produces *delirium*—a state of extreme confusion, excitement, disorientation, and difficulty focusing attention. Distortions in the sensing of time and space, feelings of unreality, distorted perceptions of body image and the outside world, and vivid, sometimes frightening, hallucinations can occur. It may seem that there is some invisible barrier separating oneself from the world. This may be a pleasant or engrossing experience, or a frightening one, depending on the user's expectations, mood, setting, and so forth. Physical effects can include increased heart rate and blood pressure, profuse sweating, and flushing. Users may stagger, and their speech may become garbled.

Users sometimes report that PCP makes them feel stronger, more powerful, even invulnerable. Yet it may also lead to paranoia, blind rage, and blotting out of unpleasant memories. Some PCP users have committed shootings and stabbings, or have injured themselves. Bizarre behavior, such as lying down in the middle of busy streets, is not uncommon. Accidents, including fatal drownings, falls, and automobile crashes, have also occurred. Chronic users may develop problems with memory and perception, speech problems, impaired concentration and judgment, depression, and weight loss.

PCP is toxic in high doses. People vary in their sensitivity to the drug, making it difficult to predict when a toxic reaction may occur. Overdoses can induce drowsiness or more serious complications, including hyperexcitability, cardiovascular damage, convulsions, permanent brain damage, coma, and death.

**Talking Glossary**
Phencyclidine
G1205

**Phencyclidine (PCP)** Commonly called "angel dust," a deliriant drug with unpredictable and sometimes dangerous effects.

**Deliriant** A substance that induces delirium, or a state of gross mental confusion, excitability, and disorientation.

**Talking Glossary**
Delta-9-tetrahydro-cannabinol
**G1206**

**Marijuana** **Marijuana** ("pot," "weed," "grass," "reefer," "dope") is derived from the *Cannabis sativa* plant. The major psychoactive ingredient in marijuana is **delta-9-tetrahydrocannabinol,** or **THC.** It is found in the leaves and branches of cannabis but is most concentrated in the resin of the plant, from which the most potent form of the drug, **hashish** ("hash"), is derived. Marijuana and hashish can be ingested by eating the parts of the plant containing THC or baking them into foods such as brownies. Smoking is the most common method of use, however. The dried leaves may be rolled into "joints" and then smoked. Or a pipe may be used to smoke the crushed leaves or resin.

Marijuana became popular among young people during the 1960s who were disillusioned with society and exploring alternative lifestyles. Some of them used the drug to "drop out" of the mainstream. Marijuana remains our most widely used illegal drug.[59] Nearly 33% of people in the United States aged 12 or older have tried marijuana, and about 5% are current users.[60]

Marijuana alters perceptions and sometimes produces mild hallucinations. Lower doses can induce relaxation and a mild euphoric high. Users may experience time as passing more slowly and become more aware of bodily sensations, such as the beating of the heart. This can lead to feelings of anxiety or even panic in users who perceive that the heart is racing out of control. High doses can cause nausea and vomiting, feelings of disorientation, panic attacks, paranoia, and hallucinations.

People use marijuana for a variety of reasons. Some find it relaxing, similar in low doses to alcohol. Some users report that the drug makes them more comfortable in social gatherings. Higher doses, however, often lead users to withdraw into themselves. Some users believe that the drug increases their capacity for self-insight or creative thinking, although the insights achieved under its influence may not seem as deep when the drug has worn off. People may turn to marijuana, as to other drugs, to help them cope with stress. Of course, marijuana and other drugs provide only a temporary escape.

**Close-up**
A recurring problem
**T1210**

Prolonged use of marijuana can impair immunological functioning; depress sperm production, lower testosterone levels, and reduce sex drive in men; and disrupt menstrual cycles in women.[61] THC acts on parts of the brain that are involved in learning and memory. Chronic use can destroy nerve cells in the brain, leading to a loss of brain tissue similar to that which occurs during aging, causing memory problems.[62] Regular smoking of marijuana and hashish can scar the lungs and introduce carcinogenic compounds into the body, leading to cancers of the mouth, throat, and lungs. Marijuana smoke contains more carcinogenic tars than tobacco smoke, which may explain why chronic users of marijuana incur the same risk of lung cancer as cigarette smokers, even if they smoke less.

Marijuana can raise the heart rate to 140 to 150 beats per minute and, in some people, raise the blood pressure, posing a risk to those with cardiovascular conditions. Marijuana impairs motor coordination and alters perceptions, a dangerous combination when users operate heavy equipment or drive. Use of marijuana can disrupt performance on skilled motor tasks even 24 hours after it is used, long after the psychological effects have worn off.[63] Users who know not to drive a car when they are high may not realize that their performance remains disrupted in subtle ways the next day. Despite the medical risks, researchers are exploring alternative medical uses of the drug. Marijuana reduces nausea among cancer patients undergoing chemotherapy and among AIDS patients who suffer from wasting syndrome, the potentially deadly loss of appetite and subsequent loss of weight that afflicts patients in the advanced stages of the disease.[64] Marijuana may also be helpful in treating glaucoma by reducing fluid pressure in the eye and pain and muscle spasms in patients with epilepsy and multiple sclerosis.

**Close-up**
More on marijuana
**T1211**

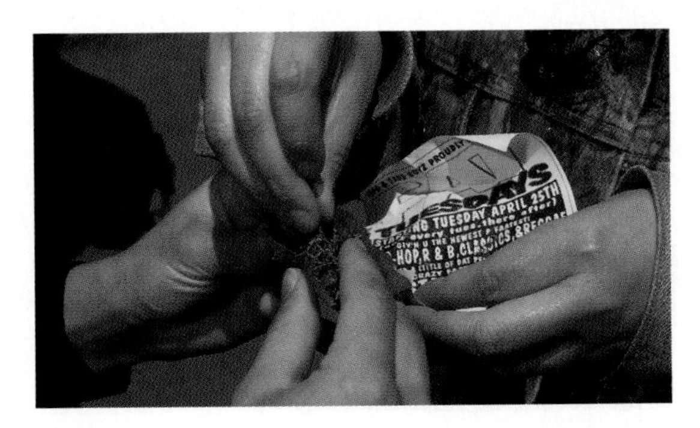

***Rolling a Joint*** Marijuana, shown here being rolled into a joint, is America's most widely used illicit drug. Chronic use can damage the immune system and lungs, as well as impair memory.

**Marijuana** A drug, derived from the *Cannabis sativa* plant, with relaxant and mild hallucinogenic effects.

**Delta-9-tetrahydrocannabinol (THC)** The psychoactive ingredient in marijuana and hashish.

**Hashish** Also known as "hash," the resin of the cannabis plant, which contains the most potent concentration of THC.

A debate is raging in many states over the issue of whether doctors should be permitted to prescribe marijuana to patients suffering from these conditions.[65]

## Other Psychoactive Drugs

Other psychoactive drugs include chemicals contained in gaseous fumes that are ingested through inhaling, and so-called designer drugs, or chemical knockoffs of illicit drugs.

**Inhalants** **Inhalants** are chemicals that emit fumes that can be inhaled to get high. Some of the more common inhalants are glues and rubber cements, gases from aerosol cans, paint thinners, spot removers, lighter fluids, gasolines and other fuels, and nitrous oxide or "laughing gas." About 17% of high school students have tried inhalants.[66] Unlike other drugs, use of inhalants is more common among younger adolescents than older adolescents. Next to alcohol and tobacco, inhalants are the most widely abused substances among eighth-graders. They appeal to young people because they are found in common household products and provide a quick "hit." Like PCP, inhalants are deliriants. They produce disorientation, dizziness, and impaired judgment. They also have depressant effects on the central nervous system.

Inhalants can be dangerous, even deadly. The chemicals that are inhaled are quickly absorbed in the bloodstream. They travel throughout the body, damaging various organs, especially the kidneys, liver, lungs, and brain. An overdose can cause unconsciousness and coma. Sustained inhalation may cause death by suffocation.

**Designer Drugs** **Designer drugs** are synthesized in secret laboratories and intended to mimic the effects of illicit drugs. Underground chemists attempt to skirt the law by ever so slightly changing the chemical structures of controlled substances to make them technically legal. Changes in the law, however, have now made these chemical knockoffs illegal.

One of the most widely used designer drugs is an amphetamine analog called **MDMA** (3,4–methylenedioxymethamphetamine), which is known on the streets as "ecstasy" or "Adam." MDMA achieved some popularity on college campuses in the 1980s because of its euphoric and hallucinogenic effects. However, use of the drug can lead to serious psychological problems, including anxiety, sleep problems, depression, and paranoia. It also can have adverse physical effects, including nausea, blurred vision, involuntary clenching of the teeth, faintness, muscle tension, and chills or sweating.[67] MDMA raises the heart rate and blood pressure, which can pose a threat to people with cardiovascular problems. It may also damage brain cells.

**Inhalants** Chemical fumes that are inhaled for their psychoactive effects.

**Designer drugs** Synthetic drugs manufactured in illicit labs that are chemical analogues (drugs having similar properties and effects) of illegal drugs.

**MDMA** Known popularly as "ecstasy," a designer drug that is an amphetamine analogue.

**Anabolic steroids** Synthetic versions of the male sex hormone testosterone.

## Anabolic Steroids

**Talking Glossary**
Anabolic steroids
G1207

**Anabolic steroids** are not used as street drugs for their psychoactive effects (to get high), but rather for their ability to foster muscle development. They are synthetic versions of the male sex hormone testosterone. They have several medical uses, such as in the treatment of osteoporosis and anemia. They are also used illicitly by bodybuilders, football players, competitive runners, and others bent on building up their muscles. These steroids may also increase the amount of available energy for peak performance. The typical user is a young man in his late teens who uses steroids to give himself an edge in athletic competition or to build up his physique in the belief that a "pumped-up" look will attract women.

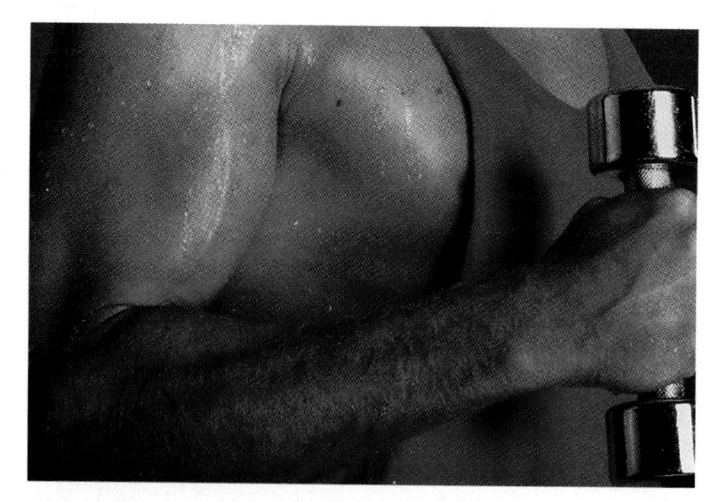

***Pumped-Up on Steroids*** Some bodybuilders and other athletes use steroids to help them build bigger muscles. However, regular steroid use can lead to serious complications, including liver disease and some forms of cancer.

Although anabolic steroids can add muscle mass, they carry serious risks. While the full range of long-term effects of anabolic steroids on health remains unclear, we know that they can damage various bodily organs and systems, especially the liver, the organ responsible for steroid metabolism. Anabolic steroid use is linked to cancers of the liver, testes, and abdomen, and to impaired reproductive functioning.[68] Steroids also reduce blood levels of "good cholesterol" (HDL), increasing the risk of cardiovascular problems. They can also lead to acne, impotence in men, and breast reduction and beard growth in women.

Anabolic steroids have some psychoactive effects, such as increasing self-confidence. They can also have disturbing behavioral effects, the most troubling of which is increasing anger and aggression ("steroid rage"). Some cases of homicide are connected with use of anabolic steroids.[69] Surveys show that 80% of teenage steroid users report aggressive crimes against people or property during the past year.[70] Psychotic symptoms and mood disturbances have also been observed among some steroid users.[71] Withdrawal from anabolic steroids can cause sleep problems, mood swings, and depression severe enough to lead to thoughts of suicide.

More than 1 million people in the United States have used anabolic steroids. About nine of ten users are male.[72] Rates of use are greatest in the 12- to 25-year age range. About 2% of high school seniors have used anabolic steroids.[73] Young people who use steroids typically do not recognize or heed the consequences of their use.

Smart Quiz
Q1206

### think about it!

- Do you use caffeine? How much? Could you stop? (Are you sure?)
- Do you know people who use marijuana or LSD? What do they report to be their effects?
- Do you know people who have used anabolic steroids to build muscle or endurance for sports? What do they report about the drug?

**critical thinking** Are you addicted to any drugs? On what evidence do you base your answer? What are you doing about it, if anything?

## DRUG TREATMENT—BECOMING DRUG FREE, REMAINING DRUG FREE

There are many ways of helping people with drug abuse or dependence problems live fuller, more productive lives free of drugs. They include clinic- or hospital-based inpatient and outpatient treatment programs, and residential and community-based rehabilitation centers. Yet, among the estimated 6.5 million drug addicts in the country, only 350,000 receive treatment.[74] Most addicts do not seek help voluntarily, or at least not until they hit "rock-bottom" or are brought to an emergency room because of a drug overdose or adverse drug reaction. Then, too, many addicts who *want* help find that there are no openings in drug treatment centers when they apply. Money to fund drug treatment centers has been increasing but is still not sufficient to meet the need, even though studies show that money for drug treatment centers is well spent. More than $11 in social costs is saved for every $1 spent on treatment.[75]

Video
Recovery from drug dependency
V1201

### Detoxification

**Detoxification** is the process of ridding the body of drugs. Detoxification may take place in a hospital so that people with chemical dependencies can be medically supervised while they withdraw from drugs. The typical program involves a stay of 28 days, during which time recovering addicts work with counselors to help prepare them for living without drugs upon discharge. Counselors attempt to break through the chemical haze and the layers of denial that prevent drug abusers from coming to grips with the consequences of their addictions. Detoxification may also take place on an outpatient basis, when it is deemed safe to withdraw addicts from drugs while they continue with their normal lives.

A variety of outpatient programs following "detox" help recovering addicts live drug free. The recovering addict may also be referred for additional help to Narcotics Anonymous, a peer-support, self-help organization fashioned after Alcoholics Anonymous (AA).

**Detoxification** The process of eliminating drugs from a person's body, usually under supervised conditions where withdrawal symptoms can be monitored and controlled.

## Therapeutic Communities

Therapeutic communities are drug-free residential treatment facilities in which recovering addicts live with strict rules. They make their own beds, prepare their own meals, and participate in daily group therapy sessions in which they are confronted with their denial of responsibility for their behavior, especially their drug abuse. The treatment philosophy is that addicts will not break the bonds of addiction until they accept responsibility for their behavior and recognize the damage caused by their drug abuse.[76] Counseling and job training are often part of the program, which may extend beyond a year. While therapeutic communities have their successes, they suffer from high dropout rates. At least 75% of newly admitted patients leave prematurely. There is also a lack of evidence as to how many recovering addicts are able to maintain abstinence after they have returned to the larger community.[77]

## Methadone Maintenance

**Methadone** is a synthetic opiate that is used as a substitute for heroin. It permits addicts to stop using heroin without developing severe withdrawal symptoms but does not produce the rush associated with heroin. However, methadone, like heroin, is addictive. Methadone also sharply reduces the rewarding effects of heroin, blocking the high that heroin normally produces. Methadone is taken orally in a single daily dose. This allows addicts on methadone maintenance to hold jobs or attend training programs after receiving their daily dose in the clinic.

Critics of methadone maintenance contend that it is a game of musical addictions. It substitutes one addiction for another. Supporters counter that methadone maintenance eliminates the need for addicts to resort to crime to support their habits and permits them to lead more functional lives. Studies bear out the belief that addicts in methadone treatment are less likely than other addicts to commit burglaries and robberies.[78] They may eventually withdraw from methadone as well. Yet critics point out that methadone maintenance programs suffer from high rates of early dropouts and relapsers. Results are better when methadone maintenance is combined with counseling.

**Methadone** A synthetic opiate that is used as a substitute for heroin in the treatment of heroin addiction.

**Naloxone** A drug that blocks the actions of opiates such as heroin, so that such drugs no longer produce a high when they are used.

## Psychological Interventions

Psychotherapy can help addicts reach a better understanding of the roots of the addictive behavior and learn more adaptive ways of handling stress and interpersonal problems. Family therapy and marital therapy can help deal with the interpersonal effects of drug abuse. Marital therapy may involve the use of a signed behavioral contract between the drug abuser and the spouse or partner. The contract might stipulate that as long as the drug abuser remains drug free, the partner agrees to refrain from negative comments about the patient's drug use or potential for relapse.

## Pharmacotherapeutic Approaches—Drugs against Drugs

Some drugs are used to treat addictions to other drugs. For example, **naloxone** is a nonaddictive drug that works as an opiate antagonist. That is, it blocks the high produced by heroin and other opiates. Heroin addicts may be placed on naloxone following detoxification. The problem with naloxone is that addicts who are bent on resuming their use of heroin can simply stop taking it.

Certain antidepressant drugs may be of value in treating cocaine addiction. The antidepressant desipramine (brand name Norpramin) has been shown to help cocaine addicts maintain abstinence in the first few weeks following withdrawal.[79] Desipramine increases the action of neurotransmitters in the brain, making it possible for addicts to derive more pleasure from life. They thus become less reliant on cocaine to experience pleasure.

## Self-Help Organizations

Many self-help organizations in the alcohol and drug abuse field offer assistance to addicts and their families. For information about the services provided by self-help organizations, such as Alcoholics Anonymous (AA) (discussed in Chapter 13), Narcotics Anonymous (NA), and Cocaine Anonymous (CA), consult the listing in Appendix A at the back of this book.

## Preventing Drug Abuse

An ounce of prevention is worth a pound of solution—in drug abuse as in other areas of life. Effective prevention involves schools, social service and law enforcement agencies, community organizations, and families.

**Close-up**
Making prevention work
T1212

**Roles for Antidrug Education** School-based antidrug education programs help make young people aware of the dangers of drugs and help them acquire skills to resist pressures from peers and dealers. While some youngsters can learn to "just say no," a broader-based approach is needed. To be effective, drug education programs must incorporate three important steps.[80]

- *Imparting basic information about drug use that is honest, factual, and complete, not exaggerated or distorted.*
- *Providing young people with behavior-change skills, especially refusal skills they can use to resist peer pressure to use drugs.* Training needs to make young people confident that they can turn down an invitation to smoke marijuana or crack with a friend or group of peers. Skills training needs to be combined with efforts aimed at changing young people's attitudes so that drug-using peers are no longer regarded as "cool."
- *Reinforcement of attitude and behavior changes.* Young people need praise, recognition, and other rewards for not using drugs. Young people need to see how drug use detracts from a healthy, attractive body.

Drug education needs to be coupled with intensive efforts to address and remediate the underlying reasons why many young people turn to drugs, such as feelings of alienation from mainstream society, lack of future directedness, and lack of hope about the future. Young people who feel that their futures count for something are less likely to throw away their prospects by turning to drugs.

**Roles for Community and Family** Social service agencies can help ensure that young people have food, shelter, and a stable family structure. Law enforcement agencies can help stop the flow of drugs into our communities and arrest and imprison drug dealers. Community residents can work with police officials to remove dealers from the streets. Many cities have designated "drug-free neighborhoods" in which citizens and shopkeepers are organized to watch for illegal drug activity and to report it to the police. Local patrols in many communities have warned drug dealers to get out of their neighborhoods. But unless more communities organize similar efforts, local citizens' groups may only succeed in moving dealers into the next neighborhood or town.

We need to face the hard reality that despite the best efforts of law enforcement agencies and community organizations, drugs will inevitably find a way into our neighborhoods as long as the demand for them exists. To cut off the supply, we need to cut off the demand. This is why educators and parents need to become involved in the effort to make children aware of the dangers of drugs. Parents need to model appropriate, drug-free ways of handling stress and tension. Parents who reach for a highball or a cigarette whenever their nerves are on edge send the wrong message to their children. Parents also need to become more directly involved in the antidrug education effort—becoming better informed themselves about the dangers of drugs and sharing this information with their children.

**Roles for Industry** Industry has important roles to play in drug prevention. Company-sponsored employee assistance programs (EAPs) can provide workers with increased access to health services, including drug and alcohol treatment and rehabilitation services. About one in three workers overall and about nine of ten in the largest companies now have access to an EAP. Drug testing is also gaining popularity as a way of identifying employees with drug problems. Most Americans believe that urine testing for drugs is appropriate under certain conditions, such as in workplaces where safety issues are paramount. Drug testing can also have a preventive effect by discouraging illicit drug use among employees who know they may be randomly tested at any time. In 1993, the federal government instituted new regulations requiring random breathalyzer tests to be used to detect alcohol use among more than 7 million transportation workers across the country, making this the largest drug-testing program in the country.[81] A combination of drug screening, workplace education focused on the dangers of drugs, and access to drug treatment and rehabilitation services offers the best chance of significantly reducing drug use in the workplace and achieving the ultimate goal of a drug-free workplace.

### think about it!

**Smart Quiz**
Q1207

- **Have you known anyone who received treatment for a drug abuse problem? What was the outcome?**
- **What do you think society can do to prevent drug abuse? What can you do to help others avoid drugs?**

**critical thinking** **Many teenagers today have parents who themselves smoked marijuana or used other drugs when they were younger. If you were one of those parents, what would you tell your kids about drugs?**

**critical thinking** **Agree or disagree and support your answer: The way to win the war against drugs is to decriminalize or legalize them.**

# Making Nondrug Choices for Healthy Living

## Take Charge

We all feel down, tense, or bored from time to time. We may also have an interest in exploring the inner parts of ourselves that remain unexplored. Perhaps we feel inadequate to meet the challenges we face. Or perhaps we see our futures as bleak and unrewarding. The question is, do we turn to drugs as an answer, or do we seek healthier, nondrug alternatives? Here are some nondrug alternatives to these problems:

*If you are . . .*

*feeling tense or anxious, try practicing relaxation or meditation, exercising, or listening to relaxing music.* If the problem persists, see a trained counselor or therapist.

*feeling bored, find a new activity or interest.* Get involved in athletics. Take up a hobby. Become involved in a political campaign or social cause.

*feeling angry, write down your feelings or channel your anger into more constructive pursuits.*

*feeling worthless, hopeless, or depressed, or putting yourself down, seek assistance from a friend or loved one.* Focus on your abilities and accomplishments, not on your deficits. If that doesn't help, seek professional assistance. You may be suffering from a treatable depression.

*wanting to probe the inner depths of your consciousness, try meditation or yoga, or seek the help of a counselor or spiritual leader.*

*pressured to use drugs by friends, learn how to say "no" politely but firmly.* If you need help saying no, take a course in assertiveness training or read a self-help book on self-assertion.

*seeking to heighten your sensations, try parachuting, in-line skating, mountain climbing, or some other way of getting your adrenaline flowing without chemical stimulants.*

*feeling stressed out, take a day or two off.* Restructure your time and establish more reasonable expectations of yourself.

*wanting to discover new insights on the human condition, take classes or workshops on philosophy and theology, attend lectures by prominent thinkers, read great works of literature, ponder great works of art, attend the symphony, and so on.* Let your mind connect with the great minds of the past and present.

*searching for deeper personal meaning in life, become more involved in spiritual activity in your church, synagogue, or mosque; explore alternative religions; do volunteer work in hospitals or charitable organizations; become involved in a cause you believe in.* Or seek personal counseling to get in touch with your inner self.

### Getting Help for a Drug Problem

Do you have a drug problem? Are you worried that you might? Or do you know someone with a drug problem but don't know where to turn for help? The National Institute on Drug Abuse (NIDA) operates a toll-free telephone service, 1-800-662-HELP, that can provide you with a referral to a drug abuse treatment program near you. You might also consult the listing of self-help organizations in the alcohol and drug abuse field in Appendix A at the back of this book.

### Helping Others Help Themselves

Does someone you know have a drug problem? Does he or she admit it? People with problems of drug abuse and drug dependence are often secretive about their drug-use habits and deny having a drug problem if directly confronted. Don't assume that if the person is really in trouble, he or she will know enough to admit that a problem exists and recognize the need for treatment. Be sensitive to the following warning signs of a possible drug problem:

- A change in behavior or habits, or a lack of attention to personal appearance.
- Taking an unusual number of days off from work or school.
- Not seeing usual friends or making new friends with whom the person doesn't seem to have much in common.
- Increased irritability or distractibility.
- Keeping more to oneself.
- Making repeated excuses for missing get-togethers.
- Seeming preoccupied when socializing.
- Seeming unusually suspicious and guarded.
- Showing signs of being high at times.
- Asking repeatedly to borrow money.
- Is discovered stealing or seems to be around when things mysteriously disappear.

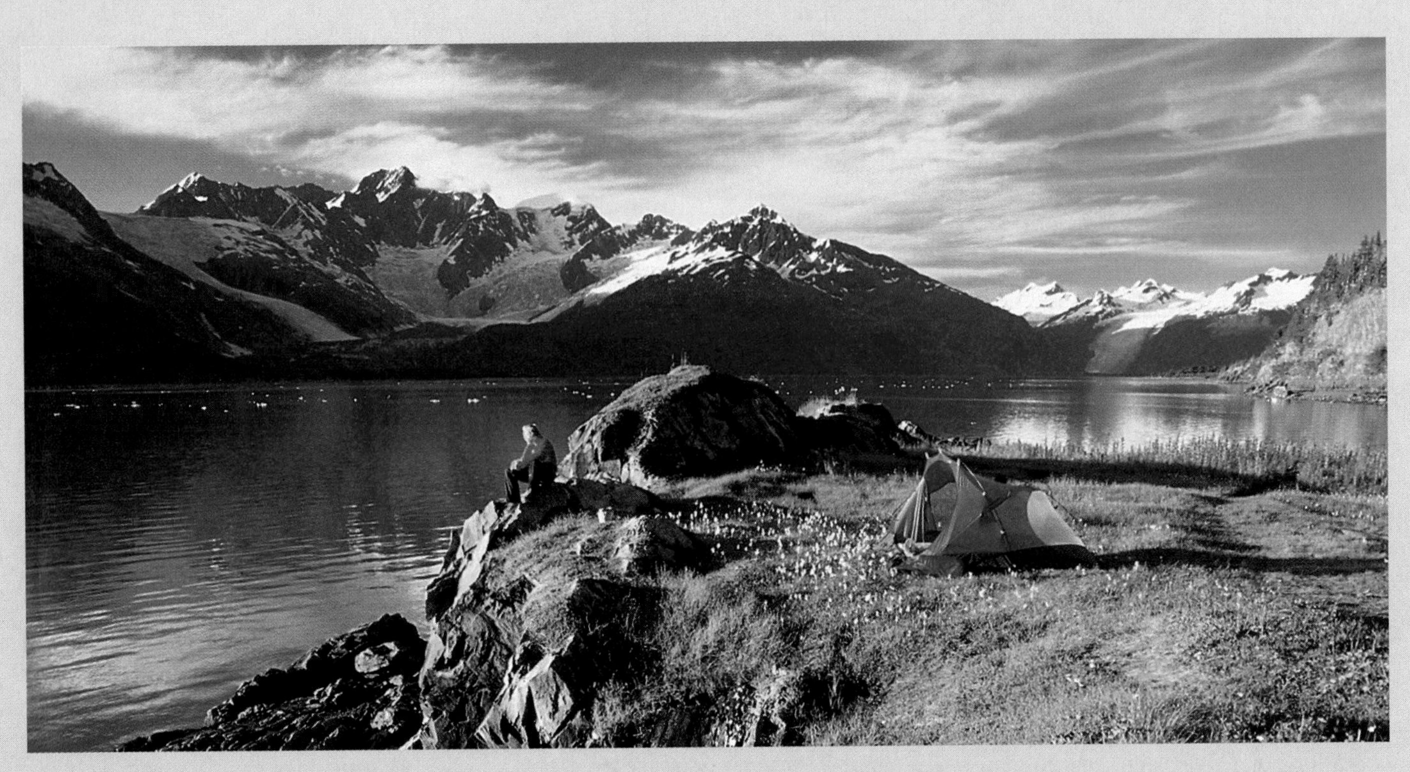

***Exploring Nature*** Mountain climbing and other outdoor adventures can get your adrenaline flowing without chemical stimulants. Many people find that spending time enjoying the natural environment helps to relieve stress.

**Confronting the Problem** What if you suspect that someone close to you has a drug problem? How should you handle it? The easiest way is also the worst way—just ignoring it and hoping that the person will come to face up to it. A person with a drug problem can wind up dead from an overdose, become a victim of drug-related violence, suffer a drug-related medical problem, or get arrested during the time you're waiting for the person to face the problem. Be gentle, but also persistent and firm. Insist that the person seek help. Avoid becoming a codependent. Set up limits and respect those limits—no excuses for the person's behavior, no loans that can be turned into drugs, no blanket acceptance of promises not meant to be kept, etc. Try to get the person to see that his or her problems are not unsolvable. Point out that treatments are available. Find the name of a drug treatment counselor and offer to accompany the person to see this individual. If the person still refuses to seek help, consult a drug treatment counselor yourself, or contact one of the self-help organizations listed in the appendix of this book. People who have had experience with this type of problem often have helpful suggestions to break through the denial that prevents the addict from beginning the process of recovery.

## Learning More about Drug Abuse

Want the latest information and research on drug abuse? You can call or write the National Clearinghouse for Alcohol and Drug Information (NCADI), Box 2345, Rockville, MD 20847 (800–729–6686). The clearinghouse distributes videos, magazine and journal articles, abstracts of the latest research results, prevention materials, and descriptions of drug abuse treatment and prevention programs throughout the United States.

Smart Quiz
Q1208

# SUMMING UP

## Questions and Answers

### TYPES OF DRUGS

**1. What are drugs?** Drugs are chemical substances that affect people's health, feelings, and behavior. *Drug misuse* is the use of a drug for the wrong reason or by the wrong person. *Drug abuse* is repeated use of a drug despite the fact that it is connected with personal, occupational, or health problems.

**2. What is the difference between over-the-counter and prescription drugs?** Over-the-counter (OTC) drugs are available without prescription. However, OTC drugs can be harmful when they are misused. OTC medications are best used for recurrent conditions that have been diagnosed by a physician.

### PSYCHOACTIVE DRUGS

**3. What are psychoactive drugs?** Psychoactive drugs act on the brain to affect one's mental state. They include depressants, stimulants, and hallucinogens.

**4. What are some medical uses of psychoactive drugs?** Opiates are used as painkillers. Sleep and diet aids help some people with insomnia and obesity.

**5. How are psychoactive drugs administered?** They can be taken orally, by inhaling (snorting), or by injection (intravenously, intramuscularly, or intracutaneously).

### EFFECTS OF DRUGS

**6. What factors enter into the effects of a drug?** These factors include the route of administration, the dosage level, the person's biological responsiveness to the drug, the person's frame of mind, the presence of other drugs in the body, and social factors.

### DRUG ABUSE AND DEPENDENCE

**7. What is physiological dependence on a drug?** This is addiction—meaning that the drug alters the person's body so that the presence of the drug becomes the normal state of affairs. Physiological dependence is known by tolerance and an abstinence syndrome.

**8. What is psychological dependence on a drug?** This means that the person comes to rely on the drug as a way of coping with stress.

**9. What factors contribute to drug dependence?** These include environmental factors (e.g., peer pressure and exposure to family members and friends who abuse drugs), psychological factors (such as feelings of hopelessness), and genetic factors (such as high tolerance for negative drug effects).

**10. What are the stages of becoming dependent on drugs?** These include the stages of experimentation, routine use, and (in the case of addictive drugs) addiction.

**11. What are gateway drugs?** These are drugs whose use often leads to use of illicit or more powerful drugs. For example, alcohol and tobacco are gateways for harder-drug use among many adolescents.

### WHO USES ILLICIT DRUGS?

**12. How common is use of illicit drugs?** As many as half of young people have used an illicit drug at least once. We also appear to be in the midst of an up-trend in the case of the school-age population.

### TYPES OF PSYCHOACTIVE DRUGS

**13. What are depressants?** Depressants lower the activity of the nervous system, produce feelings of relaxation, and provide relief from anxiety and tension. Depressants are addictive. Withdrawal from depressants is best managed by health professionals.

**14. What are stimulants?** Stimulants heighten the activity of the nervous system and can create feelings of euphoria and self-confidence. Caffeine and cocaine are known to be addictive.

**15. What are hallucinogenic drugs?** These drugs alter sensory perceptions, distorting reality and producing hallucinations. They may also produce feelings of relaxation or euphoria in some cases, or paranoia or panic in other cases. Hallucinogens are not known to be addictive. Some users experience flashbacks.

**16. What are phencyclidine and marijuana?** Phencyclidine (PCP), or "angel dust," is a deliriant that can produce states of confusion and disorientation, hallucinations, and dangerous, even violent behavior. Marijuana, the most widely used illicit drug, has a range of effects depending on dosage level. Prolonged or regular use can lead to impaired immune functioning and other adverse health effects.

**17. What are some other psychoactive drugs?** Inhalants are chemical fumes which are inhaled for their psychoactive effects. They are extremely dangerous, even deadly. So-called designer drugs are synthesized to mimic the effects of illicit drugs.

**18. What are anabolic steroids?** These are synthetic (laboratory-made) versions of the male sex hormone testosterone. They help build muscle mass but have undesirable side effects, such as reducing HDL ("good cholesterol") levels, and are connected with some kinds of cancer.

### DRUG TREATMENT—BECOMING DRUG FREE, REMAINING DRUG FREE

**19. How are problems of drug abuse and dependence treated?** A variety of treatment approaches are used, including detoxification, use of therapeutic communities, methadone maintenance programs, psychological interventions, pharmacotherapeutic approaches, and self-help organizations.

## Suggested Readings

*Physician's Desk Reference.* Montvale, NJ: Medical Economics Company. The physician's desktop compendium of drugs from A to Z—their uses, side effects, and complications—updated annually.

*The PDR Family Guide to Prescription Drugs.* (3rd Ed.). Montvale, NJ: Medical Economics Company, 1995. From the publishers of the *Physician's Desk Reference* (PDR), it provides important information to patients and their families on prescription drugs and their side effects, including special warnings and instructions for use of particular medications.

*The Complete Drug Reference.* Yonkers, NY: Consumer Reports Books, 1996. A consumer-oriented home reference for medications.

**White, J. M.** *Drug Dependence.* Englewood Cliffs, NJ: Prentice Hall, 1991. A good overview of biological, psychological, and social perspectives on drug dependence. Emphasizes the common features that underlie drug use and dependence for a wide range of drugs, including accepted drugs like caffeine, restricted drugs like alcohol, and prohibited drugs like cocaine and heroin.

# Responsible Drinking

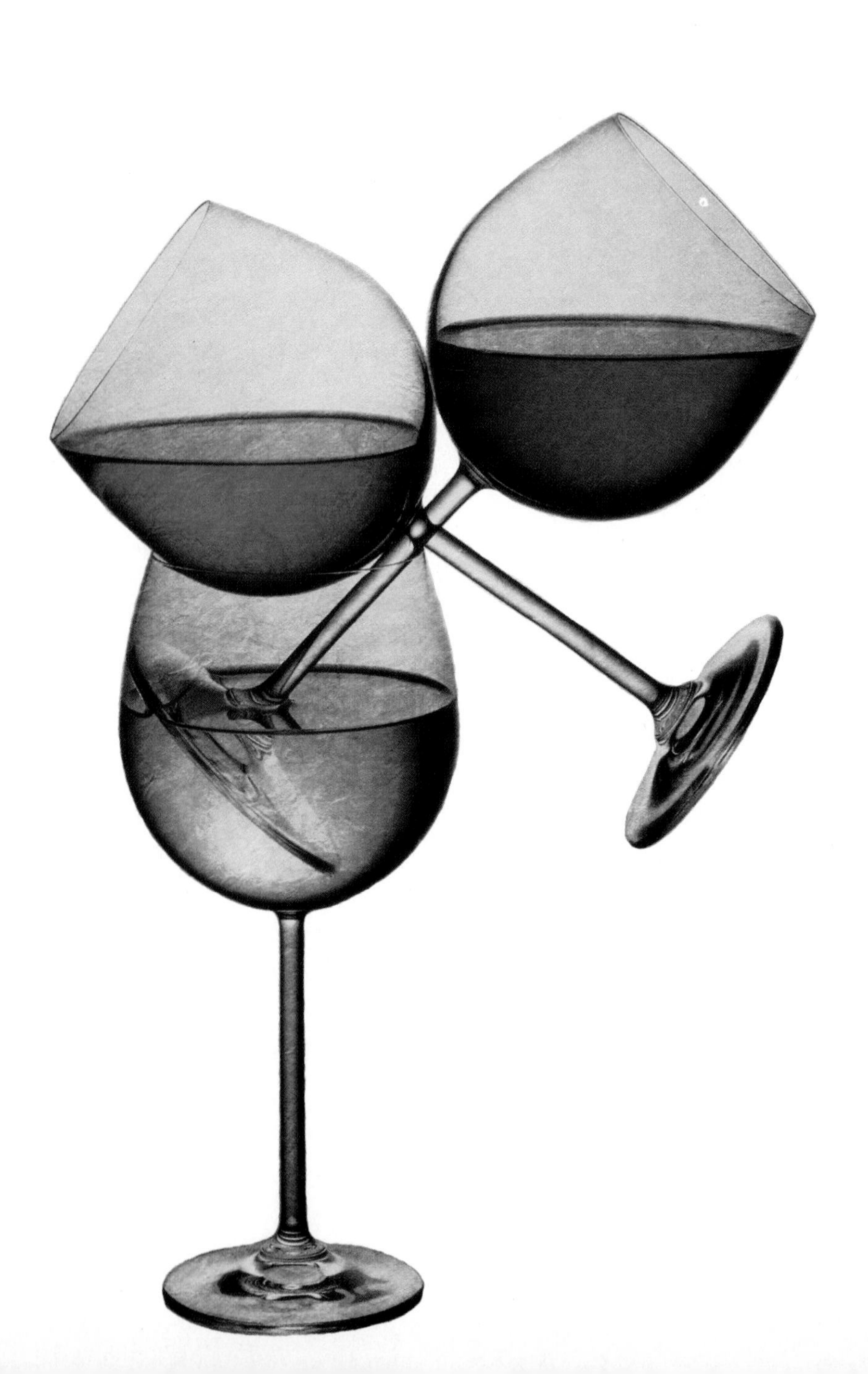

## DID YOU KNOW THAT

- People who can "hold their liquor" are at a *higher* risk of developing a drinking problem? p.348
- If you drink on an empty stomach, it will affect you more than if you drink after a meal? p.349
- In general it takes less alcohol to intoxicate a woman than a man? p.350
- As many as 10% of all deaths in the United States can be blamed on the use of alcohol? p.352
- Light to moderate intake of alcohol can reduce the risk of coronary heart disease? p.354
- More teenagers and young adults die from alcohol-related motor vehicle accidents than from any other cause? p.357
- The typical college student spends more money on alcohol than on textbooks? p.358
- It can be dangerous—indeed deadly—to let a person who blacks out from drinking too much just sleep it off? p.359
- Drinking coffee will not sober you up if you are drunk? p.371

*Alcohol is many things to many people. We use it to toast the New Year, to christen ships, to celebrate our achievements, and to salute our friends and loved ones. Offering drinks to guests is a common gesture of hospitality in our culture. Wine and beer are a staple on many dinner tables. No "fine" restaurant would be without its wine list.*

*Some people use alcohol as a bedtime relaxant to prepare for sleep. Others use it to cope with the tension of meeting new people. Some use it to quell feelings of anxiety or to take the edge off the stresses of everyday life. Because alcohol kills germs on contact, it is even found in mouthwashes.*

*Yes, alcohol is many things to many people. But alcohol is first and foremost a drug. Because alcohol is drunk, not injected like heroin or snorted or smoked like cocaine, people who drink alcohol may not think of themselves as drug users, but they are. Alcohol is the most widely used drug in the United States and the world. Next to tobacco, alcohol causes the most widespread damage to health of any psychoactive substance.*

*Most adults in our society drink alcohol at least occasionally. Most who drink do so in moderation. However, about one adult in ten, nearly 14 million people, suffers from alcoholism or alcohol abuse.*[1]

*Most people who drink do not become problem drinkers, but others cannot control their drinking. Some people are well advised to avoid alcohol altogether. They may have medical conditions that make drinking unhealthful, or alcohol may interact with their medications. Whether to use alcohol is a personal decision. Responsible drinking involves drawing the line between use and misuse and recognizing the need for help if a problem with alcohol develops.*

# 13

## WHAT IS ALCOHOL?

**Alcohol** is a chemical compound that takes the form of a colorless, flammable liquid. The psychoactive substance in alcohol is *ethyl alcohol*—**ethanol,** for short. In certain amounts, ethyl alcohol is considered safe to drink. Other kinds of alcohol have different household or medicinal uses but are toxic if ingested. Among these are isopropyl (rubbing alcohol) and methyl (wood alcohol).

Alcoholic beverages are manufactured by different processes, including **fermentation,** from which beer and wine are derived, and **distillation,** which produces hard liquors such as vodka, gin, and whiskey. Fermentation has been used to produce alcohol since the earliest agricultural societies in prehistoric times. In fermentation, yeast is used to convert sugars in plant material into ethyl alcohol and carbon dioxide.[2] Distillation is the process of boiling out alcohol from the fermentation process and condensing the vapors back into a liquid form. Distillation results in the higher alcohol concentrations found in hard liquors.

Alcoholic beverages are graded in terms of their alcoholic content, or *proof.* The proof value of an alcoholic beverage is two times the alcohol concentration of the beverage. A beverage consisting of 50% alcohol is considered 100 proof. One that is 25% alcohol is 50 proof. Hard liquors generally vary between 80 proof and 100 proof (or 40 to 50% alcohol). Wines are typically 18 to 28 proof (or 9 to 14% alcohol). Most beers contain 3 to 6% alcohol (or 6 to 12 proof). Heavier, darker beers, such as stout, are 6 to 7% alcohol. Malt liquors contain as much as 8 or 9% alcohol.

How much pure or straight alcohol (also called absolute alcohol) does the average alcoholic beverage contain? The answer depends on the size of the drink and the amount of pure alcohol it contains (see Figure 13.1). A drink consisting of a *jigger* (typically 1.5 ounces) of 80-proof liquor, such as vodka, gin, rum, or whiskey, contains about 0.5 ounces of pure alcohol. This amount of alcohol is equivalent to that found in a 5-ounce glass of wine or a 12-ounce can of beer.

**Alcohol** An intoxicating liquid that contains ethyl alcohol; other forms of alcohol include methyl (wood) alcohol and rubbing alcohol.

**Ethanol** Another term for ethyl alcohol, the psychoactive substance in alcohol.

**Fermentation** A process by which yeast is used to convert sugar into ethyl alcohol and carbon dioxide.

**Distillation** A process of boiling out the alcohol from the fermentation process and then condensing the vapors back into a liquid form.

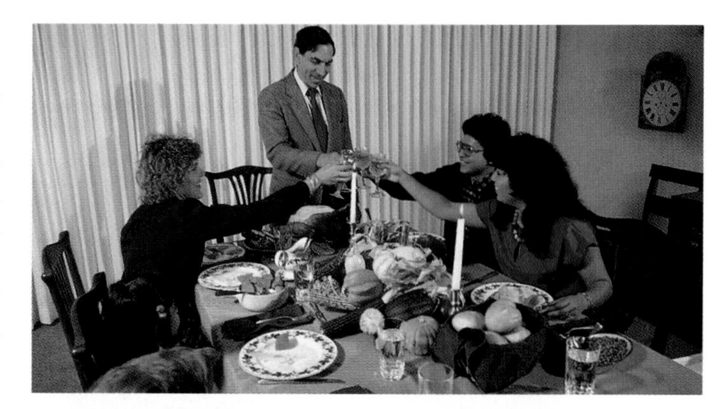

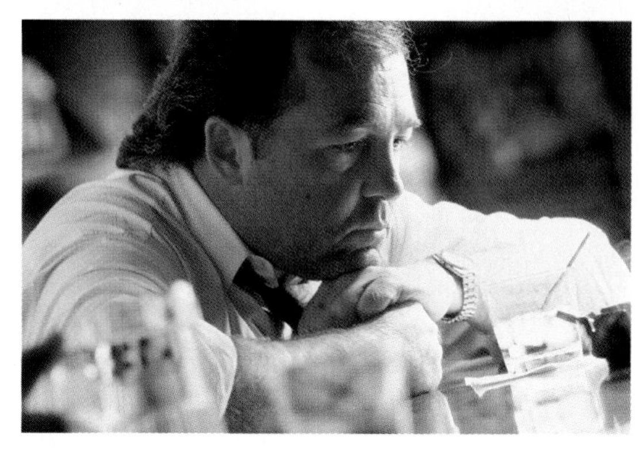

***The Different Faces of Alcohol Use—and Abuse***
Alcohol is used in many contexts, including celebrating happy occasions. However, some people turn to alcohol to drown their sorrows, which may only compound their problems by leading to patterns of abuse and dependence.

### Who Drinks?

Two of three adults in the United States drink alcoholic beverages.[3] Of those who drink, about half are light drinkers. The other half are moderate or heavy drinkers. Yet alcohol consumption is not distributed evenly within the population. About half the nation's alcohol consumption is accounted for by 10% of the population.

Younger people are more likely to drink than are older people. Alcohol use is most prevalent among 21- to 34-year-olds. Whites are more likely than blacks or Hispanics to use alcohol (see Figure 13.2). Within each of these groups, men are more likely to drink than women. Although the legal drinking age is now 21 in every state, more than half of junior and senior high school students have used alcohol during the past year, and more than a third drink weekly.[4] Young people typically have their first drink by about the age of 12 or 13.

The average drinker in the United States consumes 39 gallons of alcoholic beverages a year: 34

**Figure 13.1** *How Much Alcohol Is in That Drink?*

To figure out how much absolute alcohol is contained in an alcoholic beverage, start with the proof value of the beverage, then divide that number by half and divide again by 100. This represents the percent alcohol content. (If the percent alcohol content is shown on the label, you can skip the first step.) Now take this percent value and multiply it by the number of ounces of the alcoholic beverage. This gives you the number of ounces of absolute alcohol in the beverage. Got it? Practice using this method by calculating the amount of absolute alcohol contained in an 8 ounce can of 10-proof beer.

The answer is 0.4 ounces of absolute alcohol. This was derived by first dividing 10 (the proof level) by 2, which yields 5. This number is then divided by 100, yielding .05. This number, .05, represents the percent alcohol content. Multiplying this number by 8, the number of ounces of beer in the can, yields 0.4, the number of ounces of pure alcohol in the can of beer.

Now you should be able to figure out which of the following has more absolute alcohol.

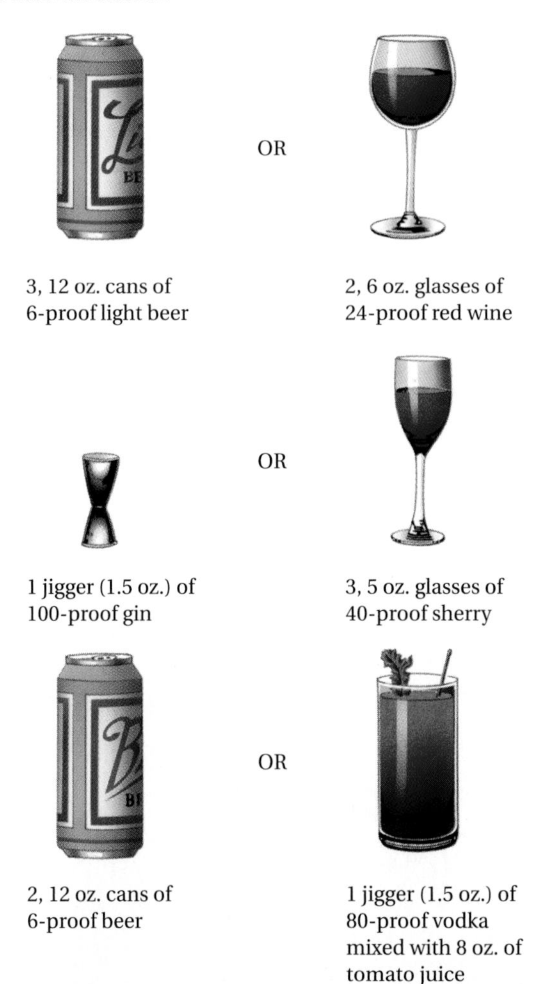


Answers: (1) The three cans of beer contain 1.08 ounces of absolute alcohol, which is less than the 1.44 ounces in the two glasses of wine. (2) The one jigger of hard liquor contains 0.75 ounces of absolute alcohol, which is less than a third of the 3 ounces contained in the three glasses of sherry; (3) the two cans of beer have 0.72 ounces of absolute alcohol, while the vodka and tomato juice drink contains 0.6 ounces. The amount of a mixer, such as tomato juice, doesn't change the alcohol content of the beverage since it does not add any alcohol.

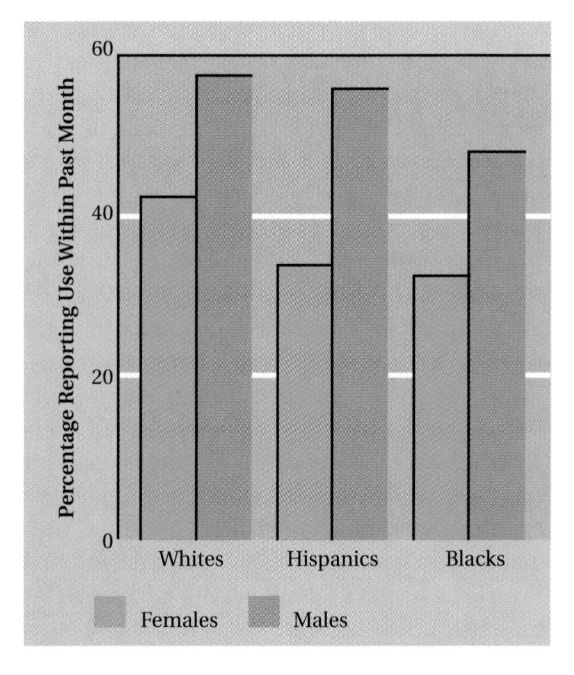


**Figure 13.2** *Who Drinks* *Source:* National Household Survey on Drug Abuse: Population Estimates 1992.

gallons of beer, 3 gallons of wine, and 2 gallons of distilled spirits such as whiskey.[5] Though consumption of alcoholic beverages remains very popular, the number of people who drink alcoholic beverages declined from 113 million in 1985 to about 100 million by the 1990s.[6] Alcohol consumption per capita (per person) also dropped.[7] Perhaps rising health awareness and greater publicity about the harmful effects of heavy drinking account for these reductions. Whatever the reasons for the decline, the proportions of men and women in their twenties who drink heavily has been rising.[8] Thus we can expect alcoholism and alcohol-related problems to increase in the future. Widespread problem drinking on college campuses and among high school and even junior high school students is a further sign that alcohol abuse remains a daunting challenge.

## Why Do People Drink?

People use alcohol for many reasons. Young people may begin drinking because their friends do, and they want to "fit in" or be accepted. Some adolescents begin drinking because it makes them feel more independent or adult. Whatever the initial reasons for alcohol use, most young people use alcohol because they enjoy the effects or to get "high," not to prove that they are adults.

The reinforcement value of alcohol has much to do with its use. Behaviors that lead to pleasant outcomes tend to be repeated. If the use of a drug makes people feel good, or relieves them of negative feelings like anxiety, they are more likely to use it again. Alcohol has direct effects on the brain. Many users report that it helps quell anxiety and produces feelings of pleasure and well-being. Alcohol can also have negative effects. It can produce unpleasant sensations when one drinks too much or too fast. It can cause a **hangover** the following day. For some people, these unpleasant sensations are a built-in deterrent to excessive drinking. But for genetic reasons, some people are less likely than others to experience unpleasant effects when they drink heavily.[9] Ironically, their ability to tolerate large amounts of alcohol may predispose them to drink heavily, which can set the stage for alcoholism.

Social factors also affect alcohol use and abuse. Many of us go out drinking with friends and offer guests alcoholic beverages when entertaining at home. When social activities regularly revolve around alcohol, use may edge into abuse.

Psychological factors are also involved in alcohol use and abuse. People who are troubled by anxiety over their jobs or social lives may be drawn to the calming effects of alcohol. Alcohol becomes a type of self-medication. Because long-term heavy drinking can lead to health problems and social problems, people who turn to alcohol to alleviate their problems may actually compound them. Positive expectations about alcohol use also affect patterns of use and abuse. People who believe that alcohol will make them more sexually responsive or sexually alluring, reduce tension, make them more outgoing or assertive, or produce or enhance feelings of pleasure are more likely to drink and to develop problems with alcohol.[10] College students who hold positive expectations about alcohol use are at greater risk of becoming problem drinkers.[11]

Smart Quiz Q1301

### think about it!

- Do you drink? Under what circumstances? Why?
- If you drink, what kinds of alcoholic beverages do you prefer? Why?

**Hangover** The unpleasant aftereffects of drinking too much alcohol, characterized by such symptoms as headache and nausea.

## EFFECTS OF ALCOHOL

Alcohol is classified as a depressant drug because it depresses, or slows down, the functioning of the body. Its biochemical effects are similar to those of a class of minor tranquilizers, the benzodiazepines, which includes the drugs diazepam (trade name Valium) and chlordiazepoxide (Librium). Alcohol is a kind of over-the-counter tranquilizer. Like other psychoactive drugs, alcohol has both physical and psychological effects.

### Physical Effects

Alcohol depresses the central nervous system and brain mechanisms regulating such bodily processes as heart rate and respiration rate. The more a person drinks, the stronger the depressant effects become. After a few drinks, the brain mechanisms controlling the sense of balance are disturbed, making it more difficult to walk a straight line or stand with one's eyes closed without swaying. Speech becomes slurred and incoherent. Heavier doses begin to act on the parts of the brain that control vital functions such as heart rate, respiration, and body temperature. In higher amounts, the slowing down of vital functions can induce a state of stupor, unconsciousness, and even death, especially if alcohol is combined with use of other depressants, such as sedatives or tranquilizers like Valium. Alcohol also has analgesic (pain-killing) properties. It dulls minor aches and pains. While alcohol may help induce sleep, larger amounts can disrupt normal sleep cycles and lead to a hangover upon awakening.

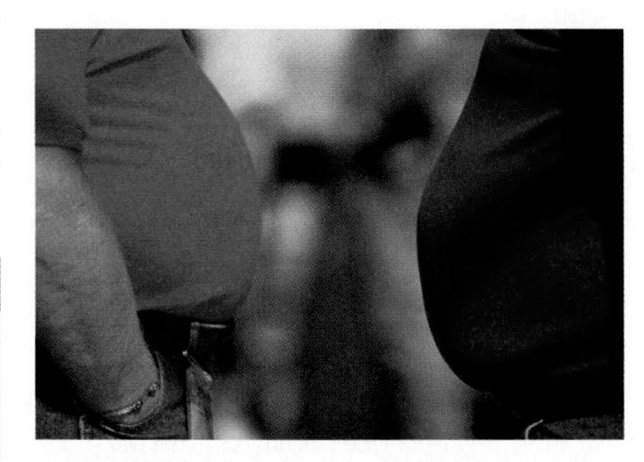

***Beer Bellies*** All alcoholic beverages, not just beer, are loaded with calories that may become stored in the body as fat. Habitual use of alcohol can also lower the body's metabolic rate, which can lead to additional fat accumulating in the hips, thighs, and, of course, the belly.

You've probably heard the expression "beer belly." There is no question that beer, which contains 140 to 150 calories per 12-ounce can, can put on the pounds. And some of it settles in that paunch in the middle called a *beer belly.* A 5-ounce glass of wine holds about 125 calories. A jigger (1.5 ounces) of an 80-proof distilled spirit like gin or vodka has about 100 calories, which doesn't count the mixer. Tonic water adds some 72 calories per 8 ounces. But it may not just be the calories in alcoholic beverages that put on the pounds. Habitual use of alcohol slows down the body's metabolic rate—the speed at which the body burns fat.[12] Fat that is not broken down during metabolism and eliminated from the body gets stored in the hips, thighs, and—you guessed it—the belly.

**Intoxication** Many psychoactive substances, including alcohol and drugs like heroin or cocaine, have chemical effects on the body that can result in **intoxication.** Alcohol intoxication or *drunkenness* is characterized by impaired coordination, motor skills, and judgment; slurring of speech; difficulty concentrating; confusion; and sometimes belligerence.

How much alcohol does it take to get a person drunk? Intoxication depends on many factors, including what is drunk, and the person's weight, gender, and ability to break down alcohol in the stomach. The more alcohol you drink, the more intoxicated you'll become. Generally speaking, the less you weigh, the less alcohol you can consume before becoming intoxicated. Heavier people have more water in their bodies, and water dilutes alcohol.

Alcohol enters the bloodstream through the stomach and small intestine. The speed of absorption into the bloodstream depends on such factors as the amount of food in the stomach and the rate of drinking. The less alcohol broken down in the stomach, the more that passes directly into the bloodstream—and the more intoxicated you become. If you down a shot of whisky on an empty stomach, it will enter your bloodstream and affect you sooner and harder than if you had sipped an after-dinner drink.

You can reduce your chances of becoming drunk if you drink slowly and limit the alcohol content of your drinks, either by diluting them or drinking beverages containing less alcohol. When you drink slowly, you give your **liver,** the organ that mainly metabolizes alcohol, more time to break it down. The liver can metabolize alcohol at a steady rate of about a half ounce an hour. That translates to about one standard alcoholic drink per hour. (A standard drink consists of 1.5 ounces of an 80-proof hard liquor, 5 ounces of wine, or 12 ounces of beer.) The liver converts about 90% of the alcohol into carbon dioxide and water, which are excreted from the body. The remaining 10% is excreted through the lungs or the urine. As you drink more than your liver is capable of metabolizing, the amount of alcohol in your bloodstream, which is called the **blood alcohol level (BAL),** rises and you become intoxicated.

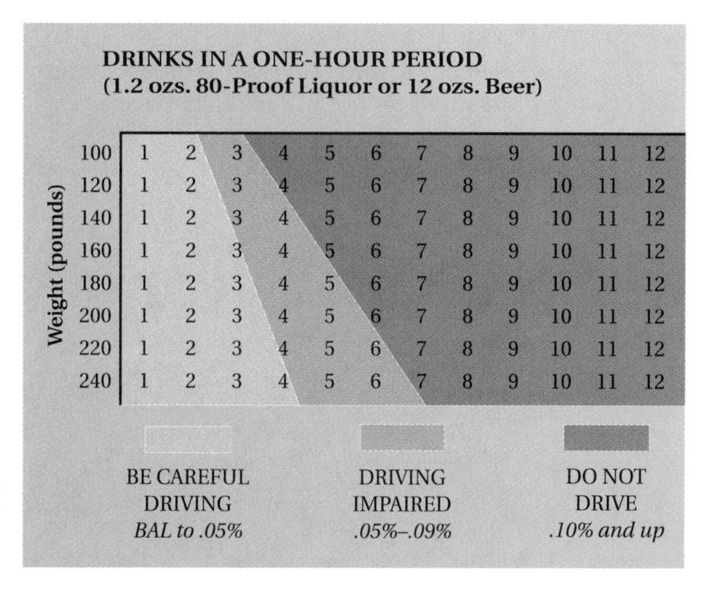


**Figure 13.3** ***BAL and Alcohol Intake*** Approximate values of BAL as a function of alcohol consumption in a 1-hour period. For example, if you weigh 180 pounds and had four beers in 1 hour, your BAL would be between .05 and .09% and your driving ability would be seriously impaired. Six beers in the same 1-hour period would give you a BAL of over .10%—the level accepted as proof of intoxication. (After National Highway Traffic Safety Administration.)

In all states, a BAL of 0.10% (10 parts alcohol to 10,000 parts of blood) is considered an illegal level of intoxication. In most states, a BAL of 0.08% is the legal limit. The average person would need to consume one drink an hour for every 35 pounds of body weight to reach a BAL of 0.10%. For a 100-pound person, this amounts to about 3 drinks; for a 150-pound person, about 4 drinks (see Table 13.1 and Figure 13.3).

Individual differences in tolerance should also be considered. Some people, alcoholics especially,

**Intoxication** A state of drunkenness brought on by the use of alcohol or other intoxicating drugs.

**Liver** The largest organ in the body. Performs a vital role in many metabolic processes, including the metabolism of alcohol.

**Blood alcohol level (BAL)** The amount of alcohol in the bloodstream, as measured in percent.

TABLE 13.1

**Percent Alcohol Content, Number of Drinks to Reach 0.10% BAL, and Calorie Content of Alcoholic Beverages**

| Alcoholic Beverage | % Alcohol (approximate) | Approximate Number of Drinks per Hour to Reach 0.10% BAL (per serving size) for 150-Pound Person | Approximate Calories (per serving size) |
|---|---|---|---|
| *Hard Liquors (whiskey, vodka, gin, tequila, rum)* | 40–50 | 4 1.5-oz. jiggers | 100 |
| *Beers (light, regular)* | 3–6 | 4 12-oz. cans or bottles | 140–150 (regular)<br>95 (light) |
| *Table wines (red or white, dry)* | 9–14 | 4 5-oz. glasses | 125 |
| *Fortified wines (sherry, port)* | 18–20 | 4 3.5-oz. glasses | 135 |

develop a higher tolerance for alcohol. They can consume large amounts of alcohol without showing obvious signs of intoxication, even though their blood alcohol level registers 0.15% or more. This doesn't mean that they are as capable of performing skilled tasks, such as driving a car, as when they are sober (although they may *believe* that they are). For people who have not built up a tolerance for alcohol, intoxication may occur with a blood alcohol level as low as 0.03%. People with a higher degree of tolerance may drink to levels that become dangerous, even life-threatening.

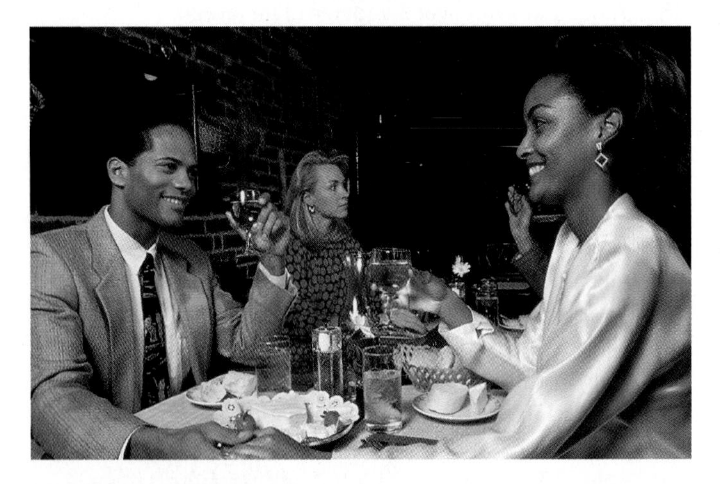

***Men, Women, and Alcohol*** Women are less likely to become problem drinkers than men, in part because of greater cultural constraints on excessive drinking in women and possibly because of women's greater biological sensitivity to the effects of alcohol. On average, women will become as intoxicated as men from drinking half as much alcohol.

**Gender Differences in Sensitivity to Alcohol** Women tend to become intoxicated by less alcohol than men. One reason is that women tend to weigh less than men. Another is that they have less of the stomach enzyme *alcohol dehydrogenase,* which breaks down alcohol in the stomach. Thus one drink may have the same effect on a woman that two drinks would have on a man. Women's greater sensitivity to alcohol may work as a biological constraint on excessive drinking among women.

American men, including college men, are more likely than women to drink, and to drink heavily.[13] Alcoholism is two to five times more common in men than women. However, the gender gap appears to be narrowing. An increasing percentage of alcoholics are women, especially younger women.[14]

**Behavioral Effects of Blood Alcohol Level** The behavioral effects of alcohol depend on the amount, or dosage, that is ingested. A person with a BAL in the range of 0.01 to 0.05% may feel mildly euphoric or somewhat relaxed (see Table 13.2). By the time the BAL climbs above 0.05%, the person may notice a reduction in alertness and feel less socially inhibited. The person may feel cheerful and more self-confident, but be less capable of exercising good judgment, which can lead to behavior that the person would ordinarily reject, such as risky sex.[15] As the BAL rises from 0.05% to 0.10%, fine motor coordination falls off and reaction time slows notably. As the BAL increases to

TABLE 13.2

**Behavioral Effects of Blood Alcohol Levels[16]**

| Blood Alcohol Level | Behavioral Effects |
|---|---|
| 0.05% | Lowered alertness; usually good feeling; release of inhibitions; impaired judgment |
| 0.10% | Slowed reaction times; impaired motor function; less caution |
| 0.15% | Large, consistent increases in reaction time |
| 0.20% | Marked depression in sensory and motor capability; decidedly intoxicated |
| 0.25% | Severe motor disturbance; staggering; sensory perceptions greatly impaired; smashed! |
| 0.30% | Stuporous but conscious; no comprehension of the world around them |
| 0.35% | Surgical anesthesia; minimal level causing death |
| 0.40% | About half of those at this level die |

0.15%, reaction time slows further and the person may not be able to stand steadily or walk in a straight line. With a BAL of 0.20 to 0.25%, the person is noticeably intoxicated and may pass out. Sensory perception is severely affected. It is difficult to see or hear clearly. Peripheral vision may be lost and speech is slurred. The person may stagger and need help moving about. If the BAL continues to increase to a level of 0.30 to 0.35%, the person becomes stuporous and drifts into unconsciousness. Deaths may occur at BALs of 0.35% or more. About half of those who reach a BAL of 0.40% die.

## Psychological Effects

Alcohol affects the brain directly. It produces feelings of euphoria and elation but also clouds judgment and impairs concentration. Some people find that alcohol boosts their self-esteem and drowns out their self-doubts, at least temporarily. But heavy, regular use of alcohol deepens feelings of depression and impairs self-esteem.

Some people feel that alcohol makes them more sexually responsive. But enhanced sexual responsiveness may reflect their expectations about alcohol or a loosening of their inhibitions, rather than the direct effects of alcohol. Alcohol is a depressant drug that may actually depress sexual responsivity and the ability to perform sexually. Yet some people may *feel* sexier because alcohol dulls their ability to perceive the consequences of their sexual behavior. As Shakespeare so aptly put it in his play *Macbeth:* Alcohol "provokes the desire, but takes away the performance."

Close-up
Alcohol and sex
T1301

The effects of alcohol vary from person to person. Different people metabolize the drug differently. They hold different attitudes toward, and expectations about, the drug. People who expect alcohol to boost their social confidence or sexual responsiveness may act the role. They may do things they might not otherwise do, such as approach a stranger at a party. Feelings of elation and euphoria may wash away their inhibitions, self-criticisms, and misgivings. Then, too, alcohol use is associated with a liberated role in our culture. People who engage in questionable behavior while drinking can later blame the alcohol.

**Alcohol and Violence** Many crimes of violence, including rape, robbery, and assault, are connected with the use of alcohol.[17] More than a third of the prison inmates in the United States were drinking heavily before committing their crimes. More than half the people convicted of murder and rape, and more than two-thirds of those convicted of manslaughter, were drinking before they committed their crimes (see Table 13.3). College administrators report that alcohol is involved in more than half of the crimes reported on campus, ranging from assaults to damage to residence halls.[18] A survey of students at a southeastern university showed that 55% of students who reported committing sexual assaults and 53% of students who had been sexually assaulted admitted to having been drinking before the assault.[19]

TABLE 13.3

**Alcohol and Violent Crime[20]**

| Crime | Percentage of Perpetrators Who Were Drinking before the Commission of Their Crimes |
|---|---|
| Murder/attempted murder | 54% |
| Manslaughter | 68% |
| Rape/sexual assault | 52% |
| Robbery | 48% |
| Assault | 62% |
| Burglary | 44% |

If alcohol tranquilizes the nervous system, how do we explain the link between alcohol and violence? Let us suggest several reasons.[21] Alcohol may reduce inhibitions that might otherwise restrain violence. People who have been drinking may be less capable of weighing the consequences of their behavior. Then, too, crimes closely linked to the use of alcohol, assault and manslaughter, frequently involve misunderstandings that escalate out of hand. Mixing alcohol with a hot temper may increase the chance of a violent outburst. Using alcohol may make it more difficult for people to read other people's motives accurately, leading them to perceive a hostile intent in other people's behavior that may trigger a violent response.

Use of alcohol can also put people at greater risk of becoming victims of crimes. Criminals choose victims who look vulnerable. People who are intoxicated may appear to be an "easy mark" or fail to take normal precautions to protect themselves in public. According to a national survey of college students, half of the respondents who had been victimized by crime had been using drugs or alcohol just beforehand.[22]

## Health Effects of Heavy Drinking

Alcohol abuse and alcoholism account for about 100,000 deaths in the United States each year. This number includes deaths due to alcohol-related diseases and motor vehicle and other accidents.[23] Following tobacco, alcohol is the second leading cause of premature death in our society. Between 3 and 10% of all deaths in the United States can be blamed on the use of alcohol.[24] Men who drink heavily stand nearly twice the risk of dying before the age of 65 as men who do not drink. Women who drink heavily are more than three times as likely to die before the age of 65 as women who do not drink.[25]

Chronic, heavy alcohol use affects virtually every organ and body system—directly or indirectly (see Figure 13.4). The health effects of alcohol depend on the amount and duration of use. Heavy alcohol use is linked to cirrhosis of the liver and cancers of the mouth, pharynx, larynx, stomach, and liver, and possibly of the breast (see Chapter 18). Some people are genetically more susceptible to some alcohol-related illnesses than others. Adding heavy smoking to heavy drinking is an even deadlier mix, increasing the risk of cancers of the mouth and pharynx by 38 times.[26] The demonstrated links between heavy drinking and cancer have not been fully explained. Chronic alcohol use weakens the immune system, making it less capable of ridding the body of cancerous cells, which then grow into cancerous lesions.[27] Heavy drinking may also directly damage cells and the DNA within them, or make cells more sensitive to chemical carcinogens (cancer-causing agents), such as those found in cigarette smoke.

**Close-up**
More on alcohol and cancer
**T1302**

Chronic, heavy drinking is also linked to coronary heart disease (CHD), ulcers, hypertension, gout, and pancreatitis, a painful inflammation of the pancreas. Generally speaking, women are only about one-third as likely as men to die young (under 55 years of age) as the result of cardiovascular disease. However, both men and women who drink heavily are about equally likely to die before age 55 from cardiovascular disease.[28]

Alcohol also affects brain cells, can trigger bleeding, can cause the heart muscle to deteriorate, and can lead to hormonal changes that dampen the sex drive in men and disrupt the menstrual cycles of women. Heavy consumption of alcohol also increases the risk of neurological problems such as seizures and dementia.

**Effects on the Liver** Heavy drinking often has its most damaging effects on the liver, the organ that primarily metabolizes alcohol. The liver is the largest organ in the body, and it has many functions. It filters the blood of toxic substances, secretes bile into the small intestine to assist in digestion and absorption of fats, stores vitamins, synthesizes cholesterol, metabolizes or stores sugars, processes fats, builds proteins from amino acids, controls the fluidity of blood and regulates blood-clotting mechanisms, and converts metabolic by-products into urea for excretion by the kidneys. Chronic, heavy consumption of alcohol is the single most important cause of illness and death from liver disease in the United States. Liver disease is the ninth leading killer in the United States and can often be prevented, because nearly half of all such deaths are due to alcohol consumption.[29]

**Close-up**
More on the liver
**T1303**

Alcohol-related liver diseases include hepatitis, fatty liver, and cirrhosis. In **alcoholic hepatitis,** widespread inflammation of the liver can have serious, life-threatening consequences. The con-

**Alcoholic hepatitis** An inflammation of the liver caused by chronic alcoholism.

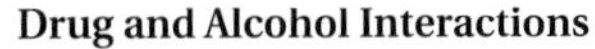

**Central Nervous System**
Alcohol speeds up the loss of brain cells. It impairs alertness, judgment, memory, coordination, and reaction time and raises the risk of falls and accidents at home and on the road. Because alcohol is a central nervous system depressant, it can cause or intensify depression.

**Heart**
Heavy drinking increases the risk of heart disease. The alcohol may mask pain that could serve as a warning signal of heart problems. Drinking can make both high blood pressure and diabetes worse—two common risk factors for heart disease.

**Sexual Functioning**
Although some alcohol may lower inhibitions, larger amounts decrease sexual interest and performance. Impotence is a common effect of alcohol in males. Even moderate intake of alcohol can lead to lower levels of the male hormone testosterone.

**Liver and Kidneys**
Alcohol interferes with the absorption and distribution of nutrients. Excessive drinking can inflame and destroy liver cells and cause cirrhosis (scarring and shrinking of the liver).

**Sleep**
Often used "to help sleep," alcohol actually aggravates insomnia, frequent awakenings, and night terrors.

**Drug and Alcohol Interactions**
Medications can intensify the effects of alcohol, leading to rapid intoxification. On the other hand, the alcohol can neutralize, lessen, or intensify the effects of drugs. Alcohol and sleeping pills may severely depress the central nervous system and lead to coma or death. Alcohol combined with insulin rapidly lowers blood sugar and with aspirin may cause stomach bleeding.

**Lungs**
Emphysema, bronchitis, and other pulmonary diseases are aggravated by alcohol abuse. Excessive drinking can cause respiratory failure and death.

**Gastrointestinal System**
Alcohol increases gastric secretions and decreases the flow of the digestive enzymes. It may lead to excess stomach acidity which can cause heartburn, ulcers, gastritis, and intestinal bleeding. Drinking also increases the risk of cancer of the mouth, throat, esophagus, and stomach.

**Nutrition**
Heavy drinking suppresses appetite and increases risk of malnutrition, which can cause confusion and impaired memory that mimic senile dementia.

**Joints**
Alcohol abuse can greatly increase the inflammation of joints caused by arthritis.



**Figure 13.4** *Effects of Heavy Drinking*

dition can usually be reversed with abstinence, although there may be some permanent scarring of liver tissue. **Fatty liver** refers to a buildup of fat that enlarges the organ. Fatty liver is a relatively benign condition that is usually reversed by abstinence. **Cirrhosis of the liver,** a serious disease that accounts for some 26,000 deaths annually in the United States, is irreversible. Cirrhosis is characterized by replacement of healthy liver cells with scar tissue. The more chronic and heavy a person's drinking, the greater the risk of the disease. Although cirrhosis is irreversible, abstinence may prolong life by reducing further deterioration of liver cells. Between 10 and 20% of heavy drinkers develop cirrhosis; 10 to 35% develop alcoholic hepatitis; nearly all develop fatty liver. Figure 13.5 shows the relationships between per capita alcohol consumption in Western countries and death rates due to cirrhosis of the liver. Note the trend: Countries with higher rates of alcohol consumption generally show higher rates of cirrhosis-related deaths.

There is some good news. Death rates from cirrhosis have been declining for the past generation. The decline may reflect declining alcohol consumption and earlier diagnosis and treatment of liver disease.

**Talking Glossary**
Cirrhosis
G1301

**Fatty liver** A condition involving an accumulation of fat in the liver, causing enlargement of the organ.

**Cirrhosis of the liver** A disease of the liver in which scar tissue replaces healthy liver tissue.

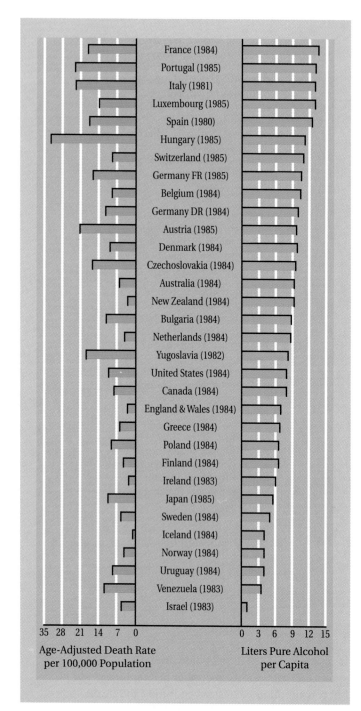


**Figure 13.5** ***Deaths due to Cirrhosis*** Death rates from cirrhosis of the liver in various countries are linked closely to level of alcohol consumption. *Source:* USDHHS, 1990, drawn from Grant, B.F., Dufour, M.C., and Harford, T.C., 1988, Thieme Medical Publishers.

**Nutritional Deficiency Disorders** Alcohol is high in calories but lacking in nutrients. Alcoholics tend to ignore their diets and obtain much if not most of their caloric needs from alcohol. Alcohol contains carbohydrates but little else of nutritional value. Heavy alcohol use also makes it more difficult for the body to absorb certain vitamins, such as vitamin $B_1$ (thiamine). For these reasons, alcoholics are prone to diseases related to vitamin and protein deficiencies, such as cirrhosis of the liver (which is linked to protein deficiencies) and a memory disorder called *Wernicke-Korsakoff's syndrome* (linked to thiamine deficiencies). People with Wernicke-Korsakoff's syndrome experience confusion, disorientation, and memory loss for recent events.

## "To Your Health"?—Is a Little Alcohol a Good Thing?

With all the concern about the health risks associated with heavy consumption of alcohol, it may come as a surprise that evidence is accumulating that suggests that drinking alcohol in moderation may actually have some healthful effects. Men who drink lightly to moderately suffer fewer heart attacks and strokes and have lower death rates overall than both heavy drinkers *and* nondrinkers.[30] A nationwide study of 85,000 female nurses showed that women who drank moderately had a lower incidence of strokes caused by blockages in blood vessels in the brain, the most common form of stroke, and fewer heart attacks than either heavier drinkers or abstainers.[31] The moderate drinkers were more likely to suffer a less common type of stroke that is related to excessive bleeding in the brain.

Researchers in Boston showed that moderate alcohol consumption (one to three drinks daily) was associated with a 50% reduction in the risk of heart attacks. Drinking more than three drinks daily did not increase the benefit. Why these apparent benefits of moderate drinking? It appears that alcohol increases levels of high-density lipoproteins (HDL), the "good" form of cholesterol that helps free blood vessels of blockage by low-density lipoproteins (LDL, or "bad cholesterol").[32]

There is growing evidence, then, that light to moderate intake of alcohol can reduce the risk of coronary heart disease (CHD). Yet health officials are cautious about recommending that people consume alcohol for its possible health benefits. The reason is that some people simply cannot limit themselves to one or two drinks a day. Drinking more than one or two drinks a day can tip the scale toward doing more harm than good. Heavy alcohol use can lead to alcohol abuse and dependence. It can damage the heart and virtually every other organ in the body. Heavy drinking can cause the heart muscle to deteriorate, leading to a poten-

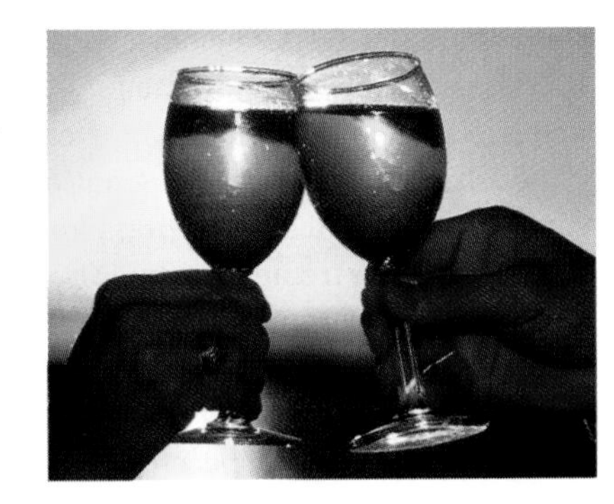

***A Toast to Your Health*** Evidence points to a beneficial effect of moderate drinking on the heart and cardiovascular system. However, health authorities are reluctant to encourage people to use alcohol because of concerns about potential alcohol abuse and health problems associated with heavy alcohol consumption.

Talking Glossary
Alcoholic cardiomyopathy
G1302

tially fatal condition called **alcoholic cardiomyopathy.** Heavy drinking is also associated with hypertension—a major risk for both CHD and stroke. In women, the incidence of hypertension is slightly less among women who drink less than a drink a day on the average compared with nondrinkers, but rises sharply among women who drink more than *three* drinks daily. In summing up their research findings, the researchers concluded: "With alcohol consumption, the differences between daily small-to-moderate amounts and large quantities may be the difference between preventing and causing disease."[33] Moreover, pregnant women and people with certain medical conditions should avoid alcohol altogether.

The benefits of moderate drinking may be obtained in other ways—ways that do not incur the risk of alcoholism or the health consequences of heavy drinking. These include quitting smoking, lowering intake of fats and artery-clogging LDL, and exercising regularly. Regular exercise, for example, increases HDL levels.

Smart Quiz
Q1302

**think about it!**

- **How does alcohol affect you physically? Have you drunk alcohol and driven? How do you feel about that?**
- **How does alcohol affect you psychologically? Have you done anything "under the influence" of alcohol that you would not have done otherwise? What? Why?**

**critical thinking** **Are you concerned about the long-term effects of drinking? Why or why not?**

**critical thinking** **Do you think it is wise to use alcohol to help prevent cardiovascular disease? Why or why not?**

# ALCOHOL MISUSE

Most people who drink do so responsibly. Use becomes misuse when it crosses the line into *alcohol abuse* or *alcohol dependence.* Misuse also occurs when people drink when it's unsafe to drink—as when they are or may be pregnant, when they drive, or when drinking prompts them to engage in risky sex. Misuse also occurs when people overdose on alcohol, which can have deadly consequences.

## Alcohol Abuse

**Alcohol abuse** is a pattern of heavy or continued drinking that becomes linked with health problems or impaired social functioning. If your drinking causes you to repeatedly miss school or work, it fits the pattern of abuse. You are abusing alcohol if your drinking causes social problems or problems on the job or at school. You are abusing alcohol if you persist in drinking although you know that it is causing or aggravating a physical problem, such as ulcers. Alcohol abuse also applies to a pattern of drinking in situations in which it is dangerous, such as driving or boating. Alcohol abuse often leads to the development of a physical dependence on alcohol, or alcoholism.

HealthCheck
Do you drink too much?
H1301

## Alcohol Dependence (Alcoholism)

**Alcohol dependence,** or *alcoholism,* is a state of physical dependence on alcohol that is characterized by a loss of control over its use. Despite the popular image of the alcoholic as a skid-row drunk, only a small minority of alcoholics, perhaps 5%, fit the stereotype. Most alcoholics are the type of people you're likely to see every day—neighbors, coworkers, friends, and family members. Alcoholics are found in all walks of life and every socioeconomic group. Many have families, hold good jobs, and live comfortably. Yet alcoholism can have just as devastating an effect on the well-to-do as the indigent, leading to wrecked careers and marriages, to motor vehicle crashes and other accidents, and to health problems.

**Alcoholic cardiomyopathy** A potentially fatal condition involving the deterioration of the heart muscle due to heavy alcohol consumption.

**Alcohol abuse** A pattern of misuse of alcohol in which heavy or continued drinking becomes associated with health problems and/or impaired social functioning.

**Alcohol dependence** An addiction to alcohol. Characterized by a loss of control over alcohol use, physiological dependence, and a withdrawal syndrome following abrupt cessation of drinking. Also called *alcoholism.*

Alcoholics increasingly turn to alcohol to deal with their problems and are unable to limit their drinking. They may go on a bender after having a drink or two or be unable to quit despite awareness that alcohol is disrupting their lives or damaging their health. Physical dependence develops when a person's body changes as the result of using a particular drug, as evidenced by the development of tolerance and/or a withdrawal syndrome when the person stops using the drug. The alcoholic, like the heroin addict, is addicted to, or chemically dependent on, the drug. The alcohol-dependent person may experience cravings for alcohol in much the same way that heroin addicts develop cravings for heroin. Tolerance may develop, such that more alcohol needs to be consumed to achieve the same effects. Thus the stage is set for chronic alcoholism and serious health consequences.

Alcoholics also tend to have a lesser sensitivity to the effects of alcohol, which makes them able to consume large amounts of alcohol without experiencing the immediate ill effects associated with heavy drinking, such as an upset stomach and nausea. They can also tolerate larger doses of alcohol without appearing intoxicated or showing signs of slurred speech.[34] This lack of sensitivity to the effects of alcohol may make them less capable of regulating their drinking intake. They may also feel more able to perform skilled tasks when they are drinking than they actually are, which can lead to tragic consequences if they combine drinking and driving.

Alcoholism tends to develop in early adulthood, usually between the ages of 20 and 40, although teens and even younger children can become alcoholics.[35] The onset of alcoholism tends to come earlier in men than women. Women alcoholics tend to suffer more serious health consequences than male alcoholics and have 50 to 100% higher death rates.[36] These differences may involve biological factors, as more alcohol is directly absorbed into a woman's body. Women may also have less access to alcoholism treatment. Until recently, the problem of alcoholism in women was largely ignored.

**Alcohol Withdrawal Syndrome** A withdrawal syndrome (sometimes called an *abstinence syndrome*) is a characteristic cluster of symptoms (which vary according to the particular drug) that develops in habitual users when drug use suddenly falls off. The withdrawal syndrome for alcohol is characterized by anxiety, nausea, sweating, shaking ("the shakes"), irritability, agitation, weakness, rapid pulse, elevated blood pressure, and, in some cases, **delirium tremens**—the DTs. The DTs usually affect only chronic heavy drinkers. The DTs are characterized by disorientation (confusion as to who or where one is, and who other people are); incoherent, rambling speech; intense autonomic hyperactivity (heavy sweating and rapid heartbeat); and terrifying auditory or visual hallucinations, sometimes of creepy, crawling insects on the skin.

**Delirium tremens (DTs)** A withdrawal syndrome in chronic alcoholics characterized by extreme restlessness, sweating, disorientation, and hallucinations.

**Patterns of Alcoholism** Some alcoholics drink heavily every day. Others binge on weekends. Others can abstain for lengthy periods but periodically "go off the wagon" and binge for weeks or months. Male alcoholics are more likely to alternate between periods of heavy drinking and periods of sobriety. Female alcoholics tend to drink more steadily and are less likely to binge.[37]

**Effects on the Family** People with alcohol problems are not the only ones who are affected by drinking. Alcoholism can devastate the family and friends of the drinker, as well as society at large through increased medical premiums and higher social costs resulting from absenteeism and lowered productivity. In the family, alcoholism wrecks marriages, impairs family life, and leaves emotional scars in children. About 43% of adult Americans, some 76 million people, have had a family member or spouse who was an alcoholic or problem drinker.[38] Nearly 30 million people in the United States are the children of alcoholics.[39] The children of alcoholics are at increased risk of abusing substances themselves, perhaps because of a combination of genetic and environmental factors. They are also at greater than average risk for developing psychological disorders such as depression. Many harbor misplaced guilt that they caused their parent's drinking.

**The Social and Economic Costs of Alcohol Abuse and Alcoholism** The personal and social costs of alcohol abuse and alcoholism exceed those for all illicit drugs combined. Health economists estimate the economic cost of alcoholism at more than $135 billion annually in the United States in terms of health-related expenses, days lost from work, and costs resulting from alcohol-related motor vehicle accidents.[42] The cost for

# Health Check

## Do You Have a Problem with Alcohol?[40]

Alcohol abuse and dependence may be fairly obvious if you shudder and shake whenever you are deprived of alcohol. Yet the signs may be more subtle. How can you know if you or someone close to you is developing a drinking problem? Here are some warning signs:[41]

- Drinking more than usual or getting drunk more often than usual.
- Gulping your drinks.
- Trying to have a few extra drinks before or after drinking with others.
- Drinking alone.
- Drinking in the morning or at times you didn't previously drink.
- Becoming noticeably drunk on important occasions.
- Drinking the "morning after" to overcome the effects of previous drinking.
- Drinking secretively.
- Drinking to relieve feelings of boredom, depression, anxiety, or inadequacy.
- Taking a drink to get through difficult situations or when you have problems.
- Binge drinking on weekends or at other times.
- Feeling uncomfortable when you are in situations in which alcohol is not available.
- Having regular Monday hangovers.
- Beginning to lose control of your drinking.
- Drinking more than you planned to drink, or getting drunk when you did not want to.
- Making promises to yourself to drink less, but failing to keep them.
- Repeatedly saying things or doing things when you are drinking that you later regret.
- Engaging in risky behavior when drinking, such as drinking and driving.
- Feeling guilty about your drinking.
- Becoming overly sensitive when others mention your drinking.
- Beginning to deny or lie about your drinking.
- Having memory blackouts or passing out while drinking.
- Finding that your drinking is affecting your relationship with friends or family.
- Losing time at work or school due to drinking.
- Staying away from people who do not drink.

If you recognize these signs in yourself, consult a health professional to learn whether you have an alcohol-related problem. If you recognize these signs in a loved one, encourage that person to seek help. Don't pester the person, as this may rouse resistance. Be patient but persistent.

medical care alone exceeds $11 billion, a cost that all of us share in one way or another in terms of health insurance premiums and taxes.[43] Between 20 and 40% of people who occupy hospital beds have medical conditions that result from alcohol abuse or alcoholism.[44] Yet the economic costs of alcoholism do not tell the story of the human toll of alcoholism. While incalculable in economic terms, this toll includes lost jobs; ruined careers and marriages; severe, even fatal, health problems; reduced productivity; and downward social mobility. Estimates are that perhaps 30 to 40% of homeless people in the nation are alcoholics.[45]

**Alcohol Misuse and Accidents** Death due to the misuse of alcohol often comes early in life, long before alcohol-related cirrhosis and other health problems become apparent. More teenagers and young adults die from alcohol-related motor vehicle accidents than from any other cause.[46] Four of ten teen deaths in this country result from automobile crashes. About one-third of drivers between the ages of 18 and 20 who become involved in fatal automobile accidents had alcohol in their bloodstreams.[47]

The average person in the United States stands a four in ten chance of becoming involved in an alcohol-related traffic accident during his or her lifetime.[48] Overall, about half of all motor vehicle crashes in the U.S. involve alcohol-impaired drivers. Alcohol is also implicated in about one in four fatal falls and accidents caused by fire and in 30 to 50% of all suicides and homicides (see Figure 13.6). Alcohol-related deaths due to unintentional injuries occur most often on weekends and during the hours of 6 P.M. to 6 A.M. All told, use of alcohol is associated with the four leading causes of death among young people: automobile accidents, homicides, suicides, and drownings.[49] Nearly half of adolescents who committed suicide had been drinking immediately beforehand.

**Close-up**
Drinking and driving
T1304

**Close-up**
Alcohol and suicide
T1305

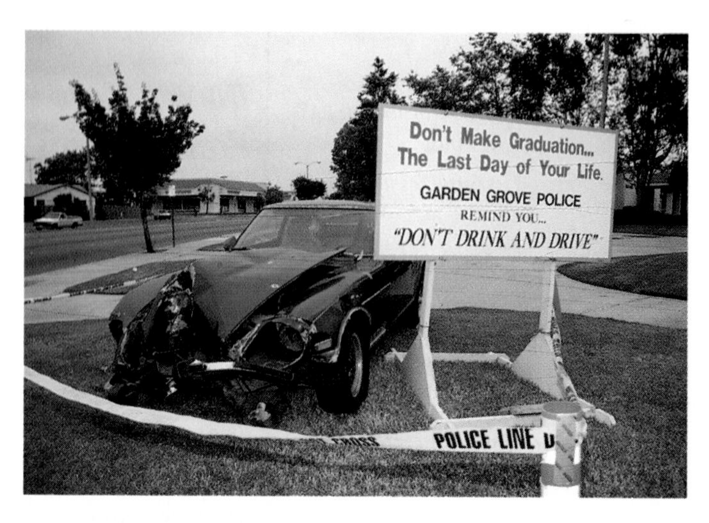
Don't Make Graduation...
The Last Day of Your Life.
GARDEN GROVE POLICE
REMIND YOU...
"DON'T DRINK AND DRIVE"
POLICE LINE

***The Deadliest Toll*** More young people die on the nation's roads in alcohol-related motor vehicle accidents than from any other cause.

Alcohol impairs coordination and balance, visual-spatial and motor skills, and also judgment. So when you drink, not only are your driving skills impaired, but so too are your coordination and balance, putting you at greater risk of accidental falls and mishaps. Alcohol also impairs your judgment, so you may take unnecessary risks or act impulsively without considering the consequences of your actions, which can lead to tragic results for yourself and others.

**Drinking and Young People—Cause for Concern** It should come as no surprise to anyone familiar with college life today that there is a lot of drinking on college campuses.[50] Alcohol, not cocaine, heroin, or even marijuana, is by far the most popular drug among college students and high school students as well. Health officials consider alcohol to be the number-one health hazard on America's high school and college campuses today.[51] Three of four college students (most of whom are underage) drink alcohol at least once a month (see Table 13.4). College students actually drink more than their peers who do not attend college. Drinking has become so integrated into college life that it has become the norm, as much a part of college as attending a football or basketball game.

How much alcohol do college students consume? The typical college student consumes more than 35 gallons of alcoholic beverages per year, mostly in the form of beer. Overall, college students in the United States consume some 4 billion cans of beer annually, which if stacked end to end would stretch to the moon and some 70,000 miles beyond![52] The typical student spends more money on alcohol than on textbooks.

Although every state prohibits drinking by people under the age of 21, about 90% of high school seniors have tried alcohol, and more than 60% drink alcoholic beverages at least once a month.[53] Some 8 million of the nation's 21 million seventh- to twelfth-graders drink weekly.[54]

Teenagers skirt drinking-age laws by finding alcoholic beverages at home or at parties in friends' homes, by using fake IDs to purchase alcohol in stores or to gain admittance to clubs that serve alcohol, or simply by purchasing alcohol in

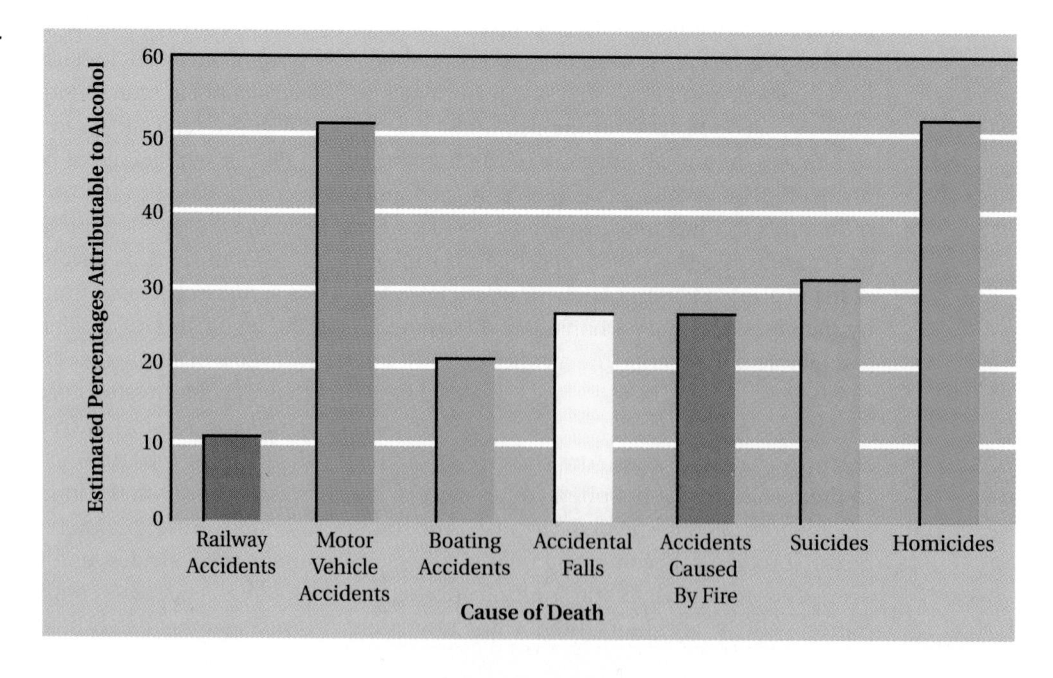


**Figure 13.6** ***Estimated Percentages of Deaths Linked to Alcohol Use*** Alcohol is implicated in about half of the deaths resulting from homicide and traffic accidents in the U.S., as well as a substantial portion of deaths due to other accidental causes and suicide.

TABLE 13.4

**Alcohol Use among College Students**

| | |
|---|---|
| Percentage who have used alcohol in their lifetime | 93.6 |
| Percentage who have used alcohol within the past year | 88.3 |
| Percentage who have used alcohol within the past 30 days | 74.7 |
| Percentage who have used alcohol daily within past 30 days | 4.1 |
| Percentage who had five or more drinks in a row during the last 2 weeks | 42.8 |

*Source:* Johnston, L. D., Bachman, J. G., and O'Malley, P. M. (1992, January 25). "Monitoring the Future: A Continuing Study of the Lifestyles and Values of Youth." The University of Michigan News and Information Services: Ann Arbor, MI.

stores that don't ask for proof of age. At a time when young people are turning increasingly against the use of cocaine and marijuana, they continue to perceive alcohol use as socially acceptable.

Most young people who drink do not become problem drinkers. But heavy or regular use of alcohol in adolescence and early adulthood foreshadows the development of alcohol-related problems later in life and is also associated with the development of other drug problems. Young people who develop problems with drugs often use alcohol first and generally continue to use alcohol along with other drugs, putting themselves at even greater risk of alcohol-related injuries and death.

**Drinking Games—A Potentially Deadly Pastime** Dangerous drinking games have been gaining popularity among high school and college students.[55] In one variation, students compete to see who can chug the most beers in a given amount of time. This game can be deadly, as people can die of acute alcohol intoxication as the result of an alcohol overdose.[56] **Blackouts** and **seizures** may also occur when large quantities of alcohol are consumed in this fashion. Yet many people remain unaware that alcohol overdoses are possible, let alone potentially fatal. In many people's minds, the worst that can happen if they drink too much is passing out. Wrong. Dead wrong. Choking on one's own vomit is a frequent cause of alcohol-induced deaths. What happens in these cases is that heavy drinking causes a person to vomit reflexively, yet the depressant effects of the drug make the person unable to vomit properly. The vomit accumulates in the air passages, causing death due to suffocation or asphyxiation.

PREVENTION

## *Preventing Death from Alcohol Overdose*

Alcohol overdose is a medical emergency that requires prompt medical attention. But how can you recognize the signs of an overdose? Here are some symptoms:[57]

- Failure to respond when talked to or shouted at.
- Failure to respond to being pinched, shaken, or poked.
- Inability to stand up without help.
- Failure to wake up.
- Purplish color or clammy-feeling skin.
- Rapid pulse rate or irregular heart rhythms, low blood pressure, or difficulty breathing.

Here are some suggestions for what you can do if you encounter someone who you suspect has suffered an alcohol overdose:

- Do not leave a person who is unresponsive or unconscious alone. Don't simply assume that he or she will "sleep it off." Stay with the person until you or someone else can obtain medical attention.
- Place the person on his or her side or, if possible, have the person sit up with the head bowed.
- Do not give the person any food or drink.
- Do not induce vomiting.
- If the person is at all responsive, find out if he or she took other drugs or had taken any medication that might have interacted with the alcohol or if the person has an underlying illness that could be contributing to the problem, such as diabetes or epilepsy.
- Reach into the person's mouth and clear the airway if the person vomits; provide artificial respiration or CPR if necessary.
- Most important, call a physician or local emergency number *immediately* and ask for advice.

It may seem easier to walk away from the situation and let the person "sleep it off." You may think you have no right to interfere. You may have doubts about whether the person is truly in danger. But ask yourself, if you were in the place of the person who showed signs of an overdose of alcohol, wouldn't you want one of your friends to intervene to save your life?

**Blackout** An episode involving a loss of consciousness.

**Seizure** A sudden attack involving a disruption of brain electrical rhythms, as in the type of convulsive seizure occurring during epileptic attacks.

**Binge Drinking on Campus** Binge drinking is a growing concern on college campuses. A Harvard University survey of nearly 1,700 students at 14 colleges in Massachusetts revealed that nearly one in three college men and one in seven college women engaged in binge drinking—drinking five or more drinks in a row—at least twice a week.[58] A national survey of college students found that more than four in ten (44% overall; 50% of the men, 39% of the women) reported guzzling more than five drinks in a row on a single occasion during the two-week period preceding the survey.[59] Overall, more than half of today's college students report getting drunk at least once a year, and between one-quarter and one-half get drunk at least once a month.[60]

Close-up
Drugs on campus
T1306

Why is binge drinking dangerous? For one thing, repeated binge drinking is a feature of alcohol abuse and can lead to more regular heavy drinking, setting the stage for chronic alcoholism. For another, binge drinkers are six times more likely to drink and drive than are their lighter-drinking peers. Moreover, students who binge drink are three times more likely to engage in unplanned or risky sexual activity, which can increase their risk of catching a sexually transmitted disease, including AIDS, as well as heighten their risk of an unwanted pregnancy.[61] Drinking alcohol may also increase the risk of infection with HIV among persons exposed to the virus.[62] As one recent AIDS prevention advertisement puts it, "First you get drunk, then you get stupid, then you get AIDS."

A survey of students from a southern university found that nearly half (47%) of the women and more than half (57%) of the men reported engaging in sexual intercourse from one to five times "primarily because they were intoxicated." Among those students over 21 years of age, only about one in five had *never* engaged in sex because of intoxication.[63]

Students who binge are also at greater risk of missing classes, falling behind in schoolwork, getting into arguments or fights with others, and getting into trouble with the police. The number-one concern of college administrators is student problems with alcohol. Many colleges have instituted "get tough" policies by prohibiting use of alcohol in dormitories or at college functions, banning alcohol in university pubs and at university-sponsored social events, expelling students who drink underage, and requiring off-campus fraternities and sororities to check IDs and control how much alcohol is served at social functions. Colleges have incorporated alcohol education as a required part of their curriculum or college orientation program. Resident assistants are being trained to recognize the signs of substance abuse.[64]

Video
Drinking on campus
V1301

Close-up
More on college drinking
T1307

**Problem Drinking in High School and Younger Children** Problem drinking is becoming an increasing problem among high school and younger children. Children are becoming problem drinkers at the ages of 9 and 10. They often sneak drinks from their parent's unlocked liquor cabinets. The younger a person starts drinking, the more likely he or she is to develop problems later in life. Among high school seniors, rates of current and heavy alcohol use are highest among white and Native American males and females and Mexican-American males. Black and Asian high school seniors have the lowest rates. About one in four 12- to 17-year-olds has experienced an alcohol-induced blackout.[65] A national survey showed that about one in four seventh- to twelfth-graders in the U.S. had binged on alcohol at least once. About one in seven reports binge drinking within the last month.[66] Among twelfth-graders, about one in three has engaged in binge drinking during the past two weeks. Beer is the alcoholic beverage favored for binge drinking.[67]

Alcohol abuse remains the most prevalent form of drug abuse across the age spectrum. The government continues to wage a war on illicit drugs, but less attention has been focused on stemming the much larger problem of alcohol misuse.

### think about it!

- **Do you know any alcoholics? What is the effect of their drinking on themselves and their families?**
- **In your experience, at what age do people start drinking? If they are underage, how do they get alcohol? What do you think should be done about it?**

**critical thinking** **Do you misuse alcohol? On what criteria do you base your answer?**

Smart Quiz
Q1303

# CAUSES OF ALCOHOLISM

After a century of research, the causes of alcoholism remain largely elusive. The most widely held view is that alcoholism is a disease that involves biological (largely genetic) and psychosocial (e.g., peer pressure, poor modeling) factors.

## Genetic Factors

The sons of alcoholics stand about a four times greater chance of becoming alcoholics than do sons of nonalcoholics. It does not appear that people inherit a specific gene or genes for alcoholism per se.[68] Instead, some people, at least some men, appear to have a genetically greater tolerance for the unpleasant effects of alcohol and a genetically greater capacity for reaping pleasure from alcohol. Both genetic tendencies may increase the likelihood of excessive drinking, leading to addiction.[69] By contrast, people whose bodies more readily "put the brakes" on excess drinking may be less likely to develop alcoholism. Other research suggests that sons of alcoholics may be unusually tense because of brain deficiencies of certain neurotransmitters.[70] They may turn to alcohol as a way to combat tension.

The strongest evidence for a genetic contribution in alcoholism comes from twin studies. Identical twins share 100% of their genes. The genes of fraternal twins, like other siblings, overlap by 50%. Higher rates of agreement for the disorder between *identical* twins compared with fraternal twins suggest a genetic contribution to the disorder. To date, evidence from twin studies on alcoholism does show greater agreement rates in identical twins, at least among men.[71] Results are inconsistent in women.

Overall, perhaps 50 to 60% of the risk of developing alcoholism is accounted for by genetic factors. The genetic risk may be greater among men than women, however.[72]

**Close-up**
More on genetics
T1308

## Psychosocial Factors

Whatever the role of genetics in alcoholism, genes don't tell the whole story. At least one in three alcoholics has no family history of the problem. Peer pressure often encourages underage and excessive drinking that can lead to problems with alcohol. Adolescents who drink heavily are also more likely than other adolescents to come from families characterized by lax control and lack of emotional support. Adolescents from one-parent homes also tend to drink more heavily than those from two-parent families. Exposure to parents or others who model heavy drinking and an environment that conveys permissive attitudes toward drunkenness also contribute to problem drinking that may lead to alcoholism.

Some people turn to alcohol as "liquid relief" from personal problems. Problem drinking may begin with using alcohol as a form of self-medication. Cultural and ethnic factors may also play contributing roles in the development of alcoholism, as the nearby ***World of Diversity*** feature illustrates. All in all, the causes of alcoholism are complex and most probably involve the interaction of biological, psychological, and sociocultural factors.

**Why Do Young People Drink?** Young people drink for many of the same reasons that older people drink—for example, to handle stress and to elevate their moods. Teenagers drink to get high and to cope with feelings of tension and boredom.

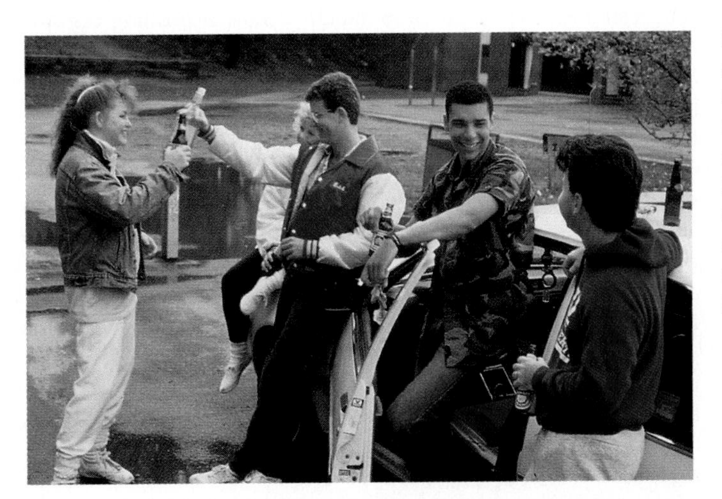

***College Students and Drinking*** Three of four college students drink alcohol regularly, even though most are underage. Though most college students who drink do not become problem drinkers, heavy or regular drinking in adolescence and young adulthood foreshadows the development of alcohol- and drug-related problems later in life.

WORLD OF *diversity*

## Ethnicity and Alcoholism[74]

Drinking is affected by social and cultural norms. Cultural beliefs and customs may encourage or discourage drinking. In some cultures, consumption of alcohol is tightly regulated and restricted to special occasions, such as religious ceremonies or weddings. In traditional Islamic cultures, alcohol is prohibited altogether.

Ethnic factors in the use and abuse of alcohol are receiving increasing attention among researchers. Here are some of the findings that have emerged:[75] Native Americans and Irish Americans have among the highest rates of alcoholism of U.S. ethnic groups. Other ethnic groups—Jews, Greeks, Italians—have lower rates of alcoholism, largely because of tight social controls imposed on excessive and underage drinking. In some groups, such as Jews, wine is incorporated within religious rituals that set an example for controlled use of the substance.

**Close-up**
Ethnicity and drinking
T1309

### Hispanic Americans

Hispanic-American men are about as likely as non-Hispanic white men to use alcohol and to develop alcohol-related problems. Yet these similarities belie some important differences. Among Mexican-American men, for example, frequent, heavy drinking is more common among men in their thirties and fifties. In general, American men in their twenties are more likely to drink heavily. Hispanic-American women are much less likely than Hispanic-American men, or non-Hispanic white women, to drink alcohol or to become problem drinkers. Cultural values may explain these differences. The traditional machismo ideal, or standard of manhood, may encourage drinking in men as a sign of masculinity. On the other hand, traditional Hispanic-American values impose severe restrictions on drinking in women, especially heavy drinking.

**Acculturation** of immigrant groups plays an important role in alcohol consumption. Alcohol consumption more closely mirrors the customs of the host culture as immigrant groups become more strongly acculturated. The more relaxed gender roles in U.S. society compared with traditional Hispanic-American cultures appear to be loosening restraints on alcohol consumption among Hispanic-American women. Drinking among Hispanic-American women has increased with each new generation born and reared in the United States. Mexican-American women who stand the greatest risk of developing drinking-related problems are those who are more acculturated, wealthier, and better educated.

### African Americans

Alcohol abuse is taking a heavy toll on African Americans, especially African-American men. They are also much more likely than white men to be diagnosed with alcohol-related diseases, including cirrhosis of the liver, alcoholic fatty liver, coronary heart disease (CHD), and oral and throat cancers. They are also more likely to experience alcohol-related accidents and homicides. However, African-American men are slightly less likely than white men to drink or to become heavy drinkers.

Why, then, do African-American men have more alcohol-related diseases? Socioeconomic factors may be involved. For example, African Americans are more likely to encounter stresses relating to unemployment and economic hardship. Stress may compound the damage caused by heavy drinking. Then, too, African Americans often have less access to health care than whites. Lack of treatment may also aggravate the problems caused by drinking.

African-American women, on the other hand, are less likely than white women to drink and develop alcohol-related problems. Cultural constraints on African Americans, like those on Hispanic Americans, discourage excessive drinking among women. Abstention from alcohol in the African-American community is strongly linked to religious identification. Church attendance and religious fundamentalism are often associated with abstinence from alcohol.

### Asian Americans

Problem drinking is less common among Asian Americans than among most other U.S. ethnic groups. Part of the reason lies in strong cultural sanctions against excessive drinking and tight family controls. Biological factors may also be involved, however. Asians are more likely than African, Hispanic, and non-Hispanic white Americans to show a **flushing response** to drinking alcohol. About 30% to 50% of Asians show this response, which involves redness and feelings of warmth on the face, and, at higher doses, nausea, rapid heart rate, dizziness, and headaches. These unpleasant reactions may help curb excessive alcohol intake. Moreover, Asian groups who show a more marked flushing response (such as Koreans, Taiwanese, and Hawaiian Asians) tend to consume less alcohol than those who show relatively less flushing.

**Acculturation** The process by which immigrant or native peoples adapt to the host or mainstream culture.

**Flushing response** A physiological reaction to the ingestion of alcohol that is characterized by reddening and warming of the face, and sometimes nausea and other unpleasant reactions.

### Native Americans

Native Americans are the U.S. ethnic group at greatest risk of incurring alcohol-related diabetes, fetal abnormalities, cirrhosis of the liver, and accident fatalities. Rates of alcohol abuse and dependence vary from tribe to tribe, and some tribes show less consumption than national averages. Yet Native Americans as a group experience more than four times the overall U.S. death rate due to cirrhosis of the liver, a direct consequence of excessive drinking. Although Native American women tend to drink less than their male counterparts, alcohol consumption among women in some tribes has been increasing dramatically. This may explain the rising rates of fetal alcohol syndrome (FAS) and of alcohol-related diseases, such as cirrhosis of the liver, in Native American women. One death in four among Native American women is caused by alcohol-related cirrhosis of the liver. This figure is 37 times higher than the rate among white women. The rate of fetal alcohol syndrome (FAS) has been reported at more than 10 per 1,000 live births among some Native American tribes, which is more than three times the overall rate. Native Americans also have much higher than average rates of death due to alcohol-related motor vehicle and other accidents. Alcoholism and drug abuse are especially acute among the young.

Sociologists see the high rate of alcoholism in many Native American communities as a consequence of the dominant culture's hostility toward tribal language and culture. The hostility leads to a loss of cultural identity that sets the stage for alcoholism, drug abuse, and depression.

In recent years, some Native American tribes have attempted to deal with these problems by emphasizing a return to traditional values and the development of native industries to serve as sources of employment for Native American youth. Several communities have also developed specialized programs to teach young people parenting skills. They also emphasize technical and scientific training to enable young people to bring new technology to the reservation and provide a new brand of tribal leadership. As one commentator notes, being a scientist does not mean "losing respect for tradition, for ceremony and ritual, and for the traditional healers and tribal leaders."

Many drink to relieve problems at home. Others drink to fit in with friends.

College students face many adjustment problems—the challenge of being on their own, the scramble for grades, pressures to make new friends or be pledged by a fraternity or sorority, and so on. Students may look to alcohol as a way of relieving the stress from these problems. College life also means greater independence from parental control. Students who live away from home tend to drink more heavily than those who do not. College also brings large numbers of young women and men together at a time when risk taking is common and peer acceptance is especially important.

Interestingly, drinking is more common among students at small colleges.[73] A survey of 56,000 students found that students at four-year colleges with enrollments of less than 2,500 consumed about 7 drinks per week, compared with about 4.5 drinks for students at four-year colleges with over 20,000 students. Why? Small schools are more often located in rural areas, leading researchers to suspect that lack of competing activities leads to heavier drinking.

There is also a link between poor grades and heavier drinking. In the same survey, students obtaining A's averaged 3.4 drinks a week. Those earning D's and F's averaged nearly 11 drinks a week. Does heavier drinking cause grades to plummet? Or do students with academic problems turn to drink? It may be difficult to identify cause and effect, but it is clear that heavy drinking and good grades don't mix.

**Attitudes toward Alcohol and Problem Drinking** Students who hold more positive attitudes toward drinking are at greater risk of developing problems with alcohol. They may believe that alcohol makes them more sociable, sexy, or in control. They may believe that they are incapable of coping with stress without alcohol. Such attitudes can lead to a pattern of behavior in which drinking becomes associated with a range of social cues (e.g., socializing or dating) and internal cues (e.g., anxiety or depression). As drinking becomes habitual, psychological as well as physical dependence may develop.

Smart Quiz Q1304

## think about it!

- **Do you know some people who can "hold their liquor" better than others? How does this "ability" affect their attitudes toward drinking and their behavior?**
- **What are the attitudes toward drinking on your campus? Toward binge drinking on weekends? Have these attitudes affected you? If so, how?**
- **What are the attitudes toward drinking in your ethnic group or cultural background? Have these attitudes affected you? If so, how?**

# TREATMENT OF ALCOHOLISM

The first step toward recovery from alcoholism is the recognition that a problem exists. Once the problem drinker breaks through denial and admits to having a problem, a range of treatment options becomes available. Among the more common interventions are psychotherapy and counseling, behavioral therapy, pharmacological treatment, and peer-support groups, such as Alcoholics Anonymous. Few can overcome alcoholism on their own. Total abstinence appears to be the only workable treatment goal for chronic alcoholics. However, some early-stage alcohol abusers may be able to learn to drink moderately and responsibly.[76]

## Detoxification

For people who are dependent on alcohol, treatment begins with **detoxification.** Detoxification permits people with chemical dependencies to be medically monitored and supervised while they withdraw from addictive substances. Detoxification often takes place in a hospital or inpatient residential treatment facility. Persons who undergo "detox" are often given tranquilizers, such as Valium or Librium, to quell anxiety and prevent dangerous withdrawal symptoms such as convulsions and seizures. They also help prevent elevated blood pressure, irregular heart rhythms, and tremors. Detoxification from alcohol generally takes about a week, although a standard stay or "drying-out period" of 28 days provides the opportunity to prepare the individual to live free of alcohol.

**Detoxification** A process of ridding the body of alcohol or other drugs under supervised conditions in which withdrawal symptoms can be monitored and controlled.

## Alcoholics Anonymous

Withdrawing from alcohol is one thing. Maintaining abstinence is another. Alcoholics Anonymous (AA) has become so synonymous with alcoholism treatment that following detox, many health care professionals refer alcoholics to AA as a matter of course. The philosophy of AA is based on the disease model of alcoholism. It holds that alcoholism is a lifelong disease as expressed in the slogan, "Once an alcoholic, always an alcoholic." AA never sees alcoholics as cured. There is no such thing as an "ex-alcoholic," only a "recovering alcoholic." Proponents of AA hold the view that alcoholics cannot drink responsibly, that just one drink creates an irresistible biologically based craving for more. They maintain that alcoholics must maintain strict sobriety if they are to control their disease.

AA helps more than 750,000 people with alcohol-related problems each year. The AA approach is part spiritual, part group therapy. The groups are run by recovering alcoholics and are offered without charge. Group participants are encouraged to appeal to a higher power to help them maintain sobriety. AA follows a 12-step program of self-reclamation and recovery. Meetings provide opportunities for group support. A buddy or sponsoring system encourages members to call one another for support if they feel tempted to drink.

AA does not appeal to everyone. Some alcoholics are put off by the spiritual basis of the AA approach (the appeal to a "higher power"). Others cannot accept the regimentation and rituals of the program.

AA has spawned spinoff organizations, such as *Al-Anon,* which supports the spouses, partners, and parents of alcoholics. Another spinoff organization, *Alateen,* offers support groups for children of alcoholics. Along with offering practical advice, Al-Anon and Alateen help those close to alcoholics to understand that they are not to blame for the alcoholic's drinking.

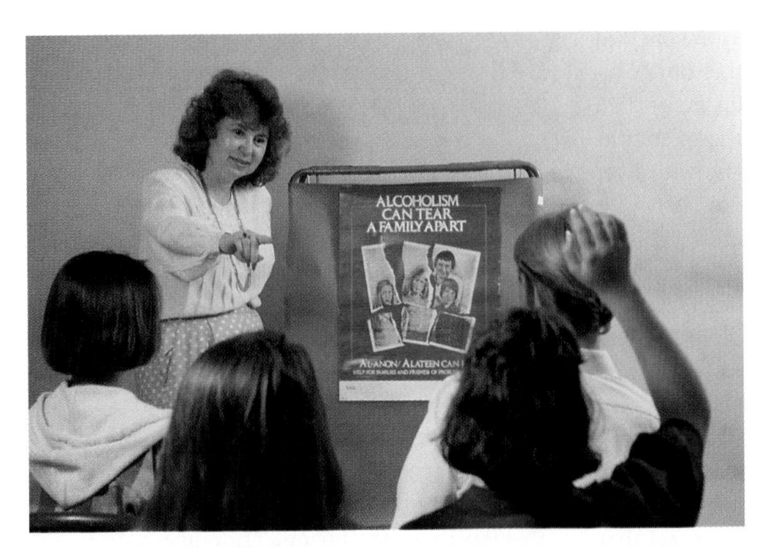


***Al-Anon and Alateen*** Al-Anon and Alateen offer support to family members and spouses of people suffering from alcoholism.

## Psychotherapy and Counseling

Psychotherapy and counseling may be used to uncover the childhood roots of substance abuse and to help individuals change self-destructive behavior. Family therapy or marital therapy may be used to deal with the effects of problem drinking on the family or the marriage.

Behavior therapists use a wide variety of other techniques to help alcoholics maintain sobriety. Assertiveness training, for example, has been used to help alcoholics learn to fend off social pressures to drink. Aversive conditioning involves the use of painful (aversive) stimuli that are paired with drinking so as to make drinking itself aversive. In one example, nausea-inducing drugs are administered when the individual drinks. As a consequence, an aversion to alcohol is conditioned that may discourage future drinking. A recent review of aversive conditioning showed an overall success (abstinence) rate of approximately 60% a year after treatment.[77] Given the usual high rate of **relapse,** a 60% abstinence rate is considered reasonably successful. However, it may be that the acquired aversion to alcohol is "unlearned" as time progresses after treatment, because the individual is repeatedly exposed to alcohol without aversive consequences.

**Relapse prevention training** describes an assortment of psychological techniques that help substance abusers maintain abstinence. Participants learn to handle temptations to drink in high-risk situations. For example, they learn to gracefully refuse drinks at social gatherings. They learn how to relax without turning to alcohol. They learn to change their attitudes toward slips or lapses (having a drink). By learning to treat a slip as a correctable and isolated problem, not as a sign of ultimate failure ("What's the use? I'm doomed to fail"), people can avoid turning a lapse into a relapse.

## Pharmacological Treatment

Researchers have learned much about the neural pathways by which alcohol exerts its influence on the brain. Their work has led to the development of chemical agents that block the pleasurable effects of alcohol or combat cravings for alcohol. Yet researchers do not expect to find a miracle drug that treats all aspects of alcoholism. Nor do they expect drugs alone to replace the need for therapy and support groups.

Naltrexone (brand name ReVia) blocks the high from alcohol as well as from opiates such as heroin. The drug doesn't prevent alcoholics from drinking, but by blocking the pleasure produced by alcohol, it may help break the vicious cycle in which one drink leads to another.[78]

Disulfiram (brand name Antabuse) has been widely used to help alcoholics maintain sobriety. Although the drug does not quell cravings for alcohol, it produces a strong aversive reaction when the person drinks alcohol. Even a single drink leads to nausea, sweating, flushing, a throbbing headache, rapid heart rate, a drop in blood pressure, and vomiting. In rare cases, drinking

**Relapse** The recurrence of a disorder or problem behavior.

**Relapse prevention training** Psychological techniques aimed at preventing relapse.

can lead to a dramatic drop in blood pressure that causes shock and, perhaps, death. One shortcoming of this approach is that people who are bent on drinking can simply stop taking disulfiram. Another is that disulfiram is toxic to people with liver disease, a frequent ailment of alcoholics.

Researchers suspect that deficiencies of the neurotransmitter serotonin may account for alcohol desires or cravings.[79] They have been focusing on whether the appetite for alcohol can be curbed by drugs called serotonin reuptake inhibitors (Prozac is an example) that increase the availability of serotonin in the brain.* The use of these drugs in the early stages of abstinence may help the recovering alcoholic maintain sobriety and continue in treatment. Researchers also suspect that another neurotransmitter, dopamine, may account for the pleasurable or euphoric effects of alcohol. Drugs that mimic dopamine may be helpful in blocking the pleasurable effects of alcohol and thus decrease motivation to drink.

Talking Glossary
Dopamine
G1303

Many treatments exist to help people with problem drinking. However, many problem drinkers do not seek help. Many who do leave treatment prematurely. High rates of relapse plague even the most comprehensive treatment programs. These facts underscore the importance of prevention. We still need to find effective ways to help young people cope with stresses and challenges without turning to alcohol. We also need to change beliefs about alcohol that give rise to problem drinking.

*These drugs are also used to treat severe depression, a psychological disorder that frequently involves deficiencies in the action of serotonin (see Chapter 4).

Smart Quiz
Q1305

## think about it!

- Do you know anyone who has overcome alcoholism? How did he or she do it?
- Have you had any personal experience with groups such as AA, Al-Anon, or Alateen? What was the experience like?

**critical thinking** Do you believe that people who were addicted to alcohol can never touch another drop without becoming addicted again? Why or why not?

**Designated driver** A person who, chosen as the driver for a group, is expected to abstain from alcohol.

**Zero tolerance laws** Laws prohibiting underage persons from driving if they have any detectable level of alcohol in their blood.

## PREVENTION

### *Combating Drinking and Driving*

Alcohol-impaired drivers kill thousands of people each year in the U.S. in automobile accidents. Many alcohol-impaired drivers are themselves killed or disabled. What can be done about it?

Organizations such as Mothers Against Drunk Drivers (MADD) have focused public attention on the issue and promoted legislation and vigorous law enforcement to crack down on people who drink and drive. Governmental initiatives to combat drunk driving have included raising the legal drinking age, implementing roadside sobriety checks, and establishing programs that train bar and restaurant workers to help them screen out underage patrons and recognize signs of alcohol impairment so that they can cut off service to people who are drunk. Some states and municipalities now mandate training programs for managers and servers in commercial establishments that serve alcoholic beverages. Fear of lawsuits also induces operators of these establishments to better police themselves. Fear of lawsuits may similarly prompt many hosts to be more careful about serving alcohol to guests.

All states have now raised their legal drinking age from 18 to 21. This change is credited with reducing the number of alcohol-related traffic deaths nationwide, especially among young people aged 16 to 24. Raising the legal drinking age has cut the number of motor vehicle fatalities in the U.S. per year by an estimated 5 to 6%, which works out to about 700 lives a year saved![80]

A notable success in the public media arena is the **designated driver** program. In this program, public service messages encourage people who go out to designate one person in their group to remain sober and serve as the driver for the others. Other media campaigns, such as one featuring the slogan, "If you drink, don't drive," have also helped alter public attitudes and perceptions toward drinking and driving.

Although designated driver and other media-based campaigns are helpful in curbing alcohol-impaired driving, they need to be combined with other initiatives to create a legal and social climate that discourages drinking and driving. Such initiatives include use of sobriety checkpoints, stricter enforcement of laws against underage drinking, advertising reforms to curtail liquor advertising (especially advertisements targeting young people), and increased excise taxes on liquor to discourage excess consumption. Authorities have also been targeting youthful drivers, for example, by instituting **zero tolerance laws** that prohibit underage persons from driving with any detectable level of alcohol in their blood.

Efforts to combat drunk driving are having an impact. Overall, the number of auto fatalities connected with drinking is down substantially from the 1980s (see Figure 13.7).

Worrisome, however, was a 4% increase in drunk-driving accidents in 1995, the first year that registered an increase since 1986. Clearly this uptick underscores the need for yet more vigorous law enforcement efforts to be brought to bear on the problem. With nearly 20,000 alcohol-related traffic deaths on the nation's roads each year, we need to find more effective ways of persuading people not to drink and drive and preventing them from attempting to drive if they have been drinking. We have a long way to go to get this message across. Nearly 60% of students polled at a northeastern university reported that they had driven a motor vehicle while intoxicated.[81]

While much of the media spotlight has been focused on drunk driving, little attention has been paid to another source of driving-impaired behavior—recreational boating. About 30% of recreational boating accident victims had blood alcohol levels that exceeded the legal limit, while another 20% had lesser amounts of alcohol in their systems.[82] The effort to prevent drinking and driving needs to be extended to include drinking and boating as well.

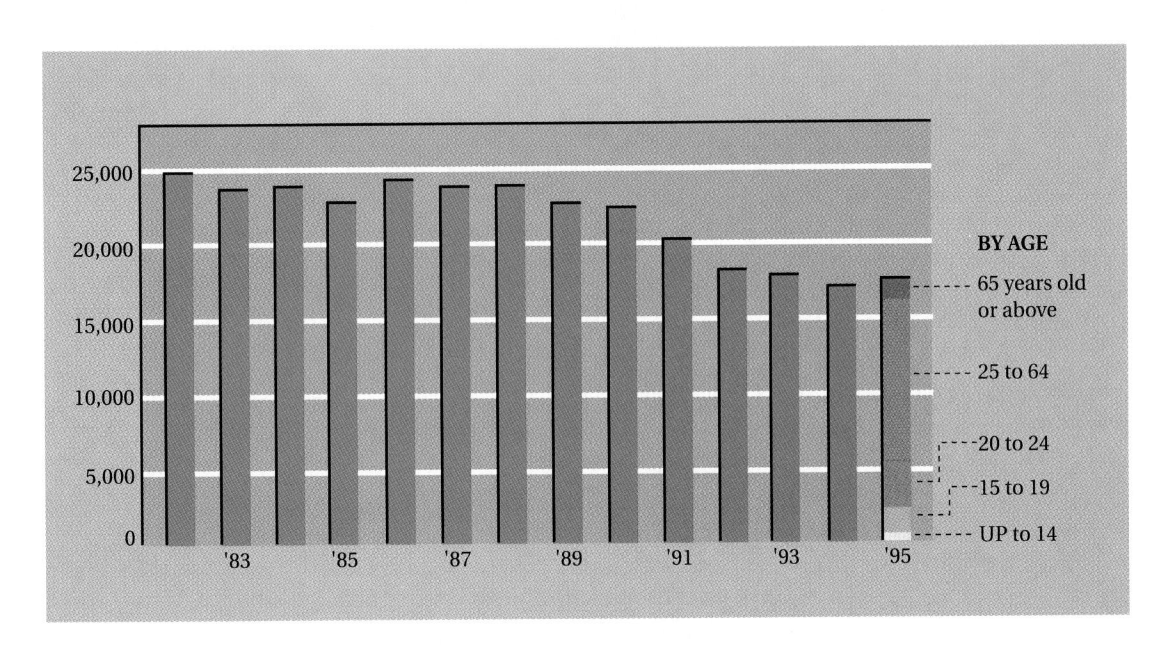


**Figure 13.7** ***Alcohol-Related Traffic Fatalities*** Alcohol-related traffic fatalities increased 4% in 1995, the first increase since 1986.

# Keys to Responsible Use of Alcohol*

## Take Charge

Alcohol is a drug—a powerful drug that can lead to addiction, health problems, and accidents when misused. Abstinence is certainly one way of controlling use, but most adults in our society drink at least occasionally. Most drinkers are able to regulate their intake because they control when, what, and how much they drink. Alcohol consumption, like eating and smoking, can be conceptualized in terms of a chain of events: the A's or *antecedent* cues that prompt or trigger the behavior; the B's or *behaviors* themselves; the rewarding or punishing C's or *consequences* that follow the behavior and serve either to encourage or discourage it:

- The **A**'s refer to the external (stimuli in the environment) or internal (feeling states) cues that trigger an urge for a drink.
- The **B**'s refer to the behaviors associated with drinking, such as stopping off at a bar after work, or consuming an alcoholic beverage.
- The **C**'s refer to the rewarding (pleasant relaxed feelings) or punishing (nausea, hangover, guilty feelings) consequences that follow drinking.

Consider an example: You finally land a date with the one person whom you feel fate has intended for you. As you are dressing for the date, you begin to feel a little anxious (an internal cue or *antecedent*). To quell this feeling, you reach for a bottle of scotch and down a jigger (a B or *behavior*), which helps calm your nerves (a reinforcing *consequence*). Though this behavior pattern may be an isolated occurrence, it can become a habit if it is repeated whenever you feel anxious or tense. Before you know it, you drink whenever anxiety strikes—in the morning before a sales call, in the afternoon when you're meeting your in-laws, in the evening when you start thinking about the hassles of the morrow.

You may be able to gain better control over your drinking behavior by changing these connections. Gaining better control of them can help avert problem drinking or help you regain control if alcohol misuse is becoming a problem for you. If misuse has become persistent and crossed the boundary into abuse, we suggest you call for a consultation with a trained professional. It may be the most important call you ever make.

**Devise a Self-Control Program** The first step in a self-control program is to identify the behaviors you wish to change. This involves taking a hard look at your behavior.

### Keep a Drinking Diary

Set up a diary to log each drink you consume. Note what you drank (for example, "a 12-ounce can of beer"), where you consumed the drink (for example, "home, living room"), what you were doing at the time (for example, "watching TV"), who you were with at the time ("alone"), and how you felt afterward (for example, "relaxed, calm"). Keep a diary for one or two weeks, or long enough to note some patterns.

### Examine Your Drinking Diary

Analyze your drinking diary. Are you drinking more than you thought you were? At what times of the day do you drink? Do you usually drink in a particular place? Do you usually drink with certain people or when you are alone? What are your feelings before drinking? How does drinking affect your feelings? Did you drink in situations where you knew it was unsafe or unwise to drink? Did you engage in dangerous behavior when you drank, such as driving? Did you notice any patterns relating drinking to negative emotional states, like anxiety, boredom, or depression? Did you drink more when you went out with certain friends? When you were worried about a test the next day? What did you learn about your drinking behavior? What goals does this assessment lead you to identify?

### Define Your Goals

What would you like to change? Be specific. First of all, set a daily consumption goal. Perhaps you will choose to limit your drinking to one glass of wine with dinner. Set some targeted goals as well. Perhaps you'd rather have a clear head when attending a party and not drink at all. Perhaps you'd like to handle negative emotions in other ways than reaching for an alcoholic drink. Perhaps you'd like to avoid socializing with friends who are heavy drinkers, at least in situations that lend themselves to heavy drinking.

### Devise a Plan for Changing Your Behavior

What do you need to do to achieve your goals? Go back and examine the ABC's of your drinking behavior.

*A basic key to responsible use of alcohol is knowing and abiding by laws regulating alcohol consumption, including laws prohibiting underage drinking and driving, or boating, under the influence of alcohol.

**Controlling the A's (Antecedents) of Your Drinking Behavior** To control your alcohol intake, break down the automatic features of your drinking habits by pulling the plug on the prompts or cues that trigger your urges for a drink.

- Limit your exposure to alcohol-related cues (A's) in your environment. Don't leave beer mugs or shot glasses lying around. Buy alcohol only in smaller quantities—a bottle of wine rather than a jug, a six-pack of beer rather than a case. Buy only as much as you need to meet your daily goals for a week. Fill your refrigerator with healthful refreshments as alternatives to alcohol.
- If you find it difficult to avoid drinking (B's) more than you should at a party or when going out with your friends, cut back or avoid those situations until you achieve a better sense of control over your drinking.
- Increase your exposure to A's that are connected with more desirable B's. Participate more often in events held in alcohol-free environments—lectures or concerts, a gym, museums, evening classes. Socialize more often with nondrinking or light-drinking friends; eat in restaurants without liquor licenses.
- Learn to handle the emotional cues that trigger excessive drinking. Develop skills in meditation, relaxation, or yoga, and practice using these skills when you feel anxious. Learn to express anger in constructive ways. Counseling or psychotherapy can help you deal with negative emotional states like depression, anxiety, or anger if they persist or become intense.

**Controlling the B's (Behaviors) of Your Drinking Behavior** Control your intake by interrupting the chain of behaviors that leads to excessive drinking.

- Break abusive habits by preventing them from occurring, such as by not bringing alcoholic beverages to school or work. Don't engage in enabling behaviors that increase the potential for abuse, such as taking a route home that just happens to pass by your favorite watering hole.
- Disrupt the behavior chain leading to the unwanted behavior by practicing a competing response. Pop a mouthful of mints or chew on sugarless gum instead of taking a drink or at any time you're exposed to a powerful drinking cue. Other competing responses include taking a shower, walking the dog, practicing relaxation or meditation, or talking to a friend or confidant for moral support.

**Controlling the C's (Consequences) of Your Drinking Behavior** Strengthen the positive consequences of drinking responsibly by rewarding yourself.

- Reward yourself for meeting your daily consumption goals and targeted goals. Pat yourself on the back when you refuse an offer of a drink. Put away a small amount of money each day you meet your goals. Don't wait until the end of the week to tally your rewards. Put each daily award aside on the day that you earned it. You may spend it on something for yourself the next day or let your funds accumulate for a few weeks or months and then buy yourself something special. You deserve it!

To shape behavior, rewards should follow three principles:

**Take Charge**
Cutting down on drinking
C1301

1. The reward (good C) must follow, rather than precede, the behavior (desired B).
2. The occurrence of the reward (good C) must be contingent on the occurrence of the behavior (B) (that is, no behavior, no reward).
3. The reward (good C) should follow the behavior (B) as quickly as possible.

**Evaluate Outcomes** Did you achieve your goals? If not, what obstacles prevented you from moving forward? How can you modify your behavior-change strategy to overcome these obstacles? Evaluation is not a final report card but a means of assessing your progress and devising alternative strategies that might be more successful.

A number of other strategies for averting alcohol-related problems follow.

## Other Strategies

**Know Your Own Limits** People vary in their sensitivity to alcohol. Some people show signs of intoxication after a few sips of wine. Others do not until they have consumed a few stiff drinks. Learn about your own reactions by examining your response when you drink, especially if you drink more than your regular amount. See how the changes in dosage affect your coordination, speech, and mental alertness. Ask a family member or roommate to give you their opinions of how the different dosages affect your behavior. Learning to gauge your own reactions can help you keep your intake at a level that does not impair your mental or motor ability.

**Keep Your Blood Alcohol Level Low** You can keep your blood alcohol content at a low level by following these guidelines:

1. *Drink slowly.* Sip, don't gulp. For the average person, it takes about an hour for the liver to metabolize the alcohol in a single drink (a jigger's worth of liquor, 5-ounce glass of wine, or 12-ounce can of beer). The more you exceed your liver's capacity to break down alcohol, the drunker you'll get.
2. *Space your drinks.* Let some time pass before ordering another round. Skip a round if your blood alcohol level begins to rise, or substitute mineral water or another nonalcoholic beverage. Alcohol tends to metabolize more slowly in people who are infrequent drinkers, so these people need to be especially aware of their limits and to space their drinks accordingly.

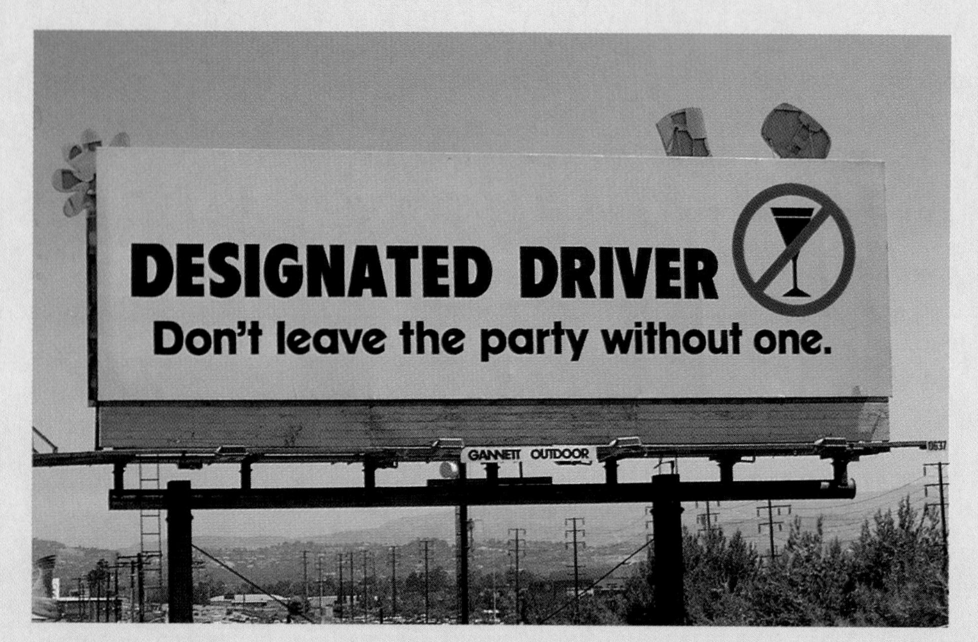
DESIGNATED DRIVER
Don't leave the party without one.
GANNETT OUTDOOR

***Combating Drunk Driving*** Initiatives to combat drunk driving, including the designated driver program, have helped reduce the carnage on the nation's roads caused by drinking and driving. Still, nearly 20,000 Americans lose their lives each year in alcohol-related motor vehicle accidents.

3. *Know when to say when.* Keep in mind how many drinks you've had and the length of time between drinks. Limit yourself to about one drink an hour. Some people, especially women and people of slighter builds, may need to drink more slowly, as alcohol tends to affect them more strongly. Also, become aware of the signs of intoxication, such as impaired coordination or balance, slurring of speech, or a slowing down of mental processes. Use these as cues to stop drinking.
4. *Judge your surroundings.* Your response to alcohol depends in part on your surroundings. Consuming a few drinks in a club or bar with blaring music and lots of activity around you has a stronger effect on you than drinking the same amount in the quiet of your home. Learn to gauge your reactions and adjust your alcohol intake accordingly.
5. *Stick to your limits.* Don't let hosts or drinking companions pressure you into exceeding your limits. Learn to politely refuse an offer of a drink when you've reached your limit.
6. *Avoid drinking on an empty stomach.* Having food in your stomach will slow the absorption of alcohol into your bloodstream. But avoid salty snacks, like pretzels, chips, and nuts, since they will make you thirstier and more likely to drink too much.
7. *Dilute your drinks, but not with carbonated beverages.* Dilute your drinks with plenty of ice or a mixer, like orange or tomato juice. But avoid using carbonated mixers, like tonic water or club soda, as these can speed the absorption of alcohol into your bloodstream.
8. *Choose lower-proof alcoholic beverages.* Ounce for ounce, you need to consume more than three times as much wine, and eight times as much beer, to equal the alcohol content in a typical distilled spirit like whiskey, vodka, rum, or gin. That's no reason to splurge on wine or beer, since either of these alcoholic beverages can quickly raise your blood alcohol level to the point of intoxication. Yet it does lead us to treat that innocent looking jigger of gin as a potent drug.

**Don't Use Alcohol as a Crutch** Don't turn to alcohol as a means of coping with your problems; relieving negative emotions like depression, anxiety, anger, or boredom; or combating loneliness. Developing a habit of using alcohol in this way, as a form of self-medication, will only compound your problems in the end, as it will set the stage for alcohol abuse. Try to develop more healthful ways of coping, such as relaxation, positive imagery, meditation, or exercise, or seek the assistance of a friend or counselor.

**Learn to Say No** College students often feel pressured to drink alcohol by their peers, especially their roommates in dormitories. They may also feel pressured to participate in dangerous drinking practices, such as drinking games. Don't let anyone pressure you to do anything you don't want to do. If "just saying no" won't do, prepare other comebacks. For instance, say, "Look, this is not my scene. Thanks, but I'd rather not." If your friends don't respect your wishes, rethink your choice of friends.

**Socialize without Drinking** You can have a good time with your friends without drinking. Don't let drinking become the focus of your social activities. If you feel more comfortable at a party holding a drink in your hand, order a tonic water or tomato juice with ice, but ask the server to hold the alcohol.

**Be a Responsible Host** The responsible use of alcohol extends to your role as a host. Keep close tabs on how much alcohol you serve your guests. Measure the amount of alcohol you serve in mixed drinks, how much wine you pour, and how many cans of beer you offer. Don't thrust alcoholic beverages on your guests by handing them drinks they haven't asked for. Don't jump to freshen guests' drinks. Don't leave open bottles of liquor lying around for guests to serve themselves. Space the drinks you serve—not more than one per hour. Avoid serving stiff drinks. Stop serving alcohol to anyone who appears noticeably intoxicated or impaired. Serve plenty of food along with alcoholic beverages and have a variety of nonalcoholic beverages available. Stop serving alcohol an hour or more before you expect guests to leave and never, never, serve "one for the road." Ask each group of people who expect to drive home together to name one person as the designated driver for the group who will abstain from drinking alcohol. Offer to call a taxi for any guest who appears intoxicated or has consumed too much alcohol but insists on driving home. Or offer to drive that person home yourself or to put him or her up for the night. Or see if someone else can drop the person off at home. Do whatever you need to do, including taking the person's car keys, to make sure the person doesn't drive. He or she may live to thank you.

**Be Aware of Alcohol-Drug Interactions** Alcohol is a powerful drug that can cause adverse effects when combined with the use of other drugs or prescription medications. Using alcohol when taking certain antibiotics can reduce their effectiveness or cause such side effects as nausea or vomiting. Combining alcohol with certain antidepressants can lead to a sudden rise in blood pressure. Alcohol can also have negative interactions with over-the-counter drugs. Combining alcohol and aspirin can lead to stomach problems or liver damage. Play it safe: Check first with your physician or pharmacist if you wish to consume alcohol while you are taking other drugs or medications.

Never use alcohol together with other psychoactive drugs, especially tranquilizers and sedatives. Combining these drugs can be dangerous, even deadly, as the combination of these drugs produces a much greater effect than the individual drugs alone.

**Be Honest with Yourself about Your Drinking** Researchers find that college students tend to have a biased view of the amount that they drink. Most students believe that their friends drink more heavily than they themselves do.[83] They tend to characterize their own drinking as "social" or "occasional" but perceive their buddies to be "heavy" or "frequent" drinkers. Of course, if you asked their buddies, the tables would likely be turned. This kind of belief is called a self-serving bias because it protects one's self-esteem by putting oneself or one's behavior in a more positive light in relation to others. While a self-serving bias may protect your self-esteem, it can prevent you from taking a realistic look at yourself and your behavior and can wind up hurting you in the end.

**Don't Depend on Coffee to Sober You Up** It is not true that a cup or two of coffee will sober you up when you have drunk too much. The caffeine in coffee does not hasten the bodily processes involved in metabolizing alcohol to sober you up. The fact is that nothing—not caffeine, not taking a cold shower, not running around the block—can speed up these metabolic processes. Only the passage of time will burn off the effects of alcohol. A good rule of thumb to keep in mind is that it takes one hour to burn off the effects of the alcohol in each 1.5-ounce jigger of liquor (or 5-ounce glass of wine or 12-ounce can of beer). Beliefs that caffeine or other remedies can adequately hasten the sobering-up process can lead to tragic mistakes, as when a person who has been drinking believes that downing a cup or two of strong, black coffee will allow him or her to get behind a wheel and drive safely even when drunk.

All in all, the key to responsible drinking is to think before you drink.

Smart Quiz
Q1306

# SUMMING UP

## Questions and Answers

### WHAT IS ALCOHOL?

1. **What is alcohol?** Alcohol is a clear, flammable liquid that contains the psychoactive substance *ethyl alcohol.* Alcoholic beverages are manufactured by fermentation and distillation.

2. **How do we define how much alcohol a drink contains?** Alcoholic beverages are graded in terms of their proof. A beverage containing 50% alcohol is 100 proof.

3. **Who drinks?** Two of three adults in the United States drink alcoholic beverages. Half are light drinkers. Younger people and men drink the most on the average.

4. **Why do people drink?** People drink for various reasons, including peer pressure, the desire to get "high," and use of alcohol as a self-medication to cope with stress.

### EFFECTS OF ALCOHOL

5. **What are the physical effects of alcohol?** Alcohol depresses the nervous system and produces intoxication. Drinking on an empty stomach is more likely to intoxicate. All states consider people to be intoxicated when their blood alcohol level reaches 0.10%. Death may occur at a blood alcohol level of perhaps 0.35% or more.

6. **What are the psychological effects of alcohol?** Alcohol produces feelings of euphoria and elation but also clouds judgment and impairs concentration. Alcohol is connected with risky sexual activity and violence, perhaps because intoxicated people are less likely to be concerned about the consequences of their behavior.

7. **What are the health effects of heavy drinking?** Heavy alcohol use is linked to liver diseases such as cirrhosis, several kinds of cancer, coronary heart disease, ulcers, hypertension, gout, pancreatitis, and Wernicke-Korsakoff's syndrome. Alcohol is also involved in half of the traffic accidents in the U.S.

8. **I heard that alcohol can be good for the heart. Is that true?** Perhaps. People who drink lightly to moderately tend to have fewer heart attacks and strokes than heavy drinkers and nondrinkers. One reason may be that light drinking appears to raise HDL ("good cholesterol") levels in the blood. But health professionals are cautious about recommending that people use alcohol for this purpose.

### ALCOHOL MISUSE

9. **When does alcohol use become alcohol misuse?** Use becomes misuse when it turns into *alcohol abuse* or *alcohol dependence.* Alcohol abuse is heavy or continued drinking that becomes linked with health problems or impaired functioning. Alcohol dependence, or alcoholism, is a state of physical dependence on alcohol that is characterized by a loss of control over its use. Alcohol dependence is also characterized by addiction and tolerance.

10. **How do we know if someone is addicted to alcohol?** People who are addicted experience characteristic withdrawal syndromes that may include anxiety, nausea, sweating, shaking ("the shakes"), irritability, agitation, weakness, rapid pulse, elevated blood pressure, and, in some cases, delirium tremens—the DTs. The personal and social costs of alcohol abuse and alcoholism exceed those for all other drugs combined.

### CAUSES OF ALCOHOLISM

11. **What are the causes of alcoholism?** We're not completely certain, but genetic factors appear to be involved. Genetic factors appear to be stronger in explaining alcoholism in men than in women. Sons of alcoholics are more likely to tolerate alcohol and become alcoholics themselves. Yet psychosocial factors such as peer pressure and problems in the home also appear to contribute to alcoholism.

### TREATMENT OF ALCOHOLISM

12. **What kinds of treatments are available for alcoholism?** If the individual is addicted, treatment usually begins with detoxification, or withdrawal from alcohol under medical supervision. Many alcoholics turn to support groups, such as Alcoholics Anonymous. Counseling and psychotherapy may help, especially when strategies are provided to help people avoid relapses. The drug disulfiram prevents people from drinking by making them nauseated if they drink. Naltrexone blocks the "high" from alcohol, while some antidepressants may reduce alcohol cravings.

## Suggested Readings

**National Institute on Alcohol Abuse and Alcoholism.** *7th Special Report to Congress on Alcohol and Health.* Rockville, MD: Author, 1990. What we know about alcohol abuse and alcoholism and how to treat these problems.

**United States Department of Health and Human Services.** *Alcohol Research: Promise for the Decade.* Public Health Service, Alcohol, Drug Abuse, and Mental Health Administration, National Institute on Alcohol Abuse and Alcoholism, Pub. No. ADM–92–1990. Washington, DC: Author. A government report on what we know and hope to learn about alcoholism.

**Clark, W. B., and Hilton, M. E. (Eds.).** *Alcohol in America: Drinking Practices and Problems.* Albany, NY: State University of New York Press, 1991. Scholarly articles on the use and misuse of alcohol in America.

**Hester, R. K., and Miller, W. R. (Eds.).** *Handbook of Alcoholism Treatment Approaches: Effective Alternatives* (2nd Ed.). Boston: Allyn & Bacon, 1995. A comprehensive review of alcoholism treatment approaches, including scientific examination of 11 of the most widely studied treatment alternatives.

*Youth and Alcohol: Selected Reports to the Surgeon General.* U.S. Department of Education. Washington, DC: U.S. Government Printing Office, 1993. An excellent resource for learning about underage use of alcohol in the U.S. This resource focuses on the dangerous and deadly consequences of youthful drinking; drinking habits, attitudes, and knowledge of young people, as well as relationships between youthful drinking and crime; and enforcement of the 21-year-old drinking age law.

DID YOU KNOW THAT

- Nearly eight times as many people die from smoking-related causes as from all types of motor vehicle accidents? p.376
- Tobacco products are the only commercially available products in the U.S. that are life-threatening when they are used in the manner in which they were intended to be used by the manufacturer? p.376
- There is no such thing as a safe cigarette? p.378
- Smoking causes wrinkles? p.378
- Second-hand smoke contains greater concentrations of carcinogens than the smoke inhaled from the cigarette itself? p.383
- Lung cancer has surpassed breast cancer as the leading cause of cancer death among women in the United States? p.389
- Smokers who quit can substantially reduce their health risks compared with those who continue to smoke, but not to the level of nonsmokers? p.390

# Cigarette Smoking and Other

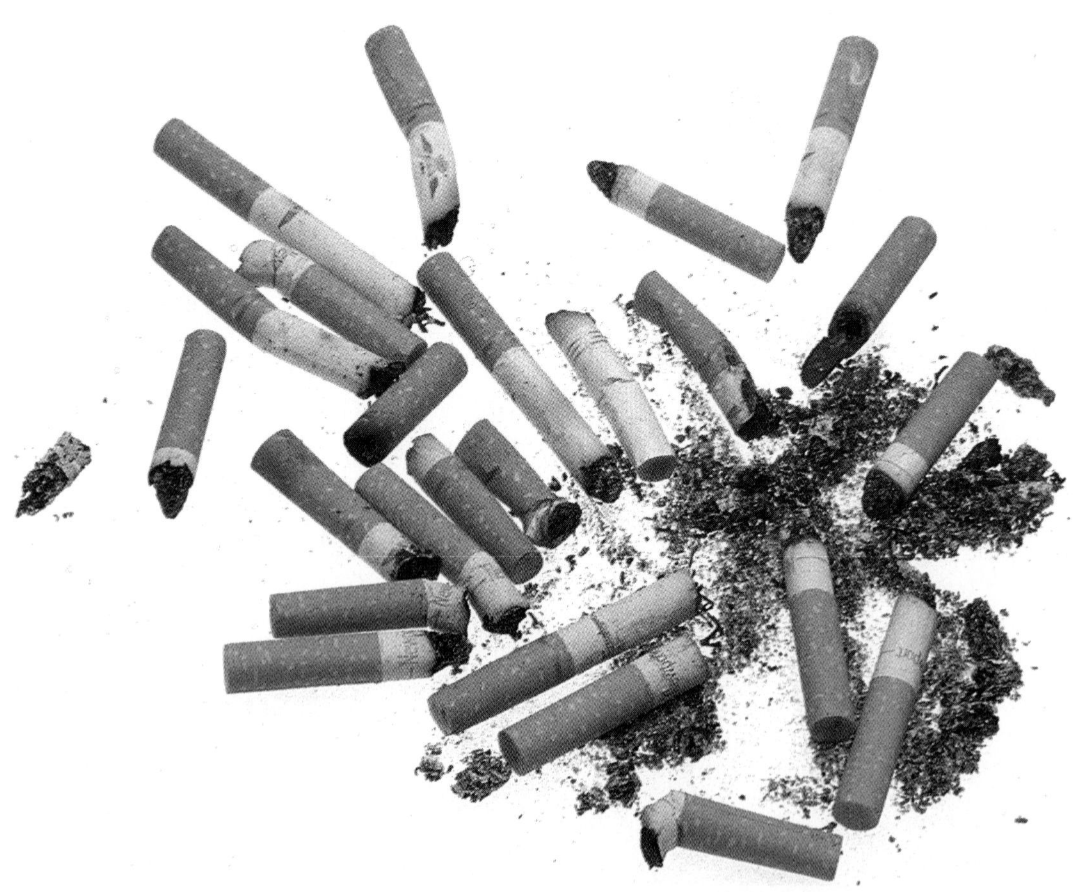

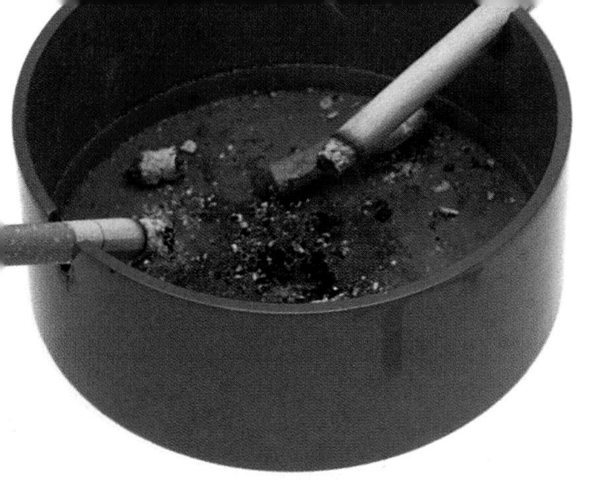

14

# Tobacco Use

*What is the major preventable cause of death today? Use of illicit drugs like cocaine and heroin? Unsafe sexual practices? Consuming a high-fat diet? Leading a sedentary lifestyle with little or no regular exercise? While all these factors are recognized health risks, the major preventable cause of death in the U.S. is cigarette smoking. It should come as no surprise that smoking is a major health risk. You only need look at any cigarette pack to see the notice, "Warning: The Surgeon General Has Determined That Cigarette Smoking Is Dangerous to Your Health."*

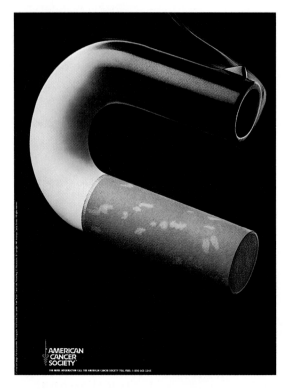


***Smoking Kills*** Smoking accounts for more than one in five deaths in the U.S., making it the nation's leading preventable cause of death.

Smoking kills. It accounts for more than one of five deaths in the United States. It claims the lives of more than 418,000 people each year, a number about equal to that of the population of Atlanta, Georgia.[1] Worldwide, smoking kills more than 3 million people a year. This means that a smoking-related death occurs somewhere every 10 seconds![2] Smoking-related deaths are expected to jump to 8.4 million worldwide by the year 2020, making it the world's leading killer.[3]

Smoking costs money as well as lives. The federal government puts the tab for direct medical costs of cigarette smoking at an estimated $50 billion annually, which represents at least 7% of the nation's total health care costs.[4] That's equivalent to more than $2 for each pack of cigarettes sold. This cost affects us all—whether we smoke or not—because of higher taxes and health insurance premiums. The total economic burden attributed to smoking, including costs resulting from sick days and premature deaths, is at least $100 billion annually.

**Tobacco** A member of a family of plants containing nicotine, its leaves are prepared for smoking, chewing, or use as snuff.

**Nicotine** A stimulant drug found naturally in tobacco.

**Snuff** A powdered form of tobacco that can be inhaled through the nose or sucked when placed inside the cheek.

**Chewing tobacco** Tobacco leaves that have been prepared for chewing or sucking when lodged between the cheek and gum.

Want some more facts?

- Nearly eight times as many people die from smoking related causes as from all types of motor vehicle accidents.
- For each death due to drunk driving, 74 premature deaths are caused by smoking.[5]
- Cigarette smoking accounts for nearly 90% of deaths due to lung cancer, the nation's leading cancer killer.
- Tobacco products are the only commercially available products in the U.S. that are life-threatening when they are used in the manner that they were intended to be used by the manufacturer.[6]
- Cigarette smoking is the leading cause of premature death in the United States and around the world.

## SMOKING AND HEALTH

**Tobacco** is a plant that contains a psychoactive drug called **nicotine.** Nicotine, a stimulant drug, is found in the leaves of the plant and is ingested in several ways. The leaves may be smoked in the form of cigarettes, cigars, or pipe tobacco, converted into a powder for inhalation as **snuff,** or ground into a chewable form called **chewing tobacco.** While the use of tobacco predated the arrival of Columbus, it wasn't until the development of specialized machinery in the 1800s that manufacturers could mass-produce large numbers of cigarettes. With mass production and marketing, the prevalence of smoking increased over time. It reached a peak by the early 1960s in the United States, when about half of the adult men and a third of the adult women smoked. Since then, smoking has declined, especially among men. This trend is largely the result of a government-sponsored antismoking campaign that began with the publication of the first Surgeon General's report on smoking in 1964 documenting the health risks of smoking. Still, Americans today consume more than 500 billion cigarettes annually, which works out to more than 2,500 cigarettes for every person 18 years of age or older, smokers and nonsmokers alike.

## Where There's Smoke, There's Trouble

When you light a cigarette, you set off a chemical reaction that changes many of the substances found in tobacco. More than 4,000 distinct compounds enter your body as the smoke fills your lungs. Many of these compounds are toxic or **carcinogenic.** Scientists have identified 43 carcinogens in cigarette smoke to date.[7] The major constituents of cigarette smoke are nicotine, carbon monoxide, and tars.

Talking Glossary
Carcinogenic
G1401

Nicotine has complex effects on the nervous system, producing a range of psychological and physical effects. It reaches the brain in about 7 to 10 seconds following a puff, which is less time than it takes for heroin to reach the brain when it is injected into the bloodstream. Nicotine causes the release of the hormone adrenaline, which increases the heart rate and produces a mild "rush" or psychological "kick." Adrenaline (epinephrine) causes reserves of sugar to be released into the blood, quelling the appetite. As a stimulant, nicotine acts on nerve cells in the brain to increase states of arousal, alertness, and concentration. Although nicotine is a stimulant, cigarette smoking may also have "paradoxical" effects, such as helping smokers relax or calming them down. In the brain, nicotine leads to the release of *endorphins,* naturally occurring hormones that function much like heroin and other opiates by producing states of pleasure and reducing pain. The direct effect of nicotine on the release of endorphins helps account for the feelings of pleasure associated with smoking.

The stimulant properties of nicotine also give rise to sensations of cold, clammy skin and nausea and vomiting in first-time users. These symptoms explain the queasiness and discomfort of novice smokers. However, the unpleasant symptoms typically disappear as the smoker's body becomes more accustomed to the drug.

Nicotine is a strongly addictive drug, but it is not as harmful as other substances found in cigarette smoke, especially tar and carbon monoxide. The **tar** in cigarette smoke is a thick, sticky residue that contains hundreds of different chemical compounds, many of which are toxic or carcinogenic. These compounds blacken the lungs and lead to the formation of cancerous growths. The compounds in tars and other constituents of cigarette smoke switch on a gene in lung cells that seems to make these compounds more likely to cause cell mutations that lead to cancer.[8]

**Carbon monoxide** is the same poisonous gas that is emitted by the exhaust systems of cars. It interferes with the transport of oxygen through the blood system by taking space in red blood cells that normally carry oxygen. This can lead to shortness of breath and deprive vital body organs, including the heart, of the oxygen they require. Carbon monoxide in cigarette smoke is at least partly to blame for the increased risk of heart attacks and stroke in people who smoke. It may directly precipitate heart attacks in smokers whose supply of oxygen to the heart is already compromised by narrowing of the arteries due to a buildup of fatty deposits.

## Health Consequences of Smoking

Smoking causes widespread damage in the body.[9] Not just the mouth, throat, and lungs are affected. The dangerous chemical compounds in tobacco smoke wend their way throughout the body, damaging many organs.

Smoking causes lung cancer.[10] People who smoke two or more packs of cigarettes daily are 12 to 25 times as likely to die from lung cancer as are nonsmokers. Smoking is also linked to many other forms of cancer, including cancers of the mouth, pharynx, larynx, esophagus, pancreas, cervix, kidney, and bladder. All told, smoking causes 30% of all cancer deaths in the United States and is the leading preventable cause of cancer. Smokers in general stand twice the risk of dying from cancer as nonsmokers. Among heavy smokers, the risk is four times as great.[11]

Close-up
Smoking and cancer
T1401

Smoking is also a major cause of **chronic obstructive pulmonary disease (COPD),** which includes chronic bronchitis and emphysema. Four of five deaths from emphysema and bronchitis are due to smoking. Smokers are also more susceptible than nonsmokers to the common cold, coughs, and respiratory infections such as influenza, bronchitis, and pneumonia. Smoking also stunts the development of the lungs of teenage smokers, even those who smoke as few as five cigarettes a day.[12] Lung damage from smoking as a teenager can set the stage for diminished respiratory health throughout adulthood.

Close-up
More on health risks
T1402

**Carcinogenic** Cancer-causing.

**Tar** The sticky residue in tobacco smoke, containing many carcinogens and other toxins.

**Carbon monoxide** An odorless poisonous flammable gas produced from the burning of carbon with insufficient air.

**Chronic obstructive pulmonary disease (COPD)** A disease process that results in diminished capacity of the lungs to perform respiration.

Smoking causes some 180,000 deaths in the United States each year due to cardiovascular disease. Smoking is associated with increased blood cholesterol levels, leading to hardening of the arteries and increasing the risks of heart attacks and strokes.[13] (When people quit, their cholesterol levels come down—yet another reason for smokers to quit.) Smoking also places an added strain on the heart by stimulating the sympathetic branch of the autonomic nervous system, leading to the release of epinephrine, which keeps the heart pumping at a higher than normal rate.[14]

Smoking in women raises additional concerns. Smoking causes women to enter menopause one or two years early.[15] Smoking during pregnancy is linked to an increased risk of birth defects in babies, low birth weights, premature births, and miscarriages.[16] As many as one in four cases of low birth weight could be prevented if mothers-to-be quit smoking during pregnancy. Simply cutting down smoking during pregnancy does not appear to offer much protection in preventing low birth weight, however. The more the mother smoked during pregnancy, the greater the reduction in the baby's birth weight. However, the sooner a pregnant woman quits smoking, the better her chances of delivering a baby who is of normal weight.

Researchers have found increased levels of a cancer-causing substance in the blood of pregnant women, and in the blood of their newborns, among women who were exposed to second-hand smoke from their spouses or other household members during pregnancy.[17] Researchers have also found an association between maternal smoking during pregnancy and the risk of sudden infant death syndrome (SIDS) in infants.[18]

Smoking depletes the body of vitamin C, a key antioxidant nutrient.[19] Smokers are more likely to develop dental problems, such as gum disease and tooth loss.

The more cigarettes you smoke and the longer you smoke, the greater your health risks. The more deeply you inhale, the greater the risks. Smoking filtered cigarettes or low-tar cigarettes may slightly reduce the health risks of cigarette smoking. But there is no such thing as a safe cigarette or a safe level of smoking. Filters do not remove many of the toxic and carcinogenic compounds in cigarette smoke. Many smokers of "light" cigarettes compensate by puffing harder or deeper, even though they may not be aware of it.[20]

**Smoker's face** A characteristic wrinkling of the face around the lips and eyes due to smoke.

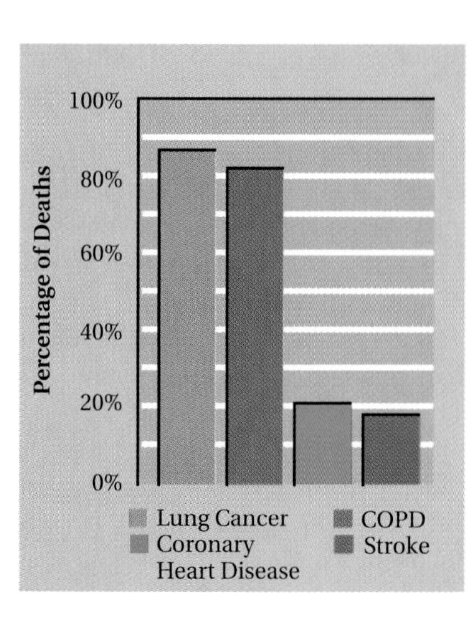


**Figure 14.1** ***Percentage of Deaths due to Smoking, by Type of Disease*** Cigarette smoking accounts for nearly 87% of deaths due to lung cancer, 82% of deaths due to chronic obstructive pulmonary disease (COPD), 21% of deaths due to coronary heart disease, and 18% of deaths due to stroke.

**If You Smoke. . .** If you smoke, you increase your chances of dying of lung cancer twelvefold if you are a woman or 22 times if you are a man.[21] You are more than ten times as likely as nonsmokers to develop cancer of the larynx, eight to ten times as likely to develop cancer of the esophagus, and twice as likely to develop cancer of the bladder, kidney, and pancreas. You stand about twice the risk of dying from coronary heart disease (CHD) or a stroke than do people who have never smoked. Figure 14.1 shows the percentages of deaths from various diseases that are due to cigarette smoking. Figure 14.2 shows the relative risk that cigarette smokers face relative to nonsmokers of dying from diseases linked to smoking. All in all, smokers may be about three times more likely than nonsmokers to die before the age of 70.[22]

## Smoking and Appearance

Need more convincing of the damage caused by smoking? Then note that smoking also causes wrinkles. Many smokers develop a **smoker's face,** with fine wrinkles radiating from the lips and eyes. The facial skin takes on a grayish, bloodless hue. Smoking also yellows the teeth. The more a person smokes, the greater the chances of developing an unsightly paunch.[23] Smokers tend to accumulate fat around their midsections and have a higher waist-to-hip ratio than nonsmokers. This pattern of weight distribution is connected with a greater risk of cardiovascular problems. The more cigarettes smoked, the greater the waist-to-hip ratio.

Next we take a closer look at tobacco—what it is, how it is used, how it becomes addictive. Then we discuss ways in which smokers can kick the habit and remain smoke-free.

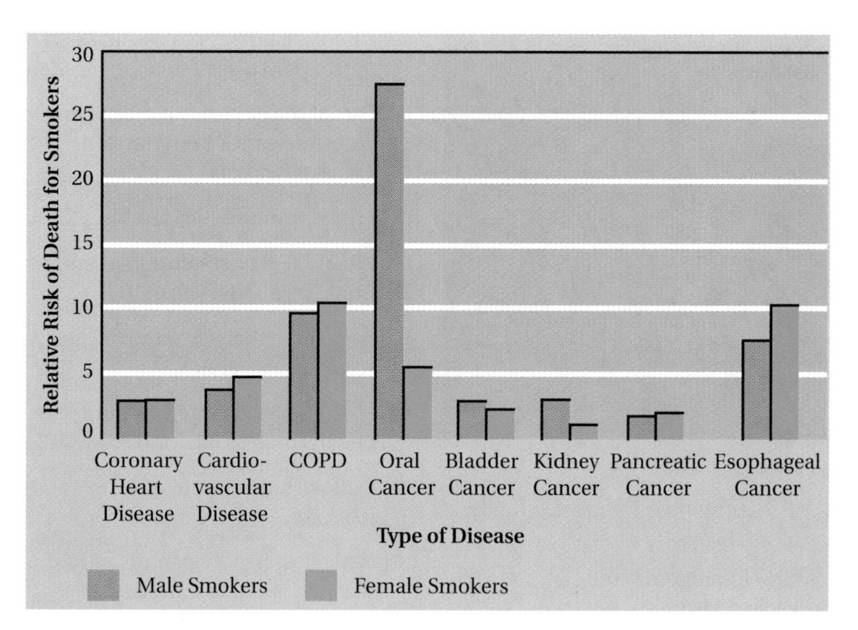


**Figure 14.2** ***Relative Risks of Death for Current Smokers by Type of Disease*** Here we compare the relative risks of death from the various diseases which cigarette smokers face. Male smokers, for example, are nearly 10 times more likely than nonsmokers to die from COPD and roughly 27 times more likely to die from oral cancers. Female smokers are 3 times more likely to die from coronary heart disease and 10 times more likely to die from cancer of the esophagus than female nonsmokers.

**Smart Quiz**
Q1401

## think about it!

- **What are the health risks associated with smoking? Knowing these risks, are you willing to commit slow suicide by smoking?**
- **Has anyone you know experienced health problems connected with smoking? What are they?**
- **Do you know anyone who smoked while she was pregnant? Did she believe that her smoking could harm the fetus?**

# WHY DO PEOPLE SMOKE?

Despite the dangers of smoking, millions of people continue to smoke, and millions more start smoking each year. *Why?*

There are many reasons why people begin smoking. Some young (and some not so young) people are ignorant of the dangers of smoking. Some young people smoke because their peers smoke and they believe that smoking helps them "fit in," or is "cool" or sophisticated. Others smoke because they find it pleasurable.

**Video**
Quitting smoking
V1401

Advertising is an important influence. Although cigarette manufacturers are no longer permitted to advertise their products on TV, they spend more than 3.5 billion dollars annually for advertising in other media, such as magazines and billboards. Many advertising campaigns are directed at the young and at minority smokers. Billboard advertisements for cigarettes proliferate in minority communities. The use of cartoon figures, like "Joe Camel," has special appeal to the young.

There are also many reasons why people continue to smoke. Some smoke for pleasure. Others smoke out of habit or because of cravings. Still others smoke because they find smoking relaxing or because it provides a lift. Some people use cigarettes as a form of self-medication, to help relieve anxiety or depression. Some people smoke for a combination of reasons. Smokers can gain some insight into their own reasons for smoking by completing the nearby ***HealthCheck*** (next page), "Why Do You Smoke?"

## Smoking—An Addiction, Not Just a Bad Habit

Though some of us may think of smoking only as a bad habit, a 1988 Surgeon General's report concluded that habitual smoking is also a form of chemical dependence or addiction.[25]

Whatever the reasons for smoking, it leads to addiction to tobacco—or more precisely, to the stimulant nicotine, which is found in tobacco. Although not every smoker becomes addicted, most do, and quickly. Typically, casual experimentation—a cigarette every now and then—yields to daily smoking. Most smokers realize that smoking

# Health*Check*

## *Why Do You Smoke?*

These are some statements made by people to describe what they get out of smoking cigarettes. If you smoke, indicate how often you feel the way described in the statement by circling the appropriate number.[24] Then check the scoring key in Appendix B to interpret your responses.

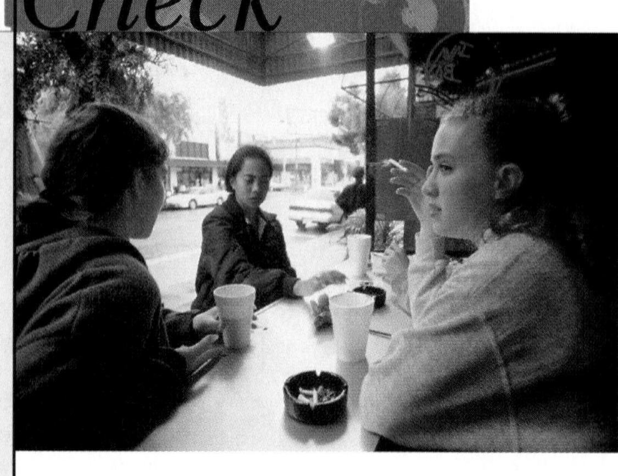

*Important: Answer every question.*

1 = never 2 = seldom 3 = occasionally
4 = frequently 5 = always

A. I smoke cigarettes in order to keep myself from slowing down. 1 2 3 4 5

B. Handling a cigarette is part of the enjoyment of smoking it. 1 2 3 4 5

C. Smoking cigarettes is pleasant and relaxing. 1 2 3 4 5

D. I light up a cigarette when I feel angry about something. 1 2 3 4 5

E. When I run out of cigarettes, I find it almost unbearable until I get them. 1 2 3 4 5

F. I smoke cigarettes automatically without even being aware of it. 1 2 3 4 5

G. I smoke cigarettes to stimulate me, to perk myself up. 1 2 3 4 5

H. Part of the enjoyment of smoking a cigarette comes from the steps I take to light up. 1 2 3 4 5

I. I find cigarettes pleasurable. 1 2 3 4 5

J. When I feel uncomfortable or upset about something, I light up a cigarette. 1 2 3 4 5

K. I am very much aware of the fact when I am not smoking a cigarette. 1 2 3 4 5

L. I light up a cigarette without realizing I still have one burning in the ashtray. 1 2 3 4 5

M. I smoke cigarettes to give me a lift. 1 2 3 4 5

N. When I smoke a cigarette, part of the enjoyment is watching the smoke as I exhale it. 1 2 3 4 5

O. I want a cigarette most when I am comfortable and relaxed. 1 2 3 4 5

P. When I feel blue or want to take my mind off cares and worries, I smoke cigarettes. 1 2 3 4 5

Q. I get a real gnawing hunger for a cigarette when I haven't smoked for a while. 1 2 3 4 5

R. I've found a cigarette in my mouth and didn't remember putting it there. 1 2 3 4 5

is harmful and damages their health. Yet they have difficulty breaking the habit because they have acquired a physical dependence—an addiction—to nicotine.

We're accustomed to thinking of a drug addict as someone injecting heroin in some darkened alleyway, not someone lighting up a cigarette. Yet the greatest number of addicts in our society are people who hold jobs, pay taxes, and are just like the people next door. They supply themselves with a "fix" of a drug every time they light up a cigarette. Each puff on a cigarette introduces a highly addictive stimulant drug, nicotine, into their bloodstream. Smoking is the leading form of addiction in our society and accounts for more deaths than all other drugs combined, legal or illegal. A nicotine addict smokes cigarettes as a means of administering the drug, just as a crack addict uses a pipe or a heroin addict a syringe. Physical dependence on tobacco doesn't develop overnight. The addiction builds gradually, usually over a period of a year or more, involving a progression from occasional experimentation to regular use.[26]

In 1996, the federal government brought tobacco under the regulatory authority of the Food and Drug Administration (FDA) as an addictive drug. The move was the linchpin of the government's effort to curb the use of tobacco by young people, since it gave the FDA wider powers to regulate tobacco. The nearby questionnaire may give smokers insight into whether they are addicted to cigarettes.

## HealthCheck

### Are You Addicted To Smoking?

Compulsive use of a substance is a hallmark of addiction. If you would like to quit smoking but feel compelled to pick up that next cigarette, you are probably hooked. If you would like to quit but feel powerless to resist the urge to smoke, you are probably addicted. But just how addicted are you? The following quiz may help give some insights into whether your smoking habit is an addiction.[27]

| Do You. . . | Yes | No |
|---|---|---|
| Find that the first cigarette smoked during the day is the most satisfying? | ____ | ____ |
| Smoke heavily early in the morning? | ____ | ____ |
| Find it difficult to resist smoking in no-smoking areas? | ____ | ____ |
| Find yourself unable to cut down or abstain from smoking when you are ill? | ____ | ____ |
| Prefer high-nicotine or unfiltered cigarettes? | ____ | ____ |
| Inhale deeply on each puff? | ____ | ____ |
| Smoke each cigarette down to the butt? | ____ | ____ |
| Chain smoke—light up a cigarette immediately after finishing another? | ____ | ____ |
| Have extreme anxiety about running out of cigarettes? | ____ | ____ |
| Have significant withdrawal symptoms if you abruptly stop smoking? | ____ | ____ |
| Find it difficult to stop smoking, even for a short period? | ____ | ____ |
| Find that you are always aware of the location of your cigarette pack? | ____ | ____ |
| Never leave home without cigarettes, except by accident? | ____ | ____ |

*Did you answer yes to any of these questions? If so, then you are probably addicted to nicotine. The more questions to which you answered yes, the stronger your addiction is likely to be.*

### Addictive Properties of Smoking

What makes smoking an addiction, not just a bad habit? For one thing, regular smoking has a compulsive quality. Addicted people feel compelled to light up even if they know that smoking is harmful and want to quit. Cigarette smoking is also associated with the two cardinal features of addiction, a tolerance effect and physical dependence. Tolerance is shown by the need for more of the drug over time to achieve the same effect, which leads smokers to increase the number of cigarettes they smoke to a certain level, usually a pack or two a day. Physical dependence on a drug is characterized by the development of an *abstinence syndrome* (also called a withdrawal syndrome), which occurs when use of the drug ceases abruptly or is sharply reduced (see Chapter 12). With smoking, going "cold turkey" produces characteristic withdrawal symptoms such as nervousness, irritability, light-headedness, dizziness, restlessness, difficulty concentrating, loss of energy, headaches, fatigue, irregular bowel movements, insomnia, cramps, sweating, palpitations, and intense cravings for cigarettes.

We know that heroin addicts regulate their intake of heroin to maintain a fairly steady level in their bloodstreams. In a similar way, smokers regulate their blood levels of nicotine by smoking about the same number of cigarettes day after day, week after week. Smokers will also adjust their smoking rate if conditions change. For example, when smokers are given drugs that speed the passage of nicotine from the body in the urine, they adjust by smoking more.[28] We also know that when smokers are switched to lower-nicotine brands, they tend to compensate by smoking more, taking more puffs, inhaling harder or more deeply, or smoking cigarettes down to the butts.[29]

#### think about it!

- **Have you heard smokers claim that they could give up their habit any time they want to? Do you believe them? Why or why not?**
- **Are you or an acquaintance addicted to cigarettes? How do you know?**
- **How did you or your acquaintance get started smoking? Were you aware of the health risks of cigarettes when you began?**

Smart Quiz
Q1402

## OTHER TOBACCO USE

Cigarette smoking is not the only means of using tobacco. Some people smoke pipes or cigars. Others use smokeless tobacco.

### Pipe and Cigar Smoking

Though pipe and cigar smokers may not inhale, or inhale as deeply as cigarette smokers, they still draw carcinogens into their body with each mouthful of tobacco smoke. They face an increased risk of cancer of the lips, mouth, and esophagus.[30] All told, the rate of cancer deaths among men who smoke cigars is 34% higher than among nonsmokers. Oral cancers are actually more prevalent among pipe and cigar smokers than among cigarette smokers. In terms of health, the trendiness of cigar smoking and cigar bars is a step backward. Second-hand smoke from cigars actually fouls the air with more cancer-causing particles than cigarette smoke inhaled by smoking—something to think about if you enter a cigar bar.

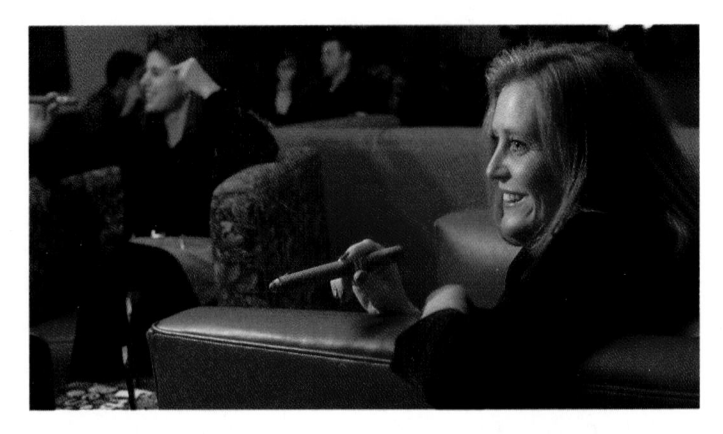

***The Cigar Bar, a Step Backward*** Cigar smoking has become trendy, even among women. Trend or no trend, cigar smokers face an increased risk of oral cancers even if they don't inhale the smoke into their lungs (not to mention the stained fingers and teeth).

### Smokeless Tobacco

Some people use tobacco without lighting up. Snuff is a powdered form of tobacco that can be inhaled through the nose. It may also be placed inside the cheek, where it is sucked. Chewing tobacco, another smokeless tobacco product, is used by lodging a pinch between the cheek and gum and then chewing or sucking. The use of snuff or chewing tobacco allows nicotine to pass through the mucosal membranes of the nose or mouth into the bloodstream.

Many people operate under a false assumption that smokeless tobacco is a safe or relatively harmless substitute for cigarette smoking. Studies show that one in four adults does not believe that chewing tobacco or using snuff is harmful to one's health.[31] The fact is that smokeless tobacco in snuff or chewable form contains some of the most powerful carcinogens in tobacco and is responsible for about three of four cases of oral cancer (cancers of the mouth, lips, and pharynx) in the United States.[32] Smokeless tobacco can also cause cancer of the esophagus as well as noncancerous conditions of the oral cavity. It also delivers about the same level of nicotine to the user as cigarettes, so it's no surprise that the use of smokeless tobacco can lead to nicotine addiction.

Oral cancers are among the most devastating forms of cancer, not only because of the risk of death, but also because of the disfiguring operations on the face and jaw that may be needed to halt the spread of the disease. Unlike some slow-forming types of cancer that don't usually strike until later in life, oral cancers brought on by the use of smokeless tobacco often strike early, at the outset of adulthood, as in the following case:

> *Eighteen-year-old Sean Marsee had used smokeless tobacco—chewing tobacco briefly, then snuff—since he was 12. But then an angry red spot with a hard white core the size of a half dollar appeared on his tongue. When the spot was removed, a biopsy found that is was cancerous and that radiation therapy would be necessary. However, soon after the operation, a newly swollen lymph node was found on Sean's neck, a sign that the cancer had spread. The best chance of stopping the cancer would be to remove the lower jaw on the side of the lesion as well as all lymph nodes, muscles, and smaller blood vessels in the area.*
>
> *Sean underwent a second operation to remove all this tissue but the jaw bone, which he insisted on keeping. He did well for five months but then he began having headaches and a CAT scan showed that the tumor had spread to his brain and back. Further, even more radical, surgery failed to stop the spread of the tumor and Sean died several months later. Just before he died, Sean, unable to speak, wrote two brief messages to share with other young people. One was a declaration of his faith. The other was a plea: Don't dip snuff.*[33]

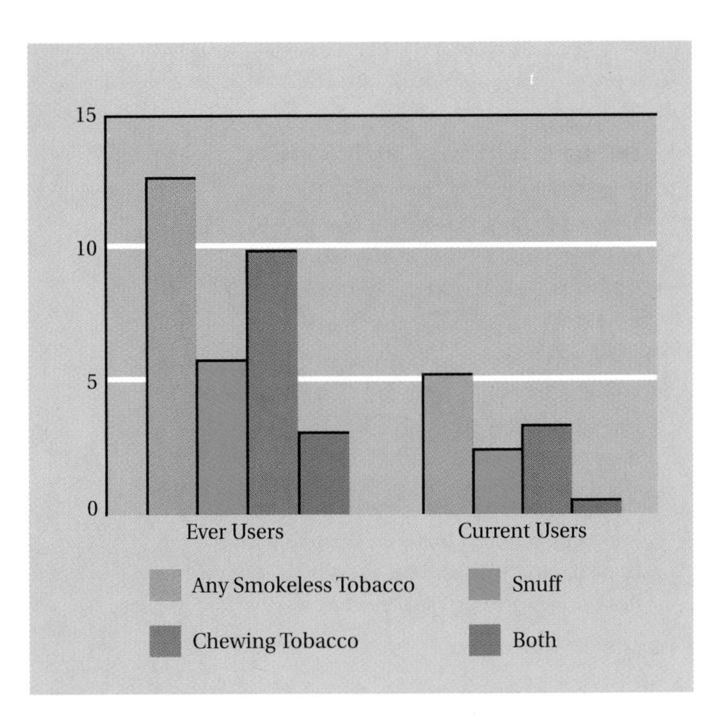


**Figure 14.3** ***Prevalences of Smokeless Tobacco Use by Males (17+ years)*** Use of smokeless tobacco is greatest among men, especially younger men. More than 12% of men have used a smokeless tobacco product at some point in their lives; 5% are current users.

While use of smokeless tobacco products has declined among people over the age of 21, about 12 million people in the United States continue to use them.[34] More than nine of ten (91%) users of smokeless tobacco are men; use by women is rare. About one in five high school boys had used chewing tobacco or snuff in the early 1990s, an eightfold increase since the mid-1970s. The habit is especially popular among young men, especially white males (see Figure 14.3). In fact, the use of snuff increased fifteenfold between 1964 and 1986, and the use of chewing tobacco increased more than fourfold among young men in the 17 to 19 age bracket.

## Second-Hand Smoking

How often have you heard a cigarette smoker ask, "Do you mind if I smoke?" While it was once a matter of social etiquette for nonsmokers to extend permission, mounting evidence of the dangers of second-hand smoke may well lead people to answer the question with a resounding "Yes, I do mind." **Second-hand smoking** (also called *passive smoking*) involves exposure to second-hand smoke from other people's cigarettes, cigars, or pipes. Regular exposure to second-hand smoke in the home or workplace nearly doubles the risk of heart attacks and deaths in nonsmokers. Because of this and other health risks, smoking has been banned in most public places, including schools, hospitals, elevators, and aboard domestic airplanes.

Second-hand smoking increases the risk of coronary heart disease (CHD), respiratory diseases including lung cancer, and other illnesses in nonsmokers.[35] Second-hand smoke contains even greater concentrations of potent carcinogens than the smoke inhaled from the cigarette itself. The amount of exposure to these carcinogens varies with proximity to the smoker and room ventilation, but we can generally assume that people who are close to the smoker will inhale some amount of second-hand smoke.

**Close-up**

Exposure widespread
T1403

Environmental tobacco smoke
T1404

Exposure to second-hand smoke is recognized as a cause of lung cancer in nonsmokers. The risk of lung cancer in nonsmokers exposed to second-hand smoke increases with the amount and length of exposure.[36] Male nonsmokers whose wives smoke stand a 1.62 greater chance of developing lung cancer than do nonsmokers whose wives do not smoke. Female nonsmokers who are exposed to smoking by their husbands have a 1.32 greater chance of developing lung cancer than do nonsmoking wives of nonsmoking men.

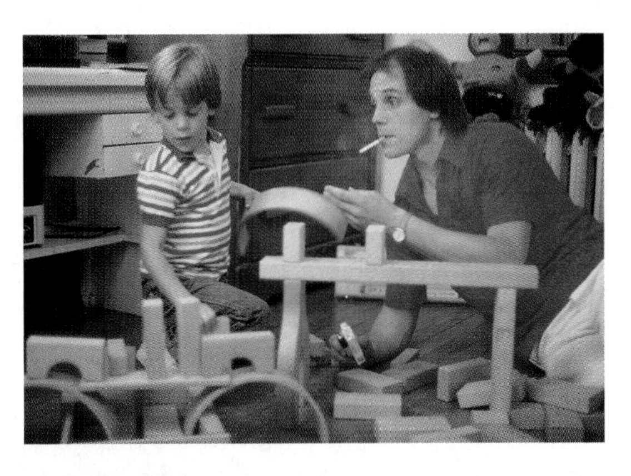

***Dangers of Second-Hand Smoke*** Children exposed to second-hand smoke are at greater risk of developing asthma and other respiratory diseases in childhood and lung cancer later in life. Nonsmokers whose spouses smoke have an increased risk of lung cancer, and a 30% greater risk of dying from coronary heart disease, than spouses of nonsmokers.

**Second-hand smoking** Ingestion of tobacco smoke from other people's lit cigarettes.

Cardiovascular deaths may well account for the greatest number of deaths due to exposure to second-hand smoke. Studies show that nonsmokers who are married to smokers incur a 30% increased risk of dying from CHD.[37] Second-hand smoke is especially dangerous to people with heart problems or respiratory conditions such as asthma.

**Dangers to Children** Children who are repeatedly exposed to cigarette smoke stand an increased risk of asthma and other respiratory diseases in childhood and are at increased risk of developing lung cancer later in life.[38] As many as one in four cases of childhood asthma is caused by exposure to maternal smoking.

### think about it!

- **Do you know any pipe or cigar smokers? Do they believe that their habits are dangerous? Why or why not?**
- **Second-hand smoke is dangerous. Would you feel comfortable asking someone not to smoke in your presence? Why or why not?**

**critical thinking** **Agree or disagree and support your answer: Tobacco should be regulated by the government as a drug.**

**critical thinking** **Agree or disagree and support your answer: Exposing children to cigarette smoke should be looked upon as a form of child abuse.**

Smart Quiz
Q1403

## PREVENTION

### *Reducing Exposure to Second-Hand Smoke*

Despite the restrictions on public smoking, many people are still regularly exposed to second-hand smoke, especially at home. Nonsmokers who live with smokers are at special risk, especially in homes that are not well ventilated. If you live with a smoker or have friends or relatives who smoke when you are around, consider yourself at risk. Here are some ways you can reduce, if not eliminate, your exposure to second-hand smoke:

- Establish no-smoking zones in your home.
- Establish a no-smoking rule in your home. Smokers who wish to smoke can politely be asked to step outside to smoke or to go into another, preferably well-ventilated, room.
- Post no-smoking signs around the house. These cues may prevent your getting into arguments.
- If you can't completely prohibit smoking in your residence, restrict it to well-ventilated rooms.
- Avoid being in these rooms when others are smoking.
- Request that smokers switch to cigarettes lower in tar and nicotine.
- Restrict smoking to times when nonsmokers are not present.
- Install fans to remove smoke that may waft through the house.

## WHO SMOKES?

Let's begin with some good news. More than 35 million smokers in the U.S. have quit since the landmark Surgeon General's report in 1964.[39] By 1987, nearly half of all people who had ever smoked had quit. Smoking rates among adults declined from about 40% in 1964 to about 25% today. By the 1990s, cigarette smoking had declined to the lowest levels since the government first started tracking smoking in 1955. The federal government estimates that about 3 million smoking-related deaths were delayed or avoided as a result of people quitting smoking or deciding not to start.

Close-up
Tobacco use: CDC Report
T1405

More and more smokers are joining the ranks of nonsmokers every day. Smokers who are better educated are more likely to quit than their less well-educated peers. Nearly six in ten (57%) college-educated people who once smoked no longer do so.

Yet the news is not all good. Smoking rates in the general population leveled off during the early to mid-1990s. They have also begun to climb sharply among teenagers, reversing an earlier steady decline.[40] By 1995, nearly 35% of teenagers 17 years of age or younger reported smoking dur-

Close-up
Children and tobacco: The facts
T1406
Children and tobacco: The problem
T1407

ing the past month. This was an increase of about 25% since 1991.[41] Estimates are that 3,000 young people take up smoking each day. A third of these will eventually die of smoking-related diseases.

In total, nearly 50 million people in the United States continue to smoke regularly. That is about 25% of the adult population. The leveling off of smoking means that the nation may not meet the national health goals set by the Healthy People 2000 project of limiting smoking to 15% of the population by the year 2000, let alone achieving the ultimate goal of a completely smoke-free society.

What are we to learn from these trends? One lesson is that young people may not be fully aware of how dangerous cigarette smoking and other uses of tobacco are to them. Images of older people dying of emphysema or lung cancer as the result of smoking may have less of an impact on younger people than highly publicized media reports of cocaine overdoses killing college athletes and other young people. If the antismoking campaign is to be effective with young people, better ways of reaching them are needed.

**Close-up**
Children's future at risk
**T1408**

## Smoking Demographics

Though smoking is still more prevalent among men overall, women under 30 are now the fastest-growing group of smokers. Smoking is also more prevalent among some ethnic minorities, especially African-American men (see the nearby ***World of Diversity*** feature, "Smoking and Ethnic Minorities"). Moreover, the sharpest rise in teenage smoking is among African-American males, portending more dire health problems in the future.[42]

Smoking is increasingly becoming a problem of the socially and economically disadvantaged in our society. Smoking is more prevalent, and rates of quitting lower, among people with less education and lower incomes. Figure 14.4 shows the prevalence of smoking broken down by gender, race, and educational level.

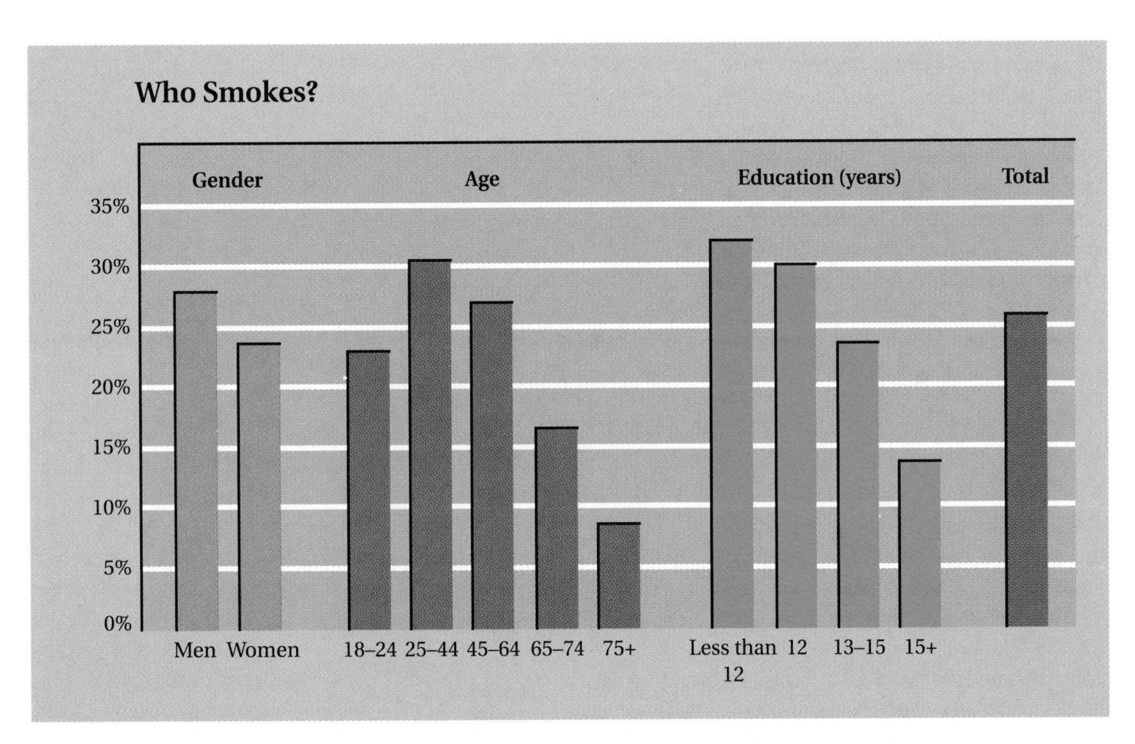


**Figure 14.4** ***Percentages of People Who Smoke by Gender, Age, and Educational Level*** Smoking is most prevalent among men, among young adults 25 to 44 years of age, and among people with less than 12 completed years of schooling. Overall, one in four people in the U.S. smokes. How about you?

WORLD OF *diversity*

## Smoking and Ethnic Minorities

Antismoking campaigns have been less effective in promoting smoking cessation among people of color than among whites. Cigarette companies have also targeted much of their advertising effort toward minority communities, especially African-American and Hispanic-American communities. Smoking is also associated with lower socioeconomic status, and people of color tend to be overrepresented in these lower strata. Taken together, it is not surprising that cigarette smoking is more prevalent among some ethnic minorities, especially African-American men, Native Americans, and some Hispanic-American subgroups such as Puerto Ricans.

Smoking, especially among men, is a worldwide health problem of staggering proportions. The World Health Organization estimates that more than 60% of men in China, Indonesia, Korea, and the Philippines smoke, compared with 28% of men in the United States.[43] Across Latin America and East Asia, about one in two men smokes.[44] In China alone, 300 million people smoke, which is more than the entire U.S. population!

Let us take a closer look at smoking among minority groups in the United States.

### African Americans

African-American men have the highest smoking rates among the major racial/ethnic groups in the U.S. (see Figure 14.5). Yet African-American women smoke at a rate similar to that of the general female population. African-American men also have the highest rates of death due to lung cancer of any group in our society.[45] African Americans overall have more than six times the incidence of lung cancer as white Americans.[46] Factors linked to higher smoking rates, such as lower socioeconomic status, less formal education, blue-collar work, and unemployment, affect African Americans disproportionately, especially those living in depressed inner-city neighborhoods. Not surprisingly, smoking is a major contributor to shorter life expectancy among African-American men in inner-city neighborhoods.[47]

According to the National Cancer Institute, if antismoking campaigns are to achieve widespread success among African Americans, especially those of lower socioeconomic status, several barriers will need to be overcome:[48]

- Reliance on cigarettes as a way of coping with the stresses and social disadvantages associated with lower socioeconomic status and pervasive discrimination.
- Less use of primary health care providers, who might serve to encourage smoking cessation and provide helpful advice. Limited access to health care in general and to smoking-related services and resources in particular.

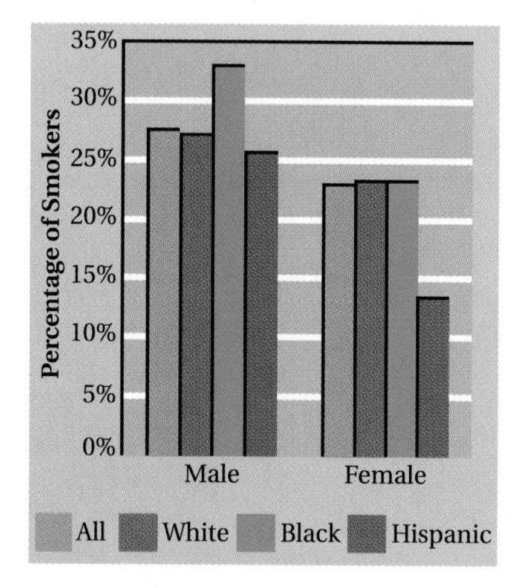


**Figure 14.5** ***Percentages of Adults Who Smoke by Gender and Racial/Ethnic Group*** Smoking is more prevalent among black men than white or Hispanic men in our society. For women, smoking prevalences are comparable between blacks and whites, but much lower among Hispanics.

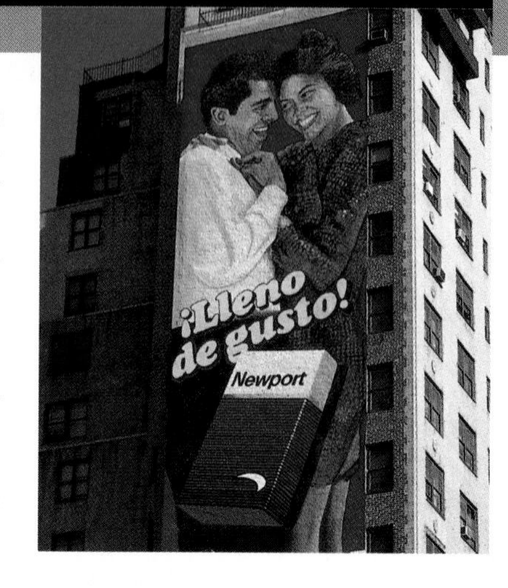


- Attitudes in African-American communities that may encourage smoking.
- Considering smoking to be less critical than other pressing social problems such as drugs, unemployment, racism, and crime.
- Powerful advertising tailored to African-American consumers that not only glamorizes and legitimizes smoking but also downplays the health risks. (Billboard advertisements are particularly prominent in minority communities.)

### Hispanic Americans

Overall, Hispanic men smoke about as much as non-Hispanic white men, while Hispanic women smoke less than non-Hispanic white women and Hispanic men (see Figure 14.5).[49] Smoking has declined among Hispanic groups overall, but it has remained stable among some Hispanic subgroups and has increased among others, such as young Puerto Ricans.

Acculturation affects smoking patterns among Hispanic Americans, especially Hispanic women.[50] Traditional Hispanic-American cultures discourage smoking among women but not among men, which may explain the traditional gender gap in smoking rates among Hispanics. Yet mainstream U.S. culture has less rigidly defined gender roles. Not surprisingly, smoking rates among more acculturated Hispanic-American women in the United States tend to be higher than those among less acculturated Hispanic women.

### Native Americans

Overall, 28% of Native American men and 35% of Native American women smoke.[51] However, there is much variability across Native American subgroups. Some groups, such as Northern Plains Indians (42 to 70% across tribes) and Alaskan Natives (56%),[52] have higher than average smoking rates. Others, such as Southwestern Indians (13 to 28%), have lower rates. Use of smokeless tobacco is also higher among some Native Americans, especially among the young.

### Asian Americans

We lack national survey data on smoking among Asian Americans. Nevertheless, local surveys of specific Asian groups show variable smoking rates. For example, a recent survey in Hawaii showed smoking rates of 25% for Filipinos and 21% for Japanese, compared with 29% for white and Native Hawaiians.[53] Men who recently immigrated from Southeast Asia have among the highest reported smoking rates of any ethnic group in the United States.[54]

### Smoking Cessation Programs for Minority Smokers

Given the diversity of smoking patterns that exists in the United States, no one approach to smoking cessation is likely to be effective for all smokers.[55] Antismoking programs need to be tailored to groups they are intended to reach. They need to take into account the distinguishing cultural characteristics of the groups. For example, Hispanic-American smokers are more likely to connect smoking with socializing with friends than are smokers from other groups. Therefore, learning how to politely refuse a cigarette takes on importance in helping Hispanic Americans quit smoking. Hispanics are also more likely to express concern about the social or interpersonal consequences of smoking, such as setting a bad example for their children, damaging their children's health, or provoking criticism from family members, and about the short-term consequences of smoking, such as bad breath and burning holes in clothing.[56] Incorporating these concerns in antismoking messages may be more effective than a campaign that focuses only on long-term health consequences. The central reference points in the Hispanic communities, such as the churches, *bodegas* (neighborhood grocery stores), community health clinics, and community organizations, need to be used as distribution points for health information.

Health organizations have begun to meet the need for smoking cessation programs that target minority smokers. In the Bedford-Stuyvesant area of Brooklyn, New York, a predominantly African-American community, the New York State Healthy Heart Program sponsored a quit-smoking contest in which people who quit smoking for a month were eligible to participate in a drawing for various prizes. In New York's Washington Heights community, an area with a predominantly Dominican population, the local Healthy Heart Program sponsored a "Burial of Joe Camel" day.

Your first author was principal investigator on a federally funded research project involving the development of a culturally sensitive smoking cessation program for Hispanic smokers, the "SI, PUEDO" ("Yes, I Can") program.[57] This eight-week-long stop-smoking program was offered in a predominantly Hispanic community in Queens, New York. It incorporated as part of a broad-ranging behavior modification program the use of videotaped vignettes of smoking-related situations enacted by Hispanic actors. Culturally laden values such as *machismo* (masculinity), *familiarismo* (responsibility to family), and *respeto* (respect for self and others) were used in these vignettes to convey antismoking messages.

In another federally funded program, the American Indian Health Care Association directed a smoking cessation program at Native Americans through Indian health clinics in the upper Midwest and Northwest.[58] At Ohio State University, the federal government funded a program in which Asian Americans were trained to help Southeast Asian men quit smoking, a group composed largely of recent immigrants from Vietnam and Cambodia among whom smoking rates are especially high.[59]

One recent example of a successful communitywide antismoking effort involved a grass-roots campaign waged in Philadelphia against the test marketing of "Uptown" cigarettes, a new brand that targeted the African-American community. Organizers were able to mobilize community residents and put enough pressure on the cigarette maker to force withdrawal of the brand.[60]

Cigarette advertising has been increasingly directed at African Americans, which has created something of a backlash. Many community organizers in African-American communities have taken action to prevent the display of cigarette advertisements on community billboards. In New York City and elsewhere, clergy and other community leaders have attempted to prohibit billboard advertising of cigarettes (in some cases, even "whitewashing" billboards) and to ensure stricter enforcement of restrictions against selling cigarettes to minors.

Antismoking organizers have also made use of churches, recreational centers, and barbershops in African-American communities as settings for stop-smoking programs. In East Baltimore, Maryland, the "Heart, Body &

Soul Project" involved a collaboration between African-American clergymen and the Johns Hopkins Center for Health Promotion in which the clergymen delivered smoking cessation messages as part of their sermons and sponsored health fairs and special programs for smoking cessation within their churches.[61]

Voluntary health organizations, including the American Lung Association, the American Heart Association, and the American Cancer Society, have become involved in spearheading stop-smoking initiatives targeting minority smokers. For example, the American Lung Association has developed a pamphlet, "Don't Let Your Dreams Go Up in Smoke," that addresses the problem of smoking in the African-American community.[62] With this increased attention focused on smoking cessation in all segments of our society, "Joe Camel's" days may well be numbered.

## PREVENTION

### *Preventing Smoking*

Smoking initiation among teenagers is a critical health issue. Most smokers take up the habit as teenagers, usually before they graduate from high school. If young people do not take up the habit, we can go a long way toward achieving the goal of a smoke-free society.

Preventing smoking, like preventing other forms of substance abuse, is a daunting challenge. People, especially young people, are often more influenced by the immediate reinforcing effects of smoking—the "kick" from nicotine, the self-image of doing something that seems "mature" or perhaps "dangerous"—than by the thought of eventual health consequences. Yes, the attitudes of many young people have shifted against smoking. However, many are still subjected to peer pressures to smoke. The approval of peers is often a stronger influence than are the health warnings of parents, teachers, and writers of health books like this one. Adolescent smokers also tend to hold certain misconceptions about smoking. For example, they overestimate the numbers of smokers among their peers and minimize the addictive properties of smoking.

Virtually all young people have heard about the dangers of smoking, but for many, especially younger women, the message goes in one ear and out the other. Effective smoking prevention programs attempt to debunk the notion that smoking is "cool" or "sexy." They help young people think critically about the hype of cigarette ads compared with the grittier realities of smoking as an addiction. Given the importance of peer influences, health professionals recognize that programs must provide youngsters with the skills they need to fend off social pressures to smoke, such as learning what to say and do when offered a cigarette. Many of the more successful programs rely on peer-counseling models. That is, they involve young people as models and tutors to help classmates learn how to refuse cigarettes.

**Close-up**
Tips for teens
T1409

In one example of a smoking prevention program with a predominantly Hispanic student population in the New York City schools, researchers achieved a nearly 30% reduction in the rates of smoking and smoking initiation compared with a control group that did not receive the prevention program.[69] Among the techniques used was an educational component that focused on providing information about the short-term consequences of smoking and the addictive nature of smoking; a decision-making component that trained students to think critically and independently when making decisions; and a rehearsal component that provided training in assertiveness skills and rehearsal opportunities for resisting peer group influences to smoke.

**Close-up**
More on prevention
T1410

Smoking prevention efforts must also focus on the use of smokeless tobacco and debunking the chic image that has lately come to be associated with cigar smoking. We could go a long way toward changing the attitudes of young people if leading movie stars shunned cigarettes and cigars and Hollywood producers refrained from glamorizing smoking in movies.

### *think about it!*

- **What is the incidence of smoking within your ethnic group? Your gender?**

**critical thinking** **What factors in your own life have influenced you to smoke or not to smoke?**

**Smart Quiz**
Q1404

WORLD OF *diversity*

## "You've Come a Long Way, Baby"? On Women and Smoking

> Girls seem to adopt smoking not because they are pressured to, but because they seek to identify themselves as independent, successful and glamorous—precisely the image projected by cigarette advertisers.
>
> National Cancer Institute, 1991, pp. 226–227

When a cigarette manufacturer uses the slogan "You've come a long way, baby" to promote tobacco products to women, the purpose is clear—to associate smoking with the feminist movement. Cigarette manufacturers have made a special effort to attract young women to smoking by piggybacking on the feminist movement. Unfortunately, when it comes to cigarette smoking, coming "a long way" toward achieving parity with men has landed many women in early graves.

*Smoking is as much of a health risk for women as for men.* Lung cancer deaths in women increased nearly sixfold from 1950 to 1987, a direct result of increased smoking rates (see Figure 14.6).[63] Lung cancer is now the leading cause of death from cancer among women, surpassing even breast cancer.

In the early twentieth century, smoking was almost an exclusively male preserve. By the 1930s and 1940s, however, smoking had become more popular among women. Smoking was spurred in large part by the images of glamorous actresses smoking or having their cigarettes lit for them by their dashing leading men. Smoking rates among women peaked at 32% by the mid-1960s and have since declined only slightly, to about 27%, in contrast to the larger declines among men.[64] Moreover, though smoking initiation (the rate of new smokers) declined in both men and women over the past 20 years or so, it dropped four times more rapidly among men than women. If present trends continue, experts expect that by the new millennium, women smokers will outnumber their male counterparts. Among college students, this crossover has already occurred. Smoking rates are especially high among poorer, less educated women.

While men have had higher rates of lung cancer deaths than women over the years, gender differences are fast disappearing. Women smokers also face a higher risk of uterine, cervical, and breast cancers than do women nonsmokers.[65] Women smokers have nearly a four times greater chance of suffering a heart attack than nonsmokers. The relative risk increases with the number of cigarettes smoked daily. Smoking a low-nicotine cigarette does not appear to decrease the risk of a heart attack.

Antismoking campaigns may have been less effective in reducing smoking among women in part because the influential Surgeon General's 1964 report highlighted the risks of CHD and lung cancer, two diseases to which women were traditionally less susceptible. CHD now claims the lives of more women than any other cause, and lung cancer has become the leading cancer killer among women, as it is among men.

Some people, especially women, smoke to control their weight.[66] Nicotine depresses the appetite and raises the metabolic rate.[67] People also tend to eat more when they stop smoking, which leads some people who have quit to return to smoking.[68]

Winds of change are in the air. Some magazines, such as *Ms.* and *Good Housekeeping,* refuse advertisements from cigarette manufacturers. It remains to be seen whether the media at large will boycott tobacco advertisers.

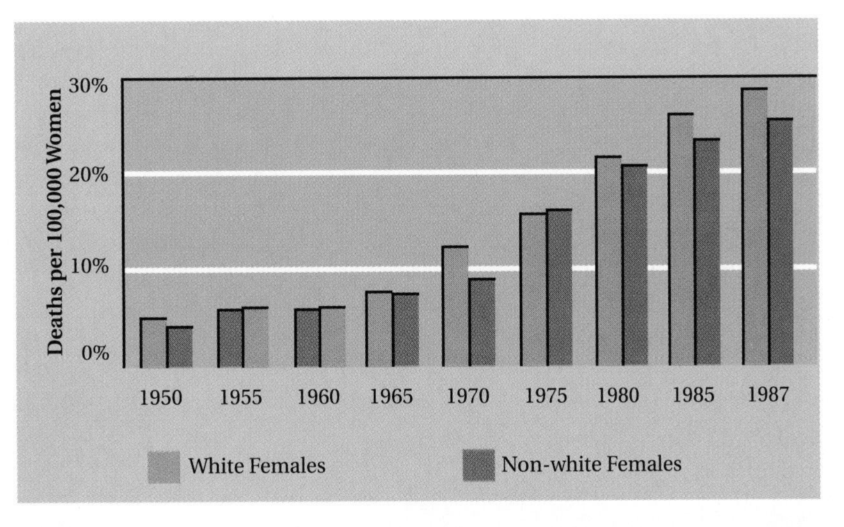


**Figure 14.6** ***Rise in Number of Deaths due to Lung Cancer among Women*** Sadly, the increased prevalence of smoking among women in the latter half of the twentieth century has led to a sharp rise in lung cancer mortality rates. The rise is especially steep among white females.

# Quitting Smoking

## Take Charge

Whether you've smoked for one year or 30, smoke now and then, or have a three-pack-a-day habit, there are considerable health benefits to quitting.[70] The sooner you quit, the sooner you begin reaping them. When you quit, your excess risk of CHD relative to people who continue to smoke is cut in half within a year. Your excess risk of suffering a heart attack disappears within either 2 or 3 years (for women) or 5 years (for men) of quitting. By 10 years after quitting, your risk of suffering lung cancer is reduced by as much as half. Quitting smoking also cuts in half the risk of cancers of the mouth and esophagus within 5 years. Greater reductions occur as abstinence continues. The risk of bladder cancer is halved only a few years after quitting. The risks of cervical and pancreatic cancer are reduced. The risk of dying from stroke returns to the level of nonsmokers in 5 to 15 years after quitting. The risk of respiratory diseases like emphysema and chronic bronchitis declines. Whereas smoking accelerates the onset of menopause in women, women who quit smoking enter menopause at an age similar to that of nonsmokers. Smokers who quit before the age of 50 cut their risk of dying during the next 15 years in half compared with those who continue to smoke. On average, male smokers between the ages of 35 and 39 who quit add 5 years to their lives. Female smokers in the same age range add 3 years to their lives. Figure 14.7 shows the reduction in the increased risk of early death for former smokers in relation to years since quitting.

While quitting smoking clearly reduces health risks, it does not return risks to presmoking levels. The risk of dying from lung cancer declines following smoking cessation but not quite to the level of people who never smoked (see Figure 14.8). Still, the earlier the smoker quits, the greater the reduction in risk. Compared with current smokers, former smokers who quit during their thirties reduce their risk of dying of lung cancer by at least 90%. Yet they are still more than twice as likely to die from lung cancer by the age of 75 as are nonsmokers. But smokers who wait until their early fifties to quit have five to six times the risk of dying from lung cancer as people who have never smoked. The lessons are clear: If you don't smoke, don't start. If you smoke, quit as soon as possible.

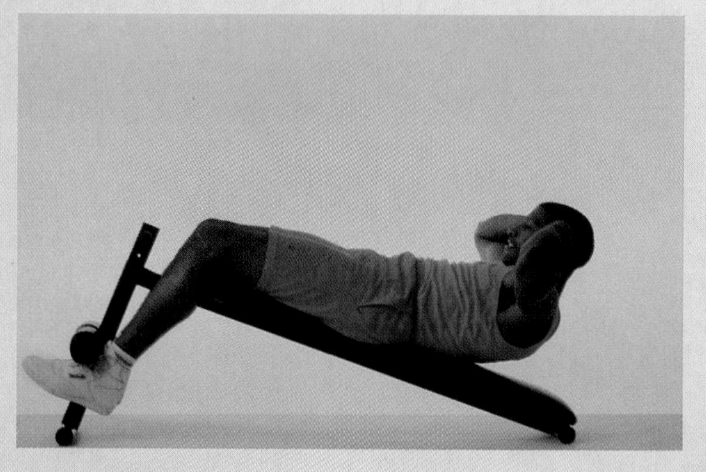

***Working It Out*** Regular exercise can help keep your mind off smoking and rebuild your stamina.

### Becoming an Ex-Smoker

Mark Twain once quipped that quitting smoking was easy—he'd done it at least a dozen times.

Why is it so hard to quit smoking? It isn't lack of willpower that keeps most smokers lighting up. Rather, most are addicted to tobacco, or rather, to the nicotine in tobacco smoke. They crave nicotine in much the same way that other addicts crave heroin or cocaine. Overcoming any addiction means breaking the body's dependence on the drug. Addicted smokers who quit are likely to experience unpleasant withdrawal symptoms. The symptoms vary from person to person, but most addicted smokers have some symptoms. The good news is that they tend to fade rapidly, within a few days to a week.

The threat of unpleasant withdrawal symptoms should not deter would-be quitters. For one thing, cutting back gradually may help lessen them. For another, nicotine replacement in the form of nicotine chewing gum or a nicotine patch is available. (Ask your physician or pharmacist.) Nicotine replacement provides the body with the nicotine it is missing following smoking cessation. It can reduce or eliminate withdrawal symptoms. Doctors can also prescribe the antidepressant, *Zyban,* which reduces the craving for nicotine.

Another reason why quitting smoking is so difficult for many people is the role of conditioning or smoking by habit. Smoking becomes associated with many cues or stimuli in everyday

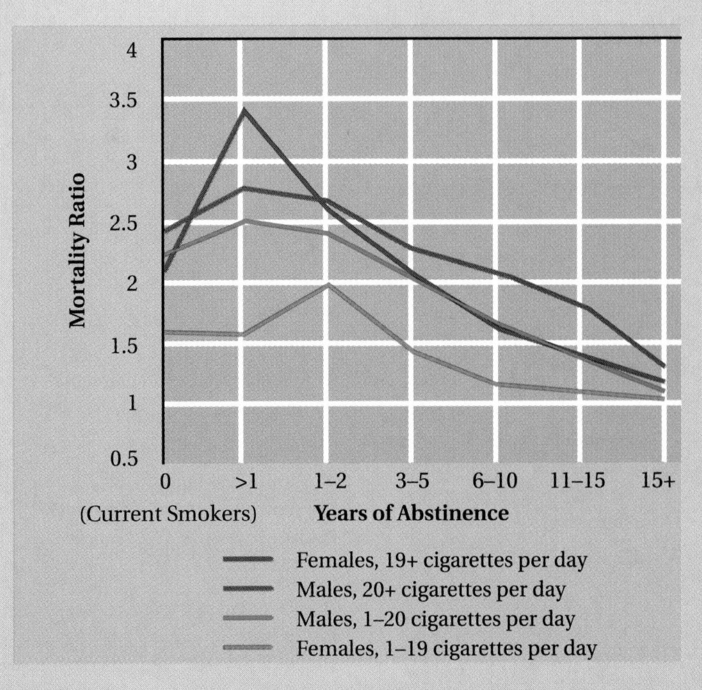


**Figure 14.7** ***Mortality Ratios of Current and Former Smokers by Length of Abstinence*** Here we see the mortality ratios of former smokers in relation to years of abstinence. The mortality ratio represents former smokers' risks of death from various causes relative to people who never smoked (a ratio of 1 represents a risk equal to that of never-smokers). The increased risk of dying relative to nonsmokers is nearly erased after 15 years for former light smokers (less than a pack a day) and is greatly reduced for former heavier smokers.

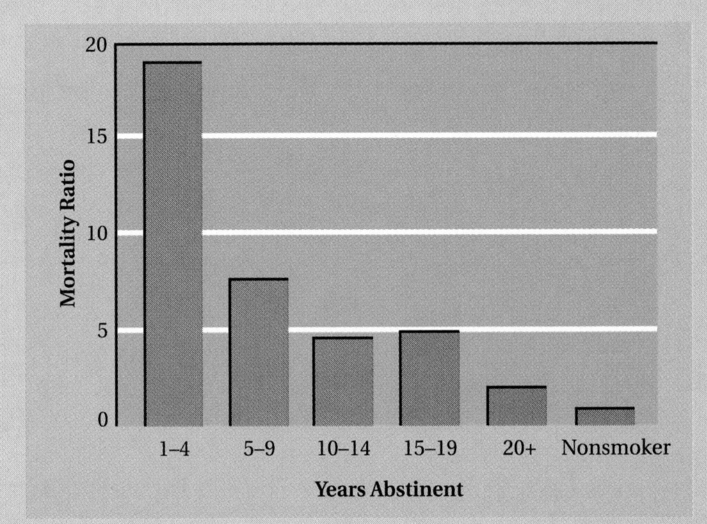


**Figure 14.8** ***Lung Cancer Mortality Ratios of Male Former Smokers Relative to Nonsmokers by Years of Abstinence*** If you quit smoking, you greatly reduce your risk of dying from lung cancer. Unfortunately, quitting does not reduce your risk to the level of nonsmokers even 20 or more years after quitting. Here we see that male former smokers who quit 20+ years earlier still stand double the chance of dying from lung cancer as male nonsmokers. But male smokers stand nearly 20 times the risk of dying from lung cancer as male nonsmokers. Some messages bear repeating: If you don't smoke, don't start. If you do smoke, stop.

life—drinking coffee, finishing a meal, watching TV, waiting for the bus, and so on. Smokers may encounter strong cravings when they find themselves in these situations.

Thus, cravings have a biological component (addiction) and a psychological component (habit). People can also become psychologically dependent on nicotine when they use it to help them cope with the stresses of everyday life. Nicotine can relax us when we're feeling tense or pick us up when we need a lift. The more often we light up to help us cope with negative emotions such as anxiety, anger, or depression, the more psychologically dependent we become.

Most people quit without assistance from professionals or smoking cessation programs. But you needn't go it alone. Many programs are offered by health organizations such as the American Lung Association and the National Cancer Institute. Many of these are offered free of charge or for a modest fee. Most programs, like the National Cancer Institute's "Fresh Start" program, help people understand their reasons for smoking, assist them in handling withdrawal symptoms, and offer tips on how to resist temptation. Those who are seeking to go it alone may profit from some of the suggestions for quitting listed below.

## Quitting Cold Turkey or Cutting Down Gradually

Deciding to quit is the first step toward becoming a nonsmoker. Once you've made that decision, you need to decide whether to quit "cold turkey" or cut down gradually before tossing away your cigarettes for good. If you shudder at the idea of going cold turkey, cutting down gradually may be a better alternative. Yet if you're the type of person who likes to take decisive steps, then you may prefer to quit all at once. In either case you may encounter withdrawal symptoms. The suggestions below can help you cope with them. Or you may discuss quitting with your physician, who may assist you by monitoring your progress or prescribing medication or nicotine replacement to help you through withdrawal.

## Suggestions for Quitting Cold Turkey[71]

1. *Set a quit date and stick to it.* Tell your family and friends that you're quitting—make a public pronouncement of your commitment. You are more likely to stick to a plan of action if you feel that you would lose face if you changed your mind.
2. *Think of things to tell yourself when you feel the urge to smoke.* Tell yourself how you'll be stronger and healthier, have greater stamina, reduce your risk of serious illness and chances of dying before your time, etc.
3. *Tell yourself that the first few days are the hardest—after that, withdrawal symptoms will subside dramatically.*
4. *Remind yourself how much better off you'll be as a result of removing these poisons from your body.*
5. *Quit in the morning, after you've gone a night without nicotine.* Doing so gives you a head start on getting beyond withdrawal symptoms.

6. *Time quitting to coincide with a cold or a vacation.* A good time for quitting cold turkey may be when you come down with a cold or the flu and don't have your usual hankering for a cigarette. Then again, if you get sick only infrequently, don't use good health as an excuse for not quitting. Some people time their quit dates to coincide with a vacation period that allows them to get away from the places and situations associated with their habits. You'll return a new person—a nonsmoker.
7. *Rearrange your furniture, get new furniture, or get rid of that old chair in which you always smoked.* Remove as many cues as possible that were associated with your smoking habit.
8. *Throw out all your smoking paraphernalia—ashtrays, cigarette lighters, matches (except kitchen matches), etc.* Tolerate no exceptions.
9. *Ask other people not to smoke in your presence or in your house.* Tell your guests that you have recently quit smoking and would appreciate their cooperation. If they must smoke, ask them to step outside.
10. *Don't carry matches or light other people's cigarettes.*
11. *Sit in nonsmoking sections of restaurants and trains.*
12. *Fill your days with new activities—things you can enjoy that won't remind you of your smoking habit.*
13. *Exercise regularly.* Exercise can help keep your mind off smoking and rebuild your stamina.
14. *Be especially good to yourself.* Set aside a small monetary reward each day you maintain abstinence. Use the money to treat yourself to something special—something you wouldn't ordinarily buy for yourself. You deserve it!
15. *Ask others to be patient with you in the days following your quit day.* Tell friends and family members that you're likely to be irritable for a while.
16. *Use sugar-free mints, gum, carrot sticks, celery sticks, or some other low-calorie snacks as substitutes for cigarettes or whenever you feel the urge to smoke.*
17. *Perform the mental exercise of reinterpreting withdrawal symptoms as signs that your body is cleansing itself of the poisons of smoking.* Tell yourself that each day without smoking makes you stronger and healthier.

Table 14.1 offers some Do's and Don'ts to follow during those first few weeks or months after quitting smoking.

**TABLE 14.1**

**Do's and Don'ts for the First Weeks of Freedom from Smoking**

| Do's | Don'ts |
|---|---|
| If you desire to go out, DO find a new restaurant and ask to sit in the nonsmoking section. | DON'T socialize with friends who smoke. |
| DO request that others around you not smoke in your presence. Explain to them that you have just quit smoking and would appreciate it if they wouldn't smoke when you are around. | DON'T go to bars, restaurants, or bowling alleys in which you used to smoke regularly. |
| If your spouse smokes, DO ask him or her to kindly not smoke when you are around or leave ashtrays or cigarettes lying around. | DON'T leave cigarettes, matches, ashtrays, and other smoking paraphernalia lying around the house. Remember: out of sight, out of mind. |
| DO frequent new places in which you have no history of smoking. | DON'T resist asking nonsmoking friends and loved ones for support and help. If quitting smoking were easy, you would have done so long ago. Reach out to someone to help you through the bad times. |
| DO frequent nonsmoking places, such as museums, libraries, schools, churches, etc. | |

## Suggestions for Cutting Down Gradually

1. *Count your cigarettes for a week or two to establish a baseline.* Smoke as you normally would, neither increasing nor decreasing your usual smoking rate.
2. *Set concrete goals for tapering off.* Reduce your smoking rate each day or each week. Set attainable goals for yourself. One typical strategy to follow is cutting back your smoking rate by 25% each week for three weeks before quitting completely during the fourth week.
3. *Gradually lengthen the amount of time between cigarettes to keep your smoking rate down to your daily limit.*
4. *Don't settle for cutting down.* Make the commitment to give up those last few cigarettes. Set a quit date and stick to it. Use the strategies listed above for quitting cold turkey.

Here are some additional suggestions for tapering down:

- Restrict the locations in which you allow yourself to smoke. Make a pact with yourself not to smoke in the car, in the living room, in the office, etc. Narrow the range of settings daily.
- Spend more time in settings where smoking isn't allowed or practical. The library is an example. What other examples can you think of?
- Switch to a low-nicotine brand, but don't allow yourself to drag harder or longer to compensate for lower nicotine. Better yet, switch each day or each week to brands with progressively lower nicotine levels. This will help your body adjust to lower nicotine levels.
- Keep around only enough cigarettes to meet your daily limit. Never buy more than a pack at a time.
- Use sugar-free mints or gum as substitutes for cigarettes or whenever you feel the urge to smoke.

- Exercise when you feel the urge to smoke. Exercise helps distract you from smoking. You're also unlikely to smoke while you're exercising. Exercise has yet another benefit: As you become more fit, you'll be less likely to want to damage your body by smoking.
- Socialize more with nonsmokers.
- Pause before lighting up. Put the cigarette in an ashtray between puffs. Ask yourself before each puff if you really want more. If not, put the cigarette out and throw it away.
- Put the cigarette out before you reach the end.
- Imagine living a longer, healthier, noncoughing life. Ah, freedom!
- As you smoke, picture your lungs becoming blackened, filling with poisons. Picture yourself becoming old before your time, your health draining away, cancer spreading through your body.

## Learn to Cope, Not Smoke

Smokers who succeed in quitting and remaining abstinent learn to handle the triggers that prompt them to smoke. They cope rather than smoke. You too can become a coper, not a smoker, by becoming aware of the cues that trigger your own urge to smoke. A smoking trigger is any signal, event, or cue that prompts an urge to smoke. We can diagram the process as follows:

Smoking Trigger → Urge to Smoke → Smoking a Cigarette

What are smoking triggers? Cues in the environment (seeing someone else's lit cigarette, or engaging in certain activities like watching television) are *situation triggers.* Emotional states that prompt an urge to smoke, like feelings of boredom or anxiety, are *bodily reaction triggers. Thought triggers* are thoughts or ideas that prompt you to smoke.

You may be waiting for the bus when someone next to you lights up a cigarette and suddenly feel an urge to smoke. Before you know it, you reach for a cigarette and start smoking. Or you may be tense and experience a sudden craving for a cigarette. The sight of the lit cigarette and the feelings of tension are triggers that prompt an urge to smoke. To control your smoking habit, you need to learn ways of coping with these situations without reaching for a cigarette.

Here are some common smoking triggers. How many of these cues prompt your urge to smoke?

| | |
|---|---|
| Situation Triggers | Drinking coffee; talking on the telephone; driving the car; waiting for the bus; noticing someone else smoking; drinking alcohol; watching TV; attending a sports contest; finishing a meal; talking with or visiting your friends. |
| Bodily Reaction Triggers | Feeling angry, tense, bored, lonely, sad, hungry, irritable, happy, excited. |
| Thought Triggers | Thinking you must have a cigarette right now; telling yourself that you won't be able to cope without a cigarette; thinking that a cigarette will make you feel better; thinking that a cigarette will make whatever you're doing more enjoyable. |

Now, let's consider alternative ways of avoiding or handling these smoking triggers to control temptations.

**Step 1. Avoiding Powerful Smoking Triggers** Identify cues that trigger your smoking, such as those listed above. Reduce or avoid these triggers. As noted earlier, avoid people, situations, and household objects that are associated with smoking.

**Step 2. Develop Coping Responses to Smoking Triggers You Can't Easily Avoid** Develop coping responses so you can resist the urge to smoke. Think of a coping response as a healthy substitute for smoking. There are basically two types of coping responses that can substitute for smoking: (1) coping behaviors (things you do or say to others that compete with the act of smoking) and (2) coping thoughts (things that you think or say to yourself to help you cope). When faced with an urge to smoke, remind yourself of the slogan, *Cope, don't smoke!* Here are some examples of coping behaviors you can use whenever the urge to smoke strikes:

*COPING BEHAVIORS*

- Calling a friend or stop-smoking buddy to help you cope with smoking urges.
- Taking a hot bath or shower.
- Taking a walk around the block.
- Practicing relaxation or meditation until the urge passes.
- Exercising vigorously to allow the urge to pass.
- Chewing sugarless mints or gum.
- Learning to just say no when someone offers you a cigarette. Say, "No, sorry, I don't smoke anymore."

*COPING THOUGHTS*

- Tell yourself that you can handle the situation without smoking.
- Tell yourself that the urge to smoke will pass.
- Remind yourself of your reasons for quitting.
- Remind yourself of the effects of smoking on health.
- Tell yourself how great you'll feel by coping with a difficult situation without smoking.

Here are some additional coping responses:

- Develop alternate strategies for handling anger or frustration. For example, write down your feelings in a diary or talk to a nonsmoking friend on the phone, rather than reach for a cigarette.
- If you typically finish a meal with a cigarette, make yourself get up from the table and do something else instead of smoking—clear the table, walk the dog, sort through your mail—anything that breaks the habit of smoking after a meal.

- If you're used to smoking while watching TV or talking on the phone, keep handy substitutes (like sugarless gum or mints, or carrot or celery sticks or other low-calorie substitutes) nearby. Learn to reach for a substitute rather than a cigarette.
- Learn to handle states of anxiety or tension without smoking. Practice relaxation. Read an absorbing book. If negative emotions persist, talk things over with a counselor at your school or consult a mental health professional.

Can you think of other coping behaviors and thoughts?

### Getting Help

When it comes to quitting smoking, you needn't go it alone. Organized stop-smoking programs are offered in many communities, generally at no cost or modest cost, through local hospitals, universities, and voluntary health agencies like the American Lung Association, the American Cancer Society, and the American Heart Association. Check the phone book listings for these or other health organizations to learn more about the availability of stop-smoking clinics in your area. Or ask your college health instructor or student health services for referral information.

### Nicotine Replacement Therapy

Nicotine replacement therapy provides the body with an alternative source of nicotine to help reduce the withdrawal symptoms that dependent smokers might encounter when quitting smoking or cutting back abruptly. Nicotine replacement is administered in the form of nicotine gum, the nicotine skin patch, and now, the latest version, nicotine nasal spray. Nicotine nasal spray, which came to market in 1996, appears to speed the delivery of nicotine relative to the patch or the gum.

Nicotine replacement therapy should be monitored by a physician and used only when the smoker stops smoking completely. (The person who smokes while using nicotine gum or the nicotine patch risks overdosing on nicotine.) Nicotine replacement should be used only during a limited period of time to prevent the substitution of one addiction (nicotine replacement) for another (cigarette smoking). It should also be used in conjunction with a behavior-change program to break the cigarette habit, not as a treatment by itself.[72]

In one study, one in four smokers who used the patch quit for at least six months. This was more than twice as many as among those who received a dummy patch.[73] Yet nicotine replacement therapy isn't for everyone. People with certain heart conditions, such as life-threatening cardiac arrhythmias, a history of a recent heart attack, or severe or worsening angina should not receive nicotine replacement. Persons with other medical conditions should consult their physicians before using either nicotine gum or the nicotine patch.

### Preventing Relapses

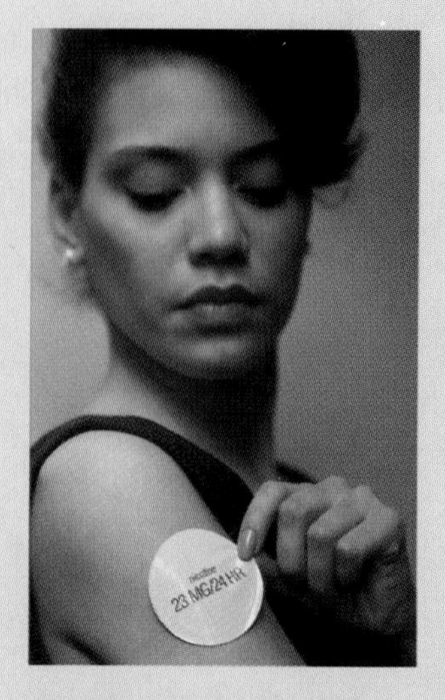

***Nicotine Patch*** Nicotine replacement in the form of the nicotine patch or nicotine-based chewing gum or nasal spray can help smokers break their dependence on nicotine. However, nicotine replacement should not be used by itself, but should be combined with a behavior-change program designed to break smoking habits.

Quitting smoking is no guarantee of remaining abstinent. Most people who quit eventually relapse, often within six months. As the length of abstinence increases, the likelihood of relapse declines, but the risk is always there. Thus ex-smokers need to be on their guard to handle temptations. They need coping strategies ready at a moment's notice when temptation strikes. High-risk situations include negative emotions, such as depression, anger, or anxiety; interpersonal problems, such as marital conflict; job problems; and social situations that trigger smoking, such as getting together after work with "buddies" who smoke.

The ex-smoker also needs to be aware of tendencies to overreact to a lapse (smoking a first cigarette after quitting) with feelings of guilt and a sense of resignation that then triggers a full-blown relapse. The person who relapses after a lapse is one who is likely to attribute the lapse to a personal flaw or weakness rather than to factors relating to the particular situation (such a social pressure or marital conflict). To avoid turning a lapse into a relapse, keep these thoughts in mind:

- A slip is a mistake, not a failure or defeat. Everyone makes mistakes from time to time, and smoking one cigarette does not make you a failure or a weakling.
- A lapse is *not* a relapse, unless you make it into one. Renew your commitment to quitting smoking.
- Use a slip as a learning experience. Learn to prevent the same kind of slip from happening in the future.
- Tell yourself that regaining abstinence is only a moment away. Tell yourself, "No more cigarettes."
- If you need help, ask for it. Call someone you trust to talk things over.

Smoking is the number-one preventable cause of illness and premature death. Don't let yourself become another statistic.

Smart Quiz
Q1405

# SUMMING UP

## Questions and Answers

### SMOKING AND HEALTH

1. **What are the effects of smoking on health?** Cigarette smoke contains many toxic or carcinogenic compounds. Smoking is linked to many forms of cancer, not just lung cancer. Smoking is also connected with respiratory diseases, cardiovascular diseases, birth defects, dental problems, even wrinkles. Smoking during pregnancy can result in low birth weight and higher infant mortality rates.

2. **What are the effects of nicotine?** As a stimulant, nicotine acts on nerve cells in the brain to increase states of arousal, alertness, and concentration. Nicotine may also have paradoxical effects, such as helping smokers relax. Nicotine is the addictive chemical in tobacco.

### WHY DO PEOPLE SMOKE?

3. **Why do people smoke?** Some are ignorant of the health risks of smoking. Some smoke because of the "cool" image of the smoker. Some smoke for pleasure or to relax. Smoking is *maintained* by addiction to nicotine. The primary features of addiction are tolerance and an abstinence syndrome.

### OTHER TOBACCO USE

4. **What other kinds of tobacco use are there?** Some people smoke pipes or cigars. Others snort or chew tobacco. Still others breathe in second-hand smoke.

5. **Are health risks associated with these other kinds of tobacco use?** Most definitely. Pipe and cigar smokers and people who snort or chew tobacco are at high risk of oral and some other types of cancers. Second-hand smoking increases the risk of coronary heart disease, respiratory disease, lung cancer, and other health problems.

### WHO SMOKES?

6. **Who smokes?** About 25% of the adult population in the United States smokes. The incidence of smoking is relatively higher among men than women, younger than older adults, African-American men and some other ethnic minority groups, poorer people, and people with less education.

7. **What are current trends in smoking among young people?** Smoking is rising among young people, most rapidly among young African-American males.

## Suggested Readings

**U.S. Department of Health and Human Services (USDHHS), Public Health Service, National Institutes of Health, National Cancer Institute.** *Strategies to Control Tobacco Use in the United States: A Blueprint for Public Health Action in the 1990's.* (NIH Publication No. 92–3316). Washington, DC: National Cancer Institute, 1991. A government report on approaches to reducing tobacco use in the U.S.

**USDHHS.** *Reducing the Health Consequences of Smoking: 25 Years of Progress. A Report of the Surgeon General.* [DHHS Publication No. (CDC) 89–8411]. Public Health Service, Centers for Disease Control, Center for Chronic Disease Prevention and Health Promotion, Office on Smoking and Health. Washington, DC, 1989. Twenty-five years after the original Surgeon General's report on the health consequences of smoking, a progress report.

**Taylor, C. B., Killen, J., D., and Editors of Consumer Reports Books.** *The Facts about Smoking.* Yonkers, NY: Consumer Reports Books, 1991. A readable and scholarly review of the addictive basis of smoking and how smokers can kick the habit.

**USDHHS.** *The Health Benefits of Smoking Cessation: A Report of the Surgeon General.* [DHHS Publication No. (CDC) 90–8416]. Rockville, MD: Centers for Disease Control, Office on Smoking and Health, 1990. A review of the scientific evidence on the health benefits of quitting smoking.

**USDHHS.** *Smoking Addiction. A Report of the Surgeon General, 1988.* [DHHS Publication No. (CDC) 88–8406]. Washington, DC. Centers for Disease Control, Office on Smoking and Health, 1988. A scientific review of the addictive bases of smoking.

# Understanding Infection and Immunity

DID YOU KNOW THAT

- Stress can cause infections that lie hidden in our bodies to flare up? p.399
- Receiving a weakened form of a virus or other pathogen can help you develop an immunity to it? p.404
- "Ringworm" is not a worm but a fungus? p.404
- Sweat helps keep bacteria and fungi from growing on the skin? p.406
- Some immune system cells stand at the ready to defend us against reinfection by infectious agents we encountered earlier in life? p.409
- About 200 different viruses cause the "common cold"? p.418
- Most common colds are "caught" by touch, not by inhaling infected droplets in the air? p.418
- Prolonged kissing, especially deep kissing, is a common way of transmitting infectious mononucleosis? p.422
- Cold viruses can live for hours on some objects or surfaces, where they can be transferred to your hands and from there to your nose, mouth, or eyes? p.426

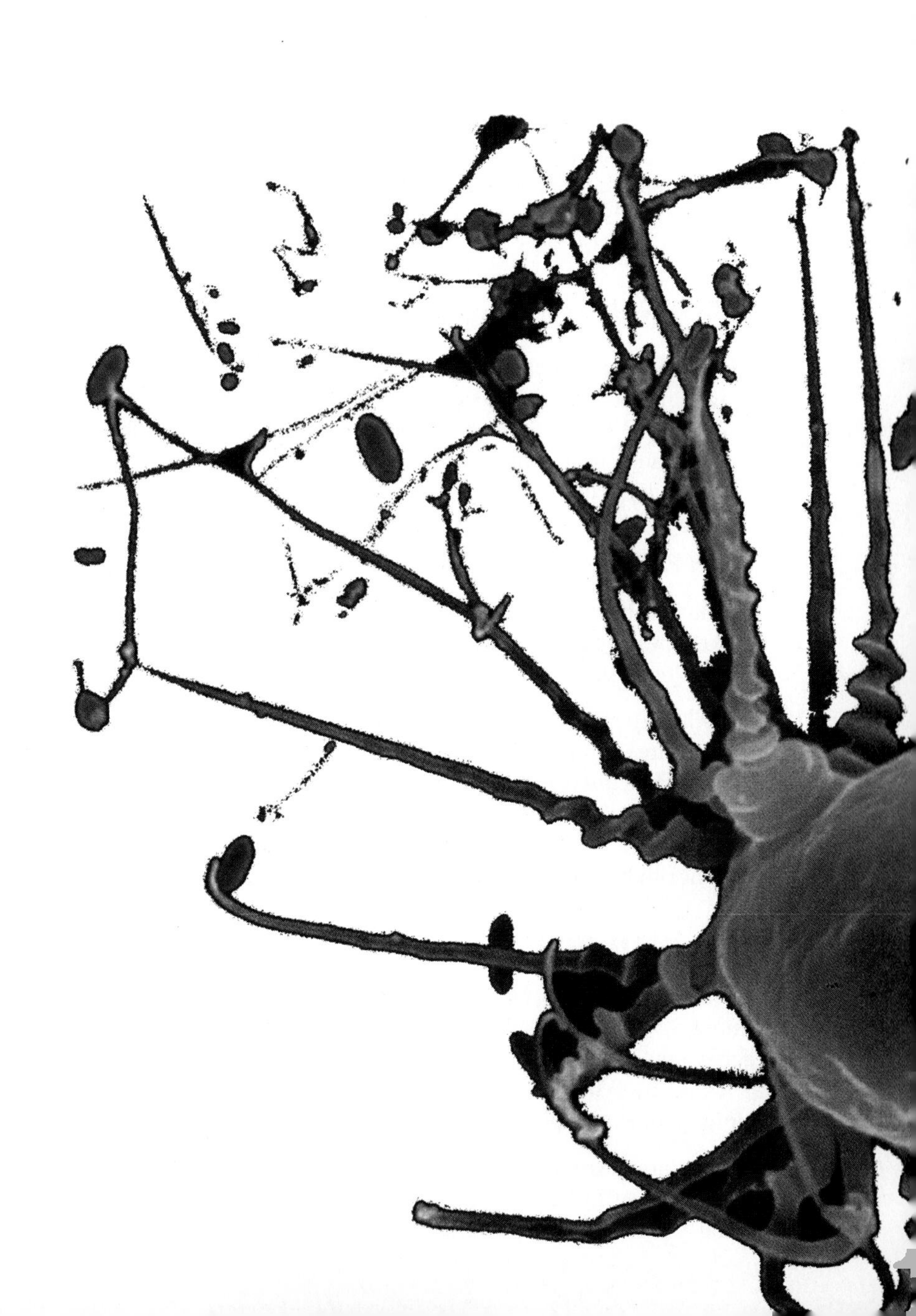

*On a sunny spring day several years ago, 20,000 students streamed out of their dorms and the library (it was finals week) and took their place in a massive line winding across the University of Connecticut campus. They weren't lining up to get tickets for a rock concert or for a UConn basketball game. They were obtaining vaccinations for a bacterial form of* ***meningitis,*** *an inflammation of the membranes (meninges) surrounding the spinal cord and brain. Three of their fellow students had been stricken with the potentially fatal infectious disease. None died, and the vaccination program stemmed the outbreak. Meningococcal meningitis is spread through the air, by sneezing or coughing. Contagion occurs through repeated and prolonged exposure to the airborne meningococcus bacterium. Symptoms begin with a fever, sore throat, or stiff neck. If not treated quickly, bacterial meningitis can lead to blood poisoning, shock, and death within 24 hours.*

Talking Glossary
Meningitis
G1501

# 15

The outbreak of bacterial meningitis at UConn reinforces the very real dangers of infectious **diseases.** Many of the most lethal infectious diseases of earlier times, such as diphtheria, cholera, and polio, no longer pose a public health threat in the United States or Canada. Others, both old and new, have taken their place. The best-known of the new breed of infectious diseases is AIDS.

Infectious diseases are the leading causes of premature death worldwide.[1] Infectious diseases like tuberculosis (TB), malaria, and childhood gastroenteritis (diarrheal disease) remain among the world's greatest killers, especially in developing countries. The world is also threatened by emerging killer diseases such as Ebola and Hantavirus pulmonary syndrome (HPS). Though they originate in other parts of the world, these diseases may be brought to our shores by infected people or animals.

**Talking Glossary**
Ebola, Hantavirus pulmonary syndrome
G1502

Although infectious organisms like bacteria and viruses cause a staggering number of cases of disease and death, perhaps most remarkable is the fact that so many of us manage to avoid or survive them. That we can remain free of disease or fight off **infections** is a testament to the amazing vigilance of our **immune system,** the network of cells and organs that defends the body against invading organisms. But the immune system is not "immune" to failure. In some infectious diseases, such as AIDS, the immune system itself succumbs to attack.

**Disease** A disruption of bodily functions linked to an identifiable group of signs and symptoms.

**Infection** The contamination and injury caused by multiplying pathogens.

**Immune system** The system that recognizes and destroys disease-causing agents and rids the body of diseased or worn-out cells.

**Infectious diseases** Diseases caused by direct or indirect contact with an infectious agent. Also called *communicable diseases.*

**Pathogens** Disease-causing organisms, including bacteria, viruses, fungi (yeasts and molds), and animal parasites such as insects and worms.

**Microorganism** Any microscopic entity capable of carrying on life processes.

**Host** Person, plant, or animal that provides a hospitable environment for a pathogen.

## INFECTIOUS DISEASES

**Infectious diseases** are also referred to as *communicable diseases.* Infectious diseases are caused by contact with **pathogens** that multiply within the body. Pathogens are disease-causing organisms, including bacteria, viruses, fungi (yeasts and molds), and parasites such as insects and worms. Most pathogens are **microorganisms**—entities capable of carrying on life processes but too small to be seen by the naked eye. Infectious organisms reproduce within a **host**—a plant or animal that unwillingly provides them with a fertile breeding ground. Pathogens enter the body through ports such as tiny pores or sores in the skin, or through oral or nasal cavities. Unchecked, they can establish beachheads within the body. They can use the body's own resources to reproduce and multiply and produce illness. Infectious organisms are transmitted in a number of ways, including contact with infected people or animals, insect bites, and contaminated food, air, soil, or objects (see Figure 15.1).

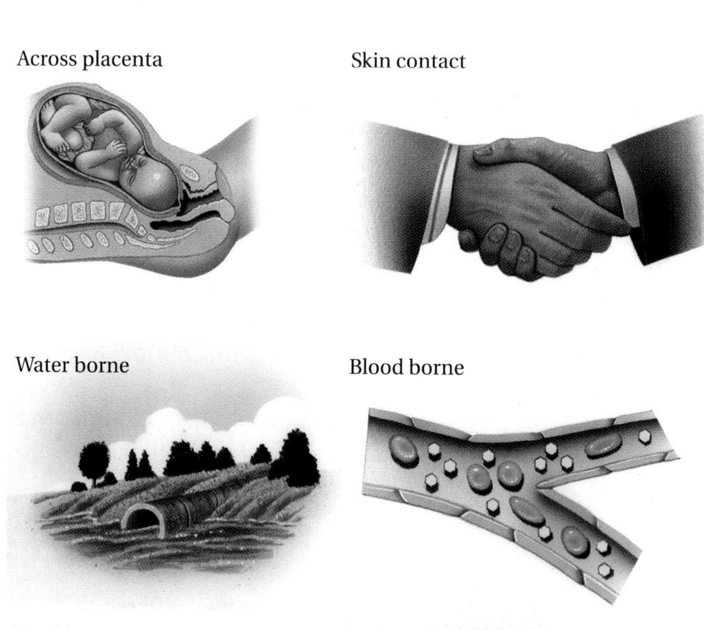


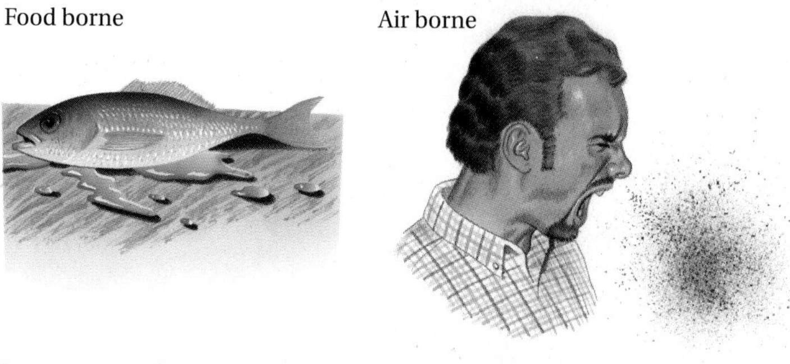


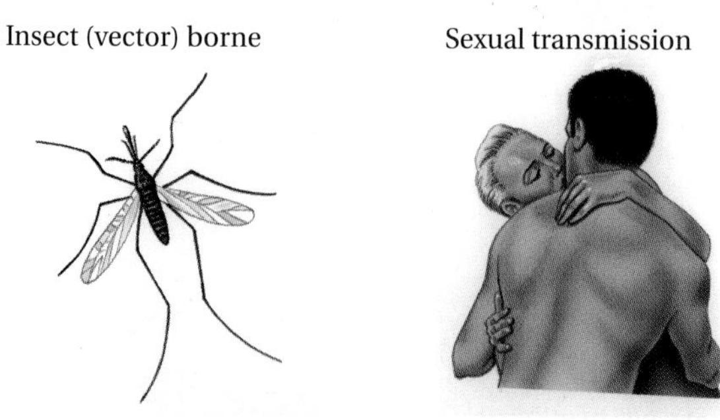


**Figure 15.1** *How Infectious Diseases Are Transmitted*

**Figure 15.2**
***Pathogens***

Viruses

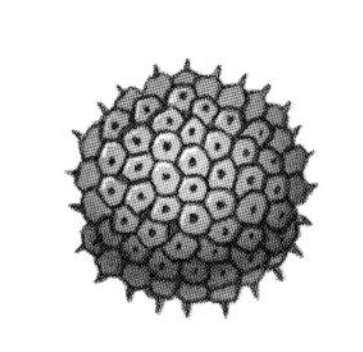

Bacteria

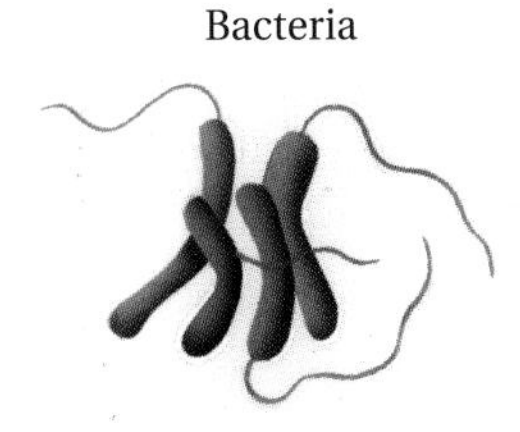

Fungi

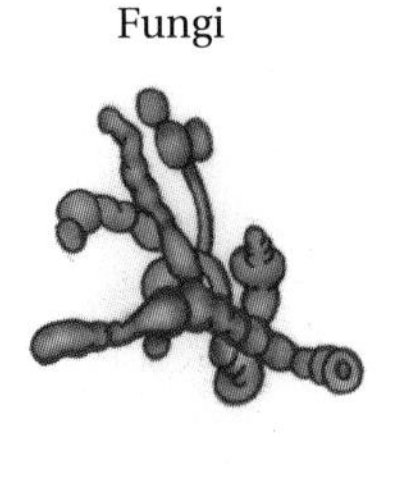

Protozoa

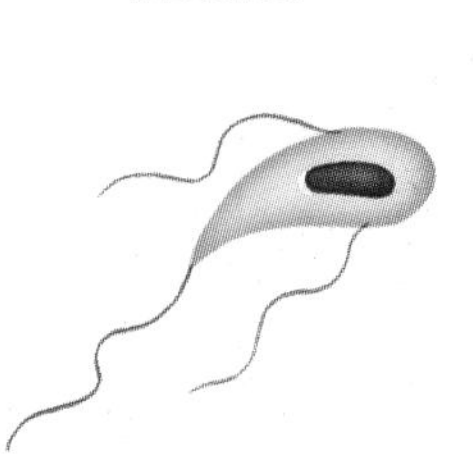

Parasitic Worms

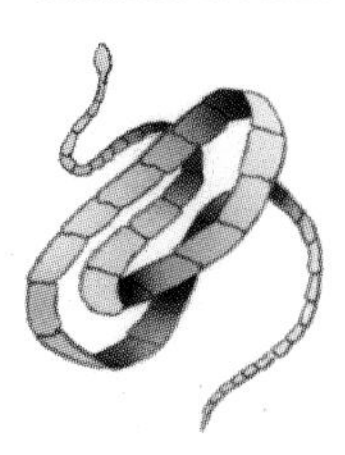

Talking Glossary
Pathogenic
G1503

Some microorganisms are normally found in the body. They become infectious or **pathogenic** only when they "overgrow," or sprout colonies in parts of the body where they are not normally found. Figure 15.2 illustrates some of the more troublesome pathogens.

## Types of Infection

Infectious diseases may be *localized,* or restricted to a particular area or part of the body, as in some skin infections, or they may be *generalized* or *systemic,* involving many body organs and systems. We can distinguish too between **acute infections,** which hit us with an immediate wallop by producing fever and assorted unpleasant symptoms, and **chronic infections,** which develop slowly and produce less dramatic but longer-lasting symptoms. Acute infections are usually short-term, like the common cold or the flu, which run their course in a matter of days or weeks as the body destroys the invading pathogens. Some acute infections, like bacterial meningitis, can overcome the body's ability to defend itself, leading in some cases to death. Moreover, some chronic infections can turn into acute infections, while some acute infections may progress to chronic infections.

Still other infections can take months or even years between the time pathogens enter the body and the time any symptoms occur. These so-called **latent** ("hidden") **infections** are symptom-free but can become suddenly active, especially when the person's physical health is compromised by stress, other diseases, or emotional disorders. The virus that causes genital sores *(herpes simplex II)* can lie dormant after its initial outbreak for long periods before producing a recurrence; HIV can remain in the body for years before producing symptoms.

## The Course of Infections—What Happens When We Get Sick

Whether you suffer a common cold or a life-threatening illness, infections progress through a sequence of common stages leading (hopefully) to recovery. Some fast-acting infections pass through each stage in a matter of days. Others take longer to run their course.

**Incubation Period** The time between the entry of a pathogen into the body and the development of initial symptoms is called the **incubation period.** Though the pathogens are not yet producing symptoms, they begin multiplying during the incubation stage. Some fast-acting pathogens, like the viruses that cause the flu, take as little as one to two days to incubate. Others, such as the virus that causes rubella (German measles), incubate for two or three weeks before any symptoms appear.

**Prodromal Stage** The period when symptoms first appear is called the **prodromal stage.** At first, symptoms are largely nonspecific and could be due to many kinds of infectious diseases. Common symptoms are low-grade fever, fatigue, and generalized aches and pains. The prodromal stage is the time at which we are generally most **contagious.**

Talking Glossary
Prodromal stage
G1504

**Clinical Stage** The development of full-blown symptoms characterizes the clinical stage. Symptoms specific to the infection appear. For rubella, for example, a characteristic red rash appears.

**Decline Stage** Though some infections can be disabling or even fatal, most eventually run their course once the immune system gains the upper hand. The infection declines and symptoms subside. Though we feel better, we are not yet 100%.

**Pathogenic** Disease-causing.

**Acute infection** Infection in which pathogens cause an immediate set of symptoms; usually short-term.

**Chronic infection** Long-term infection.

**Latent infection** "Hidden" or inactive infection in which pathogens are not active enough to produce symptoms.

**Incubation period** The time between the entrance of the pathogen and the first symptoms.

**Prodromal stage** The initial stage of a disease before the onset of acute symptoms.

**Contagious** Describes a person who harbors an infectious organism and is capable of transmitting it to others.

**Close-up**
Styles of coping with illness
**T1501**

**Convalescence and Recovery Stage** *Convalescence* is the period between the end of the disease state and the return to health. Though the infection no longer rages, the pathogen has not necessarily been eliminated from the body. In some infections, such as herpes, hepatitis, and syphilis, some of the pathogen remains in the body in a dormant or latent state. **Passive carriers** are persons who are currently symptomless but harbor a latent or chronic infection. Though they are free of symptoms, they may be capable of passing along the pathogen to others.

Always consult a health care provider if you suspect that you may not be fully recovered from an infection. For many kinds of infections, a simple culture, stain, or blood test can verify whether you remain infected.

**Smart Quiz**
**Q1501**

## think about it!

- **Why do you think it is important to understand what the incubation period of an infectious disease is?**

**critical thinking** **Some infections are *latent,* or hidden. Why is it useful to know if you are infected with them?**

**critical thinking** **Why do you think it is important to consult a health care provider if you suspect that you may not be fully recovered from an infection?**

**Passive carriers** Persons who harbor infectious organisms, do not exhibit symptoms, but are capable of infecting others.

**Endogenous microorganisms** Organisms that normally live within the body; disturbances in their growth can cause infection.

**Exogenous microorganisms** Organisms that do not normally inhabit the host.

**Flora** Plant life indigenous to specific environments.

**Fauna** Animal life, including microscopic organisms, living within a particular area.

**Immunosuppression** Weakened or suppressed immune system.

# SOURCES OF INFECTION—THE PATHOGENS

We live in a world awash with microorganisms, a virtual microbial soup. Countless numbers of microorganisms surround us each day. Many of them are not pathogenic. Some are actually helpful; indeed we couldn't survive without them. Some bacteria, for example, play important roles in our digestive processes. Microorganisms also degrade waste material. Yet many microbes are dangerous to our health, and some, like HIV, are deadly.

## Endogenous vs. Exogenous Microbes

**Talking Glossary**
Endogenous, Exogenous
**G1505**

Microorganisms are classified as endogenous or exogenous. **Endogenous microorganisms** normally live within the body. **Exogenous microorganisms** do not normally inhabit the body. Endogenous microorganisms generally live peacefully, making up our body's natural **flora** and **fauna.** *Candida albicans,* a common yeastlike fungus, is normally present in the intestinal tract and other sites in healthy persons. The bacteria *Escherichia coli (E. coli)* normally lives in the colon. In balanced amounts, these organisms serve important functions. *E. coli* breaks down foods into usable components, while *Candida albicans* keeps other potentially harmful fungi and bacteria (including *E. coli*) from growing excessively and causing infection.

Imbalances in the body's normal flora and fauna can arise when the immune system becomes weakened, allowing normally benign (harmless) endogenous organisms to overbreed and turn pathogenic or grow in parts of the body where they don't normally belong. An overgrowth of *Candida,* for instance, can cause vaginal infections or systemic infections affecting the whole body. *E. coli* may start growing in the urethra, causing a urethral infection (urethritis) and possibly spreading to involve the bladder and even the kidneys. **Immunosuppression,** a weakening of the immune system, can occur for many reasons, including overuse of antibiotics, exposure to environmental pollutants, tobacco use, excessive alcohol intake, use of other drugs, poor dietary habits, stress, and exposure to pathogens like HIV.

Exogenous microorganisms pose the greatest risk of infectious disease. These are organisms that normally live outside the host. When they invade the body, they cause acute, sometimes severe infections (tuberculosis and influenza, for example). In many cases, our only defense against such invaders is to stay out of their path. Yet, as with endogenous microorganisms, a weakened immune system can increase susceptibility to infection.

Next we consider various types of infectious organisms and the kinds of infections they cause.

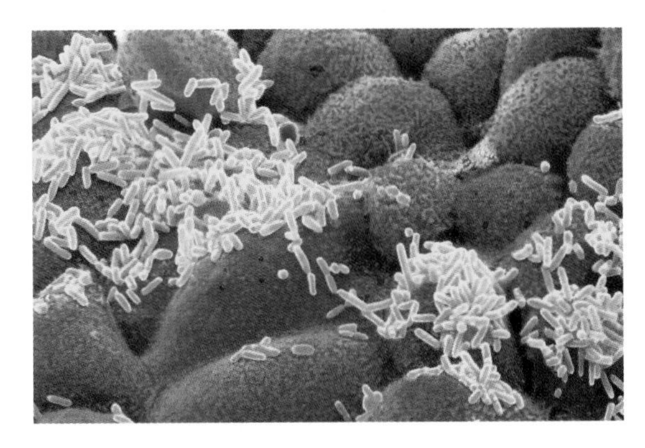

***Bacteria*** Bacteria (stained yellow) on the human nasal lining (stained pink).

## Bacteria

**Bacteria** (singular: bacterium) are microscopic, single-celled organisms that live in air, soil, food, plants, animals, and humans. In the body, bacteria thrive in warm, moist conditions, like those that line the mucous membranes of the mouth, throat, and nasal passages. Elsewhere they can survive in virtually any environment, from subarctic to desert settings. Tuberculosis, some kinds of pneumonia, urinary tract infections, Lyme disease, dysentery, botulism (food poisoning), and periodontal (gum) disease are just a few of the many diseases caused by bacteria.

Some bacteria *(cocci)* are shaped like a sphere, others *(bacilli)* resemble a rod, while still others *(spirochetes)* have a spiral shape. Each bacterium reproduces itself using nutrients from the host organism.

Bacteria cause infection by releasing **toxins**—poisonous chemical substances that damage body cells, tissues, and organs, and that produce fever and shock. Bacteria can also invade body cells directly, killing body tissue or multiplying so quickly that their numbers block the functions of the organs they inhabit. Bacteria are grouped according to the family to which they belong, including staphylococci, streptococci, and chlamydia.

Talking Glossary
Staphylococci
G1506

**Staphylococci** **Staphylococci** ("staph") are normally present in large numbers on the skin. Usually, endogenous staphylococci bacteria are harmless. However, if they get into the bloodstream, spinal fluid, bladder, or other sites in the body, they can produce serious "staph" infections. Among the major types of staph infections are urinary tract infections, acne, and blood infections.

One type of staphylococcus, *Staphylococcus aureus,* normally lives on the skin and hair. When it enters the body, it can cause wound infections, pneumonia, toxic shock syndrome (TSS), and food poisoning. Food-borne illnesses, many caused by *Staphylococcus aureus* and other bacteria, such as *E. coli* and *Salmonella,* affect some 7 million people annually in the United States (see Chapter 5).

**Toxic shock syndrome (TSS)** is a rare and sometimes fatal infection that is linked in some cases to the use of superabsorbent tampons. The plugging of the vagina with a highly absorbent tampon that remains in place for six hours or more may create an ideal breeding ground for staph bacteria. Signs of TSS include fever (102°F or greater), headache, sore throat, vomiting, diarrhea, muscle aches, rash, and dizziness. Peeling skin, disorientation, and a plunge in blood pressure may follow.[2] Although TSS can strike women and men, those at greatest risk are women who regularly use superabsorbent tampons or who leave a diaphragm in the body for prolonged periods. With the removal from the market of superabsorbent tampons, the number of TSS cases has declined dramatically in recent years.[3]

**Streptococci** Like staphylococci, a number of harmless strains of **streptococci** ("strep") are part of the normal human fauna. We find them normally in the throat, tonsils, skin, and anal area. Some strains, such as *Group A streptococci,* are pathogenic, causing **strep throat, rheumatic fever, scarlet fever,** and **impetigo.** These harmful strains of strep replace the normal fauna and when present in large enough numbers cause disease. *Group B streptococci* can cause urinary tract infections, wound infections, and *endometritis.* Another strain, *Streptococcus pneumoniae,* causes a form of bacterial pneumonia.

**Bacteria** Microscopic, single-celled organisms that live in air, soil, food, plants, animals, and humans.

**Toxins** Poisonous chemical substances that damage cells, tissues, and organs.

**Staphylococci** A type of bacteria that causes infections such as food poisoning, urinary tract infections, and toxic shock syndrome.

**Toxic shock syndrome (TSS)** A rare and sometimes fatal bacterial infection linked to tampon use.

**Streptococci** A type of bacteria, some of which cause various infections, including strep throat and certain types of pneumonia.

**Strep throat** A bacterial infection caused by streptococcal bacteria; characterized by a painful and reddish sore throat, fever, ear pain, and enlarged lymph nodes. May occur without noticeable symptoms.

**Rheumatic fever** An inflammatory disease that may follow a streptococcal infection; may damage the heart valves and kidneys.

**Scarlet fever** A contagious streptococcal infection characterized by sore throat, scarlet rash, and fever.

**Impetigo** A contagious bacterial skin disease, primarily affecting the skin around the mouth and nose.

Fortunately, most strains of staph and strep bacteria are very responsive to antibiotic therapy. There are exceptions, however. A newly identified strain of *Group A streptococci* has recently appeared: In 1990, it caused the sudden death of the famed creator of the Muppets, Jim Henson.

**Chlamydia** Strains of **chlamydia** cause respiratory tract infections, eye disease, and genital tract infections. One type, *Chlamydia pneumoniae,* is linked to a form of "walking pneumonia," a common form of pneumonia in the United States, especially among young adults. *Chlamydia trachomatis* can cause a condition called **trachoma,** which is a leading cause of preventable blindness worldwide, especially in Africa. In parts of the southwestern United States, Native Americans also suffer high rates of trachoma. *Chlamydia trachomatis* can also be transmitted sexually, causing infections of the urethra and reproductive organs in both men and women. Chlamydial infections are the most common bacterial sexually transmitted disease, or STD (see Chapter 16).

**Rickettsiae** **Rickettsiae** are bacterialike organisms that grow inside insects and other parasites; they are transmitted to humans via bites by lice, fleas, ticks, and mites. Most rickettsial diseases, including the ancient scourge of **typhus,** are now uncommon in industrialized nations but remain a threat elsewhere. **Rocky Mountain spotted fever,** however, which accounts for 90 percent of all rickettsial diseases in the United States, remains a health threat in the southeastern portion of the country. It is caused by *Rickettsia rickettsii,* an organism transmitted from dogs (or other small wild animals) to humans by way of ticks. Symptoms include a high fever lasting for many days and a skin rash. Symptoms usually last for about two weeks; then either the fever suddenly disappears or the patient suddenly worsens and dies. Diagnosis must therefore be accurate and rapid. Rickettsial diseases are treated with antibiotics such as tetracycline.

**Talking Glossary**
Rickettsiae
G1507

**Diagnosis and Treatment of Bacterial Infections** Though some bacterial infections can be identified by their characteristic symptoms, a definitive diagnosis is made on the basis of laboratory tests. A sample of blood can be analyzed under a microscope to detect the presence of particular bacteria. In the **culture method,** a throat swab, urine or blood sample, or another body fluid specimen is placed on a plate with special nutrients that allow bacteria to multiply. The presence of a particular strain is then identified by its shape and growth pattern. In the **staining method,** special stains composed of colored dyes are mixed with bacteria-laden cells on a microscope slide. Depending on the type of bacterium, the stains will bind to the cells in characteristic ways, allowing for identification.

Bacterial infections are treated with **antibiotics,** a category of drugs that inhibit the growth of bacterial organisms. Some antibiotics, such as penicillin, destroy bacteria outright; others, such as tetracycline, inhibit their rate of reproduction. Some bacterial infections, such as diphtheria, whooping cough, and tetanus, can be prevented through injection with a vaccine (see discussion of vaccination later in the chapter).

## Viruses

The tiniest of all pathogens, **viruses** are microscopic particles, perhaps a hundred times smaller than bacteria. Viruses consist of just two basic elements: a core of nucleic acid that contains genetic material (DNA or RNA) and a surrounding coat of protein. Since a virus has no independent metabolic activity (it doesn't burn food or carry on other life functions, except reproduction), it may replicate only within a cell of a living plant or animal (including human) host. The virus provides the genetic code for replication; the host cell provides the necessary energy and raw materials for replication.

When a virus invades a host cell, it injects its genes into the cell. The virus genes then take over the host cell's reproductive mechanisms and pro-

**Chlamydia** Bacteria that cause infections of the eyes and urogenital tract.

**Trachoma** A chronic form of conjunctivitis (inflammation of the mucous membrane of the eyelids) caused by a strain of chlamydia.

**Rickettsiae** Bacterialike organisms that grow inside insects and other parasites; transmitted to humans via bites by lice, fleas, ticks, and mites.

**Typhus** A group of infectious diseases especially prevalent among people living in unsanitary conditions; characterized by weakness, severe headache, and fever.

**Rocky Mountain spotted fever** A tick-borne disease caused by *Rickettsia rickettsii;* produces fever, skin eruptions, and pain in the joints, bones, and muscles.

**Culture method** A body fluid specimen containing unidentified bacteria is placed in a plate with special nutrients that allow bacteria to multiply. The bacterial strain can be identified by its shape and growth pattern.

**Staining method** Colored dyes are mixed with bacteria-laden cells. The way a stain binds to cells helps with bacterial identification.

**Antibiotics** Drugs that inhibit the growth of bacterial organisms.

**Virus** Particles consisting of a core of nucleic acid and a coat of protein; incapable of replicating outside living cells.

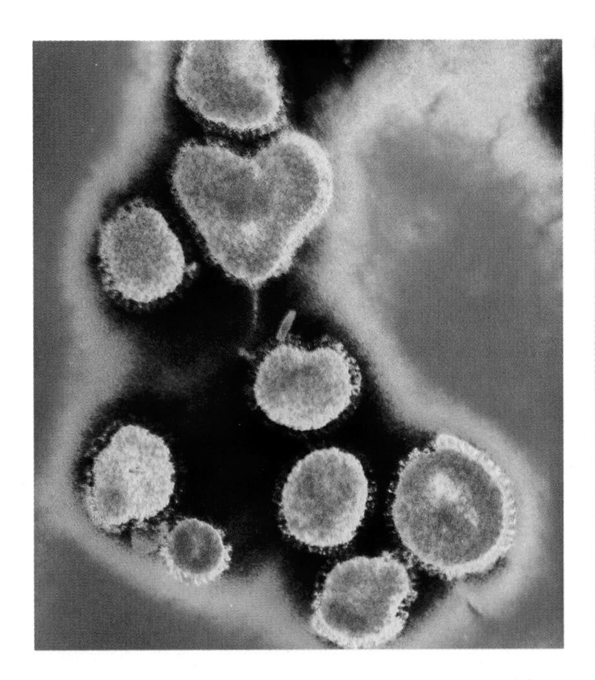

***Influenza Virus*** The virus that causes a type of flu called the Beijing flu.

TABLE 15.1

**Virus Families and Associated Illnesses**

| Virus Family | Infections They Cause |
|---|---|
| Adenovirus | Respiratory and eye infections, including the common cold |
| Arenavirus | Lassa fever, meningitis |
| Coronavirus | Common cold, possibly infectious bronchitis |
| Herpesvirus | Cold sores, genital herpes, infectious mononucleosis (Epstein-Barr virus), chicken pox |
| Orthomyxovirus | Influenza |
| Papovavirus | Papilloma (genital warts) |
| Paramyxovirus | Mumps, measles, parainfluenza |
| Picornavirus | Poliomyelitis, common colds |
| Poxvirus | Cowpox, smallpox (eradicated) |
| Reovirus | Diarrheal disease |
| Retrovirus | HIV infection/AIDS, human T-cell leukemia |
| Rhabdovirus | Rabies |
| Rhinovirus | Upper respiratory infections like the common cold |
| Togavirus | Rubella, yellow fever, dengue, equine (horse) encephalitis |

gram it to make new viruses. Some viruses remain dormant within host cells for long periods, producing latent infections with no noticeable symptoms. Others reproduce quickly and burst out of cells with a vengeance, producing acute infections (influenza, or the "flu," is an example). Some viruses produce relatively mild effects, such as cold sores or warts, whereas others, such as HIV, produce some of the most deadly diseases known to humankind. We now know of 20 different large families of viruses, consisting of some 400 known viruses. Table 15.1 lists several families of viruses and the infections they cause. These virus families include *adenoviruses,* responsible for some respiratory and eye infections, and *retroviruses,* which cause AIDS and other illnesses.

Talking Glossary
Infectious mononucleosis G1508

The **Epstein-Barr virus (EBV),** a type of herpes virus, causes **infectious mononucleosis,** a disease primarily affecting children and young adults that is spread by close contact, including kissing. EBV was also suspected of causing **chronic fatigue syndrome (CFS).** This condition lasts from six months to several years and is characterized by extreme fatigue that persists despite adequate rest, muscle or joint pain, headache, sleep problems, depression, low-grade fever, sore throat, and swollen lymph nodes.[4] Health professionals now doubt that EBV is responsible for CFS. The cause remains a mystery.

**Means of Transmission** Viruses can enter the body by all possible entry routes—the skin, eyes, nose, mouth, and genital tract. They can be inhaled, ingested, or passed into the mucous membranes of the genital tract during sexual intercourse. Many viruses that cause respiratory infections are transmitted by contact with airborne droplets or with virus-infected nasal secretions. Some viruses are sexually transmitted or contracted by contamination with infected bodily fluids, such as blood and semen. Others, like **rabies,** a disease that is often fatal if not treated immediately following infection, are passed through punctures in the skin through bites from rabid animals that carry the infectious organisms.

**Epstein-Barr virus (EBV)** A virus that causes infectious mononucleosis.

**Infectious mononucleosis** A viral disease caused by the Epstein-Barr virus; acute stage characterized by fever, sore throat, and enlarged lymph nodes and spleen.

**Chronic fatigue syndrome (CFS)** A long-term condition involving extreme fatigue and a variety of other symptoms.

**Rabies** A viral disease that primarily affects the central nervous system; can lead to paralysis and death if not treated immediately.

**Diagnosis and Treatment** Diagnoses of viral infections are made on the basis of observation of characteristic symptoms and laboratory analysis of bodily specimens that are examined for the presence of specific molecules (antibodies) that indicate exposure to particular viruses. (HIV is tested, for example, by examining a blood sample for the presence of HIV antibodies.) Viruses live only within cells, which makes them difficult to treat without also damaging the cells they infect. Antibiotics are useless against viruses, which is why they are not used against viral infections like the common cold and the flu. Some drugs do have specific antiviral properties, such as acyclovir (used in treating herpes) and amantadine (used in treating influenza). These drugs can often lessen the symptoms and length of infection.

The best weapons we have against viruses are **vaccines,** or disease-specific immunizations. Vaccines contain weakened or killed forms of viruses or other pathogens that are capable of activating the body's production of specific antibodies against them but do not produce a full-fledged infection. The immune system uses these antibodies to fend off future attacks by the particular virus. The development of vaccines against such viral diseases as polio, whooping cough, mumps, and measles has virtually eliminated these diseases in the U.S. and other developed countries where vaccination programs are widespread.

## Fungi

**Fungi** are primitive vegetable organisms such as yeasts and molds. Most fungal infections occur on skin surfaces.

**Vaccine** A substance containing killed or weakened bacterium, virus, or toxoid that stimulates the production of antibodies against these substances.

**Fungi** Primitive plant organisms such as yeasts and molds.

**Ringworm** A fungal skin infection characterized by red patches, itching, and scaling.

**Protozoa** Self-contained single-cell parasites that thrive in water.

**Parasites** Organisms that live within or on the surface of other organisms; they do not benefit their host.

**Giardiasis** A diarrheal disease caused by a protozoan parasite.

**Malaria** Potentially deadly protozoal disease transmitted by mosquitoes.

**Ringworm** Dermatomycosis, or **ringworm,** is a class of fungal infections of the hair, skin, or nails caused by the fungus *Dermatophyte.* About one in ten Americans develops ringworm each year. Among the most common types of ringworm infections are athlete's foot, jock itch, and scalp itch. Ringworm infections are characterized by itching, scaling, and, occasionally, painful lesions. Treatment includes the use of powders to dry the affected area and topical antifungal medications such as Whitfield's ointment and the antifungal drugs miconazole and clotrimazole.

## Protozoa

**Protozoa** are the largest microorganisms. Some are visible to the naked eye. Protozoa are self-contained single-cell **parasites** that thrive in water. Protozoal diseases such as malaria and diarrhea are a major health problem in tropical climates and in developing nations.

**Talking Glossary**
Giardiasis
G1509

**Giardiasis** **Giardiasis** is a highly contagious diarrheal disease that occurs most commonly in the United States among children. It accounts for a form of "traveler's diarrhea" and frequently affects children in day-care centers and people with impaired immune systems.

Giardiasis is an even more serious threat in the developing world, where 4 to 5 million children die of this or other forms of diarrheal disease each year.[5] The parasites that cause giardiasis are spread by contaminated water and oral-fecal contact. Travelers visiting and returning from developing countries often suffer its effects, especially if they have consumed water contaminated with sewage. Giardiasis is treated with the antiprotozoal drugs quinacrine or metronidazole.

**Malaria** With the invention of potent antimalarial drugs such as chloroquine in 1943 and the pesticide DDT a few years later (the protozoal parasite causing malaria is transmitted by mosquitoes, which are killed by DDT), many public health professionals in the 1950s believed that the ancient scourge of **malaria** was poised for elimination. Developed countries such as the United States and Canada are largely free of this potentially deadly disease, but worldwide about 300 million people are infected each year, many with a strain that is now resistant to antimalarial drugs such as chloroquine. Of these, between 1 and 3 million (most of whom are children) die.[6] Prevalences are strikingly high in countries in Africa, Southeast Asia, and Latin America.

Malaria is transmitted to humans by bites from the female mosquito of the genus *Anopheles.* The protozoal parasite travels to the liver and then circulates to red blood cells, where it reproduces and periodically bursts into the bloodstream. Symptoms include flulike aches and fever; if untreated, death can result. Travelers to high-risk areas are often advised to take antimalarial drugs as a precaution.[7] Insect repellents and protective clothing are essential, and travelers are advised to avoid going out between dusk and dawn, when the disease-carrying mosquitoes are most likely to bite.

### Parasitic Worms

**Parasitic worms** (technically, *helminths*) are flat or round worms that flourish in the intestines. They are multicellular parasites ranging in size from tiny microscopic flukes to tapeworms, which can be several feet long. Common infections caused by helminths include pinworms and schistosomiasis.

**Pinworms** In the United States, the most common parasitic worm infestation is by the **pinworm.** At any given time about 20 to 30% of children and perhaps half as many adults are infected with these parasites.[8] They hatch in the intestines and are transmitted by oral-anal contact (such as by scratching or touching the anal cavity and bringing the fingers to the mouth). The entire family, not just the apparently infected member, should be treated with an antihelmintic drug. Fortunately, pinworms do not multiply in the host. Even without treatment, most cases of pinworm disappear within a month or so.

**Schistosomiasis** **Schistosomiasis** is a water-borne disease caused by a type of worm called a fluke. Flukes lay their eggs in snails. When they hatch, they burrow into the skin of bathers or people working in infested water. Once in the body, they can live for five or more years within the intestines or bladder, where they produce up to 3,500 eggs each day. Eventually, these eggs clog the veins of many organs, causing obstruction and sometimes death.

Of all the parasitic diseases, only malaria causes more disability and death than schistosomiasis. Globally, some 200 million people are affected, especially those living in tropical and subtropical climates.[9] Its appearance in the United States and Canada is rare, however, Most reported cases involve people who contracted it elsewhere. Drugs used to combat this disease have a high cure rate.

**think about it!**

- **What are some of the agents that cause illness in people?**

**critical thinking** **Why is it important for you to know what kinds of organisms cause infectious diseases?**

Smart Quiz Q1502

## THE BODY'S DEFENSES AGAINST INFECTION

Our best defense against infection is not some new miracle drug. It is the body's own multilayered defense system. First-line defenses include physical and chemical barriers such as skin surfaces, saliva, and tears. Far more complex is the immune system.

Cells in the immune system recognize and destroy invasive disease-causing agents ("germs") such as bacteria and viruses. The immune system marshals the resources of an army of specialized cells that seek out, attack, and destroy infectious agents and rid the body of worn-out cells and cancerous cells that it recognizes as alien to the body. Immune system cells serve much the same function as sentries at a gate—protecting and defending the inhabitants inside.

### First-Line Defenses against Infection—Physical and Chemical Barriers

Many pathogens never make it past the body's physical and chemical barriers, which include the skin, moist body-lining tissue called mucous membranes, "sweeping" hairlike structures called *cilia* that line certain body passageways, and chemical secretions produced by the body that wage chemical warfare against invading pathogens. Infections can occur when these first lines of defense are breached, or penetrated, as when the skin is penetrated via lacerations, puncture wounds, burns, or insect bites; organisms are inhaled into and penetrate the mucous membranes of the respiratory system; an organism is ingested (via food or water) and penetrates the mucous membranes of the gastroin-

**Parasitic worms** *(helminths)* Multicellular parasites or worms.

**Pinworm** A helminth that causes an infection of the intestines and rectum.

**Schistosomiasis** A water-borne infection caused by a worm called a *fluke.*

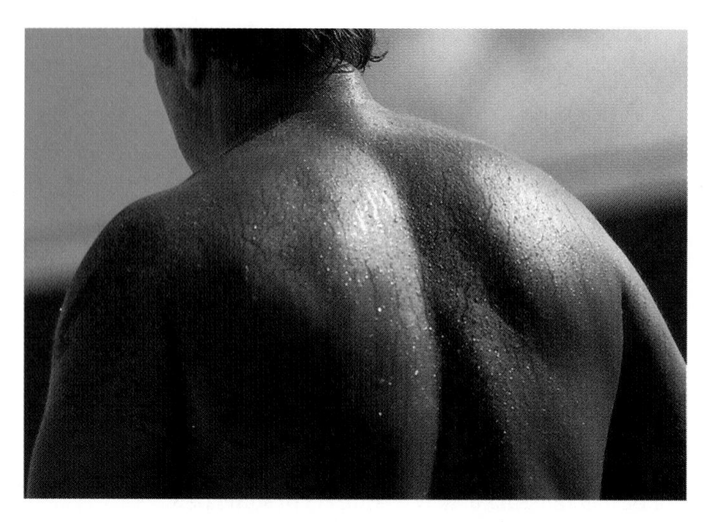

***Sweat*** Did you know that sweat not only helps keep the body cool when it is overheated but helps prevent the growth of bacteria and fungi on the skin?

testinal tract; or an organism breaches the lining of the reproductive or urogenital systems.

**Skin** Skin is composed of several layers of tightly knit cells that provide a waterproof covering that deflects pathogens. Additional protection is provided by skin secretions such as sweat and **sebum.** Sebum is an oily substance secreted by **sebaceous glands** under the skin's surface. Sweat and sebum keep both bacteria and fungi from growing on the skin.

**Mucous Membranes** The **mucous membranes** lining various body openings—including the eyes, mouth, nose, and respiratory, gastrointestinal, reproductive, and urogenital tracts—are barriers against pathogens. **Mucus** contains disease-fighting immune cells. In addition to protecting the membranes from drying out, mucus traps and disposes of many contaminants.

**Cilia** **Cilia** are tiny hairlike projections on the surface of cells. They literally "lash out" at invading organisms and sweep them away before they can invade tissue lining. The respiratory tract is lined with cilia that constantly remove (via mucus that is coughed or blown away) foreign particles from the lining of the lungs and windpipe.

**Sebum** A fatty secretion of the sebaceous glands of the skin.

**Sebaceous glands** Glands in the skin that produce oily secretions.

**Mucous membranes** Membranous linings of bodily passageways or cavities.

**Mucus** Thick, sticky fluid containing immune cells secreted by the mucous membranes.

**Cilia** Tiny hairlike projections on the surface of cells in the nose, respiratory tract, and other sites that sweep away invading organisms.

**Urogenital tract** Organs constituting the urinary and reproductive organs.

**Vectors** Animal or insect carriers of infectious agents.

**Chemical Defenders** Chemical substances in the digestive tract, saliva, and tears also destroy pathogens. Acids in the digestive tract routinely kill many kinds of bacteria. The enzyme muramidase, found in tears and in the **urogenital tract,** kills many kinds of pathogens.

**Talking Glossary**
Muramidase
G1510

## Breaching the Barriers—Six Stages to Infection

Pathogens may breach the physical and chemical barriers the body throws in their path but still not produce an infection. Infection is a multistage process. Getting past the body's sentries is merely stage one. For infection to occur, all six factors must be present.

To illustrate these six stages, we use the example of Lyme disease, an infectious disease transmitted by ticks:

1. *First, a pathogen must be present.* In the case of Lyme disease, the pathogen is the bacterium *Borrelia burgdorferi.*
2. *The pathogen must find a reservoir, or place to breed.* Deer and white-footed mice harbor the bacterium that causes Lyme disease.
3. *The pathogen must find a portal of exit, or way to escape from its breeding ground.* Feeding ticks ingest the bacterium *Borrelia burgdorferi* from the host's bloodstream, thus removing it from its breeding ground.
4. *The pathogen must find a way to transmit itself to the host.* It may, for instance, use a **vector** (an insect or animal carrier) which has contact with the host. The tick attaches itself to a host (such as a dog or person) to feed again.
5. *The pathogen must find a portal of entry, or a way to enter the host.* As the tick feeds on the new host, it transmits the bacteria via its saliva to the host's bloodstream.
6. *The pathogen must find a host that is susceptible to it.* To become infected, the host must be susceptible to the pathogen. Such factors as a history of exposure to specific pathogens, age, heredity, nutritional status, general health status, stress, and environmental factors all come

into play in determining susceptibility to infection. Susceptibility also depends on the host's level of **immunity,** or protection against specific infections and diseases. Let us now take a look at the specific functions of one of the most intricate and most important body systems, the immune system.

## The Immune System—The Body's Arsenal of Defense

When the body's external barriers have been breached, the immune system stands ready to take defensive action. Sometimes it vanquishes pathogens so quickly that we are barely aware that an infection has occurred. In other instances, the time between the onset of an infection and its resolution takes longer and we "get sick." We bear the brunt of symptoms associated with each stage of infection.

**Talking Glossary** Lymphocytes, Antigen **G1511**

The immune system commands an army of billions of specialized **white blood cells** called **lymphocytes.** Lymphocytes circulate constantly throughout the body, ever alert to foreign agents or **antigens** (literally *anti*body *gen*erators). An antigen is any substance that the immune cell recognizes as foreign to the body, such as a bacterium, virus, foreign protein, or body cell that has turned cancerous or become worn out. Chemically, antigens are proteins on cell surfaces that stimulate an immune response.[10]

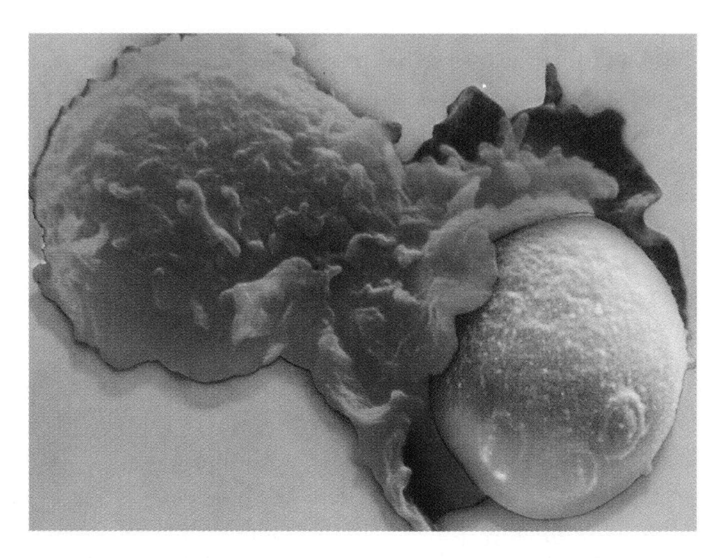

***Lymphocyte*** Here we see a human lymphocyte, a specialized type of white blood cell, engulfing an invading pathogen (a yeast cell).

### Lymphocytes and the Lymphatic System

Lymphocytes are produced in the **bone marrow** and in various organs of the **lymphatic system,** including the **lymph nodes,** the **spleen,** and the **thymus.** The lymphatic system is the body's other circulatory system. It carries **lymph,** a bodily fluid that is collected from tissues throughout the body, through its network of vessels. Lymph passes through the lymph nodes, or glands, where lymphocytes cleanse it of infectious agents and debris. This is why your lymph nodes become swollen when you come down with an infection. Lymphocytes are also released into the bloodstream, where they battle invaders. From the bloodstream, lymphocytes then return to the lymphatic system. Figure 15.3 (following page) shows the structure of the immune system.

**The Immune Response** The **immune response** is the sequence of events that takes place when lymphocytes detect antigens and target them for destruction. Some lymphocytes directly attack and destroy antigens. Others produce **antibodies.** Antibodies are protein molecules that belong to a family of large molecules called *immunoglobulins.* A particular antibody fits an invading antigen like a key fitting a lock (see Figure 15.4, following page). By locking into an antigen, the antibody marks it for destruction by other immune cells.[11] When immune cells directly attack and kill antigens without the aid of antibodies, the response is called **cell-mediated immunity.** When antibodies join the fray, the response is called **antibody-mediated immunity.**

**Immunity** Protection against specific infections and diseases.

**White blood cells** *(leukocytes)* Specialized blood cells.

**Lymphocytes** White blood cells that defend the body against antigens.

**Antigen** Substance recognized by the immune system as foreign; induces the production of antibodies.

**Bone marrow** Soft material within bones.

**Lymphatic system** The system of vessels, nodes, ducts, organs, and cells that manufacture and store lymphocytes and help destroy infectious agents.

**Lymph nodes** Lymphatic glands located throughout the body; produce and store lymphocytes and filter out infectious agents.

**Spleen** A lymphatic organ that produces lymphocytes, destroys worn-out red blood cells, and acts as a reservoir for blood.

**Thymus** A lymphatic organ in which T-cells mature.

**Lymph** The clear fluid found in lymphatic vessels.

**Immune response** The sequence of events that occurs when the immune system detects antigens.

**Antibodies** *(immunoglobulins)* Protein molecules that mark antigens for destruction by other cells.

**Cell-mediated immunity** White blood cells destroy antigens without the aid of antibodies.

**Antibody-mediated immunity** Antibodies, along with other white cells; disarm and dispose of antigens.

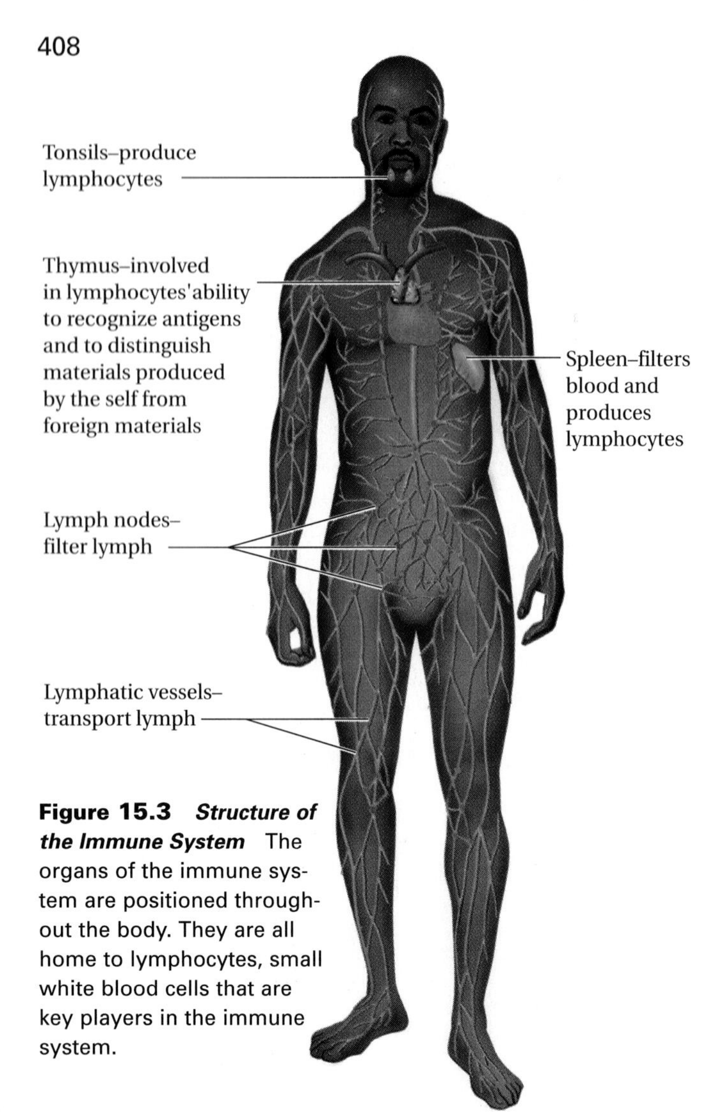


**Figure 15.3** ***Structure of the Immune System*** The organs of the immune system are positioned throughout the body. They are all home to lymphocytes, small white blood cells that are key players in the immune system.

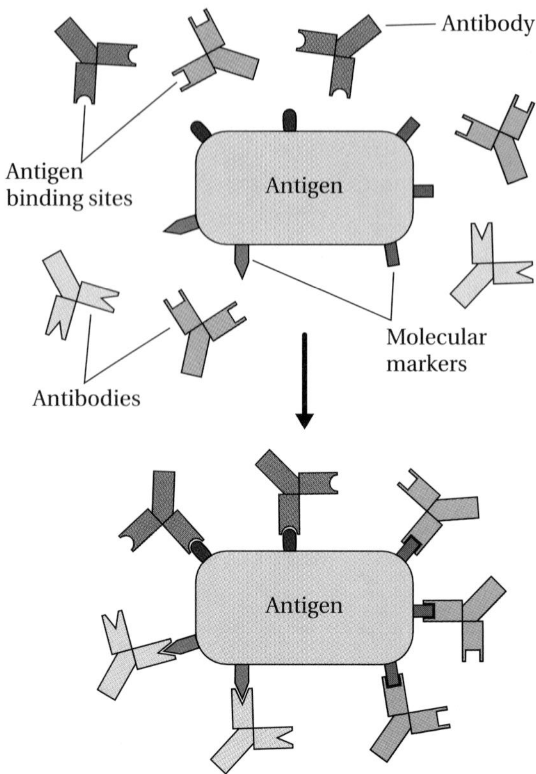


**Figure 15.4** ***Like a Key in a Lock*** A particular antibody fits a particular antigen like a key fitting a lock. Once locked in, the antibody marks the antigen for destruction by other immune cells.

Talking Glossary
Phagocytes G1512

**Phagocytes and NK Cells** When the body is invaded by a pathogen, the first line of defense is the action of **phagocytes** (large white blood cells called "cell eaters") and **natural killer (NK), cells.**

Phagocytes—"cell eaters"—and NK cells are referred to as *scavenger cells* because they continuously roam the bloodstream and body tissues hunting foreign microbes and cellular debris. When phagocytes encounter antigens, they eliminate them by swallowing and digesting them.[12] **Macrophages,** or "big eaters," are phagocytes that enter body tissues. They devour antigens as well as scavenge for worn-out cells and cellular debris.

NK cells also attack antigens and destroy them by filling them with a lethal burst of poisonous chemicals. NK cells destroy antigen-infected cells and potentially cancerous cells. To defend itself, the body must consume its own diseased parts, and NK cells perform this function.

Phagocytes also play a key role in **inflammation**—the body's largely nonspecific defense reaction to tissue damage (such as cuts, burns, or splinters) caused by invading pathogens. When an area is infected, capillaries (small blood vessels) at the site enlarge to allow more phagocytes and other white blood cells to flow to the injury. This activity causes the redness, swelling, warmth, and pain characteristic of inflammation. The **pus** that often accompanies inflammation contains the "aftermath" of the battle between these immune cells and antigens. It consists of dead cells and fluids that participated in the fight.

**Phagocytes** A major class of white blood cells that seek out and destroy antigens in the bloodstream.

**Natural killer (NK) cells** White blood cells that can destroy viruses and tumor cells.

Talking Glossary
Macrophages G1513

**Macrophages** Phagocytes that enter body tissues and scavenge for worn-out cells and cellular debris.

**Inflammation** The nonspecific defense reaction to pathogen-induced tissue damage.

**Pus** A yellowish liquidy substance that results from inflammation.

Tough as they are, some antigens are too powerful (for instance, they multiply too rapidly) to be killed by the early response team alone, consisting of phagocytes and NK cells. Phagocytes signal lymphocytes, called **helper T-cells,** to move into action. Helper T-cells act as "field generals" of the immune system, calling on other white blood cells to mount a more vigorous response to the invader. These other white blood cells act in concert with phagocytes to disarm and destroy antigens.

**HealthCheck**
Check your blood IQ
**H1501**

**T-Cells and B-Cells** The two major types of lymphocytes are *T-lymphocytes* (or simply **T-cells**) and *B-lymphocytes* (or **B-cells**). Both T-cells and B-cells attack and disarm antigens, but in different ways.

T-cells, of which there are several kinds, mature in the thymus gland. Helper T-cells prowl the bloodstream for antigens, much like free-floating phagocytes. Once they find them, they secrete chemical messengers called **cytokines.** Cytokines alert other T-cells, called **killer T-cells,** and phagocytes to swing into action. Killer T-cells are equipped with a receptor that matches one, and only one, antigen. When it finds that antigen, it "locks" into the antigen and injects it with lethal chemicals. At birth, each of us is endowed with enough T-cells to recognize at least one million different kinds of antigens—from dust mites to viruses and bacteria.[13]

Helper T-cells also trigger production of B-cells—immune cells that produce antibodies that attack antigens. Antibodies do not kill antigens themselves. They act as "vises" that hold antigens in place so that T-cells and other immune cells can destroy them. Each B-cell makes only one kind of antibody that targets a particular antigen. Some produce antibodies that target viruses that cause the common cold. Others produce antibodies that attack bacteria that cause pneumonia. Surrounded by phagocytes, T-cells, and antibodies, most antigens don't stand much of a chance.

**Memory cells** are specialized lymphocytes that remain long after the battle against a specific antigen is over, even for a lifetime. They are called memory cells because they produce antibodies that have a "memory" for the antigens to which they were exposed. This allows them to react swiftly when the same antigens invade the body again. Because of them, you will not come down with chicken pox twice. Memory cells specific to the chicken pox virus remain poised in your body, ready to rapidly disarm it should it reappear.

A group of T-cells called **suppressor T-cells** regulate the activities of B-cells and other T-cells. Suppressor cells ensure that the immune response doesn't get out of hand and damage healthy cells in the vicinity of the infection. Suppressor T-cells also signal the various T- and B-cells to cease activity when the infection has been eradicated.

**think about it!**

- **How do skin surfaces, saliva, and tears protect us from infections?**
- **What is meant by the *immune system?* What is the difference between an *antigen* and an *antibody?***
- **What is meant by terms such as *memory cells, cell eaters,* and *natural killer cells?***

**critical thinking** **Agree or disagree and support your answer: People provide their own best defense against most infectious illness.**

**Smart Quiz**
**Q1503**

## IMMUNITY AND IMMUNIZATION

The word *immunity* derives from the Latin *immunio,* meaning "to protect." The human body is capable of several kinds of immunity, or ways of protecting itself against disease.

### Innate Immunity

Inborn or **innate immunity** results from transmission of the mother's antibodies to the fetus. (Following birth, additional antibodies are passed to the baby in breast milk.) With rare exceptions, each of us is born with a certain amount of innate immunity. As we develop, we acquire more lasting immunity to many kinds of pathogens. Babies are

**Helper T-cells** White blood cells that search for antigens and signal other lymphocytes to gather at the site of infection.

**T-cells** Lymphocytes that mature in the thymus and aid the body's response to antigens.

**B-Cells** Immune cells that produce antibodies.

**Cytokines** Chemicals involved in growth regulation; help coordinate the immune response.

**Killer T-cells** White blood cells with a receptor that matches a specific antigen; killer T-cells lock onto that antigen and kill it.

**Memory cells** T-cells or B-cells that recognize and dispose of reintroduced antigens, sometimes years after initial infection.

**Suppressor T-cells** Immune cells that regulate the activities of T- and B-lymphocytes; prevent damage to healthy cells.

**Innate immunity** Immunity acquired by transfer of mother's antibodies to the fetus, through her bloodstream and, later, via breast milk.

protected for only a limited number of pathogens, and even this protection is temporary. To survive the continuous onslaught of pathogens, acquired immunity is required.

## Acquired Immunity

**Acquired immunity** develops after birth. Acquired immunity may be either active or passive.

**Active Immunity** **Active immunity** can develop naturally, as when we contract a disease and the immune system produces antibodies against the pathogen. It can develop artificially, as by vaccination. In **naturally acquired active immunity (NAAI),** foreign agents cause an infection and trigger memory lymphocytes to develop antibodies. The antibodies protect us from reinfection. However, many viral and bacterial organisms mutate, or change their form. Such is the case in influenza, which is why a single bout with the flu does not mean that we won't come down with another strain next year.

**Artificially acquired active immunity (AAAI)** develops after an artificial exposure to antigens. The antigens are usually contained in an immunizing agent such as a vaccine that is intentionally administered to the body to build up immunity. A vaccine (also called an "immunization") contains a killed or weakened pathogen and stimulates the production of antibodies. Many vaccines, such as those for diphtheria, measles, and mumps, are administered between the ages of 2 months and 6 years and provide long-term, sometimes lifelong, immunity. Often, teenagers and adults are given "booster" shots to strengthen an immune response. Some vaccines are given by injection. Others are taken by mouth.

**Acquired immunity** Immunity produced when the body makes its own antibodies against infectious agents; may be acquired naturally by contracting an infection or by vaccination.

**Active immunity** Immunity acquired through developing antibodies by contracting an infection or in response to vaccination.

**Naturally acquired active immunity (NAAI)** Immunity that follows illness; results from the natural production of antibodies against specific pathogens.

**Artificially acquired active immunity (AAAI)** Immunity that develops after an artificial, or intentional, exposure to antigens contained in vaccines or toxoids.

**Passive immunity** Temporary immunity created by introducing antibodies from another person or animal; also present at birth for about six months.

**Gamma globulin** Antibody-rich serum from the blood of another person or animal used to induce passive immunity.

**Vaccination** A means of introducing a weakened or partial form of an infectious agent into the body so as to produce immunity without producing the full-blown illness.

**Diphtheria** Acute upper-respiratory-tract bacterial infection of the tonsil area transmitted by inhaled droplets.

**Passive Immunity** Some infections—such as those produced by snake-bite toxin—act so quickly that they can prove lethal unless **passive immunity** is induced. Passive immunity is a short-lived form of protection against infections that can cause severe damage or death well before the immune system is able to produce antibodies. It is used in the treatment of snake bites, rabies (along with a vaccine), and other diseases for which there are no vaccines, such as some kinds of hepatitis.

Passive immunity can be transferred from one person to another through injecting antibody-rich blood serum *(antiserum)* called **gamma globulin** into the person needing protection. This serum is taken from the blood of a person or animal with antibodies against the targeted disease. Once in the recipient's bloodstream, the antibodies in the injected serum immediately attack antigens. Unlike active immunity, passive immunity is temporary. The "borrowed" antibodies provide protection for only a few weeks or months. The innate immunity present at birth is another form of passive immunity. It, too, is temporary (it lasts about six months).

**Talking Glossary**
Gamma globulin
**G1514**

## Immunization and Preventable Diseases

**Vaccination** prevents many infectious diseases. Most people suffer few if any adverse effects from vaccines, although people about to be vaccinated should discuss allergies or potentially complicating conditions with their health care providers. Some vaccines are recommended only for travelers and others at high risk of exposure. Others are recommended for all infants and young children (see Table 15.2). However, as discussed in the nearby ***World of Diversity*** feature, only about 40 to 60% of preschool children in the United States receive the recommended immunizations.

Immunizations prevent a number of infectious illnesses. If some of the following diseases are unknown to you or seem only vaguely familiar, it is probably because of the success of immunizations against them, which has made them rare.

**Diphtheria** **Diphtheria** is an acute upper-respiratory-tract bacterial infection of the tonsil area. It is transmitted by inhaled droplets. As a result of routine administration of the diphtheria-pertussis-tetanus (DPT) vaccine in infancy, fewer than five cases have been reported each year in the United States.[15] Worldwide, however, diphtheria remains a significant health problem, especially among children aged 2 to 5.[16]

**Talking Glossary**
Diphtheria
**G1515**

WORLD OF *diversity*

## Children and Immunizations—Many Aren't Protected

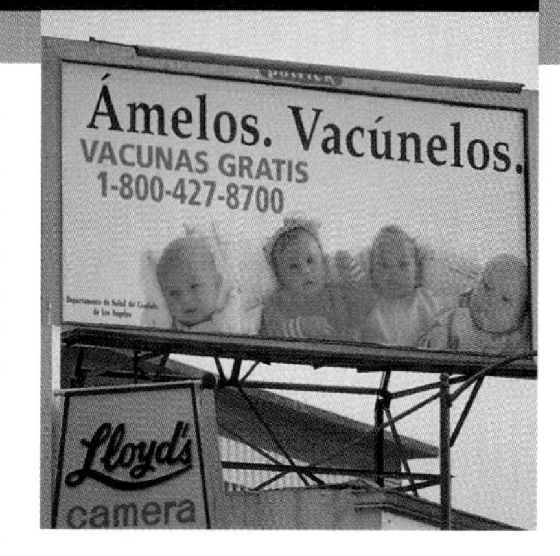


The development of safe and effective vaccinations ranks among the most important contributions of modern medicine. However, this life-saving gift of science fails to reach many people in the United States. Many preventable diseases continue to afflict large numbers of children, especially preschoolers. Why do children fail to get immunized? Reasons include lack of medical insurance, parental attitudes, poor health care delivery, or lack of access to medical care, especially among poor people.

Nearly all states require a schedule of vaccines for children entering kindergarten, and 95% of entering children are immunized. Not so with preschoolers. With the exception of licensed day-care centers, no controls currently exist for preschool children. The federal government estimates that only 40 to 60% of preschool-age children receive the recommended vaccinations.[14] In fact, children under 5 in the United States are immunized at a lower rate than children in such developing countries as India, Nigeria, and Mexico. Children without health insurance represent the single largest category of those who do not receive the recommended vaccinations. About one in five children and young adults under the age of 18 in the United States does not have insurance. Poor people and members of minority groups are disproportionately represented among them. Parental factors also affect whether children receive vaccinations. Many parents are unaware of the importance of vaccines or have negative attitudes toward them. Many find it difficult to take time off from work to take their children to the clinic. Many cannot afford medical visits but are not eligible for public assistance. Among recent immigrants, language and cultural barriers often stand in the way. Many poor parents' sole use of health care is emergency care. Emergency room workers focus on the immediate problem rather than issues such as whether children have been vaccinated.

Studies show that Hispanic-American preschoolers are more likely to contract diseases that are preventable through immunization, such as tetanus and pertussis. They are nearly ten times as likely as African-American children, and about seven times as likely as non-Hispanic white children, to come down with measles. Although only a small number of cases of tetanus and pertussis occur in the United States, Hispanic-American children are at greater risk than other groups of contracting them.

**TABLE 15.2 Immunizations Children Should Receive**

| Vaccine | Number of Shots | Ages Typically Given |
|---|---|---|
| Hepatitis B | 3 | At birth, 1 to 2 months, 6 months |
| DPT (diphtheria, pertussis, and tetanus) | 5 | 2, 4, 6, and 15 to 18 months, and 4 to 6 years |
| OPV (oral polio vaccine) | 4 | 2, 4, 15 to 18 months; booster at 4 to 6 years |
| HIB (influenza B, bacterial meningitis) | 3 | 2, 4, and 12 to 18 months |
| MMR (measles, mumps, rubella)* | 2 | 15 months, 11 to 12 years |

*May be given at 4 to 6 years where required by public health authorities for school entry.

*Source*: U.S. Food and Drug Administration, *FDA Consumer,* December 1995, p. 7.

**Pertussis** **Pertussis,** or "whooping cough," is an acute upper-respiratory disease of childhood (and more rarely, of adults) caused by the bacterium *B. pertussis.* Pertussis produces a hacking cough, along with sneezing and nasal congestion. Like diphtheria, it is transmitted by inhaling airborne droplets. The widespread use of the DPT vaccine has reduced the number of cases in the United States to about 5,000 annually.[17] Globally, pertussis remains a major health problem, killing some 1 million children each year.[18]

Talking Glossary
Pertussis
G1516

**Tetanus** **Tetanus** is an acute infectious disease resulting from the entry of bacteria-laden spores through breaks in the skin. Stepping on nails, dog bites, and other wounds can cause tetanus, especially if the wound is deep and remains uncleaned for

**Pertussis** *(whooping cough)* Acute upper-respiratory childhood disease caused by the bacterium *B. pertussis.*

**Tetanus** An acute infection caused when bacteria-laden spores enter the body through breaks in the skin.

four or more hours. The *C. tetani* bacterium that causes tetanus is found everywhere in the environment, especially in soil. *C. tetani* produces a toxin that attacks the nervous system, leading rapidly (often within hours) to paralyzing muscle spasms, including the jaw spasms characteristic of "lockjaw." Penicillin destroys the tetanus organism. The diphtheria-pertussis-tetanus (DPT) vaccine prevents tetanus, but adults need tetanus boosters every ten years to maintain immunity. (When did you last have a tetanus booster?)

**Polio** Before the introduction of a vaccine in the 1960s, **polio** was a leading cause of death and disability. The vaccine program has been so successful that by the early 1990s, no cases of polio were reported anywhere in the U.S. In 1995, the worldwide incidence of polio was the lowest ever (6,169 cases).[19]

Polio affects the "gray matter" of the spinal cord and brain. If the virus passes through the bloodstream and becomes localized in the *meninges,* membranes that surround the spinal cord and brain, paralysis of the arms, legs, and trunk may result. In its most severe form, the virus infects the brain and nerves to the upper body, resulting in paralysis of the diaphragm muscle, which prevents the person from breathing on his or her own.

Talking Glossary
Meninges
G1517

**Measles** A viral disease spread by airborne transmission of respiratory droplets expelled by an infected person, **measles** is the most contagious of vaccine-preventable infectious diseases.[20] The success of the vaccination program has been such that by 1995, only 301 confirmed cases were reported throughout the United States.[21] Along with a high fever, hacking cough, sneezing, and nasal discharge, measles causes a red rash and small red spots on the inside of the mouth. It usually passes in one to two weeks but can lead to other complications such as ear infections and pneumonia. Children should receive the measles-mumps-rubella (MMR) vaccine at 16 months, followed by a booster shot at the age of 12.

**Polio** *Poliomyelitis,* a viral disease affecting the spinal cord and the brain; can lead to muscular degeneration, paralysis, and deformity.

**Measles** Highly contagious viral infection of the respiratory tract, characterized by red spots.

**Hepatitis** An inflammation of the liver caused by various viruses or exposure to toxins.

**Rubella** Rubella, or "German measles," is a viral disease usually transmitted by respiratory droplets or direct contact. Symptoms are similar to those of measles. Rubella in pregnant women can cause birth defects. Children and unimmunized women, before becoming pregnant, should be vaccinated to protect them from the disease.

**Mumps** Mumps is a viral disease characterized by fever, headache, and swollen salivary glands. Though it usually passes without any long-term effects, it may lead to serious complications, such as deafness, meningitis, and, in adults, damage to the reproductive system. Because of these risks, inoculation in childhood with the measles-mumps-rubella (MMR) vaccine is important. (Adults cannot be vaccinated against mumps.)

**Hepatitis** **Hepatitis** is an inflammation of the liver. It can be caused by various factors, including chronic alcoholism and ingestion of toxic substances. *Viral* hepatitis is caused by exposure to one of several different types of related, but distinct, viruses. The major types of viral hepatitis are hepatitis A, B, C, and D.

Hepatitis affects millions of Americans. Some cases of hepatitis are mild. Others are severe, occasionally causing death. Symptoms range from practically none to mild fever, headache, muscle aches, fatigue, loss of appetite, nausea, vomiting, and diarrhea. Full-blown hepatitis often results in dark urine and light-colored feces, stomach pain, and yellowing of the skin and whites of the eyes (jaundice).

There is no cure for viral hepatitis. Treatment involves rest, intake of fluids, and proper nutrition. The acute stage of the disease usually subsides in a few weeks, although recovery may take months. There may be recurrent episodes or chronic damage to the liver. Though it does not cure the disease, the drug alpha interferon may prevent liver damage in people with hepatitis C. Vaccines are now available for both hepatitis B and hepatitis A. The Centers for Disease Control and Prevention has called for the vaccination of all infants and adolescents with the hepatitis B vaccine, as well as for high-risk individuals and health care workers.

Close-up
More on hepatitis
T1502

Hepatitis A, which accounts for about one in three cases of hepatitis, is usually spread by fecal-oral contact or by ingesting contaminated food and water.[22] Eating uncooked or undercooked contaminated shellfish such as clams and oysters is a major route of transmission. Concern about the spread of the hepatitis A virus (HAV) is a primary reason why restaurant employees are required to wash their hands after using the bathroom. Sexual practices involving oral-anal contact

**Take Charge**
Preventing hepatitis A
C1501

are yet another route of transmission. Most people who develop hepatitis A do not experience symptoms. Others develop flulike symptoms. Only rarely does jaundice develop.

Hepatitis B accounts for about half of hepatitis infections in the United States—about 300,000 each year.[23] The hepatitis B virus (HBV) is transmitted either through sexual contact or contact with infected blood. HBV is found in semen, vaginal secretions, and saliva. Unprotected sex is a major conduit of infection. Coming into contact with infected blood, as through sharing contaminated syringes, razors, or toothbrushes or through transfusions, is another mean of transmission.

HBV often strikes silently and can lead to chronic liver disease, even cancer of the liver. Many people with HBV are unaware of having it. Others become very ill and are beset by nausea, weight loss, abdominal pain, dark urine, and jaundice. Chronic infection can cause cirrhosis of the liver. Infected people can transmit HBV or other hepatitis viruses even if they are symptom-free.

**Take Charge**
Preventing hepatitis B
C1502

Hepatitis C is primarily contracted by contact with contaminated blood, usually via needle sharing but occasionally through blood transfusions with contaminated blood supplies. Some cases are contracted sexually. Recently developed tests that screen blood donors have greatly reduced the risk of contracting the virus through transfusions.

Approximately 4 million Americans are affected with hepatitis C.[24] Many infected people remain symptom-free or have mild symptoms. Some recover spontaneously. Others go on to develop chronic, potentially fatal liver disease, such as cirrhosis or cancer of the liver, often 20 or 30 years after infection.[25] Hepatitis C accounts for about 8,000 deaths annually from liver disease—more deaths than from hepatitis A and B combined. The number of deaths from hepatitis C is expected to triple by the year 2017. There is no vaccine at present for hepatitis C.

**Take Charge**
Preventing hepatitis C
C1503

Hepatitis D, or *delta hepatitis,* occurs only in people with hepatitis B. Like hepatitis B and C, it is transmitted sexually or by contact with contaminated blood. The hepatitis B vaccine also prevents hepatitis D.

You can protect yourself from hepatitis by practicing safer sex (see Chapter 16), avoiding needle sharing, avoiding fecal-oral contact (always wash your hands after using the bathroom), avoiding undercooked or raw shellfish, and consulting your health care provider about available vaccines.

**Take Charge**
More on prevention
C1504

## Immune System Disorders

Immune system disorders occur when the immune system overreacts to normally harmless antigens, when it misidentifies the body's own cells as foreign, or when it is unable to protect the body from common pathogens.

### Allergies—An Overly Sensitive Alarm

One out of every five Americans—about 50 to 60 million people—has allergies. An **allergy** is a hypersensitivity to normally harmless substances like dust, foods, mold, pollen, animal dander, and insect bites. An allergic reaction occurs when the immune system mounts too vigorous a response to substances that actually pose no threat to the body. Substances that trigger allergic reactions are called **allergens.**

For reasons not fully understood (genetics is believed to play a role), the immune systems in people with allergies respond to allergens with overproduction of a specific type of antibody called **immunoglobulin E,** or simply **IgE.** IgE antibodies attach themselves to the surface of millions of connective tissue cells called **mast cells.** Mast cells are spread throughout the body. They line mucous membranes and connective tissue such as skin and body-lining tissue. When IgE antibodies encounter an allergen, they trigger mast cells to release a powerful inflammatory chemical called **histamine,** which is responsible for the runny nose or other symptoms associated with allergies. Depending on the site at which the histamine is released—for instance, in the nose, chest, skin, or intestines—the allergic response induced by the release of histamine may involve sneezing, itchy skin, hives, eczema, diarrhea, nasal congestion, or lung constriction (see Figure 15.5).

**Talking Glossary**
Immunoglobulin E
G1518
Histamine
G1519
Allergic rhinitis
G1520

**Allergic rhinitis,** or "hay fever," is one of the most common kinds of allergies. It affects some 35 million

**Allergy** A hypersensitivity disorder of the immune system; ordinarily harmless substances cause an allergic response in sensitive people.

**Allergens** Commonly occurring, normally harmless antigens that trigger an allergic reaction.

**Immunoglobulin E (IgE)** An antibody produced in response to allergens. Triggers mast cells to release an inflammatory chemical, histamine, which causes reactions such as itching and sneezing.

**Mast cell** Cell that lines the mucous membranes and connective tissue, such as skin and body-lining tissue; secretes histamines in response to allergens.

**Histamine** Powerful inflammatory chemical that causes symptoms of allergies and asthma.

**Allergic rhinitis** *(hay fever)* A common allergy caused when airborne allergen particles (pollen, dust, mold, animal dander, etc.) enter the noses and throats of allergic persons.

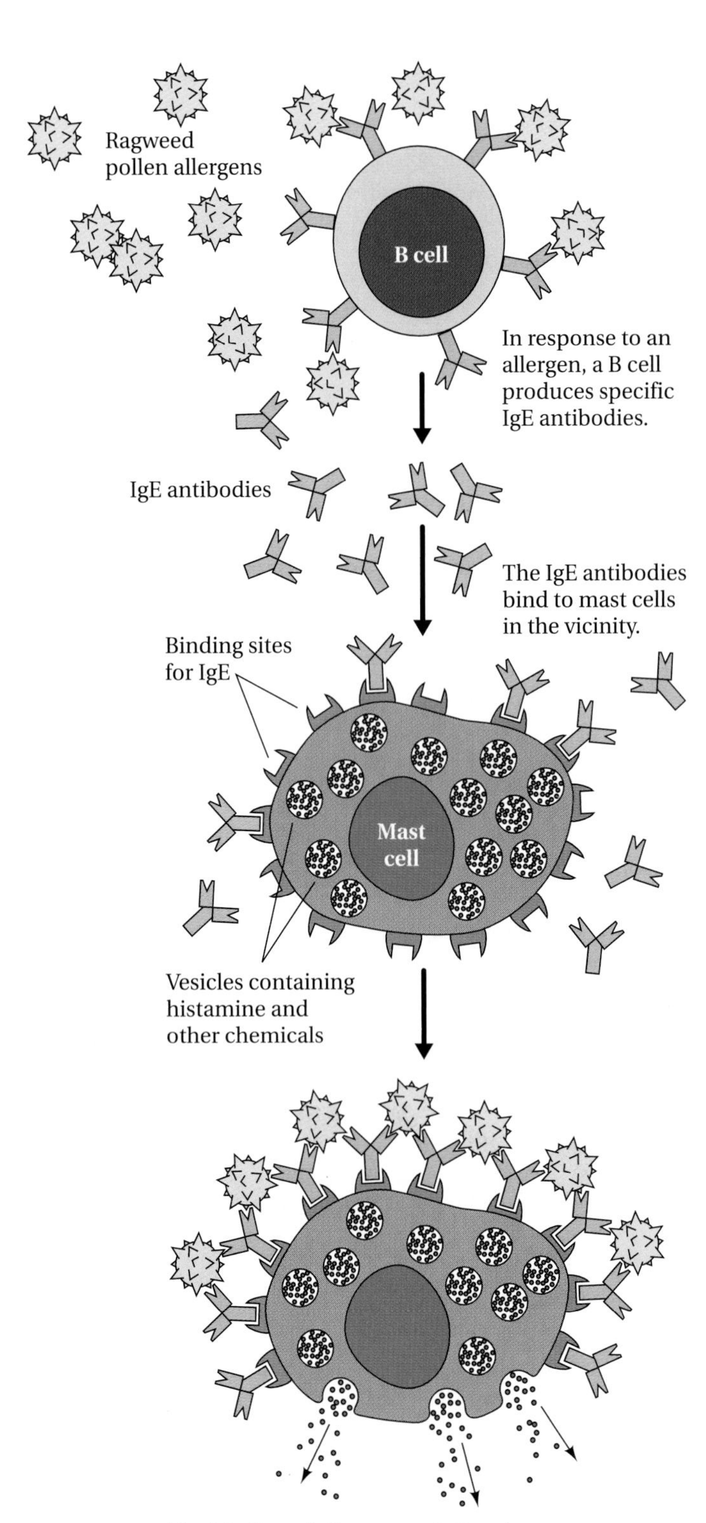
Ragweed pollen allergens
B cell
In response to an allergen, a B cell produces specific IgE antibodies.
IgE antibodies
The IgE antibodies bind to mast cells in the vicinity.
Binding sites for IgE
Mast cell
Vesicles containing histamine and other chemicals
The binding of allergens to IgE antigens on mast cells causes the release of histamines and leukotrines, which cause the inflammation, swelling, redness, and other allergy symptoms.

**Figure 15.5** ***What Makes You Sneeze—The Biology of Allergic Reactions***

**Anaphylaxis** A severe allergic reaction; treated with injections of adrenaline.

people in the United States. Allergic rhinitis occurs when tiny airborne allergens such as pollen, dust, mold, and dried dog and cat saliva particles enter the nose and throat of an allergic person. Common symptoms include puffy and itchy eyes, a runny or stopped-up nose (or both), and sneezing. People who are sensitive to pollens and ragweed suffer most during the pollination seasons of spring and fall. For those sensitive to dust or mold spores, allergic rhinitis can be a yearlong problem, although mold allergies are generally most troublesome in midsummer.

Mold allergies are caused by the spores of a group of plants in the fungus family. Molds thrive anywhere there is moisture, from piles of fallen leaves to damp basements. Dust allergies are actually caused by the feces of microscopic bugs called dust mites that live in household dust.

In some persons, insect bites, stings, and certain foods can cause a severe, life-threatening allergic reaction called **anaphylaxis** or *anaphylactic shock.* The throat may swell and shut down, and fluid may fill the lungs. Anaphylaxis is treated with injections of epinephrine (adrenaline).

**Talking Glossary**
Anaphylaxis
G1521

## PREVENTION

### *Protecting Yourself against Allergies*

Allergies are diagnosed through a test in which a drop of the suspected allergen is injected just beneath the skin. Skin tests take just a few minutes. Depending on the type of allergy, you can take steps to control it or reduce discomfort:

***Minimize Contact with Allergens*** Avoiding allergens is the most direct way of preventing an allergic response. But avoidance is not always possible, at least not without seriously compromising your lifestyle. It is more realistic to minimize contact with allergens.

If you are sensitive to pollen, check the daily pollen count in the local news. When the pollen count is especially high, minimize outdoor activity. If you are allergic to dust mites, keep your living quarters and work space dust-free. Avoid using venetian blinds, which are natural dust collectors, as well as down-filled blankets, feather pillows, and wall-to-wall carpeting. Cover your bedding with allergen-proof coverings, and wash them weekly. Dust furniture but keep vacuuming to a minimum, as it tends to raise more dust than it removes. If you do vacuum, use a machine rated by *Consumer Reports* as a low (dust) emissions model. You might also use cleaning products containing *acaricides,* chemicals that kill dust mites. They are available in most drugstores. If possible, have

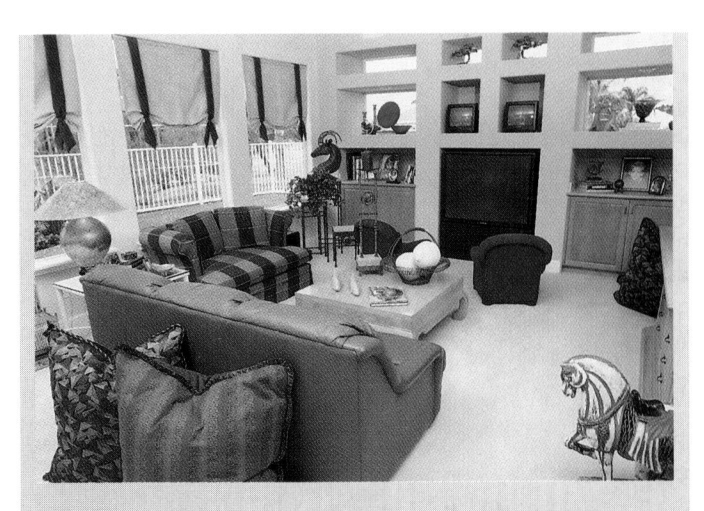

***How Clean Is This Room?*** Looks clean, yes, but wall-to-wall carpeting, overstuffed pillows and upholstery, and drapes may harbor dust and other allergens that can trigger allergic reactions in susceptible people.

someone else do the cleaning. Consider the cost a health insurance premium.

***Use Allergy Medications Prudently*** Allergy medications help control the symptoms of allergies. Your primary health care provider or allergist can help identify the nature of the allergen(s) causing your symptoms and the appropriate course of treatment. **Antihistamines** counteract the effects of histamine and treat rhinitis symptoms such as sneezing, runny nose, and itchy eyes and throat. **Decongestants** help unclog stuffy noses (see ***HealthCheck,*** next page, for further information on antihistamines and decongestants). Don't overuse these drugs (ask your health care provider how frequently and for how long you should take them). Follow the instructions on the label. Many antihistamines can cause drowsiness and should not be taken if you are driving or need to maintain full alertness.

Close-up
Allergy relief
T1503

Steroid nasal sprays take a week or longer to take effect but offer greater relief of nasal congestion than nasal decongestants do.[26] Another type of nasal spray contains cromolyn sodium. This is an anti-inflammatory drug that combats nasal congestion but takes even longer than steroid sprays to become fully effective.

***Consider Desensitization Shots*** Allergy shots contain tiny amounts of an offending allergen that gradually desensitizes the individual. Allergy shots are available for some types of allergens, ranging from animal danders to certain foods to various pollens. Though they are effective in about 85% of cases, they must be taken regularly (usually weekly) for many months to achieve a response. Persons who cannot avoid an allergen, such as veterinarians who are allergic to animals—yes, they exist—are particularly good candidates for allergy shots.

**Asthma—A Potential Killer** More than 12 million Americans, including nearly 5 million children, suffer from **asthma.** Asthma is a chronic, noninfectious lung disease that is characterized by temporary obstruction of the bronchial airways, or **bronchi,** the tubes in the lungs through which we breathe. Normally, air is exhaled from the lungs effortlessly. In an asthma attack, the muscles in the walls of the bronchial tubes tighten and go into spasm in response to an irritant or allergen, making breathing difficult. The bronchial tubes also become inflamed, swollen, and blocked with mucus, further impairing the flow of air. Asthma can result from many causes, including allergies, respiratory infections (such as bronchitis), and exposure to environmental pollutants (such as soot and cigarette smoke). Asthma attacks may last from a few minutes to a few hours. They produce such symptoms as wheezing, shortness of breath, coughing, and tightness in the chest. In severe cases respiratory blockage can be lethal.

Most cases of asthma in children, about 90%, are reactions to allergens such as dust, molds, feathers, animal dander, pollens, and some foods. For those between ages 11 and 30, the figure falls to about 70%, and to about half for those age 30 and over.[27] Some forms of asthma are genetically based.[28] Stress, strong emotions, exposure to cigarette smoke and air pollution, and even strenuous exercise can play a role in the development or course of asthma.[29] While exercise can induce an asthmatic reaction in susceptible people, people with asthma need not, nor should they, stop exercising. Rather, they should consult their health care provider about the kind of exercise that is best for them and whether they should use medication to prevent attacks.

HealthCheck
Check your asthma IQ
H1502

***Who Is Affected?*** Members of minority groups and the elderly are particularly hard hit, with death rates among African Americans, both young and old, at least three times higher than among non-Hispanic whites.[30] Asthma can develop at any age but usually begins in childhood. Though some children outgrow it, it may persist into adulthood. Asthma affects more boys than girls in childhood. By adulthood, equal numbers of men and women are affected.

**Antihistamines** Medications designed to counter the effects of histamine.

**Decongestant** Medication that eases stuffy noses and reduces mucus buildup.

**Asthma** Chronic, noninfectious lung disease characterized by a temporary obstruction and spasms of the bronchial airways or bronchi.

**Bronchi** The tubes leading from the windpipe to the interior of the lungs.

# HealthCheck

## How Much Do You Know about Cold and Flu Remedies?[38]

The over-the-counter cold remedy industry is a $2 billion a year enterprise. That's a lot of pills and potions. The following ***HealthCheck*** will help you become more aware of treatment options and will help you prepare for the next time the cold bug strikes or you get the flu. After answering each item, check your knowledge by turning to the answer key at the end of this chapter.

**True or False**

T F **1.** Antibiotics kill cold and flu viruses within a day or two.

T F **2.** Treating a common cold will shorten its duration.

T F **3.** It is always best to treat the common cold.

T F **4.** You should use a multisymptom cold remedy that treats as many symptoms as possible.

T F **5.** By using a cold remedy, you not only reduce your suffering but can help prevent a recurrence.

T F **6.** An antihistamine is good for clearing your stuffy nose, while a decongestant is good for stopping a runny nose.

T F **7.** Fortunately, most antihistamines on the market today do not induce drowsiness, so they are safe to use when driving.

T F **8.** You should not use nasal sprays or drops for longer than a few days.

T F **9.** Chicken soup is of absolutely no value in treating a common cold.

T F **10.** Always check the ingredients on cold remedies, especially if you have sensitivities to certain chemicals.

T F **11.** Any of the major over-the-counter pain relievers or analgesics—acetaminophen, aspirin, ibuprofen—work about equally well in relieving the pain and fever of a cold.

T F **12.** All cough medicines have the same effects.

T F **13.** Feed a cold; starve a fever.

***Controlling Asthma*** Asthma cannot be cured, but it can be controlled. As with allergies, reducing exposure to allergens helps prevent attacks. Avoiding smoking or second-hand smoke is a must, because tobacco smoke irritates the lungs and can induce attacks. Allergy shots can also help the person become desensitized to particular allergens. Muscle relaxation techniques may help asthmatics improve their breathing.[31]

**Take Charge** More on controlling asthma **C1505**

There are two major types of asthma medications: bronchodilators and anti-inflammatories. **Bronchodilators** are used to stop an asthma attack once it has started. They open bronchial passages by relaxing the muscles surrounding the air tubes, making it easier to breathe. **Anti-inflammatories** help prevent asthma attacks from occurring by keeping bronchial tubes open. They accomplish this by reducing swelling in the air tubes and decreasing the amount of mucus that accumulates. Anti-inflammatories come in different forms—inhalants, liquids, and pills. Cromolyn, nedocromil, and corticosteroids (steroidal agents that fight allergic reactions) are examples.

**Talking Glossary** Bronchodilators **G1522**

With proper management, people with asthma can lead full, productive lives and participate in virtually any activity, including vigorous exercise.[32] Several Olympic medalists had asthma, but it did not deter them.[33]

**Bronchodilators** Drugs that dilate (open) clogged airways and ease shortness of breath.

**Anti-inflammatories** Drugs that combat inflammation.

**Autoimmune disorders** "Self-against-self" diseases in which the immune system mistakenly attacks the body's own cells.

**Autoimmune Disorders—Self against Self** Sometimes our bodies become their own worst enemies. In **autoimmune disorders,** the immune system attacks healthy cells in the body as though they were foreign. This battle of self against self results in autoimmune disorders such as rheumatoid arthritis and multiple sclerosis. Just why this occurs is not completely understood, although heredity, hormones, and pathogens (such as viruses that alter normal body cells, making them appear foreign) may be involved.

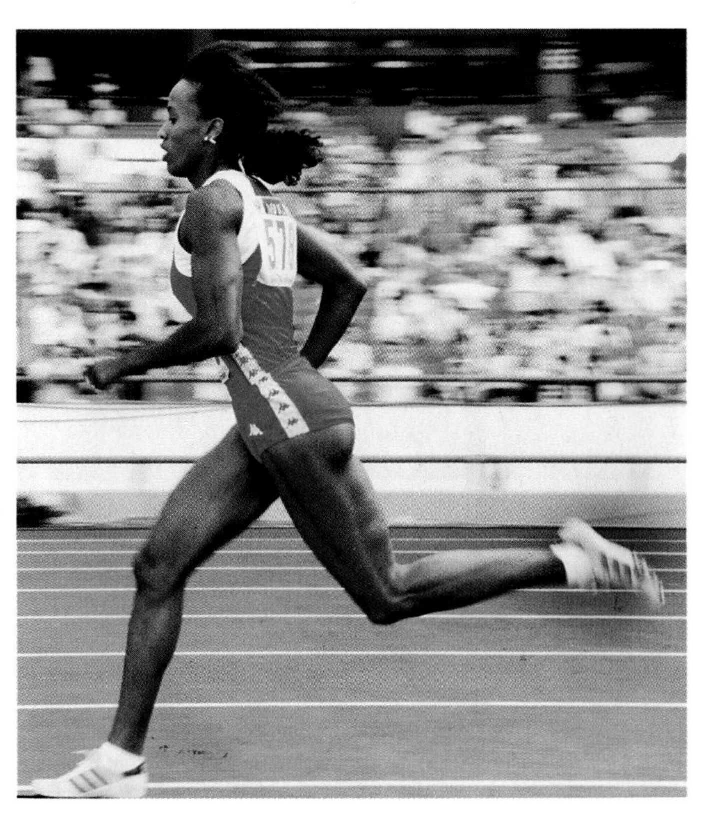

***Jackie Joyner Kersee*** The Olympic medalist Jackie Joyner Kersee suffers from asthma but has not let it prevent her from participating and succeeding in athletic competition.

Talking Glossary
Rheumatoid arthritis, Lupus erythematosus
G1523

Two of the more prevalent autoimmune disorders are **rheumatoid arthritis,** a painful, potentially disabling condition involving a chronic inflammation of the membranes that line the joints, and **lupus erythematosus,** a chronic inflammatory disorder of connective tissue. Both diseases strike women far more often than men. Though there is no cure for these diseases, they are treated with varying degrees of success with drugs that regulate or suppress the immune system response.

Talking Glossary
Myelin
G1524

**Multiple sclerosis (MS)** is a chronic and often crippling nervous system disorder in which the **myelin,** the fatty covering that insulates nerve cells in the brain and spinal cord, becomes damaged or destroyed. When myelin is damaged, the transmission of nerve impulses between the brain and spinal cord breaks down, leading to symptoms that can range from mild to severe, which can result in the person becoming unable to speak, walk, or write.[34] The disease afflicts about 350,000 Americans and strikes women about twice as often as men.

MS may be a type of autoimmune disease in which white blood cells react against the body's own nerve cells, causing inflammation that leads to a loss of myelin. A viral infection may trigger this autoimmune response, but no specific causal agent has been found. Genetic factors may also play a role in susceptibility to MS. There is no cure for the disease, but a few drugs help control the symptoms. The disease typically strikes people in the prime of life, between the ages of 30 and 50.

Close-up
More on MS
T1504

**Immune Deficiencies** In rare instances, generally resulting from a genetic defect, children are born with immune systems that fail to protect them from common pathogens. They must live in a sterile environment to prevent exposure to viruses and other pathogens that children with normal immune systems can fight off. In the case of AIDS—*acquired immunodeficiency syndrome*—a virus, HIV, attacks the immune system, crippling it and leaving the person vulnerable to **opportunistic infections** (see Chapter 16). Immune system deficiencies have also been implicated in the development of cancer. Cancer cells that would normally be eradicated may grow out of control if the immune system is weakened by age or other factors.

## think about it!

- **Do you or someone you know have allergies or asthma? If so, how do they affect your life or the other person's life? What are you or the other person doing about them?**
- **How do vaccines protect us from disease?**
- **What vaccines or immunizations have you had throughout your life? How can you find out?**
- **Are your vaccines up to date? Are you sure? If not, what will you do about it? Why?**

Smart Quiz
Q1504

**Rheumatoid arthritis** Arthritis involving inflammation, swelling, stiffness, and pain in the joints.

**Lupus erythematosus** A chronic autoimmune disease involving inflammation of the connective tissue; can affect many body organs and systems.

**Multiple sclerosis (MS)** A central nervous system disorder; the myelin coating that insulates nerve cells is damaged or destroyed.

**Myelin** The fatty material that covers and insulates nerve cells.

**Opportunistic infections** Infections caused by organisms that flourish because of a weakness in the immune system.

# COMMON INFECTIOUS DISEASES—SYMPTOMS AND TREATMENT

## Respiratory Tract Infections

Respiratory tract infections range from the common cold and milder cases of flu to more serious conditions like pneumonia and tuberculosis. Though bacteria and viruses are most often the pathogens involved, smoking and exposure to pollutants increase susceptibility to these infections.

**The Common Cold** The **common cold** is a contagious viral infection of the upper respiratory tract. Colds are the most common infectious illness. Most adults get two or three colds each year, and children suffer them even more often.[35]

About 200 different viruses cause the common cold, with **rhinoviruses** (from the Greek *rhino,* meaning "nose") the most frequent culprits.[36] Cold symptoms include nasal congestion, sore throat, fatigue, headache, and sometimes a low-grade fever.[37] Colds generally last from 2 to 14 days, but not usually longer than a week. Some colds are transmitted by airborne exposure to viruses expelled by an infected person through sneezing, coughing, or just talking. Most common colds, however, are contracted by touch, by contact with a surface (e.g., a tissue, doorknob, or hand) that contains nasal secretions left by an infected person.

The best way to recover from a cold is to rest and drink plenty of fluids. No medications or vaccines prevent or cure the common cold, but many medications alleviate cold symptoms.

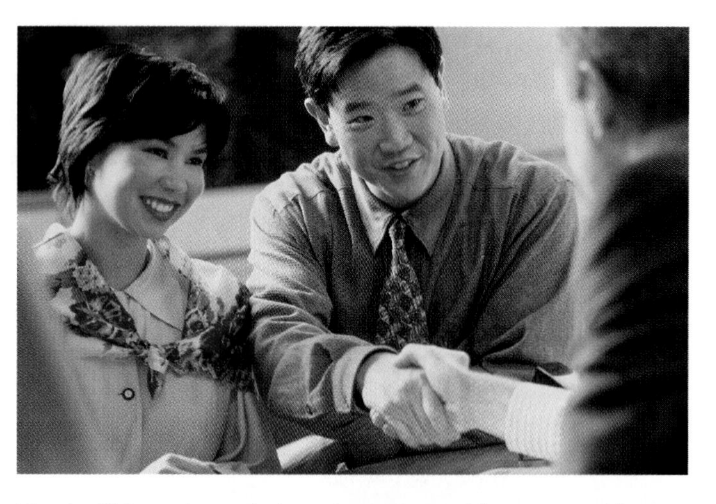

***Touch*** Did you know that most common colds are spread by touch, not by airborne exposure? Protect yourself by keeping your hands away from your nose and eyes and washing them frequently to remove viruses and other infectious agents.

**Common cold** A mild, short-lived, contagious viral infection of the upper respiratory tract.

**Rhinoviruses** A class of small RNA viruses that are the major causes of the common cold.

**Influenza (flu)** An acute viral lower-respiratory-tract infection.

**Epidemic** The rapid spread or increased prevalence of a disease within a group or population.

**Pandemic** An epidemic affecting a whole country, a continent, or the entire world.

**Bronchitis** An inflammation of the bronchial tubes; characterized by excess mucus production, a phlegmy cough, fever, and impaired breathing.

**Influenza** **Influenza** or **flu** is a highly contagious viral disease that affects the lungs and other parts of the body.[42] Like the common cold, the flu is spread by inhaling droplets expelled into the air when an infected person coughs, sneezes, or talks. It may also be contracted by touching objects used by an infected person and then bringing the hand to the mucous membranes of the eyes, nose, or mouth.

The flu is caused by viruses belonging to three families of influenza viruses: type A, type B, and type C. Within each family are a number of specific strains of flu viruses. Type A influenza is most common and typically associated with severe outbreaks. Type B influenza is typically milder, although some strains can produce severe infections. Type C influenza rarely affects people over the age of 16.

Every ten years or so, a strain of influenza virus appears that differs markedly from other strains within its family. These strains usually lead to worldwide **epidemics,** or **pandemics,** because relatively few people have antibodies against the strain. One pandemic swept the world in 1918 and accounted for more than 20 million deaths.[43]

All flu viruses produce similar symptoms that vary in severity. After an incubation period of one to three days, people with flu experience an abrupt onset of a fever between 102 and 104°F, chills, headache, general aches and pains, fatigue, weakness, and possibly a sore throat, dry cough, nausea, and burning eyes. The fever usually subsides after two or three days, but chest and nasal congestion may develop. In most healthy persons, flu symptoms disappear in about a week. In vulnerable groups, however, such as children, older people, and people with other health problems, the flu can lead to serious complications like **bronchitis**

## HealthCheck

### Is It a Cold or Is It the Flu?

Though the symptoms of the common cold and flu may be similar, here are some guidelines to distinguish between them.[45] Allergies may also mimic a cold, but they are less likely to produce a fever and don't produce the aches and pains associated with colds.

| Symptoms | Common Cold | Flu |
|---|---|---|
| Fever | None or low-grade (less than 100°) | Typically high (102–104°F); sudden onset; usually lasts 3–4 days |
| Headache | Rare | Prominent |
| General aches and pains | Slight | Typical, often quite severe |
| Fatigue and weakness | Quite mild | Extreme; can last up to 2–3 weeks |
| Prostration (need to lie down) | Uncommon | Early and prominent |
| Runny, stuffy nose | Common | Sometimes |
| Sneezing | Usual | Sometimes |
| Sore throat | Common | Sometimes |
| Chest discomfort, cough | Mild to moderate | Common, but can become severe |
| Complications | Sinus congestion or earache, possibly bronchitis and pneumonia | Bronchitis, pneumonia; can be life-threatening |
| Prevention | None at present; some vaccinations in experimental stage | Annual vaccination for specific strains |
| Treatment | Temporary symptomatic relief only | Temporary symptomatic relief and also oral antiviral amantadine for type A |

or pneumonia. Older people and people with chronic health conditions may be advised to take a flu vaccine ("flu shot") before flu season.

As with colds, the flu is best treated with rest, fluids, and pain and fever relievers like acetaminophen. When taken one to two days after the onset of infection, the antiviral drugs amantadine and rimantadine may shorten the duration and intensity of type A influenza. A new experimental drug has shown promise in preventing the flu and even stopping it in its tracks in laboratory animals.[44] Human tests were expected in 1997.

**Talking Glossary**
Alveoli
G1526

**Pneumonia** **Pneumonia** is a serious lung infection in which invading pathogens cause the air sacs in the lungs—the **alveoli**—to fill with pus and other liquid, making it difficult for oxygen to reach the blood. Lack of oxygen may cause death. There are more than 30 different causes of pneumonia, including bacteria, viruses, fungi, and protozoans. About 500,000 Americans experience a bout of bacterial pneumonia each year. A roughly equal number suffer viral pneumonia.[46] Pneumonia may also result from irritation to the lungs due to pollutants, or, in hospitalized patients, from lung irritation caused by anesthesia or intravenous foods and liquids. Symptoms of pneumonia vary depending on the agent of infection, but there are usually fever and chills, chest pain, a cough with rust, yellow, or greenish sputum (mucus-laden material coughed up from deep inside the lungs), and difficulty breathing. Pneumonia is especially dangerous in older people and the very young. Regardless of age or physical condition, pneumonia is a serious disease that requires immediate medical attention.

Bacterial pneumonia is treated with antibiotics such as penicillin

**Pneumonia** Acute infectious disease of the respiratory tract; causes fluids to collect in air sacs in the lungs.

**Alveoli** Air sacs of the lungs.

and erythromycin. Though there are no effective drugs for viral pneumonia, most cases resolve on their own. Rest, fluids, proper diet, and avoidance of smoking are crucial in the treatment of pneumonia. A vaccine is available for *pneumococcal pneumonia,* a bacterial form of pneumonia that is one of the most serious forms of the disease.[47] Older people and people with other health problems are advised to obtain it.

**Legionnaire's Disease** Legionnaire's disease is a type of bacterial pneumonia first recognized in 1976, when 29 people attending an American Legion convention became mysteriously ill and died. After a frantic search for the source of this mystery disease, the bacterium *Legionella pneumophila* was isolated in the water of the air-conditioning system of the hotel in which the conventioneers had stayed. Microbiologists soon realized that the disease had caused many epidemics in previous years.

Legionnaire's disease is transmitted by airborne droplets of *Legionella.* The bacterium apparently breeds in industrial air-conditioning units, lakes, stagnant pools, and puddles of water. Symptoms appear within a week of inhalation. Person-to-person transmission is rare. Symptoms include headache, muscular and abdominal pain, diarrhea and vomiting, and a dry cough. Pneumonia soon follows, with high fever, shaking chills, sputum, and drowsiness. Legionnaire's disease can be treated with the antibiotic erythromycin, but early detection and treatment are critical.

**Talking Glossary**
Tuberculosis
G1527

**Tuberculosis** Until the 1940s and 50s, when antibiotic drugs capable of curing the disease were finally discovered, **tuberculosis (TB)** was perhaps our most dreaded disease. Tuberculosis is a chronic infection caused by the bacterium *Mycobacterium tuberculosis.* The infection usually affects the lungs and sometimes other parts of the body, including the brain, kidneys, or spine. Symptoms include a racking cough, fever, fatigue, hoarseness, chest pain, weight loss, and blood in the sputum.

In the nineteenth and twentieth centuries alone, literally hundreds of millions of people—far more than those felled to date by AIDS—were disabled and killed by TB. By 1985, the number of cases in the United States had fallen to just 22,000, the lowest in modern times.[48] Thousands of sanatoriums and clinics closed their doors, and it seemed that the disease might well be brought under control or eliminated. Since 1986, however, TB cases have risen at an alarming rate among some groups, especially intravenous substance users, people with AIDS, homeless people, and people in confined living conditions.[49] Worldwide, about 8 million people develop TB and about 3 million die of it each year.[50]

Tuberculosis is primarily an airborne disease. Infected people cough up sputum when they sneeze, speak, sing, or even laugh, throwing bacteria-infected droplets into the air, which are inhaled by others. Once the *tubercle bacilli* (rod-shaped TB bacteria) reach the air sacs in the lungs, they slowly multiply. Eventually, they form characteristic cheeselike clumps or lesions called "tubercles." These lesions slowly spread to nearby airways, forming additional clumps. If untreated, the entire lung becomes scarred with them and eventually ceases to function. There is good reason why TB used to be called "consumption": the disease consumes people.

TB is certainly contagious, but most people who are exposed to TB bacteria don't become infected. Infection usually requires prolonged exposure—typically months of close contact with a person with the active disease. Of people who become infected, most have a latent form of the infection, which does not produce symptoms or spread to others. Fully a third of the world's population, including about 10 million people in the United States, are believed to be infected with a latent form of TB. Though most people with latent infections never develop active TB, the infection can enter an active state at some time, generally because of factors like a suppressed immune system, aging, other illness, or alcoholism.[51]

The presence of the TB bacterium is detected by a *tuberculin skin test* (or Mantoux test), in which a substance called purified protein derivative (PPD) is injected under the skin of the forearm. If a red welt appears 48 to 72 hours later, TB may be present. The tuberculin skin test is a useful first-step method of detecting TB. But because so many tests result in false positives (untrue positive findings), additional diagnostic tests (culturing a sputum specimen and chest X-ray) are necessary. But cultures take at least three weeks to process. If

**Tuberculosis (TB)** Bacterial infection that usually affects the lungs and sometimes other parts of the body, including the brain, kidneys, or spine.

TB is suspected, treatment should begin immediately. About 40 to 60% of untreated people with TB die from it.[52]

TB is treated over a period of at least six months with antibiotic drugs. If these drugs are taken properly, TB is usually cured. Many people, however, especially those who are homeless and drug addicted, fail to take medications reliably. Failure to complete drug therapy often leads to relapse and, potentially, the development of drug-resistant organisms.

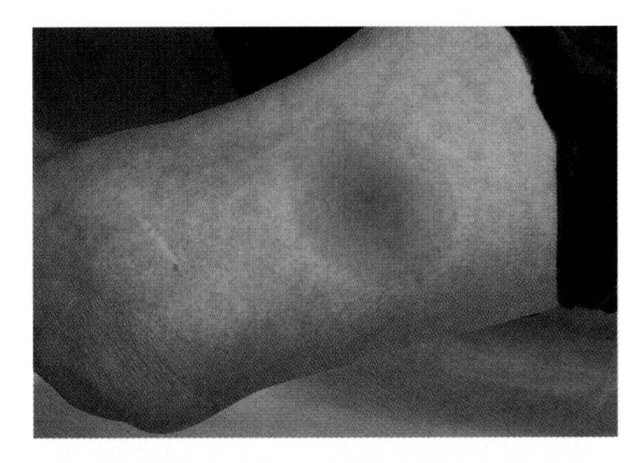

**Figure 15.6** ***Rash Associated with Lyme Disease on Adult Arm*** A reddish bull's-eye or ring-shaped rash spreading outward from the bite may appear in the early stages of Lyme disease. However, not all people who contract the disease develop the characteristic rash.

## Lyme Disease

When summer comes again, Americans will head outdoors, to the mountains and countryside, or to stroll through wooded areas close to home. Today, many of us are filled with trepidation as we or our children venture into wooded areas or even into our own backyards. The fear is of a danger that may be lurking around every tree and bush: **Lyme disease.** Lyme disease is named after a town on the Connecticut seaboard, but it is now found in nearly every state, Canada, Europe, even Asia.[53] The disease was discovered in 1975, and by 1994, some 13,000 cases were reported in the United States.[54] People in the Northeast and the Upper Midwest (Minnesota and Wisconsin) are at greatest risk. The tick season begins in April in the Northeast and Midwest, when juvenile ticks called nymphs emerge and feed voraciously. It ends in the late fall, when full-grown ticks become dormant.

**Close-up** Lyme disease, U.S. **T1505**

Lyme disease is caused by a spiral-shaped bacterium (spirochete) named *Borrelia burgdorferi,* which is spread to people and animals by ticks that inhabit the fur of deer and mice in wooded areas. When an infected tick bites, the bacterium can enter the host's blood. (When pregnant women are infected, the Lyme disease bacterium can cross the placenta and infect the fetus as well.) Between 2 and 28 days after being bitten—but usually after about 8 or 9 days—a slowly expanding circular, triangular, or oval-shaped red-ringed rash (see Figure 15.6) may develop around the bite. Within days or weeks of infection, flulike symptoms may appear, such as fever and swelling of the lymph nodes. There may be painful or swollen joints. If left untreated, the disease can progress to cause serious heart or nerve damage, crippling arthritis, or other serious medical problems[55] As if Lyme disease weren't bad enough, now we have word that many of the ticks carrying the Lyme bacterium also carry a second and sometimes even a third infectious organism, which can result in a two-way or three-way punch that makes the symptoms of the disease more severe and may make it last two to three times longer than in people infected only with Lyme.[56]

**Close-up** More on Lyme disease **T1506**

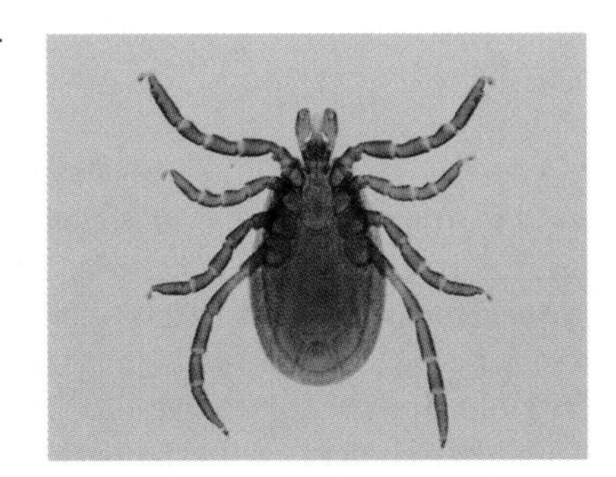

***Deer Tick*** The tiny deer tick, shown here magnified many times, harbors the pathogen that causes Lyme disease.

Lyme disease is almost always cured by penicillin or other antibiotics—that is, when it is detected early. But the tick bite and early symptoms may go unnoticed, in which case chronic symptoms may develop. Blood tests to detect antibodies for Lyme disease are available but are not always reliable.

**Lyme disease** An infectious disease spread by ticks; caused by the bacterium *Borrelia burgdorferi.*

PREVENTION

## Preventing Lyme Disease

In the spring, the world is reborn, and—especially in the Northeast and the Midwest—so is the Lyme disease season. Here are some strategies to reduce your risk of infection:

- *Engineer your environment.* Ticks like it damp, so if you live in the suburbs, you can make your yard inhospitable by clearing away leaf litter and mulches. The greatest danger is from tall grasses, moist foliage, and decaying leaves—sites that are hospitable to the ticks. Keep the grass mowed. Create as much open space between wooded areas and the house as possible.
- *Wear "body armor" when hiking.* If you hike through the woods or tall grass, wear body armor: socks and shoes, pants with the bottoms tucked into socks or boots, a light-colored hat, and a long-sleeve shirt tucked into the pants. Light-colored clothes render ticks more visible. Limit hiking to trails rather than plodding through grasses, brush, and piles of leaves.
- *Shower after outings.* This helps wash away unattached ticks.
- *Examine your body.* When you venture into tick territory, do daily body examinations. Nymphs are only the size of the head of a pin before they begin feeding, so look closely. Likely sites include the groin, buttocks, armpits, lower legs, backs of the knees, navel, neck, and hairline. (Ticks like the faces and ears of furry pets).
- *Use insect repellents.* To repel ticks, you can use insect repellents containing the chemical DEET. Products containing the chemical premethrin (permanone) kill ticks but should be applied only to clothes, not directly to the skin. Infants and young children may be especially at risk for adverse reactions to DEET. Check with your doctor or pharmacist before using an insect repellent or insecticide. Pregnant women in the first trimester may be advised not to use insect repellents.[57]
- *Remove ticks promptly.* Removing an infected tick within 24 hours prevents infection.[58] To remove ticks, use fine-point tweezers. Apply the tweezers as close to the skin as you can and pull slowly and steadily upward. Do *not* use matches, kerosene, nail polish, or petroleum jelly on the ticks. These methods may cause the tick to inject bacteria and make it more difficult to remove. Wash the site and your hands with soap and water. Then swab the site with alcohol or hydrogen peroxide and bandage it. Call the doctor if you suspect that you or your children have been exposed. Early treatment with antibiotics can prevent serious complications.

**Video**
Lyme disease prevention
V1501

## Infectious Mononucleosis

Infectious mononucleosis, also called "mono" or "kissing disease," is a viral infection caused by a virus belonging to the herpes virus family called Epstein-Barr virus. There is good reason why "mono" is referred to as the kissing disease: The Epstein-Barr virus (EBV) reproduces in the salivary glands, making the infected person's saliva especially contagious. Prolonged kissing is thought to be a primary means by which the disease is transmitted. However, mononucleosis can also be transmitted via shared toothbrushes and eating utensils.

Most people who get "mono" are between the ages of 16 and 30. Symptoms develop after an incubation period of between two and seven weeks and can range from the practically nonexistent to severe. Early ("prodromal") symptoms often include unusual fatigue, headaches, chills, and loss of appetite. The full-blown, or clinical, stage is often accompanied by fever of between 101 and 105°F, painful sore throat (caused by enlarged, often pus-covered tonsils), and swollen lymph glands in the neck, arm, and groin. The spleen becomes enlarged in about half of the cases, while an enlarged liver occurs in about one case in five.[59] The clinical stage typically lasts for about two or three weeks, although it may linger for several months. During the recuperation or convalescence stage, people may experience occasional depression and lack of energy.

A blood test is used to detect EBV, based on finding antibodies to the virus in the blood. No drugs or vaccines are available to cure or prevent "mono." Rest, ample fluids, and a balanced diet are the surest route to recovery.

## Emerging Infectious Diseases—New Threats to Health

In the late 1950s, many public health officials believed that the war on infectious diseases was nearly won. Their optimism was fueled by the development of new vaccines, powerful antimicrobial drugs, and the widespread availability of safe drinking water. Scourges like polio, tetanus, **smallpox, cholera,** and diphtheria were all but eliminated from the U.S. and other developed nations. Similar victories against other menaces lay just around the corner.

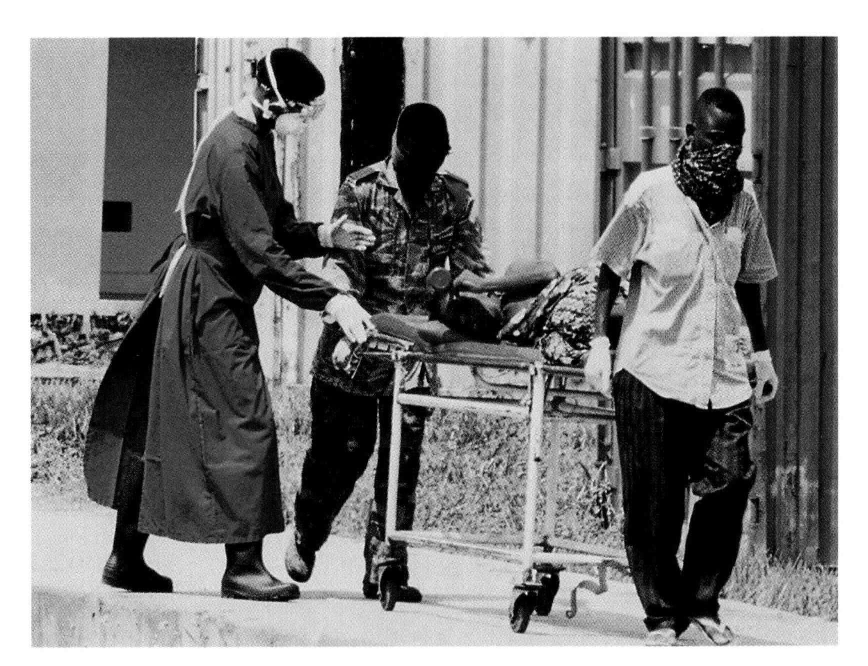

***Ebola*** Ebola is among the world's deadliest viruses. Here, during a recent outbreak in Zaire, a soldier and a civilian worker carry a patient infected with the Ebola virus as a doctor follows them.

Today, immunization and water purification prevent many illnesses, and medicines control or cure many others. Yet total victory in the war against infectious agents is nowhere in sight. To date only one infectious disease—smallpox—has actually been eradicated. At least 50 different infectious agents pose new threats to world health.[60] These agents are responsible for **emerging infectious diseases.** Some emerging infectious diseases are new to the human scene (such as Legionnaire's disease, Lyme disease, Ebola, toxic shock syndrome, and AIDS). Others have reemerged or appeared in new, sometimes more dangerous, strains, such as tuberculosis, malaria, cholera, and influenza.

One such agent is the **Ebola** virus. Ebola first entered public awareness following an epidemic in Zaire in 1976. Several more epidemics in Africa have followed. Another one occurred in Zaire in 1995 and affected 316 people, 245 of whom died. Because of the ease of moving people and goods worldwide, outbreaks of exotic diseases threaten us all. As Nobel laureate Dr. Joshua Lederberg observed, "The microbe that felled one child in a distant continent yesterday can reach yours today and seed a global pandemic tomorrow." Several factors, some natural and some of our own making, are linked to the emergence of new infectious diseases and the recurrence of old threats in new forms (see Table 15.3, following page).

**Close-up**
More on Ebola
T1507

**Smart Reference**
Shaking the Ebola tree
R1501

**Increase in World Travel** More people than ever travel about the globe, bringing infectious agents with them. Many don't realize that they harbor disease-causing agents. New populations become exposed to these agents, leading to outbreaks in new places. Some microbes hitch rides on imports and exports. The Asian tiger mosquito, which can transmit a rare but fatal brain disease called Eastern equine encephalitis, entered the United States in 1991 in watery recesses of shipments of tires bound for U.S. ports.[61]

**Changes in Ecological Conditions** From the decimation of the world's rain forests to the mushrooming of large urban centers, the natural environment has undergone extensive changes. Changes in ecological conditions bring *vectors* (insect or animal carriers of infectious agents) into contact with human populations. When the Aswan High Dam was constructed in Egypt, for instance, the new lake it created became a breeding ground for virus-bearing mosquitoes.[62] As rural land disappeared in the United States, the

**Smallpox** A devastating viral disease, now eradicated, that produced high fever and skin eruptions.

**Cholera** An infection of the small intestine that produces diarrhea and vomiting; can lead to life-threatening loss of fluids and electrolyes.

**Emerging infectious diseases** Infections seemingly new to the human scene and those that have reemerged or appear in new strains.

**Ebola** A highly fatal viral disease spread to humans by monkeys.

TABLE 15.3

## Some Recent Emerging Diseases[65]

| Illness/Causative Agent | Symptoms | Means of Transmission | Treatment | Prevention |
|---|---|---|---|---|
| *Dengue hemorrhagic fever,* caused by one of several related kinds of dengue viruses. The disease occurs in tropical, mosquito-infested areas throughout the world. | Fever, debilitating pain, and bleeding from the skin, gums, and internal organs, sometimes leading to death. | From a bite by an infected mosquito; no evidence of person-to-person transmission. | No cure or vaccine exists. Treatment consists largely of supportive therapy that replenishes body fluids and maintains electrolyte balances. | Persons traveling in tropical areas inhabited by the mosquitoes that carry dengue should take precautions to avoid mosquito bites, e.g., using insect repellant, keeping the body covered, and avoiding outdoor activities as much as possible, especially during the day (the infected mosquitoes are day-biters). |
| *Hantavirus pulmonary syndrome (HPS),* caused by a family of viruses called hantaviruses; found principally in East Asia but has spread to parts of Europe and North America, including some isolated cases in the U.S. | Fever, chills, muscle aches, headache, and respiratory problems can progress to severe lung disease, which may be fatal. | Spread by airborne transmission of viral particles in dust containing rodent excreta that has been disturbed by sweeping floors or shaking rugs. No evidence exists of person-to-person transmission. | Supportive treatment aimed at maintaining blood pressure and adequate cardiac output. No cure or effective vaccine exists. | Avoid contact with wild rodents, alive or dead. Ensure adequate ventilation and use latex or rubber gloves when cleaning areas where rodent droppings may be found. Disinfect any surfaces with Lysol or bleach and water where rodents may have been or left excreta. Further precautions needed where large numbers of rodents may be found. Protect your house from rodents by sealing holes of entry and preventing access to food by closing all food storage cabinets and keeping food in sealed containers. |
| *Ebola,* among the world's deadliest diseases, kills about 80% of its victims. Caused by the Ebola virus, it is named after a river of the same name in Zaire where it was first discovered. The disease affects monkeys, apes, and humans and involves a form of viral hemorrhagic fever. | Fever, chills, aches and pains that progress to vomiting, diarrhea, abdominal pain, sore throat, chest pain, and internal bleeding and bleeding from injection sites, which leads to death in most cases. | Monkeys are victims of, and vectors for, the disease. Among humans, Ebola is spread by close personal contact with the blood or body fluids of someone who is very ill with the disease. There is no evidence of airborne transmission among humans. | No cure or vaccine exists. Treatment is supportive in nature, involving careful management of fluids and electrolyte balances, but does not directly attack the disease. | Avoid contact with body fluids (blood, feces, urine, vomit, etc.) of infected people. Quarantining infected people can help prevent the spread of the disease. |

natural predator-prey balance shifted, and animals such as deer proliferated. Because many deer carry ticks, suburbanites in some parts of the country are now at risk for contracting Lyme disease.[63]

**Rise of Drug-Resistant Infectious Organisms** Many infectious organisms **mutate,** or vary in their genetic makeup across generations, especially when they are under siege by antimicrobial drugs. These drugs represent double-edged swords. They are necessary, often life-saving, yet their widespread use has led to the emergence of drug-resistant strains. We have so overused antibiotics that weaker strains of bacteria have been killed off and been replaced by more resistant ones. Some resultant infections are nearly impossible to treat.[64] The Centers for Disease Control and Prevention now instructs hospitals to use certain antibiotics only as a last resort. The development of drug-resistant strains has occurred in organisms causing such diseases as malaria, tuberculosis, and gonorrhea. There are also drug-resistant strains of pneumococcal and staphylococcal bacteria. Drug-resistant strains of disease can also arise when people stop using medicines prematurely or take them erratically.

Smart Reference
Beating bacteria
R1502

**Changes in Population Composition and Lifestyle** Until recently, most of the world's population was concentrated in rural areas. Today, a third of all people live in cities, often under crowded and unsanitary conditions that promote the transmission of infectious diseases. The population in many countries, including the United States, is also aging. Older people, along with children, are most susceptible to infectious illnesses. Many older people require long periods of hospitalization, giving rise to **nosocomial infections,** or infections that develop in hospitals. Nosocomial infections are often caused by the prolonged use of devices such as catheters (tubes used to pass fluid into or out of the body) that allow entry of infectious organisms.

Smart Reference
Mysterious maladies
R1503

Talking Glossary
Nosocomial infections
G1528

Substance abuse, unsafe sex, and the AIDS epidemic have increased the number of people in the population with impaired immune systems. They are thus more susceptible to opportunistic infections—infections caused by pathogens that people with healthy immune systems usually fend off.

## think about it!

- **Do you believe that you get fewer, more, or about the same number of colds as most other people? Why?**
- **Do you get flu shots when flu season is coming around? Why or why not? Are you satisfied with your answer?**
- **Do you consider yourself at risk of being infected with TB, Lyme disease, or infectious mononucleosis? Why or why not?**
- **Do you do anything to prevent Lyme disease when you go for an outing in the woods? If not, why not?**

**critical thinking** **Do you have the attitude that some or most of the diseases discussed in this chapter are someone else's problem, not yours? If so, why?**

Smart Quiz
Q1505

**Mutate** To undergo mutation, a change in genetic structure.

**Nosocomial infections** Infections acquired in hospitals.

# Protecting Yourself from Infectious Diseases

## Take Charge

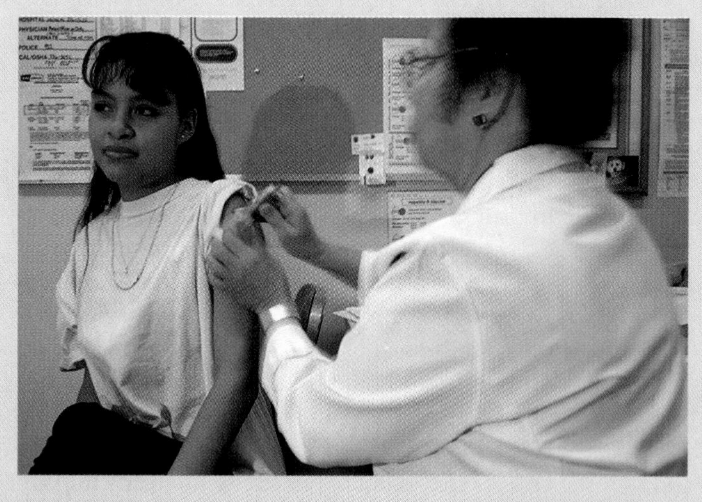

*Vaccinations* Keeping your vaccinations up to date is among the most important ways of protecting yourself from infectious disease.

Though our immune systems and modern medicine help us fight invading pathogens, healthwise behaviors can help keep infectious agents at bay.

### Avoiding Exposure to Infectious Agents

For infections to occur, pathogens must find a route of entry into your body. They may enter through body openings or through a break in the skin. Some enter the nasal cavity. Others may be ingested in food or drink. Though there is no surefire way to prevent infection, these precautions will improve your chances of staying well.[66]

- *Wash your hands frequently.* Cold germs and other infectious agents can be transferred to your hands by touching objects used by infected persons. Use warm soapy water to remove cold viruses and other infectious agents. Wash several times a day. This is especially important if you've been exposed to an infected person or have used public facilities such as restrooms, elevators, and escalators where you might have come into contact with germs. Cold viruses can survive for several hours on doorknobs, countertops, and other surfaces.
- *Keep your hands away from your nose.* Cold viruses and some bacteria cling to your hands and are transferred to the base of your nose by scratching your nose or inserting a finger into your nose. They are then inhaled into your upper nasal passageways and infect your whole body.
- *Keep your hands away from your eyes.* What goes for the nose also goes for the eyes. Rubbing your eyes can transfer germs such as cold and flu viruses from your hands to your tear ducts, and from there into your upper airways. If you must touch your eyes or nose, wash your hands first.
- *Avoid touching any object used by a person with an active infection.*
- *Avoid contact with infected people.* Move away from people who are sneezing, coughing, or blowing their noses. Cold viruses spewed into the air could wind up in your nasal cavity.
- *Use tissues rather than handkerchiefs.* Use tissues and throw them away. Cloth handkerchiefs can harbor cold and influenza viruses.
- *Keep your immune system humming.* Get enough sleep, learn to manage stress, avoid excessive alcohol intake, exercise regularly, and follow a balanced diet.
- *Practice safer sex.* People who are sexually active can protect themselves from sexually transmitted diseases, including AIDS, by following the safer sex suggestions outlined in Chapter 16.
- *Don't overuse or misuse antibiotics.* Overuse or misuse of antibiotics can give microorganisms the opportunity to develop more resistant strains. Never use an antibiotic unless you are directed to do so by your physician. Take them as directed for the full course of treatment. Discard leftover pills. Don't store them in the back of your medicine cabinet for later use.
- *Avoid irritants.* Don't smoke and avoid second-hand smoke. Exposure to tobacco smoke increases susceptibility to respiratory infections and bronchitis. Limit your exposure to air pollution from insecticides and other chemicals that can irritate your respiratory tract.

## Keep Your Vaccinations Up to Date

Vaccinations are not just for kids. Adults too need to keep their vaccinations up to date. Obtain a tetanus booster every ten years. Health care workers and veterinarians need vaccinations against infectious organisms with which they may come into contact. Health officials recommend that all young adults in their teens and twenties receive an HBV (hepatitis B) vaccination. Your student health service or primary health care provider can provide you with information about the HBV and other vaccines.

If you are uncertain about which vaccines you have received, ask your doctor, parents, or other caretakers. Log your findings. Get any needed boosters. Table 15.4 lists recommended immunizations and boosters for adults.

**Should You Get a Flu Shot?** Anyone can get the flu. The best protection against the flu is an annual flu shot. Vaccinations provide immunity in about 60 to 70% of people who receive them. Their effects last for perhaps 3 to 6 months.[67] Health professionals strongly recommend annual vaccinations for persons aged 65 and over; those with other diseases or in general poor health; children 6 months and older with respiratory disorders; and health care and other workers who come in close contact with high-risk patients. If you are uncertain whether you should receive a flu shot, check with your primary health care provider (but don't wait until the flu season strikes).

## Meet the Challenges Posed by Emerging Infectious Diseases

The past complacency shown toward the threat posed by infectious diseases has given way to a new state of heightened awareness. As individuals, we can help protect ourselves from these emerging threats by following proper hygiene, practicing safer sex, obtaining immunizations, and keeping our immune systems operating at peak levels through diet, rest, and stress management. At the societal level, vigilance includes monitoring and controlling the spread of infectious diseases, providing the public with appropriate drugs and vaccinations, and disseminating educational materials about disease prevention.

Smart Quiz
Q1506

TABLE 15.4

**Recommended Immunizations and Boosters for Adults***

| Vaccine | Who Should Receive? | How Frequently? |
|---|---|---|
| Tetanus | Everyone | Booster shots every 10 years |
| Hepatitis B | Teenagers and young adults in their 20s<br>Sexually active persons<br>Persons who practice unprotected sex<br>Persons who have another STD<br>Infants of women with the infection<br>Persons needing blood transfusions<br>Persons who share needles<br>Persons who have prolonged, close contact with carriers<br>Health care and laboratory workers<br>Residents of or frequent visitors to Alaska, the Pacific Islands, Africa, Asia, and the Amazon region of South America | Two shots 1 month apart; booster at 6 months |
| Influenza | Persons over 65<br>Persons with chronic ailments and compromised immune systems | Annually |
| Pneumococcal pneumonia | Persons 65 and older<br>Persons with chronic illnesses | One time; repeat as recommended by physician |
| Rubella | Unimmunized men and nonpregnant women | One time only |
| Rabies | Those who have been exposed to the rabies virus; veterinarians and health care workers | Every 2 years |

*This table does not include all of the recommended immunizations for travelers to other countries. Always check with your physician before traveling to another country to determine what vaccinations you may need.

# SUMMING UP

## Questions and Answers

### INFECTIOUS DISEASES

**1. What are infectious diseases?** These are diseases caused by contact with disease-causing organisms, called pathogens, that multiply within the body.

**2. What kinds of infection are there?** Some infections are localized; others are generalized or systemic (found through the body). Some are acute; others are chronic (long-lasting). Infections can also be latent (hidden) or active, causing symptoms.

**3. What is the course of infectious diseases?** We can identify five periods or stages: the incubation period, the prodromal stage, the clinical stage, the decline stage, and the convalescence and recovery stage.

### SOURCES OF INFECTION—THE PATHOGENS

**4. What kinds of organisms cause infections?** These include: bacteria, viruses, fungi, protozoa (one-celled animals), and parasitic worms. Common sources of bacterial infections include staphylococci, streptococci, and chlamydia. Viral infections cause influenza and many STDs, including AIDS. Ringworm is a common fungal infection. A protozoan causes malaria.

### THE BODY'S DEFENSES AGAINST INFECTION

**5. What are the body's defenses against infection?** These include physical and chemical barriers, such as skin, saliva, and tears, and the immune system. The immune system contains billions of white blood cells that attack invading pathogens in various ways, including specialized immune cells that produce antibodies that specifically target particular antigens (literally *anti*body *gen*erators) for destruction.

**6. What kinds of immune responses are there?** In cell-mediated immunity, immune cells such as phagocytes and NK cells directly attack and kill antigens without the aid of antibodies. When antibodies join the attack, the response is called antibody-mediated immunity.

**7. What are lymphocytes?** Lymphocytes are white blood cells produced in the bone marrow and in various organs of the lymphatic system, including the lymph nodes, spleen, and thymus. There are two major types of lymphocytes: *T-lymphocytes* (or T-cells) and *B-lymphocytes* (or B-cells). Helper T-cells help coordinate the attack against antigens. They stimulate production of antibody-secreting B-cells and release *cytokines* that alert other T-cells (killer T-cells) and phagocytes to join the fray.

### IMMUNITY AND IMMUNIZATION

**8. What kinds of immunity are there?** Immunity can be innate (passed from mother to fetus) or acquired, active or passive. Active immunity is the long-lasting sort produced by vaccination. Passive immunity is short-lived and can be transferred from one person to another through injecting antibody-rich blood serum (*antiserum*).

**9. What is vaccination?** Vaccines create active immunity to infectious diseases by administering weakened or dead forms of pathogens that trigger the body's production of specific antibodies against them, but do not produce a full-fledged infection.

**10. What are immune system disorders?** Immune system disorders occur when the immune system overreacts to normally harmless antigens, when it misidentifies the body's own cells as foreign, or when it is unable to protect the body from common pathogens. Allergies, asthma, autoimmune disorders, and immune system deficiencies are examples of immune system disorders.

### COMMON INFECTIOUS DISEASES—SYMPTOMS AND TREATMENT

**11. What are some respiratory tract infections?** These include the common cold, influenza, pneumonia, Legionnaire's disease, and tuberculosis. The common cold is the most common infectious illness. Tuberculosis is a chronic infection caused by the bacterium *Mycobacterium tuberculosis.*

**12. What is Lyme disease?** Lyme disease is caused by the *Borrelia burgdorferi* bacterium, which is spread by deer ticks in wooded areas. Lyme disease ofter produces a characteristic rash and is usually cured by antibiotics if treated promptly. Left untreated, it can produce arthritis and other health problems.

**13. What is "mono"?** Infectious mononucleosis—"mono" or "kissing disease"—is caused by the Epstein-Barr virus. Treatment for "mono" consists of adequate rest and ample fluids.

**14. What are emerging diseases?** These include Ebola, drug-resistant strains of pneumococcal and staphylococcal bacteria, and infections that develop in hospitals. These diseases have become threats because of global travel, changes in ecological conditions, the rise of drug-resistant pathogens, and changes in population composition and lifestyle.

**Answer Key to *HealthCheck*, p. 416**

p. 416

1. *False.* Antibiotics are ineffective against cold (and influenza) viruses. No medication or cold remedy can cure a cold. Taking antibiotics for the common cold or flu not only is ineffective, but may reduce their effectiveness when they needed to combat bacterial infections.
2. *False.* Colds will run their course whether you treat their symptoms or not.
3. *False.* Treat a cold if you wish to relieve some of the unpleasant symptoms, but don't feel you must. Your best weapons against the common cold are drinking plenty of fluids (to counteract the dehydration caused by fever) and resting to allow your body's own defenses to combat the infection.
4. *False.* As a general rule, select a cold remedy that targets the symptoms you want to treat—pain, fever, stuffy or runny nose, cough, etc. Don't automatically reach for the cold remedy that treats the most symptoms. Not only will you be paying more for ingredients you may not need, but some ingredients may have undesirable side effects (for example, most antihistamines induce drowsiness).
5. *False.* Unfortunately, treating or not treating a common cold has no bearing on preventing future recurrences.
6. *False.* Antihistamines, such as *chlorpheniramine* and diphenhydramine, are good for drying up runny noses, while decongestants help clear nasal congestion.
7. *False.* Though some antihistamines do not induce drowsiness (the prescription antihistamine Allegra is one), most do. Always check the product label and follow the directions and safety precautions.
8. *True.* For most nasal sprays or nose drops, three days is the limit. Using them for longer periods can constrict the membranes in the nostrils, making the nose more rather than less stuffy. Check the directions on the product label.
9. *False.* Chicken soup may not cure the common cold, but the warm vapors from the soup may help reduce nasal congestion while the liquid itself may soothe a scratchy throat.
10. *True.* This falls in the "should go without saying" category. People may have differing sensitivities to particular ingredients or health conditions that preclude using certain medications.
11. *True.* The leading over-the-counter pain relievers **(analgesics)**—acetaminophen (Tylenol, Panadol), aspirin (Bayer, Bufferin, Anacin), ibuprofen (Advil and Nuprin), naproxen sodium (Aleve), and ketoprofen (Orudis KT, Actron)—are effective, and about equally so, in relieving fever and headache. Ibuprofen, ketoprofen, and naproxen reduce inflammation and are preferred when pain is accompanied by inflammation, as in muscle sprains, some forms of arthritis pain, and dental pain. Aspirin is also an anti-inflammatory agent, but has side effects such as an increased risk of bleeding.[39]

Talking Glossary
Analgesics
G1525

Aspirin, ibuprofen, naproxen, and possibly ketoprofen may upset the stomach, while acetaminophen does not. Buffered aspirin or enteric-coated aspirin (Ecotrin) that dissolves in the intestines rather than the stomach may prevent or lessen stomach upset. In rare cases, aspirin, in combination with high fever and the flu, can cause Reye's syndrome, a neurologic disease that generally affects children. Over-the-counter analgesics and alcohol should not be mixed.[40]

12. *False.* Cough relievers are usually syrups that contain **expectorants** and **suppressants.** Expectorants (such as ammonium chloride and guaifenesin) are designed for coughs accompanied by phlegm. They loosen phlegm to make it easier to cough up. Suppressants (e.g., dextromethorphan and codeine) work on the brain's cough center to control the coughing reflex. Cough syrups may also contain alcohol, which tends to suppress coughing.
13. *False.* There is no scientific basis to this homespun saying. Should you *treat* a fever? It is possible that fever helps the body fight infection. Unless your fever is very high, it may be wise to allow it to run its course.[41] Check with your physician.

## References and Suggested Readings

### SMART REFERENCES FROM SCIENTIFIC AMERICAN

**Sinha, G. and Powell, C. S. Shaking the Ebola Tree.** "Explorations," *Scientific American* www site, August 26, 1996. **R1501**

**Nemecek, S. Pathology: Beating Bacteria.** *Scientific American,* 276(2) (Feburary 1997), 38. **R1502**

**Nemecek, S. Disease: Mysterious Maladies.** *Scientific American,* 275(3) (September 1996), 24. **R1503**

### SUGGESTED READINGS

**Preston, R.** *The Hot Zone.* New York: Random House, 1994. An engrossing but frightening look at the dangers of emerging infections.

**Garrett, L.** *The Coming Plague, Newly Emerging Diseases in a World Out of Balance.* New York: Farrar Strauss Giroux, 1996. An examination of the risk of emerging diseases and the government's response or lack of response to the threat.

**National Cancer Institute (NCI) and National Institute of Allergy and Infectious Diseases (NIAID).** *The Immune System—How It Works.* NIH Publication No. 94–3229, Revised December 1993. A useful booklet that gives you the fundamentals about the workings of the immune system and how it protects us from disease.

**Mizel, S. B., and Jaret, P.** *In Self Defense: The Human Immune System—The New Frontier in Medicine.* San Diego: Harcourt Brace Jovanovich, 1985.

**Analgesic** A pain reliever such as aspirin, ibuprofen, or acetaminophen.

**Expectorant** A cough remedy ingredient that helps to expel phlegm.

**Suppressant** A cough remedy ingredient that inhibits the coughing reflex.

# AIDS and Other Sexually Transmitted Diseases

## DID YOU KNOW THAT

- More people in the United States are infected with human papilloma virus each year than with the organisms that cause syphilis, genital herpes, and AIDS combined? p.432
- Although a syphilitic sore goes away by itself, the infection still requires treatment? p.437
- The most common bacterial STD often has no symptoms? p.438
- Vaginal yeast infections are actually caused by a fungus? p.440
- Most people who are infected by HIV remain symptom-free and appear healthy for years? p.444
- The use of new drug therapies has fueled hope that AIDS may become a manageable disease, rather than a terminal illness? p.446
- Genital herpes can be transmitted at any time, not only during flare-ups of the disease? p.447
- Pubic lice may be referred to as "crabs," but they are not of the same family of animals? p.449

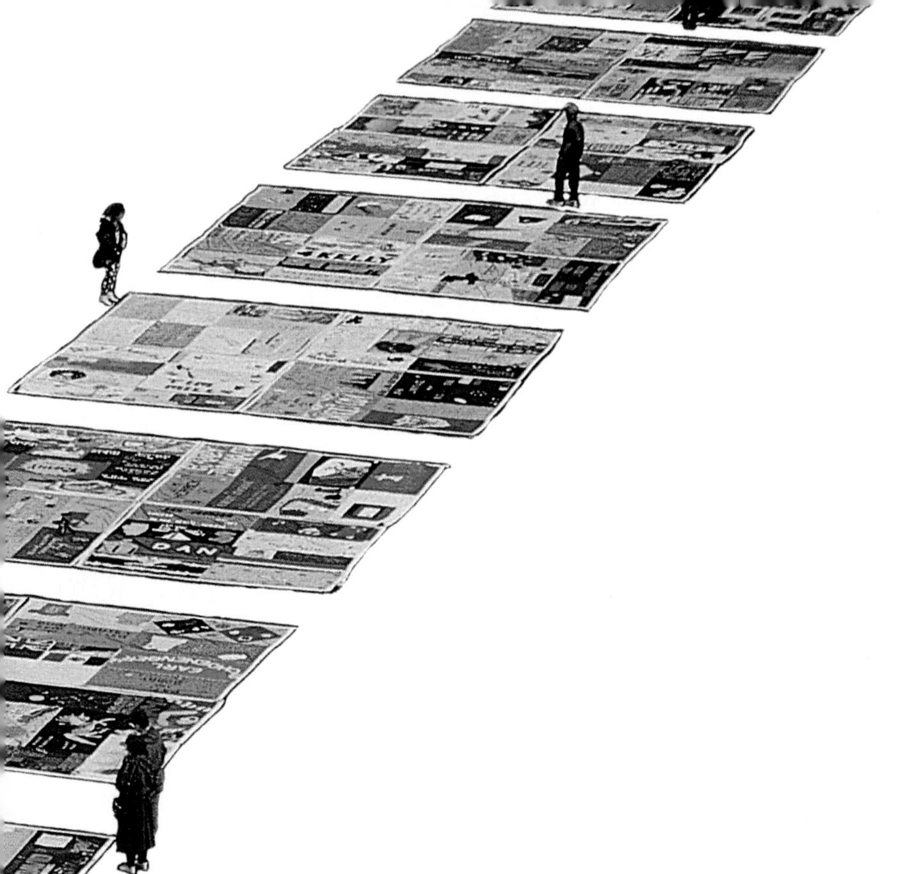

# 16



*Today, for the first time, a generation of young people have become sexually active with the threat of a lethal disease, AIDS, hanging over every sexual encounter. AIDS is a scary thing, a very scary thing. Yet other sexually transmitted diseases (STDs) pose much wider threats. In a study of more than 16,000 students on 19 U.S. college campuses, HIV (the virus that causes AIDS) was found in 30 blood samples, or 0.2% of the students in the sample.*[1] Chlamydia trachomatis *(the bacterium that causes chlamydia) was found in 1 sample in 10, or 10% of the college population.* Human papilloma virus *(HPV) (the organism that causes genital warts) is estimated to be present in one-third of college women and 8% of men aged 15 to 49.*[2]

*The U.S. has the unfortunate distinction of leading the world in the rates of STDs.*[3] *STDs represent an epidemic in the U.S., but it is largely a hidden epidemic since many people with STDs, especially those with chlamydia, have no symptoms and are unaware that they are infected. About one in four Americans is believed to have, or to have had, a sexually transmitted disease.*[4]

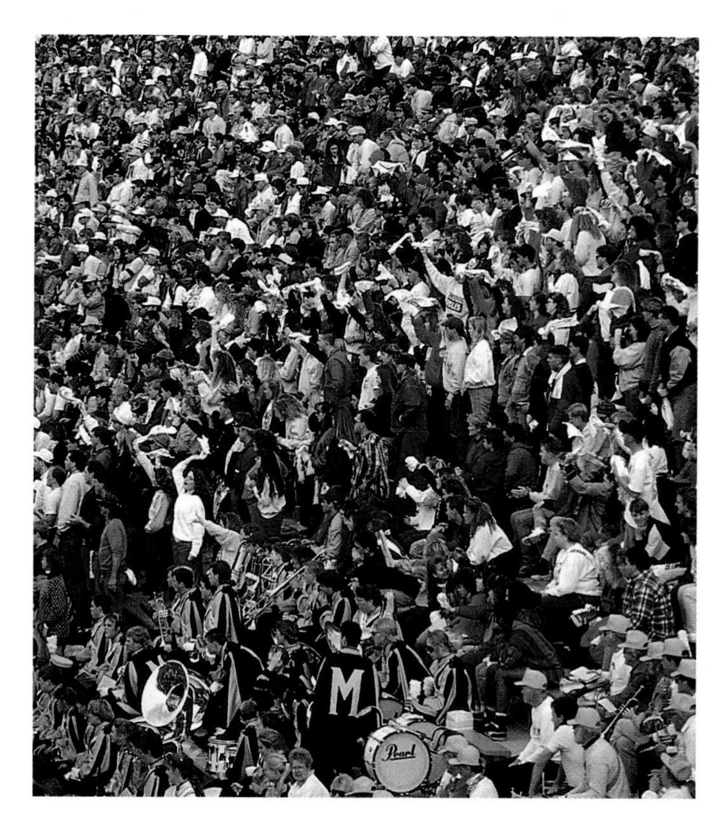

***One in Ten*** One in ten college students in a recent study was found to be infected with chlamydia. Do you know if you are infected? Do you know if your partner is?

College students are reasonably well versed about AIDS, but many don't know that chlamydia can go undetected for years. If left untreated, however, chlamydia can cause pelvic inflammatory disease (PID) and infertility in women. Many, perhaps most, students are unaware of HPV, which is linked to cervical and penile cancer.[5] Yet as many as 1 million new cases of HPV infection occur each year in the United States—more than syphilis, genital herpes, and AIDS combined.

This is not to diminish the threat posed by AIDS. But AIDS is only one of many STDs, albeit the most deadly and frightening. **Sexually transmitted diseases (STDs)** are transmitted mainly through vaginal or anal intercourse or oral sex. They were formerly called *venereal diseases* (VDs)—after Venus, the Roman goddess of love. In this chapter we discuss STDs caused by agents such as bacteria, viruses, protozoa, and parasites. Before proceeding, however, why not complete the nearby ***HealthCheck*** to assess your current knowledge about STDs?

**Sexually transmitted diseases (STDs)** Diseases that are communicated through sexual contact.

**Gonorrhea** Caused by the gonococcus bacterium; characterized by a discharge and burning urination. Can give rise to PID and infertility.

**Pharyngeal gonorrhea** A gonorrheal infection characterized by a sore throat.

**Ophthalmia neonatorum** A gonorrheal infection of the eyes of newborns; contracted by passing through an infected birth canal.

**Close-up**
More on STDs
T1601

## BACTERIAL STDs

Bacteria are one-celled microorganisms that cause many diseases such as pneumonia, tuberculosis, and meningitis—along with the common STDs: gonorrhea, syphilis, and chlamydia.

### Gonorrhea

Nearly a million cases of **gonorrhea**—also known as "the clap" or "the drip"—are reported each year.[6] Many cases go unreported, however. Gonorrhea is caused by the *gonococcus* bacterium (see Table 16.1, pp. 434–437).

**Transmission** Gonococcal bacteria require a warm, moist environment, like that found along the mucous membranes of the urinary tract in both sexes or the cervix in women. Outside the body, they die in about a minute. Gonorrhea is almost always transmitted by unprotected vaginal, oral, or anal sexual activity, or from mother to newborn during delivery.[7]

A person who performs fellatio on an infected man may develop **pharyngeal gonorrhea,** which produces a throat infection. Mouth-to-mouth kissing and cunnilingus are less likely to spread gonorrhea. The eyes provide a good environment for the bacterium. Thus, a person whose hands come into contact with infected genitals and who then inadvertently touches his or her eyes may infect them. A baby can contract gonorrhea of the eyes **(ophthalmia neonatorum)** when passing through the birth canal of an infected mother. This disorder may cause blindness but has become rare because the eyes of newborns are treated routinely with silver nitrate or penicillin ointment, which are toxic to gonococcal bacteria.

A gonorrheal infection may be spread from the penis to the partner's rectum during anal intercourse. A cervical gonorrheal infection can be spread to the rectum if an infected woman and her partner follow vaginal intercourse with anal intercourse. Gonorrhea is less likely to be spread by vaginal than penile discharges.

**Talking Glossary**
Pharyngeal gonorrhea
G1601

**Talking Glossary**
Ophthalmia neonatorum
G1602

# Health*Check*

## *STD Attitude and Belief Scale*

We have devised the following brief quiz to help you evaluate whether your beliefs and attitudes about STDs lead you to take risks that might heighten your risk of contracting an STD. Choose whether the following items are true or false. Then consult the answer key at the end of the chapter.

T F **1.** You can usually tell whether someone is infected with an STD, especially HIV.

T F **2.** Chances are that if you haven't caught an STD by now, you probably have a natural immunity and won't get infected in the future.

T F **3.** A person who is successfully treated for an STD needn't worry about getting it again.

T F **4.** So long as you keep yourself fit and healthy, you needn't worry about STDs.

T F **5.** The best way for sexually active people to protect themselves from STDs is to practice responsible sex.

T F **6.** The only way to catch an STD is to have sex with someone who has one.

T F **7.** Talking about STDs with a partner is so embarrassing that you're best off not raising the subject and hoping that the other person will.

T F **8.** STDs are a problem mainly for people who are promiscuous.

T F **9.** You don't need to worry about contracting an STD so long as you wash yourself thoroughly with soap and hot water immediately after sex.

T F **10.** You don't need to worry about AIDS if no one you know ever came down with it.

T F **11.** When it comes to STDs, it is all in the cards. Either you're lucky or you're not.

T F **12.** The time to worry about STDs is when you come down with one.

T F **13.** As long as you avoid risky sexual practices, like anal intercourse, you're pretty safe from STDs.

T F **14.** The time to talk about safer sex is before any sexual contact occurs.

T F **15.** A person needn't be concerned about an STD if the symptoms clear up on their own in a few weeks.

**Symptoms** Most men experience symptoms within two to five days after infection. Symptoms include a penile discharge that is clear at first. Within a day it turns yellow to yellow-green, thickens, and becomes puslike. The urethra becomes inflamed, and urination is accompanied by a burning sensation. About 30% to 40% of males have swelling and tenderness in the lymph glands of the groin. Inflammation and other symptoms may become chronic if left untreated.

**Close-up**
Fact sheet: Gonorrhea
**T1602**

The initial symptoms of gonorrhea usually abate within a few weeks without treatment. Thus many people think of gonorrhea as being no worse than a bad cold. However, the gonococcus bacterium will usually continue to damage the body even though the early symptoms fade.

In women the primary site of the infection is the cervix, where it causes **cervicitis.** Cervicitis may cause a yellowish to yellow-green puslike discharge that irritates the vulva. If the infection spreads to the urethra, women may also note burning urination. About 80% of women who contract gonorrhea are **asymptomatic** during the early stages of the disease, however. Unfortunately, therefore, many infected women do not seek treatment until more serious symptoms develop. They may also innocently infect another sex partner.

**Talking Glossary**
Cervicitis
**G1603**

When gonorrhea is not treated early, it may spread to the internal reproductive organs. In men, it can lead to **epididymitis,** which can cause fertility problems. Swelling and feelings of tenderness or pain in the scrotum are the principal symptoms of epididymitis. Fever may also be present. Occasionally the kidneys are affected.

**Talking Glossary**
Epididymitis
**G1604**

In women, the bacterium can spread through the cervix to the uterus, Fallopian tubes, ovaries, and other parts of the abdominal cavity, causing **pelvic inflammatory disease (PID).** Symptoms of PID include cramps, abdominal pain and tenderness, cervical tenderness and discharge, irregular menstrual cycles, coital pain, fever, nausea, and vomiting. PID may also be asymptomatic. PID can scar the Fallopian tubes, leading to infertility. PID is treated with antibiotics or surgery to remove infected tissue.

**Close-up**
More on gonorrhea
**T1603**

**Cervicitis** Inflammation of the cervix.

**Asymptomatic** Without symptoms.

**Epididymitis** Inflammation of the epididymis.

**Pelvic inflammatory disease (PID)** Inflammation of the pelvic region that can be caused by organisms such as the gonococcus bacterium; may lead to infertility.

## Major Sexually Transmitted Diseases (STDs)[8]

| STD and Pathogen | Modes of Transmission | Symptoms |
|---|---|---|
| **Bacterial Diseases** | | |
| Gonorrhea ("clap," "drip"): Gonococcus bacterium (*Neisseria gonorrhoeae*) | Transmitted by vaginal, oral, or anal sexual activity, or from mother to newborn during delivery | In men, yellowish, thick penile discharge, burning urination<br>In women, increased vaginal discharge, burning urination, irregular menstrual bleeding (most women show no early symptoms) |
| Syphilis: *Treponema pallidum* | Transmitted by vaginal, oral, or anal sexual activity, or by touching an infectious chancre | In primary stage, a hard, round painless chancre or sore appears at site of infection within 2 to 4 weeks. May progress through secondary, latent, and tertiary stages, if left untreated |
| Chlamydia and nongonococcal urethritis (NGU): *Chlamydia trachomatis* bacterium; NGU in men may also be caused by *Ureaplasma urealycticum* bacterium and other pathogens | Transmitted by vaginal, oral, or anal sexual activity; to the eye by touching one's eyes after touching the genitals of an infected partner, or to newborns passing through the birth canal of an infected mother | In women, frequent and painful urination, lower abdominal pain and inflammation, and vaginal discharge (but most women are symptom-free)<br>In men, symptoms are similar to but milder than those of gonorrhea—burning or painful urination, slight penile discharge (most men are also asymptomatic)<br>Sore throat may indicate infection from oral-genital contact |
| **Vaginitis** | | |
| Bacterial vaginosis: *Gardnerella vaginalis* bacterium and others | Can arise by overgrowth of organisms in vagina, allergic reactions, etc.; also transmitted by sexual contact | In women, thin, foul-smelling vaginal discharge; irritation of genitals and mild pain during urination<br>In men, inflammation of penile foreskin and glans, urethritis, and cystitis<br>May be asymptomatic in both genders |
| Candidiasis (moniliasis, thrush, "yeast infection"): *Candida albicans*—a yeastlike fungus | Can arise by overgrowth of fungus in vagina; may also be transmitted by sexual contact, or by sharing a washcloth with an infected person | In women, vulval itching; white, cheesy, foul-smelling discharge; soreness or swelling of vaginal and vulval tissues<br>In men, itching and burning on urination, or a reddening of the penis |
| Trichomoniasis ("trich"): *Trichomonas vaginalis*—a protozoan (one-celled animal) | Almost always transmitted sexually | In women, foamy, yellowish, odorous vaginal discharge; itching or burning sensation in vulva. Many women are asymptomatic<br>In men, usually asymptomatic, but mild urethritis is possible |
| **Viral Diseases** | | |
| Acquired immunodeficiency syndrome (AIDS): Human immunodeficiency virus (HIV) | HIV is transmitted by sexual contact; by infusion with contaminated blood; from mother to fetus during pregnancy, or through childbirth or breast-feeding | Infected people may initially be asymptomatic or develop mild flulike symptoms which may then disappear for many years prior to the development of AIDS. AIDS is symptomized by fever, weight loss, fatigue, diarrhea, and opportunistic infections such as rare forms of cancer (Kaposi's sarcoma) and pneumonia (*Pneumocystis carinii* pneumonia, or PCP) |
| Oral herpes: Herpes simplex virus—type 1 (HSV-1) | Touching, kissing, sexual contact with sores or blisters; sharing cups, towels, toilet seats | Cold sores or fever blisters on the lips, mouth, or throat; herpes sores on the genitals |
| Genital herpes: Herpes simplex virus—type 2 (HSV-2) | Almost always by means of vaginal, oral, or anal sexual activity; most contagious during active outbreaks of the disease | Painful, reddish bumps around the genitals, thighs, or buttocks; in women, may also be in the vagina or on the cervix. Bumps become blisters or sores that fill with pus and break, shedding viral particles. Other possible symptoms: burning urination, fever, aches and pains, swollen glands; in women, vaginal discharge |
| Viral hepatitis: hepatitis type A, B, C, and D viruses | Sexual contact, especially involving the anus (especially hepatitis A); contact with infected fecal matter; transfusion of contaminated blood (especially hepatitis B and C) | Ranges from being asymptomatic to mild flulike symptoms and more severe symptoms including fever, abdominal pain, vomiting, and "jaundiced" (yellowish) skin and eyes |

TABLE 16.1

| Diagnosis | Treatment |
| --- | --- |
| Clinical inspection, culture of sample discharge | Antibiotics |
| Primary-stage syphilis is diagnosed by clinical examination and by examination of fluid from a chancre in a dark-field test. Secondary-stage syphilis is diagnosed by blood test (the VDRL) | Antibiotics |
| The Abbott Testpack analyzes a cervical smear in women; in men, an extract of fluid from the penis is analyzed | Antibiotics |
| Culture and examination of bacterium | Oral treatment with metronidazole (brand name: Flagyl) |
| Diagnosis usually made on basis of symptoms | Vaginal suppositories, creams, or tablets containing miconazole, clotrimazole, or terconazole; modification of use of other medicines and chemical agents; keeping infected area dry |
| Microscopic examination of a smear of vaginal secretions, or of culture of the sample (latter method preferred) | Metronidazole (Flagyl) |
| Blood, saliva, or urine tests detect HIV antibodies. The Western blot blood test may be used to confirm the results when HIV antibodies are present. The diagnosis of AIDS is usually made on the basis of antibodies, a low count of CD4 cells, and/or presence of indicator diseases | Reverse transcriptase inhibitors such as AZT, ddI, ddC, d4T, and 3TC may delay the progress of HIV infection to AIDS. Protease inhibitors in combination with reverse transcriptase inhibitors have decreased the amount of HIV in the blood to undetectable levels in many cases. |
| Usually clinical inspection | Over-the-counter lip balms, cold-sore medications |
| Clinical inspection of sores; culture and examination of fluid drawn from the base of a genital sore | The antiviral drugs acyclovir (brand name Zovirax) and valacyclovir (brand name Valtrex) may provide relief and prompt healing over but are not a cure; people with herpes often benefit from counseling and group support as well. |
| Examination of blood for hepatitis antibodies; liver biopsy | Treatment usually involves bed rest, intake of fluids, and sometimes antibiotics to ward off bacterial infections that might take hold because of lowered resistance. Alpha interferon is sometimes used in treating hepatitis C. |

*(Continued on next page)*

| STD and Pathogen | Modes of Transmission | Symptoms |
|---|---|---|
| Genital warts (venereal warts): Human papilloma virus (HPV) | Transmission is by sexual and other forms of contact, such as with infected towels or clothing | Appearance of painless warts, often resembling cauliflowers, on the penis, foreskin, scrotum, or internal urethra in men; or on the vulva, labia, wall of the vagina, or cervix in women. May occur around the anus and in the rectum of both genders. |
| **Ectoparasitic Infestations** | | |
| Pediculosis ("crabs"): *Pthirus pubis* (pubic lice) | Transmission is by sexual contact, or by contact with an infested towel, sheet, or toilet seat | Intense itching in pubic area and other hairy regions to which lice can attach. |
| Scabies: *Sarcoptes scabiei* | Transmission is by sexual contact, or by contact with infested clothing or bed linen, towels, and other fabrics | Intense itching; reddish lines on skin where mites have burrowed in; welts and pus-filled blisters in affected areas. |

**Diagnosis and Treatment** Gonorrhea, when diagnosed and treated early, clears up rapidly in over 90% of cases. Diagnosis of gonorrhea involves clinical inspection of the genitals by a physician and the culturing and examination of a sample of genital discharge.

Antibiotics are the standard treatment for gonorrhea. Penicillin was once the favored antibiotic, but the rise of penicillin-resistant strains of gonorrhea has required that alternative antibiotics be used. Since gonorrhea and chlamydia often occur together, persons infected with gonorrhea are usually also treated for chlamydia through the use of another antibiotic. Sex partners of people with gonorrhea should also be examined.

## Syphilis

No society wanted to be associated with the origins of **syphilis.** In Naples they called it "the French disease." In France it was "the Neapolitan disease." Many Italians called it "the Spanish disease," but in Spain they called it "the disease of Española" (modern Haiti).

In 1905 the German scientist Fritz Schaudinn isolated the bacterium that causes syphilis (see Figure 16.1). It is *Treponema pallidum* (*T. pallidum,* for short). The name contains Greek and Latin roots meaning a "faintly colored (pallid) turning thread"—a good description of the corkscrewlike shape of the microscopic organism. Because of the spiral shape, *T. pallidum* is also called a *spirochete,* from Greek roots meaning "spiral" and "hair."

**Syphilis** Caused by the *Treponema pallidum* bacterium; may progress from a chancre to a skin rash to damage to the cardiovascular and central nervous systems.

**Chancre** A sore or ulcer.

**Congenital syphilis** A syphilis infection that is present at birth.

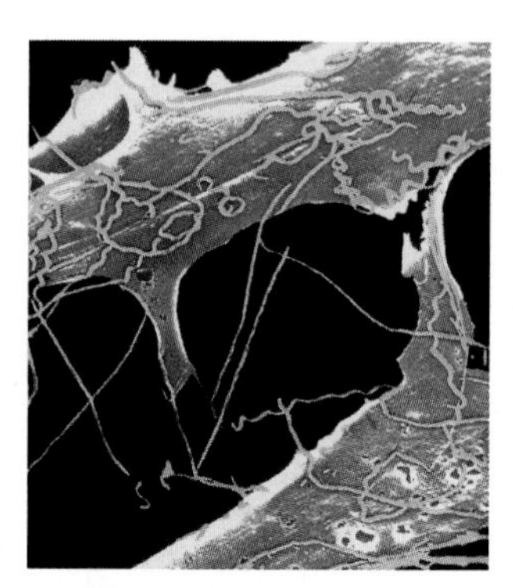

**Figure 16.1** ***Treponema Pallidum*** (shown here in orange) The bacterium that causes syphilis. Because of the spiral shape, *T. pallidum* is called a *spirochete.*

The incidence of syphilis decreased in the United States with the introduction of penicillin and then rose during the 1980s[9] before declining again in the 1990s. The increase in syphilis in the 1980s was linked to increased use of cocaine.[10] Cocaine users risk contracting syphilis not through cocaine use per se but because they often have sex with multiple partners or with prostitutes.

**Transmission** Syphilis, like gonorrhea, is most often transmitted by vaginal or anal intercourse, or oral-genital or oral-anal contact with an infected person. The spirochete is usually transmitted when open lesions on an infected person come into contact with the mucous membranes or skin abrasions of the partner's body during sexual activity. Syphilis may also be contracted by touching an infectious **chancre,** but not from using the same toilet seat as an infected person.

Talking Glossary
Chancre
G1605

A pregnant woman may transmit syphilis to her fetus, because the spirochete can cross the placental membrane. Miscarriage, stillbirth, or **congenital syphilis** may result. Congenital syphilis may impair vision and hearing or deform bones and teeth. Blood tests are administered routinely during pregnancy to diagnose syphilis in the mother

| Diagnosis | Treatment |
|---|---|
| Clinical inspection | Methods include cryotherapy (freezing), podophyllin, burning, surgical removal |
| Clinical examination | Lindane (brand name Kwell)—a prescription shampoo; nonprescription medications containing pyrethrins or piperonal butoxide (brand names RID, Triple X) |
| Clinical inspection | Lindane (Kwell) |

so that congenital problems in the baby may be averted. The fetus will probably not be harmed if an infected mother is treated before the fourth month of pregnancy.

**Symptoms and Course of Illness** Syphilis develops through several stages. In the first or *primary stage,* a painless chancre (a hard, round, ulcerlike lesion with raised edges) appears at the site of infection two to four weeks after contact. When women are infected, the chancre usually forms on the vaginal walls or the cervix. It may also form on the external genitalia, most often on the labia. When men are infected, the chancre usually forms on the penile glans. It may also form on the scrotum or penile shaft. If the mode of transmission is oral sex, the chancre may appear on the lips or tongue. If the infection is spread by anal sex, the chancre may develop on the rectum. The chancre disappears within a few weeks, but if the infection remains untreated, syphilis will continue to work within the body.

**Close-up**
Fact sheet: Syphilis
T1604

The *secondary stage* begins a few weeks to a few months later. A skin rash develops, consisting of painless, reddish, raised bumps that darken after a while and burst, oozing a discharge. Other symptoms include sores in the mouth, painful swelling of joints, a sore throat, headaches, and fever. A person with syphilis may thus wrongly assume that he or she has the flu.

These symptoms also disappear. Syphilis then enters the *latent stage* and may lie dormant for decades. But spirochetes continue to multiply and burrow into the circulatory system, central nervous system (brain and spinal cord), and bones. The person may no longer be contagious to sex partners after several years in the latent stage, but a pregnant woman may still pass the infection to her newborn.

**Close-up**
More on syphilis
T1605

In many cases, the disease eventually progresses to the late or *tertiary stage.* A large ulcer may form on the skin, muscle tissue, digestive organs, lungs, liver, or other organs. This destructive ulcer can often be successfully treated. Still more serious damage can occur as the infection attacks the central nervous system or the cardiovascular system (the heart and the major blood vessels). Either outcome can be fatal. **Neurosyphilis** can cause brain damage, resulting in paralysis or the mental illness called **general paresis.** The primary and secondary symptoms of syphilis disappear. Infected people may thus be tempted to believe that they are no longer at risk and fail to see a doctor. However, failure to eradicate the infection may lead to serious health problems.

**Talking Glossary**
Neurosyphilis, General paresis
G1606

**Diagnosis and Treatment** Primary-stage syphilis is diagnosed by clinical examination. If a chancre is found, fluid drawn from it can be examined under a microscope. The spirochetes are usually quite visible. Blood tests are not definitive until the secondary stage begins. The most frequently used blood test is the **VDRL** (named after the Venereal Disease Research Laboratory of the U.S. Public Health Service). The VDRL tests for the presence of antibodies to *T. pallidum* in the blood.

Penicillin is the treatment of choice for syphilis, although other antibiotics are sometimes used. Sex partners of people with syphilis should also be evaluated by a physician.

**Neurosyphilis** Syphilitic infection of the central nervous system; can cause brain damage and death.

**General paresis** Mental illness caused by neurosyphilis; characterized by gross confusion.

**VDRL** A test for the presence of antibodies to *Treponema pallidum* in the blood.

## Chlamydia

Although you may be more familiar with gonorrhea and syphilis, chlamydia, another bacterial STD, is more common in the United States.[11] Chlamydial infections are caused by the *Chlamydia trachomatis* bacterium. This bacterium can cause several types of infection, including *nongonococcal urethritis (NGU)* in men and women, *epididymitis* (infection of the epididymis) in men, and *cervicitis* (infection of the cervix), *endometritis* (infection of the endometrium), and PID in women.

As many as 4 million chlamydial infections occur annually in the U.S. The incidence of chlamydial infections is especially high among teenagers and college students. Researchers estimate that between 8 and 40% of teenage women become infected.[12]

Close-up
Fact sheet: Chlamydia
T1606

**Transmission** *Chlamydia trachomatis* is usually transmitted through intercourse—vaginal or anal. *C. trachomatis* may also cause an eye infection if a person touches his or her eyes after handling the genitals of an infected partner. Oral sex with an infected partner can infect the throat. Newborns can acquire potentially serious chlamydial eye infections as they pass through the cervix of an infected mother. Even newborns delivered by caesarean section may be infected if the amniotic sac breaks before delivery. Each year more than 100,000 infants are infected with the bacterium during birth.[13] Of these, about 75,000 develop eye infections and about 30,000 develop pneumonia.

**Symptoms** Chlamydial infections may produce symptoms similar to, but milder than, those of gonorrhea. In men, *C. trachomatis* can lead to nongonococcal urethritis (NGU). **Urethritis** is an inflammation of the urethra. NGU refers to forms of urethritis not caused by the gonococcal bacterium, but by other agents, including *C. trachomatis.* (NGU is generally diagnosed only in men. In women, an inflammation of the urethra caused by *C. trachomatis* is called a chlamydial infection or simply chlamydia.) NGU was formerly called nonspecific urethritis or NSU. Many organisms can cause NGU. *C. trachomatis* accounts for about half of the cases among men.

Close-up
More on chlamydia
T1607

NGU in men may give rise to a thin, whitish discharge from the penis and some burning or other pain during urination. These contrast with the yellow-green discharge and more intense pain produced by gonorrhea. There may be soreness in the scrotum and feelings of heaviness in the testes. NGU is about two to three times as prevalent among American men as gonorrhea.[14]

In women, chlamydial infections usually give rise to infections of the urethra or cervix. Women, like men, may experience burning when they urinate, genital irritation, and a mild (vaginal) discharge. Women are also likely to encounter pelvic pain and irregular menstrual cycles. The cervix may look swollen and inflamed. Yet as many as 70% of cases of chlamydia show no symptoms.[15] For this reason, chlamydia has been dubbed the "silent disease." People without symptoms may go untreated and unknowingly pass along their infections to their partners. In women, an untreated chlamydial infection can spread throughout the reproductive system, leading to PID and to scarring of the Fallopian tubes, resulting in infertility. About half of the more than 1 million annual cases of PID are attributed to chlamydia. Women with a history of exposure to *C. trachomatis* also stand twice the normal chance of developing an ectopic (tubal) pregnancy.[16]

Close-up
More on PID
T1608

Untreated chlamydial infections can also damage the internal reproductive organs of men. About 50% of cases of epididymitis are caused by chlamydial infections. Yet only about 1 or 2% of men with untreated NGU caused by *C. trachomatis* go on to develop epididymitis. The long-term effects of untreated chlamydial infections in men remain undetermined.

**Diagnosis and Treatment** The Abbott Testpack permits physicians to verify a diagnosis of chlamydia in women. The test analyzes a cervical smear (like a Pap smear) and identifies 75 to 80% of infected cases. There are relatively few **false positives** (incorrect positive findings). In men, a swab is inserted through the penile opening, and the extracted fluid is analyzed to detect the presence of *C. trachomatis.*

Antibiotics other than penicillin are highly effective in eradicating chlamydial infections. (Penicillin, effective in treating gonorrhea, is ineffective against *C. trachomatis.*) Treatment of all sex partners of infected persons is advised regardless of whether the partners show any symptoms, so as to prevent the infection from spreading or bouncing back and forth.[17]

**Urethritis** Inflammation of the urethra.

**False positive** An erroneous positive test result or clinical finding.

## Other Bacterial STDs

Talking Glossary
Chancroid
G1607

There are several other, less common, bacterial STDs. These include chancroid and shigellosis.

**Chancroid** **Chancroid,** or "soft chancre," is caused by the bacterium *Hemophilus ducreyi.* It is more commonly found in the tropics and Eastern nations than in Western countries. The chancroid sore consists of a cluster of small bumps or pimples on the genitals, perineum (the area of skin that lies between the genitals and the anus), or the anus itself. These lesions usually appear within seven days of infection. Within a few days the lesion ruptures, producing an open sore or ulcer. Several ulcers may merge with other ulcers, forming giant ulcers. There is usually an accompanying swelling of a nearby lymph node. In contrast to the syphilis chancre, the chancroid ulcer has a soft rim (hence the name) and is painful in men. Women frequently do not experience any pain and may be unaware of being infected. The bacterium is typically transmitted through sexual or bodily contact with the lesion or its discharge. Diagnosis is usually confirmed by culturing the bacterium, which is found in pus from the sore, and examining it under a microscope. Antibiotics (erythromycin or ceftriaxone) are usually effective in treating the disease.

**Shigellosis** **Shigellosis** is caused by the *Shigella* bacterium and is characterized by fever and severe abdominal symptoms, including diarrhea and inflammation of the large intestine. It is often contracted by oral contact with infected fecal material, which may occur as the result of oral-anal sex with an infected partner. It can be treated with antibiotics, such as tetracycline or ampicillin.

Close-up
Other important STDs
T1609

Smart Quiz
Q1601

### think about it!

- **Do you think you should be more concerned about chlamydia or AIDS? Why?**
- **What are you doing to be sure that you are free of STDs?**

**critical thinking** **Why is it a problem rather than a benefit that some bacterial infections may be symptom-free?**

**critical thinking** **Agree or disagree and support your answer: Gonorrhea is no worse than a bad cold.**

# VAGINAL INFECTIONS

Talking Glossary
Vaginitis
G1608

**Vaginitis** refers to any vaginal infection or inflammation. Women with vaginitis may experience genital irritation or itching and burning during urination, but the most common symptom is an odorous discharge. Most cases of vaginitis are caused by organisms that reside in the vagina or by sexually transmitted organisms. Organisms that normally reside in the vagina may overgrow and cause symptoms when the environmental balance of the vagina is upset by factors such as birth-control pills, antibiotics, dietary changes, excessive douching, or nylon underwear or pantyhose. Still other cases are caused by sensitivities or allergic reactions to various chemicals.

Close-up
Fact sheet: Vaginitis
T1610
More on vaginitis
T1611

Most vaginal infections involve bacterial vaginosis (BV), candidiasis (commonly called a "yeast" infection), or trichomoniasis ("trich"). Bacterial vaginosis is the most common form of vaginitis, followed by candidiasis, then by trichomoniasis, but some cases involve combinations of the three.[18]

Take Charge
Reducing the risk of vaginitis
C1601

The microbes causing vaginal infections in women can also infect the man's urethral tract. In some cases, a "vaginal infection" can be passed back and forth between sex partners.

## Bacterial Vaginosis

Talking Glossary
Bacterial vaginosis
G1609

**Bacterial vaginosis** (**BV**—formerly called *nonspecific vaginitis*) is most often caused by the bacterium *Gardnerella vaginalis.* The bacterium is primarily transmitted through sexual contact. The most characteristic symptom in women is a thin, foul-smelling vaginal discharge, but infected women are often asymptomatic. Accurate diagnosis requires culturing the bacterium in the laboratory. Besides causing troublesome symptoms of its own, BV may increase the risk of other gynecological problems, including infections of the reproductive tract. Oral treatment with metronidazole (brand name Flagyl) for seven days is recommended and is effective in the great majority of cases. Recurrences are common, however.

**Chancroid** An STD caused by the *Hemophilus ducreyi* bacterium. Also called *soft chancre.*

**Shigellosis** An STD caused by the *Shigella* bacterium.

**Vaginitis** Any type of vaginal infection or inflammation.

**Bacterial vaginosis (BV)** Vaginitis usually caused by the *Gardnerella vaginalis* bacterium.

## Candidiasis

Also known as moniliasis, thrush, or, most commonly, a yeast infection, **candidiasis** is caused by a yeastlike fungus, *Candida albicans.* Candidiasis commonly produces soreness, inflammation, and intense (sometimes maddening!) itching around the vulva accompanied by a white, thick, curdlike vaginal discharge.

Yeast generally produces no symptoms when the vaginal environment is normal. Infections most often arise from changes in the vaginal environment that allow the fungus to overgrow. Factors such as the use of antibiotics or birth-control pills, pregnancy, and diabetes may alter the vaginal balance, allowing the fungus that causes yeast infections to grow to infectious levels. Wearing nylon underwear and tight, restrictive, poorly ventilated clothing may also help induce a yeast infection.

Diet may play a role in recurrent yeast infections. Reducing foods that produce excessive excretion of urinary sugars (such as dairy products, sugar, and artificial sweeteners) apparently reduces the frequency of recurrent yeast infections. In one study, daily ingestion of one pint of yogurt containing active bacterial *(Lactobacillus acidophilus)* cultures helped reduce the rate of recurrent infections.[19]

Candidiasis can be passed back and forth between sex partners through vaginal intercourse. It may also be passed back and forth between the mouth and the genitals through oral-genital contact and infect the anus through anal intercourse. However, most infections in women are believed to be caused by an overgrowth of "yeast" normally found in the vagina, not by sexual transmission. Still, it is advisable to evaluate both partners simultaneously. Most men with *Candida* do not have symptoms. However, some may develop NGU or a genital thrush that is accompanied by sensations of itching and burning during urination or a reddening of the penis. Candidiasis may also be transmitted by nonsexual means, as between women who share a washcloth.

About 75% of women will experience an episode of candidiasis at some point during their reproductive years.[20] About half of them will have recurrent infections. Treatment with vaginal suppositories, creams, or tablets containing miconazole (brand name Monistat), clotrimazole (brand names Lotrimin and Mycelex), or terconazole (brand name Terazol) is usually recommended. Some medications for yeast infections are available over the counter. Even so, women with vaginal complaints are advised to consult their physicians to ensure that they receive proper diagnosis and treatment.

**Candidiasis** Vaginitis caused by a yeastlike fungus, *Candida albicans.*

**Trichomoniasis** Vaginitis caused by the protozoan *Trichomonas vaginalis.*

## Trichomoniasis

**Trichomoniasis** ("trich") is caused by *Trichomonas vaginalis,* a one-cell parasite (technically, a protozoan). Trichomoniasis is the most common parasitic STD, accounting for an estimated 8 million cases a year among women in the United States. Symptoms in women include burning or itching in the vulva, mild pain during urination or coitus, and an odorous, foamy whitish to yellowish-green discharge. Lower abdominal pain is reported by some infected women. Many women notice symptoms appearing or worsening during, or just following, their menstrual periods. Trichomoniasis is also linked to the development of tubal adhesions that can result in infertility.[21] As with many other STDs, about half of infected women do not have symptoms.

Candidiasis most often reflects an overgrowth of organisms normally found in the vagina. However, trichomoniasis is almost always sexually transmitted. Because the parasite may survive for several hours on moist surfaces outside the body, trich can be communicated from contact with infected semen or vaginal discharges on towels, washcloths, and bedclothes. This parasite is one of the few disease agents that can be picked up from a toilet seat, but it would have to directly touch the penis or vulva.

*Trichomonas vaginalis* can cause NGU in the male, which can be asymptomatic or cause a slight penile discharge that is usually noticeable before urinating in the morning. There may be tingling, itching, and other irritating sensations in the urethral tract. Yet most infected men are symptom-free. Therefore, they may unwittingly transfer the organism to their sex partners.

Except during the first three months of pregnancy, trichomoniasis is treated in both sexes with metronidazole (brand name Flagyl). Both partners are treated, whether or not they report symptoms. When both partners are treated simultaneously, the success rate approaches 100%.

Smart Quiz Q1602

## think about it!

- What is the likelihood that you, or someone you care about, will experience a vaginal infection?
- Why is someone with a vaginal infection well advised to see a doctor even though medicine for the infection may be available over the counter?
- How can women help prevent vaginal infections?

## PREVENTION

### *Talking to Your Partner about STDs*

Many people find it hard to talk about STDs with their partners. As one young woman put it:

> *It's one thing to talk about "being responsible about STD" and a much harder thing to do it at the very moment. It's just plain hard to say to someone I am feeling very erotic with, "Oh, yes, before we go any further, can we have a conversation about STD?" It's hard to imagine murmuring into someone's ear at a time of passion, "Would you mind slipping on this condom or using this cream just in case one of us has STD?" Yet it seems awkward to bring it up any sooner if it's not clear between us that we want to make love.*[22]

Because talking about STDs with sex partners can be awkward, many people wing it. They assume that their partners are free of STDs and hope for the best. Some people act as if not talking about AIDS and other STDs will cause them to go away. But the microbes causing AIDS, herpes, chlamydia, genital warts, and other STDs will not simply go away if they are not talked about.

Imagine yourself in this situation: You've gone out with Chris a few times and you're keenly attracted. Chris is attractive, bright, witty, shares some of your attitudes, and, all in all, is a powerful turn-on. Now the evening is winding down. You've been cuddling, and you think you know where things are heading. Something clicks in your mind. You realize that as wonderful as Chris is, you don't know every place Chris has "been." As healthy as Chris looks and acts, you don't know what's swimming around in Chris's bloodstream. Chris may not know either. In a moment of desire, Chris may also (how should we put this delicately?) lie about not being infected or about past sexual experiences.

What do you say now? How do you protect yourself without turning Chris off? Ah, the clumsiness! If you ask about condoms or STDs, it seems a verbal commitment to have sex, and perhaps you're not exactly sure that's what your partner intends. And even if it's clear that's where you're heading, will you seem too straightforward? Will you kill the romance? The spontaneity of the moment? Sure you might—life has its risks. But which is riskier: an awkward moment or being infected with a fatal illness? Let's put it another way: Are you *really* willing to die for sex? Given that few verbal responses are perfect, here are some things you can try:

1. You might say something like this: "I've brought something and I'd like to use it . . . " (referring to a condom).
2. Or you can say, "I know this is a bit clumsy" (you are assertively expressing a feeling and asking permission to pursue a clumsy topic; Chris is likely to respond with "That's OK," or "Don't worry—what is it?") "but the world isn't as safe as it used to be, and I think we should talk about what we're going to do."

The point is that your partner hasn't been living in a cave. Your partner is also aware of the dangers of STDs, especially of AIDS, and ought to be working with you to make things safe and unpressured. If your partner is pressing for unsafe sex and is inconsiderate of your feelings and concerns, you need to reassess whether you want to be with this person. We think you can do better.

## VIRAL STDs

Viruses are tiny particles of DNA coated with protein. They cannot reproduce on their own. When they invade a body cell, however, they can direct the cell's own reproductive machinery to spin off new viral particles that spread to other cells, causing infection. In this section, we discuss three major types of STDs caused by viral agents: HIV/AIDS, herpes, and genital warts. Viral hepatitis can also be spread sexually (see Chapter 15).

### HIV/AIDS

**AIDS** is the acronym for **acquired immunodeficiency syndrome.** AIDS is a fatal disease that is caused by the **human immunodeficiency virus (HIV).** HIV attacks and disables the immune system, the body's natural line of defense. Thus it

**Acquired immunodeficiency syndrome (AIDS)** A condition caused by the human immunodeficiency virus (HIV); characterized by destruction of the immune system.

**Human immunodeficiency virus (HIV)** A sexually transmitted virus that destroys the immune system.

**HealthCheck**
AIDS awareness inventory
**H1601**

strips the body's ability to fend off disease-causing organisms. No one knows where HIV originated, but some investigators suspect that it may be a variant of viruses found in monkeys and chimpanzees.

### Prevalence of HIV Infection and AIDS

Fewer than 100 Americans had died of AIDS in 1981 when the syndrome was first described in the medical journals. By January 1997, more than 580,000 Americans would be diagnosed as having AIDS. More than 360,000 would die from it.[23] AIDS had become the second leading killer of Americans of ages 25 to 44, just behind accidents.

By 1996, an estimated 700,000 people in the U.S. were believed to be infected with HIV.[24] The World Health Organization (WHO) estimated that 20 million people around the world were infected with HIV in 1995. Nearly 4.5 million of them had developed AIDS.[25] WHO estimates that the number of persons infected with HIV may soar to 30 to 40 million by the year 2000.

**Smart Reference**
African AIDS epidemic
**R1601**

In 1981, when AIDS-related problems were first described in medical journals, they were labeled as problems that affected gay men. For many years, at least three out of four cases of AIDS were found among the gay male population. Between July 1995 and June 1996, however, only 41% of the new cases of AIDS were reported to be due to male-male sexual contact.[26] During the same one-year period, another 26% of new cases were infected by sharing contaminated needles when injecting illicit drugs (see Figure 16.2a). Male-female sexual contact is the fastest-growing exposure category. Among women, 40% of the new cases of AIDS reported between July 1995 and June 1996 were attributed to male-female sexual contact (see Figure 16.2b).

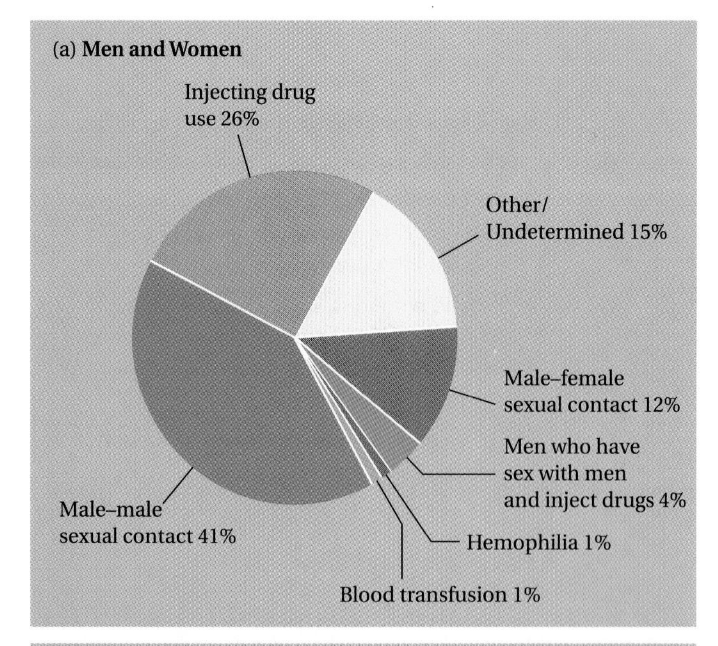


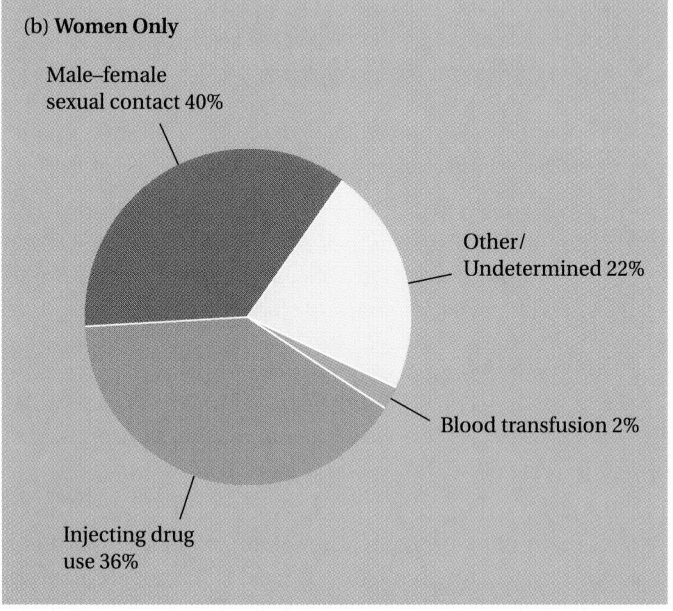


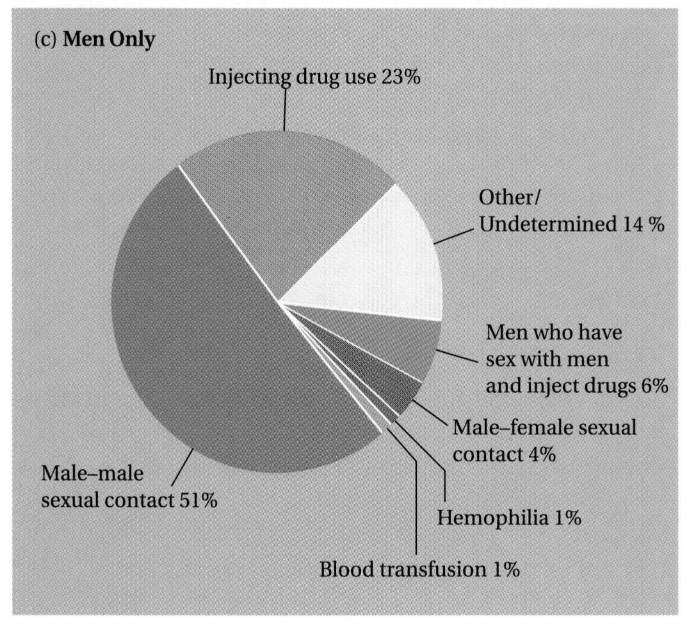


**Figure 16.2** ***AIDS Cases by Exposure Category*** This figure shows the percentage of AIDS by exposure category for cases reported between July 1995 and June 1996. For men and women (a), 12% of cases of AIDS reported between July 1995 and June 1996 were believed to have been transmitted by male-female sexual contact. Among women (b), however, two cases in five (40%) were attributed to male-female sexual contact. By contrast, only 4% of cases of AIDS among men (c) were attributed to male-female sexual contact.

WORLD OF *diversity*

## Ethnicity and AIDS in the United States

AIDS can strike anyone—rich or poor, black or white. However, the AIDS epidemic has taken a disproportionately greater toll on African Americans and Hispanic Americans. Of those diagnosed with AIDS in the U.S., 48% of the men and 76% of the women are African American or Hispanic American.[27] Yet these groups make up only 21% of the population. Figure 16.3 shows the cumulative totals for men and women combined, through June 1996, according to ethnic background. Death rates from AIDS among African Americans and Hispanic Americans (especially Hispanic people of Puerto Rican origin) are more than twice as great as among white Americans.

**Close-up**
AIDS and people of color
**T1612**

Ethnic differences in rates of transmission of HIV/AIDS reflect the drug epidemic in America's impoverished communities. Injectable drug users who share needles with HIV-infected people can become infected and pass the virus to their sex partners. Needle sharing now accounts for about one in four AIDS cases.[28] Injectable drug use and the related problem of prostitution occur disproportionately in poor, largely minority communities. Thus, it is not surprising that HIV infection and AIDS have affected these groups disproportionately.

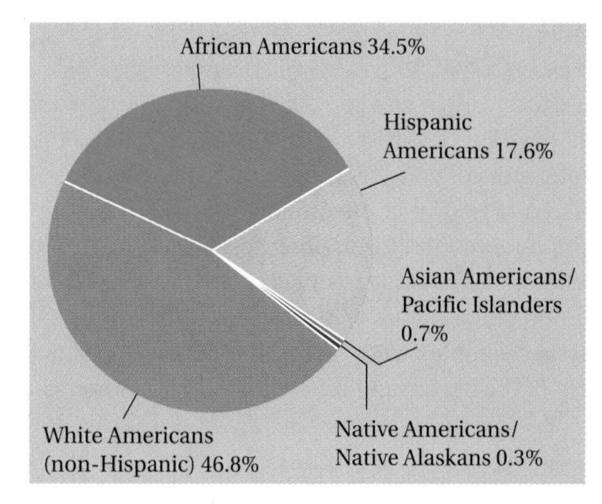


**Figure 16.3** ***AIDS Cases by Race*** The figure reflects cumulative totals for cases of AIDS for men and women combined, through June 1996.

**The Immune System and AIDS** Like other viruses, HIV uses the cells it invades to spin off copies of itself. HIV uses the enzyme *reverse transcriptase* to cause the genes in the cells it attacks to make proteins that the virus needs in order to reproduce.

HIV attacks the body's immune system—the body's natural line of defense against disease. It invades and destroys a type of lymphocyte called the CD4 cell (or helper T-cell).* The CD4 cell is the quarterback of the immune system. CD4 cells recognize invading pathogens and signal B-lymphocytes or B-cells—another kind of white blood cell—to produce antibodies that inactivate pathogens and mark them for annihilation. CD4 cells also signal another class of T-cells, the killer T-cells, to destroy infected cells. By attacking and destroying helper T-cells, HIV disables the very cells that the body relies on to fight off this and other diseases.

*CD4 cells are also known as T4 cells. The terms are synonymous and interchangeable.

The blood normally contains about 1,000 CD4 cells per cubic millimeter. The numbers of CD4 cells may remain at about this level for years following HIV infection. Many people show no symptoms and appear healthy while CD4 cells remain at this level. Then, for reasons that are not clearly understood, the levels of CD4 cells begin to drop off, although symptoms may not appear for a decade or more. As the numbers of CD4 cells decline, symptoms generally increase, and people fall prey to diseases that their weakened immune systems are unable to fight off. People become

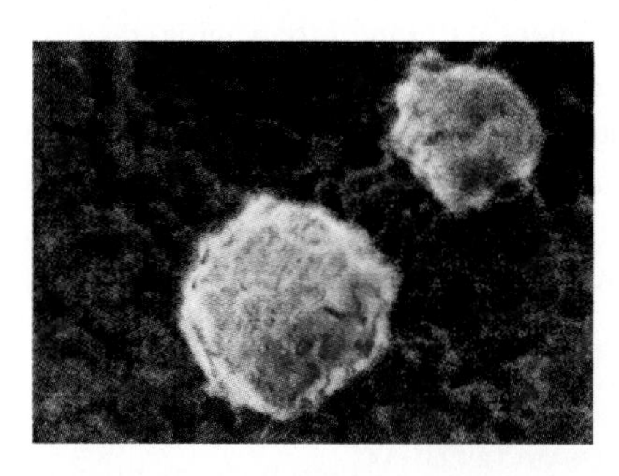

***HIV—Close-Up of a Killer*** Enlargement of two HIV particles on the surface of an immune system cell

most vulnerable to opportunistic infections when the level of CD4 cells falls below 200 per cubic millimeter.

**Progression of HIV Infection and AIDS** Most people who are infected with HIV remain symptom-free for years. Some have symptoms such as chronically swollen lymph nodes and intermittent weight loss, fever, fatigue, and diarrhea. The severity of symptomatic HIV infection depends on various factors, such as the person's general health. This symptomatic state does not constitute full-blown AIDS, but shows that HIV is undermining the integrity of the person's immune system.

The beginnings of full-blown cases of AIDS are often marked by such symptoms as swollen lymph nodes, fatigue, fever, night sweats, diarrhea, and weight loss that cannot be attributed to dieting or exercise. People with AIDS develop opportunistic diseases such as a rare form of pneumonia, *Pneumocystis carinii* pneumonia (PCP); other forms of recurrent pneumonia; Kaposi's sarcoma (an otherwise rare form of cancer); a parasitic infection of the brain; herpes simplex with chronic ulcers; invasive cancer of the cervix; and tuberculosis.

Close-up
More on HIV/AIDS
T1613

**Transmission** HIV can be transmitted by contaminated bodily fluids—blood, semen, vaginal and cervical secretions, or breast milk. The first three of these may enter the body through vaginal, anal, or oral-genital intercourse with an infected partner. Other avenues of infection include sharing a hypodermic needle with an infected person (as do many people who inject illicit drugs), transfusion with contaminated blood, transplants of organs and tissues that have been infected with HIV, artificial insemination with infected semen, or being stuck by a needle used previously on an infected person (a hazard for health care workers). HIV may also be spread by sharing needles used for other purposes, such as injecting steroids, ear piercing, or tattooing.

HIV may enter the body through tiny cuts or sores in the mucosal lining of the vagina, rectum, even the mouth. The cuts or sores may be so tiny that you may not be aware of them. Transmission of HIV from health care providers to patients is rare—extremely rare. As of this date, only two cases have been reported, one involving a dentist, the other involving a surgeon.[29]

HealthCheck
Are you at risk?
H1602

**Hemophiliacs** Persons with a hereditary blood coagulation disorder characterized by excessive bleeding.

What of kissing? There need be no concern about closed-mouth kissing. Moreover, saliva does not transmit HIV. However, deep (open-mouth) kissing may pose a potential threat because blood mixed with saliva may be transmitted from person to person if there is blood in the infected person's mouth (e.g., from gum disease or tooth brushing) and cuts or sores in the partner's mouth. Though the risk of HIV transmission from deep kissing is extremely small it may be prudent to avoid the practice with partners who are not known to be HIV negative.

HIV may also be transmitted from mother to fetus during pregnancy or from mother to child through childbirth or breast-feeding. Transmission is most likely to occur during the birth process.

Male-to-female transmission through vaginal intercourse is about twice as likely as female-to-male transmission,[30] partly because more of the virus is found in the ejaculate than in vaginal secretions. A man's ejaculate may also remain for many days in the vagina, providing greater opportunity for infection to occur. Male-female or male-male anal intercourse is especially risky, particularly to the recipient, since it often tears or abrades rectal tissue. Tears facilitate entry of the virus into the bloodstream.[31] Worldwide, male-female sexual intercourse accounts for most cases of HIV infection. In the United States, male-female transmission of HIV accounted for about 12% of AIDS cases reported between July 1995 and June 1996.[32]

Close-up
Gay men and HIV prevention
T1614

In the early years of the AIDS epidemic, HIV spread rapidly among **hemophiliacs** who had unknowingly been transfused with contaminated blood. In 1985, the test to detect HIV antibodies (revealing the presence of HIV infection) became available, and blood banks began universal screening of donor blood. Health professionals today consider the risk of HIV transmission through transfusion of screened blood to be negligible.[33]

HIV apparently enters cells in the immune system through certain receptors. About 1% of people of Western European descent have inherited a gene from both parents that prevents development of these receptors and are apparently immune to HIV infection. Perhaps 20% of individuals of Western European descent have inherited the gene from only one parent. HIV disease appears to progress more slowly in these people. Some prostitutes in Thailand and Africa, where HIV infection has been running rampant, also appear to be immune to HIV infection.[34]

Close-up
Resistance to HIV
T1615

## PREVENTION

### *How HIV Is* Not *Transmitted*

There is much misinformation about the transmission of HIV. Although knowledge about transmission of HIV is valuable, even life-saving, many people have needless concerns. Let us set aside some of these concerns by considering some of the ways in which HIV is *not* transmitted:

1. *Closed-mouth kissing.*
2. *Donating blood.* AIDS cannot be contracted by donating blood because needles are discarded after a single use.
3. *Casual contact.* There is no evidence of transmission of HIV through hugging someone, shaking hands, bumping into strangers on buses and trains; handling money, doorknobs, or other objects that have been touched by infected people; sharing drinking fountains, public telephones, public toilets, or swimming pools; trying on clothing that has been worn by an infected person; or receiving a massage.
4. *Airborne germs; contact with contaminated food; insect bites.* People do not contract HIV from contact with airborne germs, as by sneezing or coughing, or by contact with contaminated food or eating food prepared by a person infected with HIV, or by insect bites.
5. *Sharing work or home environments.* HIV has not been shown to be transmitted from infected people to family members or others they live with through any form of casual contact, such as hugging or touching, or through sharing bathrooms, food, or eating utensils, so long as there is no exchange of blood or genital secretions. But do *not* share razor blades or toothbrushes with an infected person.

**AIDS Education** How knowledgeable are you about HIV/AIDS? Do you know the risks? What steps are you taking to protect yourself?

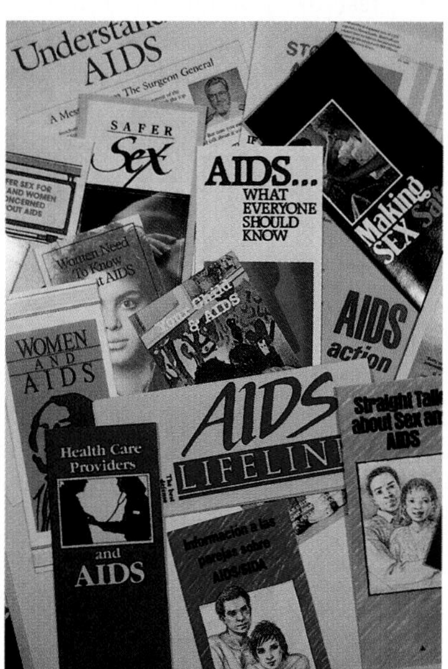


**Diagnosis of HIV Infection** The most widely used test for HIV infection is the enzyme-linked immunosorbent assay (ELISA, for short). ELISA detects HIV antibodies in the blood, saliva, or urine.* Saliva and urine tests are not as accurate as blood tests, but they are less expensive and may encourage people who avoid blood tests to be tested. Positive ELISA results may be confirmed by another test, the Western blot test, which detects a pattern of protein bands that is linked to the virus. Home tests for HIV infection were recently approved for use. They are not only highly reliable but also protect the user's anonymity.[35]

**HealthCheck** HIV testing: Questions to ask yourself **H1603**

**Close-up** Fact sheet: HIV testing **T1616**

FDA approves home test **T1617**

### Treatment of HIV Infection and AIDS

> *We can really say "Get tested, get into care." We have more to offer people, so the concept of getting into care and getting treatment becomes more important.*
>
> Margaret Chesney, Center for AIDS Prevention Studies, University of California–San Francisco[36]

**Take Charge** What to do if you test positive **C1602**

For many years, researchers were frustrated by failure in the effort to develop effective vaccines and treatments for HIV infection and AIDS. There is still no safe, effective vaccine, but recent developments in drug therapy have raised hopes about treatment.

**Close-up** AIDS vaccine research highlights **T1618**

*Zidovudine* (AZT) has been the most widely used HIV/AIDS drug. AZT is one of a number of so-called *reverse transcriptase inhibitors* because they block replication (reproduction) of HIV by inhibiting an enzyme, reverse transcriptase, that HIV needs to replicate. Other drugs of this type include ddI, ddC, d4T, and 3TC. Most studies suggest that AZT can delay the progression of infection from the asymptomatic to the symptomatic state and increase the blood count of CD4 cells.[37]

**Take Charge** Preventing AIDS **C1603**

Although AZT is helpful, the effectiveness of the drug gradually wanes as HIV becomes resistant to it. Combining AZT with similar drugs, such as didanosine (ddI) and zalcitabine (ddC), keeps the pressure on HIV and can delay the progression from HIV infection to AIDS compared with AZT alone.[38] Even more promising is a new generation of drugs that strike at a different phase of the life cycle of HIV, the *protease inhibitors*.[39] These include the drugs saquinavir and ritonavir. A cocktail of antiviral drugs that includes a combination

*HIV itself is not found in measurable quantities in saliva or urine. However, HIV *antibodies* may be.

*Living with AIDS*
Jim Howley, a 35-year old psychologist in Santa Barbara, has been living with HIV since 1983. In 1989 he was diagnosed with AIDS, seven years before this picture was taken. In 1995, Howley began receiving the new combination of drugs, the so-called AIDS cocktail, that has raised hopes that AIDS may become a manageable rather than a terminal condition.

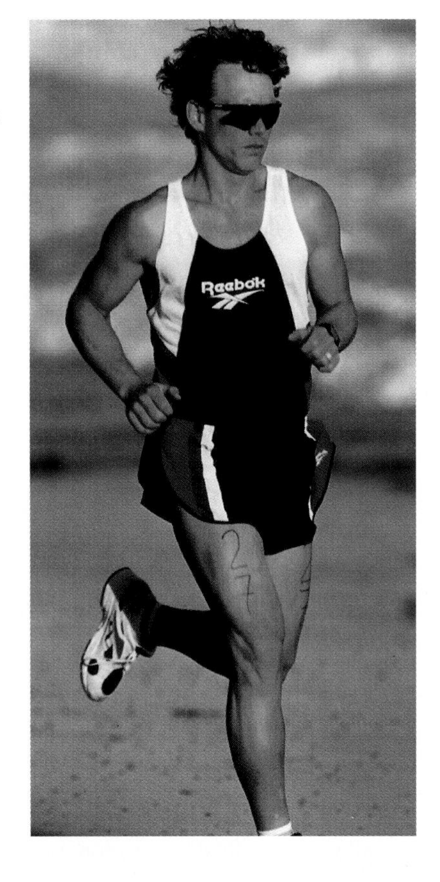


**Smart Reference**
HIV's Achilles' heel
R1602

**Video**
Advances in AIDS treatment
V1601

AIDS and the immune system
V1602

**Take Charge**
Living with AIDS
C1604

of reverse transcriptase inhibitors, such as AZT and 3TC, along with a protease inhibitor, has produced dramatic results in many cases, reducing HIV in the bloodstream to undetectable levels.[40] Scientists caution that even though HIV may not be detected in the blood it may still be lurking in other body tissue. Only time will tell whether the remarkable progress seen in many patients treated with the "AIDS cocktail" will be maintained over time. Perhaps other drugs now on the planning table will be needed to rout HIV if it returns in force.

The advent of these new drug combinations has fueled hope that AIDS may become a manageable disease, as opposed to terminal illness.[41] Some respected scientists have even expressed hopes of a possible cure.[42]

Already we are seeing a significant impact of this new approach to treatment. The number of AIDS deaths nationwide dropped 13% in the first half of 1996, as compared to the same period in 1995, the first drop since the epidemic began in 1981.[43] The Centers for Disease Control and Prevention (CDC) credits the drop to the advent of new drug therapies and increased access to treatment. A doctor in Georgia who treats AIDS patients commented that a few years ago he would see people die from AIDS in a few months. Now, he sees them leaving the hospital and going back to work. Still, AIDS continues to claim more than 44,000 lives annually in the U.S.

**Herpes simplex virus type 1 (HSV-1)**
The virus that causes oral herpes; characterized by cold sores or fever blisters on the lips or mouth.

The new drug therapy also has its limitations. For one thing, it is very expensive, averaging between $10,000 and $15,000 per year.[44] Many people who might benefit from the drug regimen may not receive it because they lack the financial resources or health insurance coverage needed to foot the bill. Moreover, we don't know whether the AIDS cocktails will maintain their effectiveness over time.

**Video**
New AIDS hope, but not for all
V1603

Researchers also find that AZT administered to HIV-infected pregnant women reduces the rate of HIV infection in their newborns by two-thirds.[45] Only 8% of the babies born to the AZT-treated women became infected with HIV, compared with 25% of the babies born to women in the placebo group.

Promising results are also reported in treating the opportunistic infections, such as PCP and fungal infections that take hold in people with weakened immune systems. Although there is more hope than there has been, make no mistake: AIDS is a killer.

## Herpes

There are some 500,000 new cases of genital herpes each year.[46] Once you get herpes, it's yours for life. You can also pass it along to sex partners for the rest of your life. After the initial attack, it remains an unwelcome guest in your body. It causes recurrent outbreaks that often happen at the worst times, such as around final exams. This is not just bad luck. Stress can depress the functioning of the immune system and heighten the likelihood of outbreaks. On the other hand, some people have no recurrences. Still others have mild, brief recurrences that become less frequent over time.

**Close-up**
Fact sheet: Herpes
T1619

Different types of herpes are caused by variants of the *Herpes simplex* virus. The most common type, **Herpes simplex virus type 1 (HSV-1),** causes oral herpes. Oral herpes is denoted by cold sores or fever blisters on the lips or mouth. It can also be transferred to the genitals by the hands or by oral-genital contact. Genital herpes is caused by a related but distinct virus, the **Herpes simplex virus type 2 (HSV-2).** This virus produces painful shallow sores and blisters on the genitals. HSV-2 can also be transferred to the mouth through oral-genital contact. Both types of herpes can be transmitted sexually. It is estimated that more than 100 million people in the United States are infected with oral herpes and perhaps 30 million with genital herpes.[47]

**Transmission** Herpes can be transmitted through oral, anal, or vaginal sex with an infected person. The herpes viruses can also survive for several hours on toilet seats or other objects, where they can be picked up by direct contact. Oral herpes is easily contracted by drinking from the same cup as an infected person, by kissing, even by sharing towels. But genital herpes is generally spread by coitus or by oral or anal sex.

**Close-up** More on genital herpes T1620

Many people do not realize that they are infected. They can thus unknowingly transmit the virus through sexual contact. Though genital herpes is most contagious during flare-ups, it may also be transmitted when an infected partner has no symptoms (genital sores or feelings of burning or itching in the genitals). Any intimate contact with an infected person carries some risk of transmission, even if that person is between flare-ups or hasn't had a flare-up in years.

Herpes may also be spread from one part of the body to another by touching the infected area and then touching another body part. One potentially serious result is a herpes infection of the eye: **ocular herpes.** Washing with soap and water after touching an infected area may reduce the risk of spreading the infection to other parts of the body.

Women with genital herpes are more likely than the general population to have miscarriages. Passage through the birth canal of an infected mother can infect babies with genital herpes, damaging or killing them. Obstetricians thus often perform caesarean sections if the mother has herpes. Herpes also appears to place women at greater risk of genital cancers, such as cervical cancer.

**Symptoms** Genital lesions or sores appear about six to eight days after infection with genital herpes. At first they appear as reddish, painful bumps along the penis or the vulva. They may also appear on the thighs or buttocks, in the vagina, or on the cervix. These bumps turn into groups of small blisters that are filled with fluid containing infectious viral particles. The blisters are attacked by the body's immune system. They fill with pus, burst, and become extremely painful, shallow sores or ulcers that are surrounded by a red ring. People are especially infectious during such outbreaks, as the ulcers shed millions of viral particles. Other symptoms may include headaches and muscle aches, swollen lymph glands, fever, burning urination, and a vaginal discharge. The blisters crust over and heal within one to three weeks. Internal sores in the vagina or on the cervix may take ten days longer than external (labial) sores to heal completely.

Although the symptoms disappear, the virus burrows into nerve cells in the base of the spine, where it may lie dormant for years or a lifetime. The infected person is least contagious during this dormant stage.

Recurrences may be related to factors such as infections (as in a cold), stress, fatigue, depression, exposure to the sun, and hormonal changes, such as those that occur during pregnancy or menstruation. Recurrences tend to be milder than the initial episode and to affect the same part of the body.

**Diagnosis and Treatment** Genital herpes is first diagnosed by clinical inspection of herpes sores or ulcers in the mouth or on the genitals. A sample of fluid may be taken from the base of a genital sore and cultured in the laboratory to detect the growth of the virus.

There is no cure or safe, effective vaccine for herpes. Viruses do not respond to antibiotics. The antiviral drugs acyclovir (brand name Zovirax) and valacyclovir (brand name Valtrex) can reduce the severity, frequency and duration of outbreaks but are not a cure.[48]

**Take Charge** Coping with herpes C1605

## Genital Warts

The human papilloma virus (HPV) causes **genital warts** (formerly termed *venereal warts*). HPV is extremely widespread, possibly infecting as many as 20 to 30% of sexually active people in the United States. The warts may appear on visible areas of the skin. In perhaps the majority of cases, however, they are found in areas that cannot be seen, such as on the cervix in women or in the urethra in men.

**Herpes simplex virus type 2 (HSV-2)** The virus that causes genital herpes.

**Ocular herpes** A herpes infection of the eye.

**Genital warts** Caused by the human papilloma virus; takes the form of warts around the genitals and anus.

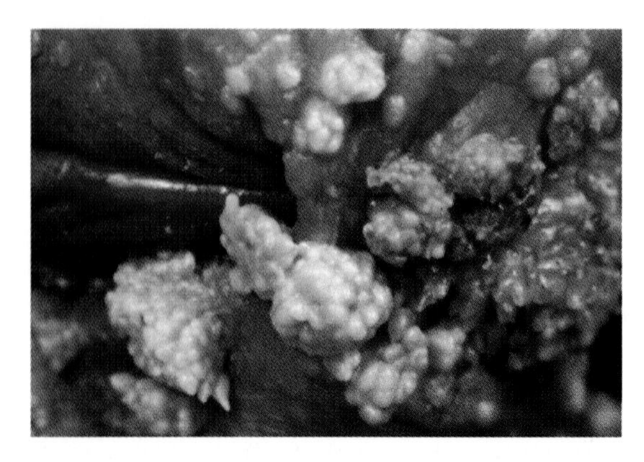

***Genital Warts*** A magnified view of cauliflower-shaped genital warts.

Within a few months after infection, the warts are usually found in the genital and anal regions. Women are more susceptible to HPV infection because cells in the cervix divide swiftly, facilitating the multiplication of HPV. Women who become sexually active before the age of 18 and who have many sex partners are particularly susceptible to infection. A study of University of California at Berkeley women revealed that nearly half—46%—had contracted HPV.[49] Similarly, it is estimated that nearly half of the sexually active teenage women in some U.S. cities are infected with HPV.[50]

**Close-up**
More on HPV
**T1621**

Genital warts are similar to common plantar warts—itchy bumps that vary in size and shape. Genital warts are hard and yellow-gray when they form on dry skin. They take on pink, soft, cauliflower shapes in moist areas such as the lower vagina. In men they appear on the penis, foreskin, and scrotum, and within the urethra. They appear on the vulva, along the vaginal wall, and on the cervix in women. They can occur outside the genital area in either gender—for example, in the mouth, on the lips, eyelids, or nipples, around the anus, or in the rectum.

Genital warts may not cause any symptoms, but those that form on the urethra can cause bleeding or painful discharges. HPV itself is believed to be harmless in most cases, but it has been implicated in cancers of the genital organs, particularly cervical cancer and penile cancer. Cervical cancer is strongly linked to certain strains of HPV (discussed further in Chapter 18).[51] Moreover, women whose husbands visit prostitutes or have many sex partners are many times more likely than other married women to develop cervical cancer, presumably because their husbands bring home HPV contracted from their other partners.

**Close-up**
HPV and cancer
**T1622**

**Ectoparasites** Parasites that live on the outside of the host's body (*endo*parasites live *within* the body).

HPV can be transmitted sexually through skin-to-skin contact during vaginal, anal, or oral sex. It can also be transmitted by other forms of contact, such as touching infected towels or clothing. The incubation period may vary from a few weeks to a couple of years.

Freezing the wart *(cryotherapy)* with liquid nitrogen is the preferred treatment. Although treatment may remove the warts, it does not rid the body of HPV. There may thus be recurrences.

Unfortunately, no vaccine against HPV exists or appears to be in the offing. Latex condoms help reduce the risk of contracting HPV. They do not eliminate the risk entirely because the virus may be transmitted from areas of the skin not protected by condoms, such as the scrotum.[52] People with active warts should probably avoid sexual contact until the warts are removed and the area heals completely.

***think about it!***

- **How does HIV strip the body of its ability to fight off disease-causing organisms?**
- **Would you find it difficult to confess to a partner that you have genital herpes? What might you say?**
- **Why is HPV a major health problem?**

**critical thinking** **Do you believe that you are at risk of being infected with HIV? Why or why not?**

**Smart Quiz**
**Q1603**

## ECTOPARASITIC INFESTATIONS

**Ectoparasites,** as opposed to *endoparasites,* live on the outer surfaces of animals (*ecto* means "outer"). *Trichomonas vaginalis,* which causes trichomoniasis, is an endoparasite (*endo* means "inner"). Ectoparasites are larger than the agents that cause other STDs. In this section we consider two types of STDs caused by ectoparasites: pediculosis and scabies.

**Talking Glossary**
Ectoparasites
**G1610**

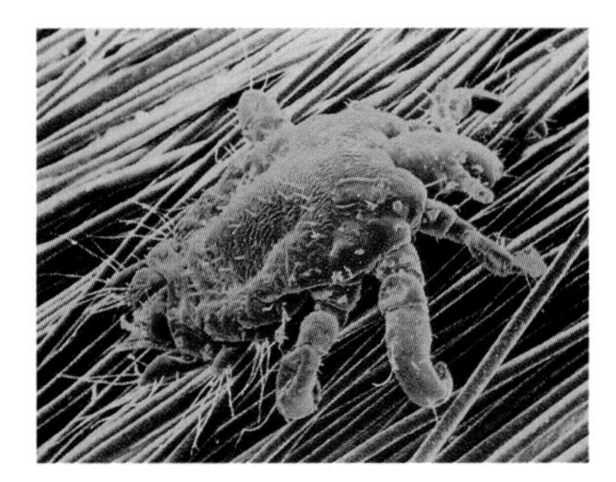

**Figure 16.4** ***Pubic Louse*** Pediculosis is an infestation by such pubic lice *(Pthirus pubis)*. Pubic lice are commonly called "crabs" because of their appearance under a microscope.

## Pediculosis

Talking Glossary
Pediculosis
G1611

**Pediculosis** is caused by *Pthirus pubis* (pubic lice). Pubic lice are insects better known as "crabs" because under the microscope they are similar in appearance to crabs (see Figure 16.4). In the adult stage, pubic lice are large enough to be seen with the naked eye. They are spread sexually but may also be transmitted by contact with an infested towel, sheet, or—yes—toilet seat. They can survive for only about 24 hours without a human host, but they may deposit eggs that can take a week to hatch in bedding or towels. Therefore, all bedding, towels, and clothes that have been used by an infested person should be washed in hot water and dried on the hot cycle or dry-cleaned. Fingers may also transmit the lice from the genitals to other hair-covered parts of the body, including the scalp and armpits. Sexual contact should be avoided until the infestation is eradicated.

Itching, ranging from the mildly irritating to the intolerable, is the most prominent symptom of an infestation. An infestation can be cured with a prescription medication, a 1% solution of lindane (brand name Kwell), which is available as a cream, lotion, or shampoo. Nonprescription medications containing pyrethrins or piperonyl butoxide will also do the job. Kwell is not recommended for use by women who are pregnant or breast-feeding.

## Scabies

Talking Glossary
Scabies
G1612

**Scabies** (short for *Sarcoptes scabiei*) is a parasitic infestation caused by a tiny mite that may be transmitted through sexual contact or contact with infested clothing, bed linen, towels, and other fabrics. The mites attach themselves to the base of pubic hair and burrow into the skin, where they lay eggs and live out their 30-day life span. Like pubic lice, scabies mites are often found in the genital region and cause itching and discomfort. They are also responsible for reddish lines (created by burrowing) and sores, welts, or blisters on the skin. Unlike lice, they are too tiny to be seen by the naked eye.

Scabies, like pubic lice, may be treated effectively with 1% lindane (Kwell). Clothing and bed linen used by the infected person must be washed and dried on the hot cycle or dry-cleaned. As with "crabs," sexual contact should be avoided until the infestation is eliminated.

### think about it!

- **How would you feel if a sex partner informed you that he or she discovered that he or she was infected with "crabs"? Why?**

**critical thinking** **Is there such a thing as "safe sex"? Explain your answer. Then read further.**

**critical thinking** **Why do you think that many people who are knowledgeable about STDs do little or nothing to prevent them? (Are you one of these people?)**

Smart Quiz
Q1604

**Pediculosis** A parasitic infestation by pubic lice (*Pthirus pubis*); causes itching.

**Scabies** A parasitic infestation caused by a tiny mite *(Sarcoptes scabiei)*; causes itching.

# Protecting Yourself and Others from AIDS and Other Sexually Transmitted Diseases

## Take Charge

Make no mistake about it. Although new drugs in the fight against AIDS have brought hope to infected people, AIDS remains a deadly disease. Other STDs are also connected with serious health problems. Protecting yourself and others from these diseases involves taking steps to prevent their transmission and making sure you get appropriate medical treatment if you suspect you have contracted an STD.

### Preventing STDs

What can you do to protect yourself from AIDS and other STDs? Given that many STDs have no vaccine or cure, prevention is our best hope. Most prevention efforts focus on education. Sexually active people have been advised to alter their sexual behavior either by practicing abstinence, by limiting their sexual experiences to a lifelong monogamous relationship, or by practicing "safe sex"—which, as we shall see, could be more accurately dubbed "safer sex."

**Take Charge**
Talking to kids about AIDS
**C1606**

1. *Consider abstinence or monogamy.* The only fully effective strategies to prevent the sexual transmission of STDs are abstinence or maintaining a monogamous sexual relationship with an uninfected partner.
2. *Be aware of the risks involved in sexual behavior.* Don't engage in denial. Many of us try to put the dangers of STDs out of our minds—especially in moments of passion. Refuse to play the dangerous game of pretending that you are immune to the threat of STDs.
3. *Stay sober.* Alcohol and some other drugs increase the likelihood of engaging in risky sexual behavior.
4. *Avoid high-risk sexual behaviors, unless you are absolutely certain that your partner is not infected.* Use latex condoms ("protection") during anal, oral, and vaginal sex. Latex condoms block nearly all sexually transmissible organisms, including HIV. Latex condoms may be even more effective in preventing STDs when used along with spermicides containing the ingredient nonoxynol-9, which kills STD-causing microorganisms including the viruses that cause AIDS and genital herpes.

   Unprotected anal intercourse is one of the riskiest practices. Other high-risk behaviors include unprotected oral-genital activity, oral-anal activity, insertion of a hand or fist into someone's rectum or vagina, or any activity in which you or your partner would come into contact with the other's blood, semen, or vaginal secretions.
5. *Be selective.* Choose partners carefully. Avoid sexual contact with someone who has engaged in high-risk sexual or drug-use practices and is not known to be uninfected with STDs.
6. *Limit your number of sex partners.* The more sexual contacts you have, the greater your risk of exposing yourself to STDs. Also avoid sex with a partner who has had multiple partners.

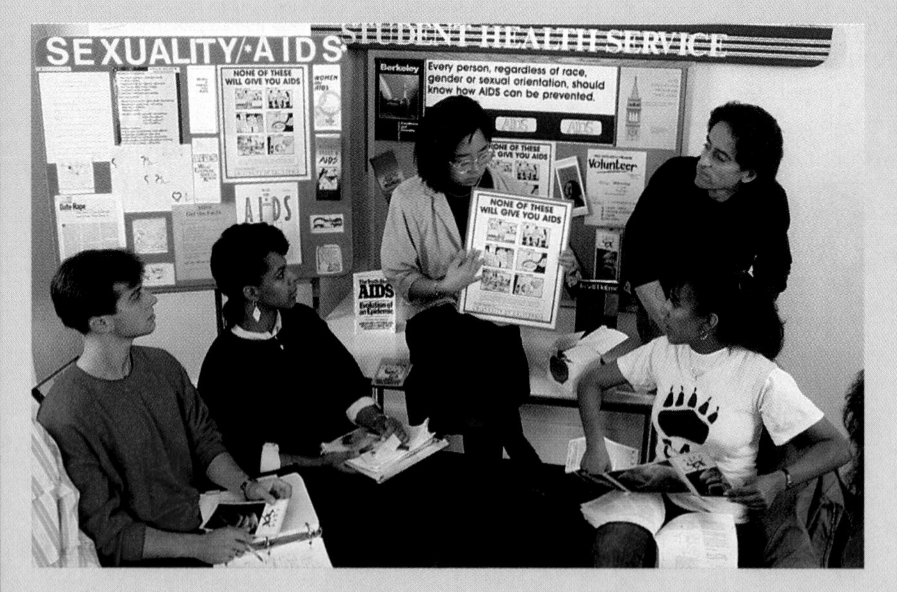
SEXUALITY/AIDS
STUDENT HEALTH SERVICE
Every person, regardless of race, gender or sexual orientation, should know how AIDS can be prevented.
Berkeley
NONE OF THESE WILL GIVE YOU AIDS
AIDS
Volunteer

***AIDS Prevention Class*** AIDS prevention programs are offered on many college campuses, including this one at the Student Health Center of UC Berkeley.

7. *Inspect your sex organs and those of your partner.* Though not all STDs have visible signs (AIDS being a prime example), you should be concerned about the presence of any discharges, bumps, rashes, warts, blisters, chancres, sores, or foul odors. To be safe, it is best for you or your partner to check out any unusual feature with a physician before engaging in sexual activity.
8. *Engage in "outercourse," not "intercourse."* Hugging, massage, caressing, mutual masturbation, and rubbing bodies together without vaginal, anal, or oral contact are low-risk ways of finding sexual pleasure, so long as semen or vaginal fluids do not come into contact with mucous membranes or breaks in the skin. These activities have been termed "outercourse" to distinguish them from sexual intercourse.
9. *Use barrier devices when practicing oral sex (fellatio or cunnilingus).* Use a condom before practicing fellatio and a dental dam (a square piece of latex rubber used by dentists during oral surgery) to cover the vagina before engaging in cunnilingus.

Close-up
Update: Barrier protection
T1623
Condoms and STD prevention
T1624

10. *Wash the sex organs before and after sex.* Washing removes many potentially harmful agents but is not an effective substitute for safer sex.
11. *Have regular medical checkups.* Many people are symptomless carriers of STDs, especially of chlamydial infections. Medical checkups enable them to learn about and treat "silent" diseases.
12. *Consult your physician if you suspect that you have been exposed to an STD.* Early intervention may prevent serious health problems.
13. *Avoid sex when in doubt.* None of the previous practices guarantees protection. Avoid sex when you are in doubt.
14. *Avoid other high-risk behaviors that might put you in contact with someone else's bodily fluids.* Avoid contact with bodily substances (blood, semen, vaginal secretions, fecal matter) from other people. Do not share hypodermic needles, razors, cuticle scissors, or other implements that may contain another person's blood. Be careful when handling wet towels, bed linen, or other material that may contain bodily fluids.

## What to Do If You Suspect You Have Contracted an STD

First, contact your personal physician right away. If you can't afford your own physician, call your local health department to see if there is a low-cost clinic in your community that offers STD treatment. This book may make you better aware of the signs and symptoms of various STDs, but it does not qualify you to diagnose yourself. Second, follow your physician's directions or seek a second medical opinion if you have any questions or doubts about the recommended treatment.

## If You Are Being Treated for an STD . . .

1. *Take all medication as directed.* Do not skip any doses or combine dosages. If you should inadvertently skip a dose, call your physician for instructions. Discuss any side effects with your physician. Although the medication may relieve symptoms in a day or two, it may be necessary to continue to take the medication for a week or more to ensure that the infection is completely eliminated.
2. *Understand how to use medication correctly.* Some medication calls for you to abstain from alcohol or to avoid certain foods, like dairy products. Some medications should only be taken before or after meals. Check with your physician or your pharmacist to determine the correct way to take any medication.
3. *Abstain from sexual contact during an active infection.* Although using a latex condom combined with a spermicidal agent containing nonoxynol-9 may provide some protection against disease transmission, it is best to abstain from sexual activity until the infection clears. Consult your physician regarding the recommended duration of abstinence.
4. *Contact sexual partners who may have infected you or whom you may have infected.* Suggest that they seek a medical evaluation to see if they too are infected. It is possible that they are infected and are unaware of the problem because of a lack of symptoms. Remember that STDs can cause internal damage and be passed along to others even if they do not produce any noticeable symptoms.
5. *Return for follow-up visits if your physician instructs you to do so.* Although the symptoms of the infection may be relieved after a few days, return for any requested follow-up visits to ensure that you are free of the infection. Your physician may also request that your partner be evaluated so that the two of you do not bounce the STD back and forth.
6. *If you have a continuing STD, such as herpes or HIV, share the information with your partner or partners. Don't keep it a secret.* Your sexual partners have a right to know about your infection status before initiating or resuming sexual relations. Make sure that both you and they understand the risks and the necessary precautions that may need to be taken. If you have any doubts about the safety of engaging in sexual relations, consult your physician before engaging in any sexual contact. It may be helpful for both you and your partner to sit down with your physician and discuss the risks you face and the concerns that either of you may have. Unfounded fears and concerns can often be allayed by receiving corrective information.

Smart Quiz
Q1605

# SUMMING UP

## Questions and Answers

### BACTERIAL STDs

**1. What are the major bacterial STDs?** These include gonorrhea, syphilis, and chlamydia. They are caused, respectively, by the *gonococcus* bacterium, *Treponema pallidum,* and the *Chlamydia trachomatis* bacterium.

**2. How are these STDs transmitted?** These STDs are usually transmitted by vaginal, anal, and oral sexual activity.

**3. What are the symptoms of the major bacterial STDs?** Gonorrhea and chlamydia are characterized by burning urination (mainly in males) and vaginal discharges. Syphilis causes a chancre that then disappears, but the later stages of syphilis have symptoms that mimic many kinds of infections. Bacterial STDs can result in infertility. Syphilis can be fatal.

**4. How are bacterial STDs treated?** Bacterial diseases, including STDs, are treated by antibiotics. They should be treated even when they produce no symptoms.

### VAGINAL INFECTIONS

**5. What are the major forms of vaginitis?** These include bacterial vaginosis, candidiasis ("yeast infection"), and trichomoniasis ("trich"). They are caused, respectively, by the *Gardnerella vaginalis* bacterium (and other bacteria), the *Candida albicans* fungus, and a protozoan (one-celled animal) called *Trichomonas vaginalis.*

**6. How do these health problems develop?** Bacterial vaginosis and candidiasis can develop by overgrowth of organisms normally found in the vagina. All three diseases can also be transmitted sexually.

**7. What are the symptoms of vaginitis?** Women with these health problems usually experience irritation or itching. Some women with trichomoniasis have no symptoms.

**8. How is vaginitis treated?** Bacterial vaginosis and trichomoniasis are usually treated with Flagyl. Candidiasis is usually treated with miconazole, clotrimazole, or terconazole.

### VIRAL STDs

**9. What are the major viral STDs?** These include AIDS, herpes, genital warts, and viral hepatitis. They are caused, respectively, by human immunodeficiency virus (HIV), the herpes simplex virus (oral herpes is caused by type 1; genital herpes is caused by type 2), human papilloma virus (HPV), and the hepatitis type A, B, C, and D viruses.

**10. How are these STDs transmitted?** HIV is blood-borne and transmitted by sexual contact, injecting contaminated blood, childbirth, and breast-feeding. Oral and genital herpes are transmitted by sexual contact; oral herpes is also spread by touching or kissing sores or blisters. HPV can be spread sexually or by touching contaminated fabrics.

**11. What are the symptoms of viral STDs?** HIV may have no symptoms or mild flulike symptoms at first. AIDS is symptomized by fever, weight loss, fatigue, and opportunistic diseases, which develop as HIV kills CD4 cells in the immune system. Oral herpes is usually symptomized by cold sores or fever blisters on the lips or mouth. Genital herpes is usually symptomized by painful, reddish bumps around the genitals, thighs, or buttocks. Genital warts are usually painless.

**12. How are viral STDs treated?** HIV infection and AIDS are usually treated by combinations of antiviral drugs. Oral herpes is treated by over-the-counter lip balms and cold-sore medications. Genital herpes is treated with antiviral drugs. Genital warts are removed by a health professional.

### ECTOPARASITIC INFESTATIONS

**13. What are the major ectoparasitic infestations?** These include pediculosis (caused by pubic lice, or "crabs") and scabies (caused by *Sarcoptes scabiei*). These diseases can be transmitted sexually or by contact with infested bedding or other objects. The major symptom is intense itching. Treatment is by lindane (Kwell), although pubic lice can also be treated with nonprescription medications containing pyrethrins or piperonal butoxide (RID, Triple X, etc.).

**Answer Key to *HealthCheck,* p. 433**

1. *False.* While some STDs have telltale signs, such as the appearance of sores or blisters on the genitals or disagreeable genital odors, others do not. Several STDs, such as chlamydia, gonorrhea (especially in women), internal genital warts, and even HIV infection in its early stages, cause few if any obvious signs or symptoms. You often cannot tell whether your partner is infected with an STD. Many attractive and well-groomed people carry STDs, often unknowingly. The only way to know whether a person is infected with HIV is by means of an HIV test.

2. *False.* If you practice unprotected sex and have not contracted an STD to this point, count your blessings. The thing about good luck is that it eventually runs out.

**3.** *False.* Successful treatment does not give immunity against reinfection. You still need to take precautions to avoid reinfection, even if you have had an STD in the past and were successfully treated. If you answered true to this item, you're not alone. About one in five college students polled in a recent survey of more than 5,500 college students across Canada believed that a person who gets an STD cannot get it again.[53]

**4.** *False.* Even people in prime physical condition can be felled by the microbes that cause STDs. Physical fitness is no protection against these microscopic invaders.

**5.** *True.* If you are sexually active, practicing responsible sex is the best protection against contracting an STD.

**6.** *False.* STDs can also be transmitted through nonsexual means, such as by sharing contaminated needles or, in some cases, through contact with disease-causing organisms on towels and bed sheets or even toilet seats.

**7.** *False.* It's understandable that you might feel embarrassed raising the subject with your partner. But don't let embarrassment prevent you from taking steps to protect your own and your partner's welfare.

**8.** *False.* While it stands to reason that people who have numerous sexual partners stand a greater chance of contracting an STD, all it takes is one infected partner to pass along an STD to you, even if he or she is the only partner you've had or even if the two of you only had sex once. STDs are a problem for anyone who is sexually active.

**9.** *False.* While washing the genitals immediately after sex may have some limited protective value, it is no substitute for practicing responsible sex.

**10.** *False.* You can never know whether you might be the first one among your circle of friends and acquaintances to become infected. Moreover, symptoms of HIV infection may not appear for years after initial infection with the virus, so you may have sexual contacts with people who are infected but don't know it and who are capable of passing the virus to you. You in turn might then pass it to others.

**11.** *False.* Nonsense. While luck may play a part in determining whether you have a sexual contact with an infected partner, you can significantly reduce your risk of contracting an STD by following the guidelines discussed in the chapter.

**12.** *False.* The time to start thinking about STDs (thinking helps, but worrying only makes you more anxious than you need be) is now, not after you have contracted an infection. Some STDs, like herpes and AIDS, cannot be cured. The only real protection you have against them is prevention.

**13.** *False.* Any sexual contact between the genitals, or between the genitals and the anus, or between the mouth and genitals, is risky if one of the partners is infected with an STD.

**14.** *True.* Unfortunately, too many couples wait until they have commenced sexual relations to have "a talk." By then it may already be too late to prevent the transmission of an STD. The time to talk is before any intimate sexual contact occurs.

**15.** *False.* Several STDs, notably syphilis, HIV infection, and herpes, may produce initial symptoms that clear up in a few weeks. But while the early symptoms may subside, the infection is still at work within the body and requires medical attention. Also, as noted previously, the infected person is capable of passing the infection to others, regardless of whether noticeable symptoms were ever present.

*Interpreting Your Score.* First add up the number of items you got right. The higher your score, the lower your risk. The lower your score, the greater your risk. A score of perhaps 13 correct or better may indicate that your attitudes toward STDs would probably decrease your risk of contracting them. Yet even one wrong response on this test may increase your risk of contracting an STD. You should also recognize that attitudes have little effect on behavior unless they are carried into action. Knowledge alone won't protect you from STDs.

## References and Suggested Readings

### SMART REFERENCES FROM SCIENTIFIC AMERICAN

**Caldwell, J.C., and Caldwell P. The African AIDS Epidemic.** *Scientific American*, 274(3) (March 1996), 62–68. **R1601**

**Beardsley, T. In Focus: HIV's Achilles' Heel.** *Scientific American*, 275(3) (September 1996), 16. **R1602**

### SUGGESTED READINGS

**Mann, J., Tarantola, D., and Netter, T. (Eds.).** *AIDS in the World: A Global Report.* Cambridge, MA: Harvard University Press, 1993. The global epidemic of AIDS—how it is spreading and what we can expect in the next millennium, according to an influential Harvard University report.

**Langston, D.** *Living with Herpes.* Garden City, NY: Doubleday & Co., 1983. A sensitive, practical guide that will be useful to people coping with herpes and to their sexual partners.

**Holmes, K. K., and others.** *Sexually Transmitted Diseases.* (2nd ed.). New York: McGraw-Hill, 1990. A scholarly, technical resource book on sexually transmitted diseases.

**Nevid, J. S.** *Choices: Sex in the Age of STDs.* (2nd ed.). Boston: Allyn & Bacon, 1998. Information about the features, diagnosis, and treatment of various STDs presented in a concise question-and-answer format, along with ways of protecting yourself from infection.

**Shilts, R.** *And the Band Played On: Politics, People, and the AIDS Epidemic.* New York: Viking Penguin, 1987. A national best-seller. Investigative reporter Randy Shilts, who later died of the disease, provides a compelling account of the chronology of the AIDS epidemic and the lack of governmental response to the AIDS crisis.

# Cardiovascular Health

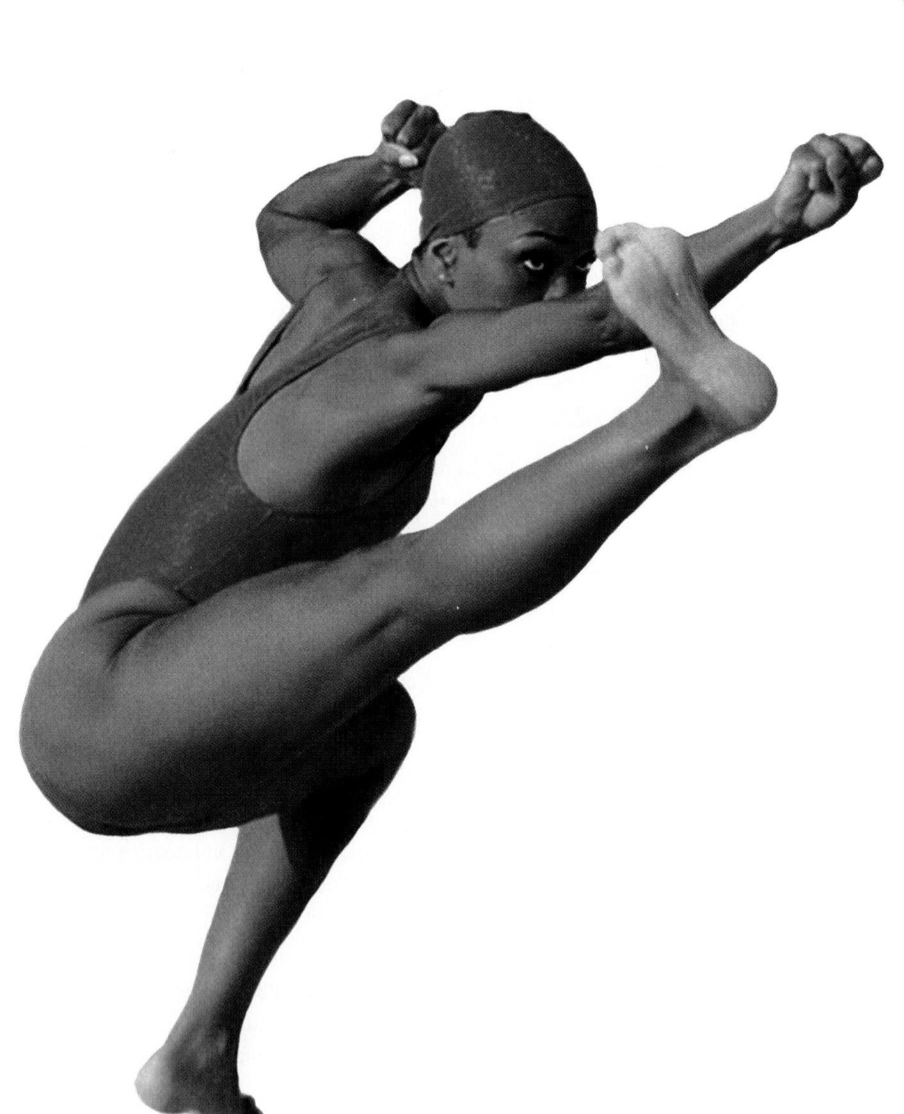

## DID YOU KNOW THAT

- If you laid all the blood vessels in an adult's body in a straight line, it would be nearly 100,000 miles long? p.458
- If we did not have platelets in the blood, we would bleed to death from the slightest wound? p.459
- Heart tissue literally dies in a heart attack? p.460
- You can have a heart attack without experiencing chest pain? p.460
- You can have high blood pressure for years and not know it? p.461
- Surgeons can clear a blocked artery by inflating a balloon inside it? p.469
- Sexual intercourse is safe for most people who have had a heart attack? p.471
- There is a kind of cholesterol that *decreases* the risk of coronary heart disease? p.473
- Chronically angry people may be at greater risk of cardiovascular disease? p.476

*This chapter is about your highway of life—your cardiovascular system. The term* cardiovascular *derives from the roots* cardio *(from the Greek* kardia, *meaning "heart") and* vascular *(from the Latin* vasculum, *meaning "vessel"). Your cardiovascular system is the network that connects your heart and blood vessels. This highway furnishes the cells in your body with oxygen and nutrients and also trucks away their wastes.*

*But there are accidents along this highway. Many of them are in the form of* cardiovascular disease. *Cardiovascular disease (heart and artery disease), or CVD, is the leading killer in the United States. It claims about 1 million lives annually and accounts for more than 40% of deaths, most often as the result of heart attacks or strokes. It leaves millions more disabled or impaired. More people die of cardiovascular disease than from all forms of cancer combined. In this chapter, we will emphasize accident prevention through adopting a heart-smart lifestyle. We will show you how you can substantially reduce your risk of CVD.*

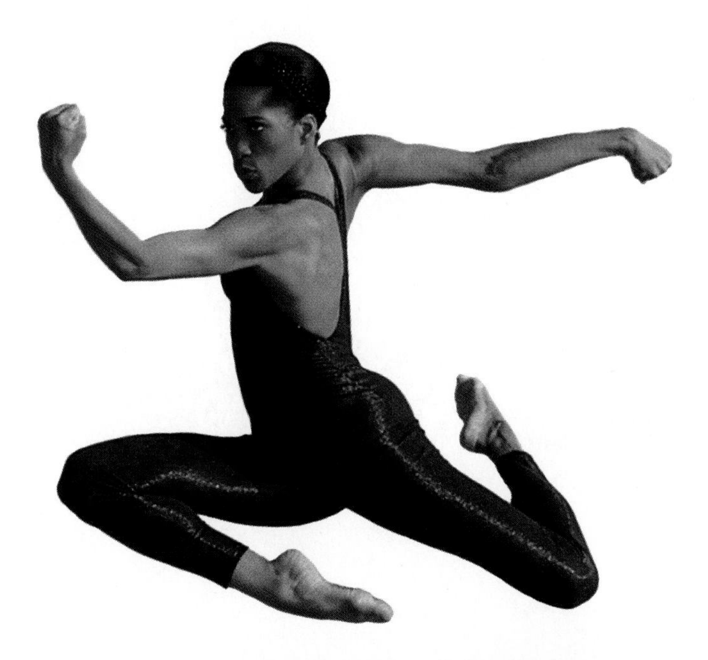

# 17

# THE CARDIOVASCULAR SYSTEM

The cardiovascular system consists of the heart, the circulatory system, and the blood.

## The Heart

The heart is no more than a pump—an efficient, remarkably engineered pump. It is small, only about the size of a clenched fist. It weighs only about 11 ounces. Yet it pumps 5 or more quarts of blood through your circulatory system per minute, or about 2,000 gallons a day.[1]

Your heart starts beating a few weeks after conception. It then continues without pause for the 70 or 80 years in the average lifetime. It beats about once every second while your body is at rest and faster when you exert yourself. Over the course of your life, your heart will beat more than $2\frac{1}{2}$ billion times. Once it stops beating for a few short minutes, life ends.

**Places in the Heart** Despite the popular image of the heart shaped like a valentine, it really looks more like an upside-down pear (see Figure 17.1).[2] It is located between the lungs in the middle of the chest. It lies in a moistened sac called the **pericardial cavity.** This cavity is well protected. It lies behind the breastbone and is surrounded by the rib cage.

Your heart itself consists of three layers of tissue:

- a thin *outer* layer, the **epicardium** (from the Greek root *epi,* meaning "outer");
- a *middle* layer, the **myocardium** (*myo* is Greek for "muscle"), which consists of the heart muscle itself; and
- a thin, smooth *inner* layer, the **endocardium** (from the Greek *endon,* meaning "within").

**Talking Glossary**
Epicardium, Myocardium, Endocardium
G1701

The interior of the heart contains open spaces called chambers. On each side of the heart there is an upper chamber called an **atrium** (plural, *atria*) and a lower chamber called a **ventricle.** The atria receive blood from the veins. The four chambers

**Figure 17.1** ***Places in the Heart*** The heart is composed of four chambers. The upper chambers are called atria and the lower chambers are ventricles. Unoxygenated blood enters the right atrium. It then passes into the right ventricle, from where it is pumped through the pulmonary artery into the lungs. In the lungs, the blood releases carbon dioxide and picks up oxygen. The oxygenated blood then enters the left atrium and from there is pumped into the left ventricle, the heart's most powerful pump, which forces the blood into the aorta. Blood vessels branch off from the aorta, eventually reaching every cell in the body.

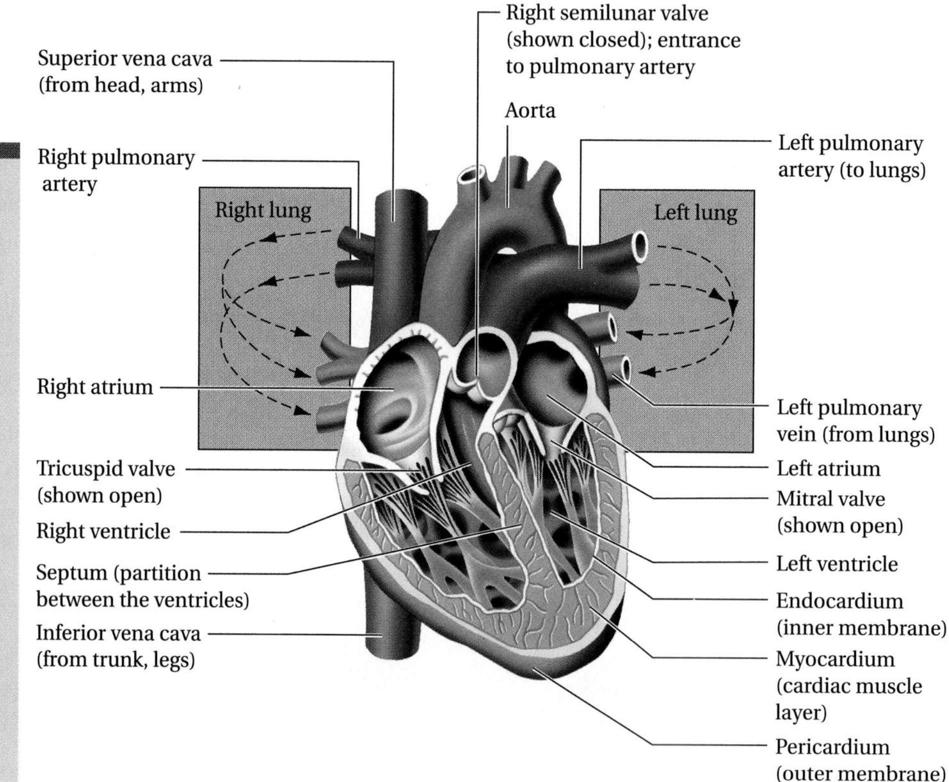


**Pericardial cavity** The moistened sac that contains the heart.

**Epicardium** The outermost layer of the wall of the heart.

**Myocardium** The middle layer of the heart, consisting of the heart muscle.

**Endocardium** The inner layer of the heart.

**Atrium** The upper chamber in each half of the heart.

**Ventricle** The lower chamber in each half of the heart.

**Pulmonary artery** The artery carrying deoxygenated blood from the right ventricle of the heart to the lungs.

**Aorta** The main artery in the body; carries oxygen-rich blood from the left ventricle to smaller blood vessels for delivery throughout the body.

are connected by valves that allow blood to pass through. Under normal circumstances, the valves allow the blood to move in one direction only.

Unoxygenated blood enters the heart from the veins through the right atrium (see Figure 17.1). It moves through valves into the right ventricle. The right ventricle pumps the blood into the **pulmonary artery,** from which it enters the lungs. In the lungs it picks up oxygen for cells and drops off carbon dioxide to be exhaled. The heart's pumping action moves oxygenated blood from the lungs into the left atrium, which gently pumps it through another set of valves into the left ventricle. The left ventricle is the heart's most powerful pump. It forces the blood into the **aorta,** the main artery. The aorta branches into smaller blood vessels that carry oxygen-rich blood throughout the body.

The pumping of the heart is controlled by the nervous system. Electrical impulses direct the chambers of the heart to contract or pump rhythmically in a coordinated fashion. Nerves connected to the heart regulate the speed at which the chambers of the heart pump. This interior guidance system functions automatically. The normal heart rate is about 72 beats per minute in the resting state. At this pace, the heart beats some 100,000 times per day. When you exert yourself, as by walking up stairs, your nervous system directs the heart to beat faster to supply your muscles with the additional oxygen they need. When you relax, the rate of electrical impulses slows down, returning your heart to its resting rhythm.

The nervous system is influenced by hormones such as epinephrine and norepinephrine. Stress due to physical exertion or strong emotions leads to the release of these hormones, stimulating the heart to beat faster. For this reason, epinephrine and norepinephrine are called *stress hormones.* Your heart "pounds" due to stress hormones when you are frightened or angry. Other strong emotions, like love and sexual attraction, can also quicken the heart rate.

## Health*Check*

### *Heart Quiz[3]—Are You Heart Smart?*

How much do you know about your heart and overall cardiovascular health? Find out by answering the questions in this quiz. Answers are in the key at the end of the chapter.

| Yes | No | |
|---|---|---|
| ___ | ___ | 1. Can people under 40 develop heart disease? |
| ___ | ___ | 2. Are there many kinds of heart and blood vessel diseases? |
| ___ | ___ | 3. Do most people who have a heart disease die suddenly? |
| ___ | ___ | 4. If your heart sometimes skips a beat, is this a positive sign of heart disease? |
| ___ | ___ | 5. Do more people die of heart disease than of any other cause? |
| ___ | ___ | 6. Do people know when they have high blood pressure by the way they feel? |
| ___ | ___ | 7. If a baby is born with a defective heart, can anything be done to remedy the defect? |
| ___ | ___ | 8. Is it possible to have a heart murmur without having heart disease? |
| ___ | ___ | 9. Can rheumatic fever be prevented? |
| ___ | ___ | 10. Should employers refuse to hire people who are known to have heart disease? |
| ___ | ___ | 11. Is there a relationship between cigarette smoking and heart disease? |
| ___ | ___ | 12. Are overweight people more likely to have high blood pressure than people of normal weight? |
| ___ | ___ | 13. When a person has a blood clot blocking a portion of his coronary artery (coronary thrombosis), must he be an invalid for the rest of his life? |
| ___ | ___ | 14. Is a pain on the left side of the chest a positive sign of heart disease? |
| ___ | ___ | 15. Does treatment for high blood pressure reduce the chance of having a stroke? |
| ___ | ___ | 16. Do you know what services there are in your community for people with heart disease? |

## The Circulatory System

The **circulatory system,** also called the blood system, consists of the network of blood vessels that bring oxygen and nutrients to the organs and tissues of the body and cart away cellular waste products. The entire blood system is so complex that if you laid all the blood vessels in an adult's body in a straight line, it would be nearly 100,000 miles long!

When blood leaves the heart through the aorta, it begins a journey that takes it from larger to smaller blood vessels. Eventually it reaches every cell in the body. Along the way, cells deposit their waste products into the bloodstream. Some wastes are filtered through the liver and kidneys before being eliminated from the body as urine. Carbon dioxide, a by-product of oxidation, is brought to the lungs and exhaled from the body.

The blood system also performs other critical functions. It carries hormones that help organs carry out their functions. It also transports armies of disease-fighting white blood cells and antibodies that enable the body to defend itself against invading microorganisms and rid itself of diseased, cancerous, and worn-out cells.

**Circulatory system** The network of blood vessels that carries blood throughout the body.

**Arteries** Vessels that carry blood from the heart and that connect to capillaries.

**Capillaries** Tiny vessels that carry blood from the smallest arteries directly to cells.

**Veins** Blood vessels that carry blood back to the heart.

**Vena cavae** The largest veins; carry blood directly into the heart.

**Blood** The circulatory system fluid that carries nutrients and oxygen to cells as well as substances such as hormones and antibodies; also removes waste products and carbon dioxide.

**Blood plasma** The liquid part of the blood.

**Erythrocytes** Red blood cells; carry oxygen to cells.

**Hemoglobin** Iron-containing pigment in red blood cells that gives blood its reddish color; transports oxygen to tissues.

**Leukocytes** White blood cells; combat infection.

**Platelets** Round or oval disks in the blood that help blood clot when there is a wound or injury.

**Coagulation** The process of blood clotting.

**Types of Blood Vessels** There are three types of blood vessels. **Arteries** carry oxygen-rich blood from the heart and branch into increasingly narrower arterial vessels that eventually connect to **capillaries.** Capillaries are the smallest blood vessels and bring blood directly to cells. Capillaries allow oxygen and nutrients absorbed from the intestines to be taken up by the cells from the blood. Carbon dioxide and waste products are deposited by the cells into other capillaries. These capillaries are connected to **veins,** which transport the blood back to the heart, widening as they near the heart.

Talking Glossary
Vena cavae
G1702

The largest veins, the **vena cavae** (literally "hollow veins"), carry the oxygen-poor blood into the right atrium of the heart, whence it begins again its journey (see Figure 17.1). The *superior vena cava* carries blood from the upper body. The *inferior vena cava* carries blood from the lower body. On the way to the heart, the blood passes through the liver and kidneys, where cellular waste products are removed for excretion in the urine.

## Blood

**Blood** is the fluid that travels through the heart and circulatory system (see Figure 17.2). The straw-colored or yellowish liquid part of blood is called **blood plasma.** Suspended in blood plasma are two types of solid blood cells, red and white; platelets, which help the blood clot; nutrients such as glucose; hormones; gases such as oxygen and carbon dioxide; and various other substances such as antibodies.

Talking Glossary
Erythrocytes
G1703
Leukocytes
G1704

Red blood cells, or **erythrocytes,** carry oxygen to cells. Red blood cells contain **hemoglobin,** the red, iron-rich substance that gives blood its reddish color. In the lungs, hemoglobin binds to oxygen, which is transported by the bloodstream to body tissues. In the capillaries, hemoglobin releases oxygen so that it can pass directly into body cells. White blood cells, or **leukocytes,** make up part of the immune system. They protect the body by destroying invading microbes.

**Platelets** are small, colorless bodies that accumulate when the wall of a blood vessel is damaged or punctured. They form clots that plug holes in the walls of the injured blood vessels. The process of clot formation (or **coagulation**) is completed by

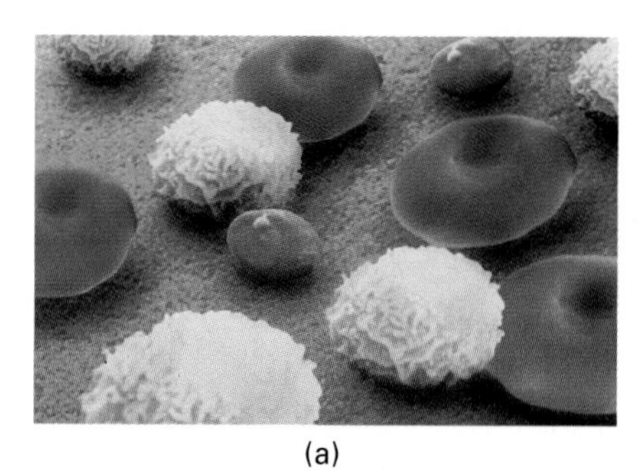
(a)

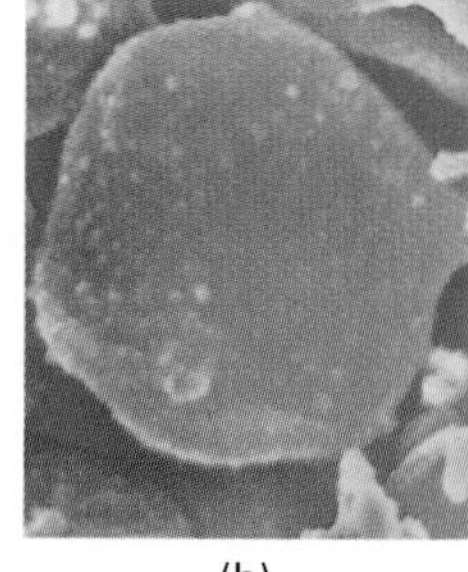
(b)

**Figure 17.2** ***Blood*** (a) Here we see a magnified view of red and white blood cells together. (b) A colorized image of a platelet. Platelets gather together to form clots that plug holes in the walls of injured blood vessels.

specialized proteins called *clotting factors,* which are also carried in the plasma. Without platelets we would bleed to death from the slightest wound.

New blood is continuously manufactured by the body to replace old or defective blood cells and blood lost through injury. However, if loss of blood from an injury is severe, a transfusion may be necessary. Most blood cells are manufactured in the bone marrow, the soft material that fills the inner cavities of bones. Some white blood cells called lymphocytes are produced in lymph glands and other organs in the lymphatic system (see Chapter 15).

Smart Quiz
Q1701

## think about it!

- **What are the parts of the heart?**
- **What is the difference between arteries and veins?**
- **What is blood made up of? What is the difference between *blood* and *blood plasma?***

**critical thinking** **Your heart has been beating and serving you for many years. Do you think it is important to know how your heart works? Why or why not?**

# MAJOR FORMS OF CARDIOVASCULAR DISEASE

The major forms of **cardiovascular disease (CVD)** include coronary heart disease (CHD), hypertension, rheumatic fever, congenital heart disease, arrhythmias, and stroke.

## Coronary Heart Disease

HealthCheck
Check your healthy heart IQ
H1701

The heart is made of muscle tissue, which like other body tissue requires oxygen and nutrients carried by the blood. The harder the heart works, the more oxygen it needs. In **coronary heart disease (CHD;** also called *coronary artery disease*), the flow of blood to the heart is insufficient to meet its needs. The word "coronary" derives from the Latin *corona* (meaning "crown") and suggests the way in which the arteries encircle the heart like a crown. CHD usually results from **arteriosclerosis** or "hardening of the arteries," a condition that makes artery walls thicker, harder, and less elastic.

Talking Glossary
Arterio-sclerosis
G1705

**Atherosclerosis** The major form of arteriosclerosis is **atherosclerosis.** In atherosclerosis, fatty deposits called **plaque** build up along the inner walls of arteries (see Figure 17.3). Atherosclerosis narrows the arterial passageways through which blood flows, which can impair circulation. The word "atherosclerosis" is derived from the Greek *athero* (meaning "paste") and *sclerosis* (meaning "hardness"), which is an apt description of the "hardening" of this artery-clogging "paste" (plaque).

Talking Glossary
Athero-sclerosis
G1706

In CHD, plaque builds up in the *coronary arteries,* the small blood vessels that provide oxygen and nutrients to the heart. The arteries no longer are able to supply the heart with enough blood, especially during physical exertion, which can lead to chest pain, or angina. Blood clots are more

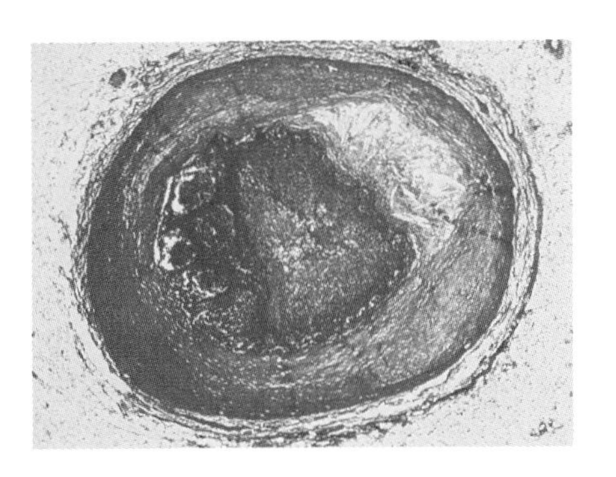

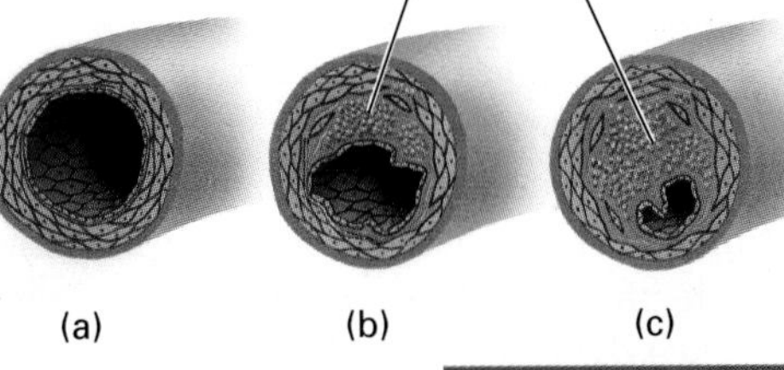


**Figure 17.3** ***Atherosclerosis*** Atherosclerosis, the major form of arteriosclerosis, refers to the formation of fatty deposits or plaque along artery walls. As a result, arteries become narrower, which can impair circulation and increase the risk of a blood clot becoming lodged in an affected artery. If the blood clot chokes off the blood flow, a heart attack or stroke can result.

**Cardiovascular disease (CVD)** A disease of the heart or blood vessels.

**Coronary heart disease (CHD)** A disease usually caused by damage to coronary arteries; the heart's blood supply becomes insufficient.

**Arteriosclerosis** ("hardening of the arteries") A condition in which the walls of arteries become thicker and harder and lose elasticity.

**Atherosclerosis** A form of arteriosclerosis characterized by the thickening of artery walls and narrowing of the arterial passageways due to the buildup of fatty deposits or plaque.

**Plaque** Fatty deposits that accumulate along the inner walls of arteries.

**Talking Glossary**
Angina, Thrombus
G1707

likely to become lodged in arteries narrowed by atherosclerosis. If a blood clot **(thrombus)** should form in a coronary artery narrowed by atherosclerosis, it may nearly or completely block the flow of blood to a part of the heart, resulting in a **heart attack.** If the blood vessel services the brain, the result can be a **stroke.**

The medical term for heart attack is **myocardial infarction,** or **MI.** The word "myocardial" derives from the Greek roots *myo* ("muscle") and *kardia* ("heart"). An **infarct** is an area of dead or dying tissue. A myocardial infarction involves the death of heart tissue arising from an insufficiency of blood supply (called **ischemia**). Within minutes of a disruption of its blood supply, the heart tissue served by the blocked artery dies. As the area of the infarct expands, the heart may no longer be able to pump enough blood to sustain life. Brain death can occur within minutes if the heart fails to pump enough blood. Though CHD typically develops slowly over a period of years, the first sign may be a heart attack.

**Talking Glossary**
Ischemia
G1708

Atherosclerosis is involved in most heart attacks. However, blood vessels not clogged by atherosclerosis may sometimes go into spasm, which if severe enough can choke off the supply of blood to the heart and also result in a heart attack. Whether one survives a heart attack depends on the extent of damage to heart tissue and to the electrical system that controls the heart rhythm.

**Close-up**
Facts about CHD
T1701

CHD, which affects about 22 million Americans, about 9% of the population, is the leading cause of death in the United States. It kills more than 700,000 Americans annually, most often as the result of heart attacks.[4] More than 4,000 Americans suffer a heart attack each day. The good news is that death rates from heart disease have declined steadily during the past 50 years, in part because fewer people are smoking (smoking is a major risk factor) and because of improvements in the treatment of heart patients.[5]

**Thrombus** A blood clot that blocks a blood vessel or cavity of the heart.

**Heart attack** The common term for a *myocardial infarction.*

**Stroke** Blockage of blood to a part of the brain or bleeding in the brain.

**Myocardial infarction (MI)** A condition involving damage or death of heart tissue due to an insufficient blood flow to the heart; usually the result of a blockage in one or more coronary arteries.

**Infarct** An area of dead or dying tissue as the result of an insufficient blood supply to the tissue.

**Ischemia** An insufficiency of blood supply to a part of the body.

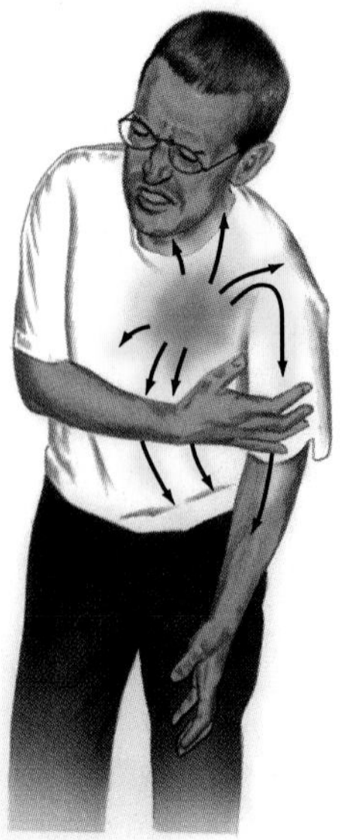

**Figure 17.4** ***Signs of a Heart Attack*** Signs of a heart attack include pain in various parts of the body, not just the chest, as well as shortness of breath; fainting or weakness; heavy perspiration, nausea, or vomiting; and intense anxiety and fear. Anyone experiencing these signs should seek immediate medical attention.

**Signs of a Heart Attack** Heart attacks are medical emergencies that require immediate attention. The first minutes and hours are critical to survival, as most people who die of heart attacks succumb within two hours. Yet about half of the people who suffer a heart attack wait two hours or more before getting help. Many heart attack victims minimize their symptoms or attribute them to more benign causes, like indigestion or heartburn. Becoming aware of the signs of a heart attack can save lives, perhaps even yours (Figure 17.4). Though not all of the following symptoms need be present, the signs of a heart attack include:

- Intense, prolonged chest pain, described as crushing, not sharp, which may be experienced as a feeling of heavy pressure or tightness in the chest. Some describe a squeezing sensation in the chest, or a sensation like a giant fist enclosing the heart. Yet some people have heart attacks without experiencing any chest pain.
- Pain extending beyond the chest to the left shoulder and arm, the back, even into the jaws and gums.
- Prolonged pain in the upper abdomen.
- Shortness of breath.
- Fainting or weakness.
- Heavy perspiration, nausea, or vomiting.
- Anxiety and fear.

**What to Do in Case of a Heart Attack** If you experience the signs of a heart attack or are with someone who does, seek medical attention immediately. Call 911 or your local emergency operator and follow their instructions. If the person stops breathing, administer CPR if you have been trained in the procedure. If not, an emergency technician may be able to guide you in CPR over the phone until help arrives.

## Angina Pectoris

Although the first signs of CHD may be a sudden heart attack, many heart attacks are preceded by a series of attacks of chest pain called **angina.** Angina is similar to, but less severe and prolonged than, the pain of a heart attack. Angina is experienced below the breastbone and may extend to the left jaw and shoulder and down the left arm. It may feel like an ache or pressure. There may also be feelings of heaviness or tightness in the chest, or a burning sensation. Sometimes the pain is mistaken for heartburn or indigestion. The technical term for angina is *angina pectoris* (from the Latin *angere,* meaning "choke," and *pectoralis,* meaning "chest").

**Close-up**
Facts about angina
T1702

Angina is a symptom, not a disease. It is caused by insufficient blood reaching the heart, the same process that can result in a heart attack. In angina, however, the restriction of blood is not as complete or prolonged as in a heart attack. Sometimes the obstruction of blood flow is caused by a spasm in an artery serving the heart, but most cases are caused by a buildup of plaque, the same process that leads to heart attacks.

Angina attacks usually occur during periods of exertion, as during exercise, when more oxygenated blood is needed by the heart. Yet they may occur at other times, during sleep, strong emotion, or exposure to extreme cold. Angina attacks typically last a few minutes and are generally relieved by rest. (If you should experience chest pain during exercise or when walking up the stairs, stop the activity immediately and call your doctor.) Angina attacks may also be relieved by the drug nitroglycerine, which dilates (opens) coronary arteries, allowing blood to flow more freely to the heart. It is usually taken in tablet form and dissolves under the tongue. Nitroglycerine is also available in a skin patch.

Angina attacks usually subside in a few minutes without lasting damage to the heart. Many people with angina never experience a heart attack, but many heart attacks are preceded by angina. Thus, angina should be treated seriously.

## Hypertension

**Hypertension,** or high blood pressure, can lead to heart attacks, congestive heart failure, kidney damage, stroke, even blindness. Blood pressure (BP) is the force or pressure applied by the blood against the walls of a blood vessel.

Blood pressure is defined by two numbers. The numerator or upper number is the *systolic* blood pressure. It is a measure of the blood pressure when the heart contracts. The denominator or bottom number represents the *diastolic* blood pressure. It shows the blood pressure when the heart relaxes between beats. A blood pressure level of 120/80 ("120 over 80") mm Hg (millimeters of mercury) is considered normal. A systolic BP that is consistently equal to or greater than 140 mm Hg and/or a diastolic BP consistently equal to or greater than 90 mm Hg indicates the presence of hypertension. More than 50 million people in the United States have high blood pressure. Some cases can be traced to an identifiable physical problem or defect, such as kidney malfunction. In *essential hypertension,* which accounts for about 90% of cases, the cause remains unknown.

Hypertension accelerates atherosclerosis, increasing the risk of heart attacks and strokes. It also forces the heart to work harder since blood does not flow as freely through stiffened arteries. This added stress can eventually weaken the heart.

**Take Charge**
What you need to know if you have high BP
C1701

The dangers of hypertension are often overlooked, because high blood pressure doesn't usually cause any symptoms until problems appear. Moreover, deaths resulting from high blood pressure are mainly credited to other causes, such as heart attacks and strokes. Yet hypertension is a killer disease and should be treated as such. Hypertension can damage the heart and blood vessels for years but have no noticeable symptoms. Therefore, it is important to routinely monitor your blood pressure.

## Congestive Heart Failure

In **congestive heart failure,** damage to the heart prevents it from pumping out all the blood it receives from the veins. Blood thus backs up or pools (congests) in the veins and elsewhere, such as the

**Angina** Heart pain arising from insufficient blood flow to the heart.

**Hypertension** High blood pressure; generally, a blood pressure reading of 140 (systolic)/90 (diastolic) or higher.

**Congestive heart failure** A condition in which the heart is unable to pump out as much blood as it receives, leading to a backing up or pooling of blood in the veins, lungs, and extremities.

WORLD OF *diversity*

## Combating High Blood Pressure among African Americans[6]

More than 40% of African-American adults have high blood pressure, compared with 20% of adults in the general population (see Figure 17.5). Why do African Americans face a greater risk?

Several factors may be involved. African Americans have higher rates of obesity and diabetes than the general population, and both of these factors are linked to an increased risk of high blood pressure. Possible genetic differences in sodium (salt) sensitivities may be involved. African Americans are also more likely to have high blood pressure than groups that have common ancestry, such as black Africans, suggesting that factors *other* than a common genetic ancestry are involved. Dietary patterns and life experiences of African Americans, especially the stresses of racial discrimination and economic hardship, high-fat diets, and high levels of smoking (among men) may mix in with genetic vulnerability to increase the risk of hypertension and other cardiovascular problems.[7] Inadequate access to health care is yet another factor. Fewer than half of African-American men with hypertension receive treatment. Lack of regular exercise may be yet another factor.

Several researchers have examined differences in physical activity between African Americans and white Americans. One of these, Barbee C. Myers of Arizona State University, found that white women were two to three times as physically active as African-American women during their leisure time. Myers and other researchers believe that the reasons for these differences involve socioeconomic status rather than race. Economic disadvantage falls disproportionately on African Americans and other minorities in our society. Affluent people tend to exercise more than poor people, perhaps because they have more free time, can better afford exercise classes or equipment, and have more access to gyms, swimming pools, and tennis courts. They may also be better informed about the need for exercise.

Exercise is an important component of an overall program to reduce high blood pressure and other risk factors for cardiovascular disease. Outreach programs that stress exercise are beginning to emerge in African-American communities. These programs typically promote vigorous walking and other forms of mild aerobic exercise and offer dietary advice.

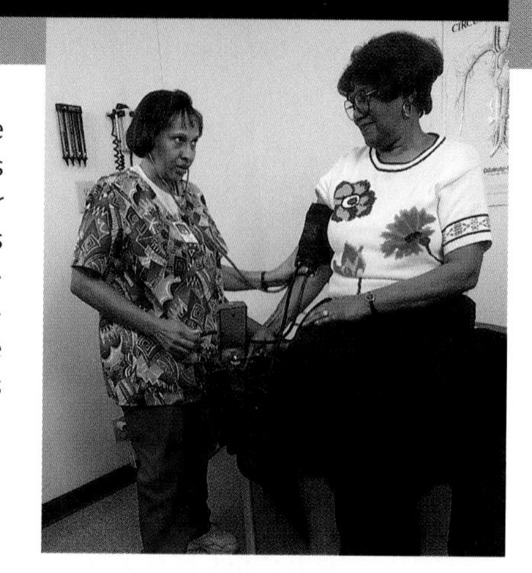

In a novel Baltimore program, health care workers taught barbers how to measure blood pressure and where to refer customers with hypertension for treatment. The barbershops in the program were also equipped with "exercycles" in addition to waiting room chairs. Customers were encouraged to exercise before and after their haircuts.

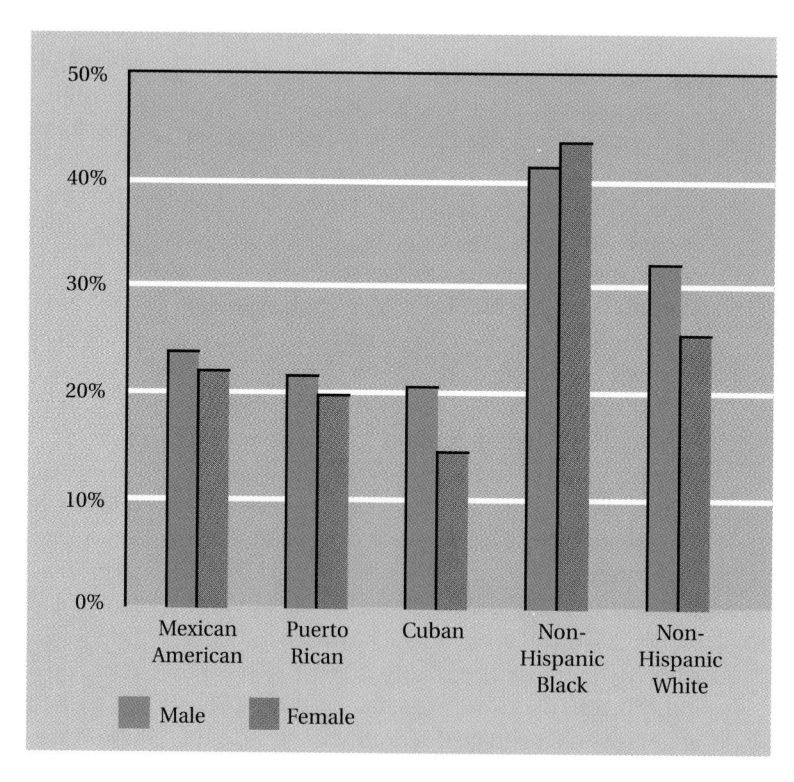


**Figure 17.5** ***Hypertension in the United States among People Age 20 to 74*** Non-Hispanic black Americans have the highest rates of hypertension among racial/ethnic groups in the U.S. Except for non-Hispanic black Americans, hypertension is more common among men than women.

lungs and the lower extremities. Congestive heart failure claims some 50,000 lives each year in the United States. It may result from a congenital heart defect, loss of muscular tissue in the heart due to a heart attack or disease, rheumatic fever, or high blood pressure.

The signs of congestive heart failure include edema (swelling), especially in the ankles and legs, and shortness of breath, which results from congestion in the lungs. If the kidneys fail to get an adequate supply of blood, excess fluid can build up in the body, contributing to edema and weight gain. Inadequate blood flow to the muscles may lead to a loss of muscular endurance, causing early fatigue during physical exertion. Though congestive heart failure is a serious and life-threatening condition, it is treatable in most cases. With proper treatment, the person may be able to maintain an essentially normal lifestyle. Treatment may involve rest and modified daily activities to conserve energy; a carefully monitored exercise program to strengthen the heart; proper diet; avoidance of alcoholic beverages; and weight control.

Drugs may bring down swelling (edema) and improve the heart's pumping efficiency. **Diuretics** (sometimes called "water pills") reduce edema by increasing the secretion of urine. **Digitalis** preparations, such as digoxin, are drugs derived from the digitalis plant. They improve the heart's pumping ability by increasing the force of contractions. **Vasodilators** make it easier for the heart to pump blood by expanding the arteries. They also reduce blood pressure. Surgery may be required to repair or replace a damaged or diseased heart valve that may be allowing blood to back up. In extreme cases, when the heart is damaged beyond repair, a heart transplant may be needed.

Talking Glossary
Diuretics, Digitalis, Vasodilators
G1709

## Rheumatic Fever

**Rheumatic fever** is an inflammatory disease accompanied by fever that can cause serious damage to heart valves and kidneys. Typically it affects children and develops on the heels of a streptococcal infection, such as a "strep throat." The disease appears to be caused by the body's own immune reaction to streptococcal bacteria if a streptococcal infection is not treated successfully. The heart valves may become inflamed, causing permanent damage. In some cases, surgery is needed to correct or replace damaged heart valves.

Talking Glossary
Rheumatic fever
G1710

Rheumatic fever has become rare because physicians routinely treat streptococcal infections aggressively with antibiotics. Treatment of rheumatic fever typically involves vigorous antibiotic treatment of any remaining streptococcal bacteria and use of anti-inflammatory drugs to control the body's immunological reaction.

## Congenital Heart Defects

The word "congenital" (from the Latin *congenitus*, meaning "with birth") means inborn or innate. **Congenital heart defects** are thus present at birth. In cases of congenital heart defects, the heart or the connections among the heart, lungs, and blood vessels fail to develop normally.

A congenital heart defect is the most common type of birth defect. It affects about one child in a hundred.[8] The cause in most cases remains unknown, but some cases can be traced to a viral infection experienced by the mother during pregnancy, such as rubella (German measles). Other common causes include maternal use of alcohol or other drugs, such as cocaine, during pregnancy and Down syndrome, a chromosomal disorder that produces mental retardation and characteristic features such as a rounded face and a wide, flattened nose.

Some congenital heart defects are relatively minor. Others are life-threatening. The most common involve obstructions in heart valves and in veins or arteries, constricting the flow of blood between the heart and the lungs or between the heart and the aorta. In some cases, a baby is born with a "hole in the heart," which is literally an opening in the wall separating the right and left chambers of the heart that allows seepage of blood between the chambers.

Most heart defects require surgery. Open-heart surgery is riskier with newborn babies, so surgeons prefer to wait until early childhood to operate. Drugs that increase the heart's pumping ability may help the heart work until corrective surgery can be performed. In many cases, the defect can be repaired and the person can lead a normal life.

**Diuretics** Agents that increase the rate of excretion of urine from the body; used in treating congestive heart failure, hypertension, and other cardiovascular problems.

**Digitalis** A drug, such as digoxin, that improves the heart's pumping ability by increasing the force of cardiac contractions.

**Vasodilators** Agents that expand (dilate) blood vessels, allowing blood to flow more freely.

**Rheumatic fever** An inflammatory disease that may occur following a streptococcal infection; sometimes causes serious damage to the heart valves and kidneys.

**Congenital heart defects** Heart defects present at birth.

## Arrhythmias

**Talking Glossary**
Arrhythmia, Tachycardia, Bradycardia
G1711

An **arrhythmia** is an abnormal heartbeat or rhythm. An abnormally fast heartbeat is called **tachycardia.** An abnormally slow beat is termed **bradycardia.** Sometimes the heart beats irregularly. Or sometimes the chambers of the heart contract in an uncoordinated fashion, reducing the heart's efficiency.

Some arrhythmias are common and hardly noticed. Most people occasionally skip a heartbeat, which is not usually a problem unless it becomes recurrent or persistent. So too with occasional attacks of tachycardia, in which the heart suddenly speeds up to about 160 beats per minute. Tachycardia may be experienced as "palpitations" or a fluttering sensation. The heart also normally speeds up during exercise and slows down during sleep.

**Close-up**
Facts about arrhythmias
T1703

Some arrhythmias are dangerous, even life-threatening. Most dangerous arrhythmias result from heart disease, although some are due to congenital defects. Loss of consciousness or death may result if the heart beats too slowly. Heart attacks can damage the heart muscle and lead to a disruption in the electrical impulses that regulate the heartbeat, causing potentially fatal arrhythmias such as **ventricular fibrillation.** Most deaths resulting from heart attacks are actually caused by ventricular fibrillation, in which the two ventricles, or lower chambers of the heart, contract irregularly and are unable to pump effectively. Ventricular fibrillation may be stopped by an electrical device called a **defibrillator,** which shocks the heart through electrodes placed on the chest and restores the normal heartbeat (a technique familiar to viewers of medical dramas on TV). Ventricular fibrillation can trigger **cardiac arrest,** in which the heart stops completely, resulting in loss of consciousness and cessation of breathing.

**Talking Glossary**
Ventricular fibrillation, Defibrillation
G1712

**Arrhythmia** An irregular heart rhythm.

**Tachycardia** An abnormally rapid heart rate.

**Bradycardia** An abnormally slow heart rate.

**Ventricular fibrillation** Irregular contractions of the two ventricles of the heart; impairs the heart's ability to pump blood effectively.

**Defibrillator** An electrical device that stops heart fibrillation by applying electrical countershocks to the heart through electrodes placed on the chest.

**Cardiac arrest** A condition in which the heart stops beating; results shortly in death.

**Cardiopulmonary resuscitation (CPR)** Emergency medical treatment used to restore coronary and pulmonary functioning following cardiac arrest.

**Atrial fibrillation** Too-rapid contractions of the atria; disrupts the coordination of the ventricles.

**Atrial flutter** Overly rapid atrial contractions, but at a somewhat slower and more regular rate than is the case in atrial fibrillation.

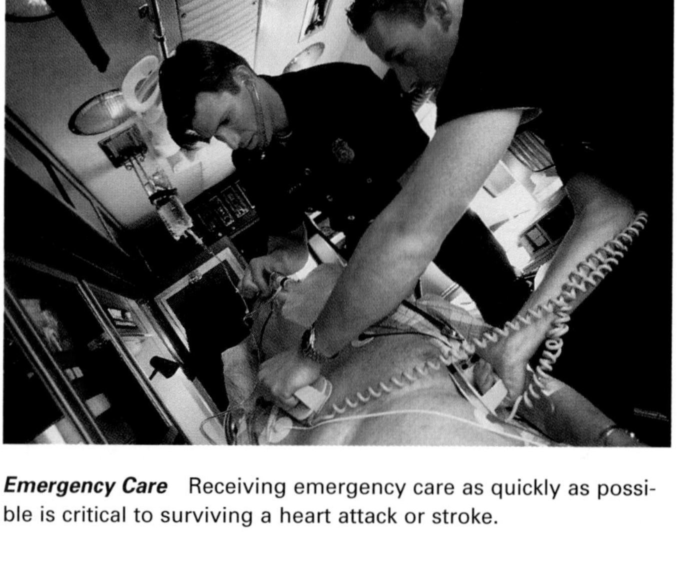

***Emergency Care*** Receiving emergency care as quickly as possible is critical to surviving a heart attack or stroke.

Death occurs shortly as the brain and other vital body organs fail to receive blood. The defibrillator can help jolt the stopped heart back to a normal rhythm.

**Cardiopulmonary resuscitation (CPR)** techniques, including cardiac massage, may be able to restart the heartbeat of someone in cardiac arrest. (CPR is a life-saving technique that everyone should learn *before* a life-threatening emergency occurs. Classes that train laypeople in CPR techniques are offered in most communities. Contact your local health department or hospital center.)

**Talking Glossary**
Cardiopulmonary resuscitation
G1713

Two other types of arrhythmias are atrial fibrillation and atrial flutter. In **atrial fibrillation,** the upper chambers of the heart, the atria, contract too fast and irregularly for the ventricles, the lower chambers, to respond in a coordinated fashion. In **atrial flutter,** the atria also contract too rapidly, but at a somewhat slower and more regular rate. In these arrhythmias, the heart's internal electrical control system falls out of synch. Therefore, the heart is unable to pump blood efficiently, resulting in symptoms such as weakness, fatigue, and faintness. Atrial fibrillation can also lead to the formation of blood clots in the atria. (The quivering contractions of the atria fail to pump enough blood into the ventricles, allowing blood to pool and clot.) A stroke may occur if a clot breaks away and becomes lodged in an artery that supplies blood to the brain. Atrial fibrillation and flutter tend to occur periodically, with normal heart rhythms occurring between episodes. Treatment may involve the use of digitalis, which strengthens ventricular contractions and helps compensate for the inefficient atrial contractions. Anticoagulants (agents that delay or prevent blood coagulation) may help prevent the formation of blood clots.

**Talking Glossary**
Atrial fibrillation, Atrial flutter
G1714

## Stroke

Strokes strike some 500,000 people and claim 150,000 lives each year in the United States.[9] They are the third leading killer of Americans, after CHD and cancer. The brain, like other body tissue, needs a constant flow of blood to supply it with oxygen and nutrients (glucose) and cart away metabolic waste products. A stroke (also called a *cerebrovascular accident,* or CVA) occurs when the flow of blood to an area of the brain is blocked by an obstruction in an artery serving that part of the brain. Deprived of its blood supply, even for a few minutes, the affected parts of the brain may be damaged or destroyed. In some strokes, brain tissue is destroyed by blood seeping out of a ruptured blood vessel. Because brain tissue does not regenerate, the functions controlled by affected parts of the brain may be lost or severely impaired.

**Types of Strokes** There are three major types of strokes (see Figure 17.6):

1. *Cerebral thrombosis.* This is the most common type of stroke. It occurs when a blood clot (a *thrombus*) blocks an artery (called a *cerebral artery*) that supplies blood to the brain. In most cases, the thrombus becomes lodged in a blood vessel narrowed by the buildup of fatty deposits (atherosclerosis).
2. *Cerebral embolism.* An **embolism** is an obstruction of a blood vessel. In a cerebral embolism, a blood clot or some other particle that forms in another part of the body travels through the circulatory system and lodges in an artery that serves the brain, blocking the flow of blood. These emboli usually form in the heart as the result of atrial fibrillation, a condition that increases the risk of stroke.
3. *Hemorrhagic stroke.* A hemorrhagic stroke, or **cerebral hemorrhage,** is the least common but most severe type of stroke. Hemorrhagic strokes result in death about half the time. They occur when a blood vessel in the brain ruptures or bursts, so that blood leaks into brain cavities, damaging sensitive brain tissue. Hemorrhagic strokes are often linked to high blood pressure. A hemorrhage (bleeding) in the brain can also result from a head injury or a burst **aneurysm.** An aneurysm is a blood-filled sac or pouch that balloons out from an artery wall due to a weakness in the wall.

**Talking Glossary**

Embolism, Cerebral hemorrhage G1715

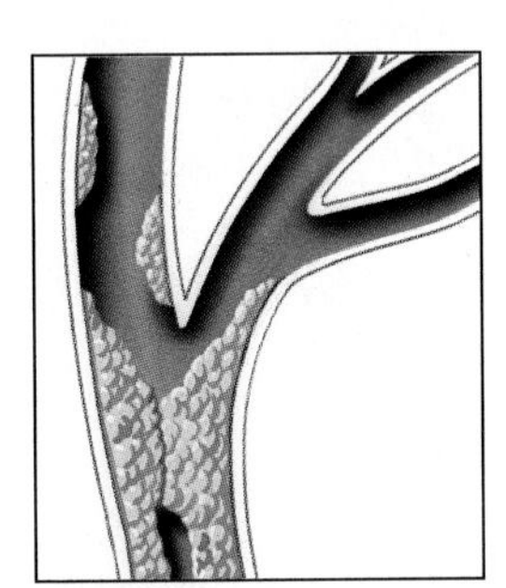

a. Thrombus

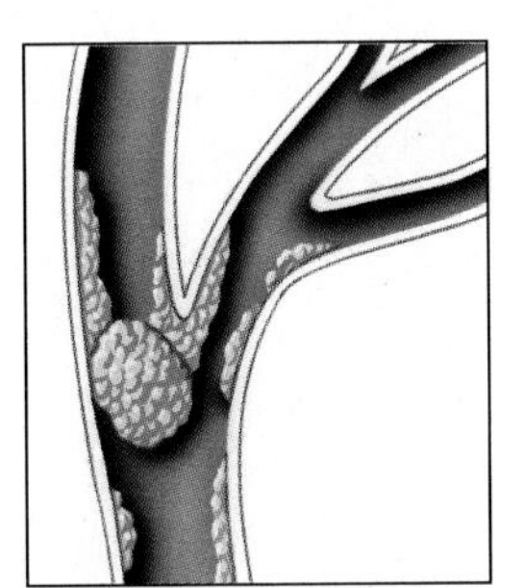

b. Embolism

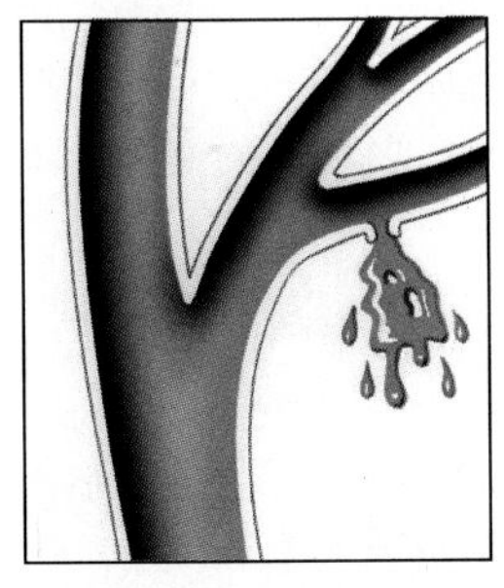

c. Hemorrhage

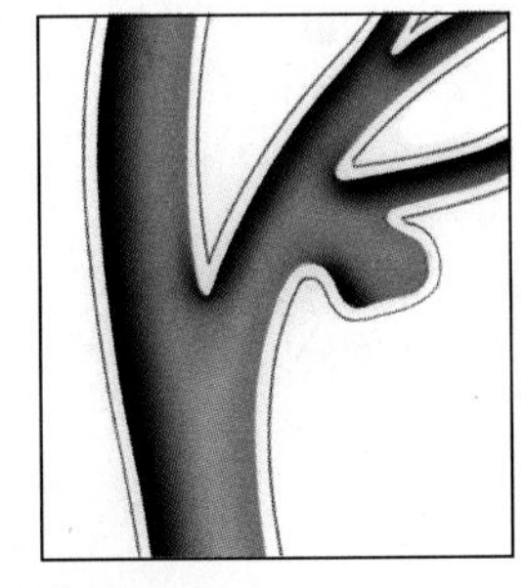

d. Aneurysm

**Figure 17.6** ***Types of Strokes*** There are three types of strokes: thrombosis, embolism, and cerebral hemorrhage. Though any stroke is a potential killer, the least common type, the cerebral hemorrhage, is the most lethal.

Strokes can affect anybody and occur without warning. However, for cerebral thrombosis, which accounts for about 75% of all strokes, the stage is set over many years by atherosclerosis.

**Effects of Stroke** Stroke is expressed in symptoms such as loss of speech or difficulty understanding speech; loss of feeling, numbness, weakness, or paralysis of a limb or the face; or sudden loss of consciousness. There may also be unexplained severe headaches, blurred or double vision, and dizziness or loss of balance or coordination. Stroke usually affects one side of the brain. The resulting loss of sensation or movement is limited to the other side of the body, because each side of the body is controlled by the opposite side of the brain.

Depending on the site and extent of the damage, the effects of a stroke can be relatively minor or involve crippling disabilities, coma, and death. If the sensory or motor areas of the brain are affected, survivors may lose sensation or develop paralysis. Damage to the speech centers can lead to a general loss of speech or to problems

**Embolism** An obstruction of a blood vessel, usually caused by a blood clot.

**Cerebral hemorrhage** Rupture of a blood vessel in the brain.

**Aneurysm** A ballooning out of an artery wall.

Smart Reference
Mind over body
R1701

with articulation. There may also be declines in cognitive abilities involving memory, reasoning, and judgment.

About 3 million people in the United States are living with the consequences of stroke.[10] With advances in stroke management, only about 10% need long-term care in institutional settings.

**Transient Ischemic Attacks (TIAs)** Transient ischemic attacks (TIAs) are brief strokelike episodes that result from an insufficient blood supply, or *ischemia,* to the brain. They occur when a small blood clot or other particle temporarily clogs an artery serving the brain. Symptoms of TIAs include numbness, weakness, tingling, dizziness, headache, blurred or double vision, and temporary blindness. There may be momentary loss of motor function on one side of the body or difficulty speaking. Unlike a stroke, the symptoms quickly pass, usually within five minutes, and the person returns to normal.

TIAs should be taken seriously. They are often early warning signs of stroke. About one in ten strokes is preceded by TIAs. About one in three people who have TIAs eventually have strokes, about half of them within a year.[11] Timely medical treatment following a TIA may prevent a stroke. Anticoagulants may be used to thin the blood and prevent the formation of clots. Surgery may remove fatty deposits that clog arteries.

Smart Quiz
Q1702

### think about it!

- **What is meant by the terms *arteriosclerosis* and *atherosclerosis?* Do you think it is important to understand the meanings of these terms? Why or why not?**
- **What is the difference between coronary heart disease (CHD) and a heart attack?**
- **Why is hypertension considered a "silent killer"?**
- **What is the difference between systolic and diastolic blood pressure?**
- **Do you know anyone whose legs are swollen because of congestive heart failure? What is he or she doing about it?**

**Heart murmur** Abnormal heart sound resulting from some disturbance in the normal flow of blood through the heart.

## DIAGNOSIS AND TREATMENT OF CARDIOVASCULAR DISORDERS

A wide range of techniques are used to diagnose and treat cardiovascular disorders.

### Diagnostic Tests

Doctors use various techniques to probe the cardiovascular system for abnormalities. The doctor may push against the patient's chest to feel for an enlarged heart. A stethoscope is used to listen for irregular heart rhythms or other unusual sounds in the chest, such as a **heart murmur.** A heart murmur occurs when blood passes through a heart valve that is normally closed. Blood tests provide information about the blood levels of fats such as cholesterol and triglycerides that are associated with coronary artery disease. Blood is also analyzed for the level of thyroid hormone, since overactivity of the thyroid gland is implicated in some arrhythmias. Abnormal blood sugar levels may suggest diabetes, a major risk factor for CHD.

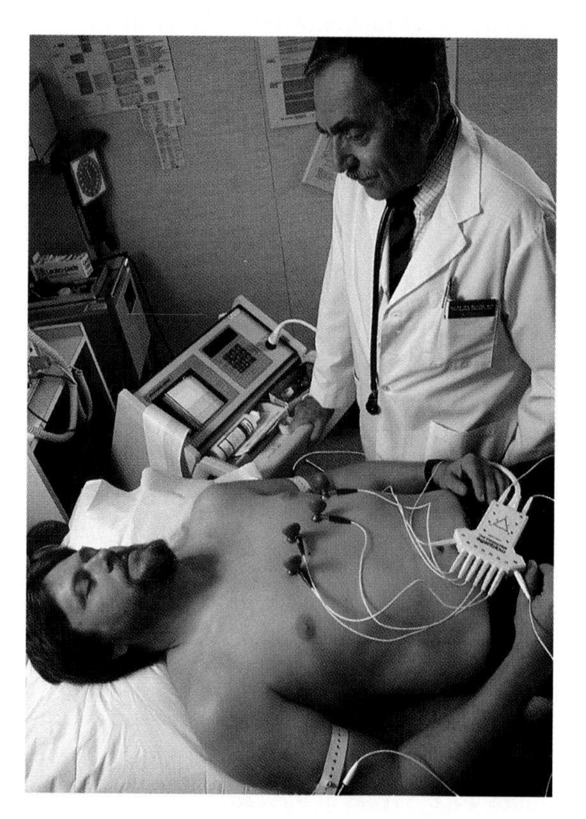

***Electrocardiogram*** The electrocardiogram (EKG) machine prints a record of the heart's electrical activity. It can reveal irregular heart rhythms caused by heart attacks or other heart problems.

**Talking Glossary**
Electrocardiogram
G1716

A chest X-ray may reveal abnormalities in the heart or the blood vessels that serve the heart. The **electrocardiogram (ECG or EKG)** prints out a record of the heart's electrical activity. In an EKG, electrodes are attached to the skin at various sites on the body to measure the electrical discharges emanating from the heart when it beats. The EKG reveals abnormal heart rhythms that may be caused by congenital birth defects, CHD, or heart attacks. Sometimes abnormal heart rhythms may not be detected unless the heart is stressed. Therefore, an **exercise electrocardiogram** ("stress test") may be used to chart the heart's activity while the person exercises on a treadmill or stationary bicycle. The stress test helps reveal heart problems, but as many as one in four people with CHD produce normal stress test results. Some arrhythmias are fleeting and don't show up at the time of the EKG. To detect intermittent arrhythmias, people may wear a portable 24-hour EKG, called a *Holter monitor,* which continuously records the heart's electrical activity as they go about their daily activities.

**Talking Glossary**
Echocardiogram
G1717

**Talking Glossary**
Radionuclide imaging
G1718

Specialized scanning techniques reveal the structure and functioning of the heart without surgery. Only as a last resort do surgeons perform open-heart surgery to detect abnormalities of the heart and arteries. The **echocardiogram** uses the reflection or "echo" of high-frequency sound waves bounced against the chest to create an image of the heart on a monitor. The echocardiogram can reveal damage to the heart muscle, the presence of tumors or blood clots, valve disorders, and aneurysms.

**Radionuclide imaging** detects blockages in the blood flow in and around the heart. Small amounts of radioactive substances called radionuclides are injected into a vein in the arm, usually as the person is exercising on a treadmill. A scanning device creates pictures from their movement into the heart. The technique may also reveal damage caused by heart attacks.

**Magnetic resonance imaging (MRI)** uses magnets to generate a computerized image of the structure of the heart or of other parts of the body. It can be used to detect congenital heart defects, heart damage from previous heart attacks, and abnormalities in the blood vessels around the heart.

**Talking Glossary**
Coronary angiography
G1719

A more invasive procedure called **coronary angiography** (or *angiogram*) provides more detailed information about blockages in coronary arteries. Through a procedure called a *cardiac catheterization,* a catheter (a thin, flexible tube) is inserted into an artery, typically in the groin. The catheter is threaded into the heart from the main artery, the aorta, and from there into a coronary artery. A dye is injected through the catheter, which can be detected by a specialized X-ray that reveals the shape, size, and location of plaque deposits within coronary arteries. The procedure takes from 30 minutes to an hour and is performed under local anesthesia. More than 1 million angiograms are performed each year in the United States. The angiogram can reveal the location and type of blockage and suggest the most appropriate treatment. Because of the costs and possible risks of the angiogram, its widespread use is debated among health professionals. It has not been proved that heart patients who receive angiograms are more likely to survive than those who do not.[12] Before undergoing angiograms, people are advised to discuss the risks, costs, and benefits with their health care providers.

**Video**
Angiograms: Finding the blockages
V1701

**Talking Glossary**
Electroencephalogram, Computerized axial tomography, Digital subtraction angiography
G1720

Specialized diagnostic tests are used to determine the causes of strokes, the extent of damage, and the most appropriate treatment. An **electroencephalogram (EEG)** measures brain waves and can reveal abnormal brain wave activity that results from damage to the brain. Imaging techniques such as magnetic resonance imaging (MRI) and **computerized axial tomography scan (CAT scan)** may reveal the areas of the brain damaged by a stroke. The CAT scan is a specialized X-ray machine that takes pictures from different angles to display a three-dimensional image of the brain. These imaging techniques can help doctors determine whether a stroke was caused by a blood clot (thrombus) or a hemorrhage. Anticoagulants that "thin the blood" and prevent further blood clots from forming can cause damage when strokes

**Electrocardiogram (ECG or EKG)** A device for recording and graphing the electrical activity of the heart.

**Exercise electrocardiogram** *(stress test)* An electrocardiogram taken when the heart is stressed during exercise.

**Echocardiogram** A device that uses reflected sound waves ("echoes") to create an image of the internal structure and movement of the heart.

**Radionuclide imaging** A specialized scanning device; detects blockages of blood flow in and around the heart by tracking the movement of radioactive substances injected into the bloodstream.

**Magnetic resonance imaging (MRI)** The use of magnets to generate a computerized image of internal body structures.

**Coronary angiography** ***(angiogram)*** Rapid-sequence X-rays detect a radioactive dye as it passes through the coronary arteries; provides information on blockages restricting blood flow to the heart.

**Electroencephalogram (EEG)** A device that uses electrodes on the scalp to measure and display brain wave activity.

**Computerized axial tomography scan (CAT scan)** An X-ray machine that passes a narrow X-ray beam through the body at different angles and generates a computer-enhanced image of internal structures.

are caused by a cerebral hemorrhage. Another technique used with stroke victims is **digital subtraction angiography (DSA).** DSA provides images of the major blood vessels in the brain, which allows detection of blockages. A dye is injected into a vein in the arm and its passage through the blood vessels in the neck and brain is captured in a series of pictures taken by a specialized X-ray machine.

## Treating Heart Disease

Major advances have been made in the treatment of heart disease in recent years. In most cases, people with heart disease can be successfully treated with medication or with such techniques as balloon angioplasty, coronary bypass surgery, artificial pacemakers, and heart transplantation. The general goals of treatment are to reduce pain, improve circulation, and regulate the heart rhythm.

**Medication** Heart medications can help regulate the heart rhythm by suppressing abnormal firing patterns. Anticoagulants help prevent the formation of blood clots in people with narrowed arteries. Clot-dissolving drugs, called *thrombolytic agents* (streptokinase is one), can dissolve blood clots following a heart attack. *Beta-blockers* reduce the pumping demands placed on the heart, which is useful in treating angina. *Vasodilators* expand blood vessels narrowed by fatty deposits, which increases the blood flow to the heart. *Calcium-channel blockers* interfere with the normal flow of calcium through the channels in the heart muscle. This can have several beneficial effects: expanding the coronary arteries, allowing more blood to flow to the heart; reducing blood pressure; and reducing the pumping demands on the heart. Nitroglycerine dilates coronary arteries, increasing blood flow to the heart and relieving angina attacks. Pain-killing drugs (analgesics), such as morphine, may relieve intense chest pain.

Drugs may also help lower blood cholesterol levels.[13] Diet modification is generally recommended as the first step in reducing blood cholesterol. However, diet may not always be successful in itself, especially in people with extremely high cholesterol levels. In hospital settings people's diets can be carefully monitored. Hospitalized people on highly restrictive low-fat diets are able to reduce their cholesterol level by about 50%. However, when outpatients are put on cholesterol-lowering diets, they typically achieve a reduction in the 5 to 10% range. Apparently they do not rigidly adhere to the diet. On the other hand, cholesterol-lowering drugs can sharply reduce levels of artery-clogging LDL cholesterol while slightly increasing HDL cholesterol, the "good cholesterol" that lowers the risk of CHD.[14]

**Digital subtraction angiography (DSA)** An angiogram that detects blockages in the major blood vessels in the neck and brain.

**Coronary artery bypass graft (CABG) surgery** A surgical technique that grafts pieces of vein from elsewhere in the body to direct the flow of blood around a blocked or narrowed coronary artery.

Cholesterol-lowering drugs can save lives. In a Scandinavian study, people with moderate to high cholesterol levels and a history of heart attacks or angina were put on a cholesterol-lowering drug. They had 30% lower death rates (and 42% fewer deaths from CHD) over five years than people who were given a dummy pill.[15] A study in Scotland showed a lower rate of heart attacks and deaths from heart disease in apparently healthy men with high cholesterol who received cholesterol-lowering medication compared with men who received a placebo.[16]

Cholesterol-lowering drugs are now used by millions of apparently healthy people who are unable to control their high blood cholesterol levels by diet alone. But should people who don't yet have evidence of heart disease be using these drugs? They carry some potential risks, such as a possible risk of cancer. Therefore, some health professionals believe that the drugs should be used only by people who face such a high short-term risk of CHD that it offsets any potential long-term risk.[17]

**Coronary Bypass Graft Surgery** In **coronary artery bypass graft (CABG) surgery,** surgeons take a piece of a vein from elsewhere in the body, usually a leg, and construct grafts that direct the flow of blood around a blocked or narrowed coronary artery. One end of the graft is attached to the artery just above the blockage. The other end is connected to the artery just below the blockage. Typically, four or five bypasses are needed. The bypass allows blood to circumvent the blockages and flow more freely to the heart. Bypass surgery is typically recommended when blockages are severe or when the symptoms of coronary artery disease do not respond to other forms of treatment.

**Video** Advances in coronary bypass grafting V1702

Like any form of major surgery, CABG carries some risk, but the risk of dying is less than 1% for patients who are otherwise healthy. There are other potential drawbacks to the procedure, however. Fatty deposits may later develop in the bypass segments, causing new blockages that require further surgery. The grafted segments may be even more susceptible to fatty deposits than the coronary arteries themselves. Nor does CABG correct the underlying disease process, atherosclerosis. The person must still follow a strict regimen consisting of proper diet, regular exercise, and avoidance of smoking.

**Talking Glossary**
Percutaneous transluminal coronary angioplasty
G1721

**Percutaneous Transluminal Coronary Angioplasty** **Percutaneous transluminal coronary angioplasty** (**PTCA,** also called *balloon angioplasty*) is used to clear coronary arteries of fatty deposits that obstruct the flow of blood to the heart (see Figure 17.7). Under local anesthesia, a catheter is inserted into a leg artery and threaded into a blocked coronary artery. Once it reaches its destination, a tiny balloon is inflated. The balloon widens the blocked artery by flattening the blockage against the artery wall. Widening improves circulation to the heart. Through a procedure called an *atherectomy,* blockages are surgically removed rather than just compressed as in traditional angioplasty. A laser may also be used to clear away blockages.[18]

Many people in coronary care undergo angioplasty rather than CABG. Angioplasty is less costly, avoids the trauma of open-heart surgery, and shortens recovery.[19] However, angioplasty is not problem free.[20] It generally succeeds in widening arteries, but blockages often return, requiring bypass surgery or repeat angioplasty. A variation on the procedure involves the use of a *stent,* a device that reopens a clogged artery and remains in place to keep it open. Stenting appears to substantially reduce the need for a repeat procedure.

Angioplasty is generally more successful in clearing some blockages than others, depending on the location and shape of the blockage. People facing the need for angioplasty or coronary bypass surgery need to sit down with their surgeons and carefully weigh their comparative risks and benefits. The surgeon should be able to cite evidence for the use of any procedure recommended for the type of blockage in the patient's case. The decision as to which procedure to use often comes down to how much narrowing has occurred, the size and shape of the plaque deposits, and the arteries involved.

**Heart Transplants** **Heart transplant** operations are the most dramatic and risky of the procedures used to treat heart disease. The defective or diseased heart is replaced with a healthy heart from a donor whose death did not damage the heart. The donor's heart is preserved for transport in a special solution and is inserted in the recipient's chest cavity once the recipient's heart is removed.

**Smart Reference**
Pump it up
R1702

People who are not expected to live more than two or three years with their present hearts may be candidates for a heart transplant. These include people whose hearts have been severely damaged by previous heart attacks or by **cardiomyopathy,** a weakening of the heart muscle due to disease, and those with severe congestive heart failure. Though never routine, heart transplantation has become accepted medical practice as a treatment of last resort for people who otherwise have little or no hope for survival. More than 2,000 heart transplants are performed each year in the United States. About four out of five recipients live for at least a year following the procedure. Many have survived for a decade or more with their new hearts. The major problem with heart transplants is the risk that the body will reject the new heart. Drugs that suppress organ rejection increase patients' chances of survival.

**Talking Glossary**
Cardiomyopathy
G1722

**Figure 17.7** ***Tools for Unclogging Arteries***
Source: Harvard Health Letter, January 1996, p. 4.

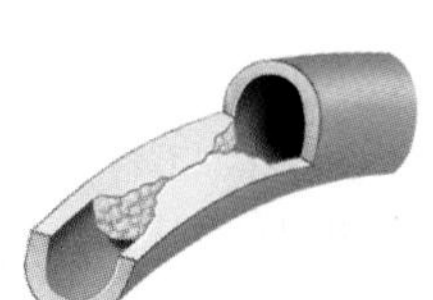

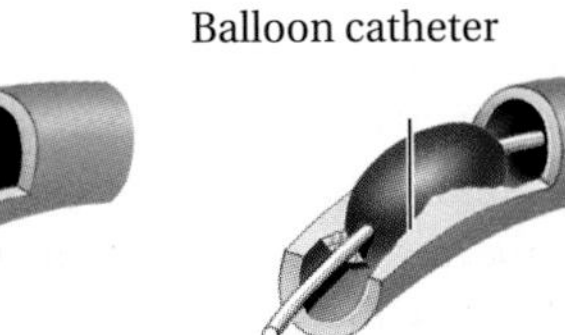


a. Balloon angioplasty
A balloon catheter is used to flatten plaque and stretch artery walls.



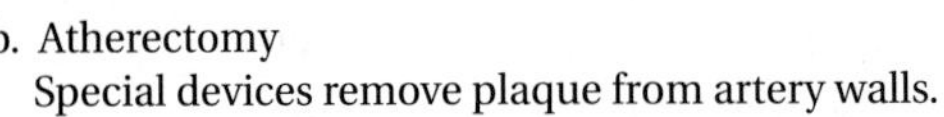

b. Atherectomy
Special devices remove plaque from artery walls.

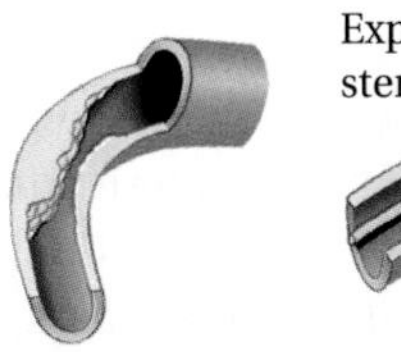

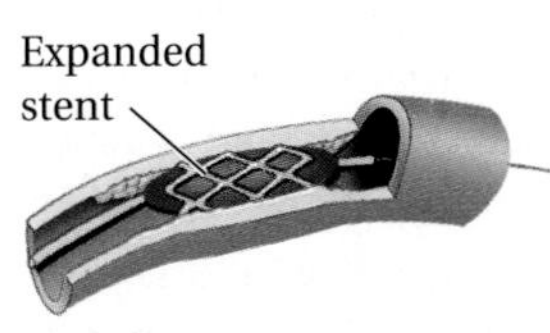


c. Coronary stenting
A device called a stent is placed inside the artery and props it open.

**Percutaneous transluminal coronary angioplasty (PTCA)** *(balloon angioplasty)* Widening a blocked artery by inflating a tiny balloon within the artery, compressing the blockage against the artery wall.

**Heart transplant** The replacement of a diseased heart with a healthy donor heart.

**Cardiomyopathy** A disease of the heart muscle or myocardium.

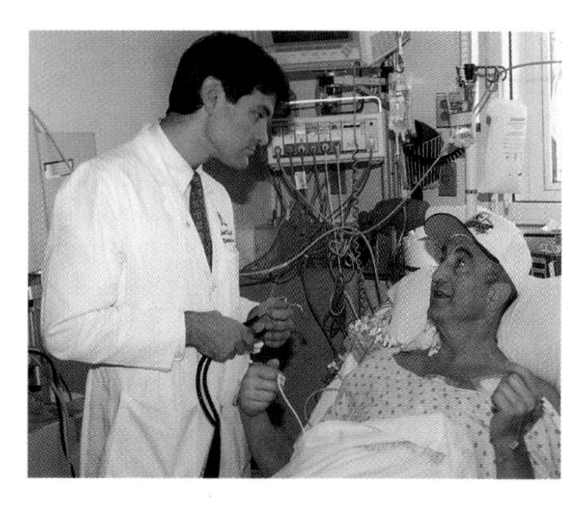

***A New Lease on Life*** Frank Torre, the older brother of New York Yankees manager Joe Torre, shown here with his heart surgeon the day after receiving a new heart. The operation took place while brother Joe's team was battling the Atlanta Braves in the 1996 World Series.

**Artificial Pacemaker** Implanted under the skin, an **artificial pacemaker** is a small electrical device, about $1\frac{1}{2}$ ounces in weight and about the size of a silver dollar. Leads from the device extend to the heart and transmit electrical impulses at a given rate to maintain a normal heartbeat. The device replaces the heart's own internal control system and is used when the heart is unable to maintain a normal rhythm on its own. At times when the heart beats fast enough on its own, the device automatically switches to a standby mode. Artificial pacemakers are powered by lithium batteries that can last for 10 years or more before replacement.

**Artificial pacemaker** A small device that transmits electrical impulses to the heart to maintain a normal heartbeat.

PREVENTION

## *Aspirin—Not Just for Headaches Anymore*

The common aspirin in your medicine cabinet not only reduces headache and fever. It is also helpful in preventing and treating blood clots, including clots that can cause heart attacks when they become lodged in arteries narrowed by fatty deposits. A Harvard University study showed that aspirin can lower the risk of heart attacks in middle-aged and older men. Other studies find a substantial reduction in heart attacks and deaths in people with CHD who take a low dosage of aspirin daily.[21] Even if a heart attack does happen, aspirin may reduce its severity.[22]

Aspirin reduces the stickiness of platelets, the bodies in blood that clump together to form clots when bleeding occurs. Aspirin may prevent unnecessary clots, such as those that can form in coronary arteries and trigger a heart attack. Aspirin is so effective that the American Heart Association recommends that it be used routinely in low doses by people with CHD and those who have survived a heart attack.[23] It is also becoming increasingly common for aspirin to be administered immediately after a heart attack. For people who can't tolerate aspirin, other anticoagulants may be used to reduce the risk of life-threatening blood clots.

Should aspirin be taken regularly by healthy people to reduce their risk of a heart attack? The question remains under study. Meanwhile, the Food and Drug Administration (FDA) has taken a cautious approach. It endorses the daily use of low-dose aspirin only for people who have suffered a heart attack or have known heart disease.[24] Aspirin can cause bleeding problems and may slightly increase the chance of a stroke. The risks for the general population in taking an aspirin a day may outweigh the benefits. If you have hypertension, a family history of stroke, a bleeding disorder, an ulcer, or liver or kidney problems, you should avoid aspirin. In any event, discuss the benefits and risks with your physician before undertaking any drug regimen, including over-the-counter drugs like aspirin. Nor should you assume that a daily dose of aspirin can substitute for practicing CHD-preventive behaviors, such as following a proper diet, exercising regularly, and avoiding smoking and excessive use of alcohol.

## Treating Heart Attacks

Delays in health care following a heart attack cost lives. About one in three people who have a heart attack dies before receiving medical attention.[25] Not so long ago only one in two survived. The increased rate of survival is due largely to improvements in emergency medical care. Today, emergency medical system (EMS) teams in most cities can reach people with heart attacks in minutes, apply life-saving techniques such as CPR, and stabilize them enroute to the hospital. Most people who die before receiving medical help either ignore their symptoms or delay seeking help. Of those who reach the hospital alive, more than 90% survive.[26]

**In the hospital . . .** Various tests are used to diagnose a heart attack and determine the extent of the damage. An electrocardiogram (EKG) reveals patterns of electrical impulses that indicate whether a heart attack has occurred and any irregular heart rhythms that may have resulted.

Blood tests detect enzymes that are released by damaged heart tissue. An angiogram may be performed to diagnose blocked arteries.

Blood clots that lodge in arteries already choked off by fatty deposits cause heart attacks. Doctors race against the clock to dissolve the clot before the blockage leads to permanent damage or death. They may try to dissolve the clot by use of a drug like streptokinase. Or they may use balloon angioplasty or a related procedure to clear a blocked coronary artery. Angioplasty, which is widely used in treating people with chest pain before they suffer a heart attack, is now coming into greater use after a heart attack. Health professionals continue to debate the relative merits of clot-dissolving drugs versus angioplasty.[27]

Nitroglycerine may be administered through a vein during or following a heart attack to increase the blood flow to the heart and decrease the heart's need for oxygen. Beta-blockers may be used to reduce the oxygen requirements placed on the heart by slowing down the heart rate and reducing the force of heart contractions. Aspirin is also becoming a standard part of treatment for heart attack victims (see the nearby ***Prevention*** feature on aspirin therapy).

People who remain alive two hours after a heart attack are more likely than not to survive. (As a rule of thumb, the more time that elapses after the heart attack, the greater the chances that the person will live a long life and avoid another attack.) Nevertheless, there may be complications. Damage to the heart muscle may affect the electrical system that controls the heartbeat, leading to life-threatening arrhythmias (irregular heart rhythms). In some cases the heart beats abnormally slowly, which may require the implantation of an artificial pacemaker. In some cases, the damage to the heart muscle is so severe that congestive heart failure develops.

**After the hospital . . .** Most people who recover from a heart attack are able to resume their normal lives within a few weeks. However, they need to make lifestyle adjustments if they want to improve their chances of living a long life and avoiding another attack. The adjustments apply to anyone who wishes to reduce the risk of heart disease: quitting smoking, decreasing intake of dietary cholesterol and fat, losing excess weight, exercising regularly, and keeping blood pressure under control.

People who have had a heart attack often ask when, or if, they may safely resume having sexual relations. It is generally safe for people who have had heart attacks to resume sexual activity within 3 to 6 weeks after returning home from the hospital.[28] Sexual intercourse is about as vigorous as taking a brisk walk and poses virtually no danger to most people, even those who have suffered a heart attack or undergone cardiac surgery. Of the very few deaths linked to sexual intercourse, more than three of four involve extramarital sex. Therefore, anxiety or guilt rather than sex itself may be responsible. Of course, any sign of recurrence of chest pain or shortness of breath should be taken as a sign to stop any physical activity and seek medical guidance at the first opportunity.

## Treating Stroke Victims

As with a heart attack, delays in seeking medical attention following a stroke can be fatal. There is perhaps a three- to six-hour window of opportunity during which treatment has its greatest benefits.[29] Unfortunately, the average stroke victim does not receive medical assistance for about a day.

**In the hospital . . .** Diagnostic tests can help pinpoint the cause of the stroke. If the stroke was due to a thrombus, clot-dissolving drugs such as tissue-plasminogen activator (t-PA) may be used to disperse the clot or prevent it from growing. If clot-dissolving drugs are used within the first few hours, the flow of blood to the brain can be restored and brain tissue may be saved or the damage minimized.[30] However, clot-dissolving drugs may cause more bleeding and further brain damage if the stroke was due to a cerebral hemor-

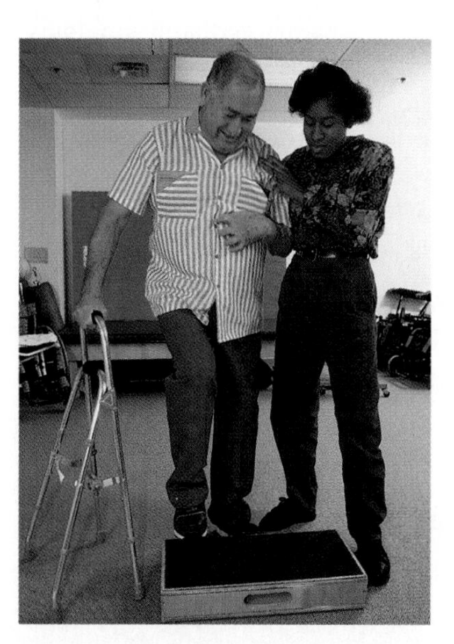

***The Road Back*** Physical therapists and other rehabilitation specialists help stroke victims recover as much function as possible following a stroke.

**Smart Reference**
A strike against stroke
R1703

rhage. Therefore, health professionals need to diagnose the *type* of stroke. If an embolism is suspected, doctors may attempt to track down its source and remove it surgically. Surgery may also be used to widen narrowed arteries in order to improve the blood supply to the brain.

**After the hospital . . .** Changes in diet and lifestyle may help reduce the risk of recurrent strokes: avoiding smoking, restricting intake of saturated fat and dietary cholesterol, and controlling blood pressure. In some cases, blood thinners (anticoagulants) may be needed indefinitely to prevent clotting.

Rehabilitation after a stroke depends on the nature of the disability. Physical therapy can improve muscle strength and coordination and help the person use mechanical aids, such as crutches or walkers, to compensate for loss of motor function. Occupational therapy can help improve eye-hand coordination and improve skills needed for daily living, such as bathing, dressing, and cooking. Speech and language therapy can help people whose speech has been affected. Rehabilitation typically begins in the hospital stay and continues as needed. The rate of progress varies. Some people experience nearly complete recovery within days or weeks. Most improvement occurs within the first 30 days. For many stroke victims, the road to recovery is tedious, and coping with permanent disability is a lifetime challenge.

## PREVENTION

### *Warning Signs of a Stroke*[31]

**Close-up**
Stroke warning signs
T1704

Anyone who experiences these symptoms should treat them as a medical emergency and call for help or dial 911 fast. Immediate treatment for a stroke can spell the difference between life and death, or between rapid recovery and permanent disability.

- Sudden, severe, unexplained headache.
- Sudden blurring of sight or loss of vision in one eye.
- Sudden loss of speech or trouble speaking.
- Sudden difficulty understanding simple statements.
- Sudden dizziness or loss of balance or coordination.
- Sudden weakness, numbness, or paralysis of an arm, leg, or the face, especially on one side.

**Risk factors** Factors that indicate an increased risk of developing a particular disease or disorder.

### *think about it!*

**Smart Quiz**
Q1703

- **Have you or has anyone you know been diagnosed or treated for a cardiovascular condition? What procedure or procedures were used? What was the experience like?**
- **Do you know anyone who has had a heart attack? What were the symptoms? What happened in the ambulance or hospital?**
- **Do you know anyone who has had a stroke? What were the symptoms? Are there any sensory or motor problems as a result?**
- **Have you or has anyone you know made lifestyle changes to prevent cardiovascular disorders? In what ways?**

## RISK FACTORS FOR CARDIOVASCULAR DISEASE

Knowledge of the **risk factors** (see Figure 17.8) for cardiovascular disease will tell you whether you are at special risk and would be well advised to take preventive measures. You have no control over some risk factors, such as your age, gender, family history, and ethnic background. You do have control over others, by making changes in your lifestyle or obtaining appropriate treatment. Even if you are healthy and have no present risk factors, taking preventive measures now may help avert cardiovascular disease later.

### Things You Can't Control

**Age** With men, the risk of CHD rises sharply with age after about age 40. Among women, it rises slowly until menopause, and then accelerates. Stroke most often affects people over the age of 65.

**Gender** Men face a greater risk of cardiovascular disease (CVD) than women. However, for CHD, which accounts for most deaths due to CVD, the relative risks for men and women even out by about age 65 and then remain even (see the nearby ***World of Diversity*** feature).

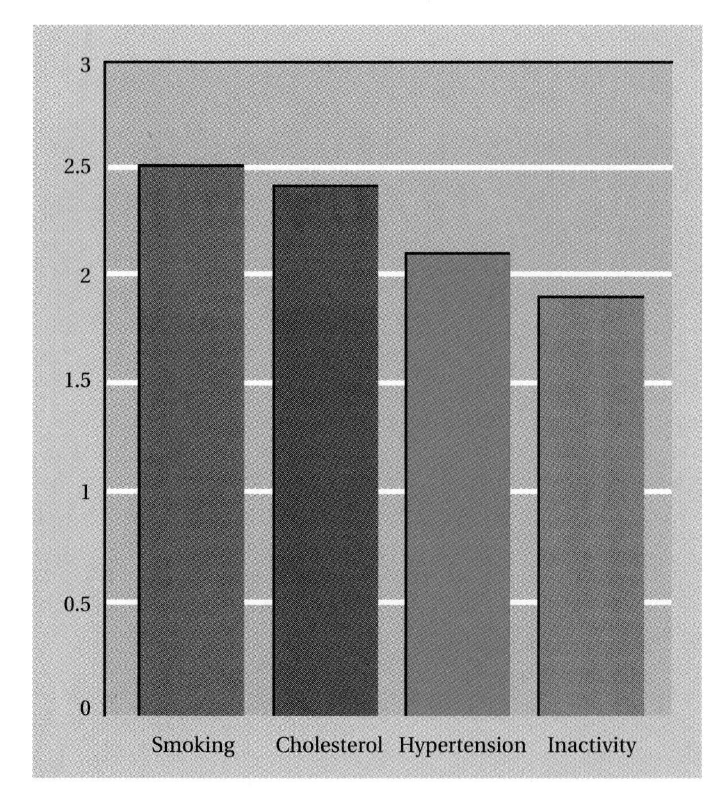


**Figure 17.8** ***Risk Factors for Coronary Heart Disease*** Several major risk factors for coronary heart disease are smoking, high cholesterol, hypertension, and inactivity. This chart shows the increased risk of CHD for people with these risk factors.

**Heredity** CVD tends to run in families, so people with a family history of cardiovascular disease are at greater risk than other people. This is especially so for people with a close male relative who had a heart attack or died suddenly before the age of 55, or a close female relative who suffered these consequences before the age of 65.

**Race/Ethnicity** African Americans are about 75% more likely to die from CHD and about 60% more likely to suffer strokes than are white Americans. The greater prevalence of hypertension and diabetes among African Americans is largely responsible for their elevated risks of cardiovascular disorders. Economic differences may also be involved. Poorer people have more risk factors for cardiovascular disease, including smoking, obesity, high-fat diets, inactivity, and stress.[32] African Americans as a group face greater economic hardships than white Americans do.

Blacks are also less likely than whites to receive aggressive treatments such as coronary artery bypass surgery and angioplasty, resulting in many needless deaths.[33] This dual standard of care may reflect discrimination and possible cultural factors, such as mistrust of black patients toward the medical establishment.

## Things You *Can* Control

**Hypertension** Hypertension is a major risk factor for CHD and stroke. For every one-point drop in diastolic blood pressure, there is an estimated 2 to 3% reduction in the risk of heart attacks.[34] Control of hypertension is largely credited with a reduction of about 60% in the incidence of strokes in recent years. Table 17.1 shows the blood pressure levels corresponding to normal BP and high blood pressure and the follow-up recommendations based on these classifications.

**Close-up**
Preventing stroke
**T1705**

**Blood Cholesterol** Another prominent risk factor for CVD is high blood cholesterol, especially high levels of low-density lipoproteins (LDLs), the type of cholesterol that clings to artery walls. Excess cholesterol is deposited in blood vessels, where it forms plaque that can eventually choke off blood flow, causing heart attacks or strokes. (See Chapter 5 for suggestions for cutting back on dietary cholesterol and fat.)

Another type of cholesterol, HDL, lowers your risk of CHD by carrying excess cholesterol to the liver for elimination from the body. The higher your HDL level, and the greater the proportion of HDL cholesterol in relation to total blood cholesterol, the lower your risk of CVD.

In terms of blood cholesterol, how high is too high? A blood cholesterol level lower than 200 milligrams per deciliter (mg/dl) is associated with a low risk of CHD. A level of 240 or greater is associated with twice the risk.[36] The cholesterol level of the average middle-aged American is 215 mg/dl, which is higher than the recommended maximum level of 200 established by the National Heart,

**HealthCheck**
Check your cholesterol and CHD IQ
**H1702**

**TABLE 17.1**

**Classification of Blood Pressure Levels[35]**

| Classification | Systolic BP | Diastolic BP | Recommendations |
|---|---|---|---|
| Normal | Below 130 | Below 85 | Recheck in 2 years |
| High normal | 130–139 | 85–89 | Recheck in 1 year |
| Mild hypertension | 140–159 | 90–99 | Confirm within 2 months |
| Moderate hypertension | 160–179 | 100–109 | See physician within a month |
| Severe hypertension | 180 or above | 110 or above | See physician immediately |

WORLD OF *diversity*

## Women and Heart Disease

Heart disease is not for men only:

*Fact 1:* Nearly half of the 500,000 Americans who die from heart attacks each year are women.

*Fact 2:* Heart disease takes the lives of more American women than any other cause. More than ovarian cancer, more than lung cancer, even more than breast cancer (see Figure 17.9, next page).

Heart disease eventually affects one in two to three women, as opposed to one in eight who develops breast cancer. CHD typically develops more gradually in women than in men. Before the age of 65, women's risk of dying from a heart attack lags behind that of men by about ten years. That is, the average 60-year-old woman stands about the same chance of dying of a heart attack as the average 50-year-old man.[41] At around 65, women's risk level for CHD and heart attacks is about the same as men's.

**Close-up**
Women and CHD: Are you at risk?
T1706

Younger women may stand a lesser risk than men of CHD and heart attacks because of the protective effect of high estrogen levels. Estrogen helps keep levels of HDL cholesterol high. After menopause, however, estrogen production is cut and the risk of CHD rises. Artery-clogging LDL cholesterol also tends to increase after menopause and with advancing age.

Elevated blood pressure may also help raise the risk of CHD in older women. Blood pressure tends to rise with age. Though men have a greater risk of hypertension until age 55, the risks then equalize until age 65. Thereafter, the risks are actually greater among women.[42]

**Close-up**
Controlling hypertension
T1707

### Estrogen Replacement—Weighing the Benefits and Risks

The risk of CHD and heart attacks may be reduced by half or more in postmenopausal women by replacing the estrogen the woman's body is no longer producing. Studies show that postmenopausal women who obtain hormone-replacement therapy that provides them with estrogen have significantly lower risks of CHD and other cardiovascular disorders, such as stroke.[43] Estrogen replacement is also associated with lower risks of osteoporosis and colon cancer.[44] Moreover, researchers find the overall death rate from all causes is 46% lower in women receiving estrogen replacement.

On the other hand, estrogen-replacement therapy may increase the risk of breast cancer and uterine cancer.[45] Taking progestin, a synthetic form of progesterone, along with estrogen eliminates the increased risk of uterine cancer.[46] But the increased risk of breast cancer may not be as great as people had feared. The National Institutes of Health recently reviewed the scientific literature and concluded that hormone-replacement therapy posed only a slightly increased risk of breast cancer.[47] Still, estrogen replacement is not recommended for women with a family history of breast cancer.

### Why Do Women with Heart Disease Fare More Poorly Than Men Do?

Women who develop heart disease do not do as well as men. They are twice as likely to die after a heart attack, are more likely to have a second heart attack, and are less likely to survive after CABG and balloon angioplasty. Several factors may account for these worse outcomes. For one thing, women with heart disease tend to be older than their male counterparts, and age tends to worsen the outlook.[48] For another, heart disease tends to be recognized sooner and treated more aggressively in men than in women. This may reflect the traditional bias that heart disease is essentially a male problem. Complaints of chest pain in women may not be taken as seriously by women or their doctors as are such symptoms in men. This bias may explain why women are less likely to be referred for angiograms that can diagnose blockages in coronary arteries. Then, too, the drugs used to treat heart disease have been largely tested on men and may not work as well with women.

Risk factors that predict the risk of heart attacks in women parallel those for men: high blood pressure, smoking, inactivity, a combination of high LDL and low HDL, diabetes, and obesity. These conditions are either avoidable or controllable. For example, women with established heart disease can significantly reduce their risk of dying from a heart attack by lowering their cholesterol levels.[49] Regular use of low-dose aspirin may further reduce the risk of heart attacks in women with heart disease as well as in men.

**Close-up**
CHD and women: Be physically active
T1708

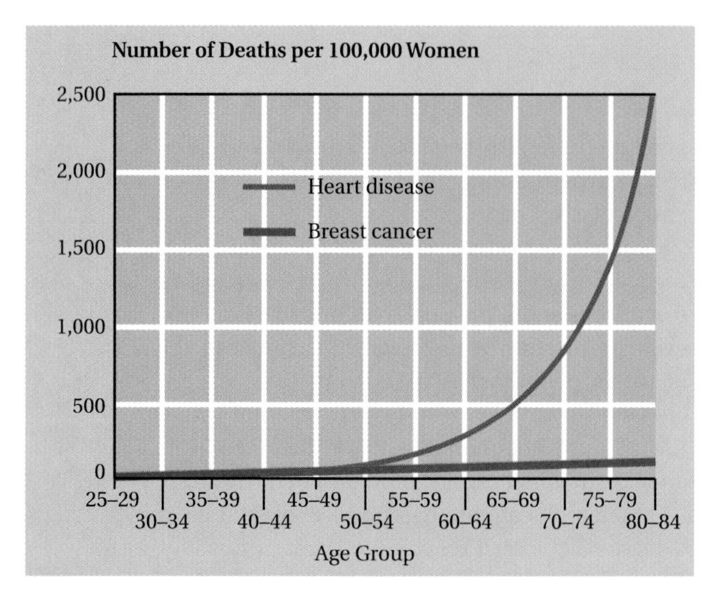


**Figure 17.9** ***Rates of Heart Disease vs. Breast Cancer in Women*** Though most women believe that breast cancer is the greatest threat to their lives, heart disease takes the lives of five times as many women as breast cancer.

Lung, and Blood Institute. A blood cholesterol level in the 201 to 239 range is associated with moderate increased risk.

Total blood cholesterol levels tell only part of the story. A more complete indication of risk comes from comparing levels of LDL and HDL and calculating the ratio of total cholesterol to HDL. Even people with low levels of total cholesterol are at elevated risk of heart disease if their HDL levels are too low.[37] A range of 130 to 160 mg/dl for LDL cholesterol falls in a borderline high range, while levels greater than 160 are associated with high risk. For HDL, a level at or below 35 mg/dl is considered undesirable. Ask your health provider to test your blood cholesterol and inform you of your total cholesterol and your levels of HDL and LDL. Then compute the ratio of total cholesterol to HDL cholesterol to assess your risk potential for CHD, as shown in Table 17.2.

High blood cholesterol is linked to an increased risk of CHD among older as well as younger people, although not as great.[38] Blood cholesterol may have less of an impact on people in advanced old age because their survival may indicate more resistance to the artery-clogging effects of high blood cholesterol. Nonetheless, controlling cholesterol is a good idea at any age.

**TABLE 17.2**

**Blood Cholesterol and CHD Risk Potential**

| Coronary Heart Disease Risk Potential | Total Cholesterol/HDL Ratio |
|---|---|
| Below average risk | 3.0–4.0 |
| Average risk | 4.1–5.0 |
| High risk | > 5.0 |

*Note:* For example, if your HDL cholesterol is 36 mg/dl and your total cholesterol is 200, your risk ratio would be 200/36, or 5.55. A ratio this large is associated with a high CHD risk.

**Triglycerides** **Triglycerides** are the most common form of dietary fat in the bloodstream. They are derived from fats and carbohydrates in the foods we eat. High triglyceride levels increase the risk of heart disease, perhaps because they are often connected with obesity and high blood cholesterol.[39] The National Heart, Lung, and Blood Institute has set a trigylceride cutoff of 250 mg/dl of blood serum or higher for identifying people at risk of CHD.[40] Other researchers set the cutoff at about half that level or even less.

**Diabetes Mellitus** Diabetes mellitus is an endocrine disorder that stems from an insufficient production or utilization of the hormone insulin. It increases the risk of CHD, hypertension, and stroke. Diabetes increases the risk of CHD by two to three times in men and three to seven times in women.[50] Diabetes damages blood vessels, hastens the process of atherosclerosis that can lead to heart attacks and strokes, and contributes to hypertension.

**Obesity** Obesity increases the risk of cardiovascular disorders such as CHD, stroke, and hypertension, in large part because obesity is associated with other risk factors such as high blood cholesterol. The risks of excess fat also depend on how it is distributed on the body. People with excess fat around their midsections ("apples") have a greater risk of cardiovascular and other chronic diseases like diabetes, and higher mortality rates, than do "pears" (see Chapter 5). Pears carry excess weight in the lower parts of their bodies, such as their hips, buttocks, and thighs. HDL cholesterol levels are lower in people who are apple-shaped than those who are pear-shaped.[51] Men are more likely than women to be "apples." Therefore, it is not surprising that men have higher rates of CHD than do women, at least until menopause, when women lose the protective benefits of estrogen. Whatever your shape, losing excess weight can help reduce your risk of cardiovascular disease.

**Smoking** Smoking more than doubles the chances of having a heart attack and is

**Triglycerides** Common fats found in the bloodstream, derived from fats and carbohydrates in food.

linked to more than one of five deaths due to CHD.[52] Smokers also have twice the risk of nonsmokers of having a stroke. Smokers are also much less likely to survive a heart attack than nonsmokers.

Tobacco smoke contains thousands of chemical compounds that are absorbed through the lungs and eventually enter the blood vessels, where they damage the lining of artery walls, making them more receptive to the formation of plaque. Tobacco smoke contains nicotine, which accelerates the heart rate and blood pressure. Smoking also increases total blood cholesterol while reducing levels of HDL. The carbon monoxide in tobacco smoke also competes with the hemoglobin in the blood for oxygen, reducing the supply of oxygen reaching vital body organs, including the heart. Smoking also raises blood pressure and increases the risk of blood clots by making platelets stickier.

The added risk of cardiovascular disease from smoking increases with the number of cigarettes smoked daily and the levels of tar and nicotine. Regular exposure to second-hand smoke in the home also increases the risk of CHD to nonsmokers.

The good news is that the excess CHD risk associated with smoking can be eliminated within two years of quitting smoking. The sooner you quit, the sooner you lower your risk of dying from heart disease. Quitting also helps protect people who live and work with you.

**Inactivity** Sedentary people have about twice the risk of heart disease as their more active peers and are also at increased risk of having strokes.

**Personality** The Type A personality is characterized by such traits as competitiveness, impatience, and hostility. Evidence shows a connection, albeit a modest one, between the Type A pattern and the risk of CHD.[53] If the Type A behavior pattern matches yours, consider following the steps outlined in Chapter 3 for changing your behavior.

**Emotional Arousal** Mental stress, especially strong negative emotions like anger and anxiety, may damage the cardiovascular system. Occasional feelings of anger or anxiety may not hurt your health if you are generally healthy. Yet chronic anger—the sort of anger you see in people who seem to be angry all the time—may be as dangerous to the heart as obesity, smoking, heredity, and a high-fat diet.[54] High levels of anxiety in middle-aged men are also associated with an increased risk of hypertension, a major risk factor for CHD and stroke.[55]

Laboratory evidence shows that mental stress, the kind of stress encountered when we are asked to perform under pressure, can provoke ischemic events (episodes of restricted blood flow to the heart) in people with CHD. People who experienced ischemia in response to mental stress turned out to be more likely to experience heart attacks and other cardiac problems in the future.[56]

Much of the attention given to stress and heart disease has focused on chronic anger or hostility. Anger or hostility appears to be the component of the Type A personality most strongly related to heart disease. Many Type A people have "short fuses" and get angry easily and often. This may cause them to have problems getting along with others and may put them at a higher risk of developing cardiovascular problems.

How might the emotional stress associated with anxiety, anger, or other negative emotions damage the cardiovascular system? One possibility is that emotional stress triggers release of the stress hormones epinephrine and norepinephrine. They, in turn, speed up the heart rate and raise the blood pressure. Oversecretion of these stress hormones over a long period might damage the heart and blood vessels, setting the stage for cardiovascular disease. Stress hormones also increase the stickiness of blood platelets, which increases the risk of blood clots.[57]

Acute episodes of anger may also have damaging effects on the cardiovascular system, perhaps even triggering a heart attack in vulnerable people.[58] In one study, researchers interviewed heart attack victims about their emotional state before their heart attacks. Heart attacks were more than twice as likely to occur in the two hours that followed episodes of anger than at other times of the day.[59] This finding underscores the connection between psychological states and cardiovascular disease. Avoiding "flying off the handle" may not only help you get along better with others, it may also protect your heart.

**Environmental Stress** Environmental stressors, such as chronic family conflict, poverty, and unemployment, can also take a toll on cardiovascular health. Job-related stress is linked to a higher risk of CHD, especially overtime work, conflicting demands, and a combination of high strain and low control, as found in waiting tables and assembly-line work.[60]

# HealthCheck

## Are You at Risk for Cardiovascular Disease?

This ***HealthCheck*** can help you determine whether you have any of the identified risk factors for cardiovascular disease. The more factors you possess, the greater your risk of having a heart attack or stroke.

| Yes | No | |
|---|---|---|
| ___ | ___ | 1. You are a male over the age of 45 or a female over the age of 55. |
| ___ | ___ | 2. You have or had a male relative under the age of 55, or a female relative under the age of 65, who suffered a heart attack or sudden death. |
| ___ | ___ | 3. You are overweight (weighing 20% or more than your recommended weight). |
| ___ | ___ | 4. You now smoke cigarettes, pipes, or cigars or quit smoking within the past 2 years. |
| ___ | ___ | 5. You live with a heavy smoker and are exposed regularly to tobacco smoke in the home. |
| ___ | ___ | 6. You have a total blood cholesterol level above 200 mg/dl, and/or an HDL level below 35 mg/dl, and/or an LDL level above 130 mg/dl, or a total cholesterol-to-HDL ratio of 5.0 or greater. |
| ___ | ___ | 7. You have hypertension (blood pressure of 140/90 or higher). |
| ___ | ___ | 8. You don't follow a regular aerobic exercise program or incorporate at least 30 minutes of moderately vigorous physical activity into your daily routine. |
| ___ | ___ | 9. You are often angry and hostile toward others or continually feel overstressed. |
| ___ | ___ | 10. You have diabetes. |
| ___ | ___ | 11. You are unaware of your blood pressure, cholesterol level, or family history of CVD, or are unable to answer any of the above questions. |

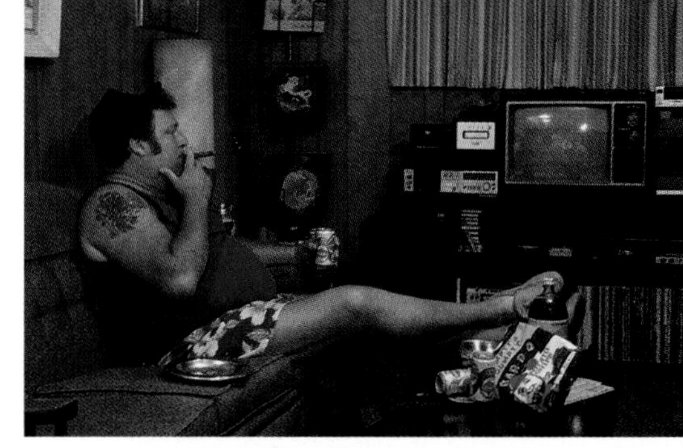

***How Many Risk Factors Can You Identify?*** Many of the risk factors for CHD are controllable, a message that seems to have been lost on this man.

If you answered "yes" to any of these questions, consider yourself at risk. The more "yeses," the greater your risk and the more important it is to take steps to reduce your risk potential—steps such as those in the ***Take Charge*** section of this chapter. If your present risk potential is low, you can *keep* it low by following that advice.

Frequent work shift changes may also be damaging to the heart, at least among women. A Harvard study of women nurses found that those who worked irregular work shifts over a six-year period had up to a 70% greater risk of suffering heart attacks than those working regular shifts.[61] As an investigator of the Harvard study put it, "Shift work is a type of stress. . . . If you disrupt the body's daily biological clock, the body responds by pouring out stress-related hormones. . . . These things generally do bad things for the body" (p. A28).

Smart Quiz
Q1704

### think about it!

- **What risk factors do you have for cardiovascular disease that you *cannot* control?**
- **What risk factors do you have for cardiovascular disease that you *can* control?**

**critical thinking** **What is your blood pressure? If you don't know the answer, what will you do to find out? If your blood pressure is too high, what will you do to lower it?**

**critical thinking** **What are your blood levels of total cholesterol and HDL? If you don't know the answer, what will you do to find out? If you have a cholesterol problem, what will you do about it?**

- **Agree or disagree and support your answer: "Since I have some uncontrollable risk factors for cardiovascular disease, it is useless to try to prevent it."**

# PROTECTING YOUR CARDIOVASCULAR SYSTEM

## Take Charge

It is never too early to make changes in your lifestyle to protect your cardiovascular system. If you're in your teens, twenties, or thirties, you may wonder why you need to be concerned about your cardiovascular health. After all, few people in your age group have heart attacks or strokes. The reason is that the seeds of a heart attack or stroke are planted many years earlier, sometimes in childhood. Silently, slowly, atherosclerosis and unrecognized hypertension may be laying the groundwork for cardiovascular problems. By taking steps now, you may well prevent a future heart attack or stroke. These steps are especially important for people with identified risk factors, such as family history of CHD or stroke, or with medical conditions such as diabetes or hypertension that place them at risk. The American Heart Association offers seven steps to help you protect your cardiovascular system.

### Don't Smoke (Stop If You Do)

Smoking is a major risk factor for CHD. It damages artery walls, which can accelerate atherosclerosis, and increases total blood cholesterol while reducing levels of HDL. Over time, these and other consequences of smoking impair cardiovascular functioning. The message is clear: Don't smoke. If you smoke, quit. If you live with someone who smokes, insist that they step outside to smoke. Better yet, encourage them to quit.

**Lower Intake of Saturated Fat and Cholesterol** The National Cholesterol Education Program recommends that all healthy Americans over the age of two follow these dietary recommendations to lower their blood cholesterol levels:

Take Charge
Lowering your blood cholesterol
C1702

1. Fewer than 10% of all calories consumed should come from saturated fat.
2. 30% or less of calories should come from fat.
3. Consume less than 300 mg a day of dietary cholesterol.

These recommendations apply to an average daily intake. If you exceed the recommended levels on a given day (a holiday, for example), reduce your intake below the recommended levels over the next few days to compensate. Table 17.3 offers some suggestions for cutting cholesterol levels through diet.

### Maintain a Healthy Weight

Keep your weight within a healthy range for your age, sex, and height. If you are overweight, use the weight-management techniques described in Chapter 6 or seek professional counseling. Develop healthy eating habits and make them a permanent part of your lifestyle. That's the best way to take pounds off and keep them off. Since fats contain more than twice the calories of proteins and carbohydrates, lowering your fat intake is a good start. Losing excess weight can also have other healthful benefits, such as lowering high blood pressure and total blood cholesterol while raising levels of HDL.[63]

### Control Your Blood Pressure

High blood pressure is a silent killer. It usually produces no symptoms and may go unnoticed until problems develop. Check your blood pressure regularly, at least once a year. If it is high, your physician may recommend lifestyle changes, such as cutting salt intake, avoiding smoking and excess alcohol, reducing excess weight, practicing relaxation or meditation, and engaging in regular exercise. Many people, especially those in the mild hypertensive range can control their blood pressure through lifestyle changes, without medication. Even if antihypertensive medication is needed, healthful lifestyle changes may reduce the amount required.

Close-up
Diet lowers BP
T1709

For people with high blood pressure, the American Heart Association recommends the following:

1. Know your blood pressure. Have it checked regularly.
2. Keep your weight at a healthy level.
3. Use less salt. Avoid salty foods or excessive amounts of salt in cooking.
4. Follow a low-fat diet.
5. Don't smoke. If you do, quit.
6. Take medications exactly as prescribed. Don't skip prescribed medication, even for a day.
7. Keep appointments with your doctor.
8. Follow your doctor's recommendations for exercise.
9. Lead a normal life in every other way.
10. Have family members check their blood pressure regularly.

## Check for Diabetes (Control It, If You Have It)

If left uncontrolled, diabetes can damage the blood vessels and increase the risk of heart attacks and stroke. If you have diabetes, your physician will help you control it through weight management, exercise, and, if necessary, insulin replacement.

## Manage Stress

When you're under stress, your body pumps out stress hormones that increase your heart rate and blood pressure. When the stress is relieved, your body returns to its normal state. But if stress becomes persistent or recurrent, your body can remain in an overaroused state for prolonged periods, which may eventually impair your cardiovascular system. You can help bring stress under control by avoiding unnecessary sources of stress and learning to manage unavoidable stress (see Chapter 3).

## Exercise

Regular exercise can strengthen the heart, improve circulation, reduce blood pressure, and help achieve and maintain a healthy body weight. Exercise can increase healthful HDL levels and relieve stress. See Chapter 7 for suggestions on incorporating physical activity into your daily routine. The American Heart Association recommends that people should engage in regular aerobic exercise: dancing, bicycling, cross-country skiing, hiking uphill, running, swimming laps, rowing, or stair climbing.

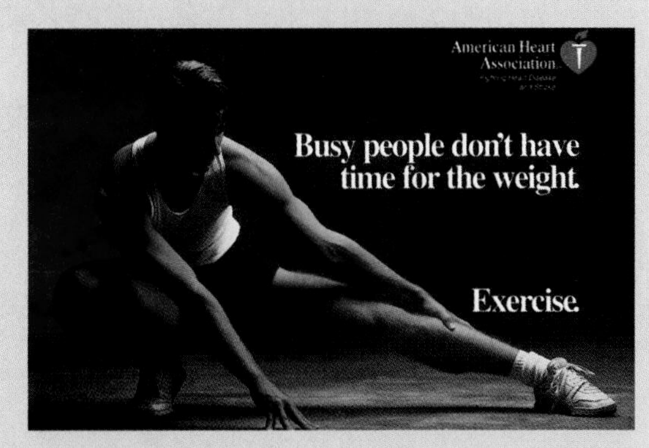
American Heart Association
Busy people don't have time for the weight.
Exercise.

## In Addition . . .

You may also wish to consider a daily regimen of 400 mg of the B vitamin folic acid and a low daily dose of aspirin. Folic acid may protect the heart by reducing levels of an artery-blocking amino acid homocysteine in the blood.[64] Aspirin may reduce the risk of heart attacks, especially after age 40 or 45. Some health professionals recommend a moderate level of alcoholic beverages (no more than one drink a day for women; no more than two drinks daily for men). There doesn't appear to be any advantage to the heart of any one type of alcoholic beverage (wine, beer, or spirits) over another, so long as alcohol is used in moderation.[65] Some health professionals fear that the potential health benefits of moderate drinking are offset by the threat of alcoholism and by a possible increased risk of cancer.* Check with your health care provider before using folic acid, aspirin, or alcohol.

It sounds corny to say that if you take care of your heart, it will likely take care of you, but it's true.

*Even as little as two drinks a day may raise the risk of some cancers, according to the American Cancer Society—see Chapter 18.

TABLE 17.3

**Cutting Your Cholesterol Level: What to Do, What Not to Do[62]**

| What to Buy More Often | What to Buy Less Often | What to Do Preparing Food | What to Snack On | What Not to Snack On |
|---|---|---|---|---|
| Lean cuts of meat, poultry, fish | Fatty cuts of meat, breaded poultry or fish | Trim the fat from meat before cooking | Air-popped popcorn (no butter); pretzels | Popcorn with butter |
| Skim or 1% milk | Whole milk, cream | Bake or broil meat; do not fry | Hard candy, jelly beans | Chocolate bars or other chocolate treats |
| Low-fat cottage cheese, low-fat yogurt | Cheese spreads and cheese | Cook meat on a rack so the fat will drip off | Bagels, raisin toast, or English muffins with margarine or jelly | Doughnuts, Danish pastry |
| Part-skim-milk cheese (like part-skim mozzarella) | Lard, butter, fat back, salt pork, shortening | Use fat or oil sparingly | Low-fat cookies (like Fig Newtons, vanilla wafers, gingersnaps, or Snack-wells) | Cake, cookies, brownies |
| Vegetable oils low in saturated fats and squeezable margarine | Toppings (like butter, cheese sauce, gravy, sour cream) | Take the skin off chicken and turkey | Fruits, vegetables | Milkshakes, eggnogs, floats |
| Baked potatoes, rice, pasta | Vegetables in cream or cheese sauces | Pack fruits and low-fat cookies as ready-to-eat snacks | Fruit juices and drinks | Ice cream (except low-fat ice cream or frozen desserts) |
| Plain fresh, frozen, or canned vegetables and fruit (without syrup) | French fries or hash browns | | Frozen yogurt, sherbet, popsicles | |
| English muffins, bagels, breads, tortillas, pita; cold and hot cereals | Doughnuts; Danish pastry; desserts like many cakes, cookies, and pies | | | |

Smart Quiz Q1705

# SUMMING UP

## Questions and Answers

### THE CARDIOVASCULAR SYSTEM

1. **What is the cardiovascular system?** The cardiovascular system consists of the heart, the circulatory system, and blood.

2. **What are the parts of the heart?** The heart consists of three layers: the *outer* layer (epicardium), the *middle* layer (myocardium), and the *inner* layer (endocardium). The heart contains two upper chambers *(atria)* and two lower chambers *(ventricles)*. The atria receive blood from the veins. The right ventricle pumps the blood into the pulmonary artery, and from there it travels to the lungs to pick up oxygen. The left ventricle pumps into the aorta (main artery), which branches into smaller vessels that carry oxygen-rich blood throughout the body.

3. **How is the heart rate controlled?** Pumping is controlled by the nervous system. Electrical impulses direct the chambers of the heart to contract rhythmically.

4. **What is the circulatory system?** This system is the network of blood vessels that bring oxygen and nutrients to the body and remove cellular wastes. Arteries carry oxygenated blood from the heart into increasingly narrower arterial vessels, which eventually connect to capillaries. Veins return oxygen-poor blood to the heart.

5. **What is blood?** Blood is the fluid that travels through the heart and circulatory system. Blood plasma (the liquid) contains red and white blood cells, platelets (which form clots), hormones, gases, antibodies, and other substances. Hemoglobin transports oxygen.

### MAJOR FORMS OF CARDIOVASCULAR DISEASE

6. **What is coronary heart disease (CHD)?** In coronary heart disease, the flow of blood to the heart is insufficient to meet the needs of the heart. CHD usually results from arteriosclerosis or "hardening of the arteries," a condition that makes artery walls thicker, harder, and less elastic. The major form of arteriosclerosis is atherosclerosis, in which fatty deposits called plaque build up along the inner walls of arteries.

7. **What is hypertension?** Hypertension is high blood pressure, which can lead to heart attacks, congestive heart failure, kidney damage, and stroke. Hypertension is defined as a systolic BP that is consistently equal to or greater than 140 systolic, or a diastolic BP consistently equal to or greater than 90 (140/90, or greater). Hypertension accelerates atherosclerosis. High blood pressure usually does not cause symptoms until problems appear.

8. **What is congestive heart failure?** In congestive heart failure, damage to the heart prevents it from pumping out all the blood it receives from the veins. Blood thus backs up or pools (congests) in the veins and elsewhere, such as the lungs and lower extremities.

9. **What is rheumatic fever?** Rheumatic fever is an inflammatory disease accompanied by fever that can damage the heart valves and kidneys.

10. **What are congenital heart defects?** These conditions are present at birth. The heart or the connections among the heart, lungs, and blood vessels fail to develop normally.

11. **What is an arrhythmia?** An arrhythmia is an abnormal heartbeat or rhythm. An abnormally fast heartbeat is called tachycardia. An abnormally slow beat is termed bradycardia. Other arrhythmias include ventricular fibrillation, atrial fibrillation, and atrial flutter.

12. **What is a stroke?** A stroke *(cerebrovascular accident)* occurs when the flow of blood to an area of the brain is blocked by an obstruction in an artery serving that part of the brain. The three major types of strokes are cerebral thrombosis, cerebral embolism, and hemorrhagic stroke.

### DIAGNOSIS AND TREATMENT OF CARDIOVASCULAR DISORDERS

13. **How are cardiovascular disorders diagnosed?** Health providers use instruments such as the stethoscope, blood tests, X-rays, electrocardiograms, stress tests, echocardiograms, radionuclide imaging, magnetic resonance imaging (MRI), angiograms, CAT scans, and digital subtraction angiography (DSA).

14. **How are cardiovascular disorders treated?** People with heart disease are usually treated with medication, balloon angioplasty, coronary artery bypass surgery, artificial pacemakers, or heart transplantation. Medicines include clot-dissolving drugs, beta-blockers, vasodilators, calcium-channel blockers, and pain-killing drugs (analgesics). Drugs may also lower blood cholesterol levels. Artificial pacemakers transmit electrical impulses that maintain a normal heartbeat.

15. **What happens when people have heart attacks?** Emergency medical system (EMS) teams in most cities reach people with heart attacks in minutes, apply life-saving techniques such as CPR, and stabilize them en route to the hospital. Blood tests are used to detect damage. Nitroglycerine may be used to increase the blood flow to the heart. Beta-blockers may be used to reduce the oxygen requirements of the heart. After the emergency is over, people who have had heart attacks are encouraged to make lifestyle adjustments that include quitting smoking, eating a low-fat diet, losing excess weight, exercising, and controlling blood pressure.

**16. What happens when people have strokes?** If the stroke was due to a thrombus (clot), clot-dissolving drugs may be used to disperse the clot or prevent it from growing. Rehabilitation is used to try to restore lost functioning.

## RISK FACTORS FOR CARDIOVASCULAR DISEASE

**17. What are the risk factors for cardiovascular disease?** Factors you *can't* control include age, gender, heredity, and race. Factors you *can* control include hypertension, blood cholesterol levels, triglycerides, diabetes, obesity, smoking, inactivity, the Type A (hostile) personality, and stress.

**Answer Key to *HealthCheck*, p.457**

1. *Yes.* People of any age may have diseases of the heart or blood vessels.

2. *Yes.* There are many diseases of the heart and of the arteries and veins. These affect various parts of the body besides the heart, including the kidneys and brain.

3. *No.* In most types of heart disease, death, when it comes, is not sudden.

4. *No.* Many people with normal hearts sometimes feel their hearts skipping a beat or beating faster or slower than usual. However, such events (may) be a sign of heart disease. In your own case, ask the doctor.

5. *Yes.* People of any age may have diseases of the heart or blood vessels.

6. *No.* The majority of people with high blood pressure have no specific warning symptoms. The only way to know is to have your blood pressure checked.

7. *Yes.* Often surgery can help or cure the child.

8. *Yes.* Some people with perfectly good hearts have slight murmurs. Your doctor can tell you when a murmur is a sign of heart disease.

9. *Yes.* Rheumatic fever is an inflammation that follows a streptococcal infection, usually of the throat ("strep throat"), and that may affect the heart. Doctors can usually prevent rheumatic fever by promptly and thoroughly treating streptococcal infections. Because susceptibility to rheumatic fever is greatly increased after the first attack, doctors frequently prescribe regular, continuous medication to prevent repeat streptococcal infections and subsequent attacks of rheumatic fever.

10. *No.* If the employer checks with a physician to make certain that an employee with heart disease can work at a particular job, there is no special risk.

11. *Yes.* Cigarette smokers have both a higher rate of heart attack and a higher death rate from heart attack than nonsmokers have.

12. *Yes.* Since overweight is a general health hazard, you are acting to protect your health by losing weight. Reducing weight may also lower blood pressure in some people.

13. *No.* Many patients recover and are able to lead normally active lives.

14. *No.* A pain in the left side of the chest is usually *not* due to heart disease, but should be checked by a physician.

15. *Yes.* High blood pressure is one of the most important risk factors in stroke.

16. If your answer is "yes," award yourself a medal of merit—but don't stop there. Work with your local American Heart Association to

a) let others know what help is available

b) improve and extend present services for people with heart and blood vessel diseases.

# References and Suggested Readings

## SMART REFERENCES FROM SCIENTIFIC AMERICAN

**Horgan, J. Mind over Body. "Explorations" from Scientific American's www site** (September 23, 1996). **R1701**

**Sinha, G. Cardiology: Pump It Up.** *Scientific American*, 275(5) (November 1996), 44. **R1702**

**Nemecek, S. Stroke Damage: A Strike against Stroke. "Explorations" from Scientific American's www site** (April 30, 1996). **R1703**

## SUGGESTED READINGS

**Diethrich, E. B., and Cohan, C.** *Women and Heart Diseases.* New York: Times Books, 1992. Focuses on the frequently overlooked problem of heart disease in women, with a step-by-step guide that women can use to evaluate their own risk.

**McGoon, M. D.** *Mayo Clinic Heart Book.* New York: William Morrow, 1993. Covers the anatomy of the heart and the fundamentals of diagnosis and treatment of heart disease, and offers suggestions for reducing your risk.

**American Heart Association and American Cancer Society.** *Living Well, Staying Well: Big Health Rewards from Small Lifestyle Changes.* New York: Times Books, 1996. From two of the leading health organizations in the country, the book offers suggestions for achieving maximum health by making small changes in your life.

**Zaret, B. L., and others (Eds.).** *Yale University School of Medicine Heart Book.* New York: Hearst Books, 1992. An authoritative and comprehensive guide to the heart and heart disease, presented in clear, understandable language, written by members of the Yale medical school faculty and staff.

# Combating Cancer and

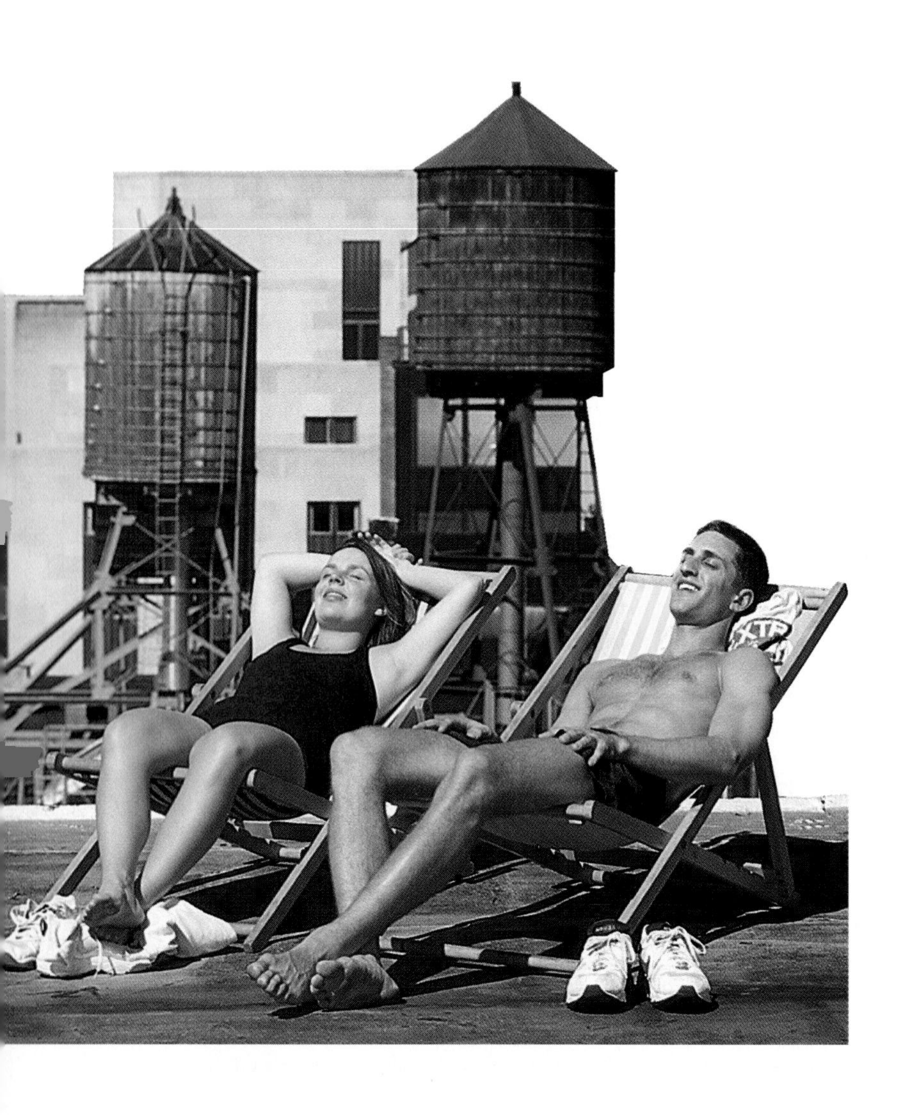

## DID YOU KNOW THAT

- Cancer is not one disease, but a group of more than 100 distinct diseases? p.484
- Some genes suppress cancer by curbing cell division? p.485
- Assuming you do not die from other causes, you are more likely than not to survive at least five years after a diagnosis of cancer? p.486
- Some kinds of cancer are often curable? p.486
- Smoking and diet account for nearly two of three cancer deaths in the United States? p.487
- Viruses and other disease-causing organisms may play a role in the development of about one case of cancer in six? p.488
- Colon cancer kills more women than cervical and ovarian cancers combined? p.495
- Tomato sauce may help prevent prostate cancer? p.499
- Viruses have been used to ferry corrective genes directly into the tumors of cancer patients? p.504
- Vaccines against several types of cancer are being developed? p.505
- Native Americans have the highest rates of diabetes in the world? p.508

# 18

# Other Major Chronic Diseases

Cancer *may be one of the most feared words in English or any other language. Fear is understandable. Nearly everyone knows people who have had cancer or who have died from it.*

*The statistics are not reassuring either. More than 1 million Americans are diagnosed with cancer each year, and about half a million die from it. One of every five deaths in the U.S. is caused by cancer. Cancer is the nation's second leading killer, after heart disease. If present trends continue, by the year 2000, cancer will become the leading cause of death.*[1]

Yet this chapter is not about doom and gloom. Cancer remains a life-threatening disease. But in many cases, cancer can be controlled. Some cancers can even be cured, especially when they are detected early. By following the advice in this chapter, you will achieve two health goals:

1. You will place yourself in lower risk categories for developing cancer.
2. By learning about the warning signs of cancer and screening methods for early detection, you will be better able to detect cancer at its earliest and most treatable stage.

**Cancer** is a chronic, noncommunicable (noninfectious) disease. Despite the threat of infectious diseases like influenza, pneumonia, and STDs, the leading causes of death in the U.S., Canada, and other industrialized countries are chronic, noncommunicable diseases such as heart disease, cancer, bronchitis/emphysema, and diabetes[2] (see Figure 18.1).

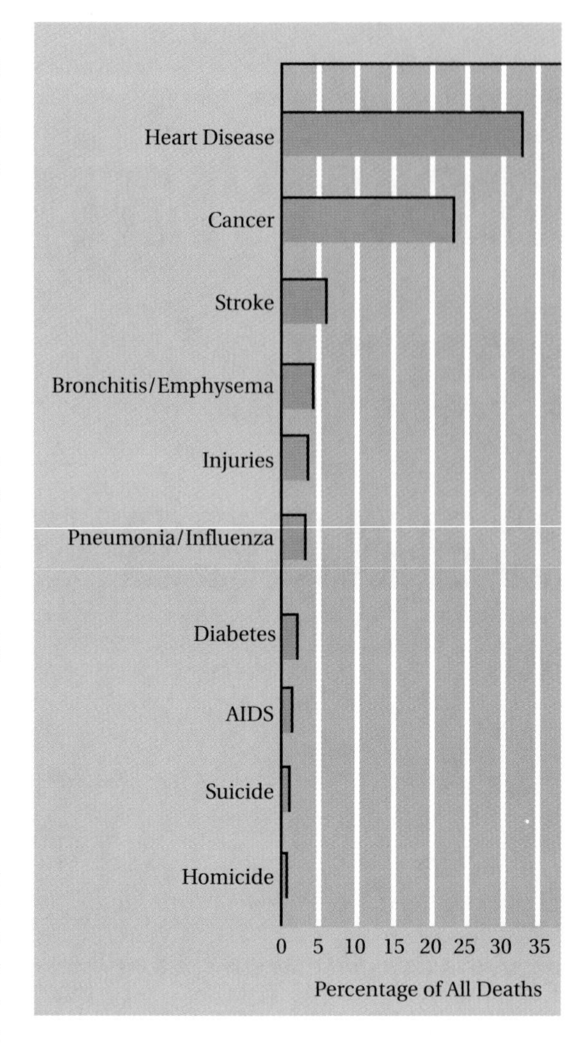


**Figure 18.1** ***Chronic Diseases—America's Leading Killers*** Chronic diseases are America's leading killers, with heart disease and cancer topping the list. Other killer chronic diseases include chronic bronchitis/emphysema and diabetes.

# WHAT IS CANCER?

**Close-up**
What is cancer? **T1801**
Metastatic cancer: Q & A **T1802**

Cancer is not one disease but a group of more than 100 distinct diseases characterized by uncontrolled growth of body cells.[3] Normally, new cells are formed by cell division only when the body needs them. Genes cause them to replicate themselves in an orderly way. In some cases, cells lose the ability to regulate their growth. They multiply when new cells are not needed, forming masses of excess body tissue called **tumors.** Tumors can be **benign** (noncancerous) or **malignant** (cancerous). Benign tumors do not spread to surrounding tissues. Only rarely do they pose a threat to life. They can generally be removed surgically and don't recur. Malignant tumors invade and destroy surrounding tissue. Cancerous cells in malignant tumors may also break away from the **primary tumor** and travel through the bloodstream or lymphatic system to form new tumors, called **metastases** or secondary tumors, in other parts of the body. They damage vital body organs and systems and in many cases lead to death. Figure 18.2 shows the ten leading cancer killers of men and women.

**Cancer** Diseases characterized by the development of malignant tumors, which may invade surrounding tissues and spread to other sites in the body.

**Tumor** A mass of excess body tissue or growth, which may or may not be cancerous.

**Benign** Noncancerous.

**Malignant** Cancerous growths capable of invading surrounding tissue and spreading to other sites.

**Primary tumor** The original site of a tumor or growth.

**Metastases** Secondary tumors that arise from the primary growth and spread to another part of the body.

**Mutations** A change in a cell's genetic structure that replicates in each cell division.

**Carcinogens** Cancer-causing substances.

**Talking Glossary**
Metastasis **G1801**

## How Does Cancer Develop?

Cancer begins when a cell's DNA, its genetic material, changes in such a way that the cell divides indefinitely. The change is triggered by **mutations** (from the Latin *muto,* "to change") in the DNA. Mutations are caused by internal or external factors. Internal factors include heredity, immune conditions, and hormonal influences. External cancer-causing agents are called **carcinogens** and

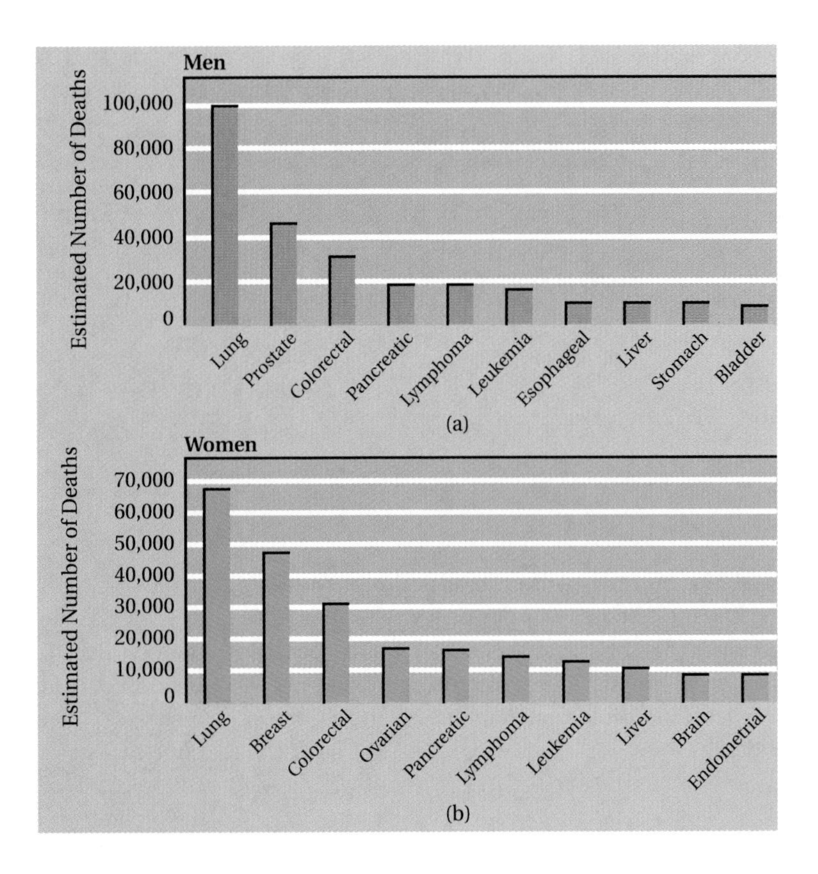


**Figure 18.2** ***Ten Leading Cancer Killers in Men and in Women*** Lung cancer is the nation's leading cancer killer of men (a) and women (b), surpassing the number two cancer killers—breast cancer in women and prostate cancer in men—by a wide margin. Reprinted by permission of the American Cancer Society.

include some viruses, chemical compounds in tobacco, and ultraviolet solar radiation. A combination of these factors may foster **carcinogenesis,** which may occur for ten years or more before cancer is detected.

Two types of genes play important roles in the development of cancer. One type are **oncogenes**—genes that normally induce cell division. The prefix *onco* is from the Greek *onkos,* meaning "bulk" or "mass." This is the same root as in the term **oncology,** the study of cancer. Physicians who specialize in the treatment of cancer are called **oncologists.**

The other type are **suppressor genes,** which normally curb cell division and suppress the development of tumors. The balance between the two types of genes helps regulate cell reproduction. Mutations on these genes can lead to overpromotion or undersuppression of cell division. Either path leads to the runaway cell growth (like a car with a stuck accelerator pedal and no brakes) that characterizes the development of cancerous tumors.[4]

## Cancer Trends

Cancer rates rose sharply during the 1970s and 80s, rising overall by 22% between 1973 and 1991.[5] Because the risk of cancer increases with age, part of the rise can be explained by the aging of the population. Part of the increase also reflects more widespread screening and detection. Other factors, too, underlie the increase, including a sharp rise in smoking-related lung cancer cases, especially among women.

On a more hopeful note, the overall cancer *death* rate has been declining.[6] Reasons for the decline include increased early detection, advances in treatment, and a reduction in smoking rates, especially among men. If we exclude lung cancer,

**Carcinogenesis** The process by which cancer arises and develops.

**Oncogenes** Genes involved in normal processes of cell growth and regulation; may give rise to cancerous growths if subjected to mutations or viral influences.

**Oncology** The branch of medical science dealing with the study of cancer.

**Oncologists** Medical doctors who specialize in the diagnosis and treatment of cancer.

**Suppressor genes** Genes that curb cell division and suppress tumor development.

TABLE 18.1

**Five-Year Survival Rates for Selected Cancer Sites[7]**

| Chance of 5-Year Survival | Selected Cancer Sites |
|---|---|
| Less than 10% chance | Esophagus, liver, pancreas |
| 10% to 29% chance | Brain & nervous system, lung & bronchus, stomach |
| 30% to 59% chance | Colorectal, kidney, leukemias, non-Hodgkin's lymphoma, oral cavity & pharynx, ovary |
| 60% to 89% chance | Breast (females), cervix, endometrial, Hodgkin's disease, larynx, melanoma of skin, urinary bladder |
| 90% or better chance | Testes, thyroid |

**Close-up**
10 important facts about cancer
T1803

death rates from cancer overall declined 3.4% from 1973 to 1992 and 14% from 1950 to 1990. Even lung cancer deaths have begun to decline, because more people have been quitting smoking. Smoking is responsible for about nine of ten lung cancer deaths.

## Surviving Cancer

At the turn of the century, few people diagnosed with cancer survived longer than a few years. By the 1930s, the odds of surviving five years had improved, but were still less than one in five. By the 1940s, the five-year survival rate jumped to one in four. By the 1960s, it was one in three. Today, about four of ten people with cancer survive five years or longer. Yet six out of ten people with cancer die within five years. Some die from other causes unrelated to the cancer, however. If we exclude those deaths, the odds of surviving cancer rise to more than half (54%) at five years.

Surviving five or more years is a widely used measure of success in the war against cancer, but reaching this threshold doesn't mean that cancer is cured. Some cancers return in people whose bodies have shown no evidence of the disease for five, ten, or more years. Breast cancer, for example, can recur in ten, twenty, even thirty years. For some cancers, five-year survival is a good benchmark for long-term survival. If there are no traces of lung cancer, pancreatic cancer, or stomach cancer five years after treatment, they will probably not recur.

The American Cancer Society considers a person to be cured of cancer if he or she shows no further evidence of the disease and has the same life expectancy as a person who has never had cancer. According to this standard, several million people are cured. Some cancers that had a bleak outlook decades ago can often be cured today, including Hodgkin's disease, testicular cancer, most skin cancers, some forms of lymphoma, bone cancer, and leukemia and kidney cancer in children. In addition to the millions who have been cured of cancer are millions more who are surviving day to day and year to year.

**PREVENTION**

### *Warning Signs of Cancer[9]*

Cancer often causes symptoms that you can watch for. The word CAUTION can remind you of the most common warning signs of cancer:

C Change in bowel or bladder habits.

A A sore that does not heal.

U Unusual bleeding or discharge.

T Thickening or lump in the breast or any part of the body.

I Indigestion or difficulty swallowing.

O Obvious change in a wart or mole.

N Nagging cough or hoarseness.

These symptoms are not always warning signs of cancer. They can also be caused by less serious conditions. It is important to see a doctor if you have any of these symptoms. Only a doctor can make a diagnosis. DON'T WAIT for pain: Cancer usually does not cause pain in the early stages of development.

**Smart Reference**
What causes cancer?
R1801

WORLD OF *diversity*

**Breast Cancer in African-American Women**

Close-up
Surviving breast cancer: Racial differences
T1807
Mammography and African-American women
T1808
Mammography and Hispanic-American women
T1809

Though white women are more likely to develop breast cancer than African-American women, African-American women are more likely to die of it. Why? African-American women are less likely than white women to obtain mammograms and breast examinations, which are the most effective ways of detecting breast cancer early, when it is most treatable. Despite a recent increase in breast cancer screening among American women in general, many African-American women, especially those who are poor, do not obtain screenings.

The National Cancer Institute (NCI) and other organizations have begun targeting breast cancer prevention programs toward ethnic minorities.[10] One example is the Save Our Sisters (SOS) program in New Hanover County, North Carolina, which forges links between health care providers and minority women. An older African-American woman from the community served as project director and conducted focus groups to identify the concerns of local African-American women. Many felt uncomfortable talking about cancer and felt detached from the health care system. Many had experienced discrimination when they had sought health care in the past. Women were more likely to turn to each other than to health professionals for support for "female problems." The SOS program identified people in the community to encourage friends and relatives to obtain screening for breast cancer. Such programs not only raise awareness of breast cancer and the importance of screening; they also provide access to health professionals.

Close-up
Mammography and Native American women
T1810
Mammography and white American women
T1811

## Racial Differences in Cancer

Close-up
Prostate cancer: Racial differences
T1804
Lung cancer: Racial differences
T1805

Cancer is not an equal opportunity destroyer. African Americans face an 8% greater risk of developing cancer than white Americans and are more than twice as likely to die of cancer.[8] Much of the difference in mortality rates is attributable to late diagnosis. Many African Americans lack health insurance or access to health care facilities. Many have negative attitudes toward the health care system, which may be seen as impersonal, insensitive, and racist. Therefore, they do not receive regular cancer screenings that could promote early detection and treatment. Early detection can be a life-saver for cancers such as breast cancer and colorectal cancer. There may also be differences in the underlying biochemical mechanisms involved in tumor growth between races. African-American men are also more likely than white men to smoke (African-American men have the highest smoking rates in the nation). Consuming a high-fat diet, implicated in colorectal and prostate cancer, is also more common among African Americans than other groups.

Hispanic Americans generally have lower cancer prevalence and mortality rates than non-Hispanic white Americans.

## Causes of Cancer

Close-up
More on signs and symptoms
T1806

There are many causes of cancer. However, smoking and diet account for nearly two of three cancer deaths in the United States.[11] The good news is that these causes are correctable.

**Smoking** People who smoke two or more packs of cigarettes daily are 12 to 25 times as likely to die from lung cancer as nonsmokers. Cigarette smoking is also linked to many other forms of cancer, including cancers of the mouth, pharynx, larynx, esophagus, pancreas, kidney, bladder, and, possibly, the prostate. All told, cigarette smoking causes 30% of all cancer deaths. Second-hand smoking also accounts for several thousand cancer deaths per year.[12] There may also be connections between smoking and breast and cervical cancer.[13] Other forms of tobacco use, including pipe and cigar smoking and smokeless tobacco, also cause cancer (see Chapter 14).

**Diet** Diet accounts for another 30% of cancer deaths in the United States. The prime culprit is saturated fat, especially animal fat, which is linked to some forms of cancer, including prostate cancer and colorectal cancer.[14] Following a diet low in saturated fat and rich in fruits, vegetables, and whole grains can reduce your risk of cancer.

An analysis of seven studies involving more than 300,000 women found *no* relationship between fat intake and breast cancer.[15] The mineral selenium taken in small amounts may help prevent cancer.[16] Traces of selenium are found in fish, whole grains, meat, and vegetables. Researchers caution that large doses of selenium can be toxic.

**Alcohol** Heavy alcohol consumption raises the risk of several cancers and is responsible for an estimated 2 to 4% of all cancers.[17] Heavy alcohol use is believed responsible for 75% of esophageal cancers and nearly 50% of cancers of the mouth, pharynx, and larynx. It may also play a role in stomach cancer and primary liver cancer, a rare but often deadly form of cancer.[18] It also appears that heavy drinking of alcohol raises the risk of breast cancer.[19] The American Cancer Society believes that the risk of cancer may begin to rise with as little as two drinks a day (10 oz. of wine, 24 oz. of beer, or 3 oz. of distilled spirits).

**Environmental Factors** Some chemicals are known to cause cancer in humans, including benzene, asbestos, vinyl chloride, and arsenic. Other chemicals are classified as probable carcinogens, including chloroform, DDT, formaldehyde, PCBs, and some hydrocarbons. Many of these chemicals are found in industrial settings and in household chemicals and pesticides. Another environmental hazard that can cause cancer is **ionizing radiation,** a form of radiation found in X-rays and **radon** gas (See Chapter 22).

It is prudent to limit exposure to known or probable carcinogens and to be vigilant about the quality of our air and water. However, exposure to environmental pollutants and sources of radiation (apart from the sun) is believed to account for but a small number of cancers. Most people are not exposed to heavy doses of these hazards. Moreover, their harmfulness pales in comparison to the cancer risks posed by smoking and unhealthy diets.

The federal government sets safety standards for chemical or radiation exposure in the environment and the workplace. Setting cancer safety standards involves a process called **risk assessment.** Evidence of risk derives from observations of people exposed to high doses of suspected carcinogens and from experiments with animals. Researchers prefer to err on the side of caution and set safety standards that minimize risks that may be small to begin with. With respect to cancer safety standards, the "acceptable risk" is the level of exposure that would be expected to increase the risk of one or fewer additional cases per million people.

**Sun Exposure** One form of radiation that does pose a significant cancer risk is **ultraviolet (UV) radiation** in the form of sunlight. Exposure to the sun is the main cause of a worldwide increase in all forms of skin cancer among whites.[20] Prolonged exposure can lead to the development of **basal cell carcinoma (BCC)** and **squamous cell carcinoma (SCC).** These are the most common forms of skin cancers that tend to occur later in life. They are relatively benign and can be removed surgically. Sunburns are believed to play a major role in the development of **malignant melanoma,** the most deadly form of skin cancer.

**Obesity** Obesity is recognized as a risk factor in breast cancer, at least for postmenopausal women, and may play a role in other cancers, such as cancer of the colon, rectum, prostate, gall bladder, kidney, and endometrium.[21] Preventing obesity, especially in middle age, may well reduce the incidence of cancer.

**Microbes** Cancer is not contagious, but infectious agents such as viruses, bacteria, and parasites play a role in the development of some cancers. Perhaps as many as 15% of all cancers (about one in six) are due to infectious agents.[22] Viruses—especially those that are sexually transmitted—are the major microbial culprits. For

**Ionizing radiation** Powerful, high-energy radiation capable of causing atoms to become electrically charged or ionized. Includes X-rays, cosmic rays, uranium, and radium.

**Radon** An invisible, odorless radioactive gas emitted from the natural decay of uranium; may pass from the soil into our homes.

**Risk assessment** A procedure for assessing the relative health risk of various hazards.

**Ultraviolet (UV) radiation** Part of the radiation spectrum of sunlight.

**Basal cell carcinoma (BCC)** A form of nonmelanoma skin cancer; easily curable if treated early.

**Squamous cell carcinoma (SCC)** Another form of nonmelanoma skin cancer; easily curable if treated early.

**Malignant melanoma** A potentially deadly form of cancer that forms in melanin-forming cells; most commonly found in the skin but sometimes in other parts of the body.

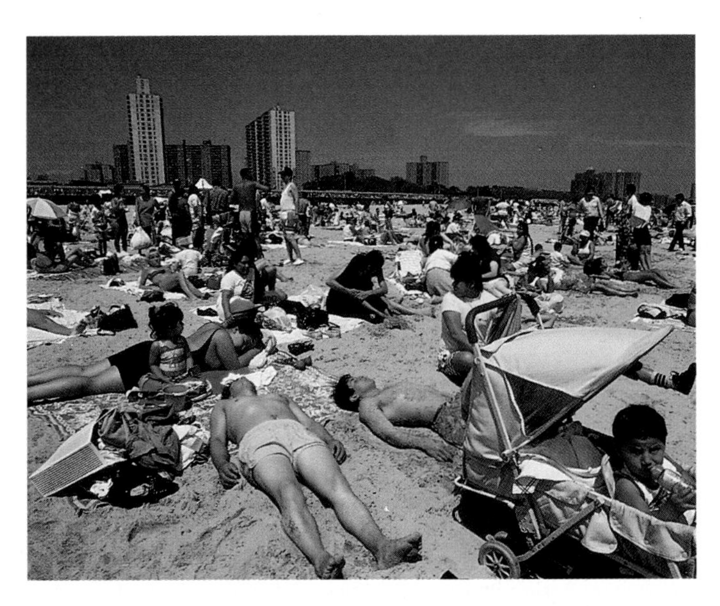

***Sun Exposure*** Increased exposure to the sun is the primary contributor to the rising incidence of skin cancer among light-skinned people worldwide. What are you doing to protect yourself when you go out into the sun?

example, husbands who frequent prostitutes or have affairs may bring home the human papilloma virus (HPV) to their wives, which not only causes genital warts but can also lead to cervical cancer. HPV far outweighs all other known risk factors for cervical cancer.

HIV, the virus that causes AIDS, frequently leads to Kaposi's sarcoma, a rare soft-tissue cancer that is characterized by the development of purplish spots on the body. HIV is also implicated as a risk factor in non-Hodgkin's lymphoma. Other sexually transmissible organisms, the hepatitis B and hepatitis C viruses, can cause liver cancer. The Epstein-Barr virus, which causes mononucleosis, is believed to contribute to some cases of cancer of the pharynx, cancer of the stomach, and several forms of lymphoma. Human T-cell leukemia/lymphoma virus-1 (HTLV-1) has been implicated in forms of leukemia and lymphoma.

**Close-up**
More on viruses and cancer
**T1812**

Some viruses inject themselves into the cell's DNA and activate genes that lead to tumor growth or *de*activate genes that suppress tumors. Viruses like HIV also weaken the immune system, making it less capable of ridding the body of cancerous cells.

The only bacterium known to be linked to cancer, *Helicobacter pylori,* is associated with stomach cancer. It apparently causes stomach ulcers, which may contribute to the development of the cancer.

**Genetic Factors** Hereditary factors are responsible for some cancers, perhaps 5 to 10%. People may inherit defective or mutant genes that lead to the development of cancer, including some forms of colon cancer, skin cancer, and breast cancer. Investigators have identified about a dozen genes that play roles in the development of cancer.[23]

One gene stands guard against basal cell carcinoma, the most frequent type of skin cancer, and suppresses development of these tumors. If the gene is defective, either because of an inherited mutation or a mutation caused by an external influence, basal cell cancers may develop unchecked. Damage to two other genes, BRCA1 and BRCA2, is linked to an increased risk of breast cancer and ovarian cancer. They may also be involved in pancreatic cancer, prostate cancer, cancer of the larynx, and breast cancer in males. These genes are suppressor genes that normally keep cellular growth in check. Defects in these genes can lead to the uncontrolled growth found in the development of tumors.

**Close-up**
More on genes and cancer
**T1813**

Other mutant genes are linked to other forms of cancer, including colon cancer, cancer of the pancreas, and prostate cancer. Men who carry a particular defective gene stand an 88% chance of developing prostate cancer by the age of 80, compared with 50% of the general male population.[24]

Genetic susceptibility to breast cancer is greatest in the early-onset form of the disease that affects women under the age of 35. About one in three women in their twenties who have breast cancer has an inherited form of the disease, as opposed to about 2% of cases of cancer in women in their seventies.

Knowledge about specific cancer-predisposing genes has opened the doors to genetic testing to identify people at higher risk of developing certain types of cancer. One researcher remarks, "With the explosive developments in molecular biology, physicians can now determine a patient's cancer destiny with a simple blood test."[25] But who should be tested, and why? Would you want to know if you were carrying a cancer gene? Would knowing you have a cancer gene make you more vigilant about screening or demoralize you enough that you'd avoid screening? Would the information stay between you and your doctor or be passed along to others? These questions are taking center stage in a developing debate about genetic testing (see nearby ***HealthCheck,*** "Should You Be Tested for a Cancer Gene?")

**Video**
Are you at risk? Testing for cancer genes
**V1801**

# HealthCheck

## Should You Be Tested for a Cancer Gene?[26]

It was once the stuff of science fiction. Now health professionals can peer into people's DNA and predict whether they're likely to develop some kinds of cancer. Only about 5 to 10% of cancers are thought to be inherited. But that percentage translates into about 50,000 deaths a year.

Tests can now detect mutations linked to an increased risk of breast, colon, and thyroid cancers and melanoma. The hope is that people who learn they are at risk may derail fate through medical treatment, diet, and vigilant screening for signs of the disease at its earliest, most curable stage.

Some diseases, like Huntington's disease, are linked to a single gene. But cancer may involve a combination of many genes along with environmental factors such as diet, smoking, and exposure to carcinogens. Inheriting a defective gene may increase the odds that one may develop cancer, but is not a guarantee. Nevertheless, some women with the inherited breast cancer genes have opted to have their breasts removed as a preventive measure. Conversely, the *absence* of such genes may not mean that the individual can throw caution to the winds and smoke or eat a high-fat diet with impunity.

**HealthCheck**
Should you be tested?
**H1801**

There are many questions about genetic testing: Should people be tested for diseases if they cannot be prevented or treated successfully? What of the costs of testing everyone concerned about his or her personal risk of cancer? Presently, doctors do not recommend genetic screening for anyone with a fear of developing cancer. But for people with an inherited predisposition to colon cancer, genetic testing can be a lifesaver. They can be screened early and frequently to detect cancerous growths.

**Close-up**
Benefits of gene testing
**T1815**
Limitations of gene testing
**T1816**

Society needs to deal with the health care implications of widespread testing to ensure that genetic information is not misused. For example, people who inherit "cancer genes" may risk losing their medical insurance or find it impossible to get life insurance. At least a dozen states have now passed laws that bar health insurers or employers from discriminating on the basis of genetic information.

Should you be tested? The decision is personal and should be made after thoughtful consideration of the benefits and risks associated with testing. Why not discuss the risks and benefits of genetic testing with a knowledgeable health care provider? If your health care provider isn't familiar with genetic testing, you can ask for a referral to someone who is.

**Inactivity** A sedentary lifestyle is believed to contribute to an estimated 3% of all cancers.[27] Sedentary workers have higher rates of colon cancer than physically active workers. But in some cases, workers in sedentary jobs may have other risk factors, such as obesity, that account for their increased risk. Thus, cause and effect remain somewhat unclear.

**Psychosocial Factors** Whether stress, personality, and social factors affect the risk of cancer remains a subject of debate. A recent study found no relationship between stress and the development of breast cancer.[28] However, psychological factors may be important in helping people survive cancer. Studies of people with breast cancer and melanoma found that social support helped increase chances of survival.[29]

Will you get cancer? Your risk depends on many factors, especially diet, smoking, exposure to the sun, and family history. Table 18.2 shows the risks faced by the average American for various cancers at selected ages. The nearby ***HealthCheck*** can help you assess your personal risk potential.

**TABLE 18.2**

**Risk of Being Diagnosed with Most Common Cancers[30]**

| Age | All Sites (Males) | All Sites (Females) | Breast (Females) | Colorectal (Males) | Colorectal (Females) | Prostate | Lung (Males) | Lung (Females) |
|---|---|---|---|---|---|---|---|---|
| By age 39 | 1 in 58 | 1 in 52 | 1 in 213 | 1 in 1,667 | 1 in 2,000 | <1 in 10,000 | 1 in 2,000 | 1 in 3,333 |
| By age 59 | 1 in 13 | 1 in 11 | 1 in 26 | 1 in 108 | 1 in 139 | 1 in 78 | 1 in 66 | 1 in 93 |
| By age 79 | 1 in 3 | 1 in 4 | 1 in 14 | 1 in 23 | 1 in 30 | 1 in 6 | 1 in 15 | 1 in 27 |
| From birth to death | 1 in 2 | 1 in 3 | 1 in 8 | 1 in 16 | 1 in 17 | 1 in 5 | 1 in 12 | 1 in 19 |

*Note:* These risks are based on the general population. Your individual risks may vary in relation to your personal risk factors, including family history and lifestyle.

Smart Quiz
Q1801

## think about it!

- Did you know what cancer was before reading this section? How do the facts differ from your earlier ideas?
- Why is it important to detect cancer early?
- Do any of the risk factors for cancer apply to you or to people in your family? How?

**critical thinking** Agree or disagree and support your answer: People should be tested to see if they carry any cancer genes.

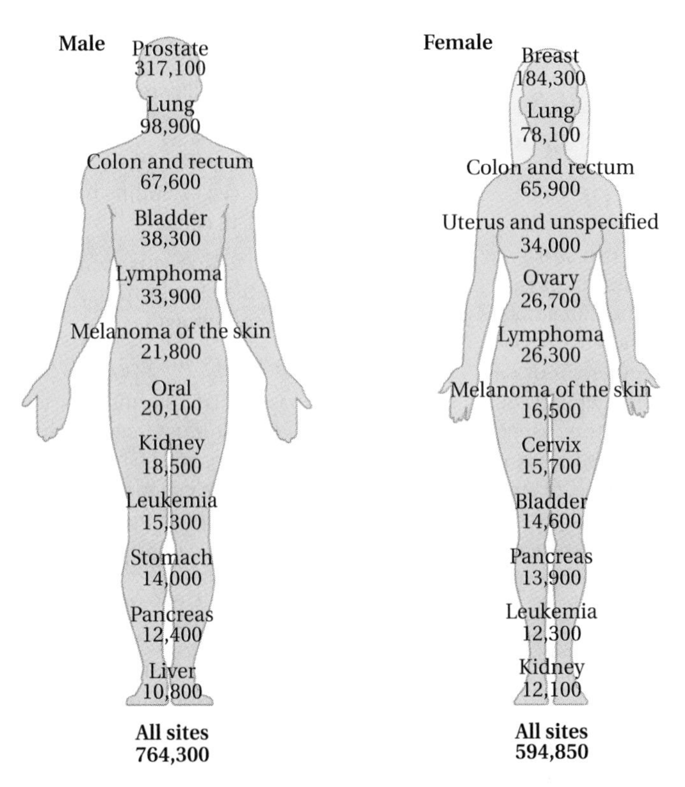


**Figure 18.3** ***Leading Sites of New Cancer Cases by Site and Sex, 1996 Estimates*** Though lung cancer is the leading cancer killer, breast cancer in women and prostate cancer in men account for the most new cases of cancer (excluding basal and squamous cell skin cancer and in situ carcinomas except bladder cancer). Reprinted by permission of the American Cancer Society.

# TYPES OF CANCER

Talking Glossary
Carcinoma
G1802

Cancer can develop in any organ or tissue of the body:

- **Carcinoma** is the most common type of cancer. It refers to malignant tumors that form in **epithelial tissue,** the tissue that covers body surfaces and lines body cavities. The most common sites for such cancers include the epithelial layers of the skin, the large intestine, the lungs, and the prostate gland in men and breast in women.
- **Sarcoma** is a malignancy of the connective tissue in the body, such as the muscles or bones.
- **Lymphoma** refers to cancer that forms in the lymph system.
- **Leukemia** is cancer that arises in the blood and blood-forming tissues of the body.
- **Melanoma** is cancer of the melanin-containing cells of the skin.

Most cancers are named after the organ or type of cell in which the cancer originally forms. The original site of a cancer is called the *primary cancer* or *primary tumor.* If the cancer spreads elsewhere in the body, these sites are called *secondary tumors.* For example, breast cancer begins with the formation of small tumors in the breast. It can spread to other parts of the body, such as the liver. The disease is called metastatic breast cancer, not liver cancer. Some parts of the body are more likely than others to become sites of secondary tumors, including the lymph nodes, brain, lungs, liver, and bones. Because of the risk that cancer may spread, it is important to detect it early, while it remains *in situ* (localized), where it formed. Figure 18.3 shows the leading sites of new cancer cases for men and women.

## Breast Cancer

One in eight women will develop breast cancer if she lives to advanced old age. Breast cancer is the second leading cancer killer among women, after lung cancer. It accounts for about one in three cases of cancer among women. Breast cancer can affect

**Carcinoma** Cancer originating in the epithelial tissues of the body.

**Epithelial tissue** Tissue that covers the outer surface of the body and lines internal body surfaces.

**Sarcoma** Cancer originating in connective tissues of the body.

**Lymphoma** Cancer forming in the cells of the lymphatic system.

**Leukemia** Cancer forming in the blood and blood-forming tissues of the body.

**Melanoma** Cancer of the melanin-containing cells of the skin.

# HealthCheck

## *Assessing Your Risk of Cancer*

Cancer can strike anyone; none of us is immune. But some of us are at greater risk than others. Your relative risk depends on many factors, especially your family history and lifestyle. Examining your risk profile can help you identify risk factors that you can change.

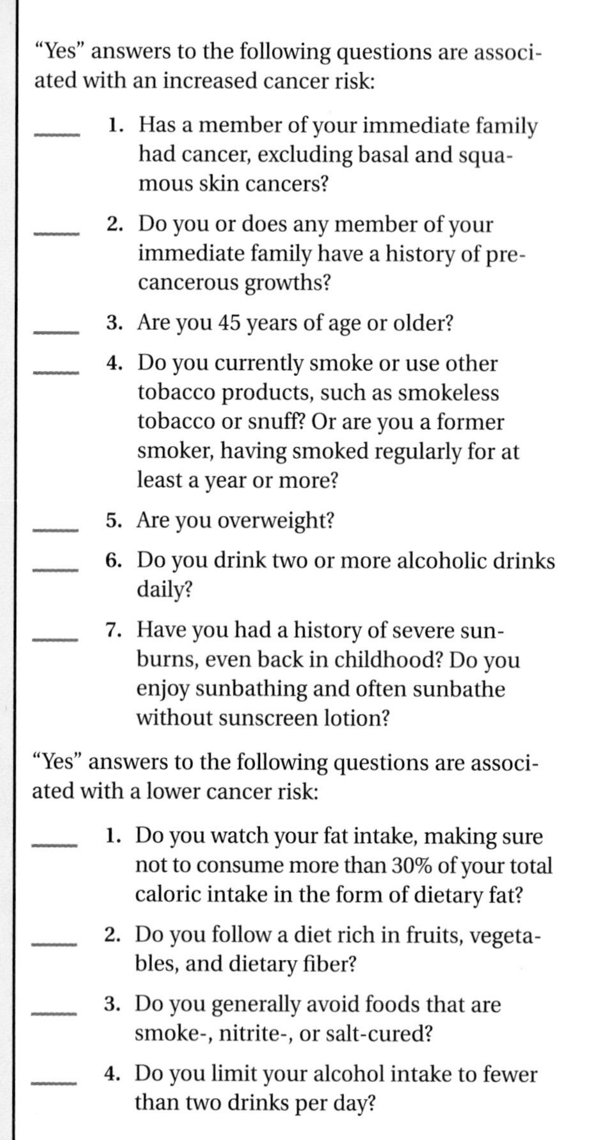

"Yes" answers to the following questions are associated with an increased cancer risk:

____ 1. Has a member of your immediate family had cancer, excluding basal and squamous skin cancers?

____ 2. Do you or does any member of your immediate family have a history of precancerous growths?

____ 3. Are you 45 years of age or older?

____ 4. Do you currently smoke or use other tobacco products, such as smokeless tobacco or snuff? Or are you a former smoker, having smoked regularly for at least a year or more?

____ 5. Are you overweight?

____ 6. Do you drink two or more alcoholic drinks daily?

____ 7. Have you had a history of severe sunburns, even back in childhood? Do you enjoy sunbathing and often sunbathe without sunscreen lotion?

"Yes" answers to the following questions are associated with a lower cancer risk:

____ 1. Do you watch your fat intake, making sure not to consume more than 30% of your total caloric intake in the form of dietary fat?

____ 2. Do you follow a diet rich in fruits, vegetables, and dietary fiber?

____ 3. Do you generally avoid foods that are smoke-, nitrite-, or salt-cured?

____ 4. Do you limit your alcohol intake to fewer than two drinks per day?

____ 5. Do you use sunscreen protection (SPF value of 15 or higher) when you go out in the direct sun for longer than a few minutes?

____ 6. Do you protect your skin from overexposure to the sun by wearing protective clothing?

____ 7. Do you avoid use of all tobacco products?

____ 8. Do you exercise regularly and take generally good care of your health?

____ 9. Do you get regular health checkups and follow recommended cancer screening guidelines given your age and family history, such as Pap smears, prostate cancer screening tests, clinical breast exams and mammography, and digital rectal exams?

____ 10. If you are a woman, do you regularly examine your breasts for lumps? If you are a man, do you regularly examine your testicles for lumps?

____ 11. Do you limit your exposure to environmental hazards such as asbestos, radiation, and toxic chemicals?

____ 12. Do you avoid tanning salons and home sunlamps?

____ 13. Is your diet rich in sources of essential vitamins and minerals?

No particular score translates into a precise risk estimate. The more "Yes" answers to the first set of questions and the fewer "Yes" answers to the second set, the greater your overall cancer risk. Examine these risk factors carefully. Ask yourself which risk factors you can change to help improve your chances of remaining healthy and cancer-free.

**Close-up**
Hair coloring products and cancer risks
**T1818**

younger women, but it usually strikes later in life. The average age at which women are diagnosed with breast cancer is 64. The average age of death from breast cancer is 67.[31] Three of four women with breast cancer are over the age of 50. Nonetheless, breast cancer is the leading cause of death of women between the ages of 35 and 54.[32] Nearly 185,000 women are diagnosed with breast cancer each year and more than 44,000 die from it.[33] Breast cancer in men is rare, with about 1,400 new cases reported annually.

The number of reported cases increased about 2% per year during the 1980s before leveling off during the early 1990s. The rise was due largely to the increased use of mammography, a form of X-ray that allows for early detection of breast cancer. Yet some portion of the increase remains a mystery. Lifestyle changes may be putting women at higher risk of breast cancer. Women today are having children later and, due to improved nutrition, girls are beginning menstruation earlier. These factors are associated with an increased lifetime

**Close-up**
Mammography: Q & A
**T1819**

exposure to estrogen, and estrogen may promote the development of breast tumors.

Though breast cancer has been on the rise, the good news is that the death rate from the disease is headed downward, thanks largely to improvements in early detection and treatment.[34] Overall, about 80% of women diagnosed with breast cancer survive at least 5 years and about 65% survive at least 10 years. The chances of survival depend largely on when the disease is detected. Women with localized breast cancer have about a 95% chance of surviving 5 years, compared with about 75% for women with regional spreading of the cancer and only about 20% for those whose cancers have metastasized to distant sites in the body.

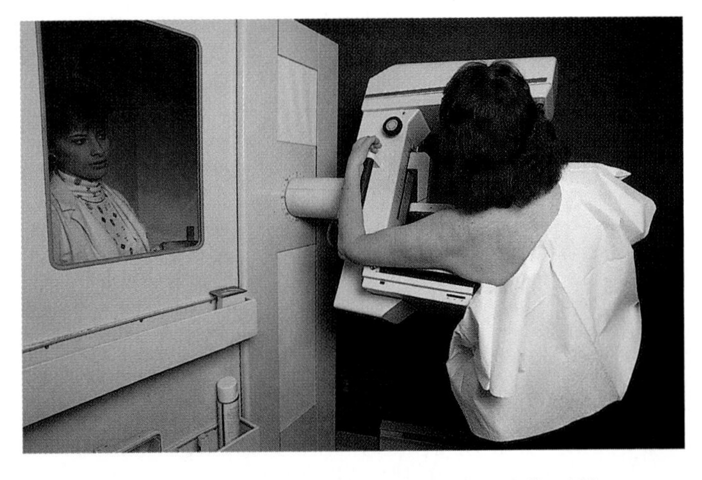

***Mammography*** Mammography involves a specialized X-ray procedure of the breast that can lead to early detection of breast cancer by identifying lumps that are too small to be felt by hand.

**Risk Factors** The primary risk factors are age and family history of the disease. The average 30-year-old woman has less than 1 chance in 2,500 of developing breast cancer. By age 40, her risk increases to about 1 in 200. Thereafter, the risk increases sharply with age, becoming 1 in 24 by age 60 and 1 in 14 by age 70.

Other risk factors include a history of benign breast disease and hormonal factors such as early age at menarche (before age 12), late completion of menopause (after age 55), few or no births, and delayed childbearing (first child after age 30).[35] These hormonal factors are related to greater exposure to the female sex hormone estrogen at a time in life when the breasts may be most susceptible to the cancer-causing properties of the hormone.[36] Though about 10% of breast cancer cases are believed to be inherited, 80% of women with breast cancer do not have a family history of the disease.

**Close-up**
More on risk factors
**T1820**
Genes and breast cancer: Q & A
**T1821**

Heavier women face an increased risk of breast cancer as they reach their forties and fifties. According to researchers at the National Cancer Institute (NCI), a 5-foot 5-inch woman in her fifties who weighs 145 pounds or more has more than twice the chance of developing breast cancer as a 118-pound woman of the same height and age. Her risk is even greater if she gained at least 10 of those pounds while she was in her forties.[37] There is a positive side to the NCI findings: Heavy women in their forties and fifties who lose weight reduce their risk of developing breast cancer.

**Close-up**
Breast cancer: What you need to know
**T1822**

Taller women also face a higher risk. Perhaps the hormonal factors that predispose them to greater height play a role in the development of breast cancer. The risks of breast cancer as well as breast cancer mortality rates also vary with racial and ethnic differences.

Some, but not all, evidence links oral contraceptives ("the pill") to a small increased risk of breast cancer in younger women.[38] This evidence cautions women who have a family history of breast cancer or other risk factors for breast cancer to carefully consider their choice of contraception in consultation with their doctors. On the other hand, long-term use of oral contraceptives reduces the risks of some cancers, including endometrial (uterine) cancer and ovarian cancer (cancer of the ovary), one of the deadliest forms of cancer affecting women.[39] Hormone-replacement therapy (HRT) is also associated with a slightly increased risk of breast cancer among postmenopausal women and with an increased uterine cancer risk in women taking estrogen without progestin (synthetic progesterone).[40]

**Close-up**
Breast cancer and "the pill"
**T1823**

**Warning Signs** Breast cancer often does not cause noticeable symptoms in its early stages or a lump sizable enough to be felt or seen, although it may be detected by mammography. Yet there are warning signs that should be brought to the attention of a physician:

- Any lump or thickening felt in the breast (see Figure 18.4, next page).
- A change in the size or shape of the breast.
- Discharge from the nipple.
- A change in the color or texture of the skin of the breast or areola (the skin around the nipple).

**Close-up**
Questions to ask your doctor
**T1824**

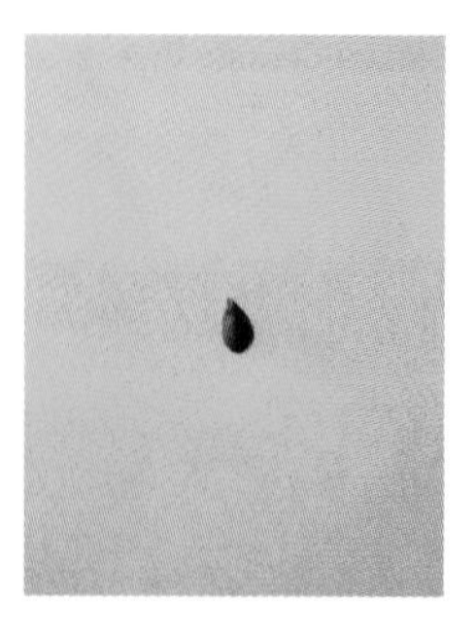

The average lump found by women getting regular mammograms is 0.3 cm. If treated when it's smaller than 0.5 cm, there's a 96% chance of cure.

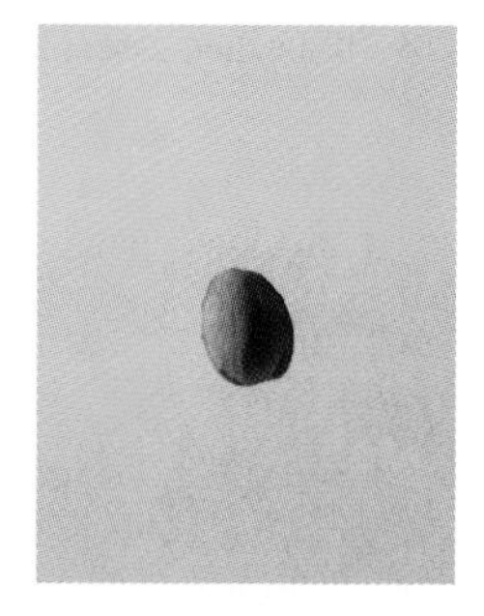

The average-size lump found by a first mammogram is 0.65 cm. If treated when it's 0.5 cm to 1 cm, there's a 90–95% chance of cure.

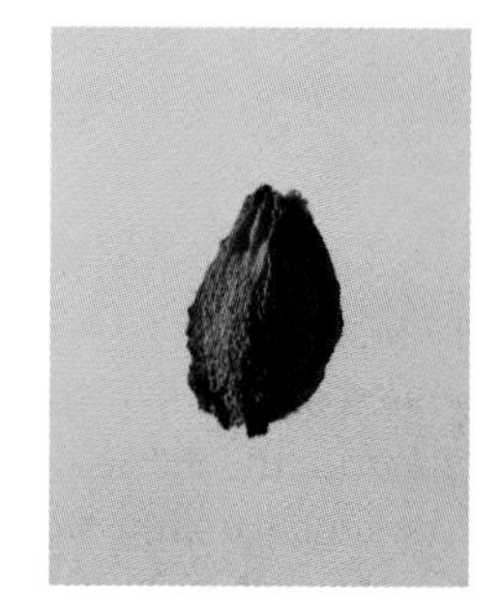

The average lump found by women practicing regular self-exam is 1.3 cm. If treated between 1 and 2 cm, there's a 85–90% chance of cure.

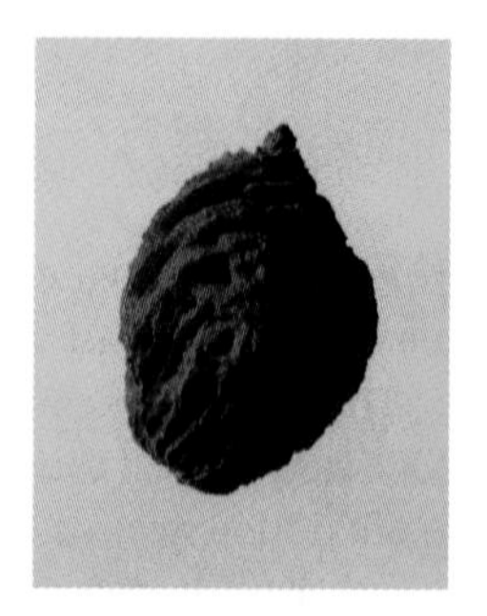

The average-size lump found by occasional self-exam is 2.6 cm. If treated between 2 and 3 cm, there's a 70–75% chance of cure.

**Figure 18.4** ***A Guide to Breast Lumps*** Source: *Self,* October 1996, p. 193.

**Treatment** The four standard ways of treating breast cancer include surgery, chemotherapy, radiation, and hormone treatment. A combination is usually used. Depending on the size and location of the tumor, treatment may involve surgical removal either of the tumor and surrounding tissue **(lumpectomy)** or of the entire breast **(mastectomy).** If the tumor has spread to the adjoining lymph nodes in the armpits, these too would be surgically removed. **Radiation therapy** (use of high-energy X-rays) and/or **chemotherapy** (use of anticancer drugs) kills cancer cells or stops their growth. **Hormone therapy** involves the use of drugs that decrease the estrogen supply to cancerous cells in the breast.

**Close-up** Treating breast cancer T1825

The decision to have a lumpectomy or mastectomy can be agonizing. Lumpectomy may be as effective as mastectomy in women with small or early breast cancers.[41] This probability underscores the value of early detection so that lumpectomy is an option.

Following a healthy diet and losing excess weight can also give breast cancer treatment a boost.[42] Overweight women with breast cancer are at greater risk of recurrences than their slimmer counterparts. Scientists suspect that enzymes in fat stimulate production of estrogen.

**Lumpectomy** A breast cancer treatment in which the tumor and surrounding tissue are surgically removed but the breast is spared.

**Mastectomy** Surgical removal of the breast.

**Radiation therapy** Use of high-energy X-rays to eradicate or shrink cancerous growths.

**Chemotherapy** The use of drugs to combat disease; the use of anticancer drugs to treat malignancies.

**Hormone therapy** The use of hormones to retard the growth of cancerous cells.

**Breast self-examination** A self-administered breast exam in which the woman feels for lumps or abnormalities.

**Clinical breast examination** A breast exam performed by a health care provider to detect lumps or abnormalities.

**Mammogram** X-ray of the breast.

**Prevention** There is no guaranteed way of preventing breast cancer. Nevertheless, researchers recognize at least two ways of lowering the risk: regular exercise and limiting alcohol consumption. Women who are 40 years old or younger and who exercise regularly are less likely than their less active peers to develop breast cancer.[43] As for alcohol, women who report having two or more alcoholic drinks a day have at least a 25% greater risk of breast cancer than abstainers. It appears that women who drink tend to have higher levels of estrogen in their bloodstream. Researchers are also studying whether tamoxifen, a drug used to treat breast cancer, may also reduce the risk of the disease in women at high risk.

## PREVENTION

### *Early Detection of Breast Cancer Saves Lives*

The American Cancer Society recommends a three-pronged strategy to help detect breast cancer in its earliest and most treatable stage.

1. *Breast self-examination.* Women should make it a regular habit to conduct a **breast self-examination** every month. (See directions in Chapter 9.)
2. *Clinical breast examination.* Women 20 to 40 years of age should receive a **clinical breast examination** by a physician or health care professional every three years and then annually after age 40.
3. *Mammograms.* A **mammogram** is a specialized X-ray that creates a picture of the internal structure of the breast.

Close-up
Importance of mammography
T1826

Smart Reference
Mammography debate
R1802

Women are advised to have regular mammograms every year beginning at age 40.[44] The National Cancer Institute recommends mammograms every one to two years for women in the fourties. Women aged 50 and over can reduce their risk of dying of breast cancer, on the average, by 30 to 40% by having regular mammograms along with clinical breast examinations.[45] Though evidence of health benefits from regular mammograms for women in their forties is less clear,[46] the American Cancer Society and National Cancer Institute believe it is prudent for women to start regular mammography by age 40.

In addition to lumps, women should also be sensitive to other changes and report them to their physicians. These include changes such as thickening, swelling, dimpling, skin irritation, pain, discomfort, or any change in tenderness of the nipple or nipple discharge.

## Lung Cancer

Lung cancer is the leading cancer killer in the United States. It is also the most preventable form of cancer. As an estimated 90% of the nearly 160,000 lung cancer deaths reported annually are directly attributable to smoking, achieving a smoke-free society would go far toward victory against this killer disease. Exposure to high levels of radon gas can also cause lung cancer, but it is unclear whether the low levels of household exposure to radon in many people's homes pose a significant risk.[47] Even so, why not test your home for radon and vent it if the levels are high?

Lung cancer is the third most frequently diagnosed cancer in men and women, after skin cancer and prostate cancer in men, and skin cancer and breast cancer in women. More than 175,000 Americans are diagnosed with lung cancer each year, most of them in the 50-to-80 age range. Though lung cancer typically occurs in middle and later life, the damage to lung tissue from smoking is generally many years in the making.

**Treatment** Lung cancer is especially deadly. The type of treatment depends on the stage of the disease and the extent to which it has spread, but it usually involves surgery to remove the tumor, together with radiation and chemotherapy. Five-year survival rates remain very low, only 13% overall. Still, there is a reasonable chance of survival (47%) if the cancer is detected and removed while it is still confined to the lungs.[48] However, since the disease produces few symptoms in the early stages, only about 15% of lung cancers are detected before they have spread.

Precancerous cellular changes can sometimes be identified before malignant tumors form. If smokers stop smoking at this early stage, lung tissues may return to normal, averting the development of cancer. Of course, smokers who wait to stop smoking until evidence of cancer develops may not be able to stop in time to prevent it. Some ex-smokers develop lung cancer years after quitting smoking.

**Risk Factors** Lung cancer rates parallel smoking rates. The disease is more common in men than women, and more common among African-American men than white men. Diet may play a role in the disease in nonsmokers. People who follow a diet rich in fruits and vegetables are less likely to develop lung cancer than others, even when the amount of smoking is held constant. Plant foods contain powerful disease-fighting compounds—phytochemicals—that may help prevent cancer. High levels of exposure to toxic substances, such as asbestos, arsenic, radon, and second-hand smoke, also raise the risk of lung cancer.

## Testicular Cancer

Testicular cancer is relatively uncommon, and it is also one of the most curable cancers if detected early. It accounts for about 10% of cancer deaths in young men in the 20-to-34 age range, mostly because of delayed diagnosis. Five-year survival rates are better than 95% when the cancer is detected and treated while it remains localized. Doctors will remove the affected testicle and may recommend chemotherapy to kill remaining cancer cells. About one-third of testicular cancer patients have an inherited predisposition to the disease.[49]

Close-up
Treating testicular cancer
T1827

## Colorectal Cancer

Colorectal cancer involves cancers of the colon and the rectum. It is the third leading cancer killer in the United States. About 55,000 Americans die each year of colorectal cancer. Colon cancer alone kills more women than cervical and ovarian cancers combined. About 7% of Americans will eventually develop colorectal cancer, which is the third most frequently occurring cancer overall, after lung cancer and skin cancer.[50]

Colorectal cancer tends to be a slow-growing cancer. It is rare in young people, with fewer than 6% of cases occurring in people under the age of 50. Overall, more than 133,000 Americans are diagnosed with colorectal cancer each year (about 70% with colon cancer and about 30% with rectal cancer).

**Risk Factors** A family history of colorectal cancer, familial disposition to develop colorectal **polyps,** male gender, advanced age, and a history of inflammatory bowel disease or polyps are risk factors for colorectal cancer. People with a family history of the disease have three to four times the risk of developing the disease than does the general population. Several genes appear to play key roles in the formation of polyps and cancerous growths. These genes normally suppress cell growth. If they become defective, they may be unable to prevent the abnormal growth pattern that leads to colorectal cancer.

Diet plays a role. The United States may be a world leader in computers and space technology, but it is also among the world leaders in colorectal cancers. Colorectal cancer is also quite prevalent in Canada and northern and western Europe, much more so than in less developed areas of Africa, Latin America, and Asia. Why? People in the developed countries consume more dietary fat, especially meat products. People in less developed countries eat more high-fiber plant and vegetable matter and less animal fat. These dietary factors—high fat consumption and low intake of dietary fiber—are linked to high rates of colorectal cancer. Fiber helps speed waste products through the colon and rectum, reducing the length of exposure to possible cancer-causing substances in the stool. Dietary fiber may also alter the natural bacterial fauna in the colon, which would affect the chemical composition of the stool. High fat intake may cause the body to secrete more bile acids needed for digestion, which may in turn irritate the lining of the bowel. Bile acids may also be converted by the body into secondary bile acids, which have been shown to produce tumors in animals.

Another risk factor is lack of physical activity. People who exercise more are less likely to develop colon cancer than their more inactive peers.[51] Exercise also helps speed the stool through the colon. No relationship has been found between physical activity and rectal cancer.

**Prevention and Treatment** The key to preventing colorectal cancer is identifying and removing precancerous polyps or growths. Colorectal cancer usually begins as benign polyps that turn cancerous after five to ten years. Since fewer than 10% of colorectal cancers are believed to be inherited, everyone needs to be screened for the presence of polyps and other bowel irregularities, not just people with a family history of the disease. The problem is that many people feel uncomfortable discussing bowel problems with their doctors, or they wish to avoid the discomfort of a rectal examination. Yet a few minutes of discomfort is a small price to pay for preventing a deadly cancer. Note the following recommended screening guidelines for colorectal cancer:[52]

1. **Fecal occult blood test (FOBT).** This is a home test for hidden blood in the stool. Fecal blood may indicate bleeding from a precancerous or cancerous polyp. However, the test may produce unreliable results, including false positives (blood from other conditions) and false negatives (some polyps do not produce regular bleeding). To detect intermittent bleeding, the test should be repeated over several days.
2. **Digital rectal examination (DRE).** This examination involves insertion of a lubricated, gloved finger into the rectum to detect the presence of abnormal growths. It is also used to check the prostate gland in men.
3. **Sigmoidoscopy.** In a sigmoidoscopy, the physician inserts a hollow flexible lighted tube to detect polyps in the rectum and lower third of the colon.
4. **Colonoscopy.** If polyps are detected or suspected from other tests, a colonoscopy may be performed. A colonoscopy allows the physician to view the entire colon and to remove

**Polyps** Bulging masses of tissue, which may become cancerous.

**Fecal occult blood test (FOBT)** A test for blood in the stool, used to detect the presence of precancerous or cancerous polyps.

**Digital rectal examination (DRE)** A test used to screen for colorectal and prostate cancer; the physician inserts a gloved finger into the rectum to feel for abnormal growths.

**Sigmoidoscopy** Insertion of a hollow, flexible lighted tube into the lower colon to detect polyps.

**Colonoscopy** The visual examination of the colon through the use of a *colonoscope,* an elongated instrument for viewing inner surfaces of the body.

**Talking Glossary**
Sigmoidoscopy
G1803

small polyps. This is typically performed as an outpatient procedure while the patient is sedated. Larger polyps may be removed in follow-up surgery.

5. **Barium enema.** A barium enema may be used in some cases to allow an X-ray to be taken of the entire intestines.

The American Cancer Society recommends an annual FOBT for people aged 50 and over, a DRE for people aged 40 and above, and a sigmoidoscopy every 3 to 5 years for people over 50. Putting off these tests can be a tragic mistake, since delays in detection and treatment can be deadly. Colorectal cancer can often be completely cured if it is detected in its early, localized stage. The disease is often "silent" in its early stages and does not produce any noticeable symptoms. Once symptoms appear—such as rectal bleeding, noticeable blood in the stool, diarrhea, and constipation—the cancer may already have spread, reducing chances of recovery. Unfortunately, only about one in three colorectal cancers is identified in the localized stage. Five-year survival rates plummet precipitously from 91% for colorectal cancer detected at the localized stage to only 7% for those in which it has metastasized to distant sites in the body.

**Close-up** Treating colon cancer T1828

Treatment for colorectal cancer involves surgical removal of any precancerous and cancerous growths. This is usually followed by chemotherapy and/or radiation to eradicate remaining cancer cells. Improvements in cancer treatment have minimized the need for a **colostomy bag,** an external bag worn to collect fecal wastes from an artificially constructed anus after surgery for colorectal cancer.

## Prostate Cancer

Prostate cancer is the second most common cancer in American men, after skin cancer. It is the second leading cancer killer of men, after lung cancer. Prostate cancer is the disease many men are reluctant to talk about or do anything about. We see public campaigns such as "Race for the Cure" bring together thousands of women to push for expanded breast cancer screening and research. Yet prostate cancer remains very much in the shadows. Few men know what the prostate gland does or where it is. Many confuse prostate cancer with an enlarged prostate, which is a noncancerous condition. Yet, like breast cancer a generation earlier, increasing public attention to prostate cancer is beginning to raise awareness.

**Close-up** Prostate cancer: Seeking answers T1829

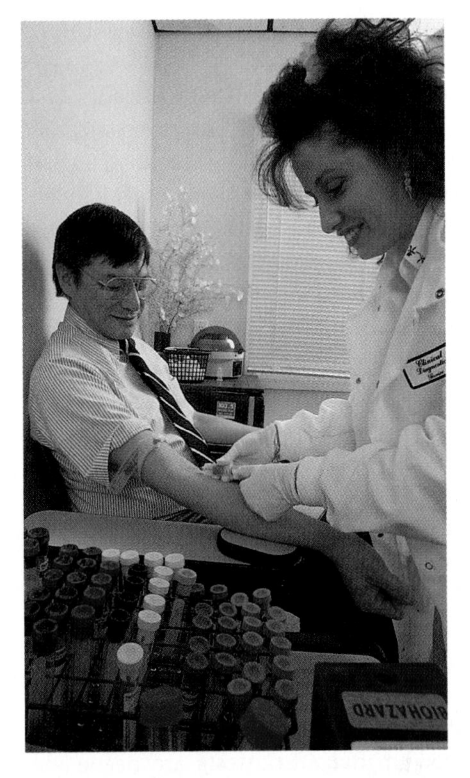


***Does This Man Have Prostate Cancer?*** The PSA test analyzes a sample of blood for levels of an enzyme, prostate-specific antigen (PSA), which is often elevated in men who have prostate cancer. However, follow-up tests are needed to pinpoint a diagnosis.

The prostate is a male sex gland. It secretes most of the seminal fluid, the milky medium that carries sperm. The prostate is about the size of a walnut. It is located below the bladder and surrounds the upper urethra, the tube through which urine passes. If it becomes enlarged, which often occurs as the man grows older, it can obstruct the flow of urine and may need to be reduced through medication or surgery.

Prostate cancer is a much more serious threat. It strikes roughly one in ten American men and claims the lives of about three men in a hundred.[53] Many men with prostate cancer don't know they have the disease, since it typically does not produce any symptoms in its early stages. Like breast cancer, prostate cancer generally occurs later in life. It usually strikes men in their seventies, although it can hit men under 55, usually in a more aggressive form.

Since prostate cancer primarily affects older men and usually grows slowly, most men with the disease eventually die of other causes. For some, the disease is far more aggressive. It spreads rapidly and causes disability and premature death. Each year about 300,000 men are diag-

**Barium enema** An enema administers radioactive barium to facilitate X-rays of the lower intestinal tract.

**Colostomy bag** A bag worn outside of the body to collect fecal waste following surgical removal of the bowel.

nosed with prostate cancer and about 40,000 die of the disease.

The good news about prostate cancer is that five-year survival rates have improved steadily during the past 50 years. Today, more than 85% of men diagnosed with prostate cancer will be alive five years later, compared with 50% 30 years ago. In men with localized prostate cancer in which the cancer has not spread beyond the prostate, the five-year survival rate jumps to 99%.

Though the incidence of prostate cancer has been rising in recent years, medical researchers believe that the increase reflects improved screening and early detection rather than changes in underlying disease patterns. Early detection received a significant boost with the introduction of a blood test that measures the levels in the blood of an enzyme, **prostate-specific antigen (PSA),** which is often elevated in men with prostate cancer. However, there are many false positive results because high PSA levels may also be caused by an enlarged prostate or other conditions. Follow-up diagnostic tests are needed to pinpoint a diagnosis, typically a biopsy in which a sample of prostate tissue is removed and examined for cancerous growths. **Ultrasound imaging** may be used to estimate the size of the prostate and guide a biopsy.

**Smart Reference**
Does screening make sense?
R1803

**Early Detection** Early, localized prostate cancer does not usually produce pain or other symptoms. Men may notice some difficulty in urination, but such symptoms are more often associated with other causes, such as an enlarged prostate or **prostatitis.** The American Cancer Society recommends annual prostate cancer screening exams for men 40 and older. Men 40 to 49 should receive a digital rectal exam (DRE). For men aged 50 and above, the annual DRE should be combined with a PSA test. The PSA test improves detection of localized prostate cancers that might otherwise go undetected, but does not distinguish men with early prostate cancer who require surgical removal of the prostate from those who might be just as well off if the physician takes a "wait and watch" approach.[54] Nor is it certain that screening reduces the mortality rate or extends the lives of people with prostate cancer.[55] Still, early detection gives men the opportunity to make treatment decisions before the cancer reaches a more advanced stage.

**Talking Glossary**
Prostatitis
G1804

**Prostate-specific antigen (PSA)** An enzyme produced in the epithelial cells of the prostate gland. Abnormally high blood levels of PSA may indicate prostate cancer.

**Ultrasound imaging** High-frequency sound waves are used to produce an image of organs or tissues.

**Prostatitis** An inflammation of the prostate gland.

**Radical prostatectomy** Surgical removal of the entire prostate gland.

**Treatment** The choice of treatment depends on the stage of development of the cancer, the man's age, and his general health. For men with localized cancers of the prostate, one treatment alternative is surgical removal of the prostate, termed **radical prostatectomy.** Removal minimizes the risk that the cancer will spread to other organs. A major study found that 87% of the men with early prostate cancer who had their prostates removed showed no evidence that the cancer had spread 10 years later.[56] But surgery sometimes produces the side effects of urinary incontinence (loss of control over urinating) and impotence (problems obtaining and maintaining erection).

**Talking Glossary**
Radical prostatectomy
G1805

**Close-up**
Treating prostate cancer
T1830

Alternative treatments include radiation therapy, which kills or shrinks cancer cells lurking within the gland, and hormone therapy. Since the male sex hormone testosterone stimulates the growth of prostate cancer cells, in hormone therapy, hormones or hormone-blocking drugs are used to reduce or suppress the body's production of testosterone. Some men with early prostate cancer may prefer a "wait and watch" approach to surgery and radiation, especially men over 65, who are not likely to experience significant disability or have their lives cut short because of these slow-growing cancers.[57] Prostate cancer that has metastasized has a poorer outcome and is usually treated with a combination of radiation therapy, chemotherapy, and hormone therapy to slow the progression of the disease.

**Close-up**
Early prostate cancer: Q & A
T1831

**Risk Factors** The primary risk factor for prostate cancer is age. Other risk factors include race, family history, and diet.[58] African-American men have the highest incidence of prostate cancer in the world—50% higher than that of white American men. They are also more than twice as likely to die of the disease, probably because of more limited access to health care and screening.[59] When African-American men with localized prostate cancer have equal access to health care, they survive as often as white men do. Biological factors may also help account for the greater rates of prostate cancer among African-American men. For example, African-American men may have higher levels of hormones that promote prostate cancer.

Genetic factors also appear to be involved. Men with a family history of prostate cancer, especially in fathers or brothers, are at higher risk of developing the disease. Dietary fat may also play a role. Men in countries like China and Japan, where low-fat, high-fiber diets are the norm, have much lower rates of prostate cancer than men in northwestern Europe and North America, where fat intake is much higher.[60] Prostate cancer rates for first- and second-generation Japanese-American men are also higher than those for Japanese men in Japan, a difference that probably reflects the higher-fat Western diet. Two other factors have emerged as possible risk factors: cigarette smoking and vasectomy.[61]

**Close-up**
Vasectomy: A possible risk factor
**T1832**

**Prevention** Since prostate cancer may be linked to dietary fat, it makes sense for men to curb their intake of fatty foods. Reducing fat intake may also help prevent other health problems, including cardiovascular disease and adult-onset diabetes. Tomatoes may also be of help. Yes, tomatoes. Men who eat more cooked tomato products, such as tomato sauce, have a lower risk of developing prostate cancer.[62] A plant chemical called *lycopene,* the carotenoid that makes tomatoes red, may be the preventive agent. And as noted in nearly every chapter in this book, if you haven't started smoking, *don't.* If you do smoke, think about quitting.

## Skin Cancer

Skin cancer is the most common and most rapidly increasing type of cancer in the United States. It affects one in six Americans.[63] Two possible reasons for the increase are the popularity of sunbathing and the thinning of the ozone layer of the atmosphere. The ozone layer surrounding the earth filters harmful ultraviolet (UV) radiation from the sun.

The three major types of skin cancer include basal cell and squamous cell carcinomas, which are highly curable, and the more threatening malignant melanoma. Over 800,000 new cases of basal and squamous cell carcinoma, and more than 38,000 cases of malignant melanoma, occur each year in the United States. Skin cancer claims more than 7,300 lives each year, with malignant melanoma accounting for more than three of four of these deaths.

Basal cell carcinoma and squamous cell carcinoma are referred to as **nonmelanoma skin cancers.** Basal cell carcinoma (BCC) is a translucent, pearly raised tumor found mostly on the skin of the face, neck, hands, and trunk. The tumor may crust, ulcerate, and bleed. Squamous cell carcinoma (SCC) is a raised red or pink nodule that generally appears on the face, hands, or ears. It may grow and spread to other parts of the body. Early detection and treatment leads to a cure in 95% or more cases of nonmelanoma skin cancers. They primarily affect older people after a lifetime of exposure to the sun.[64]

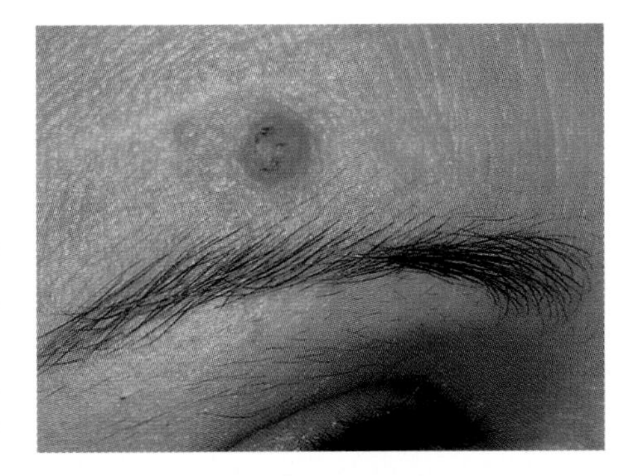
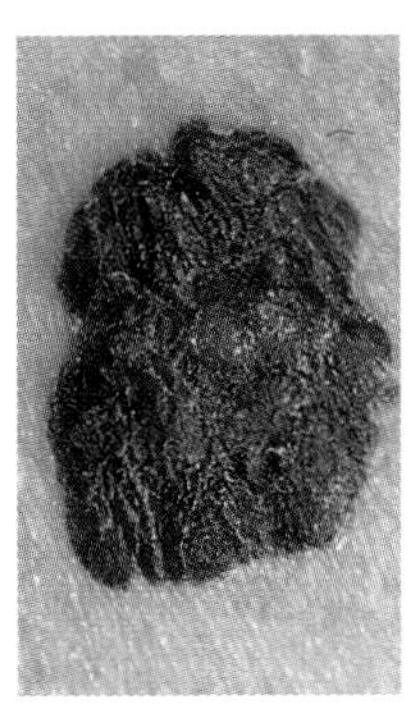

**Figure 18.5** ***Major Types of Skin Cancer*** (a) The two forms of nonmelanoma skin cancer, basal cell carcinoma (shown here) and squamous cell carcinoma, are the most common forms of skin cancer and the most easily treatable when detected early. (b) A melanoma, like the one shown here on a lower leg, is the most deadly form of skin cancer, accounting for more than 7,000 deaths annually in the U.S.

**Talking Glossary**
Malignant melanoma
**G1806**

Malignant melanoma (sometimes just called *melanoma*) has been increasing about 4% a year in the United States, due mainly to increased sun exposure. Melanomas are ten times more common in white people than in African Americans.

Melanoma usually begins as a small, molelike growth that enlarges, changes color, ulcerates, and bleeds from the slightest injuries. Melanomas may be flat or raised. They sometimes develop from existing moles. Unlike *non*melanoma skin cancers, which mainly affect older people, melanomas often occur during young and middle adulthood. If they go untreated, they can spread rapidly and invade organs such as the lungs and liver. There is an excellent chance of cure if they are detected early, but the prospects are dim after they have spread. The good news is that survival rates for melanoma are on the rise, thanks largely to better early detection.[65]

**Nonmelanoma skin cancers** Skin cancers other than melanoma, including basal cell and squamous cell carcinomas.

**Risk Factors** *Sun, sun, sun.* No, this is not a refrain from an old Beach Boys' song. It is the principal risk factor for skin cancer. The same sun that sustains life on earth and provides that popular tan can also prematurely age and wrinkle the skin, giving it a leathery appearance, and cause skin cancer. Two types of ultraviolet radiation found in sunlight, **ultraviolet A (UVA)** and **ultraviolet B (UVB),** are largely responsible for skin damage and skin cancer. UVB rays quickly redden the skin, producing dangerous sunburns. They are responsible for more than 90% of skin cancers and are especially dangerous because they can damage cellular DNA.[66] UVA rays, once thought to be harmless "tanning" rays, can also penetrate the inner layers of skin, causing premature aging. UVA rays can also damage blood vessels and impair immune system functioning. Moreover, UVA radiation makes the skin more sensitive to sunlight, so that exposure becomes yet more dangerous.

Cumulative sun exposure over many years is thought to be responsible for most nonmelanoma skin cancers. Frequent sunburns are suspected to be the major cause of melanoma. Lighter-skinned people and people with more sensitive skin who burn easily are at greater risk of skin cancer. Severe sunburns, including those you had as a child, increase your chances of developing melanoma. Parents thus need to protect children from the sun. Nearly 80% of a person's lifetime exposure to the sun occurs before age 18.

**Prevention** Preventing skin cancer and minimizing its damage rests on adoption of sun-sensible behaviors (see ***Take Charge*** section) and early detection by means of regular self-examinations and head-to-toe medical examinations. But many people remain in the dark about skin cancer. Only about half of the men and a third of the women polled by the Centers for Disease Control recognized the word *melanoma.* Even fewer, only one in four, could identify the early signs of melanoma.[67]

Many people have turned to tanning salons in the belief that they offer a safe way to tan. Wrong. Evidence links tanning lamps to skin cancer, including both basal cell carcinoma and malignant melanoma.[68] Because their lamps rely mainly on ultraviolet A (UVA) radiation and are less likely to burn the skin, tanning salons would have you believe that they are safe. They do not say (or do not know) that both types of ultraviolet radiation (UVA and UVB) can damage the skin and promote skin cancer. Save your money and your skin. Stay out of tanning salons. Home sunlamps are no safer.

**Ultraviolet A (UVA)** A form of ultraviolet radiation from sunlight that can damage the skin and eyes.

**Ultraviolet B (UVB)** A more dangerous form of ultraviolet radiation from sunlight that is principally responsible for sunburns.

In addition to sun, a high-fat diet may also promote the growth of basal and squamous cell carcinomas.[69] Practicing sun-sensible behaviors and following a low-fat diet are your best line of defense against skin cancer.

**Warning Signs of Skin Cancer** Can you identify the moles and other spots, bumps, and growths on your body? Have you given yourself a "once-over"? Examined your skin from head to toe, front and back? Awareness of moles or areas of pigmentation on your skin establishes a benchmark for evaluating changes that might raise suspicions of cancer. The warning signs and symptoms of skin cancer include any unusual skin condition, particularly a change in the size, shape, or pigmentation of moles or other dark areas of skin. Take notice of any bleeding, ulceration, scaliness, or other changes in any nodule, growth, bump, or "beauty mark." Notice any changes in sensation (pain, tenderness, itchiness) of skin marks or a spreading of pigmentation. Notify your doctor of any changes or suspicious-looking moles or growths. Finally, learn the warning signs (the ABCD's) of melanomas in the nearby ***Prevention*** feature.

## PREVENTION

### *Recognizing the ABCD's of Melanoma*

The National Cancer Institute offers a simple ABCD rule to identify the warning signals of melanoma:

*A* is for *asymmetry.* One half of the mole does not match the other half.

*B* is for *border irregularity.* The edges are ragged, notched, or blurred.

*C* is for *color.* The pigmentation is not uniform.

*D* is for *diameter greater than 6 millimeters.* Any sudden or progressive increase in size should be of special concern.

Become aware of these warning signs and report any suspicious findings to your family physician or dermatologist without delay. It may be "just a mole," but it is best to play it safe when it comes to melanoma.

**Talking Glossary**
Electrodesiccation, Cryosurgery
G1807

**Treatment** Early skin cancers are excised (removed surgically) in most cases, though other methods are sometimes used to destroy cancerous growths, such as the use of heat **(electrodesiccation),** freezing **(cryosurgery),** and radiation therapy. For malignant melanoma, the primary growth and some surrounding healthy tissue is removed surgically, sometimes along with nearby lymph nodes, which may harbor some migrating cancer cells. Though early melanomas can usually be cured, the chances of recovery are slim if they are detected after they have metastasized. The chances of surviving five years following diagnosis of melanoma are 93% if the cancer is detected and removed before it has spread, 57% if it has spread to nearby tissue, and only 15% if it has spread to distant sites in the body. Fortunately, more than four of five melanomas are detected when they are in the localized and most curable stage.

**Close-up**
Treating skin cancer
T1833
More on treating melanoma
T1834

## Ovarian Cancer

The lives of more women are lost to ovarian cancer than to any other gynecological cancer, including uterine and cervical cancer. According to present estimates, more than 26,000 women in the United States are diagnosed with ovarian cancer each year and more than 14,000 die of it.[70] Only 44% of women with ovarian cancer survive five or more years, because most cases are diagnosed only after the disease has metastasized. Five-year survival jumps to about 90% when ovarian cancer remains localized, but fewer than one in four cases are picked up this early. The survival rate declines to about 50% if the cancer has spread to the surrounding region, and to 23% if it has spread to distant sites.

Detection usually occurs late because in its early stages, ovarian cancer is often "silent" (produces no noticeable symptoms). Women over the age of 40 are advised to have an annual cancer-screening examination, which includes a pelvic examination. Even a pelvic examination may fail to pick up signs of early ovarian cancer. A newer diagnostic test, called **transvaginal sonography (TVS),** may help identify early-stage ovarian cancers that go undetected in pelvic examinations.[71]

**Talking Glossary**
Transvaginal sonography
G1808

**Risk Factors** One factor that increases a woman's risk of ovarian cancer is a family history of the disease. Women with first-degree relatives (a mother or sister) with ovarian cancer have a lifetime risk of 5%, compared with 1.4% for other women.[72] Other risk factors include age, not having borne children, and breast cancer.

Some factors appear to provide some protection against the disease, such as having had several pregnancies and having used oral contraceptives. Cutting down on dietary fat also seems to lower the risk.[73]

**Treatment** Treatment of ovarian cancer depends on the stage of the disease and may involve surgery, radiation, chemotherapy, or a combination of treatments. The extent of surgery depends on the state of the disease. It may include removal of one or both ovaries **(oophorectomy),** the uterus **(hysterectomy),** and the Fallopian tubes **(salpingectomy).** The newer drug hycamtin has shrunk tumors in a number of women with advanced ovarian cancer that has not responded to more standard chemotherapy.

**Talking Glossary**
Oophorectomy, Hysterectomy
G1809

## Cervical Cancer

Cancer of the cervix, the lower end or opening of the uterus, is among the most common gynecological cancers. It accounts for about 6% of cancers in women. More than 15,000 women are diagnosed with the disease each year, and about 5,000 die of it. Cervical cancer tends to strike women between the ages of 30 and 55, although it may occur in younger and older women. Cervical cancer is highly curable if it is detected and treated before it metastasizes. Overall, the five-year survival rate is 68%. For localized cancers, the survival rate rises to 91%.

**Detection** Because of the importance of early detection, a woman's best defense against cervical cancer is an annual **Pap test** (or **Pap smear**). In this test, a sample (called a *smear*) of cervical tissue is examined for the presence of cancerous cells. All women 18 years or older, and younger women who have been sexually active, should receive an annual Pap test. However, about one-

**Electrodesiccation** Destruction of cancerous tissues or growths by use of heat.

**Cryosurgery** Surgery using freezing temperatures produced by liquid nitrogen or carbon dioxide in order to destroy cancerous tissue.

**Transvaginal sonography (TVS)** Imaging technique using ultrasonic sound waves to assess a woman's inner reproductive organs.

**Oophorectomy** Surgical removal of one or both ovaries.

**Hysterectomy** Surgical removal of the uterus.

**Salpingectomy** Surgical removal of the Fallopian tubes. Synonymous with *tubectomy*.

**Pap test** or **Pap smear** The scraping of a "smear" of cells from the vagina and cervix for microscopic examination to reveal cancer.

third of women do not receive regular Pap tests.[74] Some physicians schedule Pap tests less often in women who show negative findings on three or more consecutive tests.

Women should also be alert to early signs of cervical cancer, including abnormal bleeding from the uterus or spotting and abnormal vaginal discharge.

**Risk Factors and Treatment** Though all women are at risk of cervical cancer, the most significant risk factor is a history of infection with HPV, human papilloma virus. Other risk factors include a high number of sex partners, young age at first intercourse, and smoking.[75] Surgery or radiation, or a combination of these approaches, is used in treating cervical cancer.

**Close-up**
Treating cervical cancer
**T1835**

## Uterine Cancer

More than 33,000 women develop uterine cancer each year in the United States. About 6,000 die of the disease. Uterine cancer is cancer of the body of the uterus, the hollow, pear-shaped organ in which the fetus develops. The cancer usually develops in the endometrium, the inner layer of the uterine wall, and is called endometrial cancer. Risk factors for uterine cancer include early menarche, late menopause, infertility, failure to ovulate, use of the drug tamoxifen (a breast cancer drug), hormone-replacement therapy, and obesity. The Pap test, so effective in detecting early cervical cancer, often fails to pick up uterine cancer. The American Cancer Society recommends that women over 40 should have annual pelvic exams to help detect uterine cancer. Moreover, women at high risk of the disease should have endometrial tissue removed at menopause and evaluated for the presence of cancerous cells. Women should also be aware of unusual symptoms that might be warning signs of endometrial cancer: uterine bleeding or discharge not connected to menstruation, painful or difficult urination, pain during intercourse, and abdominal pain.

**Treatment** Treatments for uterine cancer include surgery to remove cancerous tissue, radiation, hormone therapy, and chemotherapy. Surgery often involves removal of the uterus (hysterectomy) and nearby structures. In advanced cases, a **radical hysterectomy** may be performed, in which the surgeon removes the cervix, uterus, Fallopian tubes, ovaries, part of the vagina, and, possibly, nearby lymph nodes. Like other forms of cancer, the chances of recovery depend upon whether it has metastasized. The five-year survival rate is 83% overall. It ranges from 95% if the disease is localized to 65% if it has spread to the adjoining region and to 26% if it has spread distantly.

**Radical hysterectomy** The surgical removal of cervix, uterus, Fallopian tubes, ovaries, part of the vagina, and possibly nearby lymph nodes.

**Close-up**
Treating uterine cancer
**T1836**

## Oral Cancer

Oral cancers include cancers of the mouth, lip, tongue, and throat. More than 28,000 new cases of oral cancer and some 8,000 deaths are reported annually. The disease is most common in men, especially men over 40. Early signs of oral cancer include a sore in the mouth or on the lips that bleeds easily and doesn't heal; a lump, thickening, or persistent red or white patch in the mouth, lips, tongue, or throat; and difficulty chewing, swallowing, or moving the tongue or jaw. Oral cancer is linked to such risk factors as smoking, use of smokeless tobacco (snuff or chewing tobacco), and excessive use of alcohol. The principal methods of treatment are surgery and radiation therapy. Cancerous parts of the oral cavity and jaw may be removed surgically. With early treatment, cure rates are excellent and functional disability can be kept to a minimum.[76] Recent advances in reconstructive surgery have also helped reduce functional disability.[77] The key to fighting oral cancer, however, is prevention: avoidance of smoking, smokeless tobacco, and excessive alcohol use.

## Leukemia

Many people think of leukemia as a childhood disease. However, it affects more adults (an estimated 24,800 new cases in 1996) than children (about 2,800 new cases). There are several different types of leukemia, which collectively now account for some 21,000 deaths each year.

Leukemia is cancer of the body's blood-forming tissues, including bone marrow and lymph tissues. The cancer leads to the accumulation of abnormal white blood cells in the bloodstream, bone marrow, and lymph nodes, which can interfere with vital body organs. It also leads to a deficiency in the numbers of healthy white blood cells, which impairs the immune system, making the person more susceptible to infectious disease. If leukemia is suspected, a biopsy of the bone marrow and blood tests are used to confirm a diagnosis. Though the causes of leukemia remain a mystery in most cases, some forms of the disease are known to be caused by a retrovirus, the HTLV-1 (human T-cell leukemia/lymphoma virus-1). Exposure to certain chemicals such as benzene, a toxic chemical used in industry and found in lead-free gasoline, may also play a part. People with certain genetic abnormalities are also at higher risk. The most effective method of treatment is chemotherapy. Blood transfusions and bone marrow transplants may be used to restore healthy blood cells. Though the five-year survival rate overall remains relatively low, only 40%, some forms of leukemia show higher rates of survival. In children with acute lymphocytic leukemia, for example, 78% survive five years or longer.

## Lymphoma

Lymphomas develop in the lymphatic system. Lymph cells grow abnormally and can spread to other organs. **Hodgkin's disease** is a rare form of lymphoma that primarily affects people aged 15 to 34 or over 55. Other lymphomas are termed **non-Hodgkin's lymphomas.**

About 60,000 new cases of lymphoma are reported each year, with nearly nine of ten of these non-Hodgkin's lymphoma. The incidence of non-Hodgkin's lymphoma has increased sharply during the past two decades, while the rate of Hodgkin's disease has declined. The numbers of deaths attributed to lymphoma are nearly 25,000 each year, with about 90% of them due to non-Hodgkin's lymphoma. A few decades ago, few people survived non-Hodgkin's lymphoma. Today, advances in treatment have increased the chances of surviving five or more years to more than 50%. Five-year survival rates from Hodgkin's disease are even higher: 80%.

Early signs of lymphoma include enlarged lymph nodes, fever, and weight loss. Diagnosis is made from taking a biopsy of an enlarged lymph node. Exposure to certain viruses, impaired immune system functioning, and a history of organ transplantation (which can alter immune system functioning) increase the risk of certain lymphomas. Treatment depends on the type of lymphoma and the stage of the disease, and may involve chemotherapy, radiation therapy, and surgery.

## Pancreatic Cancer

Pancreatic cancer is most deadly. It claims the lives of nearly 27,000 people each year in the United States. It is all the more dangerous because it does not produce symptoms until it is well advanced. The disease primarily strikes people between the ages of 65 and 79. Only about 4% of patients diagnosed with the disease live five years or longer. Though little is known about the causes of pancreatic cancer, people who smoke double their risk of developing the disease. Other possible risk factors include a high-fat diet and a history of chronic infection of the pancreas, diabetes, and cirrhosis of the liver. Treatment is usually too late to affect the outcome, but involves surgery, radiation therapy, and chemotherapy.

**Close-up**
Treating pancreatic cancer
**T1837**

## Promising Approaches in Cancer Treatment

The traditional methods for treating cancer are surgery (removal of cancerous tissue), radiation (high-dose X-rays or other sources of high-energy radiation to kill cancerous cells and shrink tumors), chemotherapy (drugs that kill cancer cells or shrink tumors), and hormonal therapy (hormones that stop tumors from growing). The choice of treatments depends on factors such as age, general health, the progression of the cancer, and the type and location of the original tumor or metastasis. In many cases, a combination of treatments is used. Cancer treatments yield good results in many cases, even cures, especially for cancers that remain localized.

**Close-up**
How is cancer treated?
**T1838**

**Close-up**
More on radiation therapy
**T1839**

Tamoxifen: Q & A
**T1840**

Traditional methods also have their problems and limitations. Anticancer drugs and radiation kill healthy tissue as well as cancerous tissue and are associated with unpleasant side effects. Chemotherapy can produce nausea, vomiting, loss of appetite, and hair loss. Radiation can produce such side effects as fatigue, skin rashes, loss of appetite, and loss of white blood cells. Surgery can be painful, lead to complications, or fail to remove all cancerous cells. Present treatment techniques fail to stop the progression of many cancers, especially more advanced cancers. New anticancer drugs and bold new advances in biological therapies offer promise of boosting the odds of controlling or even defeating cancer.

**Take Charge**
Chemotherapy: How you can help yourself
**C1801**

**Hodgkin's disease** A rare type of lymphoma (cancer of the lymphatic system) characterized by enlargement of the lymph nodes.

**Non-Hodgkin's lymphomas** All forms of lymphoma other than Hodgkin's disease.

**Advances in Chemotherapy** New anticancer drugs may deliver more powerful punches to cancerous tumors yet spare surrounding healthy tissue. New drug delivery systems may also deliver more of the drug directly to cancerous cells. In one example, researchers encapsulate an anticancer drug in a lipid (fat) capsule, which tricks cancer cells into taking up more of the drug than usual, allowing for more cancer-killing action. Drug potency has also been improved by attaching antibodies to anticancer drugs. The antibodies allow the drug to home in on cancer cells by reacting with the receptors on those particular cell types.

**Gene Therapy**[78] In **gene therapy,** which is still highly experimental, the person's own genetic material is altered to enable the body to fight or prevent disease. Scientists are hopeful that altered genes injected directly into a tumor might make tumor cells more vulnerable to anticancer drugs. Since these drugs would kill only the cells containing the inserted genes, healthy cells would be spared, and side effects would be minimized. In another potential application, healthy genes might be substituted for defective or missing genes. Scientists are also experimenting with ways to genetically alter cells in the immune system to make them more effective in fighting cancer. These cells might be returned to the body in the hope that they will help the immune system mount a more forceful attack against the cancer.

**Close-up**
Gene therapy: Q & A
T1841
More on gene therapy
T1842

**Video**
Cancer genes: Key to a cure?
V1802

In one application under study for prostate cancer, genetically altered PSA genes are used to target and destroy cancerous cells.[79] The genes target the cancerous cells like "smart bombs," sparing healthy cells in the region. In another, normal copies of a gene that functions as a tumor suppressor were carried into cancerous lungs by a harmless virus. No one was cured in this experimental test, but the growth of tumors in some patients was temporarily halted. In other cases, tumors were temporarily shrunk.[80] Even though the patients eventually died, the injected genes became part of their hosts' genetic material. These findings give hope that further advances in gene therapy may alter the eventual outcome.

**Smart Reference**
Gene therapy
R1804

**Gene therapy** The alteration of a person's genetic material to fight disease.

**Immunotherapy** Treatment of disease involving efforts to boost the functioning of the immune system.

**Interferons** Proteins manufactured by the body that have antiviral and antitumor effects.

**Interleukin-2 (IL-2)** A naturally occurring growth factor that helps the immune system destroy cancer cells.

**Immunotherapy** On another front in the war against cancer, scientists are attempting to strengthen the immune system, the body's own cancer-fighting system. The immune system normally recognizes cancer cells as deviant or "alien" and dispatches armies of lymphocytes—B-Cells, T-cells, and NK cells—to kill them. Somehow, this normal housekeeping function breaks down in people who develop cancer.

In **immunotherapy** (sometimes called *biological therapy*), researchers use substances called BRMs (biological response modifiers) to give the immune system a boost in its fight against cancer.[81] BRMs occur naturally in the body and can be manufactured in the laboratory to combat tumors and strengthen healthy cells.

**Talking Glossary**
Immunotherapy
G1810

BRMs have the potential to inflict serious harm on cancerous tumors. They may make cancer cells more vulnerable to the immune system, block or reverse processes that turn normal or precancerous cells into cancerous cells, prevent metastasis, and protect normal cells from the damage caused by cancer treatments such as chemotherapy or radiation. A variety of BRMs are currently under investigation in cancer treatment, including interferons, interleukins, tumor necrosis factors, colony-stimulating factors, monoclonal antibodies, and cancer vaccines.

**Close-up**
More on immunotherapy
T1843

***Interferons*** **Interferons** are proteins manufactured in the body that can kill cancer cells or stop their growth. Interferons produced in the laboratory, such as interferon-A, may give immune system cells, B-cells and T-cells, a boost in their anticancer warfare and may stop the growth of cancer cells. They may have benefits in treating a range of cancers including leukemias, Kaposi's sarcoma, kidney cancer, melanoma, and some non-Hodgkin's lymphomas.

**Talking Glossary**
Interferon, Interleukin-2, Necrosis
G1811

***Interleukin-2*** **Interleukin-2 (IL-2)** is a naturally occurring growth factor that can help lymphocytes (disease-fighting white blood cells) destroy cancer cells. Lymphocytes drawn from the patient's blood can be mixed with synthesized IL-2 and then returned to the patient's body to stimulate a more vigorous anticancer response. IL-2 has shown the most promising results in treating advanced cases of kidney cancer and melanoma.[82] Scientists are studying the effects of combining BMRs such as interferon-A and interleukin-2 with treatments such as chemotherapy and surgery.[83]

***Tumor Necrosis Factor (TNF)*** The word *necrosis* derives from the Greek *nekrosis*, meaning "death." Necrosis refers to death of body cells, tissues, or organs resulting from irreversible damage. **Tumor necrosis factor (TNF)** destroys tumors by directly attacking tumor cells, rendering them unable to survive. Like interferon-A and IL-2, it also stimulates the body's immune system response. The problem with TNF is that it is highly toxic. The best results to date have come from injecting it directly into a tumor rather than administering it generally throughout the body.

***Colony-Stimulating Factors (CSFs)*** **Colony-stimulating factors (CSFs)** stimulate bone marrow to produce more white blood cells and other blood cells. CSFs hold the promise of protecting the bone marrow from the toxic effects of chemotherapy or radiation, which may permit patients to tolerate higher doses of these treatments. CSFs may also enhance the immune system response to cancerous tumors.

Talking Glossary
Monoclonal antibodies
G1812

***Monoclonal Antibodies (MOABs)*** **Monoclonal antibodies (MOABs)** are artificial antibodies that target antigens found on cancer cells. Since they latch onto specific cancer cells, they may be used to deliver anticancer drugs and other cancer-fighting substances (other BMRs, radioactive substances) directly to tumors.

***Cancer Vaccines*** A vaccine against cancer? Perhaps. Vaccines against several types of cancer are under study. There are promising preliminary results with malignant melanoma. Vaccines work by stimulating the immune system to develop memory lymphocytes that can recognize and destroy a particular antigen the next time the body is exposed to it. Researchers are developing cancer vaccines that work the same way: They help the body recognize and attack cancer cells before they develop into tumors.

Research is under way to develop new anticancer drugs with greater potency and less toxicity. Researchers are also finding new ways of combining cancer treatments to give a knockout punch to cancerous tumors. New methods already enable doctors to perform less extensive surgery than was required in the past.[84] Many people with early cancer of the larynx are able to retain their voice boxes. Many women with breast cancer can undergo lumpectomies rather than mastectomies. Fewer colostomies need to be done. Advances in prostate surgery have also reduced the occurrence of impotence.

With these many new advances in cancer treatment, there is hope of controlling many types of cancer that have resisted traditional treatments.

## Alternative Treatments

Many people have been discouraged that traditional medicine has little to offer them to combat their particular type of cancer. Some have turned to alternative treatments in the hope of a miracle cure. Some are taken in by swindlers who prey on their vulnerability and peddle modern-day "snake oils" as cures. Others pin their hopes on untested or controversial treatments. One example is **laetrile,** a drug derived from apricot pits, which is touted by promoters as a safe and effective cancer treatment. The National Cancer Institute tested laetrile with laboratory animals and with human cancer patients, finding no evidence that it had any anticancer effect.[85] Moreover, some serious side effects were reported.

Some cancer patients have turned to **holistic medicine.** This approach focuses on the "whole person," not just the illness. Holistic medicine uses physical, mental, emotional, and spiritual components to treat the person as a functioning whole. Holistic practitioners run the gamut from licensed physicians, nurses, osteopaths, and chiropractors to faith healers and unlicensed therapists. Some holistic approaches are based on sound nutrition and principles of stress management. These have been incorporated by many mainstream practitioners. However, some holistic practitioners make unsupported claims for unconventional cancer therapies (such as pressure-point massage or use of diet therapies alone) or offer simplistic solutions to complex health problems. Some even recommend that patients abandon medically proven techniques of cancer management.[86]

Close-up
Unconventional treatment
T1844

Untested treatments may cause serious side effects or divert patients from potentially effective therapies. On the other hand, use of safe alternative treatments,

**Tumor necrosis factor (TNF)** A naturally occurring body protein that can be lethal to cancer cells.

**Colony-stimulating factors (CSFs)** Proteins found in blood serum that stimulate the bone marrow to produce more white blood cells and other blood cells.

**Monoclonal antibodies (MOABs)** Manufactured antibodies capable of identifying antigens on cancer cells.

**Laetrile** A drug derived from apricot pits; its alleged anticancer effects are unproved.

**Holistic medicine** An approach to treatment that focuses on the whole person, including physical, emotional, spiritual, and social aspects, not just the disease.

including some nutritional and psychological approaches, may be of value to some patients.[87] They may increase the patient's sense of control and relieve some pain and anxiety, even if they do not increase the length of survival.

## Living with Cancer[88]

A diagnosis of cancer was once a virtual death sentence. Few people with cancer survived more than a few years. Because of two generations of advances in detection and treatment, a higher proportion of cancer patients are living for five, ten, or more years. Many long-term survivors are in a state of **remission.** (They show no evidence of cancer.) Some have recurrences that are controlled with treatment.

Living with cancer isn't easy. People with cancer may have trouble sleeping or eating, or they may fall into depression. They may resent people who remain well and ask, "Why me?" Anger toward the medical profession is common. Medicine sometimes has no cure or treatment. Some treatments like chemotherapy and radiation have unpleasant side effects—nausea and vomiting, mood swings, and loss of hair. There are a number of resources available to people who are living with cancer.

**Support for Cancer Patients** Many people with cancer join support groups composed of people coping with cancer or other life-threatening diseases. Group members offer emotional support and practical suggestions about whom to tell about the cancer, how to tell the children, and how to cope with symptoms and treatment. Discussing fears and concerns with others also helps many people cope with the prospect of death—for themselves and for their families.

**Take Charge**
Talking with your child about cancer
C1802

Many health organizations help cancer patients and their families by providing emotional support, home care, financial assistance, and transportation. One such organization is the American Cancer Society, a leading nonprofit health organization. To find out what services it offers in your area, contact your local chapter (see the white pages of your phone book for its telephone number, or ask your health care provider).

Cancer Care, Inc., a nonprofit social service agency headquartered in New York City, provides counseling; home visits; homemaking services; referrals to hospices, hospitals, and child care services; and financial assistance. There are no fees for their services.

**Remission** A lessening of severity or abatement of the symptoms of a disease.

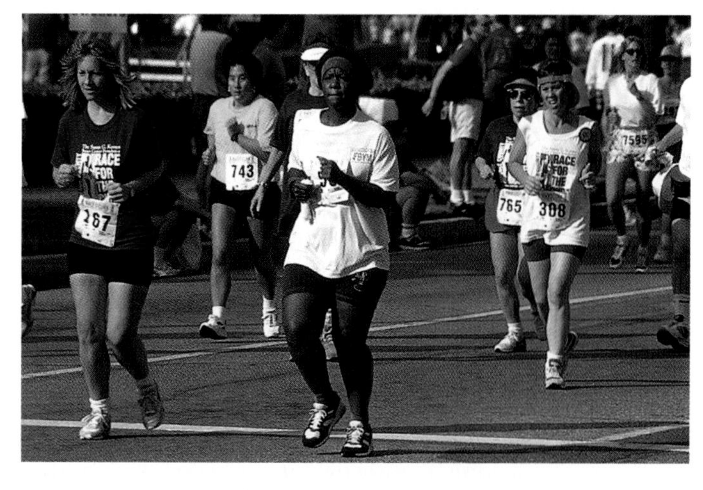


***The Race for the Cure*** Many people are involved in the fight against cancer, such as the people shown here participating in the "Race for the Cure" to raise funds to support breast cancer research. What about you?

The federal government provides several information services that can be of help to cancer patients and their families. The National Health Information Center (NHIC) puts patients and health professionals in touch with organizations that can provide answers. The Cancer Information Service (CIS) is a nationwide service supported by the National Cancer Institute. It provides information about particular types of cancer, as well as information on how to obtain second opinions and the availability of clinical trials. The toll-free number is 1-800-4-CANCER.

### think about it!

- **Which types of cancer are most common? Which are most deadly?**
- **At what ages should *you* be screened for various types of cancer? Why?**
- **Do you know anyone who has been treated for cancer? How? Was the treatment effective?**
- **Do you know anyone who sought nontraditional methods to fight cancer after traditional methods failed? What was the outcome?**

**critical thinking** **Agree or disagree and support your answer: "I am doing all I should to reduce my risk of developing cancer."**

**Smart Quiz**
Q1802

## DIABETES MELLITUS

About 16 million people in the United States have **diabetes mellitus,** but only half of them know it.[89] Ignorance of diabetes is not bliss, however. Failure to diagnose and treat diabetes can lead to serious complications and even death. Diabetes claims some 170,000 lives per year, making it the seventh leading cause of death in the United States. Diabetes mainly affects older adults, but it is also among the most common chronic disorders of children and adolescents. It affects nearly 130,000 people under the age of 20.

The cells in our body use **glucose,** a form of sugar, as the major source of fuel for growth and energy. The body converts most food into glucose and releases it into the bloodstream to circulate and be taken up by cells. **Insulin,** a hormone produced by the **pancreas,** allows cells to draw glucose from the blood. Like a key fitting into a lock, insulin opens glucose receptors on cells. The pancreas regulates the amount of insulin the body needs. In diabetes, the pancreas produces too little insulin or none at all, or cells in the body fail to make proper use of the insulin that is available. Thus too much glucose circulates in the blood. It is eventually excreted in the urine while cells remain starved for nourishment. Lacking glucose, the cells begin burning fat and even muscle as fuel. Unless diabetes is controlled, excess glucose in the blood can damage sensitive bodily organs and cause nerve damage and circulatory problems, leading to heart disease, blindness, kidney failure, sexual dysfunction, and amputation of lower extremities due to nerve damage or poor circulation.

Diabetes more than doubles the risks of coronary heart disease and strokes. Nearly two of three people with diabetes also suffer from hypertension, a leading risk factor for cardiovascular disease.

### Types of Diabetes

**Talking Glossary**
Insulin-dependent diabetes mellitus
G1813

#### Insulin-Dependent Diabetes Mellitus

**Insulin-dependent diabetes mellitus (IDDM)** is also called *juvenile diabetes* or *Type I diabetes.* In IDDM, the pancreas produces too little insulin. IDDM typically develops in children and young adults and accounts for about 1 million of the 16 million cases of diabetes in the U.S. IDDM is thought to be a type of autoimmune disorder in which the immune system attacks and destroys insulin-producing cells in the pancreas. Why does the immune system turn against the body? Perhaps genetic factors and viruses are involved. One possibility is that genetic factors make insulin-producing cells in the pancreas more susceptible to certain viruses, which can damage them and lead the immune system to attack the affected cells.

Symptoms of insulin-dependent diabetes include increased urination, which leads to extreme thirst, as well as chronic hunger, weight loss, blurred vision, and extreme fatigue. People with IDDM require daily injections of insulin. If insulin-dependent diabetes goes undiagnosed and untreated, the person can lapse into a life-threatening coma.

#### Noninsulin-Dependent Diabetes Mellitus

Far more common is **noninsulin-dependent diabetes mellitus** or **NIDDM,** also called *adult-onset* or *Type II diabetes.* NIDDM usually occurs in middle or late adulthood and among overweight people. NIDDM affects some 15 million people in the United States and accounts for 90 to 95% of cases of diabetes. NIDDM involves a breakdown in the body's use of insulin. Though the pancreas pumps out enough insulin, the body cannot use it effectively. Too little glucose gets through to the cells, and blood glucose rises to unhealthy levels. Eventually the pancreas becomes exhausted and cuts back production of insulin. The symptoms of NIDDM typically occur gradually and may go unnoticed. Symptoms include fatigue; feeling ill; frequent urination, especially at night; increased thirst; weight loss; and blurred vision.

#### Gestational Diabetes

**Gestational diabetes** is a form of diabetes that occurs among pregnant women. It usually disappears after childbirth but increases the risk that women may later develop NIDDM.

**Diabetes mellitus** A metabolic disease involving insufficient production of insulin or a failure of cells to utilize the insulin produced.

**Glucose** A form of sugar produced by digestion; transported by blood to cells.

**Insulin** A pancreatic hormone that allows cells to take up glucose from the blood.

**Pancreas** A gland located near the stomach that secretes a digestive fluid into the intestines and manufactures the hormone insulin.

**Insulin-dependent diabetes mellitus (IDDM)** *(juvenile* or *Type 1 diabetes)* Diabetes that usually develops in childhood or young adulthood; the person requires daily doses of insulin.

**Noninsulin-dependent diabetes mellitus (NIDDM)** *(adult-onset* or *Type II diabetes)* Diabetes that usually develops in middle or later life; involves a breakdown in the body's use of insulin.

**Gestational diabetes** Diabetes developed during pregnancy.

About 10% of the U.S. population has **impaired glucose tolerance (IGT),** a condition in which blood-sugar levels are too high but not high enough to be diagnosed with diabetes. People with this condition are at much greater risk of developing NIDDM.

## Risk Factors for Diabetes

Diabetes is not communicable. Nor do you get diabetes from eating too much sugar. Yet certain factors can increase your risk. People who are overweight and who have a family history of diabetes stand an increased risk of developing the disease. African Americans, Hispanic Americans, and Native Americans are at greater risk than white Americans of developing NIDDM, the most common form of diabetes. IDDM, on the other hand, is most common among white Americans. Though IDDM affects males and females about equally, NIDDM is more common among women, especially older overweight women.

**Close-up** National diabetes fact sheet **T1845**

**Diabetes and Ethnic Minorities**[90] African Americans have a 60% greater risk of developing diabetes than white people do. Mexican Americans and Puerto Ricans have twice the risk of non-Hispanic white people. Yet Native Americans have the highest rates of diabetes—not just in the United States, but in the world. Native Americans are more than four times as likely as white Americans and two times as likely as African Americans to die from diabetes-related causes. Genetic factors and differences in prevalences of obesity may explain the greater risks faced by Native Americans.

## Managing Diabetes

Diabetes is a chronic disease that requires lifelong management. Treatment emphasizes control of blood glucose levels through monitoring, sugar-restrictive diets, and regular physical activity, which helps clear excess glucose from the blood. People with insulin-dependent diabetes also need daily doses of insulin in order to survive, administered by injection, oral medication, or an insulin infusion pump. About 40% of people with NIDDM also need to take daily doses of insulin.

**Impaired glucose tolerance (IGT)** Indicates excessive levels of glucose in the blood after eating a carbohydrate-rich meal, but not high enough to be indicative of diabetes.

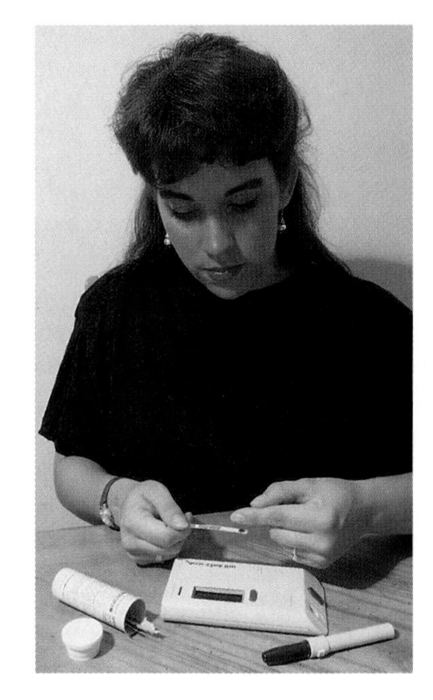

***Managing Diabetes*** Diabetes is a chronic condition that requires lifelong management, which includes taking daily blood-sugar levels (shown here) as well as following a planned diet and exercise program. With proper management, people with diabetes can lead full and productive lives.

**Hope for the Future** Alternatives to insulin injection are under development, including new forms of oral medication, nasal sprays, and even skin patches. A new drug approved in 1997, Rezulin, sensitizes cells to make better use of insulin, which may help some people with Type II diabetes eliminate the need for daily injections of the hormone while allowing others to reduce their daily dose.[91] New medical devices may also make it possible for diabetics to test their blood sugar without having to prick a finger. Researchers are also searching for the causes of diabetes to find new means of prevention and treatment. Much of this work focuses on genetic factors. We can now test for genetic markers for IDDM; they reveal whether a person is at increased risk of the disease. Researchers are testing whether IDDM can be prevented in people at risk through low doses of insulin or insulin-like agents. Perhaps the best hope for a cure lies in transplantation of the pancreas or of insulin-producing cells in the pancreas. Pancreas transplantations have yielded some success, but there are problems with organ rejection.

### think about it!

- **Do you know anyone with diabetes? Do you know what type of diabetes?**
- **How is this person being treated for diabetes? How does he or she feel about the treatment? Why?**
- **Must the person watch his or her diet? In what ways?**

**Smart Quiz** **Q1803**

# CHRONIC OBSTRUCTIVE PULMONARY DISEASE (COPD)

**Chronic obstructive pulmonary disease (COPD)** (also called *chronic obstructive lung disease* or *COLD*) is a general term for chronic lung diseases, principally emphysema and chronic bronchitis. These diseases impair the functioning of the lungs and make it difficult to breathe.[92] COPDs can cause severe disability and death. As the American Lung Association puts it, "When you can't breathe, nothing else matters."

Talking Glossary
Emphysema
G1814

## Emphysema

**Emphysema** is a progressive and disabling disease process involving the destruction of the walls of the air sacs **(alveoli)** in the lungs, reducing lung functioning. People with the disease have trouble catching their breath following exertion. They may find it difficult to walk short distances or climb a flight of stairs. Of the nearly 2 million people in the U.S. with emphysema, about 80% developed the condition because of smoking. Exposure to air pollution and dust may be other contributing factors. There is also a rare inherited form of the disorder.

Talking Glossary
Chronic bronchitis
G1815

## Chronic Bronchitis

**Chronic bronchitis** is an inflammation of the lining of the **bronchial tubes,** the airways that connect the windpipe to the lungs. The inflammation obstructs the flow of air and leads to the buildup of mucus or phlegm. As a result, people experience a hacking persistent cough, shortness of breath, and wheezing. You may have had acute bronchitis on the heels of a cold or the flu. Usually it passes within several weeks. In chronic bronchitis, which affects about 14 million people, the symptoms persist for months or years and cannot be explained by an underlying infection. It is often called a "smoker's cough" because, like emphysema, cigarette smoking is the most common cause. Prolonged exposure to air pollution also irritates the lungs, leading in some cases to bronchitis. Chronic bronchitis often leads to, or is accompanied by, emphysema.

## Treatment of COPD

Since smoking figures prominently in the development of these chronic respiratory diseases, stopping smoking is a critical element in their management. So too is the adoption of a regular exercise or conditioning program. Exercise helps improve overall fitness while also strengthening the respiratory muscles. Thus the person can breathe more easily while walking or climbing stairs. Exercises such as walking, water aerobics, and riding a stationary bicycle are generally recommended. Since people with chronic lung disorders are more prone to respiratory infections such as pneumonia and influenza, it is important for them to protect themselves by taking the appropriate vaccines. They are also advised to avoid exposure to air pollution and dusty working conditions, and to stay indoors on days when unhealthy levels of ozone (smog) are in the air. Medications such as bronchodilators may also be helpful. Bronchodilators—epinephrine is an example—may be inhaled in the form of aerosol sprays or taken as pills. They open clogged airways and reduce shortness of breath.

### think about it!

- **Do you know of someone with chronic obstructive pulmonary disease who continues to smoke? Why doesn't he or she quit?**
- **Does it seem ironic that health professionals would prescribe exercise for people who are short of breath? Why do they do so?**

Smart Quiz
Q1804

**Chronic obstructive pulmonary disease (COPD)** General term applying to chronic lung diseases, especially emphysema and chronic bronchitis, that result in impaired lung function.

**Emphysema** A lung disease involving destruction of the walls of the air sacs (alveoli) in the lungs.

**Alveoli** The air cells of the lungs where gases are exchanged during respiration.

**Chronic bronchitis** An inflammation of the lining of the bronchial tubes, producing chronic coughing.

**Bronchial tubes** The passageways through which air travels from the windpipe to the lungs.

# Protecting Yourself from Cancer and Other Chronic Diseases

## Take Charge

Close-up
Can cancer be prevented?
T1846

There is no guaranteed way to prevent diseases such as cancer and diabetes, but you can lower your risk. You cannot control risk factors such as age and heredity. But let us consider all the ones you can control.

### Avoid Tobacco

Don't smoke. If you do smoke, quit. Quitting may be difficult, but millions have done it. Chapter 14 contains suggestions for quitting smoking. Smoking and exposure to second-hand smoke are major risk factors for various cancers and for chronic lung diseases. Also avoid snuff and chewing tobacco. They are leading causes of oral cancers.

### Avoid Excessive Drinking

Excessive use of alcohol is implicated in oral cancers and liver cancer. It may play a role in other cancers. The American Cancer Society advises that the risk of some cancers may increase with as little as two drinks a day.

### Be Sun-Smart

Sun exposure is a major factor in the development of skin cancer, including potentially deadly melanomas. Here are some tips for being sun-smart:[93]

- *Limit exposure to the sun, especially during the midday hours (10 A.M. to 3 P.M.).*
- *Use the shadow method to avoid exposure to the sun when it is most dangerous.* The closer the sun comes to being directly overhead, the more dangerous are the UV rays it projects. (And the shorter your shadow is.) Avoid the sun when your shadow is shorter than you are.
- *If you can't avoid the sun, use sunscreen with a sun protection factor (SPF) of 15 or higher.* Apply sunscreen not only when you go to the beach, but whenever you and your children will be in the summer sun for longer than a few minutes. People with sensitive skin may need to use sunscreens with SPFs of 30 or higher.[94] The most sensitive people may need to use sunscreens year-round. Apply sunscreen about 30 minutes before exposure to the sun to allow it to be absorbed fully. Reapply it after swimming or perspiring heavily.
- *Wear protective clothing to shield yourself whenever you are out and about in direct sun, including a hat and a long-sleeve shirt.* Also wear protective clothing and eyewear when you are exposed to ice or snow, which reflects as much as 80% of damaging UV rays. Also, don't be misled into a false sense of security by an overcast day—high, thin clouds fail to filter out many UV rays.

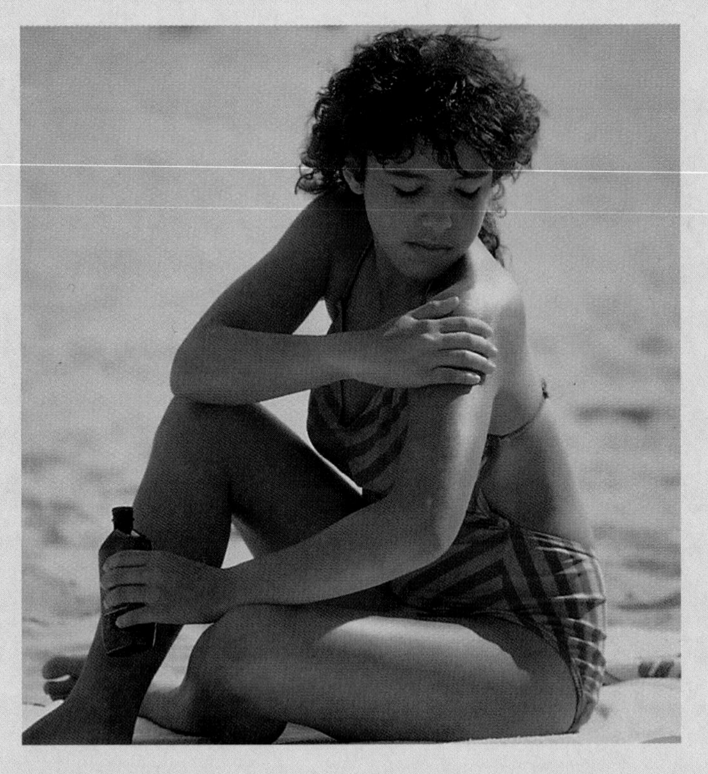

***Check that SPF*** Use a sunscreen with an SPF of 15 or higher whenever you are out in the summer sun for longer than a few minutes. Check the SPF value listed on the product label and avoid lotions containing too little or no protection.

- *Avoid tanning salons and use of home tanning lamps, which provide artificial but potentially dangerous UV radiation.*
- *Don't be lulled into a false sense of security by the use of "bronzers."* Bronzers are tanning agents that give the skin a bronzed or tanned look without the sun. However, they do not provide protection against the sun.

### Follow Cancer-Screening Guidelines

Cancer screening may do more than detect cancers when they are in the earliest, most treatable, and possibly curable stage. They may also detect precancerous conditions that may lead to cancer if they are left untreated. An example is polyps in the colon that might turn cancerous if they are not removed.

TABLE 18.3

**Cancer-Preventive Behaviors Save Lives**

| If People Practiced Cancer-Preventive Behavior | |
|---|---|
| If people protected themselves from the sun | 720,000 cases of skin cancer would be prevented |
| If people avoided tobacco use | 170,000 fewer people would die of cancer |
| If people avoided excessive alcohol use | 18,000 fewer people would die of cancer |
| If people had their cancers detected in an early stage | 100,000 fewer people would die of cancer |

### Maintain a Healthy Weight

Obesity is a risk factor for many chronic diseases, including several forms of cancer, cardiovascular disease, and diabetes. Chapter 6 contains suggestions for achieving and maintaining a healthy weight.

### Adopt a Healthy Diet

Your diet plays a role in determining your risk of certain forms of cancer. Here are some guidelines that may reduce your cancer risk. The guidelines are intended for healthy people. People with cancer or another disease should consult their physicians.[95]

- *Curb your fat intake.* Reducing your fat intake, especially fat from red meat, may reduce your risk of some cancers, including colon and prostate cancers. (Chapter 5 contains tips on cutting your fat intake.)
- *Increase your intake of dietary fiber, fruits, and vegetables.* A diet rich in dietary fiber, especially whole grains and a variety of fruits and vegetables, is associated with a lower risk of some forms of cancer, including colorectal, stomach, lung, prostate, bladder, and esophageal cancers. Scientists have also discovered a substance found in many plant foods, *resveratrol,* that blocks the development of tumors. This substance is found in rich supply in grapes and grape products, especially red wine.[96] It can be derived from eating grapes and nonalcoholic grape products without incurring the risks associated with alcohol misuse, such as alcoholism or alcohol-related health problems. We don't know yet whether consuming this substance reduces the risk of cancer.
- *Include crucifers in your diet.* One particular group of vegetables—crucifers, including broccoli, cauliflower, sauerkraut, and cabbage—may help prevent the development of colorectal and stomach cancers.
- *Limit your intake of smoked and salt-cured foods, and foods containing nitrates and nitrites.* Some of the substances found in these foods may be carcinogenic or turn into carcinogens in the body. Nitrites and nitrates are food preservatives found in processed meats such as ham, salami, sausage, hot dogs, and bacon. They are converted in the stomach into nitrosamines, which are known carcinogens.

### Avoid Exposure to Environmental Hazards

Most people have such low levels of exposure to environmental hazards that they pose a negligible cancer risk. Nevertheless, it makes sense to limit exposure to carcinogens in the environment and the workplace, especially to cancer-causing agents such as nickel, chromate, asbestos, and vinyl chloride.

### Practice Safer Sex

Viruses such as HPV, hepatitis B and C, and HIV can lead to the development of certain cancers as well as sexually transmitted diseases. Following the guidelines for safer sex listed in Chapter 16 can help reduce your risk of cancer as well as protect you from STDs.

### Get Active, Stay Active

Regular exercise can help protect you against colon cancer and may provide some protection against other cancers such as breast cancer and prostate cancer.[97] Regular exercise is also important in the prevention and management of diabetes.[98]

Adopt a steady diet of exercise equivalent to at least 30 minutes daily of moderately strenuous activity. You needn't work out in a gym. Use any activity in which you exert yourself, from gardening to vigorous walking from your car to your school or office. See Chapter 7 for suggestions for making regular exercise a part of a healthy lifestyle, one that will help guard against two major threats to your life, heart disease and cancer.

Smart Quiz Q1805

# SUMMING UP

## Questions and Answers

### WHAT IS CANCER?

**1. What is cancer?** The term *cancer* refers to a group of more than 100 distinct diseases characterized by uncontrolled growth of body cells. Tumors form when unneeded new cells multiply. Malignant tumors are cancerous. Malignant tumors become deadly when they invade and destroy surrounding tissue, or when they metastasize (when cancerous cells break away from the primary tumor to form new tumors).

**2. What are the current trends in cancer?** Cancer rates have been rising, perhaps in part because people are living longer and because of better screening for cancer. People with cancer are surviving longer, however, because of early detection and improvements in treatment.

**3. What are the causes of cancer?** The two main causes of cancer are controllable: smoking and (high-fat) diet. Other causes include excessive alcohol intake, environmental factors (e.g., industrial chemicals, excessive exposure to the sun), microbes, heredity, and inactivity.

### TYPES OF CANCER

**4. What are some of the major types of cancer?** These include breast cancer, lung cancer, colorectal cancer, prostate cancer, skin cancer, ovarian cancer, cervical cancer, uterine cancer, oral cancer, leukemia, lymphoma, and pancreatic cancer.

**5. What are some methods of detecting cancer early?** Screening methods for breast cancer include breast self-examination, clinical breast examination, and mammography. Colorectal cancer screening includes analysis of the stool for blood, rectal examination, sigmoidoscopy, or colonoscopy. Prostate cancer screening involves rectal examinations and blood tests for prostate-specific antigen (PSA). Cervical cancer is detected by Pap test. Pelvic examinations can help detect other cancers of the female sex organs.

**6. What are some methods of treating cancer?** Traditional methods for treating cancer are surgery (removal of cancerous tissue), radiation (high-dose X-rays or other sources of high-energy radiation to kill cancerous cells and shrink tumors), chemotherapy (drugs that kill cancer cells or shrink tumors), and hormonal therapy (hormones that stop tumor growth).

**7. What problems are connected with these cancer treatments?** Anticancer drugs and radiation kill healthy tissue as well as malignant tissue. They also have side effects such as nausea, vomiting, loss of appetite, loss of hair, and loss of white blood cells.

**8. What new treatment techniques for cancer are in the research pipeline?** These include more powerful drugs that better target cancerous cells (like chemical "smart bombs"), gene therapy, and immunotherapy (which uses substances called biological response modifiers to help the immune system fight cancer). Vaccines against several types of cancer are also under study.

### DIABETES MELLITUS

**9. What is diabetes mellitus?** In diabetes, the pancreas produces too little insulin (as in insulin-dependent diabetes mellitus, also called juvenile diabetes or Type I diabetes) or cells in the body fail to use insulin effectively (as in noninsulin-dependent diabetes mellitus, also called adult-onset or Type II diabetes). Therefore, glucose remains in the blood and is eventually excreted, while cells are starved for nourishment. Risk factors for diabetes include excess weight and family history of diabetes. Many people with diabetes take insulin supplements and other medications.

### CHRONIC OBSTRUCTIVE PULMONARY DISEASE (COPD)

**10. What are chronic obstructive pulmonary diseases?** These include emphysema and chronic bronchitis. In emphysema, the walls of the air sacs in the lungs are destroyed, reducing lung functioning. People with emphysema have trouble catching their breath, even following brief exertion. Chronic bronchitis is inflammation of the lining of the airways which connect the windpipe to the lungs. As a result, people have a hacking cough, shortness of breath, and wheezing. Both conditions can be caused by smoking and air pollution. Treatments involve quitting smoking, exercise, and use of bronchodilators.

## References and Suggested Readings

### SMART REFERENCES FROM SCIENTIFIC AMERICAN

**Trichopoulos, D., Li, F. P., and Hunter, D. J. What Causes Cancer?** *Scientific American,* 275(3) (September 1996), 80–87. **R1801**

**Maranto, G. Should Women in Their 40s Have Mammograms?** *Scientific American,* 275(3) (September 1996), 113. **R1802**

**Hanks, G. E., and Scardino, P. T. Does Screening for Prostate Cancer Make Sense?** *Scientific American,* 275(3) (September 1996), 113–114. **R1803**

**Anderson, W. F. Gene Therapy.** *Scientific American,* 273(3) (September 1995), 124–128. **R1804**

### SUGGESTED READINGS

**Rosenberg, S. A.** *The Transformed Cell: Unlocking the Mysteries of Cancer.* New York: G. P. Putnam, 1992. The biology of cancer.

**Korda, Michael.** *Man to Man: Surviving Prostate Cancer.* New York: Random House, 1996. A personal account of one man's battle against prostate cancer.

**Walsh, P., and Worthington, J.** *The Prostate: A Guide for Men and the Women Who Love Them.* Baltimore: Johns Hopkins Press, 1994. Helpful suggestions for men and their loved ones coping with prostate cancer.

**Harpham, W.** *Diagnosis Cancer: Your Guide through the First Few Months.* New York: Norton, 1992. Written by a physician with cancer, it provides helpful information to cancer patients about such issues as treatment alternatives and coping emotionally with a diagnosis of cancer.

**Rollin, B.** *First You Cry.* New York: Harper Paperback, 1993. Written by a TV journalist, this is a compelling first-person account of one woman's struggle to survive breast cancer.

**American Cancer Society (1-800-ACS-2345).** The American Cancer Society publishes a wide range of pamphlets and other resource materials for the general public dealing with cancer statistics, risk factors, diagnostic issues, treatment alternatives, and suggestions for prevention.

# Healthy Aging in the

## DID YOU KNOW THAT

- The older you are, the longer you're likely to live? p.519
- Men who live beyond their seventies are less likely to be poor and in ill health than women of the same age? p.520
- In colonial America, maturity was viewed so positively that men claimed to be older than they were? p.521
- As we age, we need fewer calories to maintain our ideal body weight? p.523
- African-American women are at less risk of developing osteoporosis than are white women and Asian women? p.524
- Dementia is *not* a consequence of normal aging? p.526
- Nearly half of Americans say that middle age begins when you don't know who the new music groups are? p.526
- People can enjoy sexual relations for a lifetime? p.528
- Older Americans are on the whole at least as happy as younger people? p.534
- Anxiety disorders are more common among younger than older adults? p.535

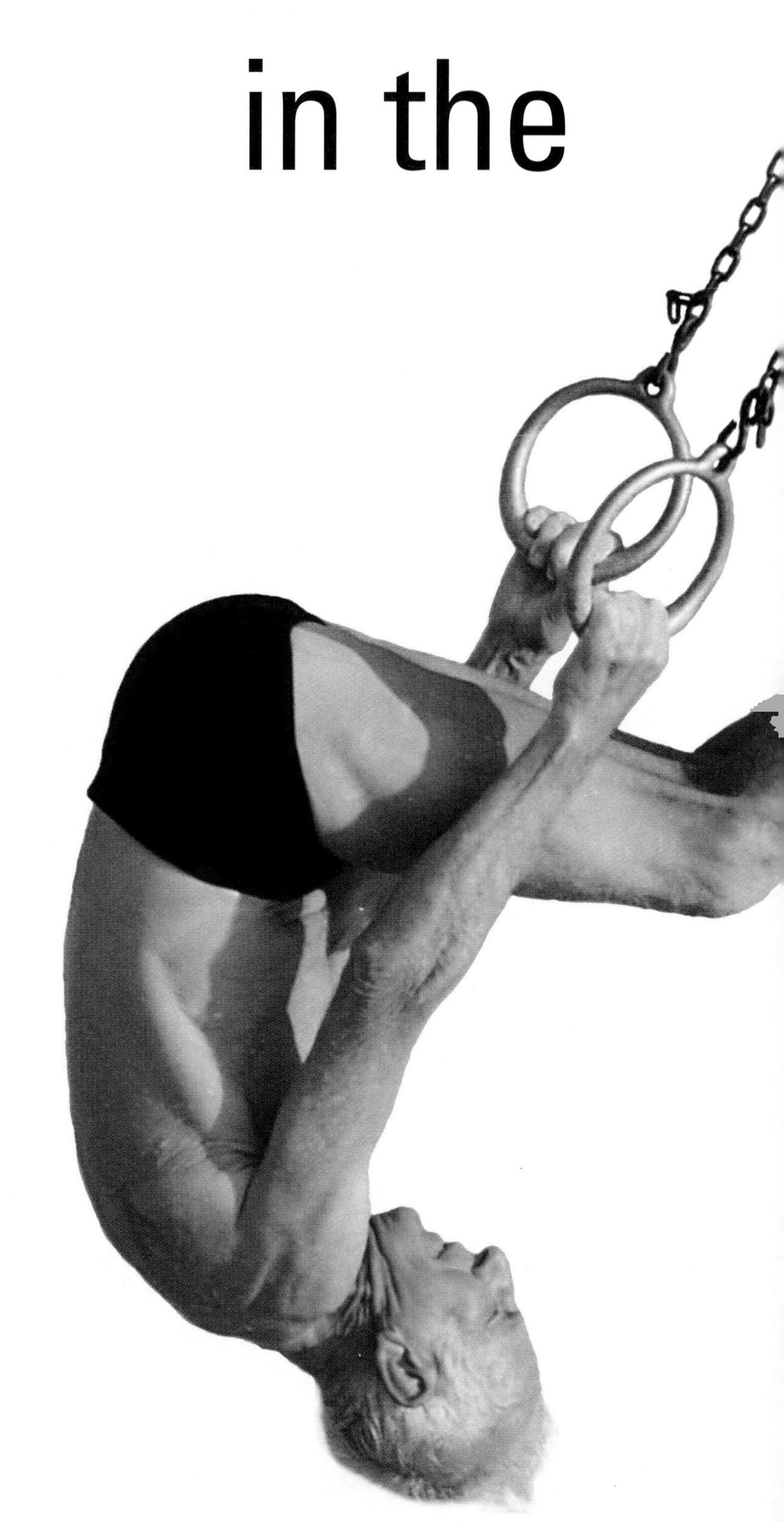

# New Millennium

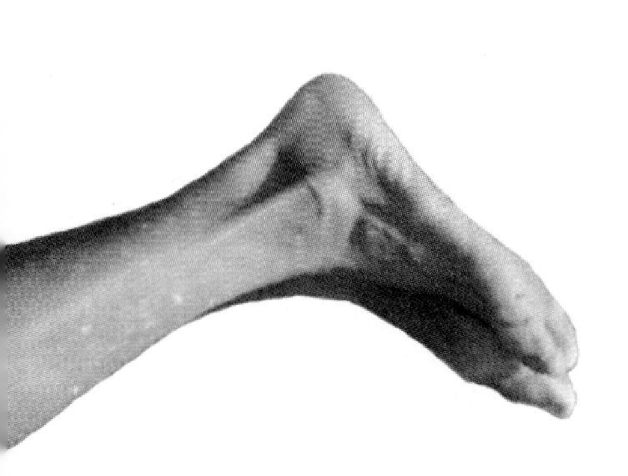

An agequake is coming. *One day, if you're fortunate enough, you will join the ranks of the most rapidly growing segment of the population—people aged 65 and above. So many people are living longer that the age of the population is shifting radically. There is a literal graying of America.*[1] *In 1900, only 1 person in 25 was over the age of 65. Today, that figure has more than tripled, to 1 in 8 of us. By the year 2030, about 1 in 4 of us will be in the 65 or over age group, more than 66 million people (see Figure 19.1).*

# 19

These are some "statistical snapshots" of the aging of America:

- Children born in the 1990s can expect to live 76 years, compared with 47 years for children born in 1900.
- In 1790, only half of the population of the newly formed United States was 16 years of age or older. By 1990, half of the population was 33 years of age or older. By the year 2030, half of the population will be over the age of 40.
- The fastest growing segment of the elderly population consists of people in the advanced elderly range, age 85 and above. The 85+ age group is 25 times larger today than 100 years ago.
- The number of centenarians—people who live to be 100 or more—is also increasing rapidly. In 1900, only 1 out of 400 persons in the United States had surpassed the century mark. In 1992, centenarians numbered 1 out of every 87 persons in the country.

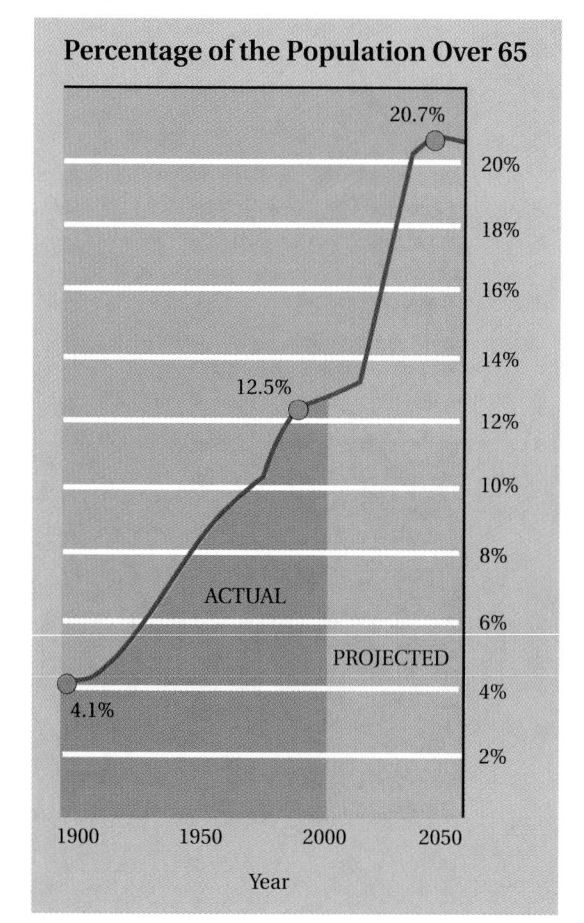


**Figure 19.1** ***The Aging of America*** America is getting grayer: Today, one in eight Americans is over 65. By 2005, it will be one in five. *Source:* U.S. Bureau of the Census. Copyright © 1995, Newsweek, Inc. All rights reserved. Reprinted by permission.

The trend toward living longer may be an "agequake . . . that will shake America as much as the youth culture of the 1960s did."[2] The aging of the population is expected to accelerate even more as the "boomers"—people born during the "baby boom" that followed World War II—approach late adulthood early in the new millennium. The age shift has already influenced the themes of TV shows and movies. Consumer products are shaped to appeal to older consumers. Leisure communities dot the Sun Belt. Yet older people today differ in many ways from their counterparts of a generation or two ago. Chronological age has become less likely to determine one's behavior and lifestyle.

**Close-up** Aging in America T1901

This chapter focuses on how and why we age. Futurists envision a day when scientists will find ways to slow or even reverse aging. But for now, **aging** remains inevitable. That doesn't mean we must throw in the towel and surrender to aging. Many older people are happier than they have ever been. There is much we can do to live healthier, more fulfilling, and longer lives. Modern medicine has made important contributions to keeping us healthy and alive. However, maintaining health and wellness also depends on adopting healthful habits long before we reach our golden years.

**Aging** The progressive changes and declines in functioning that begin after sexual maturation and continue until death.

**Longevity** The maximum number of years an organism can expect to live under the best circumstances.

**Life expectancy** The statistical average number of years that people in a given population can expect to live.

## HEALTH AND LONGEVITY

**Longevity** is the length of time an organism lives under the best of circumstances.[4] The life span of a species, including human beings, depends on its genetic programming. With the right genes and environment, with the good fortune to avoid serious accidents or illnesses, people have a maximum life span of about 115 years.

**Life expectancy** refers to the average number of years people in a given population group can expect to live. The average white child born 100 years ago in the United States could expect to live only 47 years. The average African American could expect an even shorter life, only 35.5 years.[5] Life expectancy has been rising steadily. By the 1990s, average life expectancies had jumped to 76.8 years for white Americans and 70.3 years for African Americans (see Figure 19.2). Figure 19.3 (p. 519) shows life expectancies worldwide.

**Close-up** Disability rate declining among elderly T1902

# Health Check

## *Examining Your Attitudes toward Aging*[3]

What are your assumptions about growing old? Do you see older people as fundamentally different from younger people in their behavior and outlook, or just as more mature?

To evaluate the accuracy of your attitudes toward aging, mark each of the following items true or false. Then turn to the answer key at the end of the chapter.

T F **1.** By age 60 most couples have lost their capacity for satisfying sexual relations.

T F **2.** Older people cannot wait to retire.

T F **3.** With advancing age people become more externally oriented, less concerned with the self.

T F **4.** As individuals age, they become less able to adapt satisfactorily to a changing environment.

T F **5.** General satisfaction with life tends to decrease as people become older.

T F **6.** As people age they tend to become more homogeneous—that is, all old people tend to be alike in many ways.

T F **7.** For the older person, having a stable intimate relationship is no longer highly important.

T F **8.** The aged are susceptible to a wider variety of psychological disorders than young and middle-aged adults.

T F **9.** Most older people are depressed much of the time.

T F **10.** Church attendance increases with age.

T F **11.** The occupational performance of the older worker is typically less effective than that of the younger adult.

T F **12.** Most older people are just not able to learn new skills.

T F **13.** When forced to make a decision, older people are more cautious and take fewer risks than younger persons.

T F **14.** Compared with younger people, older people tend to think more about the past than the present or the future.

T F **15.** Most people in later life are unable to live independently and reside in nursing-home-like institutions.

**Video**
Aging: Myths versus reality
**V1901**

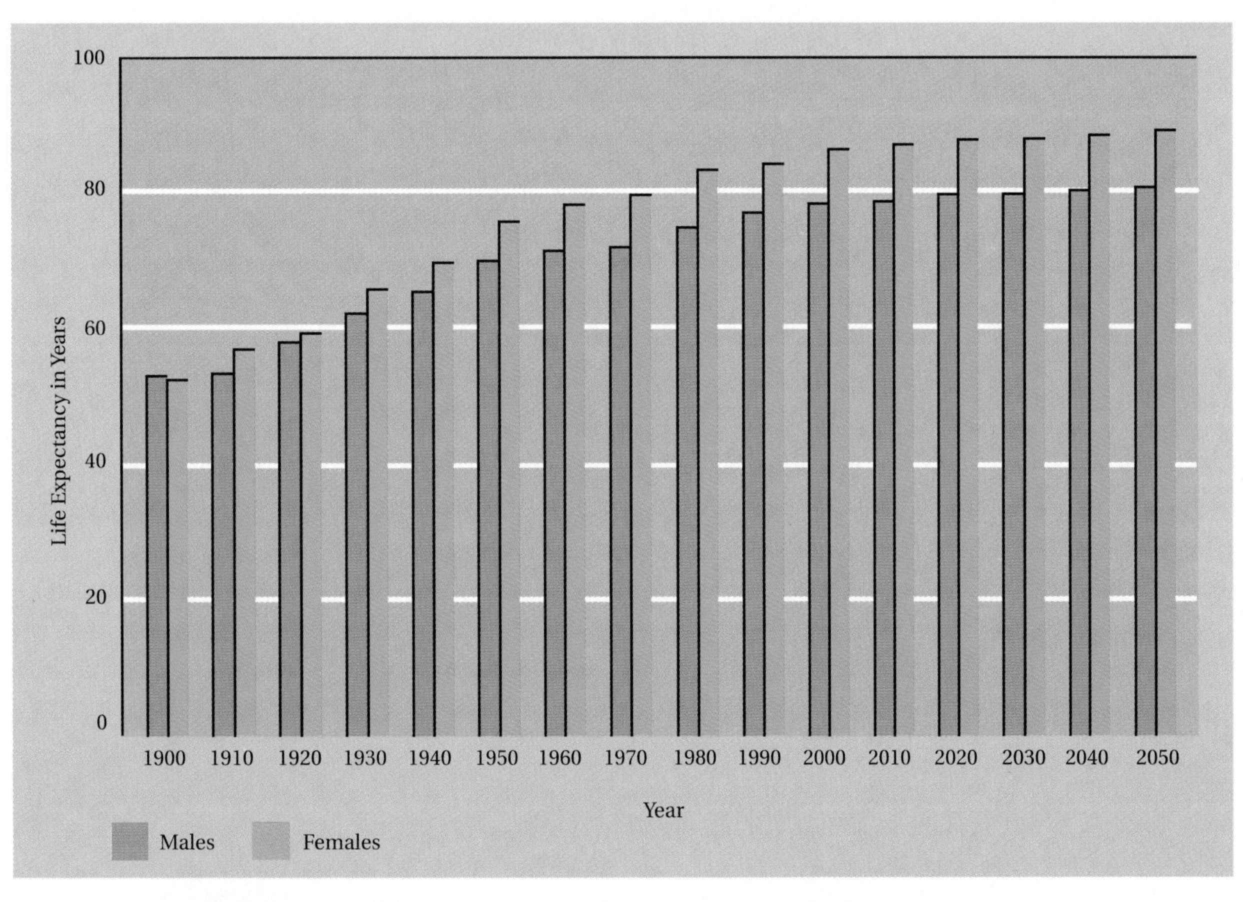


**Figure 19.2** ***Increasing Life Expectancy*** Life expectancies have been rising and are expected to continue to rise. if present trends continue, females born in the middle of the 21st century may expect to live well into their nineties, perhaps even topping 100. Males born at that time would be expected to live until perhaps 80 on the average.

# Calculate How Long You Will Live

THIS CHART WILL GIVE YOU A ROUGH IDEA OF HOW YOUR life expectancy varies from the norm. To estimate how long you'll live, begin by using the table at right to find the median life expectancy of your age group. Then add or subtract years based on the risk factors listed below (you should adjust your risk-factor score by the percentages at right if you're over 60).

| AGE | MALE | FEMALE | SCORING RISK FACTORS |
|---|---|---|---|
| 20–59 | 73 | 80 | use table as shown |
| 60–69 | 76 | 81 | reduce loss or gain by 20% |
| 70–79 | 78 | 82 | reduce loss or gain by 50% |
| 80+ | add five yrs. to current age | | reduce loss or gain by 75% |

| | Gain in Life Expectancy | | | No Change | Loss in Life Expectancy | | | start with your median life expectancy |
|---|---|---|---|---|---|---|---|---|
| HEALTH | +3 YEARS | +2 YEARS | +1 YEAR | | –1 YEAR | –2 YEARS | –3 YEARS | TALLY |
| Blood pressure | Between 90/65 and 120/81 | Less than 90/65 without heart disease | Between 121/82 and 129/85 | 130/86 | Between 131/87 and 140/90 | Between 141/91 and 150/95* | More than 151/96 | |
| Diabetes | — | — | — | None | Type II (adult onset) | — | Type I (juvenile onset) | |
| Total cholesterol | — | — | Less than 160 | 161–200 | 201–240 | 241–280 | More than 280 | |
| HDL cholesterol | — | — | More than 55 | 45–54 | 40–44 | Less than 40 | — | |
| Compared with that of others my age, my health is: | — | — | Excellent | Very good or fair | — | Poor | Extremely poor | |
| LIFE STYLE | +3 YEARS | +2 YEARS | +1 YEAR | | –1 YEAR | –2 YEARS | –3 YEARS | TALLY |
| Cigarette smoking | None | Ex-smoker, no cigarettes for more than 5 yrs. | Ex-smoker, no cigarettes for 3–5 yrs. | Ex-smoker, no cigarettes for 1–3 yrs. | Ex-smoker, no cigarettes for 5 mos.–1 yr. | Smoker, 0-20 pack-years* | Smoker, more than 20 pack-years* | |
| Secondhand-smoke exposure | — | — | — | None | 0–1 hour per day | 1–3 hours per day | More than 3 hours per day | |
| Exercise average (give yourself most positive category) | More than 90 min. per day of exercise(e.g., walking) for more than 3 yrs. | More than 60 min. per day for more than 3 yrs. | More than 20 min. per day for more than 3 yrs. | More than 10 min. per day for more than 3 yrs. | More than 5 min. per day for more than 3 yrs. | Less than 5 min. per day | None | |
| Saturated fat in diet | — | Less than 20% | 20%–30% | 31%–40% | — | More than 40% | | |
| Fruits and vegetables | — | — | 5 servings per day | — | None | — | — | |
| FAMILY | +3 YEARS | +2 YEARS | +1 YEAR | | –1 YEAR | –2 YEARS | –3 YEARS | TALLY |
| Marital status | — | Happily married man | Happily married woman | Single woman, widowed man | Divorced man, widowed woman | Divorced woman | Single man | |
| Disruptive events in the past year † | — | — | — | — | One | Two | Three | |
| Social groups, friends seen more than once/month** | — | Three | Two | One | — | None | — | |
| Parents' age of death | — | — | Both lived past 75 | One lived past 75 | — | — | Neither lived past 75 | |

*A PACK- YEAR IS ONE PACK PER DAY FOR A YEAR. †DEATHS OF FAMILY MEMBERS, JOB CHANGES, MOVES, LAWSUITS, FINANCIAL INSECURITY, ETC.
**PEOPLE WHO OFFER SUPPORT THROUGH DISRUPTIVE EVENTS (APPLICABLE ONLY IN CASE OF TWO OR MORE SUCH EVENTS). SOURCE: MICHAEL F. ROIZEN, M.D., USING DATA ABSTRACTED FROM THE REAL AGE AND AGE-REDUCTION-PLANNING PROGRAMS OF MEDICAL INFORMATICS

Your estimated life expectancy

| | Men | Women |
|---|---|---|
| **Asia and Middle East** | | |
| Cambodia | 48 | 51 |
| China | 68 | 71 |
| India | 59 | 60 |
| Iraq | 66 | 68 |
| Israel | 76 | 81 |
| Japan | 76 | 83 |
| Philippines | 63 | 69 |
| Saudi Arabia | 67 | 71 |
| South Korea | 70 | 77 |
| Turkey | 70 | 74 |
| **North and South America** | | |
| Argentina | 68 | 75 |
| Brazil | 57 | 67 |
| Canada | 76 | 83 |
| Cuba | 75 | 80 |
| Haiti | 47 | 51 |
| Mexico | 70 | 77 |
| United States | 73 | 79 |
| **Eastern Europe** | | |
| Czech Republic | 70 | 78 |
| Poland | 68 | 76 |
| Russia | 57 | 70 |
| **Western Europe** | | |
| Britain | 74 | 79 |
| France | 74 | 82 |
| Germany | 73 | 79 |
| Greece | 76 | 81 |
| Italy | 75 | 81 |
| Netherlands | 75 | 81 |
| Norway | 74 | 81 |
| Spain | 74 | 81 |
| Sweden | 76 | 82 |
| Switzerland | 75 | 82 |
| **Africa** | | |
| Egypt | 60 | 63 |
| Kenya | 56 | 56 |
| Morocco | 68 | 72 |
| Nigeria | 53 | 56 |
| South Africa | 57 | 62 |
| Zambia | 36 | 36 |
| **Pacific** | | |
| Australia | 76 | 83 |
| New Zealand | 74 | 80 |

**Figure 19.3** ***Life Expectancy Worldwide*** How long you can expect to live is partly a function of where you live. Life expectancies are higher in developed countries like the U.S., Canada, Japan, and the industrialized societies of Europe than in less technologically developed countries like Cambodia, India, and Zambia. Why?

Lower life expectancies a century ago in part reflected high infant mortality rates due to diseases such as German measles, smallpox, polio, and diphtheria. All of these have been brought under control or eradicated. Other major killers, including bacterial infections such as tuberculosis, are now largely controlled by the use of antibiotics. Other factors that contribute to longevity include public health measures, such as safer water supplies, and improved dietary habits, such as reduced intake of fat.

## Factors Affecting Longevity

Oddly enough, the older you are, the longer you're likely to live. Life expectancy tends to increase with each year you survive.[10] The typical 20-year-old African-American female, for instance, has a life expectancy of 75.3 years. For the typical *50-year-old* African-American female, life expectancy increases to 78.1 years. These are averages, of course. Your own longevity is determined by several factors. Some of them lie outside your control, such as heredity. People with a family history of heart disease and some forms of cancer are more likely than others to develop these health problems themselves.

**Video**
Fear of Aging
**V1902**

Why does life expectancy expand as people age? One reason is statistical: dying young drags the general average down. If you survive until middle or later life, you obviously have not succumbed to diseases or accidents that take many young lives. Increased longevity may also reflect other factors, such as reductions in death rates due to chronic diseases such as coronary heart disease.[11]

There is little we can do about our genetic heritage—although, given the strides made by genetic researchers, this may change. Many factors that affect longevity lie within our control. These include eating healthful foods, exercising regularly, and avoiding smoking and excessive use of alcohol. Many of the chronic diseases and physical conditions that reduce longevity, including hypertension, heart disease, some cancers, and adult-onset diabetes, occur more commonly in people with unhealthy lifestyles.

## Ethnicity and Longevity

Ethnicity is linked to life expectancy. White Americans of European background live longer on the average than do Hispanic Americans, African

## WORLD OF *diversity*

### Gender and Aging—Different Prospects

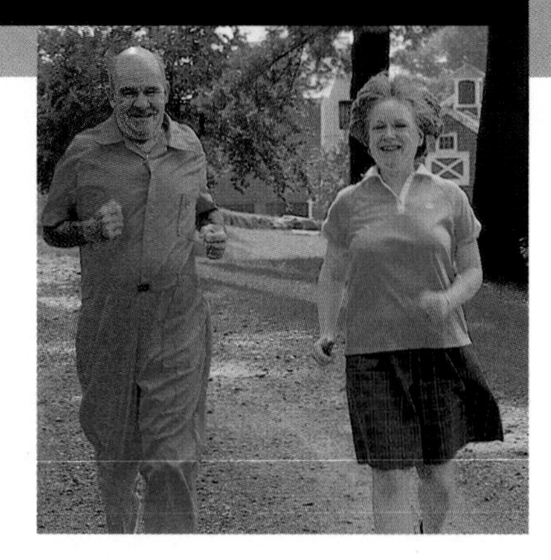

Women and men face different prospects as they age. Women tend to live longer, yet older men tend to live better than older women do.

#### Differences in Longevity

Women in the United States outlive men by about seven years. Why? For one thing, heart disease typically develops later in life in women than in men. Men are also more likely to die from accidents, cirrhosis of the liver, strokes, suicide, homicide, AIDS, and some forms of cancer.[6] Many of the deaths reflect unhealthful habits which are more typical of men, such as drinking, reckless behavior, and smoking. Unfortunately for women, the gender gap in smoking has been narrowing.

Many men are also reluctant to have regular physical examinations or to talk over health problems with their doctors. Many doctors report that men are more likely to avoid medical attention until problems that could have been easily prevented or treated become serious or life-threatening.[7] Says a representative of the Men's Health Network: "In their 20s, they're too strong to need a doctor; in their 30's, they're too busy, and in their 40's, too scared." As an example, women are much more likely to examine themselves for signs of breast cancer than men are to examine their testicles for any unusual lumps.

#### Differences in the Quality of Life of Older Men and Women

Women may live longer than men, but their prospects for a happy and healthy late adulthood are dimmer. Men who beat the statistical odds by living beyond their seventies are far less likely than women of the same age to be poor, live alone, or have chronic disabling conditions.

Women are much more likely than older men to live alone because they are five times more likely to be widowed.[8] Widows constitute half of the female population over age 65. Beyond age 75, about half of the surviving women live alone, compared with only one in five men. Among people older than 85, two-thirds of women live alone, compared with only one-third of men.[9]

Older women are also twice as likely as older men to be poor. Why? The current crop of older women were less likely to work outside the home. If they worked, they were paid much less than men and received smaller retirement benefits. Because more women than men live alone, they must more often shoulder the burdens of supporting a household alone. The problems of poverty, isolation, and ill health that face many older women represent a challenge for the new millennium.

Americans, and Native Americans. Life expectancy for Hispanic Americans falls between the figures for African Americans and white Americans. The longevity of Asian Americans falls closer to that of white Americans than African Americans. Native Americans have the lowest longevity.[12]

How do we explain these differences? Poverty most strongly accounts for reduced life span in the United States. Minority groups are more likely to be poor, and poor people tend to eat less nutritious diets and have less access to medical care. There is a seven-year difference in life expectancy between people in the highest income brackets and those in the lowest.

Other factors that may contribute to ethnic differences in life expectancies include cultural differences in diet and lifestyle, the stress of coping with discrimination, and genetic differences.[13]

## Quality of Life—Not Just How Long You Live, but How Well

Average life expectancy rose dramatically during the twentieth century, but what about the quality of health during the later years? People not only want longer lives; they also want to lead them in good health. Traditionally, health professionals distinguished longevity from health by contrasting

**Video**
Age, an elastic quality
**V1903**

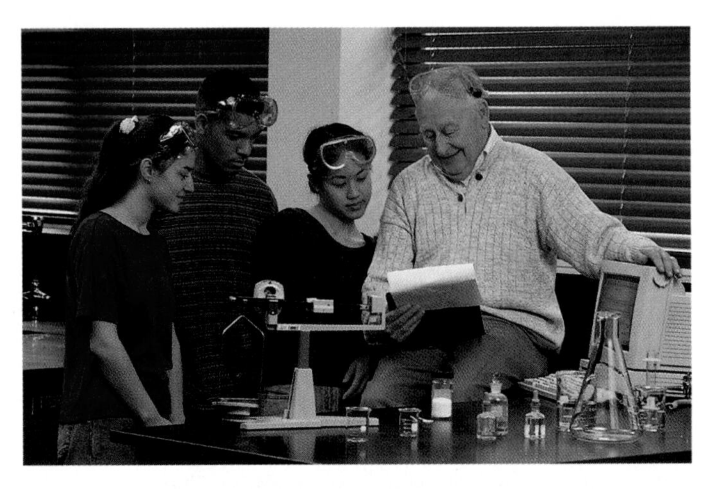

***Quality of Life*** Maintaining good health and a sense of meaning or purpose in life is important to the quality of life at any age.

**mortality,** or the rate of death in a given population, with **morbidity,** the number of sick people in a population. Today, a new measure of health has emerged. It combines length of life with quality of life. It is called **quality-adjusted life years (QALY).** It provides a better picture of the ability of your body to work efficiently.[14] QALY measures your biological age rather than your chronological age. It considers **biomarkers,** such as aerobic capacity and muscle strength, that tend to decline with age. Older people who actively maintain their health may outperform younger people on these biomarkers and may therefore have a younger biological age.

The number of quality-adjusted life years (QALY) for the U.S population on the whole is about 64, which is lower than the average life expectancy of 75.[15] In other words, many people survive for more than a decade after their bodies can no longer readily meet the demands that are placed on them. For African Americans, the QALY figure is even lower—56 years.

We can do better. Most of us prepare for retirement by saving money. We can also extend our "physical capital" into later life by better managing our physical well-being in young and middle adulthood.

Smart Quiz
Q1901

## think about it!

- **How long do you expect to live? Why?**
- **What can you do to increase your quality-adjusted life years? Will you? Why or why not?**

# HOW WE AGE

What can we expect as we grow older? What changes will there be in our health and our ability to function? Will our lives be satisfying? In what ways? Why can Mr. Cruz still play tennis at 78, while Mr. Schaefer, 10 years his junior, needs a cane to walk across the street?

Questions about aging are addressed by the field of **gerontology.** Gerontologists consider the biological, psychological, and social aspects of aging. Biological aging, or maturation, is an inevitable process that occurs in all living organisms. We humans reach our peak physical maturity by around age 30. After that, our biological functions begin a gradual decline. Aging also involves the psychological process of adapting to changing physical and social realities. "Young Turks" in the workplace become the "old guard." One-time newlyweds come to celebrate their silver and golden anniversaries. Yet aging can involve more than adjustment. It can bring about personal growth and exciting changes in direction as well. Even advanced old age can bring greater harmony and integration to our personalities. Then too, we must learn to adapt to changes in our mental skills and abilities. Though older people's memories may not be as keen, maturity and experience frequently enhance their wisdom.

Talking Glossary
Gerontology
G1901

Aging also has social aspects. Our self-concepts and behavior as "young," "middle-aged," or "old" people stem in large measure from cultural beliefs. In colonial times, "mature" people had great prestige. Men routinely claimed to be older than they were.[16] Women, however, perhaps because they had a less powerful role in society, generally did not do so. By contrast, the modern era has been marked by **ageism**—prejudice against older people.

The three dimensions of aging affect one another (see Figure 19.4, following page). Social factors such as isolation and neglect can affect psychological functioning. Psychological functioning can affect physical health. Physical well-being or illness affects people psychologically and socially.

**Mortality** Death rate.

**Morbidity** Prevalence of disease.

**Quality-adjusted life years (QALY)** Years of healthy life.

**Biomarkers** Physiological measures of aging, such as aerobic capacity and muscle strength.

**Gerontology** The study of aging and the elderly.

**Ageism** Attitudes of prejudice and discrimination toward older persons.

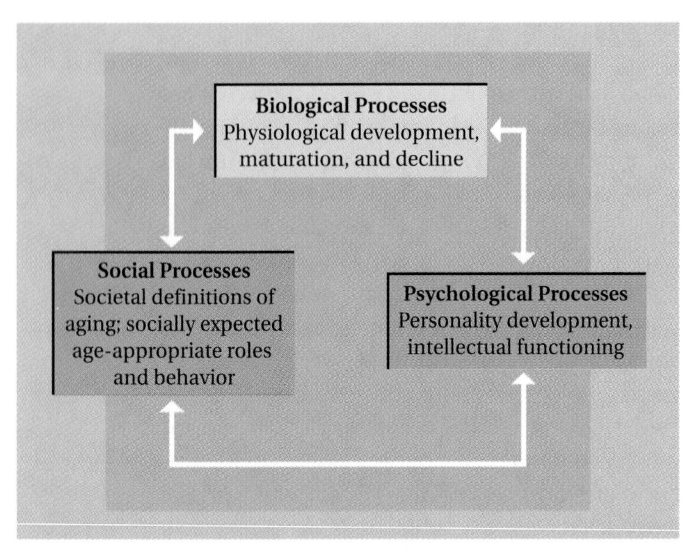


**Figure 19.4** ***Three Dimensions of Aging*** Aging can be thought of in terms of three dimensions that influence each other: social processes, biological processes and psychological processes.

## Physiological Changes

**Talking Glossary**
Integumentary system
**G1902**

No two people age in the same way or at the same rate. The older people become, the less similar they become in physical functioning.[17] However, physiological aging is defined by changes in the body's **integumentary system** (the body's system of skin, hair, and nails), senses, reaction time, and lung capacity. These changes may well be unavoidable. Other changes may be moderated, perhaps even reversed, through exercise and diet, however. These include changes in metabolism, muscle mass, strength, bone density, aerobic capacity, blood-sugar tolerance, and ability to regulate body temperature.[18]

Let's consider some of the more common changes that occur as we age.

**Integumentary system** The skin, along with its attachments, including hair and nails.

**Melanin** Pigment that gives color to skin and hair and other body tissues.

**Collagen** A fibrous protein that is the major structural component of skin, cartilage, tendon, and connective tissues.

**Elastin** A protein in connective tissue that is the basic component in elastic fibers.

**Keratinocytes** Cells in the outer layer of the skin that are regularly shed and renewed.

**Photoaging** Skin wrinkling caused by exposure to ultraviolet rays.

**Presbyopia** Loss of elasticity in the lens of the eye; diminishes ability to focus on small, close objects.

**Cataracts** A clouding of the eyes, which reduces vision; a common result of aging.

**Glaucoma** An eye disease involving a buildup of fluid pressure inside the eyeball; can damage the eye, impair vision, and sometimes cause blindness.

**Presbycusis** Hearing loss, especially in the higher frequencies, that accompanies aging.

**Changes in Skin and Hair** Despite advertising claims of cosmetics companies, we inevitably develop wrinkles and gray hair if we live long enough. Hair begins to gray as the production of **melanin,** the pigment responsible for hair color, decreases. Hair loss also accelerates with aging, especially in men.

**Talking Glossary**
Collagen, Elastin, Keratinocyte
**G1903**

Beginning (slowly) in the twenties, the body produces less **collagen** and **elastin.** These are proteins that give the skin its elasticity, making it soft and supple. The body also produces fewer **keratinocytes**—the cells in the epidermis (outer skin layer) that are regularly shed and renewed. The skin thus becomes more dry and brittle.

Yet people do not wrinkle at the same rate. Factors such as genetics, diet, hormonal balances, and, especially, exposure to the sun come into play. Much wrinkling associated with aging is actually caused by exposure to ultraviolet (UV) rays—a process called **photoaging.** Photoaging accelerates the aging of the skin. Using sunscreens and staying out of the sun, especially in midday, slow photoaging.

**Talking Glossary**
Presbyopia, Cataracts, Glaucoma
**G1904**

**Changes in Sensory Functioning** Normal age-related changes in vision generally begin to appear by the midthirties. **Presbyopia** (Latin for "old vision") refers to loss of elasticity in the lens. As a result, it is harder for the muscles of the eye to bend the lens to focus close objects or fine print.

Chemical changes involved in aging can lead to vision disorders such as **cataracts** and **glaucoma.** Cataracts cloud the lenses of the eyes, reducing vision. Today, outpatient surgery for correcting cataracts is routine. If performed before the condition progresses too far, the surgery usually has excellent results. Glaucoma is a buildup of fluid pressure inside the eyeball. Glaucoma can lead to tunnel vision (lack of peripheral vision) or blindness. Glaucoma rarely occurs before age 40 and tends to be inherited. It affects about 1 in 250 people over the age of 40. The incidence rises to 1 in 25 people over the age of 80.[19] Rates are higher among African Americans than among non-Hispanic white Americans and among diabetics. Glaucoma is treated with medication or surgery.

The sense of hearing, especially the ability to hear higher frequencies, also declines with age. **Presbycusis** ("old hearing" in Latin) is age-related hearing loss. It affects about one person in three over the age of 65.[20] Hearing ability tends to decline more quickly in men than in women. Hearing aids magnify sound and can compensate for hearing loss.

Taste and smell become less acute as we age. Our sense of smell decreases almost ninefold from youth to old age.[21] We also lose taste buds in the tongue with aging. Their number declines from about 250 as young adults to about 100 by age 70.[22] As a result, foods must be more strongly spiced to yield the same flavor.

**Slowed Reaction Time** **Reaction time** is the time it takes to respond to a stimulus. It also declines with age. It takes older people longer to dodge falling objects and to avoid other cars when driving. Reaction time slows because of changes in the nervous system. Beginning at around age 25, we begin to lose neurons, or nerve cells, involved in coordinating movements and responding to sensory signals such as sights and sounds.

**Reduced Lung Capacity** Lung tissue becomes stiffer as we age and does not expand as it did when we were younger. Between the ages of 20 and 70, breathing capacity may decline by as much as 40%.[23] Regular exercise can offset much of this loss, however.[24]

**Loss of Lean Body Mass and Increase in Body Fat** Lean body mass, especially muscle, declines with age. Beginning at age 20, we lose nearly 7 pounds of lean body mass with each decade. The rate of loss accelerates after the age of 45.[25] Fat replaces lean body mass. Consequently, the average person's body mass index (BMI) rises.

**Reduced Muscle Strength** Loss of muscle leads to a decline in muscle strength. From age 20 to about age 70, we lose almost 30% of our muscle cells.[26] On the other hand, vigorous exercise can largely compensate for the loss of muscle cells by increasing the size of remaining muscle cells—a process called **muscle hypertrophy.**

Talking Glossary
Muscle hypertrophy
G1905

**Metabolic Slowdown** Metabolism is the rate at which the body burns food to produce energy. The resting metabolic rate—also called the basal metabolic rate (BMR)—declines as we age. The decline may be largely attributed to the loss of muscle tissue and the corresponding increase in fatty tissue. Fat burns fewer calories than muscle. A person's basal metabolism drops by about 2% per decade beginning at age 20. Since we require fewer calories to maintain our weight as we age, excess calories are deposited as fat. Older people are thus likely to gain weight if they eat as much as they did when they were younger.

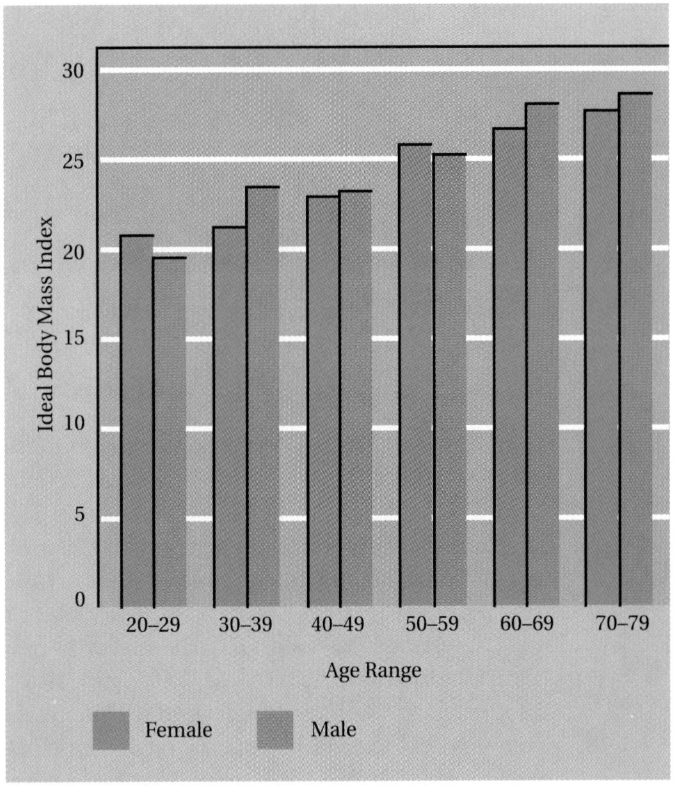

**Figure 19.5** ***Age and Ideal Body Mass Composition*** The body mass index (BMI) is a ratio of weight to height. BMIs under 25 fall in a healthy weight range for people under the age of 50. However, BMIs tend to increase as people age, as fat replaces lean body mass. See Chapter 6 for the computations to calculate whether your BMI falls within an ideal range for your age.

The lesson here is twofold: First, the more muscle you retain as you age (vigorous exercise builds muscle), the less your metabolism will slow down. Second, to maintain a steady weight over your adult life span, you should expect to reduce your caloric intake by 100 calories a day for each decade. If as a 20-year-old you maintained your body weight with 2,200 calories daily, at age 30 you should consume 2,100 calories. At 40, you'll only need 2,000 calories, and so on.

Older people may find it harder to shed extra pounds, but they need not surrender in the battle of the bulge. Regular exercise and a healthy diet help people control their weight at any age.

**Bone Loss** Bone, which consists largely of the mineral calcium, begins to lose density at

**Reaction time** Time it takes to respond to a stimulus.

**Muscle hypertrophy** Increase in the size of muscle cells, resulting in increased muscle size.

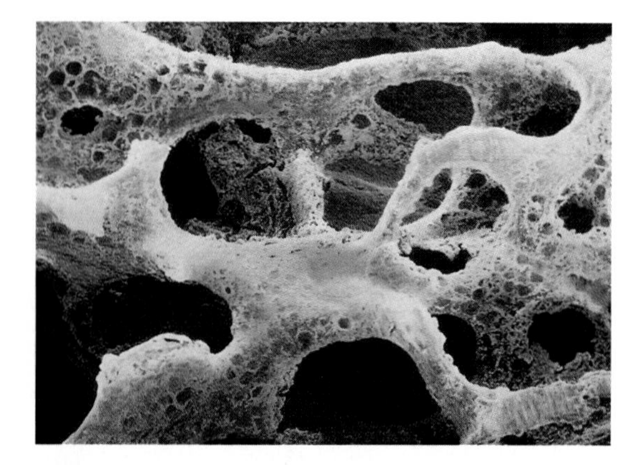

**Figure 19.6** ***Osteoporosis*** In osteoporosis, bones become spongy or more porous, which makes them more susceptible to fractures.

around age 40. The strength of bone is proportional to its density. Bone that is twice as dense is four times as strong. As bones lose density, they become more brittle and prone to fracture. Bones in the spine, hip, thigh (femur), and forearm lose the most density as we age.

Osteoporosis is bone loss that makes bones brittle and more likely to break (see Figure 19.6). Both men and women are at risk of osteoporosis, but it poses a greater threat to women. Men typically have a larger bone mass, which provides them with more protection against the disease.

About one woman in four over the age of 60 has osteoporosis. White women and Asian women are more likely to develop osteoporosis than African-American women are. So are women with smaller frames. Women's greater susceptibility to bone loss is tied to the loss of the female sex hormone estrogen following menopause. Beginning with menopause, women experience a sharp seven-year drop in bone density. They may wind up with half the bone mass they had in young adulthood. Women stand about twice the risk of hip fractures and about eight times the risk of spine fractures as men do.

Osteoporosis can shorten us by inches and lead to deformities in posture, such as the curvature in the spine known as "dowager's hump." It also results in more than a million bone fractures a year in the United States, the most serious of which are hip fractures. A hip fracture is actually a break in the upper femur, or thigh bone, which is just below the hip joint. Hip fractures often result in hospitalization, loss of mobility, and, sometimes, death from complications. More than one-fourth of the people who sustain a hip fracture die within a year.[27] Of the more than 280,000 hip fractures experienced by people in the United States in 1992, three of four occurred in women. Seven of eight occurred in people aged 65 or older.[28]

PREVENTION

## *Preventing Osteoporosis*[30]

The key to preventing osteoporosis is building strong bones, especially before the age of 35. The health of your bones depends on a number of factors, including diet and exercise.

***Diet*** Bones need calcium to maintain mineral density. Yet studies show that many of us get half or less of the daily calcium requirement. For young adults in the 19-to-24-year age range, the recommended dietary allowance for calcium is in the neighborhood of 1,200 to 1,500 mg (see Table 5.5 on page 119). An 8-ounce glass of milk, a cup of yogurt, 1.5 ounces of cheese, or 2 cups of cottage cheese each contain about 300 mg, so 4 to 5 helpings of these calcium-rich foods can be used to meet the daily calcium requirement for young adults. (For a listing of other calcium-rich foods, see Table 5.10.) When selecting calcium-rich foods, choose those that are low in fat, such as skim or 1% milk rather than 2% or whole milk, and low-fat cheese products. Keep track of your dietary intake of calcium for a week. If it falls below the recommended level for your age, ask your health care provider whether you should take a calcium supplement. If you decide to use a calcium supplement, consult with your doctor or pharmacist to select one that is best absorbed by your body.

The body needs adequate levels of vitamin D to absorb calcium. Vitamin D is manufactured by the body in response to ultraviolet light, such as sunlight. It is also available in our food supply, such as in vitamin-fortified milk products. But excesses of vitamin D can be harmful (ask your doctor). Multivitamins containing 100% of the recommended RDA of the vitamin can be taken safely, however.

***Exercise*** Exercise is even more important as you age and can help slow down, halt, or even reverse many of the effects of aging.[31] Stretching, aerobic exercise, and muscle strengthening are important throughout life. Weight-bearing exercise that makes you work against gravity helps build bone density and keep bones and muscles strong. Exercises such as walking, jogging, aerobic dance, stair climbing, and racquet sports do the trick. Even non-weight-bearing exercise, such as cycling and water aerobics, can help build bone density. Exercise also decreases the loss of calcium and other bone minerals. But you need to keep going—the positive effects of exercise last only as long as you maintain your exercise program.

***Avoid Excessive Use of Alcohol*** Excessive alcohol intake (more than two or three drinks per day) can interfere with the absorption of calcium from the small intestine into the bloodstream.

***Hormone Replacement*** Estrogen-replacement therapy for postmenopausal women can reduce their risk of osteoporosis, heart disease, and colon cancer. Estrogen replacement (use of a synthetic form of the natural hormone) reduces the risk of heart disease and stroke in postmenopausal women by 50% or more.[32] Estrogen replacement can also substantially reduce other symptoms caused by the hormonal deficiencies of menopause.

Estrogen is often combined with a synthetic form of another female sex hormone, progesterone (progestin). Yet hormone-replacement therapy remains controversial because it may increase the risk of breast cancer (and uterine cancer if estrogen is used without progestin) as well as cause other symptoms ranging from insomnia to joint aches. Both osteoporosis and cardiovascular disease are far more common than breast cancer, which may tip the scale in favor of hormone-replacement therapy for most women.[33]

What about hormone-replacement therapy for men? Men experience a decline in the production of androgen, or male sex hormone, as they age. By age 65, this deficiency can lead to loss of body strength, decreased muscle mass, declining sex drive, even osteoporosis. Androgen replacement can help reverse these effects, but there are possible increased risks of prostate cancer and cardiovascular disease. Check with your health care provider for the latest information.

Though there is no guarantee that you can prevent osteoporosis, there are steps you can take to minimize your risk, such as adopting healthy nutritional and exercise habits. Postmenopausal women also need to consult their personal physicians to carefully weigh the risks and benefits of hormone-replacement therapy in light of their personal risk profile.

**Close-up**
Osteoporosis studies
T1903

**Decline in Aerobic Capacity** As we age, the cardiovascular system becomes less efficient. Heart and lung muscles shrink. Aerobic capacity declines as less oxygen is taken into the lungs and the heart pumps less blood. The maximum heart rate declines. On the other hand, exercise can expand aerobic capacity at *any* age.

**Reduced Blood-Sugar Tolerance** Blood sugar, or glucose, is the basic fuel and energy source for living cells. The energy from glucose supports cell activities and maintains body temperature. Glucose circulates in the bloodstream and enters cells with the help of insulin, a hormone secreted by the pancreas.

As we age, the tissues in our body become less capable of taking up glucose from the bloodstream. This condition is called *impaired glucose tolerance*. Body tissues lose their sensitivity to insulin, which requires the pancreas to produce more insulin to achieve the same effect. Thus blood-sugar levels rise, increasing the risk of adult-onset diabetes. Although the rate at which our bodies metabolize glucose may decline with age, we can take steps to minimize this condition. Controlling weight, eating less fat, and exercising can help rebuild sensitivity to insulin and, perhaps, prevent adult-onset diabetes.[29]

**Decline in Ability to Regulate Internal Temperature** A stable body temperature within a degree of 98.6° F or 37.5° C is vital to health. As we age, however, the body becomes less able to maintain a steady temperature. Two factors are responsible for this: lowered metabolism and a lessened ability to generate heat by shivering—a process known as **thermogenesis.**

**Talking Glossary**
Thermogenesis
G1906

The decline in internal temperature control makes older people more susceptible to dehydration and more sensitive to heat and cold. Because the sense of thirst also declines with age, older people risk depleting their bodies of fluids.

## Changes in Mental Abilities

The brain is remarkably adaptive. Although you lose brain cells (neurons) as you age, the remaining cells develop new connections, or synapses, with neighboring cells that partially compensate for the loss. Consequently, mental abilities are largely preserved.

Yes, by about age 60, you can expect some decline in your ability to recall recent events, such as what you ate for dinner last night, and such information as names and telephone numbers. You may experience greater difficulty with tasks requiring visual-spatial skills, such as packing your trunk or using a map. By about age 70, there is usually some decline in the ability to think in abstract terms (for example, to learn geometry or physics). But most mental abilities, such as vocabulary, general knowledge, reasoning, and ability to recall important information, remain intact as we age. Many people in their eighties perform nearly as well on intelligence tests as people in their thirties and forties. Mental exercise, like physical exercise, can slow the declines of aging. People who remain mentally active are usually better able to retain

**Smart Reference**
Memories are made of . . .
R1901

**Thermogenesis** The production of heat, generally within the body.

their mental sharpness as they age.[34] Dementia (senility) is not a normal or inevitable part of aging. It is caused by degenerative brain diseases, such as Alzheimer's disease.

Health plays a role in learning and memory as we age. Diseases such as arteriosclerosis can impair mental functioning. Depression, which often goes unrecognized in older people, can also affect mental functioning, including memory. When depression is identified and treated, however, mental performance may improve.

Deficiencies in vitamins and minerals and exposure to harmful substances such as alcohol and some other drugs can also affect brain functioning among older people.

## Psychological Changes

Aging has psychological as well as physical aspects. People need to adapt to physical changes and to changes in life circumstances, such as the children's leaving home, retirement, the deaths of peers, and the approach of one's own death. Psychological theories help to account for the psychological changes that accompany aging. *Life stage theorists* explain ways in which we adapt to various stages of life from young adulthood through late adulthood. *Life transitions theorists* focus less on stages and more on how people cope with unpredictable events.

The experiences of youth and middle age help shape the later years. If we develop caring relationships when we are young, we are more likely to enjoy intimacy and companionship later on. If we develop a satisfying work life and other interests in young adulthood or middle age, we are less likely to experience boredom and inactivity later on.

### Life Stage Theories of Adult Development

Life stage theorists assume that adult development proceeds in stages from young adulthood through old age.

***Young Adulthood*** Young adulthood spans the ages of 20 to 40. The psychoanalyst Erik Erikson believed that each stage of life brings different challenges to identity. The major identity challenge of adolescence is to form a cohesive sense of *ego identity*, the sense of who you are and what role you plan to pursue in life. The identity challenge in young adulthood, according to Erikson, is *intimacy versus isolation*. Intimacy means sharing oneself with others through emotionally intimate relationships such as marriage and deep friendships. Erikson believed that people who do not develop intimate relationships risk falling into isolation and loneliness.

Erikson also believed that young adulthood was a time of increasing autonomy. People establish identities separate from their parents' and assert greater control over their lives.

Psychologist Robert Havighurst outlined tasks that confront young adults—selecting a mate, learning to live with him or her, becoming a parent, managing a home, starting a career, assuming civic responsibilities, and creating a social network.[35] Havighurst's tasks reflect societal expectations as much as individual goals. Many people choose not to marry or have children. Yet they can enhance their development in other ways.

***Middle Adulthood*** In a survey, 46% of the people questioned said that middle age begins when you realize you don't know who the new music groups are; 42% said it begins when the last child leaves home.[36] Most health professionals consider middle adulthood to roughly span the years from 40 to 60 or 65.

Erikson wrote that the major psychological challenge of the middle years is *generativity versus stagnation*. Generativity is the ability to generate or produce. It can take various forms—rearing children, advancing in a career, making things of lasting value, or contributing to civic works. Gen-

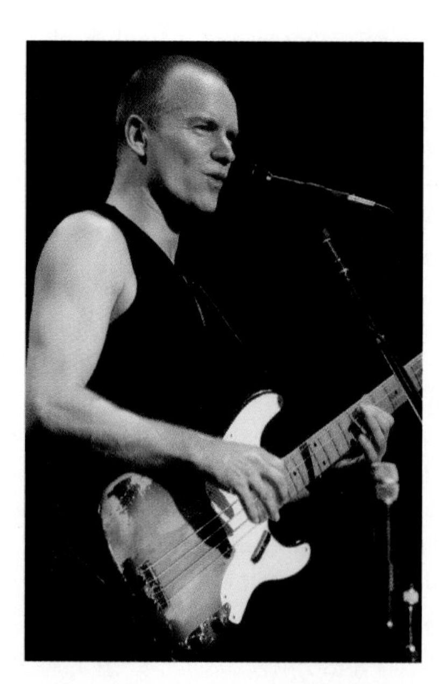

***Who's Middle-Aged?*** Veteran rock stars like Sting have led to a blurring of generational lines.

erativity enhances one's self-esteem. People who are not productive (generative) risk stagnating and falling into routines that can strip their lives of meaning and purpose.

Some people experience a *midlife crisis,* during which they fear they have more to look back upon than forward to. There may be one last attempt to deny the realities of aging: having an extramarital affair to prove to ourselves that we are still sexually attractive, buying a sports car (red, of course), or suddenly shifting careers. Yet the writer Gail Sheehy[37] terms the years from 45 onward a "second adulthood." She writes that many Americans find the middle years to be opportunities for new direction and fulfillment. For many people today, the so-called midlife crisis is imposed from the outside in the form of a career crash resulting from corporate *downsizing*—the thinning of the ranks of middle managers. But people who are flexible enough to make the transition to other careers can find increased satisfaction.

The fifties are often more relaxed and productive than the forties. Yet many people in their fifties need to adjust to the children leaving home (the "empty nest"), the effects of aging, and competition from younger workers.

***Late Adulthood*** Late adulthood is generally considered to begin at age 65. For people in good health, being 65 or older is experienced more as an extension of middle age than of late adulthood—particularly if they continue to work. A key characteristic of older people today is their more youthful self-concepts. They do not see themselves as being old, at least not until they reach advanced old age (75 or 80). Erikson characterized late adulthood as the stage of *ego integrity versus despair.* Erikson saw the basic psychological challenge of late adulthood as maintaining a sense of meaning and purpose while facing the inevitability of death. The alternative is to slip into despair. Ego integrity derives from wisdom, from coming to accept oneself and one's life, from recognizing one's place in the stream of history.

Some people age more healthily or successfully than others. "Successful agers" have characteristics that can inspire all of us to lead more healthful and enjoyable lives:[38]

- *Concentrating on what is important and meaningful.* Successful agers form emotional goals that bring them satisfaction. Rather than cast about in several directions, they may focus on their families and friends. Successful agers no longer compete in arenas best left to younger people. Instead they focus on maintaining a sense of personal control.
- *A positive outlook.* Some older people attribute occasional health problems—such as aches and pains—to temporary factors, such as a cold or jogging too long. Others attribute aches and pains to ongoing factors such as aging itself. People who attribute their problems to specific factors have a more positive outlook or attitude.
- *Self-challenge.* Many people think of late adulthood as a time for resting from life's challenges. But sitting back and allowing the world to pass by is a prescription for vegetating, not living healthfully.

Doing less is no prescription for health and adjustment among older people. Focusing on what is important, keeping a positive outlook, and meeting new challenges is as important for older people as for any of us.

**Life Transitions Theory of Adult Development** Life stage theorists focus on predictable age-related changes and their related challenges. To life transitions theorists, such as psychologist Nancy Schlossberg, adult identity is affected as much by *what* happens to us as by *when* it happens to us.

At any time, life may pose challenges that require a shift from one role or situation to another.[39] These **life transitions** can throw curve balls into the best-laid plans. Young adults may assume that they will marry once, have children, and remain in the careers they selected in their twenties. Sometimes these assumptions are borne out. Sometimes they are not. Cultural expectations of stages of life also change over time. For example, it used to be unusual, perhaps even "abnormal," to begin raising a family after the age of 30 or 35, let alone age 40 or older as many couples do today. Similarly, most people—nearly always males—were expected to select one career and stick with it until retirement at 65. Today, however, career-oriented people are more likely to change jobs 10 times or so during their working lives. Many workers not only switch jobs but careers. Some people begin college at 30, 40, or later. They go on to enjoy later careers in their chosen fields. Age-related expectations have shifted so much

**Life transitions** Changes in our roles or life situations caused by anticipated or unexpected events.

that people facing the challenges of new parenthood and college may represent different generations.

Schlossberg describes four transitions that may confront us during any stage of adult life:[40]

1. *Anticipated transitions:* Graduating from school, getting a job, getting married, and having children are examples of anticipated transitions. We expect to encounter the anticipated transitions.
2. *Unanticipated transitions:* Unplanned pregnancies, job losses or forced retirement, or being refused admission to the college of your choice are examples of unanticipated transitions. Because they are unexpected, they may require greater resilience.
3. *Nonevent transitions:* Sometimes events we expect don't materialize. We may find at age 40, for instance, that we haven't found Mr. or Ms. Right, or at age 65 or 70 that we can't afford to retire. Nonevent transitions force us to revise our expectations and find the inner resources to deal with them.
4. *Chronic hassle transitions:* Disruptive life events may occur at any time, causing us to shift course. These include personal or family illness, a difficult boss, accidents, or exposure to war.

The ways in which we cope with life's transitions depend on many factors, including our personalities, the availability of social support, and our physical and mental health.

## Changes in Sexuality

There are unfounded cultural myths to the effect that older people are sexless and that the few older men with sexual interests are "dirty old men." If older people buy into these myths, they may renounce sex or feel guilty if they remain sexually active. Older women are handicapped by a double standard that has greater tolerance of continued sexuality among men.

The fact is that older people are not asexual. They may need to adjust to age-related changes in sexual response (see Table 19.1), but healthy people can reap sexual fulfillment for a lifetime. Sexual daydreaming, sex drive, and sexual activity all tend to decline with age, but sexual satisfaction may remain high.[41] Older people with partners usually remain sexually active. The adage "use it or lose it" may contain some truth. Younger adults who have active and satisfying sex lives are more likely to continue to enjoy sex in late adulthood. Sexual *activity* may in itself help maintain sexual interest and enjoyment. Sexual *inactivity,* by contrast, may lessen sexual appetite.[42]

**Close-up**
Sexuality in later life
**T1904**

**Changes in the Female[43]** Many of the physical changes in women stem from the decline in estrogen that occurs with menopause. Older women frequently experience reduced muscle tension (of the sort connected with sexual arousal and orgasm), reduced vaginal lubrication, reduced vaginal size and elasticity, smaller increases in breast size during arousal, and reduced intensity

**TABLE 19.1**

**Changes in Sexual Response Often Associated with Aging[45]**

| Changes in the Female | Changes in the Male |
|---|---|
| Reduced pelvic muscle tension | Longer time to achieve erection and orgasm |
| Reduced vaginal lubrication | Need for more direct stimulation to achieve erection and orgasm |
| Reduced elasticity of the vaginal walls | Less semen emitted during ejaculation |
| Smaller increases in breast size during sexual arousal | Erections may be less firm |
| Reduced intensity in muscle spasms at orgasm | Testicles may not elevate as high into scrotum during orgasm |
| | Less intense orgasmic contractions |
| | Lessened feeling of need to ejaculate when aroused |
| | Longer refractory period |

of muscle spasms during orgasm. Because the vaginal walls lose elasticity, sexual intercourse can become painful—a condition known as dyspareunia (see Chapter 9). The thinning of the vaginal walls may place greater pressure against the bladder and urethra during sex, leading to urinary urgency or burning. The spasms of orgasm may become less powerful and fewer in number. Intensity or frequency of orgasmic contractions may have no bearing on feelings of sexual satisfaction, however.

**Changes in the Male**[44] Age-related physical changes occur more gradually in men than in women. They do not reflect any one biological event, as is the case with menopause in women. As men age, it takes longer for them to attain erection and reach orgasm. Erections become less firm. Less semen is emitted during ejaculation. Orgasms become less intense.

These changes may reflect declining testosterone levels. However, most men remain capable of erection throughout their lives. The refractory period (the amount of time a man needs before he can have another orgasm) lengthens with age. An adolescent may require only a few minutes to regain erection and ejaculate. A man in his thirties may require half an hour. Past age 50, the refractory period may increase to several hours, perhaps requiring a night's sleep. Testosterone production usually declines gradually from about age 40 to 60, and then begins to level off. Yet viable sperm may be produced quite late in life. Many men can still father children in their seventies and eighties.

**Adjusting to Changes in Sexuality** Acceptance of the changes of aging helps people maintain a healthy sex life. Men may feel inadequate when they take longer to become sexually aroused. Once they understand that a slower response is normal, they may experience less sexual pressure. Although men require more time to reach orgasm as they age, their partners may actually view them as better lovers. Attitudes and expectations are keys to satisfaction.

Despite the stereotype, menopause does not signal an end to a woman's sex life. Natural lubrication may be increased through more foreplay. The need for more foreplay may encourage the man to become a more considerate lover. (He too will probably need more time to become aroused.) An artificial lubricant may also be of help. Though orgasms may become less intense, women retain their ability to reach orgasm into advanced old age. Sexual satisfaction can remain very high. Age-related changes in the woman's sexual response may be slowed or reversed through hormone replacement.

Prescription medicines, alcohol, and other drugs can severely depress sexual functioning, causing alarm in males who are unaware of such side effects. Many men on medication to control high blood pressure, for instance, report a loss of sex drive. Adjusting dosages sometimes helps.

### think about it!

- **What physical and mental changes have been taking place as you have matured? How do you feel about them? Why?**
- **What physical and mental changes do you expect during the next decade? The next two decades? How do you feel about them? Why?**
- **What is your current "stage" of psychological development? Does your life fit any of the "standard" profiles? How or how not?**
- **Do you plan to be a "successful ager"? Why or why not?**

Smart Quiz
Q1902

## WHY WE AGE

Why do people grow older? Why do some people age faster than others? Perhaps if we understood the mechanisms of aging, we might learn how to slow them down or—should we dare say?—even stop or reverse them.

Current theories of aging fall into two general categories: *Programmed theories* see aging as the result of genetic instructions; and *cellular damage theories* propose that aging results from damage to cells.

### Programmed Theories of Aging

Programmed theories propose that aging and longevity are determined by a biological clock that ticks at a rate governed by the organism's genes. If these theories are correct, the seeds of our own demise lie in our genes, those bits of DNA that carry our genetic code. If we knew which genes controlled aging and could interpret them, we would know how long you would live (if you avoided serious accidents or illness). There is much evidence for a genetic component in aging. For example, longevity runs in families.

But why should organisms carry "suicidal" genes? Why would they not carry genes that enable them to live forever? Programmed-aging theorists believe that species were designed by natural selection to survive long enough to reproduce and pass along their genetic inheritance. From the evolutionary perspective, there would be no advantage to the species (and probably a disadvantage, given limited food supplies) to develop genes that function to maintain life indefinitely. It would make more sense for each generation to be better adapted than the previous generation. As a result, the body ages and eventually dies.

**Programmed Senescence** Cancer cells divide indefinitely, but normal human cells have finite life spans.[46] After dividing about 50 times, they cease dividing and eventually die. Cells from longer-lived species divide more times before they die than cells from shorter-lived species. For example, cells from newborn chickens, which can live 12 years, divide about 25 times. Cells from humans divide about 50 times. Cells from the Galapagos tortoise, which can live as long as 175 years, divide about 100 times.[47] When cells cease dividing, they enter a dormant state called **cell senescence** before they die.

Talking Glossary
Cell senescence
G1907

Another view is that cellular aging, not cell senescence, is responsible for aging. Cells become less capable of repairing themselves as we age, making us more prone to cellular breakdowns, such as cancer, and to other chronic diseases. Perhaps the finite limits on cell division—the maximum number of times a cell can divide—determine a species' longevity. If so, for humans the figure would be about 115 years. Yet only a few of us live that long. Genetic programming may underlie not only cell senescence but also cellular aging. Individual genetic differences might also largely account for differences in longevity among people.

**Endocrine Theory** Another programmed theory of aging focuses on the endocrine system—the system of ductless glands that releases hormones into the bloodstream. Hormonal changes signal age-related changes, such as puberty and menopause. Preprogrammed hormonal changes connected with aging may leave the body more vulnerable to conditions that affect older people, such as diabetes, osteoporosis, and cardiovascular disease.

**Cell senescence** A condition in which cells stop dividing and become dormant; eventually leads to cell death.

**Immunological Theory** Another programmed theory holds that the immune system is preset to decline by an internal biological clock. For example, the production of antibodies declines with age, rendering the body less able to fight off foreign substances and more likely to turn against itself.[48] Age-related changes in the immune system increase the risk of cancer and may contribute to general deterioration.[49]

## Damage Theories of Aging

Programmed theories assume that internal bodily processes are preset to age by genes. In contrast, damage theories propose that internal bodily changes and external environmental assaults (such as carcinogens and toxins) cause cells and organ systems to malfunction, leading to death.[50]

**Wear and Tear Theory** The *wear and tear theory* suggests that over the years, our bodies become less adept at repairing themselves. Like a machine whose parts wear out through use, vital organs are worn down by time.

**Free-Radical Theory** The *free-radical theory* attributes aging to damage caused by the accumulation in the body of unstable molecules called free radicals, which are produced during metabolism by oxidation. These highly reactive molecules steal electrons from other molecules, causing a chain reaction that damages cell proteins, membranes, and DNA. The damage may cause us to age faster and become more vulnerable to diseases associated with aging such as cancer, heart disease, diabetes, and arthritis.[51] Free radicals may also be produced by exposure to external environmental agents such as ultraviolet or other forms of radiation, extreme heat, pesticides, and air pollution.

Our cells constantly produce free radicals. Most are naturally disarmed by scavenger nutrients and enzymes called *antioxidants.* Some antioxidants are made by the body. Others, like beta-carotene and vitamins C and E, are found in food. As we age, the body produces fewer of its own antioxidants. People whose diets are rich in antioxidants are less likely to develop heart disease and some forms of cancer. Recently, researchers reported that vitamin E can help boost immune system response in older people.[52] It remains to be seen whether the body can better withstand the effects of aging if people increase their intake of antioxidant nutrients through diet or supplements.

**Cross-Linking Theory** Cross-links occur when cell proteins bind to one another, toughening tissues. Cross-linking stiffens collagen—the connective tissue supporting tendons, ligaments, cartilage, and bone.[53] The *cross-linking theory of aging* holds that the stiffening of body proteins, including collagen, accelerates and eventually breaks down bodily processes, leading to aging. The most obvious example is coarse, dry skin, which results from the cross-linking of collagen. The immune system combats cross-linking, but it becomes less able to do so as we age. Cross-linking may contribute to some of the effects of aging, but it is probably not the most important factor in the aging process.[54]

In considering the many theories of aging, we should note that aging is an extremely complex biological process that may not be explainable by any single theory or cause. Aging may involve a combination of factors.

## Promising New Directions

**Close-up**
Life extension: Science or science fiction
T1905

Innovative avenues of research may soon yield new insights into the aging process. One avenue involves caloric restriction. Reducing calorie intake without sacrificing nutrition has been shown to extend the lives of laboratory animals, including mice, rats, and fruit flies. Another avenue concerns the anti-aging properties of hormones that normally decline as we age: melatonin, DHEA, and human growth hormone (hGH).

**Caloric Restriction** In laboratory experiments, mice were fed a diet that was 30 to 60% lower in calories than normal but contained all necessary nutrients. The mice lived two to four years beyond their normal life spans.[55] Not only does caloric restriction extend life in lab animals; it also slows or prevents the growth of many diseases and tumors. It remains to be seen whether such severe caloric restriction will extend life in people. For the time being, it makes sense to adhere to a low-fat diet and avoid excess calories.

**Melatonin** The hormone **melatonin** is produced by the pineal gland and appears to play a role in the sleep–wake cycle. Melatonin supplements may help people with insomnia, especially in cases of jet lag and shifting work schedules. Because the pineal gland helps regulate body functions, the question has been raised as to whether it serves as a kind of "aging clock."[56] Blood levels of melatonin decline with age, but it remains unclear whether melatonin supplements affect aging. Melatonin has been shown to extend life expectancies in mice, but no studies on its effects on aging in humans have been reported.

**Talking Glossary**
Melatonin
G1908

**Smart Reference**
Melatonin mania
R1902

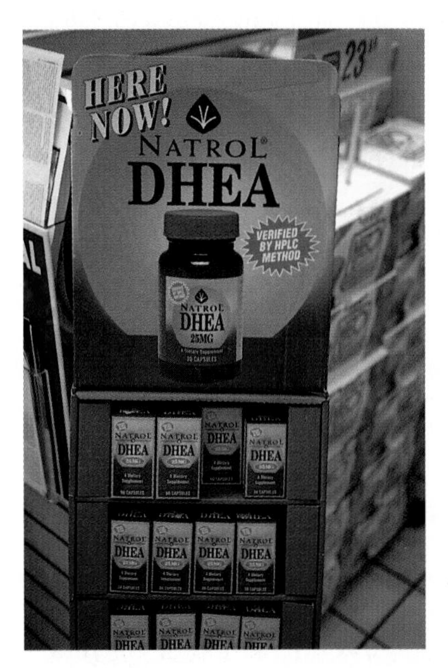


***Buyer Beware*** Claims that dietary supplements such as melatonin, DHEA, and hGH can combat aging remain unproven. We do know that these are powerful substances that can have unexpected and potentially harmful effects on the body.

**DHEA** The hormone **DHEA** (dehydroepiandrosterone) is produced by the adrenal glands. The body converts DHEA into other hormones, including the sex hormones testosterone and estrogen. DHEA production begins to decline after about age 30, dipping as low as 5 to 15% of its peak levels by age 60.[57] DHEA appears to play a role in bolstering the immune system, so lower levels of DHEA may increase our susceptibility to infectious organisms and cancer. Studies suggest that DHEA reduces the risk of some forms of cancer, improves immune functioning, and extends life in laboratory animals. However, studies with humans have yielded inconclusive or contradictory results to date.

**Melatonin** A hormone produced by the pineal gland that is believed to play a role in regulating the sleep–wake cycle.

**DHEA** A hormone produced by the adrenal glands; appears to play an important role in the production of other hormones and in the immune system.

**Human Growth Hormone** **Human growth hormone (hGH)** is a pituitary hormone. It plays a crucial role in growth and development during childhood and adolescence. The hormone regulates the growth of bones, muscles, and glands. Like DHEA and melatonin, natural production of hGH declines with age. Lower hGH levels may account for some of the effects of aging, such as loss of bone density and muscle mass. Though the hormone shows promise in reversing some effects related to aging (reducing body fat and increasing body mass), it is no fountain of youth.[58] There are also unpleasant side effects, such as swelling in the legs and ankles, and aching joints. hGH may also have dangerous complications such as cardiovascular disease and cancer. The National Institute of Aging is currently funding a number of clinical trials on hGH, so we may soon learn more about the relative risks and benefits of hGH treatment.

**Video** Anti-aging drugs: Hope or hype? V1904

**A Word of Caution** Be wary of claims that any product will combat aging or prevent disease. Many substances are just plain worthless. Others, such as melatonin, DHEA, and hGH, are powerful substances that can have unexpected effects on the body.[59]

**Close-up** Government issues warning T1906

**Smart Quiz** Q1903

### think about it!

- **Which theory or theories of aging make sense to you? Why?**
- **Do the various theories of aging suggest anything that you can do to live longer and healthier? What?**

**critical thinking** **Agree or disagree and support your views: Living forever would prevent a species from adapting to the environment.**

**Human growth hormone (hGH)** A hormone produced by the pituitary gland; involved in regulating growth and development during childhood and adolescence.

**Varicose veins** Abnormally enlarged or swollen veins, usually in the lower extremities.

**Arthritis** Inflammation of a joint, typically accompanied by pain and swelling.

**Osteoarthritis** A degenerative form of arthritis linked to wear and tear on the joints.

## HEALTH CONCERNS AND AGING

Though aging takes a toll on our bodies, many gerontologists believe that disease is not inevitable. They distinguish between *normal aging* and *pathological aging.* In normal aging, physiological processes decline slowly with age and the person is able to enjoy many years of health and vitality well into later life. In pathological aging, chronic diseases or degenerative processes, such as heart disease, diabetes, and cancer, lead to disability or premature death. In 1900, older people were more likely to die from infectious diseases such as pneumonia than is the case today. Older people today are at less risk of lethal infections. They are more at risk of developing chronic diseases such as heart disease and cancer.

### Physical Health Problems

More than four out of five people over the age of 65 have at least one chronic health problem.[60] Some, like **varicose veins,** are relatively minor. Others, like heart disease, pose more serious health risks. Figure 19.7 lists the top ten chronic conditions affecting persons 65 and older in the United States. Arthritis tops the list, followed by hypertension, hearing impairment, and heart disease. While longevity is increasing, so too is the length of time older people are living with chronic health problems.

**Arthritis** **Arthritis** is joint inflammation, which can result from more than 100 conditions affecting the structures inside and surrounding the joints. Symptoms progress from redness to heat, swelling, and pain, and finally to loss of function.[61] Arthritis can seriously limit activity as people age. About 37 million people in the United States have some form of arthritis. Even children can be affected by arthritis, but it is more likely to occur with advancing age. Arthritis is more common in women than in men and in African Americans than white Americans.[62]

Osteoarthritis and rheumatoid arthritis are the two most common forms of arthritis.[63] **Osteoarthritis** is a painful, degenerative form of arthritis linked to wear and tear on the joints. It is most likely to affect people over the age of 40. By age 60, more than half of all Americans show some signs of the disease. Among people over the age of 65, two of three have the disease. The joints most commonly affected are those in the knees, hips, fingers, neck, and lower back. Osteoarthritis is caused by an erosion of cartilage, the pads of fibrous tissue that cushion the ends of bones. As

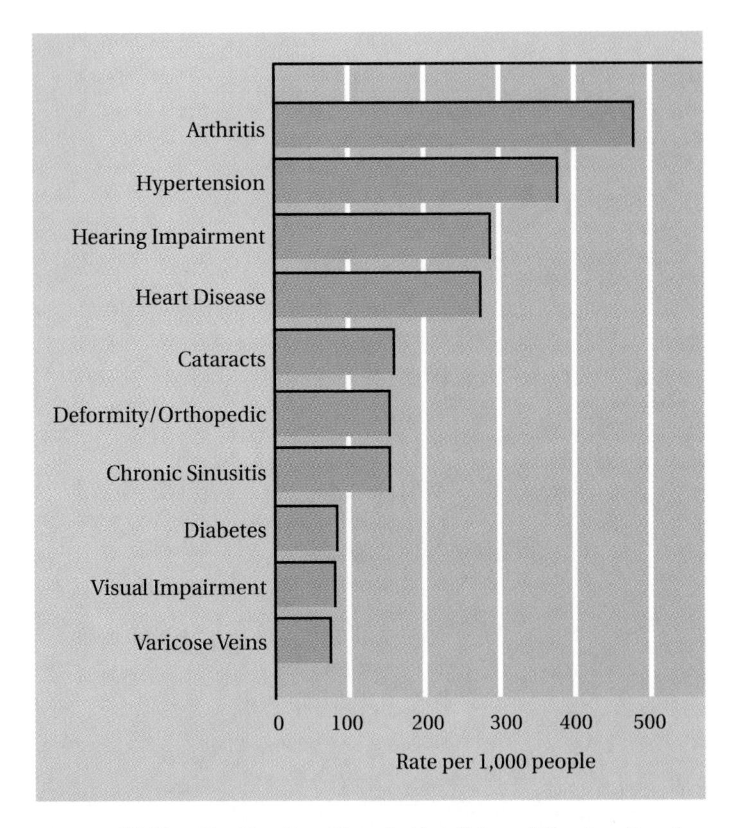


**Figure 19.7** ***The Top Ten Chronic Conditions Affecting People Age 65 and Older*** Arthritis, the leading chronic condition affecting people age 65 and over, affects nearly one in two people in this age range.

cartilage wears down, bones grind together, causing pain. Osteoarthritis is more common among obese people because excess weight adds to the load on the hip and knee joints. Doctors therefore often encourage overweight people with arthritis to lose weight. The over-the-counter drug acetaminophen (brand names Tylenol, Panadol) may help relieve pain and discomfort. If acetaminophen doesn't work effectively, nonsteroidal anti-inflammatory drugs (NSAIDs) are often used, such as two other over-the-counter drugs, aspirin and ibuprofen (brand names Advil, Nuprin). Prescription NSAIDs may also be used when pain doesn't respond to over-the-counter drugs. In severe cases, joint replacement surgery may be needed. Regular exercise may help improve joint mobility and reduce pain, especially (nonimpact) endurance exercises, such as walking, swimming, and cycling; stretching exercises; muscle-strengthening exercises (but not high-resistance exercises, like lifting heavy weights, which might increase joint inflammation); and range of motion exercises, which gently put the joint through its normal range of motion.

**Smart Reference**
Attacking arthritis
**R1903**

More than 2.5 million Americans have *rheumatoid arthritis,* which involves chronic inflammation of the membranes that line the joints. In rheumatoid arthritis, the body's immune system attacks its own tissues, causing inflammation. The condition affects the entire body. It can produce unrelenting pain and eventually lead to severe disability as the result of joint damage.[64] Bones and cartilage may also be affected. The disease usually affects people in the 30-to-50-year-old age range and strikes about twice as many women as men. Even children may develop it. Anti-inflammatory drugs are useful in treating the disease, but not all cases respond to these drugs. A new class of genetically engineered antibodies, now undergoing clinical testing, may help.

**Talking Glossary**
Rheumatoid arthritis
**G1909**

**Heart Disease, Cancer, and Stroke** The three biggest killers of Americans aged 65 and above are heart disease, cancer, and stroke (see Figure 19.8, following page). These three health problems account for 7 out of every 10 deaths among older people.[65] Cardiovascular diseases, which include heart disease and stroke, are the leading cause of death and the fourth most common form of chronic disease among persons aged 65 and above. The dominant form of heart disease among those 65 and older is coronary artery disease resulting from atherosclerosis. Other cardiovascular disorders prevalent among older persons include hypertension, heart arrhythmias, and congestive heart failure.

Note that among the top ten chronic conditions listed in Figure 19.7, several are also leading causes of death or else pose significant risk factors for mortality. For example, hypertension, the third most common chronic disease, affects about 40% of Americans over the age of 65. It is a major risk factor for both heart attacks and strokes. Diabetes, the eighth most common chronic illness, is the sixth leading cause of death. Other chronic conditions, such as cataracts, chronic sinusitis, visual impairment, and varicose veins, are rarely fatal but can lead to disability.

Many forms of cancer are also more common in people aged 50 and above. Overall, after cardiovascular disease, cancer is the second most common cause of death in older people. The risk of developing cancer increases tenfold for people aged 65 and above.[66] A key reason that the incidence of cancer is higher among older people is that the immune system becomes less able to rid the body of precancerous and cancerous cells. Unfortunately, many older people are not adequately screened

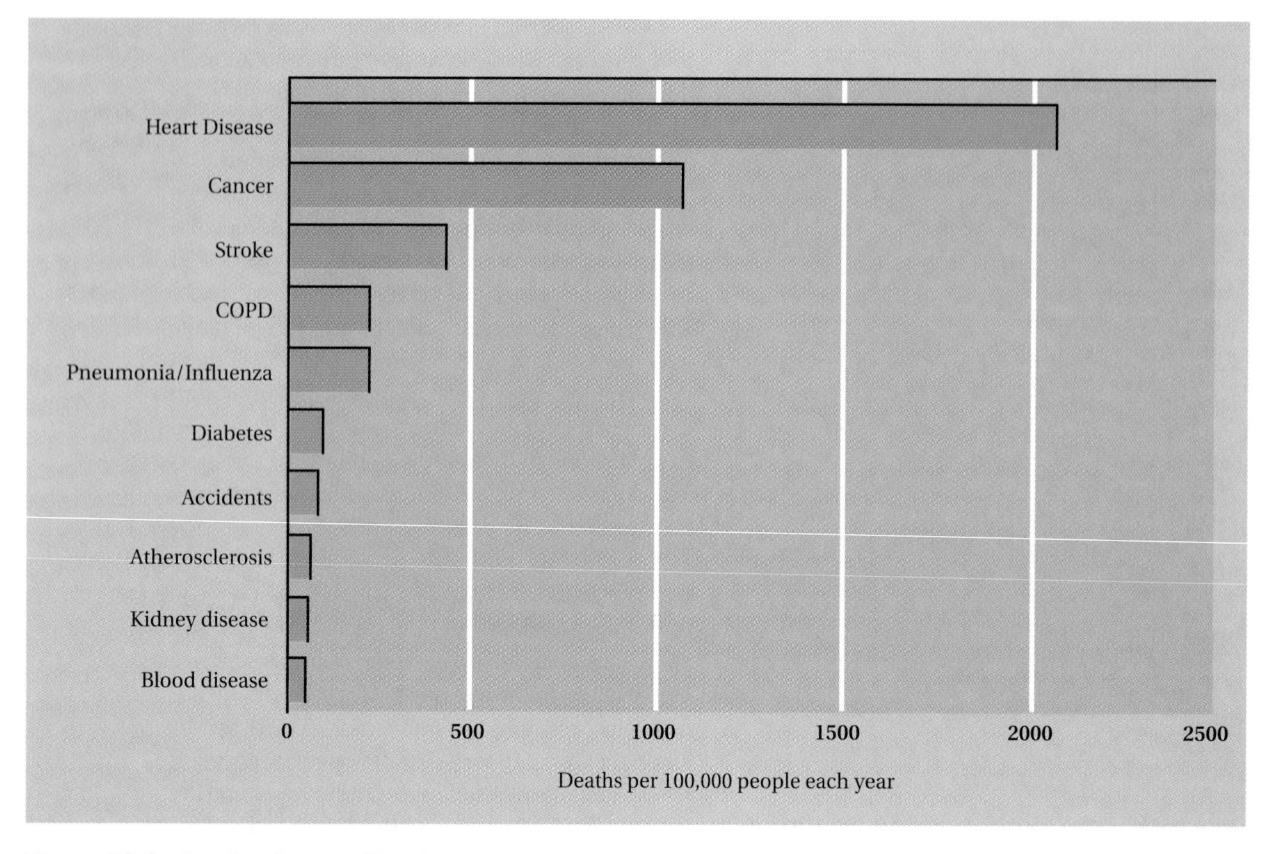


**Figure 19.8** ***Leading Causes of Death among Persons 65+*** The two leading causes of death in older people are heart disease and cancer.

for cancer, and their physicians are not as aggressive in treating them as they are in treating younger cancer patients.[67] The same is true of heart disease and other potentially fatal illnesses. One reason for the gap in diagnosis and treatment is **elder bias** on the part of some health professionals. Such attitudes may prevent older patients from receiving the same quality of health care that younger patients receive.

## Psychological Problems

For many people, the mature years are the best years, especially if they are filled with meaningful activity. The stresses involved in building and maintaining a career, selecting a mate, and rearing children may have receded into the past. Painful questions of identity may be settled. Without the pressing anxieties of youth, many older people savor life.

Older Americans are on the whole at least as happy as younger people. According to the National Health Interview Survey, most people 65 and older consider themselves to be in "excellent," "very good," or "good" overall health compared with other people of their age.[68] A *Los Angeles Times* survey found that older people worried less than their younger counterparts. Even though most were on fixed incomes, they were about three times more likely than younger persons to say they were "never depressed."[69]

**Elder bias** Discrimination against the elderly in medical practice and other institutional settings.

Not surprisingly, economic status plays a key role in psychological well-being. People with higher incomes report more satisfaction with their overall well-being than those in lower-income groups. Physically healthy people also report higher levels of psychological well-being.

Yet aging is often accompanied by difficult challenges. Older people are more likely to be bereaved by the loss of a spouse and close friends. They may need to cope with declining health, retirement, and relocation. Some must cope with decreasing mobility and independence, others with incapacitation and placement in a nursing home. Retirement, whether forced or not, can sap one's feeling of purpose in life and contribute to a loss of role identity. Problems in coping can lead to psychological problems, including depression, anxiety, and sleep disorders.

**Depression and Aging** According to the National Institute on Aging, about one in six people 65 years of age or older experience serious depression. Depression is even more common among residents of nursing homes. Depression in older people is often related to grief over the loss of loved ones; to brain disorders like Alzheimer's disease, stroke, and Parkinson's disease; or to physical illnesses like cancer or heart disease.[70] The poor, the very old, and those who lack social support are most likely to be depressed.[71] Depression can pose a risk to one's physical health as well as to one's mental health. For example, depression nearly triples the risk of stroke among older people with hypertension.[72]

Social support may act as a buffer against stress. It helps people cope with the stresses of declining health and the loss of loved ones. Yet older people may find it difficult to form new friendships and romantic relationships.

Depression in older people goes undetected and untreated most of the time.[73] Depression may be overlooked because its symptoms are masked by physical complaints (such as low energy and loss of appetite) and because health care providers tend to focus more on older people's physical health than their mental health. Many older people are reluctant to admit to depression because psychological problems carried more of a stigma when they were young.[74] Because depression can cause memory problems, some people with depression are misdiagnosed with Alzheimer's disease.[75] Depression in older people can usually be treated successfully by the same means that work in younger people—antidepressant drugs, psychotherapy, and, when needed, electroshock therapy (ECT).

**Close-up**
New hope for depressed elderly
**T1907**

Untreated depression can lead to suicide, which is most common among older people, especially white males. Suicide rates among older people jumped 9% from 1980 to 1992, reversing a four-decade decline.[76] Perhaps the increase occurred because medical advances have increased the length of life, but not necessarily the quality of life, for people with chronic health conditions. The social isolation faced by many older people also plays a role. The highest rates of suicide in older men are found among those who are widowed or otherwise isolated. Society's increasing acceptance of some forms of suicide may also increase the rate of suicide among older people.

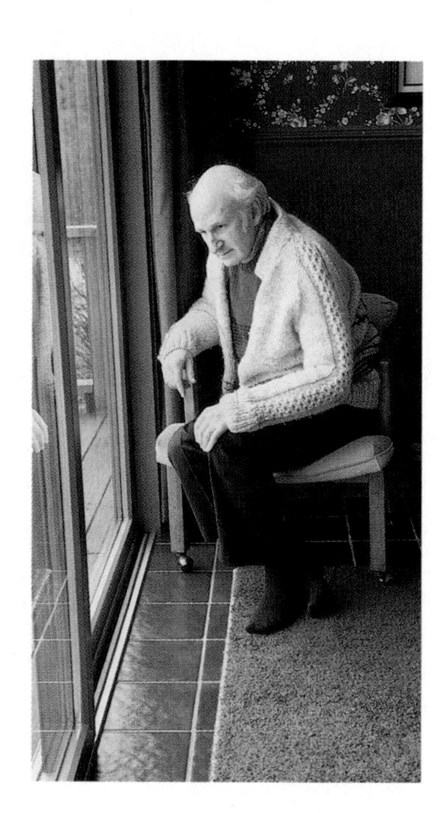

***Depression and Aging***
Clinical depression is common among older adults, though it often goes undetected and untreated. When diagnosed properly, it can usually be treated successfully with antidepressant medication, psychotherapy, or, in some cases, electroshock therapy.

**Anxiety Disorders and Aging** We might expect older people to have more than their share of anxiety disorders, as life challenges mount in later life, including coping with declining health and with the loss of family and friends, and confronting the finality of life itself. Not so. Anxiety disorders are more common among younger than older adults.[77] This is not to say that older people are immune to anxiety disorders. The most common type of anxiety disorder affecting older people is generalized anxiety disorder, which is characterized by persistent worry and tension. Panic disorder, however, is rare. Cases of agoraphobia (fear of venturing out in public) tend to follow the loss of social support systems as the result of the death of a spouse or close friends. Some older people fear venturing out not because of agoraphobia, but because of realistic fears of crime or of falling in the street. Anxiety disorders in older people (as in other age groups) frequently co-occur with other psychological problems, especially depression. Anxiety disorders in older people are commonly treated with medication (usually mild tranquilizers) and behavior therapy. Methods such as relaxation training and meditation may also help.

**Sleep Problems** Sleep disorders become more common as we age, especially insomnia and **sleep apnea.** In sleep apnea, the person stops breathing momentarily perhaps 200 to 400 times during the night, usually without knowing it. Apnea is more than a sleep problem. It is also linked to heart attacks and strokes.[78]

Sleep problems in older people sometimes involve biological changes related to aging. Sometimes they are symptoms of psychological disorders such as depression, dementia, and anxiety disorders.[79] Other contributing factors include loneliness, especially after the death of a spouse. Upsetting ideas, such as exaggerating the consequences of not getting enough sleep, can raise anxiety levels and prolong insomnia in older as well as younger people.

Sleep medications (typically mild antianxiety drugs like Halcion) are the most common treatment for insomnia. However, they can lead to dependence and withdrawal symptoms if used regularly. Older people are as capable of benefiting from psychological interventions, especially behavior therapy, as younger people.[80] Typically, the behavior therapist uses strategies such as limiting the use of the bed to sleeping (e.g., not eating or reading in bed), challenging upsetting ideas, and teaching relaxation techniques. Sleep apnea may be treated with surgery to widen the upper airways that block breathing or by the use of mechanical devices, such as a specialized nose mask that maintains pressure to keep the upper airway passages open as the person sleeps.

**Dementia and Alzheimer's Disease** **Dementia** involves a dramatic deterioration of mental ability involving such functions as thinking, memory, and reasoning. Dementia is not a consequence of normal aging, but of pathological processes that damage brain tissue. Some of the causes of dementia include brain infections such as meningitis, HIV infection, and encephalitis; chronic alcoholism, strokes, and tumors; and brain diseases, such as **Alzheimer's disease (AD).** Alzheimer's disease is the most common cause of dementia, accounting for more than half of the approximately 4 million cases in the United States (see Figure 19.9).[81] Although some dementias may be reversible, especially those caused by tumors and treatable infections, or those that result from depression or substance abuse, the dementia resulting from AD is progressive and irreversible.

**Sleep apnea** A condition characterized by a temporary cessation of breathing during sleep.

**Dementia** A broad-based impairment of intellectual ability involving disturbances of memory, reasoning, language skills, and judgment that interferes with normal functioning and is often accompanied by personality changes.

**Alzheimer's disease (AD)** A degenerative disease of the brain that leads to an irreversible, progressive form of dementia.

Talking Glossary
Alzheimer's disease
G1910

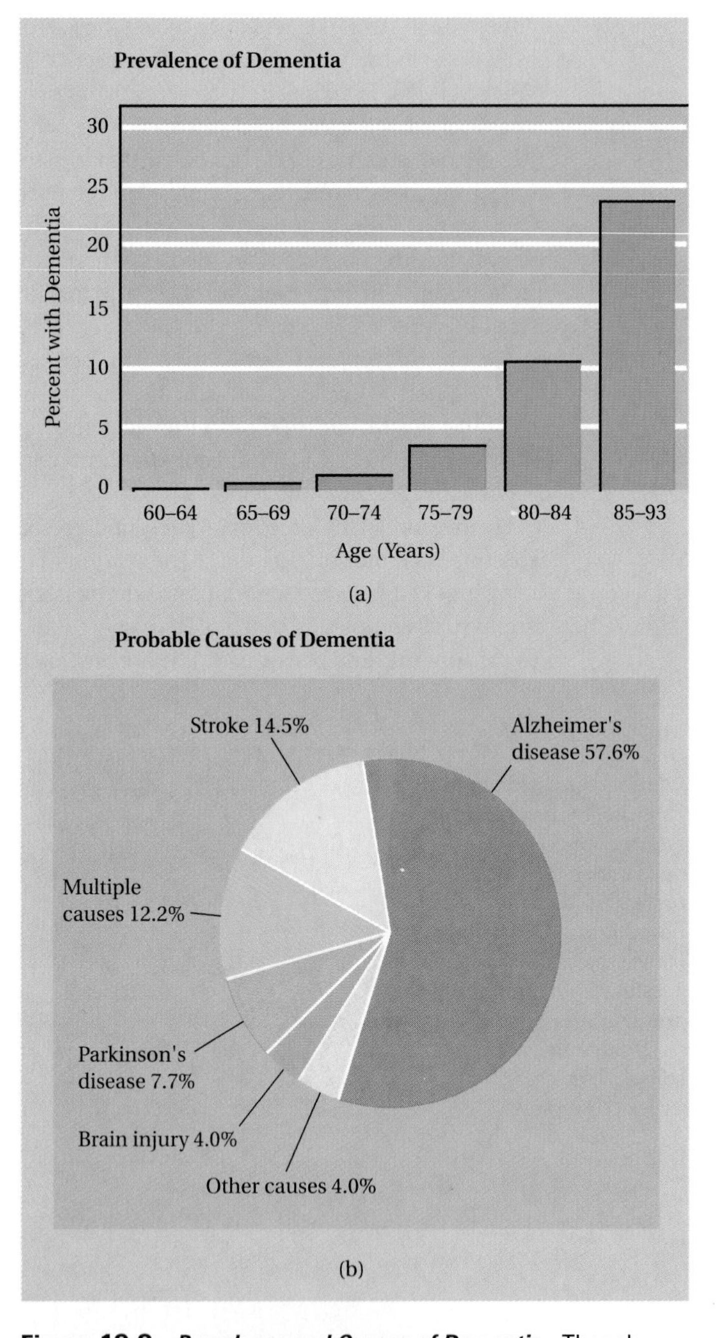


**Figure 19.9** ***Prevalence and Causes of Dementia*** Though dementia can have many causes, Alzheimer's disease is the leading cause. Though we lack any effective treatment to reverse Alzheimer's disease, some forms of dementia are treatable and may be reversed.

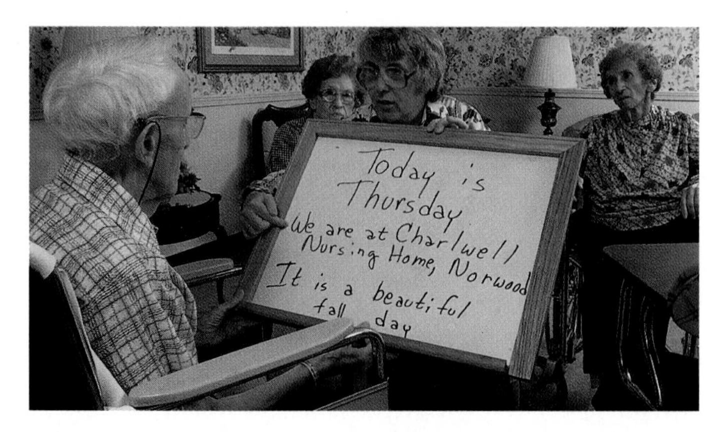
Today is
Thursday
We are at Charlwell
Nursing Home, Norwood
It is a beautiful
fall day

***Alzheimer's Disease*** In the advanced stage, Alzheimer's disease strips the mind of the ability to recall even the most basic information about one's surroundings or even to recognize one's loved ones.

AD claims the lives of more than 100,000 people annually in the United States.[82] The risk of AD rises sharply with age. The rate of AD in persons aged 65 to 74 is only 1%, but it rises to 7% in those 75 to 84 and then steeply—to perhaps as much as 50%—among people aged 85 and older.[83] It affects some younger people, but only rarely. With the population aging and medical advances helping to prolong life, AD is expected to become an even greater problem in the new millennium. Barring a medical breakthrough, 10 million Americans may develop AD by the middle of the twenty-first century.[84]

AD progresses in stages. At first there are subtle cognitive and personality changes, which eventually progress to total disability. During the early stage, people with AD may have trouble managing finances and recalling recent events. As the disease progresses, people find it harder to manage daily tasks and need help selecting clothes, recalling names and addresses, and driving. Later on, they have trouble using the bathroom by themselves and keeping themselves clean. They no longer recognize family and friends or speak in full sentences. They may become restless, agitated, confused, and aggressive. They may get lost in stores, parking lots, or even in their own homes. They may have hallucinations or paranoid delusions, believing that others are attempting to harm them. They may eventually become helpless—unable to walk or communicate—and completely dependent on others to meet their needs.

**Smart Reference**
Senile words
R1904

**Close-up**
Features of AD
T1908

A diagnosis of AD is definitively confirmed only by autopsy. To date, no definitive test for diagnosing AD in living people has been developed. In practice, diagnosis is made by process of elimination: Health professionals rule out other health problems that can mimic AD. This imperfect process leads to many misdiagnoses.

The cause or causes of AD have remained a mystery since it was first recognized by the German physician Alois Alzheimer in 1907. During the course of autopsying the brain of a woman who had severe dementia, Alzheimer found two basic signs of the disease: *neuritic plaques*, or clumps of degenerative brain tissue; and *neurofibrillary tangles*, or twisted bundles of nerve cells. The steel-wool-like neuritic plaques may destroy adjacent brain tissue, leading to the memory loss and other problems associated with AD. Still, it remains unclear whether these plaques kill brain cells or are merely an effect of the disease.[85]

Evidence of a genetic component in AD is increasing.[86] Many genes may be involved in different forms of the disease, including one that directs production of a protein that carries cholesterol through the bloodstream.[87] The protein, called *apolipoprotein E* (APOe), may be involved in promoting the development of the plaques in the brain that are associated with AD. People who inherit a particular form of the gene stand a greater chance of developing the disease. Still, the gene is believed responsible for only a small percentage of AD cases.

Research has also focused on the possible role of neurotransmitters, especially **acetylcholine (ACh),** which is found in reduced levels in people with AD. Current treatment approaches have focused on drugs which increase the availability of ACh.[88] To date, these drugs have produced some modest benefits in improving memory functioning of AD patients. On another front in the war against AD, evidence suggests that high doses of vitamin E may be helpful in slowing the progression of the disease.[89] Promising but preliminary results are also reported in using estrogen therapy to help women with AD retain more of their memories.[90] All in all, the available treatments offer at best marginal results in the battle against AD.

**Talking Glossary**
Acetylcholine
G1911

**Close-up**
New drug therapies for AD
T1909

On the prevention front, researchers have linked regular use of the common painkiller ibuprofen (brand names Advil, Motrin) to a lower risk of developing AD.[91] Anti-inflammatory drugs like ibuprofen may help prevent the brain inflammation associated with AD. Because of concerns about potentially serious side effects of taking ibuprofen over the long term, experts do not recommend taking it regularly as a preven-

**Acetylcholine (ACh)** A type of neurotransmitter, deficiencies of which have been linked to Alzheimer's disease.

tative. Perhaps other anti-inflammatory drugs can be developed that provide protection against AD without dangerous side effects.

## Prescription Drugs and Alcohol

Medication abuse, much of which is unintentional, poses a serious health threat to older Americans.[92] About 40% of all prescription drugs in the United States are taken by people aged 60 and above. More than half of these people take two to five medications daily. Among the most commonly used drugs are blood pressure medication, tranquilizers, sleeping pills, and antidepressants. Taken correctly, prescription drugs can be of help. If used incorrectly, they can be harmful. Millions of older adults are addicted to, or risk becoming addicted to, prescription drugs, especially tranquilizers.

**Close-up**
Using medicines safely
T1910

About a quarter of a million older adults are hospitalized each year because of adverse drug reactions. Reasons include the following:

1. *Doctors may prescribe an incorrect dosage.* Because bodily functions slow with age (such as the ability of the liver and kidneys to process and clear drugs out of the body), the same amount of drug can have stronger effects and last longer in older people. Yet physicians often prescribe the same dosage that would be used by a younger person.[93]
2. *Some people may misunderstand directions or be unable to keep track of their usage.*
3. *Many older people have more than one doctor, and treatment plans may not be coordinated by their primary physician.*

Although consumption of alcohol is lower among older people compared with other age groups, at least one person in ten over 60 is a heavy drinker.[94] Of these, about two-thirds are recent *(late-onset)* alcoholics. Late-onset alcoholism usually occurs in response to a life crisis, such as retirement, the death of a spouse, or impaired health. The remaining one-third began abusing alcohol earlier in life (*early-onset* alcoholics). They enter late adulthood with a likelihood of many alcohol-related health problems. For either type of alcoholic, alcoholism in later life can shorten life and impair health and well-being. The health risks of alcohol abuse increase dramatically with age. The slowdown in metabolism that accompanies aging reduces the body's ability to metabolize alcohol. As a result, intoxication becomes more likely. The combination of alcohol and other drugs, even prescription drugs, can be dangerous, even deadly. Used in combination, alcohol can also lessen or intensify the effects of prescription drugs. Alcohol abuse may also mask other physical symptoms, such as the early warning signs of heart attacks.

**Close-up**
Aging and alcohol abuse
T1911

## Accidents

Unintentional injuries—falls, motor vehicle accidents, residential fires, and nonfatal poisoning—are an important risk factor for older Americans. They constitute the seventh leading cause of death in this population. More than half a million older Americans visit emergency rooms each year because of accidents in the home. Older people often fall in bathrooms and on stairs. Such accidents are especially dangerous for older people in whom osteoporosis increases the risk of hip fractures and other broken bones. Of course, accidents can occur at any age. According to the National Safety Council, accidents kill 1 person and disable 150 more every five minutes in the United States.

Many accidents involving older people could be prevented by equipping the home with safety features such as railings and nonskid floors. Wearing proper glasses and using hearing aids can reduce the risk of accidents resulting from vision or hearing problems, including many motor vehicle accidents. Adherence to safe driving speeds is especially important among older drivers because they have slower reaction times than younger drivers. Because people over the age of 65 represent an increasingly large proportion of licensed drivers, the federal government has established the goal of improving the design of road signs to make them more visible to older drivers.[95]

### think about it!

- **Do you know people with arthritis? Does it limit their functioning? How? What do they do about it?**
- **Are the older people in your life generally happy or unhappy? How do you know? Why are they happy or unhappy?**
- **Do you know anyone with Alzheimer's disease? At what age did it strike? How did it develop? What treatment is the person receiving? How does the disease affect the family?**

**Smart Quiz**
Q1904

## HEALTH CARE FOR OLDER PEOPLE

The graying of America poses daunting challenges to society. Chief among them are providing for and paying for the costs of health care for older people.

### Needs for Health Care

Older persons typically need more health care than younger people. Though people over the age of 65 make up only about 12% of the population, they occupy 25% of the hospital beds. As the numbers of older people increase into the next century, so will the cost of caring for them.

**Close-up** Health care for the elderly **T1912**

Medicare, a federally controlled health insurance program for older Americans and the disabled, only partially subsidizes the health care needs of these groups. Another government program, Medicaid, covers a portion of the health care costs of people of all ages who are otherwise unable to afford coverage. About 33% of Medicaid spending goes to older people. The Medicare program is funded on the basis of employee and employer contributions, while federal tax dollars offset the cost of Medicaid. Yet the costs of these programs have been escalating rapidly. If present trends continue, the Medicare program may run out of funds in the first half of the next century. The difference between what these programs are now paying out and what older Americans spend on their own health care already runs into the billions of dollars.

**Video** Political power of older Americans **V1905**

On a more hopeful note, it could be that health care for older Americans may not cost as much as has been feared. Older Americans appear to be more robust than was generally believed.[96] Not only are people living longer today; they are also living healthier. Fewer older Americans each year are disabled to the point that they cannot take care of themselves, take a walk, feed themselves, or comb their hair.[97] Moreover, the rates of chronic diseases such as hypertension, arthritis, and emphysema declined steadily between 1982 and 1994. Why these improvements? One likely explanation is that people are taking better care of themselves during their younger and middle years. They are more likely to avoid or to quit smoking. They are more careful about what they eat. They are also likely to have benefited from improvements in public health, such as better water quality and food safety.

### Needs for Housing, Support, and Caregiving

Let us put to rest some misconceptions about older people's living arrangements. Relatively few older people, less than 10%, are institutionalized in nursing homes or other long-term care facilities. The population of nursing homes is made up largely of people aged 80 and above. Still, nearly half of the older population will someday require nursing or home health care. Second, most people in late adulthood are not dependent on others. More than two of three of them live in their own homes. Third, despite the proliferation of "retirement" communities in the Sun Belt, most older Americans stay in their own communities after retirement. And despite beliefs that older people are impoverished, Americans aged 65 and above are actually *less* likely than the general population to live in poverty. The percentages of older Americans living below the poverty line have declined steadily from about 33% in the 1950s to about 12% today.[98] Still, many older Americans who live on fixed incomes find it difficult to make ends meet. Among minority groups, the rate of poverty is much higher. Two of three older African Americans, for example, live below the poverty level.

Community support programs assist older people in need. These include public assistance programs, such as food stamps, and home assistance programs that provide "meals on wheels," transportation to medical facilities, visiting nurses, and home attendants. Many of these programs seek volunteers to spend time visiting older people, assisting them with cooking, cleaning, and shopping, or just socializing.

Social support—important at any age—is especially important to older people. Most older people have good relationships with their grown children and treasure their grandchildren and great-grandchildren. In many families, there is a shifting of responsibility and control of family functions to the middle generation. Some older people also entrust management of their finances or the family business to their grown children. Strains can arise, however, over such matters as inheritance and "suggestions" offered by grandparents concerning the rearing of grandchildren. Nonetheless, grandparents are generally valued for playing vital and important family roles.

Community resources provide additional sources of support for the elderly. Senior citizen centers offer activities and social life. Day treatment centers in health care facilities provide physical therapy and rehabilitation services. For older people living in nursing homes and other institutional settings, the realities can be grim. Institutions vary widely in quality. Some facilities provide excellent care, but many are drab and poorly managed; they provide little more than basic custodial care. Congress recently enacted legislation that establishes a "bill of rights" for nursing home residents, including the right to privacy, the right to file a complaint without reprisal, the right to be informed about treatment, and the right to refuse treatment.

One of the major problems in nursing homes is **elder abuse**—physical, emotional, or verbal abuse of older people. In one recent study, 40% of nursing home staff members admitted physically abusing a resident, and 10% reported psychologically abusing a resident.[99] Yet most elder abuse occurs at home at the hands of family members, most frequently spouses. It may take the form of hitting, verbal abuse, neglect, or financial exploitation.

Care of older parents falls disproportionately on the shoulders of middle-aged daughters and daughters-in-law, who often feel sandwiched between the needs of the aging parent and their own children. Gerontologists point out that today's baby boomers may spend more time caring for their aging parents than for their children. Family members can easily burn out from the stress of caring for an aging parent. Stress may be relieved by dividing responsibilities among adult family members, by taking frequent breaks from caretaking, and by taking periodic vacations.

The burdens carried by family caregivers of people with Alzheimer's disease can be highly stressful. Some family members describe adjustment to living with someone who is deteriorating before their eyes as "a funeral that never ends." If the person undergoes personality changes or no longer recognizes them, it may seem like they are caring for a stranger. As many as two-thirds of family caregivers have their demented family member institutionalized within a period of 18 months, typically because they can no longer cope with the stress of providing care. Incontinence and aggressive acting out are especially hard to take.[100] To help meet the needs of family caregivers, more than a thousand support groups have been established by members of the Alzheimer's Disease and Related Disorders Association (ADRDA) (see the Appendix A).

## think about it!

- **Are you concerned about affording health care in late adulthood? If so, what can you do about it? If not, why not?**
- **Do you know any robust older people? Why do you think that they are robust while many others are not?**
- **Which older people in your life live independently? Which live dependently? How do you account for the difference?**

Smart Quiz
Q1905

**Elder abuse** Abuse of the elderly, including physical abuse, verbal abuse, neglect, or financial exploitation.

WORLD OF *diversity*

## Older Native Americans in Urban America—An Invisible Minority[101]

The composition of the older population is rapidly changing. In 1990, European (white) Americans made up about 90% of the older population. By the year 2050, the percentage of other ethnic groups in late adulthood is expected to double to about 20%. In some states, such as California and Florida, there have already been dramatic changes in the population, with tremendous increases in the proportions of older Asian Americans and Hispanic Americans. Within 25 years, about 40% of the older population in California will be members of ethnic minorities.

Researchers are only now beginning to examine factors of ethnicity and culture in relation to health care status and needs. Historically, little attention has been focused on older people from ethnic minority groups. One of the least examined groups of all are older Native Americans.

Half of all older Native Americans live in cities. Their greatest concentration is in Los Angeles, which is home to some 11,000 older Native Americans. Most of these older people came to the city after World War II as part of a federal relocation project to move Native Americans from the reservation into mainstream communities. Later in life, many of those who were relocated are frail, lonely, and unable to enjoy their retirement years. They are dispersed widely throughout the area, and many are separated from their families and from other Native Americans in the city.

Health providers are just now beginning to discover and address the concerns of this largely invisible minority. The popular image of older Native Americans as living in multigenerational, extended families has proved to be greatly exaggerated, at least among the urban population in Los Angeles. Six out of ten older Native Americans surveyed by the Los Angeles County Agency on Aging lived alone or with a spouse. The only older adults who lived in extended or multigenerational families were those who were so impaired that they could no longer live independently. An overwhelming number said that they needed health and income assistance. But most did not know how to get it. Cataracts, arthritis, dental problems, and hypertension were reported at high rates. Diabetes was reported at four times the rate of other older Americans.

The older Native Americans expressed the desire for activities that would reduce their social and cultural isolation. They requested senior centers, with kitchens catering to Native American food preferences, where they could hold potluck dinners and powwows. Transportation, legal assistance, and space for bingo games and craft classes were also cited as major needs.

The survey also revealed underlying differences in the very concept of aging between Native Americans and others. Native Americans measure age by productive capability and performance of social roles, not by chronological age. Grandparenting or physical disability qualifies a person as elderly in the eyes of the Native American community. Reaching the age of 60 or 65 is itself meaningless. In one case, a woman with many disabilities defined herself as elderly, although she was only 37. Aging holds different meanings for different ethnic groups.

# Living Longer, Living Better

## Take Charge

Living a long and healthy life is in part a function of genetics—a factor that is beyond your control. Other factors that contribute to health and longevity are within your control. Taking charge of these factors can help extend your life and enhance your health and vitality in your later years. Chief among these factors are regular exercise, adopting a diet low in fat and cholesterol, avoiding unhealthy habits, and maintaining an active, involved lifestyle. Though people in their twenties and thirties may feel that aging is only a concern to older people, the earlier in life we start to adopt healthier habits, the greater our chances of living a longer and better life.

**Video**
Advice for healthy aging
**V1906**

### Exercise and Nutrition

The Spanish explorers who searched for the fountain of youth might have done better to stay at home and build a gym. Exercise can slow down or even reverse the effects of aging, such as losses in aerobic capacity, bone strength, muscle strength, and lean body mass. Exercise can also lower the risk of certain cancers, such as cancer of the colon, heart disease and stroke, diabetes, and osteoporosis.[102] Recent evidence shows that postmenopausal women who exercise regularly have a lower risk of death than those who do not.[103] The more frequent or vigorous the exercise, the lower the risk. Older adults who remain physically active, even just gardening or walking regularly, are also less likely than their sedentary peers to become disabled or to suffer serious falls.[104] Physical exercise even helps keep the mind sharp.

**Close-up**
Don't take it easy
**T1913**

Older as well as younger people can benefit from aerobic and isotonic (weight training and stretching) exercises. Walking, swimming, bowling, dancing, biking, and golf provide excellent aerobic workouts. But people over 40 should have a medical checkup before undertaking any exercise program and phase in their exercise routine gradually.

**Close-up**
Exercise boosts cardiac fitness
**T1914**

Good nutrition is also important at any age. Adopting a balanced diet that is low in fat and cholesterol and rich in dietary fiber and other plant nutrients can lower the risk of many diseases, including cancer, heart disease, and diabetes.

Together, proper exercise and nutrition can add years to our lives and help us retain vitality. Yet older people are the demographic group at greatest risk of malnutrition.[105] Several reasons account for this increased vulnerability:

1. As we age, the body becomes less capable of compensating for nutritional imbalances.
2. The body's ability to absorb and use various nutrients is often compromised by the use of prescription medicines, especially when taken in combination. Nearly half of all older Americans take two or more prescription drugs regularly.
3. Declining sensitivity of taste buds and the sense of smell may affect the appetite of some older persons, leading them to neglect their diets.

Like other age groups, older adults need adequate daily servings of each of the five basic food groups described in Chapter 5. They also need to limit foods high in fats, cholesterol, and sodium. Though caloric needs decline with age, the need for many

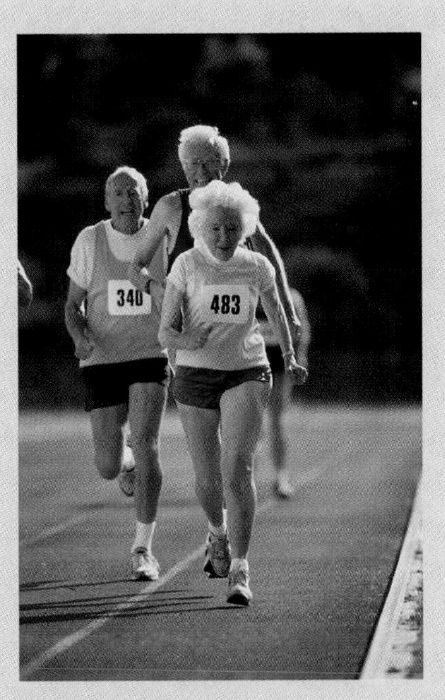


***Keeping Fit*** Keeping active and fit helps maintain good health and vitality at any age.

nutrients, such as calcium, increases. A diet rich in high-fiber foods such as whole-grain breads and cereals and fruits and vegetables is most healthful. A survey of 700 older persons showed that those in the best health had the highest intakes of vitamins A and C, riboflavin, folic acid—vitamins found in fruits and vegetables—and vitamin $B_{12}$.[106]

## Keeping Involved

Staying involved offers the best protection against psychological problems later in life. Many of us will spend up to one-fourth to one-third of our lives in retirement. Satisfaction with retirement is related to fulfilling relationships and pursuits. Activities such as returning to school, volunteering, traveling, and participating in civic clubs offer many social and intellectual opportunities. Older people who participate in volunteer organizations or who are affiliated with a religious institution are less likely to experience depression than uninvolved peers.[107]

**Close-up**
Healthy living, active living
T1915

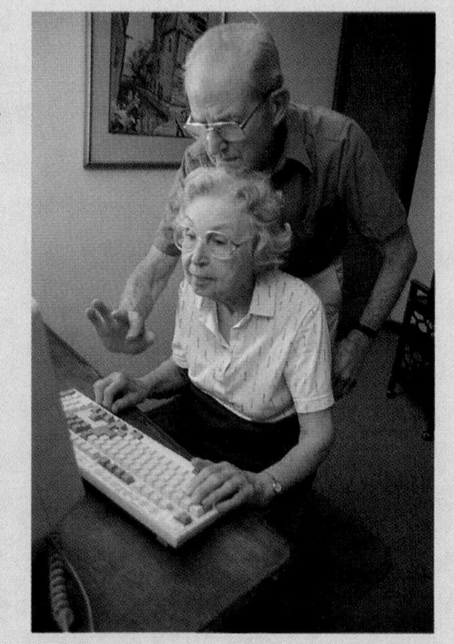

***Exercise the Mind, Not Just the Body***
Our minds need to be stretched by mentally stimulating activity to keep them sharp and alert. This 86-year-old man is helping his 80-year-old wife learn to work a computer.

## Maintaining a Healthy Weight

Obesity is a major risk factor for a number of chronic diseases that can shorten life—cardiovascular disease, cancer, and diabetes. Because metabolism naturally slows with age, losing excess weight and keeping it off becomes more of an uphill struggle. This is all the more reason to adopt good diet and exercise habits early in life. The weight management strategies outlined in Chapter 6 can help you achieve these goals.

## Avoiding Unhealthy Habits

Harmful substances can damage health, cut life expectancy, and increase the risk of suffering from painful and disabling diseases in later life. Cigarette smoking and use of other tobacco products account for more health problems than any other substance. Excessive alcohol intake can also cut life expectancy and increase the risk of disease and disability.

## Managing Stress

Prolonged or intense stress can impair vital bodily systems, including the immune system, and may contribute to the development of chronic diseases associated with aging, such as hypertension, cancer, and heart disease. The techniques described in Chapter 3 can help prevent the development of stress-related disorders.

## Exercising Your Mind, Not Just Your Body

Though we normally experience some decline in mental ability as we age, we can help maintain our mental sharpness by doing for our brains what we do for our bodies to keep them fit: exercise. Like the body, the mind needs to be worked to stay in shape. Mental exercise need not be strenuous or mentally taxing; in fact it can be fun.

What types of mental exercise help? Challenging work keeps one attuned to new knowledge and technological developments of the day. People who maintain mental fitness into later life tend to be better educated and involved in more challenging and stimulating activities.[108] Activities that can help keep the mind agile and sharp include games of mental skill and concentration like chess, crossword or jigsaw puzzles, reading and writing, and other mentally stimulating activities like painting and sculpting.

## Healthy Habits—Do They Pay Off?

Do healthy habits pay off in terms of a longer and better life? The answer is decidedly yes. People with healthier habits—who do not smoke, who stay active physically and socially, who do not drink excessively, and who control their weight—typically live longer and healthier lives. In one study, University of California researchers tracked some 7,000 people for more than 20 years. They found that men with healthier habits lived an average of 11 years longer than those with more negative traits. Among women, the difference was smaller but still substantial.[109] In another California study, people with healthier habits had fewer chronic health conditions. Healthy habits apparently count more than genetics in determining whether people in their seventies and eighties are healthy.[110] It's like saving money for your later years: Developing healthy habits when you're young and maintaining them is the best way of ensuring a longer and healthier life.

**Smart Quiz**
Q1906

# SUMMING UP

## HEALTH AND LONGEVITY

**1. What is the difference between longevity and life expectancy?** *Longevity* is the length of time an organism lives under the best of circumstances. Our life span depends on our genetic programming. *Life expectancy* is the average number of years people in a given population group can expect to live.

**2. What are some group differences in life expectancy?** Life expectancy has been increasing due to advances in medicine and the adoption of healthier lifestyles. Women tend to outlive men. White Americans of European background tend to outlive Hispanic Americans, African Americans, and Native Americans.

**3. Has the quality of life kept pace with increases in life expectancy?** Probably not. According to one measure of health—quality-adjusted life years—Americans are surviving for more than a decade after their bodies can no longer readily meet the demands that are placed on them.

## HOW WE AGE

**4. What physical changes take place as we age?** Skin wrinkles. Hair grays. Senses become less acute. Reaction time increases. Lung capacity decreases. Lean body mass, bone density, and strength decline. Metabolism slows. Blood sugar tolerance declines. Sexual response comes more slowly, but sexual relations can be as fulfilling as ever.

**5. How do mental abilities change as we age?** There are some normal declines in memory and capacity for abstract thought in late adulthood, but dementia is not a normal part of aging.

**6. What psychological changes occur as we age?** According to stage theorists, young adults face the challenges of forming intimate relationships and establishing their place in the world. The ideals of generativity and ego integrity are, respectively, the major identity challenges faced in middle and later adulthood, according to Erikson.

**7. What are *successful agers*?** Successful agers concentrate on what is important and meaningful, have a positive outlook, and challenge themselves.

## WHY WE AGE

**8. What are programmed theories of aging?** Programmed theories see aging as preordained by genetic codes present at birth.

**9. What are cellular damage theories of aging?** Cellular-damage theories hold that aging results from damage to cells. One cellular-damage theory is that cells are impaired by wear and tear due to disease, pollution, and so on.

## HEALTH CONCERNS AND AGING

**10. What is the difference between normal and pathological aging?** In normal aging, physiological processes decline slowly and people enjoy long years of health. In pathological aging, chronic health problems such as heart disease, diabetes, and cancer lead to disability or premature death.

**11. What are some common health problems among older Americans?** These include arthritis, heart disease, cancer, and stroke. Osteoarthritis is linked to wear and tear on the joints. By age 60, more than half of Americans show signs of osteoarthritis. Rheumatoid arthritis is chronic inflammation of the membranes that line the joints, resulting from an autoimmune response.

**12. What psychological problems affect older people?** Older Americans are generally as happy as younger Americans. Their most common psychological health problems are depression, anxiety, and sleep problems.

**13. What is Alzheimer's disease?** Alzheimer's disease (AD) is a degenerative disease that becomes more common as we age. It is characterized by memory problems and confusion and by the formation of neuritic plaques and neurofibrillary tangles in the brain. Genetic factors appear to play a role in the disease.

## HEALTH CARE FOR OLDER PEOPLE

**14. What are the health care needs of older people?** Older people usually require more health care than younger people do. Medicare and Medicaid do not cover all the costs. On the other hand, many older people are more robust than had been anticipated.

**15. What are some misconceptions about living arrangements for older people?** Most older Americans live independently in their own homes. Most remain in their communities after retirement.

**Answer Key to *HealthCheck*, p. 517**

1. *False.* Most healthy couples continue to engage in satisfying sexual activities into their seventies and eighties.
2. *False.* This is too general a statement. Those who find their work satisfying often are not eager to retire.
3. *False.* In late adulthood, we tend to become more concerned with internal matters—our physical functioning and our emotions.
4. *False.* Adaptability remains reasonably stable throughout adulthood.
5. *False.* Age itself is not linked to noticeable declines in life satisfaction. Of course, we may respond negatively to disease and losses, such as the death of a spouse.
6. *False.* Although we can predict some general trends for older adults, we can also do so for younger adults. Older adults, like their younger counterparts, are heterogeneous in personality and behavior patterns.
7. *False.* Older adults with stable intimate relationships are more satisfied.
8. *False.* We are susceptible to a wide variety of psychological disorders at all ages.
9. *False.* Only a minority are depressed.
10. *False.* Actually, church attendance declines, but not verbally expressed religious beliefs.
11. *False.* Although reaction time may increase and general learning ability may undergo a slight decline, older adults usually have little or no difficulty with familiar work tasks. In most jobs, experience and motivation are more important than age.
12. *False.* Learning may just take a bit longer.
13. *False.*
14. *False.* Older adults do not direct a higher proportion of thoughts toward the past than do younger people. Regardless of our age, we may spend more time daydreaming at any age if we have more time on our hands.
15. *False.* Fewer than 10% of people aged 65 and older require institutional care.

## References and Suggested Readings

### SMART REFERENCES FROM SCIENTIFIC AMERICAN

**Beardsley, T. Biotechnology: Memories Are Made of. . . .** *Scientific American,* 276(3) (March 1997), 32. **R1901**

**Beardsley, T. Melatonin Mania: Separating Facts from Hype. "Explorations," Scientific American's www site** (April 1, 1996). **R1902**

**Nemecek, S. Medicine: Attacking Arthritis.** *Scientific American,* 276(6) (June 1997), 41. **R1903**

**Wallich, P. Neuroscience: Senile Words.** *Scientific American,* 274(6) (June 1996), 26. **R1904**

### SUGGESTED READINGS

**William, M. E.** *The American Geriatrics Society, Complete Guide to Aging & Health.* New York: Harmony Books, 1995. Many topics relating to aging, including how we age, caring for parents, long-term care choices, and making wise health care decisions.

**Gruetzner, H.** *Alzheimer's: A Caregiver's Guide and Sourcebook.* New York: Wiley, 1992. A pragmatic approach to living with and caring for Alzheimer's victims.

**Hayflick, L.** *How and Why We Age.* New York: Ballantine Books, 1994. A fascinating and engaging account of the biology of aging from an eminent cell biologist—a must read for any serious student of the aging process.

**Solomon, D. H., and others.** *A Consumer's Guide to Aging.* Baltimore: Johns Hopkins Press, 1992. A comprehensive and fact-filled compendium of information about aging.

**Jong, E.** *Fear of Fifty.* New York: HarperCollins, 1994. A personal look at the challenges of aging, from a leading author.

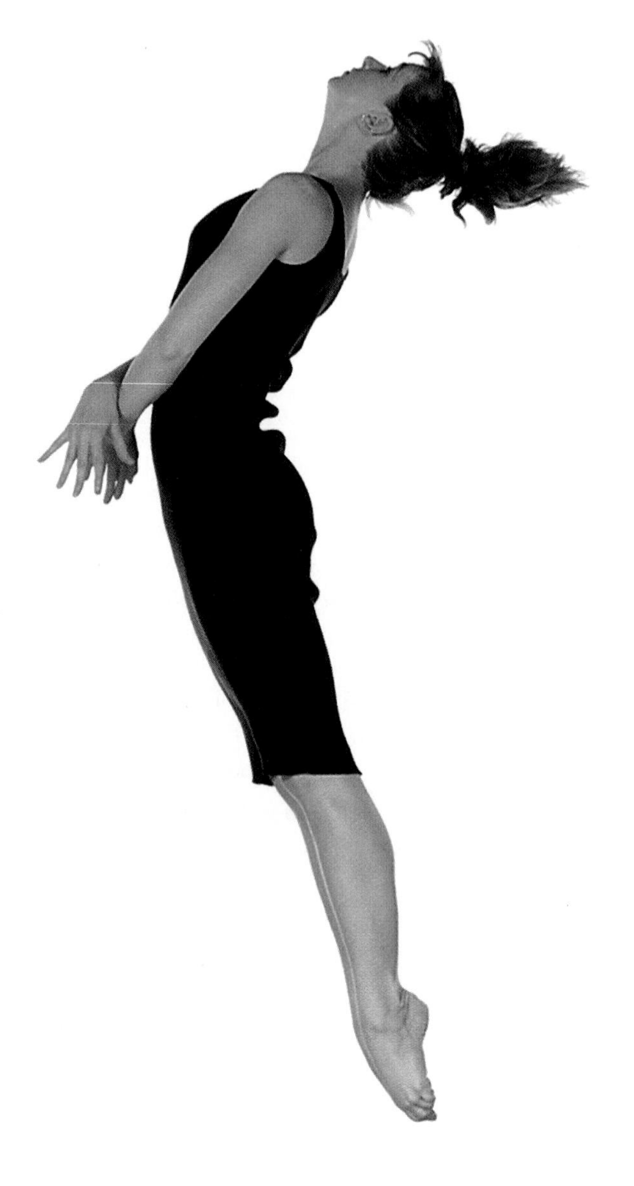

## DID YOU KNOW THAT

- A person may stop breathing and have no heartbeat but still be alive? p.548
- Some people have had near-death experiences in which they reported contacting deceased relatives "in the light"? p.552
- The great majority of people in the United States die in hospitals? p.552
- Doctors can be prosecuted for helping terminally ill patients take their own lives? p.554
- Many living wills are ignored in actual medical practice? p.558
- Grief can increase a person's vulnerability to a heart attack? p.562

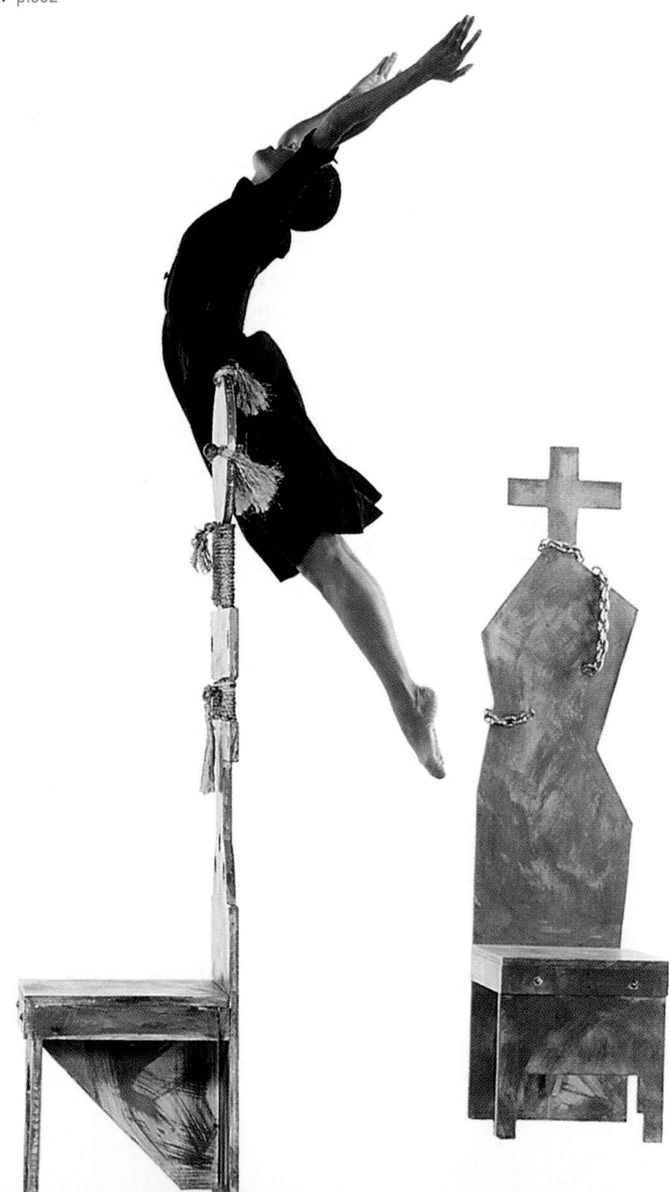

20

# Life's Final Passage

*This chapter concerns a topic that many of us would rather not think about: death. When we are young and our bodies supple and strong, we may think we will live forever. We may have but the dimmest awareness of our own mortality. We parcel thoughts about death and dying into a mental file cabinet to be opened much later in life, along with items like retirement, social security, and varicose veins. But death can occur at any age—by accident, violence, or illness. Death can also affect us deeply at any stage of life through the loss of loved ones.*

Denial of death is deeply embedded in our culture and not limited to the young. We prefer not to think about death or plan ahead for our eventual demise, as though planning for it might magically bring it sooner. The **thanatologist** Elisabeth Kübler-Ross helped us see death through the eyes of people who were dying. Yet most of us prefer not to see. As Kübler-Ross noted in her classic book, *On Death and Dying*:[1]

Talking Glossary
Thanatologist
G2001

> *We use euphemisms, we make the dead look as if they were asleep, we ship the children off to protect them from the anxiety and turmoil around the house if the [person] is fortunate enough to die at home, [and] we don't allow children to visit their dying parents in the hospitals.*

We hear people joke that nobody gets out of life alive. Facing the realities of death and dying, while not abandoning our sense of humor, may be the best way to prepare for the inevitable and to cope when those who are dear to us die. Thinking about death and dying raises questions for each of us:

Should I donate my organs after my death?

How can I protect my assets so that they will be passed along to my loved ones?

Do I want to be buried or cremated? Or should I donate my body to science?

Should I leave a living will so that doctors will not use heroic measures to prolong my life when all hope of recovery is gone?

Other questions probe the boundaries among science, morality, and the law:

Do terminally ill people have the right to die?

Should doctors be prosecuted if they help terminally ill people take their own lives?

Still other questions focus on ways of helping the bereaved cope with loss:

What can I do to help someone who has suffered a loss?

How can I help myself?

Many people seek answers to questions about death and dying in religious teachings or in works of prominent philosophers or spiritual leaders. Whatever source we draw upon, the search for answers is a highly personal one. We begin our exploration by first posing a question that may seem to have an obvious answer, "How do we know that someone has died?"

**Thanatologist** A scholar of thanatology, the interdisciplinary study of death and dying.

**Death** The irreversible cessation of vital life functions.

**Dying** The state of approaching death.

**Cardiopulmonary resuscitation (CPR)** Emergency medical care used to revive a person who is unconscious and may be in respiratory and/or cardiac arrest.

**Brain death** Complete cessation of brain activity as evidenced by an absence of brain wave activity.

**Electroencephalograph (EEG)** A device for measuring the electrical activity of the brain.

# UNDERSTANDING DEATH AND DYING

**Death** is the cessation of life. Many people think of death as a part of life, but death is the *end* of life. **Dying,** though, is a part of life, the stage during which bodily processes decline, leading to death. Yet life still can hold significance and meaning even in the face of death. Many dying people experience the meaning of life in a deeper and more personal way than they had before.

## Charting the Boundaries between Life and Death

When has a person died? When the heart no longer beats? When breathing stops? When brain activity ceases? Doctors today can often revive people whose hearts and lungs have ceased functioning by using **cardiopulmonary resuscitation (CPR).** Where, then, do we draw the line between life and death?

In most states, a person is legally dead if there is an irreversible cessation of breathing and circulation or of brain activity, including activity in the brain stem that controls breathing.[2] Health professionals use **brain death** as the standard. The most widely used measure of brain death was developed at Harvard Medical School:

1. Lack of response to external stimuli, including painful stimuli.
2. Absence of brain wave activity as recorded by an **electroencephalograph (EEG).**
3. Absence of spontaneous breathing or movement.
4. Lack of observable reflexes.

Talking Glossary
Electroencephalograph
G2002

These standards must be met in two separate tests performed at least 24 hours apart. They exclude cases in which the person's condition can be explained by *hypothermia* (extreme loss of body temperature) or use of drugs, such as barbiturates, that can depress the nervous system. Under these criteria, people are considered to be "alive" as long as their brains continue to function, even though they lie unconscious in a permanent vegetative state. Then too, some people who are clinically brain dead are kept "alive" by life-support equipment that takes over their breathing and circulation.

Another concept is that of **cellular death.** It refers to the gradual death of body cells that occurs when cells are starved for oxygenated blood after the heart and lungs stop functioning. Cellular death leads to **rigor mortis,** the stiffening of the muscles of the body that occurs several hours after death.

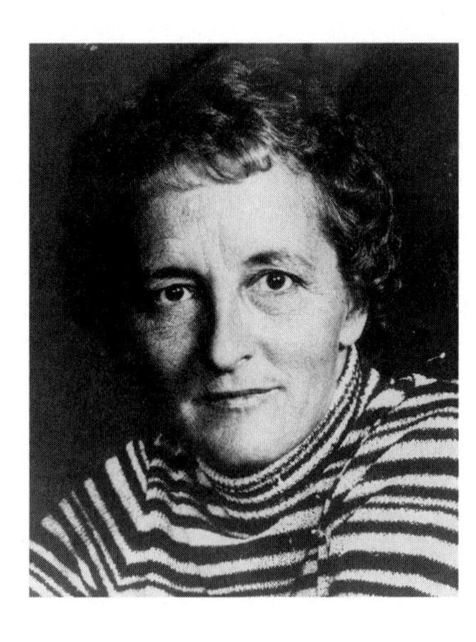

***Dr. Elisabeth Kübler-Ross***

## Stages of Dying

**Close-up** Interview with Kübler-Ross **T2001**

Our understanding of the process of dying owes a considerable debt to the pioneering work of Kübler-Ross. From her work with terminally ill people, she found some common responses to news of impending death. She identified five stages of dying through which many dying people pass. Older people who suspect that death may be near may undergo similar responses. The stages are:[3]

1. *Denial.* In this stage, people feel "It can't be me. The diagnosis must be wrong." Denial can be flat and absolute. It can also fluctuate so that the person accepts the medical verdict one minute and in the next starts chatting animatedly about distant plans.
2. *Anger.* Denial usually gives way to anger and resentment toward the young and healthy, and sometimes toward the medical establishment for failing to provide a cure.
3. *Bargaining.* Next, people may bargain with God to postpone death, promising, for example, to do good deeds if they are given another six months, another year.
4. *Depression.* With depression come feelings of grief, loss, and hopelessness—grief at the specter of leaving loved ones and life itself.
5. *Final acceptance.* Ultimately, an inner sense of peace may come with the acceptance of the inevitable. This "peace" is not contentment; it is nearly devoid of feeling. The person may still fear death but comes to accept it with quiet dignity.

Kübler-Ross suggested that hospital staff and family can help support the dying person by understanding the stages that he or she is going through, by not imposing their own wishes or expectations, and by helping the person achieve final acceptance.

The stages outlined by Kübler-Ross's theory address common experiences among dying people, but many health professionals find that not every dying person goes through them, or goes through them in the order described by Kübler-Ross. Some dying people bypass the denial stage and come to a rapid but painful acceptance of the inevitable. Some who face death become despondent. For others, the prominent emotion is terror. Some experience a rapid shifting of feelings, ranging from rage to surrender, from envying the young and healthy to yearning for the end. People's responses reflect their personalities and their philosophies of life.

## Near-Death Experiences—A Glimpse into the Beyond?

*I was coming out of the operating room—it happened in the recovery room—and I just remember going. . . . It was like going through a tunnel, like shooting through something and seeing the light at the end. I heard a sort of whooshing sound, like fast wind or something like that—a sort of whshshsh. . . .*

*At the end of the tunnel I saw floating patches of light. It was like all of those patches of light were entities of some kind, but they were all part of one thing. . . .*

**Cellular death** Complete death of cellular tissue resulting from the stoppage of blood flow.

**Rigor mortis** The stiffening of the muscles that occurs several hours after death.

# HealthCheck

## How Concerned Are You about Death?

Reproduced with permission of author and publisher from Dickstein, L. H. "Death concern: measurement and correlates." *Psychological Reports,* 1972, *30,* 563–571. © Psychological Reports 1972.

Thinking about death evokes various thoughts and feelings. Our reactions to death are affected to some degree by our philosophy about death, by what, if anything, we believe follows death. The Death Concern Scale is intended to measure people's concerns or anxieties about death.[4] After completing the questionnaire, consult the key in Appendix B at the end of this book to better understand your responses.

*The questionnaire contains two parts. Respond to questions 1 through 11 by using the code below:*

1 = Never
2 = Rarely
3 = Sometimes
4 = Often

____ **1.** I think about my own death.

____ **2.** I think about the death of loved ones.

____ **3.** I think about dying young.

____ **4.** I think about the possibility of my being killed on a city street.

____ **5.** I have fantasies of my own death.

____ **6.** I think about death just before I go to sleep.

____ **7.** I think of how I would act if I knew I were to die within a given period of time.

____ **8.** I think of how my relatives would act and feel upon my death.

____ **9.** When I am sick I think about death.

____ **10.** When I am outside during a lightning storm I think about the possibility of being struck by lightning.

____ **11.** When I am in an automobile I think about the high incidence of traffic fatalities.

*Answer questions 12 through 30 by circling one of the choices according to the code given below and then inserting the corresponding code in the blank space:*

SA = I strongly agree
A = I somewhat agree
D = I somewhat disagree
SD = I strongly disagree

____ **12.** I think people should first become concerned about death when they are old.

SA 1 A 2 D 3 SD 4

____ **13.** I am much more concerned about death than those around me.

SA 4 A 3 D 2 SD 1

____ **14.** Death hardly concerns me.

SA 1 A 2 D 3 SD 4

____ **15.** My general outlook just doesn't allow for morbid thoughts.

SA 1 A 2 D 3 SD 4

____ **16.** The prospect of my own death arouses anxiety in me.

SA 4 A 3 D 2 SD 1

____ **17.** The prospect of my own death depresses me.

SA 4 A 3 D 2 SD 1

____ **18.** The prospect of the death of my loved ones arouses anxiety in me.

SA 4 A 3 D 2 SD 1

____ **19.** The knowledge that I will surely die does not in any way affect the conduct of my life.

SA 1 A 2 D 3 SD 4

____ **20.** I envision my own death as a painful, nightmarish experience.

SA 4 A 3 D 2 SD 1

____ **21.** I am afraid of dying.

| SA | A | D | SD |
|---|---|---|---|
| 4 | 3 | 2 | 1 |

____ **22.** I am afraid of being dead.

| SA | A | D | SD |
|---|---|---|---|
| 4 | 3 | 2 | 1 |

____ **23.** Many people become disturbed at the sight of a new grave but it does not bother me.

| SA | A | D | SD |
|---|---|---|---|
| 1 | 2 | 3 | 4 |

____ **24.** I am disturbed when I think about the shortness of life.

| SA | A | D | SD |
|---|---|---|---|
| 4 | 3 | 2 | 1 |

____ **25.** Thinking about death is a waste of time.

| SA | A | D | SD |
|---|---|---|---|
| 1 | 2 | 3 | 4 |

____ **26.** Death should not be regarded as a tragedy if it occurs after a productive life.

| SA | A | D | SD |
|---|---|---|---|
| 1 | 2 | 3 | 4 |

____ **27.** The inevitable death of a person poses a serious challenge to the meaningfulness of human existence.

| SA | A | D | SD |
|---|---|---|---|
| 4 | 3 | 2 | 1 |

____ **28.** The death of the individual is ultimately beneficial because it facilitates change in society.

| SA | A | D | SD |
|---|---|---|---|
| 1 | 2 | 3 | 4 |

____ **29.** I have a desire to live on after death.

| SA | A | D | SD |
|---|---|---|---|
| 4 | 3 | 2 | 1 |

____ **30.** The question of whether or not there is a future life worries me considerably.

| SA | A | D | SD |
|---|---|---|---|
| 4 | 3 | 2 | 1 |

*Then I remember being in the light, just suddenly being totally engulfed by the light, I'm saying "engulfed," but it was very nice. . . . And suddenly I had the feeling that everything was okay, everything was perfectly all right. That was the feeling I remember most. . . . I can say it's the most beautiful thing I've felt in my life, but in saying that, it's just words. . . .*

*The next moment I was coming back, and then I was suddenly back in my body, fighting off this oxygen mask, which apparently had failed to work (laughs). I think I was made to come back. I don't think I really had any choice because I didn't have any intention of coming back, but somehow or other I ended up back here anyway (laughs). . . .* [5]

What is death like? What happens to us after we die? Since no one has died and returned to tell about it, these questions may be unanswerable. But can we learn something from people who report **near-death experiences (NDEs)?** A near-death experience is not death but an experience described by people who have come *close* to death. Though these experiences are intensely personal and meaningful, they tend to share some common threads, as noted by sociologist Cherie Sutherland (who herself had a near-death experience):[6]

*The near-death episode itself is typically characterized by a feeling of peace, an out-of-body experience, the sensation of traveling very quickly through a dark tunnel, generally toward a light, an encounter with the spirits of deceased relatives or friends or a "being of light," an instantaneous life review, and for some, entrance into a "world of light."*

Some people report out-of-body experiences, feeling as though they were floating above their bodies and looking down at the doctors struggling to revive them. Oddly, they report feeling calm and peaceful, free of pain. Some report returning to their bodies soon. Others describe a next level of the experience in which they move through an area of darkness, or tunnel, at the end of which is a magnificent, warm light that fills the entire vista. They feel drawn toward the light and become enveloped by it, experiencing what they describe as a feeling of pure love.[7] Those having this level of the experience may report sensing a presence in the light, a form

**Near-death experiences (NDEs)**
Experiences reported by people who came close to dying or who were considered "clinically dead" but survived.

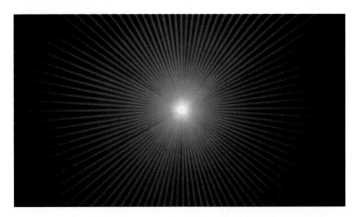

***Into The Light*** Many people who have near-death experiences report a sensation of moving through a dark tunnel toward a warm embracing light. Is a near-death experience a glimpse into an afterlife or a perceptual distortion brought about by the release of brain chemicals at the brink of death? What do you think?

they cannot see but whose consciousness is linked to their own. Some described this presence as God, Christ, or a spiritual being. Some claim to have contact with deceased relatives "in the light." Though they feel comforted and embraced by the light, they sense that they must choose whether to remain or return to their bodies. Some report being "told" that they must return for the sake of their families or to fulfill some purpose. Then they are again in their bodies, back in the hospital or where they were at the time they came to the brink of death, remembering vividly what happened to them.

Many people say that the near-death experience changes their lives, making them value life more deeply and leading them to become more compassionate and tolerant. Some people become devoted to spirituality or to helping older or terminally ill people come to terms with death. Many report that their near-death experience left them convinced of the existence of an afterlife, and that death no longer frightens them.

Not all near-death episodes are so uplifting. Some people find the experience frightening, even harrowing. Nor are all near-death experiences transforming. Some people reclaim their lives much as they left them, though thankful for another chance at living.

**Explanations of Near-Death Experiences** No one knows how many people have had near-death experiences—thousands for sure, perhaps millions. Some may be making them up, perhaps to gain attention or fame, but even critics believe that many people who had such an experience are reporting what they genuinely believe happened to them.

But what *did* happen? Some people who have had these experiences believe that they are a gateway to the afterlife, a kind of stairway to heaven. Skeptics claim that they might merely be dreams or hallucinations induced by oxygen deprivation occurring naturally at the brink of death. Or perhaps they result from the flooding of the brain in life's last moments with endorphins, those opiate-like substances that the brain produces to quell pain and produce feelings of pleasure. Perhaps the brain supplies the content of the experience from its storehouse of information about death and from religious beliefs. Perhaps the sensations of movement through a dark tunnel and approaching brilliant light are brought about by a flurry of electrical impulses in the brain that precede death.

Whether near-death experiences result from naturally occurring brain activity shortly before death or are a glimpse into an afterlife remains open to debate. Whatever the explanation, it appears to be an experience that has touched many people profoundly.

**Hospice** An approach to treating dying patients that focuses on support and understanding, rather than curative treatment; also refers to houses or facilities that provide palliative (supportive) care to dying patients.

## Caring for the Dying Person—The Role of Hospice Care

A century ago, most people died in their homes with their family members gathered around their beds. Today, most people, perhaps as many as four of five, die in hospitals. Hospitals can be impersonal, cold, and sterile places in which to die. Hospitals function to treat diseases, not help prepare people and their families for death.[8] Instead of dying in familiar surroundings, where they are comforted by loved ones and friends, people in hospitals may face death isolated and alone.

Many dying people have turned to hospices as an alternative. **Hospices** help make the dying person's final days as meaningful and free of pain as possible. The word "hospice" is derived from the Latin *hospitium,* meaning "hospitality," the same root of the words *hospital* and *hospitable.* The derivation is fitting: Hospices provide a homelike atmosphere in which people are helped to approach death with a maximum of dignity and a minimum of pain and discomfort.

**Talking Glossary**
Hospice
**G2003**

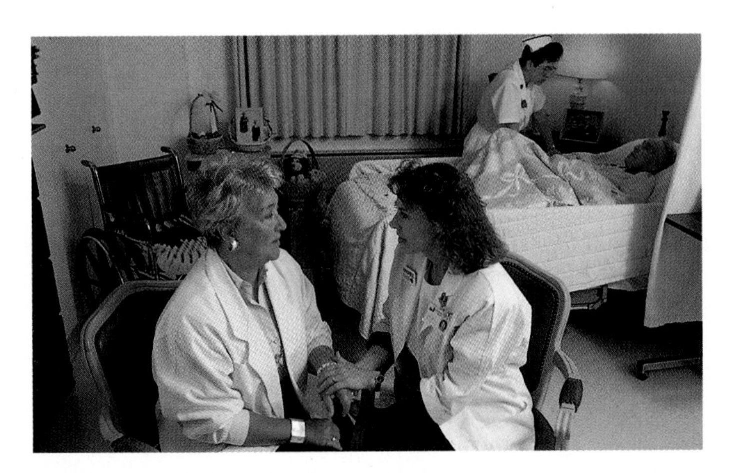

***Hospice Care*** Hospice workers provide assistance to dying patients and their families.

Hospices provide care in inpatient settings when necessary, such as a hospital, skilled nursing facility, or a hospice center. Most hospice care, however, is provided in the person's own home, where the person can be with loved ones in familiar surroundings. The focus of hospice care is to help the person make the most of each remaining day while helping to relieve pain. As Rigney Cunningham, Executive Director of Hospice Federation of Massachusetts, describes it, "Hospice comes from the heart. It is not a place, but a special kind of care that seeks to treat and comfort terminally ill patients and their families at home or in a homelike setting."[9] Ira Byock, a hospice worker in Montana, comments on the personal meaning that can be achieved in life's fading moments:[10]

> *I am continually amazed and humbled that something good can come of this last portion, however grim or painful, of a person's life. There is always that letter to be written to a daughter whose graduation the dying person will not attend, a son to be told how wonderful he is, an estranged relationship to be repaired, old stories of growing up to be tape recorded. People want their death to mean something, for accounts to be settled. For the dying, the last days can bring with them a heightened awareness, contentment, connectedness. The transition from life to death can be as beautiful and profound as the miracle of birth.*

Hospice workers typically work in teams consisting of physicians, nurses, social workers, psychologists, or counselors, and hospice home health aides. Team members provide physical, medical, spiritual, and emotional support to the whole family. Bereavement specialists help the family prepare for the loss and support them through the grieving process. In contrast to hospital procedures, hospices provide the person and the family with as much control over decision making as possible. The dying person's wishes not to be resuscitated or be kept alive on life-support equipment are honored. Patients are given ample amounts of narcotics to alleviate pain.

**Close-up**
More on hospice care
T2002

To be eligible for hospice care, a physician must certify that the person is terminally ill and not expected to live beyond six months. Hospices—especially home-based hospice care—not only provide a more supportive environment; they are also less costly than hospital treatment. Though the person may be required to pay some of the costs of hospice care, most of the costs are borne by Medicare or by insurance. While hospice care is often thought of in connection with cancer, people with other terminal diseases and conditions can also benefit when a cure is no longer the goal of care. One study found that 78% of hospice patients had cancer, and the remainder were diagnosed with a variety of terminal conditions, including heart-related illnesses, AIDS, kidney disease, and Alzheimer's disease.[11]

Hospice care often arrives too late for the dying person to reap the full benefits of the spiritual and psychological counseling.[12] The average hospice patient lives a little more than a month after admission, whereas hospice workers consider three months to be ideal. The problem is that many doctors are reluctant to refer their patients to hospices, as it signals acceptance that death is near.

To find the hospice nearest you or a loved one, or to obtain additional information about hospice, call the National Hospice Organization Hospice Helpline toll-free at 1-800-658-8898.

**Talking Glossary**
Palliative care
G2004

**How Hospice Differs from Other Types of Health Care[13]** Hospices offer **palliative care,** rather than curative treatment. Hospices use methods of pain and symptom control that enable the person to live as fully and comfortably as possible. According to the National Hospice Organization:

- *Hospice treats the person, not the disease.* The interdisciplinary hospice team is made up of professionals who can address the medical, emotional, psychological, and spiritual needs of terminally ill people and their loved ones.

**Palliative care** Treatment focused on the relief or reduction of pain and suffering rather than cure.

- *Hospice emphasizes quality, rather than length, of life.* Hospice neither hastens nor postpones death: It affirms life and regards dying as a natural process.
- *Hospice considers the entire family, not just the patient.* Patients and their families are included in the decision-making process. Bereavement counseling is provided after the death.
- *Hospice offers help and support 24 hours a day, 7 days a week.* Help is always just a phone call away. Dying people receive in-home services from nurses, aides, social workers, volunteers, and other members of the team.

**What You Can Do in Caring for a Dying Person** First of all, be there for the person. Be available to talk, to listen, to share experiences. Give the person the opportunity to talk about death and to grieve, but don't be afraid to talk about life. People who are dying often need to focus on other things than impending death. They may be comforted to hear about your life experiences—your concerns and worries as well as your joys, hopes, and dreams. But be aware of the person's emotional state on any given day. Some days are better than others. Don't attempt to minimize the person's emotional pain or need to grieve by changing the subject or refusing to acknowledge it. Be sensitive to the person's feelings, offering consolation and support.

## Euthanasia

Talking Glossary
Euthanasia
G2005

The word **euthanasia,** literally "good death," is derived from the Greek roots *eu* ("good") and *thanatos* (death). Also called "mercy killing," it refers to the act of causing a person's death through gentle or painless means to relieve unavoidable pain or suffering. There are several different types of euthanasia.

**Euthanasia** Causing a painless death in a person suffering from an incurable and painful disease or condition.

**Active euthanasia** Intentional administration of lethal drugs or other means of producing a painless death in a person with an incurable and painful disease or condition.

**Doctor-assisted suicide** Suicide, usually of a person suffering from an incurable and painful disease, in which a physician helps to administer a lethal drug.

**Active Euthanasia—Mercy Killing or Just Plain Murder?** In **active euthanasia,** a lethal treatment (usually a drug) is administered to cause a painless death. Usually a spouse or family member administers the treatment. When euthanasia is carried out with the person's consent, it is called *voluntary active euthanasia* or *assisted suicide.*

Voluntary active euthanasia, including assisted suicide, remains illegal, although legal challenges to state laws making it a crime are now working their way through the courts. It is legal in some other countries, such as the Netherlands. In 1994, Oregon became the first state to permit doctors to legally prescribe lethal drugs for terminally ill patients who request their help in ending their lives, so long as they follow guidelines, which include a waiting period of several weeks and efforts to ensure that the person is not suffering from depression or another psychological disorder that might impair his or her judgment. As of 1997, however, the law remained on the books but had not yet been implemented because of legal challenges.

*Involuntary active euthanasia* stands on much shakier moral, ethical, and legal grounds than voluntary euthanasia. In involuntary active euthanasia, a person causes the death of another without the person's informed consent. Cases of involuntary euthanasia usually involve people who are comatose or otherwise incapacitated and whose loved ones believe they would have wanted to die had they retained the capacity to make such a decision. Still, in the eyes of the law, it is considered murder.

**Doctor-Assisted Suicides** In some cases of active voluntary euthanasia, doctors have assisted people with certain terminal or incapacitating illnesses who wished to take their own lives by providing them with lethal doses of drugs or by sometimes administering the drugs when people have been too ill to take them themselves. The best known cases of **doctor-assisted suicides** involve Dr. Jack Kevorkian, a retired pathologist dubbed "Dr. Death" by the press for having assisted in dozens of suicides. As of this writing, Kevorkian had been tried several times for his actions in these cases but was acquitted each time. Unlike Dr. Kevorkian, most physicians who assist in patient suicides (about one in four admit to doing so) do so quietly and secretly. Doctor-assisted suicide, like other forms of active voluntary euthanasia, remains against the law, and doctors can be prosecuted for the act or lose their license to practice.

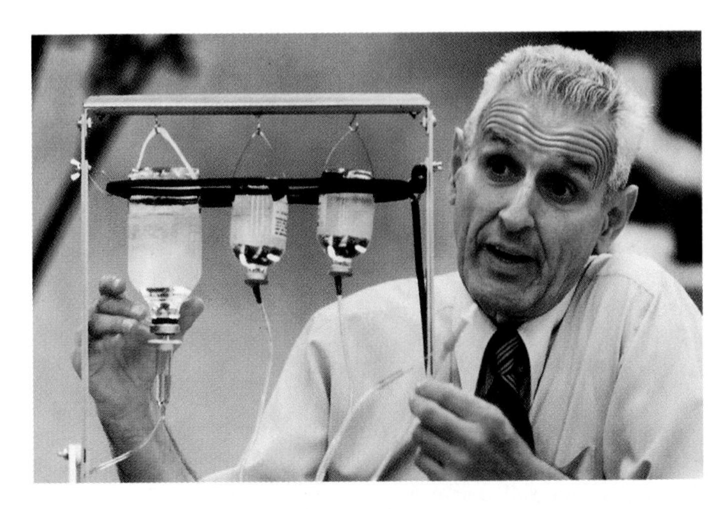

***Dr. Jack Kevorkian*** Kevorkian, shown here with his so-called death machine, gained a reputation as "Dr. Death" because of his role in assisting many terminally ill patients in ending their lives.

The issue of doctor-assisted suicide continues to be debated among physicians and the larger society. The American Medical Association opposes the practice. Doctors themselves are split on whether doctor-assisted suicide is justified. Doctors who oppose the practice often cite the belief that it flies in the face of thousands of years of medical tradition. Doctors are meant to *treat* patients, says one physician, not do away with them.[14] A recent survey of cancer specialists showed strong opposition to the practice. Only about one in seven reported having performed the procedure, although more than half (57%) reported that people had asked them to end their lives.[15] Polls in the United States and Canada show that about three of four people believe that doctors should be permitted to help a terminally ill person commit suicide.[16] More than half (54%) of the adult Americans surveyed in one poll reported that they would probably ask a doctor to administer a lethal dose of a painkiller if they had an incurable illness and were suffering a great deal of pain.[17]

Despite the medical community's opposition to assisted suicide, more than 90% of physicians (and of members of the general public) believe it is acceptable for doctors to gradually increase a patient's dose of morphine to relieve pain in a terminally ill person, even if it hastens death.[18] U.S. courts allow this practice, and the medical profession has long maintained that it falls within its ethical guidelines. It is not considered physician-assisted suicide or euthanasia because the goal is to relieve pain.[19] In actual practice, about 6,000 deaths per day are assisted in one way or another, often by doctors who prescribe pain-relieving medications to hasten death or who do *not* apply potentially life-extending treatments.[20]

**Passive Euthanasia** **Passive euthanasia** hastens death by withholding potentially life-saving treatments. For example, doctors may fail to resuscitate a terminally ill person who stops breathing, or they may withdraw medicine, food, or life-support systems, such as a respirator, from a comatose person. Physicians may accede to a dying person's request not to be resuscitated or sustained on life-support systems, but legally, they must draw the line at directly causing death or assisting in suicide.

The legal status of passive euthanasia varies with the circumstances. One form of passive euthanasia that is legal throughout the United States is the withholding or withdrawing of life-sustaining techniques in terminally ill people who make it known that they do not wish to be kept alive by aggressive or "heroic" treatment. The declaration of these wishes may be made orally or contained in a **living will.** The will is a written document that contains instructions or *advance directives* that specify the conditions under which the person desires to have life-sustaining treatment withdrawn or withheld.

## Active Euthanasia—Sorting Out the Issues

Perhaps no contemporary social issues other than abortion have sparked as much debate as active euthanasia and doctor-assisted suicides. As a society, we have been more comfortable with passive means of hastening death, such as withdrawing life-support systems, than with active means, such as assisted suicide. Many people oppose active euthanasia because it violates their religious teachings. Others believe that people should be permitted to decide the issue for themselves and that people should not impose their morality on others. To sort through these issues, let us frame the debate in terms of several of the more commonly heard arguments favoring and opposing active euthanasia.

**Video**
Dying: A matter of choice
**V2001**

**Smart Reference**
Right-to-die
**R2001**

**Passive euthanasia** The withholding or withdrawal of life-sustaining treatment to hasten death.

**Living will** A document prepared when a person is well directing termination of life-sustaining treatment under certain conditions.

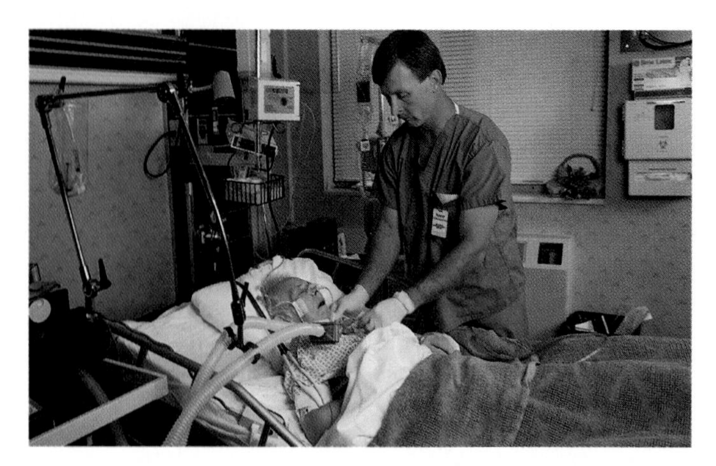

***Whose Life Is It?*** Do terminally ill patients have a right to die? Should doctors be permitted to assist them in taking their lives by giving them lethal doses of drugs? Or should a doctor's proper role be limited to relieving pain and suffering, not inducing death? Where do you stand on these troubling issues?

### Arguments Favoring Active Euthanasia

*An act of kindness.* The major justification for voluntary active euthanasia and assisted suicide is that it is merciful to agree to the wishes of people suffering from terminal disease to end their agony. In this view, mercy killing becomes justifiable when the person's fight to live clearly becomes hopeless and his or her suffering becomes unbearable.[21] We would not hesitate to end the life of a suffering animal that is beyond saving. Proponents of active euthanasia argue that we should do no less in helping people.

*The right to die as a basic human right.* Many proponents of euthanasia contend that the decision to end one's life is a private matter, not a social issue.[22] Some ethicists believe that there is a right to die that is similar to other basic rights, like rights to liberty, freedom of speech, and freedom of religion. They argue that the right to die, like other basic rights, need not be "proven" by argument.[23]

### Arguments Opposing Active Euthanasia

*Many patients who want to die are depressed and may change their minds once depression lifts.* In the first survey of its kind, Americans with cancer were polled concerning their attitudes toward euthanasia and doctor-assisted suicide. The survey found that most patients who wished to die were driven more by depression than by pain.[24] In the words of a psychiatrist, "We can treat the depression, we can bring people back from depression. We can't bring them back from the dead."[25] Even advocates of euthanasia such as Derek Humphry, author of the best-selling book *Final Exit* and founder of the pro-euthanasia Hemlock Society, do not support all forms of suicide. Humphry maintains that the right to die rests on the belief that the suicide is a **rational suicide.** Only mentally competent people can decide whether their lives have value and are worth living. As Humphry puts it,

> We do not support any form of suicide for mental health or emotional reasons. . . . But we do say that there is a second form of suicide—justifiable suicide, that is, rational and planned self-deliverance from a painful and hopeless disease which will shortly end in death.[26]

The number of presumably rational suicides that were committed by people whose judgment and reasoning ability were colored by depression or other psychological disorders is unknown.

*Pain can be successfully managed in most cases, even among terminally ill people with cancer.* Pain specialists recognize that pain can be effectively relieved in most cases, even in 90% or more of cancer patients.[27] Through the clinical management of pain with narcotics and other analgesics, terminally ill people can live out their lives in relative comfort. The problem, say medical authorities, is that too few doctors are trained in effective pain management. Doctors are accustomed to treating acute pain, such as that which follows surgery. They know little about the management of long-term pain. Moreover, some states legally prevent the regular use of pain-killing narcotics. Yet euthanasia proponent Derek Humphry argues that controlling pain misses the point:

> Most, but not all, terminal pain can today be controlled with the sophisticated use of drugs, but the point these leaders miss is that personal quality of life is vital to some people. If one's body has been so destroyed by disease that it is not worth living, that is an intensely individual decision which should not be thwarted. In some cases of the final days in hospice care, when the pain is very serious, the patient is drugged into unconsciousness. If that way is acceptable to the patient, fine. But some people do not wish their final hours to be in that fashion. There should be no conflict between hospice and euthanasia—both are valid options in a caring society. Both are appropriate to different people with differing values.[28]

**Rational suicide** Suicide based on a rational decision that life is not worth living in light of current suffering.

Consider an opposing view from Dr. Kathleen Foley, a leading cancer pain specialist. In testimony to Congress, Foley said, "It is a documented fact that those asking for assisted suicide almost always change their minds once we have their pain under control."[29] Foley believes that the proper role for physicians should be relieving pain and suffering though palliative care, not inducing death. Hospitals and hospices should coordinate their efforts to make the end of life as meaningful and pain-free as possible.

*The "slippery slope" argument.* Opponents of active euthanasia argue that helping terminally ill people kill themselves will lead to a slippery slope. That is, once active euthanasia becomes a medical option for terminally ill people, it may also be extended to other people, including those with disabilities and chronic health problems, especially when continuing care imposes a great financial or emotional burden on the family. Even Dr. Kevorkian reportedly participated in at least one suicide of a patient who suffered from a chronic though not terminal disease. Some opponents of doctor-assisted suicide fear that if the practice becomes legitimized, it may even eventually lead to involuntary euthanasia as doctors, not patients themselves, make life-and-death decisions based on their own views of the "patient's best interests." Proponents of euthanasia counter that the slippery slope argument is a scare tactic. They say that safeguards can be established to prevent such abuses.

There are compelling arguments on both sides of the euthanasia debate. The debate is now entering a new legal arena, as the Supreme Court has begun to review cases that test the constitutionality of laws against euthanasia. In a 1997 ruling, the Court allowed state laws to stand which prohibit assisted suicide. However the Court left the door open to future challenges asserting the right, in some cases, of terminally ill patients in intractable pain having a doctor assist them in hastening their deaths. The legal basis of assisted suicide remains inconclusive.

## The Living Will—Making End-of-Life Health Care Decisions

Suppose you suffered a tragic accident that left you in an irreversible coma and dependent on artificial life support to maintain your breathing (a respirator) and nutritional needs (feeding tubes that supplied your body with nutrients). Would you want your life to be maintained by whatever means were at the disposal of modern medicine, or would you want doctors to withdraw life support, allowing you to die naturally? Or suppose you suffered from a terminal disease and your heart suddenly stopped. Would you want the doctors to resuscitate you by whatever intrusive means were necessary to prolong your life for a few days or weeks? Who is to decide when it is time to die? You or the doctors managing your care?

In 1990, the U.S. Supreme Court ruled that people have a right to end life-sustaining treatment as long as they can make their wishes clearly known. The decision was brought in the case of Nancy Cruzan, a young woman who was left in a vegetative state from an automobile accident. Her parents' long legal battle to have her feeding tubes removed became the centerpiece of a widespread public debate about end-of-life decision making. Ironically, the Supreme Court decision in the *Cruzan* case did not directly lead to the removal of her feeding tubes, since she lay in a deep coma and was unable to communicate her wishes. Her parents brought in witnesses who had heard Nancy indicate that she would never want to live "like a vegetable." A local judge ruled that this constituted clear evidence of her wishes and ordered the feeding tubes removed; she died shortly thereafter.[30]

The Supreme Court decision in the *Cruzan* case provided the legal backing for the creation of a living will. This is a legal document that people can draft while they are well. It directs health professionals not to use aggressive medical procedures or life-support systems to prolong their lives in the event they become permanently incapacitated (e.g., enter an irreversible coma) and unable to communicate their wishes. There is no distinction in the eyes of the law between withholding life-support equipment (e.g., feeding tubes or respirators) and withdrawing it after it has been started.[31] Terminally ill people can insist that "Do Not Resuscitate" (DNR) orders be included in their charts, directing doctors not to use CPR if they suffer cardiac arrest.

The living will allows people to make their own end-of-life medical decisions and avoid invasive medical treatments that are unwanted, expensive, and futile.[32] A living will allows the person to die naturally, comforted by loved ones rather than rendered virtually helpless by life-support equipment. As one dying person said, "When I am breathing my last breath, it is better to be touched by a hand than violated by a tube."[33]

The withdrawal of life-sustaining treatment in accordance with the provisions of a living will is a form of passive euthanasia. Unlike active euthanasia, death is not induced by administering a lethal drug or assisting in a patient's suicide. More than 90% of the American public approve of living wills.

Living wills are also called *advance directives* because they spell out in advance the person's wishes. Though people can tell their doctors what they want, it is best to write them down. In the absence of any (written or verbal) advance directives, physicians are bound in some states to continue life-sustaining treatment no matter how futile the effort, even if family members object that the patient would have preferred to die naturally. Other states do allow surrogates such as family members to make end-of-life decisions regarding withdrawal of life-sustaining equipment for incapacitated people, even for people without living wills.

**Close-up**
More on advance directives
**T2003**

Living wills need not be complicated documents, though they must be drafted in accordance with state laws (Figure 20.1 shows a part of a living will for residents of California). The living will only takes effect if, because of illness or injury, people are unable to speak for themselves to express their wishes.

**HealthCheck**
What advance directives do you have?
**H2001**

Though living wills give people greater control over end-of-life treatment decisions, many situations are not clear-cut when it comes to emergencies. A living will may specify that extraordinary or heroic treatments be suspended, but who is to decide what treatments meet these conditions? For example, is a blood transfusion a heroic or extraordinary treatment? None of us can fully anticipate all the situations in which advance directives may be applied. For this reason, living wills usually identify some individual, or proxy, usually the next of kin, to make decisions in the event the signer becomes unable to communicate (see Figure 20.2).

Despite these safeguards, many advance directives are ignored.[34] Some are disregarded by proxies, perhaps because they don't understand the patient's wishes, perhaps because they can't bear the emotional burden of "pulling the plug."[35] Investigators find that when patients and their proxies are asked to respond to a set of hypothetical situations, there is generally a low rate of agreement as to the treatment decisions each party would make.[36] Designated proxies are more hesitant about withdrawing life-sustaining treatments than are patients themselves.[37]

Physicians, too, may not comply with living wills. Perhaps they aren't available when needed. Perhaps they are not clear regarding specific treatments that can be administered. Some doctors and nurses just ignore written directives and make the decisions they feel are best for the patient, regardless of the patient's expressed wishes.[38] Health professionals may find it difficult to "give up" on someone and allow death to take its course. Doctors who for moral or religious reasons feel unable to comply with a patient's advance directions are obliged to transfer the person to a doctor who will be able to do so.[39]

(THIS IS A PART OF A LIVING WILL DRAFTED IN ACCORDANCE WITH STATUTES IN CALIFORNIA. **THIS IS NOT A COMPLETE DOCUMENT AND SHOULD NOT BE USED FOR PURPOSES OF PREPARING A LIVING WILL.** LAWS GOVERNING LIVING WILLS VARY FROM STATE TO STATE. FOR THE FULL FORM OF A LIVING WILL IN YOUR STATE, CONSULT YOUR FAMILY ATTORNEY OR PHYSICIAN)

**CALIFORNIA DECLARATION**

If I should have an incurable and irreversible condition that has been diagnosed by two physicians and that will result in my death within a relatively short time without the administration of life-sustaining treatment or has produced an irreversible coma or persistent vegetative state, and I am no longer able to make decisions regarding my medical treatment, I direct my attending physician, pursuant to the Natural Death Act of California, to withhold or withdraw treatment, including artificially administered nutrition and hydration, that only prolongs the process of dying or the irreversible coma or persistent vegetative state and is not necessary for my comfort or to alleviate pain.

If I have been diagnosed as pregnant, and that diagnosis is known to my physician, this declaration shall have no force or effect during my pregnancy.

**Figure 20.1** ***Sample from a Living Will***

## Health Care Proxy

(1) I,______________________________

hereby appoint______________________________
(name, home address and telephone number)

______________________________

as my health care agent to make any and all health care decisions for me, except to the extent that I state otherwise. This proxy shall take effect when and if I become unable to make my own health care decisions.

(2) Optional instructions: I direct my agent to make health care decisions in accord with my wishes and limitations as stated below, or as he or she otherwise knows. (Attach additional pages if necessary.)

______________________________

______________________________

______________________________

(Unless your agent knows your wishes about artificial nutrition and hydration [feeding tubes], your agent will not be allowed to make decisions about artificial nutrition and hydration. See instructions on reverse for samples of language you could use.)

(3) Name of substitute or fill-in agent if the person I appoint above is unable, unwilling or unavailable to act as my health care agent.

______________________________
(name, home address and telephone number)

______________________________

(4) Unless I revoke it, this proxy shall remain in effect indefinitely, or until the date or conditions stated below. This proxy shall expire (specific date or conditions, if desired):

______________________________

(5) Signature______________________________

Address______________________________

Date______________________________

Statement by Witnesses (must be 18 or older)

I declare that the person who signed this document is personally known to me and appears to be of sound mind and acting of his or her own free will. He or she signed (or asked another to sign for him or her) this document in my presence.

Witness 1______________________________

Witness 2______________________________

Witness 3______________________________

Address______________________________

**Figure 20.2** ***Health Care Proxy*** Part of a health care proxy form used in New York State. You should consult an attorney before signing such an agreement.

Dr. William Knaus, a chief investigator of a study of terminally ill patients, says, "The [medical] system doesn't know when to stop"[40] Even when doctors were clearly informed about what their patients wanted, researchers found no difference in the use of life-sustaining treatments. Nor did the presence of living wills make any difference in the treatments patients received. Overall, estimates indicate that as many as one-quarter to one-half of the people with living wills cannot rely on having them carried out.[41]

How can we help ensure that dying people's wishes are carried out? For one thing, doctors are more likely to withhold treatment if the patient's advance directives refer to specific orders (e.g., "Do not resuscitate") rather than to general guidelines. For another, proxies and other family members need to make sure they clearly understand the dying person's wishes, are comfortable in executing them, and are willing to insist that health professionals follow them.

Even if advance directives are not always followed to the letter, having them in place gives people more of a say in the decision-making process than not having them. Yet only about 20% of the population has executed them.[42]

Smart Quiz Q2001

**think about it!**

- **Do you find it difficult to think about or talk about your own death or the death of someone close to you? Why or why not?**
- **Do you believe that brain death is the best standard for determining the boundaries between life and death? Why or why not?**
- **Do you tend to agree with any of the explanations for near-death experiences that have been summarized in the text? (Which one?) Why or why not?**
- **Do you believe that terminally ill people have the right to die? Why or why not?**
- **How can we help ensure that dying people's wishes are respected and carried out through living wills?**
- **Would you arrange to have your organs donated after your death? Why or why not?**

**critical thinking** **Agree or disagree and support your answer: Doctors should be prosecuted if they help terminally ill people take their own lives.**

## COPING WITH DEATH

Coping with the death of a loved one is a painful ordeal for most people. Though grief may resolve with the passage of time, in some cases a deep sense of loss and emptiness remains, especially if the loss involves the death of a child. Knowing what to expect when someone dies can help us cope.

### What to Do When Someone Dies[43]

**Coroner** A public official with responsibility for investigating deaths not clearly resulting from natural causes.

**Medical examiner** An official, trained as a physician, who performs autopsies in deaths suspected of resulting from unnatural causes.

**Autopsy** The surgical examination and dissection of a dead body to ascertain the cause and circumstances of death.

**Embalming** A process of replacing the blood and bodily fluids of a dead body with chemicals to prevent decay.

If you are present when someone dies, the first thing to do is to call the family doctor. A doctor needs to complete the death certificate and indicate the cause of death. If the cause of death cannot be readily determined, a **coroner** or **medical examiner** may become involved to determine the cause of death. Once the body has been examined by the doctor and the death certificate completed, a funeral director may be contacted to remove the body from the home or the hospital and make arrangements for burial or cremation. When death occurs unexpectedly, or when foul play is involved or suspected, an **autopsy** may be performed to determine the circumstances of death. An autopsy may also be performed with the family's consent if the person died from a rare or threatening disease and health professionals wish to gain knowledge from the procedure that might benefit others.

**Funeral Arrangements** Funerals provide an organized way of responding to death that is tied closely to religious customs and cultural traditions. The funeral is a ritual that provides family members with customary things to do when someone dies. It allows them to grieve publicly and say farewell to their departed loved ones. The funeral helps give the experience of death a sense of closure that can help family and friends begin to get on with their own lives.

Family members of the deceased discuss with the funeral director how simple or elaborate they wish the funeral to be. They decide whether they want **embalming,** a procedure in which blood and other bodily fluids are drawn out from the body of the deceased and replaced with chemicals that slow down the process of deterioration. Embalming reduces odors and makes the body more presentable for viewing prior to burial. Perhaps foremost is the decision as to whether the body should be buried or cremated. Some people

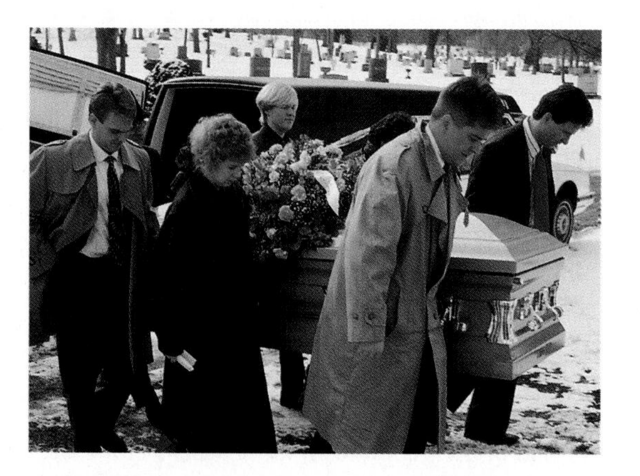

***Saying Goodbye*** Funerals are rituals that help families grieve publicly and bid farewell to their loved ones.

express their wishes concerning burial beforehand, but in many cases the decision rests on the shoulders of family members, who may be torn between "doing the right thing" and the financial obligations they may have to bear. An ethical, responsible funeral director helps families balance financial realities with the desire to fulfill the departed person's burial wishes. Unfortunately abuses can and do occur, as we see in the following ***Prevention*** feature.

PREVENTION

## *Preventing Funeral Rip-Offs*[44]

After their homes and automobiles, Americans spend more on funerals than anything else. Their average cost is nearly $6,000. Though many funeral directors are honest and sensitive to the family's needs, critics charge that others are unscrupulous and take advantage of people when they're in shock from their loss. The following guidelines can help you arrange a funeral that meets your needs.

***Have a Trusted Friend Nearby*** Get a good friend to stand by your side. Choose someone who will be swayed by reason and good sense rather than emotions or guilt. This person will help you resist the sales pitches that can drive up funeral costs. Be wary of any funeral director who says something like, "I know you want to do the best by Uncle Charley, so why don't you leave everything to me."

***Selecting a Funeral Home*** If possible, shop around. Yes, you can and should ask about the services they provide and the costs. If the body is in the morgue or the hospital, it can remain there for several hours while you make the arrangements for burial or cremation. Make sure that the funeral home you select is the one that arranges for the pickup and preparation of the body, or you may incur additional costs in using another funeral home for this purpose.

***Ground Burial*** Though cost is not the determining factor in this decision for most families, traditional ground burial is far more expensive than cremation.

A burial plot alone can range from $500 to many thousands. In addition to the plot, the costs for ground burial include the casket ($500 and up), a burial vault or grave liner ($500 and up), fees for opening and closing the grave ($350 to $2,000, depending on the time of day and day of week), the monument (about $1,200 on average), and fees for perpetual maintenance (vary widely). Despite what some families are told, no state requires the use of a burial vault or grave liner. Cemeteries, motivated to increase their profits, may require them, even though there is no evidence that they protect against moisture, roots, decay, or microorganisms.

Some cemeteries offer the plot free of charge but demand exorbitant fees for maintenance, opening and closing fees, monuments, and so on. Persons who wish to donate their bodies to science for humanitarian reasons will save their loved one's or their estate a considerable expense. Donation is free, and the cremated ashes are usually returned to the family in about a year. Veterans are entitled to a free burial plot in a national cemetery, but the family must pay to transport the body.

***Caskets—The Major Burial Expense*** Caskets are often the major burial expense but need not be. Costs for caskets can range from $500 to about $1,000 for a "respectable" steel model to around $2,000 for a walnut or oak model. Some of the more elaborate and ornate models cost five figures. Top-of-the-line models may exceed $50,000! More expensive models may look more elaborate but do not provide significantly better protection for the remains. It is illegal for funeral homes to claim that they do, but widespread flouting of the national funeral law appears to be common in the industry. Families may be driven by feelings of guilt or shame to choose higher-priced caskets. Grieving families need to remember that the type of casket makes no difference to the deceased person.

When selecting a casket, tell the funeral director to show you models that fall within your comfortable price range. If you feel uncomfortable asking about costs, have your friend say something like, "You know, I think the family wants to see something in the $500 to $1,000 range. Can we see three models in that range?" Don't fall for the sales ploy that no caskets available in your price range have seals. Seals are not necessary in caskets. Ask to see the funeral home's price list. The law requires funeral homes to provide one.

Don't allow yourself to be manipulated by a salesperson who demeans a lower-priced model or snickers when you ask for one. Many funeral directors are sensitive to the family's needs and financial situation and are genuinely concerned about how prices have risen in the industry. They are more than willing to locate a casket that falls within the family's budget. Unfortunately there are also funeral directors who are motivated more by profit than by interest in serving the public.

***Mausoleums*** Mausoleums provide above-ground burial in an indoor facility. As expenses for ground burials have risen, this once expensive option has become more affordable. Mausoleums offer the advantage of indoor visitation with protection from the weather.

***Cremation*** As many as 20 to 30% of American families opt for cremation. Increasing numbers of families are choosing cremation, in part because the costs, including funeral services, average about half of those for traditional ground burials. Cremations can cost less than $1,000 but typically fall in the $2,000 to $3,000 range. After the cremation, the family is given an urn to hold the ashes (remains). Some people direct their families to have their bodies cremated and then thrown to the wind at sea or from some other favorite place. Some families preserve the ashes in an urn.

Though there may be charges for "renting" a casket for purposes of viewing the body, there is no need to purchase a casket for cremation. Nor is the family required to purchase a special urn or container for the ashes. Any container will do, though families may prefer a dignified holder, perhaps a nice antique box, which would still be a fraction of the cost of the urns sold by funeral homes.

The major rip-off in funeral expenses is not deceptive practices but excessive markups, especially on caskets, and exorbitant fees for professional services (some funeral homes even charge for use of the parking lot). Only by shopping around, asking for recommendations, asking questions of funeral directors, and being on their toes—a difficult task at a trying time—can families protect themselves and obtain the services they want.

**Legal and Financial Matters** Many legal and financial matters usually require attention following a death. There may be issues concerning estates, inheritance, outstanding debts, insurance, and funeral expenses. It can be difficult for family members to focus on these matters during a time of grief. They should seek legal counsel if they have questions about how to handle the deceased person's affairs and to protect their own financial interests. An attorney will usually be needed to settle the estate, especially if it is sizable or complex.

## Grief and Bereavement

The death of a close friend or family member can be a traumatic experience. Typically it leads to **bereavement,** an emotional state of longing and deprivation characterized by feelings of **grief** and a deep sense of loss. **Mourning** is the culturally prescribed manner of displaying grief. Different cultures prescribe different periods of mourning and different rituals for expressing grief, such as the "Irish wake" and the New Orleans jazz funeral. In the Jewish religion, for example, it is customary for the family of the deceased to "sit *shivah*" for seven days after the burial. In sitting *shivah,* mourners stay at home and sit on the floor or on low benches or crates as a mark of bereavement and receive visitors who pay their respects. Coping with loss requires time to come to terms with the loss and move ahead with one's life. Having a supportive social network helps.

**Bereavement** The state of deprivation brought about by the loss of a close friend or loved one.

**Grief** Emotional suffering, sorrow, or distress resulting from loss or other misfortune.

**Mourning** The ways of expressing grief in accordance with the customs of a particular culture.

**Grieving** There is no one right way to grieve or fixed period of time for grief to last. In some cases, especially for parents who have lost a child, grief never ends, although it does tend to lessen over time. People grieve in different ways. Some grieve more publicly, while others reveal their feelings only in private. You may not always know when someone is grieving.

Grief usually involves a combination of emotions, especially sadness, loneliness, feelings of emptiness, numbness, apprehension about the future ("What will I do now?"), guilt ("I could have done something"), and even anger ("Why did he or she have to die?" "How could the doctors let this happen?"). Grief may also be punctuated by a sense of relief that the deceased person is no longer suffering intense pain or discomfort and by a heightened awareness of one's own mortality. There is also a physical component to grief. The person may become fatigued, have difficulty sleeping or sleep too much, lose appetite or gain weight, or have feelings of tightness in the chest, back, or throat. Grief may also compromise the immune system, leaving the person more vulnerable to disease. Moreover, the death of a loved one places the survivor at greater risk of a heart attack.[45] In some cases, heart attacks have been linked to grief in people who had no prior history of heart disease.

**Stages of Grief** Though each person grieves in his or her own way, we can identify some common stages of grief and mourning.[46] The first stage typically involves feelings of numbness and shock. In the days following the death, the bereaved may find it difficult to accept the reality of the loss and feel dazed or detached. He or she may need others to take responsibility for funeral arrangements and other necessities. The next stage is characterized by preoccupation with thoughts about the deceased and by deep feelings of grief. Finally, as grief begins to resolve, the person enters a third stage, involving an acceptance of the loss and a return to a usual level of functioning.

Bereaved people may find much social support through the funeral. The most intense grief may be experienced directly after the funeral, when the other mourners have returned home and the grieving person is finally alone. It is then that the person may begin to grasp the reality of living in an empty house, of sleeping alone, of listening to the silence left by the absence of a familiar voice. The grieving person needs support—not suffocating support, but the kind of support that recognizes that mourning takes time, sometimes needs to be done alone, and may not proceed in a straight line and that some days are better than others. Mourners may need to "rework" the events leading to the loss. That means recounting the details of the illness and the events that occurred in the hospital. There may be feelings of misplaced guilt over what one could have done, should have done, or might have done. You can help a person in mourning by listening without judging or criticizing.

Grief may resolve, but it doesn't mean that the grieving person forgets the deceased person. Rather, grief is replaced with an acceptance of the loss and commitment to resuming a full life. Some people grow more compassionate as a result of their loss. They develop a deeper appreciation of the value of life.

## How to Cope with the Loss of a Loved One

Just as there are many ways to grieve, there are many ways of coping with loss.

**Take Care of Yourself** People who are grieving can become so absorbed with their loss that they may fail to attend to their own personal needs. They may not eat or bathe. They may feel guilty doing things for themselves and avoid pleasurable experiences. One can grieve without withdrawing from life. This may be the very time when you need to take good care of yourself to avoid compounding your grief with other problems.

**Allow Yourself to Feel Your Loss** Some people grieve silently, preferring to keep their feelings bottled up. Though this may work for a while, the feelings may not disappear. Covering up feelings or trying to erase them with tranquilizers may prolong mourning. Let negative feelings surface. Turning to a trusted friend or a professional counselor may help you get in touch with your feelings.

Give yourself time. And then some more time. No two people grieve the same way. There is no fixed timetable for grieving. One person may get back to normal in a few weeks. Others may take a year or more. Recognize that you'll have good days and bad days, ups and downs. Don't expect to get back to the way you were. The loss of a person who was close to you changes your life, but it can be a change that leads you to reaffirm your commitment to life and to those who remain. Some people never get over a loss, although their feelings of grief become more bearable over time.

**Take Charge**
Understanding and moving through grief
C2001

Do not compare yourself with others and criticize yourself if your feelings seem more intense or prolonged. Don't let other people push you into moving "to the next stage" unless you are prepared to do so.[47]

**Reach Out** Don't reject offers of help from friends and relatives. If they don't know what to do—what you need and what you don't need—tell them. Grief can also be compounded by serious depression. If you suspect that you are depressed, consult a mental health professional. Signs of depression include loss of appetite, sleeping problems, lack of energy, inability to experience pleasure, extended periods of sadness or downcast mood, negative feelings about yourself, and feelings of hopelessness. If you are suicidal, call a suicide hotline, your family doctor, or a psychotherapist. Don't go it alone.

Bereavement support groups can also help. For one thing, you'll see that you are not alone in your pain. Sharing experiences with others in similar circumstances can help you cope and work through your grief. Do not allow yourself to be pushed into a group by well-meaning relatives or friends, but don't avoid a group because of worries that reaching out is a sign of weakness. To obtain information about bereavement support groups in your area, consult your family physician or local hospice.

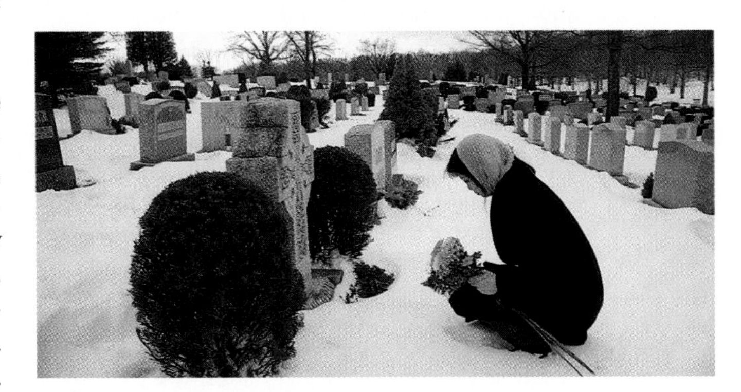

***Grieving*** People grieve in different ways and for different lengths of time. Eventually, grief resolves when people come to accept the loss and get on with their lives.

**Avoid Labeling Yourself** Our society has little tolerance for people who are grieving. We allow them a few weeks to "get over it" and then expect them to return to their normal routines. People who are grieving may be made to feel somehow abnormal or even crazy for feeling as they do, especially if bereavement is prolonged or intense. Recognizing that there is no fixed time limit for grieving and that people experience a range of intense emotions can help you see that your feelings are normal.[48]

## How to Help a Grieving Friend or Relative

When someone has lost a loved one, it is natural to want to reach out to them to help. Yet you may not know how to help or fear that you'll say the wrong thing. *Don't worry about what to say.* Just spending time with the person can help. Don't expect to have all the answers. Sometimes there are no answers. Sometimes what matters is being a good listener. Don't be afraid to talk about the deceased person. Take your cue from the bereaved person. Not talking about the departed person brings down a curtain of silence that can make it more difficult for the bereaved person to work through feelings of grief. On the other hand, don't force the person to talk about his or her feelings. Keep in touch regularly. Don't assume that the person doesn't want to talk if he or she doesn't return your calls. The bereaved person may be too depressed or lack the energy to reach out. Offer to help for a few weeks or months with shopping, errands, baby-sitting, and so on. Grieving is not done all at once or at a steady pace. Don't assume that grieving is "over" once the person reestablishes a normal routine.

The following suggestions were offered by an anonymous contributor to the Internet:

1. *Take some kind of action.* Make a phone call, send a card, give a hug, attend the funeral, help with practical matters (for example, meals, care of children).
2. *Be available.* Allow the person time so there is no sense of urgency when you visit or talk.
3. *Be a good listener.* Accept the words and feelings being expressed. Don't be judgmental. Avoid telling the person what he or she should feel or do.
4. *Don't minimize the loss and avoid giving clichés and easy answers* like, "You're young, you can have more children" or "It was for the best."
5. *Don't be afraid to talk about the loss, the deceased.*
6. *Allow the bereaved person to grieve for as long as needed.* Be patient. There are no shortcuts.
7. *Encourage the bereaved to care for himself or herself.* It is helpful for bereaved people to attend to their own physical needs, to postpone major decisions, and to allow themselves to grieve and recover.
8. *Acknowledge and accept your own limitations.* Many situations can be hard to handle but can be made easier with the help of outside resources—books, workshops, support groups, other friends, or professionals.

**Children and Grief[49]** Loss—especially the loss of a parent—is often extremely difficult for children to bear. The death strikes at the core of their sense of security and well-being. Younger children also lack the cognitive ability to understand death. Preschoolers may think that death is reversible or temporary, a belief that is reinforced by cartoon characters that die and come back to life. Older children may feel guilty, concluding that the death was a punishment for something they had done or that the person died because they had once "wished" for them to die. Their loss of security may drive them to anger, which may be directed toward surviving loved ones or acted out aggressively. Children may also show regressive or infantile behaviors, such as "baby talk" or demands for food or attention. Some children may persist in believing that the deceased person is alive. Such denial is common, but prolonged denial may herald the development of more severe problems.

How can you help a child cope with grief? First, don't force a child to go to the funeral if the child is frightened by it. Some other kind of observance may be more appropriate, such as lighting a candle, saying a prayer, or visiting the grave later on. Avoid using euphemisms that deny the reality that grieving children face—euphemisms like, "Aunt Tilly is sleeping comfortably now." Respond to children's questions and worries honestly, but reassure them that you are available to help them cope with their loss. Let them know that they can express their feelings freely without fear of criticism. Spend as much time as possible with them, providing the emotional support and reassurance

**Take Charge**
Helping children cope with grief
C2002

WORLD OF *diversity*

## A Japanese Way of Death

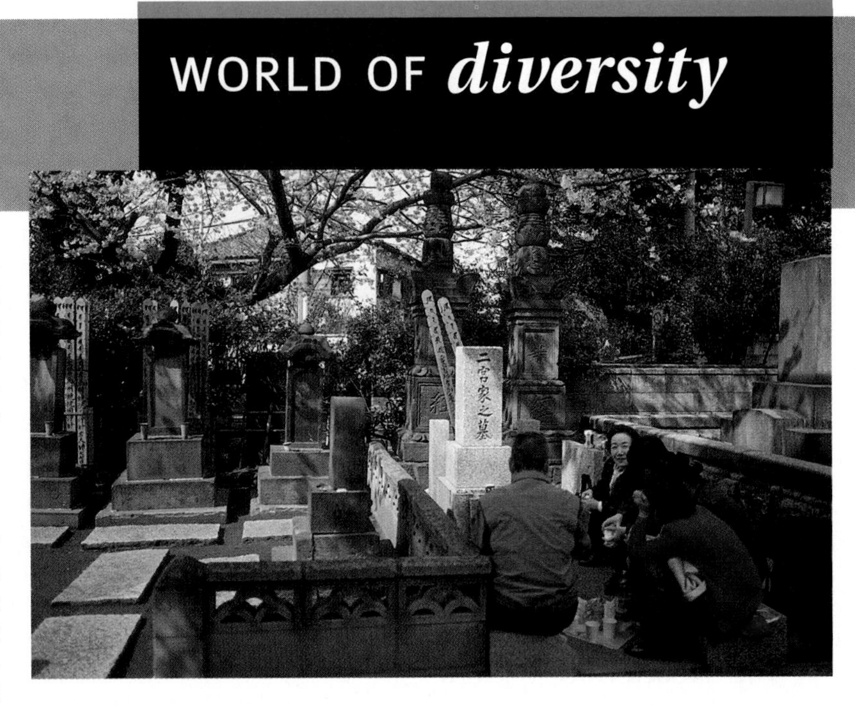

Burial customs vary from culture to culture. The following account of burial customs in Japan was written by a young Japanese woman, Etsuko Shioda.[50] She recounts her personal experience but notes that customs vary according to locations and times.

### Funeral Ceremony

The day after a person's death, family members invite a Buddhist priest to their house and have him recite a sutra (passage from Buddhist scripture). That evening, family members and close relatives burn incense sticks (called *senko*) in front of the altar all night long. This is what the Japanese call *otsuya,* meaning "all night long." The next day, they burn the body to ashes at a funeral hall and bring the ashes back to their house. Finally, the funeral service is conducted. People burn incense by turns in front of the altar while the priest recites a sutra. After the service is over, family members and close relatives go to the graveyard and lay the ashes to rest. Family members and close relatives serve meals (often feasts) to the people who come to mourn for the dead, at least twice, on the day after death and the day of cremation.

### Funeral Gifts

People bring *ko-den* (money) to either *otsuya* or the funeral service and hand it to the person at the reception. Family members prepare token gifts to be given back to the people who come to mourn for the dead.

### After the Funeral: Customs of Visiting the Grave

The family with a newly deceased member visits the family grave once a week during seven weeks starting from the funeral ceremony. On the forty-ninth day from the funeral, they offer feasts again to the close relatives and neighbors. The custom is called *Shijuku Nichi,* which literally means "the forty-ninth day."

Most Japanese people visit their ancestors' graves at least four times a year, once in each season, and twice in *obon* (Buddhist festival days). People believe that all their ancestors' souls visit their houses during *obon* days, which start on August 13 and last until August 16 in most areas in Japan. So they prepare simple altars for the deceased and offer three meals a day, fruits, and flowers. They visit the family grave to bring their ancestors' souls back to their houses, and to see them off.

Many Japanese families have a *Butsudan* (small family altar in front of which they pray to their ancestors for safety and fulfillment of other wishes and offer meals every day). Most Japanese people believe that their ancestors are always with them, watching, protecting, and guiding them.

they need. Be aware of signals that indicate that a child may need professional help. These include loss of sleep or appetite, prolonged depressed or downcast mood, development of excessive fears such as fear of being alone, withdrawal from friends, a sharp decline in school performance or refusal to attend school, or a persistent pattern of immature behavior.

**think about it!**

- **What would you do if someone close to you died? Has your reading of this chapter influenced you? If so, how?**

**critical thinking** **Agree or disagree and support your answer: Bereaved people should be left alone to grieve on their own.**

Smart Quiz Q2002

# Planning for the Inevitable

## Take Charge

When we are young, issues of mortality may be far from our minds. But since death can occur at any age, it is wise to put one's legal and financial house in order early, including drafting a will. Then there are other questions to consider: Should you draft a living will? How should you dispose of your remains? Should you become an organ donor?

### Draft a Will

No matter how large or small your assets are, a will is the only way to ensure that your possessions are disposed of in the manner you wish. Your family lawyer can help you draft a will, or you can use one of the many available legal software programs that allow you to draft a will on a personal computer. Review your will every three to five years or after any major life transition, such as a marriage, a divorce, the birth of a child, or the death of a loved one.

### Organize Your Financial Records

Gather and safely store important financial documents, such as wills, bank loans, mortgage documents, debts, college loan documents, life insurance documents, property deeds, pension and retirement documents, veteran's benefits, and names and account numbers of bank accounts. Include a copy of your federal and state income tax returns for the past few years. Make sure your spouse, parents, or other loved ones know where these records are and have access to them.

### Make Your Funeral Preferences Known

Make your preferences for ground burial, cremation, a cemetery, organ donation, and so on, known to your next of kin, the person who is most likely to be responsible for disposing of your remains. Also write your preferences in the form of a letter, which you should enclose in an envelope marked "Open in the Event of My Death." Store the envelope with your other important documents. Specifying your funeral preferences can help spare your loved ones from having to make an anguished decision. Be careful about prepaying funeral expenses, however. If you purchase a burial plot and later decide to be buried elsewhere, find out what happens to your investment.[51] If you wish to donate your organs after death, follow the suggestions given below.

### Consider Drafting a Living Will

You have a constitutional right to make your own end-of-life medical decisions. Drafting a living will puts in writing your wishes for life-sustaining medical care if you should become permanently incapacitated and unable to speak for yourself.

Should you draft a living will? Some people, including many physicians, believe that advance directives are only for people who are terminally ill or in the later years of life. Given the vagaries of life—you could be hit by a truck while crossing the street—all persons who feel strongly that they would not want life-support systems to needlessly prolong their lives if they are beyond hope of recovery should consider drafting a living will. Here are some tips for drafting a living will:[52]

- *Use the right forms.* The laws governing living wills vary from state to state. Therefore, you may want to consult an attorney who is familiar with the laws in your state. Attorneys specializing in estates and trusts are usually familiar with living wills. Or you may obtain state forms from your local or state health department or hospital. You may also download ready-made forms for your particular state from a website maintained by the nonprofit organization Choices in Dying (http://www.choices.org).
- *Appoint a proxy.* You can't anticipate every medical situation you might face. Fortunately, you can use a form of a living will called a *durable power of attorney for health care* (sometimes called a "health care proxy") to appoint someone, usually a next of kin, to make decisions you cannot make for yourself (see Figure 20.2). This document ensures that end-of-life medical decisions about you are made by the person you choose, not the doctors who happen to be caring for you at the time. Make sure that your proxy understands your wishes and is prepared to carry them out. Appoint an alternate proxy in the event that the first one is unavailable.
- *Distribute copies to anyone who may be involved in your health care.* A living will can be followed only if it is available to all the people involved in your medical care. Retain a signed copy for yourself and distribute other copies to your proxy (if you have appointed one), next of kin, family doctor, and attorney. If you should be hospitalized, give a copy to the hospital admitting clerk and insist that it be placed in your hospital chart.
- *Be specific.* Health professionals are more likely to adhere to living wills when they contain clear and specific instructions. Consult with your physician or attorney and specify the types of life-sustaining treatments you would want suspended or withheld under specific medical circumstances.

- *Keep your living will up to date.* Living wills can be revoked or changed at any time. Review your living will every year or two to make sure that it remains current with your wishes. Update your signature every several years.
- *Speak up for yourself.* Don't rely solely on the written document. Tell your doctors and your proxy what you want regarding end-of-life medical treatment and make sure they understand you.

## Organ Donation—The Gift of Life

It is called the gift of life. Donating your organs for transplant surgery after your death literally keeps a part of you alive while helping someone else in desperate need. Or you may donate your whole body to medical science, to help scientists conduct research that may lead to breakthrough cures or to help train a future generation of physicians. Your doctor can give you information about bequeathing your body to medical science.

Living donors—usually family members—can be used for some transplants, such as kidney and bone marrow transplants. But in most cases, such as those involving liver, heart, lung, and corneal transplants, organs must be taken from donors shortly after death. Only organs that were healthy at the time of death and remain intact are suitable for transplantation. The donor must also have been free of such infectious diseases as hepatitis, HIV infection, and tuberculosis.

Medical advances have greatly improved the chances of success of organ transplantation. To minimize the risk of rejection of the transplanted organ by the body's immune system, the recipient may require immunosuppressive drugs indefinitely.[53]

There is a nationwide shortage of available donor organs. Many desperately ill people are awaiting word that an organ is available for them. The federal government has instituted a system that helps ensure an equitable distribution of donated organs. Hospitals are required to inform relatives of donors about the United Network for Organ Sharing (UNOS), a central registry of available organs.[54]

**How Can You Donate Organs?** If you wish to donate your organs after death, you need to register as a designated organ donor. This can be done by drafting a living will that specifies which organs you wish to donate, or, in some states, by having an organ donor designation added to your driver's license. If this designation isn't available in your state, you may request a uniform donor card (see Figure 20.3) from the National Kidney Foundation (30 East 33rd St., New York, NY 10016). If you have any questions about becoming a donor, talk to your family physician. You should also inform your next of kin of your wish to become an organ donor. (This person will presumably be responsible for disposing of your remains.) Make sure the person understands which organs you wish to donate.

NATIONAL KIDNEY FOUNDATION

*Please detach and give this portion of the card to your family.*

This is to inform you that, should the occasion ever arise, I would like to be an organ and tissue donor. Please see that my wishes are carried out by informing the attending medical personnel that I have indicated my wishes to become a donor.

Thank you.

*SIGNATURE* *DATE*

*For further information write or call:*

NATIONAL KIDNEY FOUNDATION

30 East 33rd Street, New York, NY 10016

(800) 622-9010

UNIFORM DONOR CARD

Of ______________________

(print or type name of donor)

In the hope that I may help others, I hereby make this anatomical gift, if medically acceptable, to take effect upon my death. The words and marks below indicate my wishes.

I give: ☐ any needed organs or parts

☐ only the following organs or parts

______________________

(specify the organ(s), tissues(s) or part(s))

for the purposes of transplantation, therapy, medical research or education:

☐ my body for anatomical study if needed.

Limitations or special wishes, if any: ______________

**Figure 20.3** ***A Uniform Donor Card*** Reprinted with permission of the National Kidney Foundation.

## "Lying Down to Pleasant Dreams . . . "

Though most young people spend little if any time thinking about death, the American poet William Cullen Bryant was just 18 when he penned his best-known poem, "Thanatopsis." Though it concerns death, it is really more about life, about maintaining a sense of optimism and meeting challenges with integrity and commitment, so we can leave life with dignity when the time comes to "join the innumerable caravan" of the billions who have died before us:

Live, wrote the poet, so that

*when thy summons comes to join*
*The innumerable caravan that moves*
*To the pale realms of shade, where each*
*shall take*
*His chamber in the silent halls of death,*
*Thou go not, like the quarry-slave at night,*
*Scourged to his dungeon, but, sustained and soothed*
*By an unfaltering trust, approach thy grave*
*Like one who wraps the drapery of his couch*
*About him, and lies down to pleasant dreams.*

Smart Quiz
Q2003

# SUMMING UP

## Questions and Answers

### UNDERSTANDING DEATH AND DYING

1. **How do we know when somebody has died?** Health professionals use the standard of brain death. People can still be alive even if they stop breathing and their hearts stop beating due to conditions such as hypothermia.

2. **Are there stages of dying?** Kübler-Ross proposed that terminally ill people experience five stages of dying: denial, anger, bargaining, depression, and final acceptance. However, not all dying people experience these stages, and those who do may experience them in different order.

3. **What is a near-death experience?** This is an experience reported by people who almost die, as during a medical procedure, but who then recover. Many people report out-of-body experiences, moving through something like a dark tunnel, and then moving toward a warm, embracing light. There is no agreed-upon explanation for such experiences.

4. **What is a hospice?** A hospice cares for terminally ill people, as inpatients or at home. Hospice care helps the person maximize remaining days and avoid pain as much as possible. It also helps the family cope with the death.

5. **How can you help a dying person?** Be available to listen and to talk.

6. **What is euthanasia?** Euthanasia derives from roots meaning "good death." In active euthanasia, a lethal treatment (usually a drug) is used to cause a painless death. In passive euthanasia, death is hastened by withholding potentially life-saving treatments.

7. **What's the story on doctor-assisted suicide?** This is a form of active euthanasia in which a doctor helps an ill person commit suicide. Doctor-assisted suicide remains generally illegal, and medical organizations oppose it. Public sentiment favors the practice, however.

8. **What are the pros and cons of active euthanasia?** People who favor active euthanasia say it is an act of mercy ("mercy killing") and that people have a basic right to die. People who oppose it argue that many people who want to die are depressed and change their minds after the depression lifts, that pain can be managed in most cases, and that active euthanasia could be extended even to people who are not terminally ill.

9. **What is a living will?** A living will records a person's wishes concerning the use of aggressive or "heroic" medical treatments to sustain life if he or she becomes permanently incapacitated and cannot make choices or express them. However, many health professionals do not follow the instructions in living wills.

### COPING WITH DEATH

10. **What should you do when someone dies?** Call the doctor, arrange for a funeral that meets the person's expressed wishes (without straining family finances), gather important papers, and seek legal counsel to settle the estate. Select a trusted friend to help you make decisions.

11. **What is the difference between bereavement and mourning?** *Bereavement* is an emotional state following a death that is characterized by feelings of grief and loss. *Mourning* is a culturally prescribed manner of displaying grief.

12. **Are there stages of grief?** There are individual differences, but many bereaved people show shock or numbness soon after the death, followed by preoccupation with thoughts of the person who has died, and then acceptance and return to a more usual level of functioning.

13. **How can you cope with the loss of a loved one?** Consider these suggestions: Take care of yourself. Allow yourself to feel the loss. Do not make demands on yourself to get over it quickly. Reach out to other people, possibly by joining a support group.

14. **How can you help someone else who has experienced a loss?** Be available. Listen. Don't minimize the loss. If the person is a child, don't force him or her to go to the funeral, but encourage expression of feelings.

## References and Suggested Readings

### SMART REFERENCES FROM SCIENTIFIC AMERICAN

**Horgan, J. In Focus: Right to Die.** *Scientific American*, 274(6) (June 1996), 26. **R2001**

## SUGGESTED READINGS

**Colgrove, M., Bloomfield, H. H., and McWilliams, P.** *How to Survive the Loss of a Love.* Los Angeles: Prelude Press, 1991. Clear, practical, and sensitive guidance that can help people through each step of the process of grief and recovery from a loss.

**Kübler-Ross, E.** *On Death and Dying.* New York: Macmillan, 1969. The classic study of the final stages of life by a leading scholar, it helps us understand the anxieties, expectations, hopes, and fears of the dying patient and how professionals can help.

**Nuland, S.** *How We Die: Reflections on Life's Final Chapter.* New York: Knopf, 1994. Written by a surgeon, it helps demythologize death by helping the lay reader more clearly understand the physiology of dying—what happens to people as they die from such causes as heart disease, aging, cancer, AIDS, accidents, homicide, and suicide.

**Kushner, H.** *When Bad Things Happen to Good People.* New York: Avon Books, 1981. Spiritual advice for people whose lives have been deeply affected by painful experiences, including illness, injury, disappointment, and death, and who find it difficult to maintain their religious beliefs because of what has happened to them.

**Humphry, D.** *Final Exit.* Eugene, OR: Hemlock Society, 1991. The controversial best-seller by a leader of the right-to-die movement, it promotes the belief that suicide can be a rational choice for people with terminal or irreversible illness that is causing them great suffering. The book offers suggestions for ending one's life painlessly. Though it is not intended for people contemplating suicide who are depressed or have other mental health problems, critics contend that people with these problems may turn to the book anyway.

**Cundiff, D.** *Euthanasia Is Not the Answer: A Hospice Physician's View.* Totowa NJ: Humana Press, 1992. The case against euthanasia from the perspective of a hospice physician who offers palliative care as an alternative.

**Carroll, D.** *Living with Dying: A Loving Guide for Family and Close Friends.* New York: Paragon House, 1991. Addresses the practical and emotional concerns faced by people with loved ones who are dying. Topics include helping the dying patient cope with pain, talking to the dying person about death, talking to children about the death of a loved one, deciding to use hospice services, making funeral decisions, and learning about the grief process.

**Sutherland, C.** *Reborn in the Light* (1995) and *Within the Light* (1993). New York: Bantam Books. Personal accounts of dozens of people who have had near-death experiences and how they were affected by them, written by a sociologist who herself had a near-death experience.

# Violence and Abuse

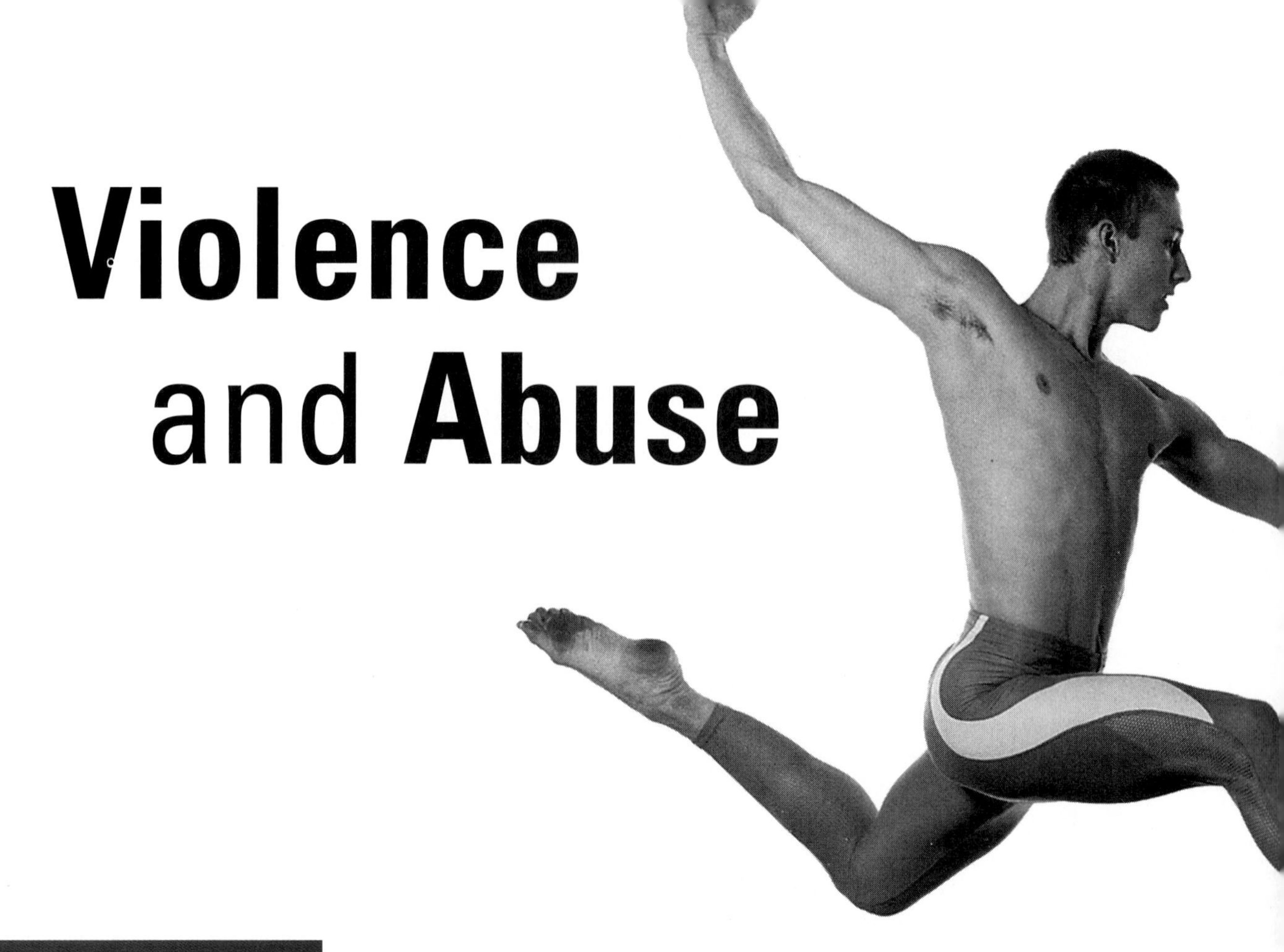

## DID YOU KNOW THAT

- Women are more likely to be attacked or killed by men they live with than by strangers? p.572
- Young men are more likely to die as the result of homicide in the U.S. than in any other industrialized nation? p.573
- Male teenagers in the United States are more likely to die from the use of firearms than from all natural causes combined? p.573
- On average, a rape occurs every three minutes in the United States? p.577
- The belief that women desire to be overpowered by men and forced into sexual relations is nothing more than an excuse for violence? p.580
- One woman in four and one man in six reports being sexually abused during childhood? p.584
- The great majority of people who sexually molest children are heterosexual men? p.584
- Sexual harassment has more to do with issues of power and control than with sexual motives? p.586

# 21



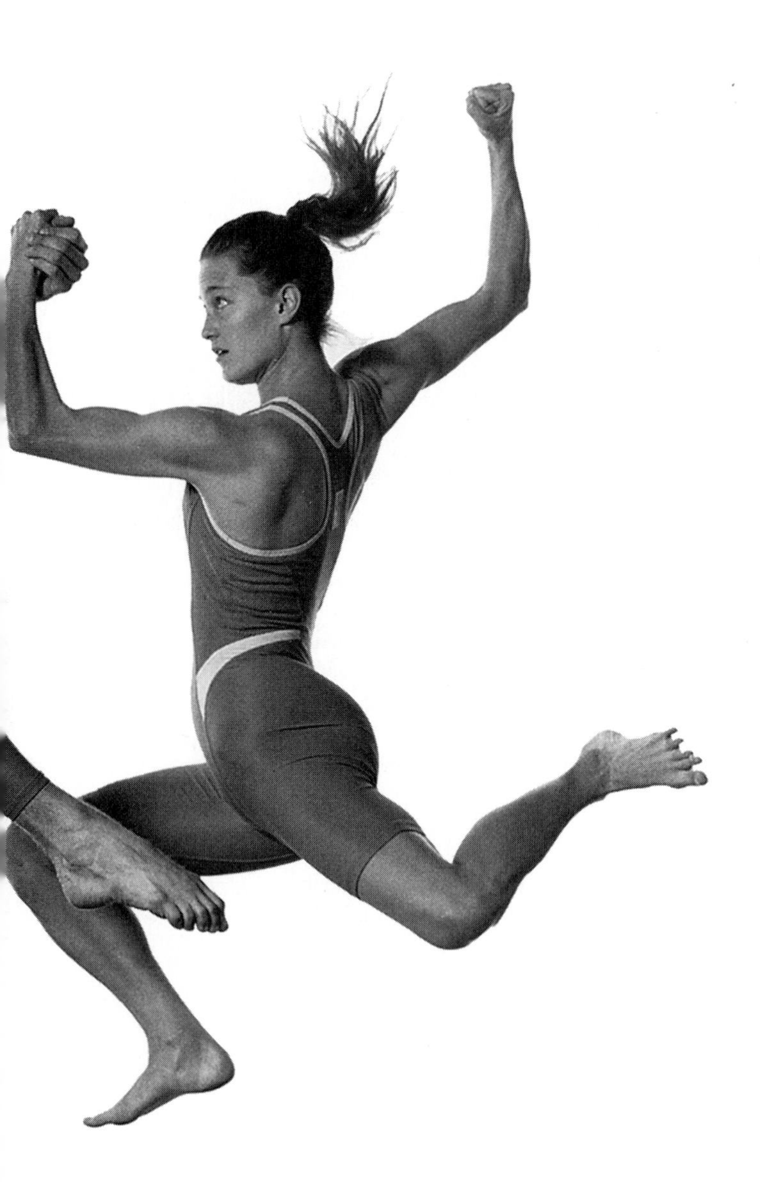

America the beautiful? *Yes, but also* America the violent. *Concerns about crime and violence have become a staple of American life. Not so many years ago we might have left our front doors open or walked through city parks late at night. Today, many of us live behind triple-bolted doors, invest thousands in home security systems, and avoid parks shrouded in darkness. With the increased incidence of carjackings, even a trip to the mall has become fraught with danger for many suburbanites. Some of us stay in at night, even in our own neighborhoods. The continual wail of car alarms is a daily reminder to city dwellers of concerns about crime.*

**Close-up**
Violence and drugs
T2101
Effects of media violence
T2102

**Take Charge**
Violence on TV: What parents can do
C2101

As a nation we are obsessed with crime. Reports of crime dominate news headlines and TV progams. The more sensational the crime, the greater the feeding frenzy of the media. Violent police dramas dot the prime-time landscape of commercial TV, and "real-life" cop shows attract a large audience. Movies feature a never-ending diet of stabbings, murders, and ever more inventive methods of mayhem.

This chapter examines the health threats posed by interpersonal violence and abuse. The U.S. Public Health Service identifies violence as a major public health problem contributing to premature death and disability. It's not just random street crime that threatens our health and safety. Most forms of aggression occur between people who know each other, often between members of the same household. We are much more likely to be attacked, murdered, raped, harassed, or abused by people we know than by strangers lurking in dark alleys.

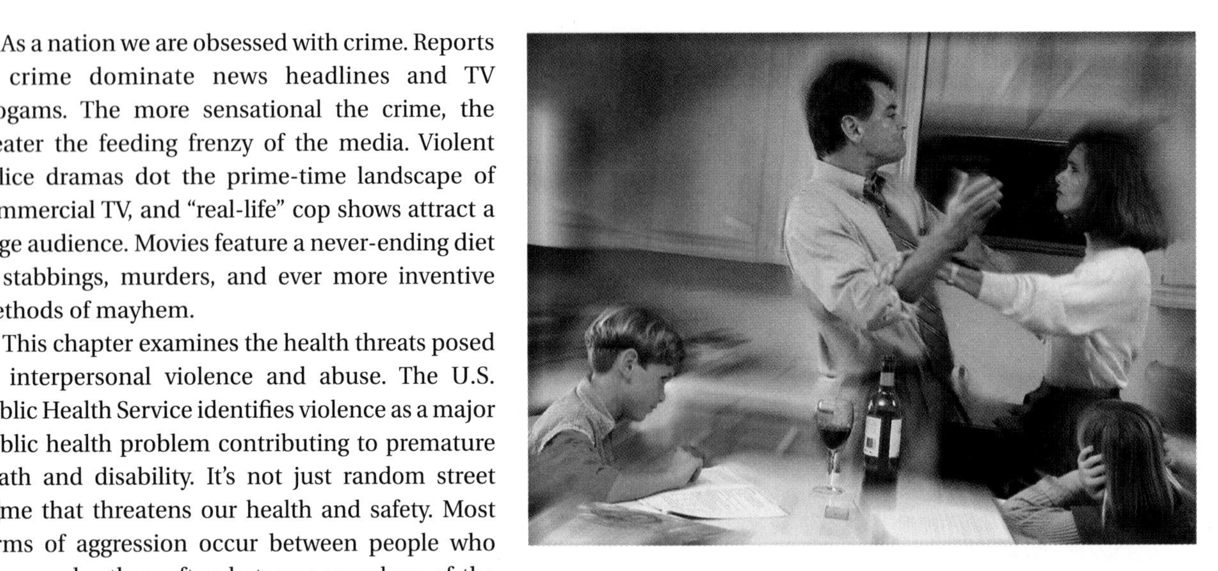

***What about the Children?*** It's not just the parents who are affected by domestic violence. Children exposed to it also suffer. Many become depressed or develop behavior problems. They may also learn that violence is an acceptable way of dealing with marital problems, which may set the stage for the perpetuation of domestic violence from generation to generation.

# SPOUSE ABUSE

The problem of spouse abuse may have been underscored by the O. J. Simpson trials, but it has long been a national crisis. The Justice Department estimates that a million American women are victims of domestic violence each year.[5] Women are more likely to be beaten, raped, and killed by men they live with than by any other type of assailant.[6,7]

Women too abuse their spouses. In fact, women are at least as likely to act violently toward their partners as men are.[8] In about half of all abusive relationships, the partners abuse each other. The big difference is that women are far more likely to sustain serious bodily harm at the hands of their partners than are men, including broken bones, damage to internal organs, even death. For this reason, we focus on the male batterer.

## Who Batters?

Batterers are found in every walk of life and income bracket. However, spousal abuse is more commonly reported among people in lower-income groups, perhaps because of the added stress that financial hardship places on already strained relationships. Or perhaps upper-income people have greater access to personal physicians who may be less inclined to report incidents of abuse to authorities than their counterparts in public facilities. Spouse abuse also cuts across all ethnic groups. In fact, ethnic differences in the prevalence of spouse abuse disappear when we take into account socioeconomic status.[9]

No one psychological profile fits all male batterers, but some common patterns have emerged.[10] Many batterers are impulsive, antisocial, and hostile. Many also have drug abuse problems and low self-esteem. They may feel personally inadequate, which leads them to become overly dependent on their partners for emotional support. Their dependence may lead them to feel threatened if they perceive their partners as growing distant, more independent, or developing interests of their own (such as school or work). They may respond to the "threat" by becoming overly demanding and violent. Typically, spousal violence follows an event that triggers the batterer. Triggering events typically touch on the man's feelings of insecurity or inadequacy, such as criticism or rejection from the partner. The use of alcohol or other drugs further raises the risk of battering.

**Close-up**
Alcohol and Domestic Violence
T2105

## WORLD OF *diversity*

### Homicide—As American as Apple Pie?

The statistics are alarming: The murder rate in the United States is nearly 10 times higher than it is in Japan. The robbery rate is more than 100 times higher.[1] The homicide rate among young men in the United States far exceeds that in all other industrialized countries (see Figure 21.1). Among young people aged 15 to 24, homicide has become the second leading cause of death, after accidents.

Most murders occur among people who know each other, who are often members of the same family or household. The great majority occur among people of the same race.

Though no one factor accounts for the high rate of homicide in the United States, the availability of firearms is one contributing factor. Male teenagers are more likely to die from the use of firearms than from all natural causes combined. Firearms are used in about three of four cases of homicide of young people in the United States, compared with fewer than one in four in other industrialized countries.[2]

Private gun ownership is virtually prohibited in Japan. Perhaps as a result, in a typical year in the 1990s, Japan recorded fewer than 40 homicides involving firearms. There were more than 16,000 such deaths in the United States in the same years. Put another way, the number of firearm deaths in Japan in one year is less than the number recorded in the United States in a single day! Guns account for an increasing percentage of homicides, rising from 60% in 1985 to 72% in 1994.[3]

**Close-up**
Preventing youth violence
T2103

Although the homicide rate in the United States remains high, there is some good news. The murder rate began to drop in 1992, and serious and violent crime overall declined steadily during the first half of the 1990s, the longest decline in 25 years.[4] It remains to be seen whether these trends are a temporary blip or indicators of lasting changes.

**Close-up**
Crime and older people
T2104

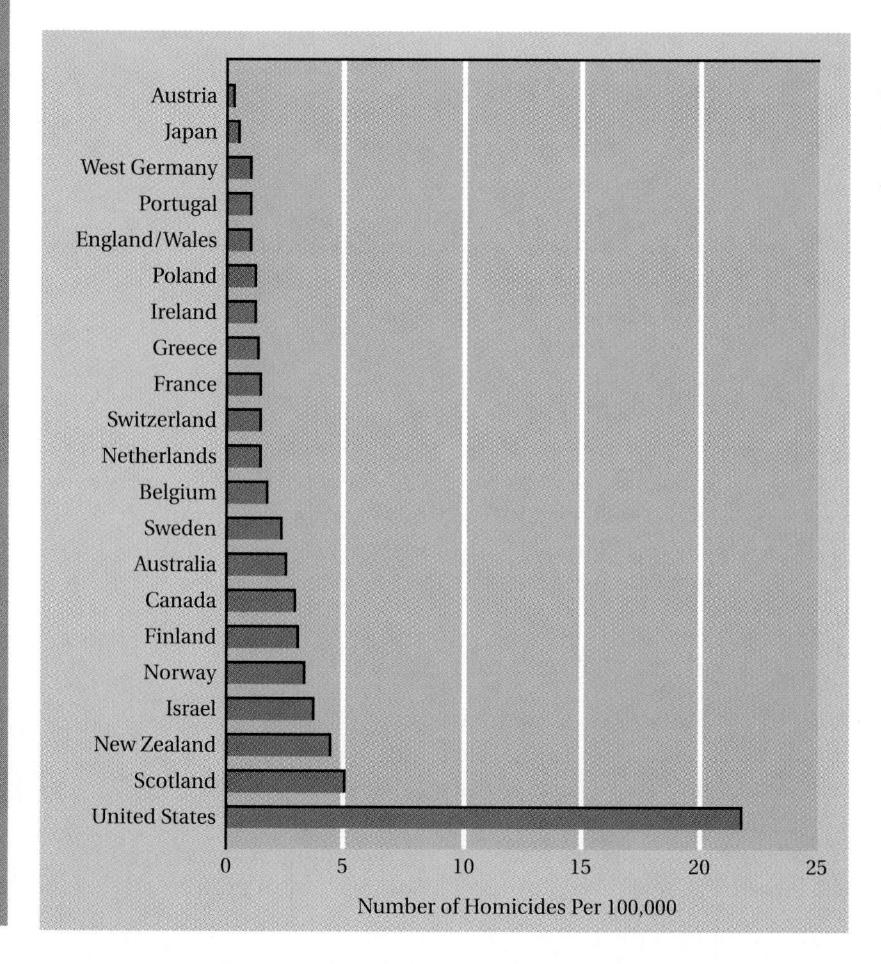


**Figure 21.1** ***Homicide Rates—U.S. versus Other Developed Countries*** The homicide rate in the U.S. among young men far exceeds the rate in other industrialized countries. What factors do you think contribute to the high murder rate in the U.S.?

Battering in marriage is usually part of a recurrent pattern that may start before marriage vows are taken. At first, battering may involve pushing and grabbing. It then escalates if nothing is done to stop it. Batterers are also more likely to abuse their children and to sexually abuse their partners than are nonbatterers.

### Health Effects of Spouse Abuse

Spouse abuse is a major health problem, especially for women. It can cause physical injury, emotional problems, even death. The bruises and broken bones are the more obvious signs of abuse, but the psychological effects can linger and include posttraumatic stress disorder (PTSD), depression, low self-esteem, alcohol and substance abuse, even suicide.[11]

More than 3 million children in the United States witness spouse abuse each year, and they too are at risk.[12] They are more likely than their peers to develop emotional difficulties such as depression and academic problems. Children exposed to aggressive parents may learn that violence is an acceptable means of solving marital conflicts. The lesson may set the stage for an intergenerational pattern in which children from violent families become batterers as adults.

### What's to Be Done?

To stop domestic violence, we need to address the larger societal context in which it occurs. In societies like ours there is an unequal power distribution between men and women. Young men are socialized to play dominant roles and to expect women to bend to their wishes.[13] Men learn that aggressive behavior is part of the masculine ideal. Aggression is glorified in sports and the movies. Though wife beating may not be part of the male curriculum, men may enter relationships believing that force is appropriate when their needs are not being met or when their power is being challenged by their partners.

We also need to take society to task for its ineffective response to domestic violence. Police officers often take the batterer aside and talk to him "man to man" rather than arrest him. They thus send a message that society is willing to look the other way so long as things are kept relatively quiet.[14] Even if the man is arrested, he may only receive a "slap on the wrist." He almost certainly receives a lesser sentence than he would if he had attacked a stranger.

Stopping domestic violence requires that children learn other lessons. By word and example, parents can demonstrate zero tolerance toward violence. Young men can be encouraged to respond to social conflicts with their heads, not their fists. Law enforcement officials can deal with domestic violence as they deal with other acts of violence, not making exceptions because the victim shares the household with the assailant.

**Close-up**
Preventing violence against women
T2106

**think about it!**

- **Why do you think the United States has the highest homicide rate among industrialized nations?**
- **Why do you think women are most likely to be abused by the men they live with?**
- **Have you witnessed or experienced spouse abuse? What were its apparent causes? Its effects?**

**critical thinking** **Agree or disagree and support your answer: Despite what we see and hear in the media, our society condones spouse abuse.**

**Smart Quiz**
Q2101

## CHILD ABUSE

More than a million cases of child abuse are reported each year in the United States.[15] More than 1,000 children die as the result of abuse or neglect. These numbers are but the tip of the iceberg, because many, probably most, child abuse cases are not reported or publicly identified. Child abuse is among the major health threats faced by children in our society.

Nearly half of the deaths from child abuse and neglect involve children under one year of age. The great majority involve children under five. But the older child is more likely to suffer physical abuse than children under two years of age.[16] Boys and girls are about equally likely to be abused.

**Close-up**
Child abuse increasing
T2107

### Characteristics of Child Abusers

Child abuse, like other forms of violence and abuse, cuts across all socioeconomic and ethnic divisions. Teenage parents, single parents, parents from lower income levels, poorly educated parents, and parents with poor parenting skills are more likely than other parents to abuse or neglect their children.[17] Parental stress due to financial

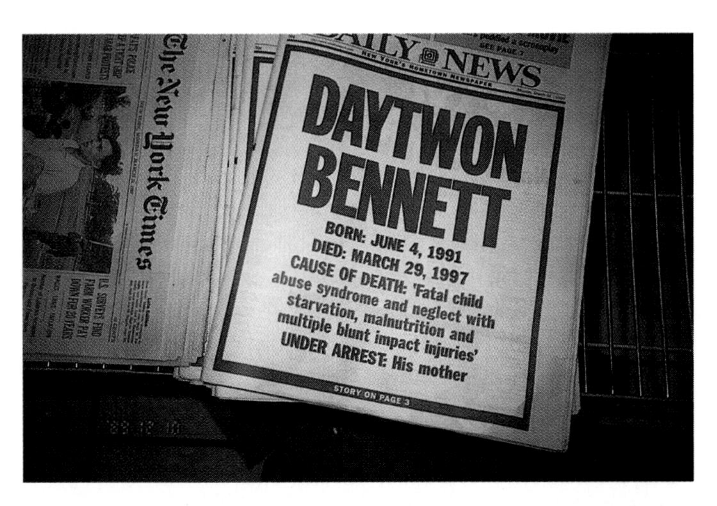
The New York Times
DAILY NEWS
DAYTWON
BENNETT
BORN: JUNE 4, 1991
DIED: MARCH 29, 1997
CAUSE OF DEATH: 'Fatal child abuse syndrome and neglect with starvation, malnutrition and multiple blunt impact injuries'
UNDER ARREST: His mother
STORY ON PAGE 3

***Child Abuse*** Each year more than 1,000 children in the U.S. die at the hands of their parents or from their parents' neglect. More than 1,000,000 cases of child abuse and neglect are reported to authorities, but many others go unreported.

problems or marital conflicts is a prominent risk factor. So is exposure to violence in one's own family of origin or being abused oneself during childhood. Abusive parents tend to have poor anger management skills and poor parenting skills, and they may have difficulty forming attachments to their children. Use of alcohol and other drugs figures prominently in many cases of child abuse and neglect, as it does in other kinds of violence and abuse. Child abusers also tend to hold rigid attitudes toward child rearing. They rely more on physical punishment and less on reasoning than other parents do.[18]

The abusive parent is often young and under stress and resorts to force to control his or her children's behavior. In a society that licenses drivers and many occupational trades, there is no license, training, or experience required to become a parent. Parenting skills do not come naturally but must be learned, a process that begins with exposure to one's own parents as models—for better or worse. Many abusive parents relate to their own children in the same destructive ways that their parents related to them. Thus they repeat a cycle of abuse that can continue for generations.

Child abuse generally becomes more severe over time. Rationalizations, such as blaming the child for the abuse (e.g., "If he didn't want to get hit, he shouldn't have left his clothes lying around"), serve to justify the abuse. Abusive parents often lack effective problem-solving skills for dealing with their children's behavior and have a low tolerance for children's demands.[19]

Child abuse often occurs in a context of family disruption.[20] Stress from financial difficulties and from parental drug and alcohol abuse often figures into family disruption. For some parents, the stress of coping with a disintegrating home situation, together with these other stressors, may lead to irrational, impulsive acts of violence directed against children.

## Types of Child Abuse

We can classify different forms of child maltreatment into four major types: physical abuse, neglect, sexual abuse, and emotional maltreatment[21] (see Table 21.1). Neglect, not physical abuse, is the most common type, involving about half (49%) of all cases.[22] Physical abuse accounts for about one in five cases (21%); sexual abuse, for about one in ten (11%). The rest involve emotion-

**TABLE 21.1**

**Types of Child Abuse[23]**

| Type of Abuse | Definition |
|---|---|
| Physical Abuse | Nonaccidental physical injury of a child caused by a parent or caretaker. The injuries may range from superficial bruises to broken bones, burns, and serious internal injuries, and may result in death in some cases. |
| Physical Neglect | Failing to provide children with, or withholding from them, adequate food, shelter, clothing, hygiene, medical care, or supervision needed to promote their growth and development. |
| Sexual Abuse | The sexual exploitation of children involving acts ranging from nontouching offenses, such as exhibitionism, to genital fondling, sexual intercourse, or involving them in the production of pornography. |
| Emotional Maltreatment | The use of constant harsh criticism of the child involving verbally abusive language, or emotional neglect, which is characterized by the withholding of physical and emotional contact needed to promote normal emotional development and, in some extreme cases, physical development. |

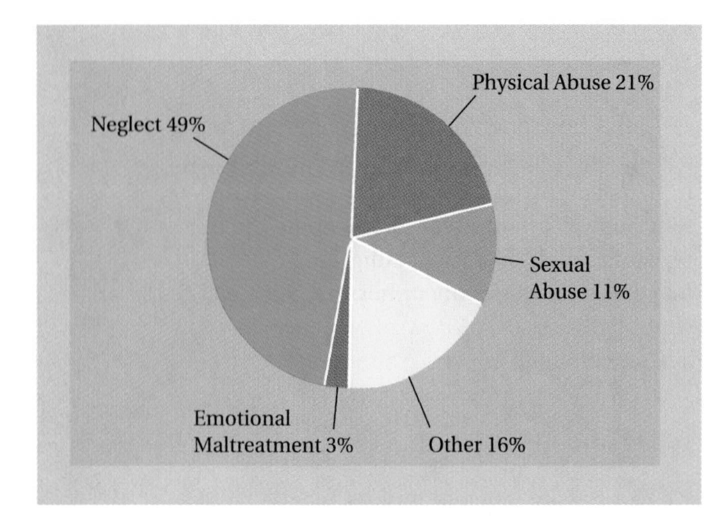


**Figure 21.2** ***Reported Cases of Child Maltreatment by Type***
Here we see a breakdown of the types of child maltreatment cases reported to child protective services agencies in 1993 and 1994 in 36 states. The most frequent case involved neglect, followed by physical abuse and sexual abuse.

al maltreatment (3%) and other forms of abuse (16%) (see Figure 21.2).

Public concerns about protecting children from abuse have led to passage of mandatory reporting laws in all 50 states. These laws require many professionals, including physicians, social workers, marriage and family counselors, and psychologists, to notify authorities when they suspect or know of abuse. Nevertheless, many cases still go unreported.

## Health Effects of Child Abuse

Child abuse can cause serious, sometimes life-threatening injuries, ranging from welts and bruises to broken bones and massive internal damage. The physical injuries may be the obvious and dramatic signs of abuse, but the emotional wounds can run deeper and last longer.[24] Neglect can have even more damaging consequences than physical abuse. Nearly half of all child fatalities due to maltreatment result from neglect.[25]

Abused or neglected children may have difficulty establishing healthy attachments and peer relationships, may lack the capacity for empathy, and may fail to develop a sense of conscience. They may act out in ways that mirror the cruelty they have endured. They may act aggressively toward smaller, more vulnerable children, torture and kill small animals, or set fires. They are more likely than nonabused children to become child abusers themselves. Child abuse and neglect also commonly lead to emotional, cognitive, and behavioral problems, including failure to thrive; immature or regressive behaviors like bed-wetting and thumb-sucking; impaired verbal, perceptual, and motor skills; lower academic achievement; lower self-esteem; depression, even suicidal behavior.

Abused children often assume that they deserved the abuse. Misplaced self-blame can lower self-esteem and set the stage for depression and self-hate. Abused and neglected children are at greater risk than nonabused children of developing disturbed personalities—in some severe cases, multiple personalities. They are at risk of behavioral problems such as bulimia, suicidal behavior, and criminal conduct. They are also likely to achieve lower incomes and educational levels.[26]

## What's to Be Done?

Child maltreatment is a major health crisis. Although billions of dollars are spent on the problem each year, progress has been limited. One encouraging development is parent-training programs that target abusive parents. These programs help abusive parents develop better parenting techniques, control anger, and manage the stress that can set the stage for abuse.[27]

Preventing child abuse is a daunting challenge. If we are to make significant progress, we must address the factors that underlie abuse, including parental stress and poor parenting skills. Economic pressures are a major contributor to parental stress, and single parents, especially teenagers, are likely to be poor. Therefore, part of the solution lies in deterring people from bearing children until they have the financial and psychological resources to support them.

### think about it!

- **Do you know anyone who was abused as a child? What were its apparent causes? Its effects?**

  **critical thinking** **Why do you think that people who were abused as children are more likely to become abusers themselves?**

  **critical thinking** **Agree or disagree and support your answer: Schools should require students to take parent-training classes to help prepare them for parenting roles.**

Smart Quiz
Q2102

## RAPE

Rape is a violent act in which sex is used as an instrument of aggression, anger, control, and power. There are two general categories of rape:

1. **Forcible rape,** which involves force or the threat of force to compel a person into having sexual intercourse.
2. **Statutory rape,** which refers to sexual intercourse with a person who is unable to give consent because of immaturity or mental disability, even if the person cooperates.

Though almost all rapes are perpetrated by men against women, rape laws in some states also apply to men who rape other men or to women who coerce men into sex or assist men in raping other women. Even if a sexual attack does not meet the legal definition of rape in a given state, it can be classified and prosecuted as a sexual assault.

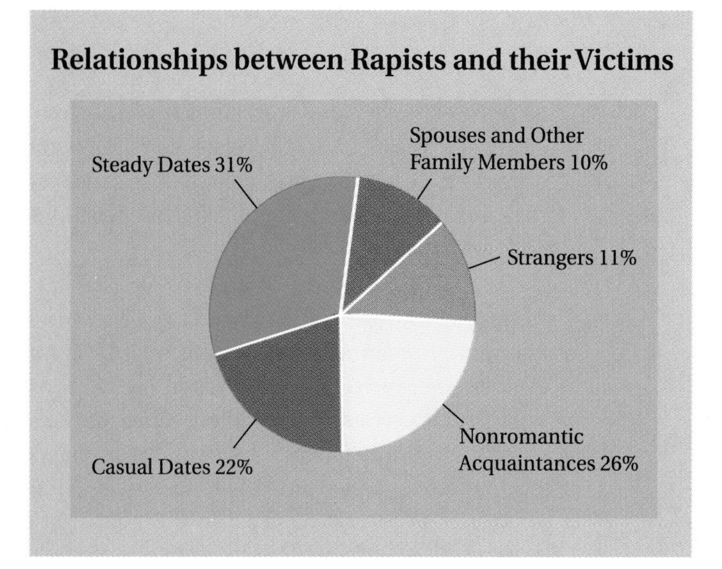


**Figure 21.3** ***Relative Percentages of Stranger Rape versus Acquaintance Rape of College Women*** The great majority of cases of rape reported by college women in a large national survey were committed by men the women knew, including dates, nonromantic acquaintances, and spouses and other family members. Only about 12% involved strangers.

### Incidence of Rape

According to the National Crime Victimization Survey, a government-sponsored survey, an estimated 500,000 women are sexually assaulted each year.[28] This includes 170,000 rapes and 140,000 attempted rapes. These figures work out to one rape occurring somewhere in the U.S. every three minutes. However, fewer than one in four rapes are reported to police. Women fail to report rapes out of fear or misplaced shame, or because they believe (incorrectly) that rape in the eyes of the law can only be committed by strangers (not by dates).

**Who Is at Risk?** Young women aged 16 to 24 are two to three times more likely to be raped than younger or older females. Most rapes are committed against girls under 18 years of age. About one in six is committed against a girl under 12.[29] Yet any woman, young or old, African American or white, rich or poor, is at risk of being raped. Although reported rapes occur more often among poorer women, the difference may partly reflect the tendency of more affluent women to forgo reporting attacks to avoid dealing with the legal system and the media.

A large, nationwide survey of more than 6,000 college students (3,187 women and 2,972 men) on 32 campuses across the United States found that 15% of the women reported that they had been raped. An additional 12% reported attempted rapes.[30] Estimates are that 14 to 25% of women in the United States will be raped at some point during their lives.[31] Like most other measures of violence, rape is more common in the United States than in other developed nations such as Canada, Great Britain, and Japan.

### Types of Rape

Most rapes are *not* perpetrated by strangers lurking in dark alleys or intruders who climb through windows in the middle of the night. Most rapes—about 80% according to the National Crime Victimization Survey[32]—are committed by men the victims knew, often by men they had come to trust. Figure 21.3 shows the relationships between women who were raped and their assailants in the nationwide college sample.[33]

There are several major types of rape: stranger rape, acquaintance rape, male rape, marital rape, and rape by women.

**Stranger Rape** **Stranger rapes** are committed by assailants who are not known by the person they attack. The stranger rapist often selects targets who seem vulnerable—women who live alone, are older or retarded, are walking deserted streets, or are asleop or

**Forcible rape** Sexual intercourse with a nonconsenting person achieved by force or threat of force.

**Statutory rape** Sexual intercourse with a person who is below the age of consent, even if the person cooperates.

**Stranger rape** Rape committed by an assailant previously unknown to the victim.

intoxicated. After choosing a target, the rapist may search for a safe time and place to commit the crime—a deserted, run-down part of town, a darkened street, a second-floor apartment without window bars or locks.

**Acquaintance Rape** An **acquaintance rape** is committed by an assailant known by the victim. Women are more likely to be raped by men they know, such as classmates, fellow office workers, even their brothers' friends, than by strangers. Acquaintance rapes are much less likely than stranger rapes to be reported to the police. One reason is that rape survivors may not perceive sexual assaults by acquaintances as rapes. Only about a quarter of the women in the national college survey who had been sexually assaulted perceived the incident as a rape. Despite increased public awareness of acquaintance rape, the belief remains common that a rapist is a stranger lurking in the shadows and that a woman should be able to resist unless the man uses a weapon. Even when acquaintance rapes are reported to police, they are often treated as "misunderstandings" or lovers' quarrels rather than violent crimes.

**Date rape** is a type of acquaintance rape. Between 10 and 20% of women report being forced into sexual intercourse by their dates.[34] In one college study, most date rapes were not committed by recent acquaintances or "blind dates," but by men whom the women had known for nearly a year on average.[35] Rapes were more likely to occur when the couple had too much to drink and then went parking or back to the man's residence. Most of the men ignored the women's protests and overcame their resistance by force. None used a weapon.

The date rapist may wrongly believe that acceptance of a date indicates willingness to engage in sexual intercourse or that women should reciprocate with sex if they are taken to dinner or treated nicely. Others assume that women who frequent settings such as singles bars are expressing tacit agreement to engage in sexual intercourse with men who show interest in them. Some date rapists believe that women who resist their advances are merely "protesting too much" so that they will not look "easy." They interpret resistance as coyness—a ploy in the cat-and-mouse game that, to them, typifies the "battle of the sexes." They may believe that when a woman says no, she means maybe. When she says maybe, she means yes. They may thus not see themselves as committing rape. But they are.

**Acquaintance rape** Rape committed by an acquaintance of the victim.

**Date rape** A type of acquaintance rape in which the assailant is the person's date.

Consider the case of Ann:[36]

*I first met him at a party. He was really good looking and he had a great smile. I wanted to meet him but I wasn't sure how. I didn't want to appear too forward. Then he came over and introduced himself. We talked and found we had a lot in common. I really liked him. When he asked me over to his place for a drink, I thought it would be OK. He was such a good listener, and I wanted him to ask me out again.*

*When we got to his room, the only place to sit was on the bed. I didn't want him to get the wrong idea, but what else could I do? We talked for awhile and then he made his move. I was so startled. He started by kissing. I really liked him so the kissing was nice. But then he pushed me down on the bed. I tried to get up and I told him to stop. He was so much bigger and stronger. I got scared and I started to cry. I froze and he raped me.*

*It took only a couple of minutes and it was terrible, he was so rough. When it was over he kept asking me what was wrong, like he didn't know. He had just forced himself on me and he thought that was OK. He drove me home and said he wanted to see me again. I'm so afraid to see him. I never thought it would happen to me.*

College men on dates frequently perceive their dates' protests as part of an adversarial sex game. One male undergraduate said "Hell, no" when asked whether a date had consented to sex. He added, "but she didn't say no, so she must have wanted it, too. . . . It's the way it works."[37] Consider the comments of Jim, the man who raped Ann:

*I first met her at a party. She looked really hot, wearing a sexy dress that showed off her great body. We started talking right away. I knew that she liked me by the way she kept smiling and touching my arm while she was speaking. She seemed pretty relaxed so I asked her back to my place for a drink. . . . When she said yes, I knew that I was going to be lucky!*

*When we got to my place, we sat on the bed kissing. At first, everything was great. Then, when I started to lay her down on the bed, she started twisting and saying she didn't want to. Most women don't like to appear too easy, so I knew that she was just going through the motions. When she stopped struggling, I knew that she would have to throw in some tears before we did it.*

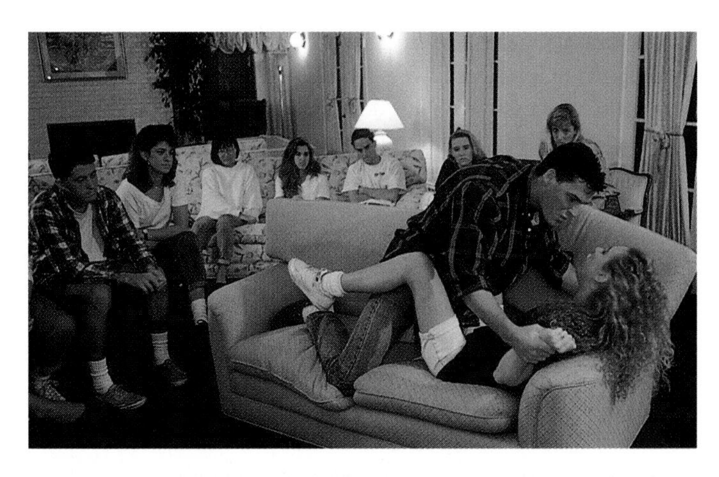

***Date Rape Prevention*** Many colleges and universities offer date rape prevention workshops, which may include simulations as seen here.

*She was still very upset afterwards, and I just don't understand it! If she didn't want to have sex, why did she come back to the room with me? You could tell by the way she dressed and acted that she was no virgin, so why she had to put up such a big struggle I don't know.*

It does not matter whether the woman wears a "sexy" outfit, is "on the pill," is treated to an expensive dinner, accompanies a man to his place, or shares a passionate kiss or embrace with him. No matter what the preceding events were, if the encounter ends with the woman being forcibly violated or threatened with force, then it is rape.[38] When a woman says no, the man is obligated to take no for an answer.

**Male Rape** In male rapes, sex is used as an instrument to dominate, to exact revenge, or to degrade the victim. Sexual motivations are generally absent. When the rape is carried out by a gang member, it may be intended to achieve or maintain status or enhance group affiliation. Most male rapes occur in prison settings, but some occur outside prison walls. Most men who rape other men are heterosexual.

**Marital Rape** A generation ago, husbands in most states could not be prosecuted for raping their wives. This marital exclusion for rape was derived from English common law, which held that a woman "gives herself over" to her husband when she becomes his wife and cannot then retract her consent.[39] Today, most states and the District of Columbia permit the prosecution of husbands who rape their wives. Although there are no precise statistics on marital rape, a committee of the U.S. Congress estimated that one wife in seven is likely to be raped by her husband. Marital rape goes largely unreported and even unrecognized as rape by survivors. Many women fail to report marital rape because of fear that no one will believe them.

Motives for marital rape vary. The husband who rapes his wife may believe that he is entitled to sexual access to his wife any time he desires it, even if she is uninterested. Some men use sex to dominate their wives. Others degrade their wives through sex, especially after arguments. They use sex to "teach them a lesson" about who's in control. Sexual coercion often occurs within a context of a wider pattern of marital violence, battering, and physical intimidation.

**Rape by Women** Rape by women is very rare. When it does occur, it often involves aiding or abetting men who are attacking another woman. Rape by women may occur in gang-rape situations in which women follow male leaders to gain their approval. In such cases, a woman may be used to lure another woman to a reasonably safe place for the rape. Or the woman may hold the other woman down while she is assaulted. Rape of men by women is even rarer, although some isolated cases have been reported of women who have physically coerced men into sex, including one case of a 37-year-old man who was coerced into sexual intercourse by two women who accosted him at gunpoint.[40] Like other rapes, these have more to do with motives of exerting power or control, or exacting revenge, than they do with sexual motivation.

## Why Do Men Rape Women?

It is common sense that rape is motivated by sexual desire. Though sexual motivation is involved in rape, the primary motives are more likely to involve power, anger, revenge, and intentional cruelty.[41]

**Anger, Power, and Sadistic Rape** The **anger rape** is a vicious, unplanned attack that is triggered by resentment against women. The anger rapist usually employs more force than is needed to obtain compliance. The woman may be coerced into degrading and humiliating acts. Typically, the anger rapist reports being humiliated by women and uses rape to gain revenge.

**Anger rape** A vicious rape motivated by anger and resentment toward women.

The **power rape** is motivated by a desire to control and dominate the victim. Sexual gratification is secondary. The power rapist uses rape as an attempt "to resolve disturbing doubts about [his] masculine identity and worth, [or] to combat deep-seated feelings of insecurity and vulnerability."[42] Only enough force is used to subdue the woman.

The **sadistic rape** is a ritualized, savage attack. Sadistic rapists often carefully plan their assaults and use a pretext to approach their targets, such as asking for directions or offering assistance.[43] Some sadists bind their victims and subject them to humiliation. They may torture, mutilate, or murder them. Sadistic rapists are often preoccupied with violent pornography but have little or no interest in nonviolent (consensual) pornography.

The great majority of rapes, perhaps 95%, are anger rapes or power rapes. Only about 5% are sadistic rapes.[44]

**What Are We Teaching Our Sons?** Many rapists—perhaps most—appear perfectly normal, except for their sexual violence against women. Their sheer ordinariness invites the question, What are we teaching our sons? Many social observers believe that our society breeds rapists by socializing young men into socially and sexually dominant roles.[45] Not every young man grows up to be a sexual predator, of course, but a surprising number do. In the national college survey, one in thirteen men reported having raped or having attempted to rape a woman. In another college study, about one in three college men reported that he would force a woman into sexual relations if he knew he could get away with it.[46]

American men are usually reinforced from an early age for stereotypically aggressive and competitive behavior. They may come to view dates not as chances to get to know their partners but as opportunities for sexual conquest in which the object is to overcome a woman's resistance by whatever means necessary. College men who more closely identify with the stereotypical masculine role more often report having engaged in forcible rape as well as verbal sexual pressure.[47]

**Power rape** A rape motivated primarily by the desire to exercise power or control over the victim.

**Sadistic rape** A savage rape in which the victim is subjected to painful and humiliating experiences and events, sometimes including ritualized acts of torture.

Cultural myths also underlie rape, such as the belief that a masculine man should be sexually aggressive and overcome a woman's resistance until she "melts" in his arms. The myth that women fantasize about being overpowered sanctions force to "awaken" a woman's sexual desires. Images from popular books and movies reinforce these themes, such as that of Rhett Butler carrying a protesting Scarlett O'Hara up the stairs to her bedroom in *Gone with the Wind.* Violent pornography, which fuses violence and erotic arousal, may also serve to legitimize rape in some men's minds.

The lessons learned in competitive sports may indirectly encourage sexual violence.[48] Coaches often urge boys to win at all costs. Boys are taught to dominate their opponents, even if it means injuring or "taking out" the opposition. This philosophy may be carried from the playing field into relationships with women. Perhaps this helps explain why student athletes commit a disproportionate number of sexual assaults.[49] Many of these are gang rapes committed by groups of student athletes who live together and bond so strongly that they even share coercive sexual encounters.

Sexual behavior and competitive sports are linked through common idioms. Friends may taunt a young man who has been on a date with such questions as, "Did you score?" or more bluntly, "Did you get in?" Consider, for example, the aggressive competitiveness with which this male college student views dating relationships between men and women:[50]

> *A man is supposed to view a date with a woman as a premeditated scheme for getting the most sex out of her. Everything he does, he judges in terms of one criterion—"getting laid." He's supposed to constantly pressure her to see how far he can get. She is his adversary, his opponent in a battle, and he begins to view her as a prize, an object, not a person. While she's dreaming about love, he's thinking about how to conquer her.*

Other myths contribute to a social climate that legitimizes and increases the potential for rape. Many people believe that "only bad girls get raped," that "any healthy woman can resist a rapist if she really wants to," and that "women 'cry rape' only when they've been jilted."[51, 52] Another myth is that rapists are not responsible for their actions; sexually provocative women unleash uncontrollable sexual urges in them. Some people even believe that deep down inside, women want to be raped. Although many women report rape fantasies, they do not wish to have the fantasy enacted in real life. The belief that they do is a rationalization for violence. Though both men and women are susceptible to rape myths, researchers find that college men show greater acceptance of them than do college women.[53] College men who endorse rape myths are more likely to see themselves as likely to commit rape.[54]

## Health Effects of Rape

Depending on the brutality and amount of force, women may suffer grievous physical injuries, even death. Victims may also be infected with sexually transmitted diseases and impregnated. The psychological effects may be more profound and long-lasting than the physical injuries.[55] Many rape survivors are distraught following the attack. They cry frequently and suffer insomnia, loss of appetite, cystitis and other gynecological problems, headaches, irritability, mood changes, and anxiety and depression.[56] Many become withdrawn, sullen, and mistrustful. Because myths about rape tend to blame the victim, some survivors experience feelings of guilt and shame. A survey of sexual assault survivors (including women and men) from Los Angeles showed that the most frequently reported emotional reactions to sexual assault were anger (59%), sadness (43%), and anxiety (40%) (see Table 21.2).

Psychological problems can linger for a year or more. For some survivors, emotional problems such as depression and anxiety last for many years. Survivors often develop sexual dysfunctions, including lack of sexual desire, fears of sex, and difficulty becoming sexually aroused. Many also develop posttraumatic stress disorder (PTSD), as evidenced by intrusive memories and nightmares about the rape. Some survivors develop problems with alcohol and other drugs.

## Treatment of Rape Survivors

Treatment of rape survivors typically involves a two-stage process of helping the victim through the crisis and then helping to foster long-term adjustment. Crisis intervention services provide the survivor with support and information to help her express her feelings and develop strategies for coping with the trauma. Longer-term psychotherapy can help the survivor cope with the emotional consequences of rape, avoid self-blame, improve self-esteem, and help her establish or maintain loving relationships. It is important to help the survivor identify supportive social networks. Family, friends, religious leaders, and health care special-

TABLE 21.2

**Reported Emotional and Behavioral Reactions to Sexual Assault: Los Angeles Community Sample[57] (in percent)**

| Reaction | Women | Men | Total |
|---|---|---|---|
| Fearful | 45.5% | 15.9*% | 35.1% |
| Stopped doing things | 31.8 | 15.2* | 25.9 |
| Fearful of sex | 21.6 | 7.9* | 16.8 |
| Less sexual interest | 32.5 | 6.9* | 23.5 |
| Less sexual pleasure | 27.1 | 8.0* | 20.4 |
| Felt dishonored or spoiled | 33.9 | 20.0* | 29.1 |
| Guilt | 35.0 | 25.9* | 31.8 |
| Sad, blue, or depressed | 50.6 | 28.8* | 43.0 |
| Anger | 72.0 | 34.8* | 59.0 |
| Tense, nervous, or anxious | 49.9 | 22.9* | 40.4 |
| Insomnia | 25.2 | 11.6* | 20.4 |
| Loss/increase in appetite | 15.8 | 8.4 | 13.2 |
| Alcohol/drug use | 5.1 | 5.9 | 5.4 |
| Fearful of being alone | 23.0 | 2.2* | 15.7 |

Responses based on sample of 447 persons who had suffered a sexual assault, which included a range of coercive acts from fondling of the breasts or sex organs to sexual intercourse. Women were more likely to report 12 of 14 listed reactions. Survivors who were physically threatened by their assailants reported greater fear and anxiety, depression, and sexual distress (reduced interest and pleasure, fear of sex). Attacks that resulted in forced intercourse were more distressing than those that did not.

*Indicates that the differences between men and women were statistically significant at the .05 level of significance; that is, there is less than a 5% chance that the differences between men and women were due to chance.

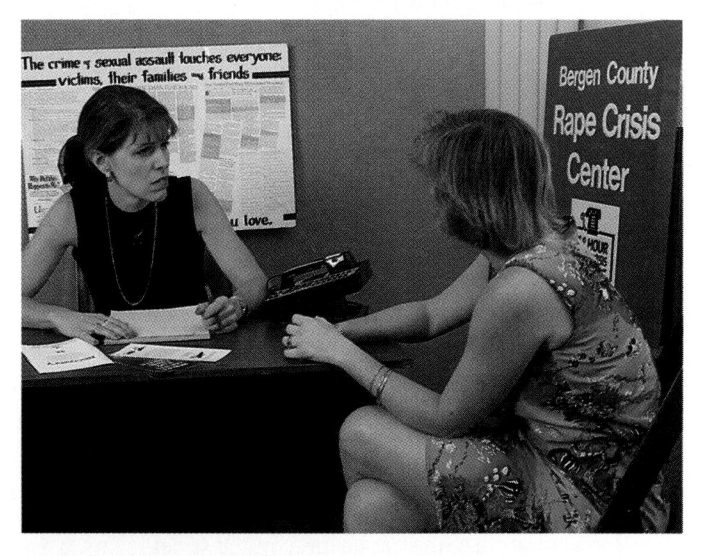
The crime of sexual assault touches everyone:
victims, their families and friends
Bergen County
Rape Crisis
Center

***Rape Crisis Counseling*** Rape crisis centers help women cope with the trauma of rape. They provide supportive counseling and help rape survivors obtain medical, legal, and psychological services.

ists are all potential sources of help. In major cities and many towns, rape crisis centers and hotlines, peer counseling groups, and referral agencies provide additional support. Phone numbers for these services can be obtained from women's organizations (for example, the local office of the National Organization for Women [NOW]), the police department, or the telephone directory.

PREVENTION

## *Rape Prevention*[58]

Rape prevention efforts should start with socializing men to be respectful of women and aware of the boundaries between consent and coercion. Young men need to learn that when a woman says "no," it means "no," not maybe, possibly, or perhaps. They need to understand that both parties must clearly and openly express consent for any physical contact. Unfortunately, many men in our society fail to either learn or abide by such lessons. How can we help get this message across? For one thing, rape prevention workshops, like those offered in many colleges, need to be incorporated in the school curriculum in high schools and lower grades. For another, society needs to send a message that sexual coercion, like any violent crime, will not be tolerated and will be punished to the fullest extent of the law.

In the meantime, it is prudent for women to take precautions to minimize their risk of being assaulted. But is not the very listing of rape prevention measures a subtle way of blaming the woman if she should fall prey to an attacker? No, providing the information does not blame the person who is attacked. The rapist is *always* responsible for the assault.

### Preventing Rape by Strangers

- Keep doorways and entries well lit.
- Keep your keys handy when approaching the car or the front door.
- Do not walk by yourself after dark.
- Avoid deserted areas.
- Do not allow strange men into your house or apartment without first checking their credentials.
- Keep your car doors locked and the windows up.
- Check out the back seat of your car before entering.
- Don't live in a risky building if you can possibly avoid it.
- Don't stop for hitchhikers (including women hitchhikers).
- Don't converse with strange men on the street.
- Shout "Fire!" not "Rape!" People are likely to flock to fires but avoid scenes of violence.

### Preventing Date Rape

- *Communicate your sexual limits to your date.* For example, if your partner starts fondling you in ways that make you uncomfortable, you might say, "I'd prefer if you didn't touch me there. I really like you, but I prefer not getting so intimate at this point in our relationship."
- *Meet new dates in public places and avoid driving with a stranger or a group of people you've just met.* When meeting a new date, drive in your own car and meet your date at a public place. When dating a person for the first time, try to date in a group. Don't drive with strangers or offer rides to strangers or groups of people. In some cases of date rape, the group disappears just before the assault.
- *State your refusal definitively.* Be firm in refusing a sexual overture. Look your partner straight in the eye. The more definite you are, the less likely your partner is to misinterpret your wishes. If kissing or petting is leading where you don't want it to go, speak up.
- *Become aware of your fears.* Take notice of any fears of displeasing your partner that might stifle your assertiveness. If your partner is truly respectful of you, you need not fear an angry or demeaning response. But if your partner is not respectful, it is best to become aware of it and end the relationship right there.
- *Trust your feelings.* Many victims of acquaintance rape said afterward that they had a "strange" feeling about the man but failed to pay attention to it.
- *Be especially cautious in a new environment, such as college or a foreign country.* You may be especially vulnerable to exploitation when you are becoming acquainted with a new environment, different people, and different customs.
- *If you have broken off a relationship with someone you don't really like or feel good about, don't let him into your place.* Many rapes are committed by ex-lovers and ex-boyfriends.
- *Stay sober.* We often do things we would not otherwise do—including sexual activity with people we might otherwise reject—when we have had too many drinks. Be aware of your limits.
- *Encourage your school to offer educational programs about date rape.* The University of Washington, for example, offers students lectures and seminars on date rape and provides women with escorts to get home. Many universities require all incoming students to attend orientation sessions on rape prevention.
- *Talk to your date about his attitudes toward women.* If you get the feeling that he believes that men are in a war with women or that women try to "play games" with men, you may be better off dating someone else.

**Video**
Rape prevention on campus
**V2101**

### Should You Fight, Flee, or Plead?

There is no one answer to whether women who face a rapist should flee, fight, or plead.[59] No one suggestion is helpful in all situations. Self-defense training may help women become better prepared to fend off an assailant. Yet many law enforcement officials caution that physical resistance may spur some rapists to become more aggressive. Federal statistics show that women who resist their assailants increase their chances of preventing the completion of a rape by 80 percent. However, resistance increases by as much as threefold the odds of being physically injured.[60]

Some women have thwarted attacks by pleading, reasoning, begging, or crying. Others have found that these less forceful forms of resistance failed to fend off an attack. In some cases they may actually heighten the probability of injury. Screaming may work in some situations, as might running away. But running may not be effective if a woman is outnumbered by a group of assailants.

The Boston Police Department recommends that whatever form of self-defense a woman intends to use, she should carefully think through and practice methods of doing so before the occasion arises.[61] Effective self-defense is built on the use of multiple strategies, ranging from attempts to avoid potential rape situations (such as by installing home security systems or by walking only in well-lit areas), to acquiescence when active resistance would seem too risky, to the use of more active verbal or physical forms of resistance in some low-risk situations.[62]

Women must make their own decisions about whether to physically resist a rapist, based on their assessment of the rapist, the situation, and their own ability to resist.

### If You Are Raped . . .

These suggestions may help women cope in those terrible minutes and hours immediately after a sexual assault:[63]

- *Don't change anything about your body—don't wash or even comb your hair. Leave your clothes as they are.* Otherwise you could destroy evidence.
- *Report the incident to police.* You may prevent another woman from being assaulted, and you will be taking charge, starting on the path from victim to survivor.
- *If you can't get an ambulance or a police car, ask a relative or friend to take you to a hospital.* If you call the hospital, tell them why you're requesting an ambulance, in case they are able to send someone trained to deal with rape cases.
- *Get help.* Seeking help is a way to assert your self-worth. Seek medical help to detect injuries of which you are unaware. Insist that a written or photographic record be made to document your condition. You may decide to file charges and the prosecutor may need this evidence.
- *Ask questions.* You have medical rights. Ask what treatments are available to you. Ask for whatever will make you comfortable. Refuse what you don't want.
- *Call a rape hotline or rape crisis center for advice.* A rape crisis volunteer may be available to accompany you to the hospital and help see you through the medical evaluation and police investigation. It is not unusual for rape survivors to try to erase the details of the rape from their minds, but remembering details clearly will help you give an accurate description of the rapist to the police, including his clothing, type of car, and so on.

**think about it!**

Smart Quiz Q2103

- **What can you do to decrease the incidence of rape in our society?**

**critical thinking** **Agree or disagree and support your answer: A woman who walks in a dangerous neighborhood or dresses provocatively bears some responsibility if she is attacked.**

**critical thinking** **Agree or disagree and support your answer: Our society breeds rapists by socializing males into socially and sexually dominant roles.**

## CHILD SEXUAL ABUSE

Few crimes are as heinous as child sexual abuse. Children who are sexually assaulted may suffer severe social and emotional problems that can persist into adulthood, affecting their self-esteem and their ability to form intimate relationships.

Any sexual contact with a child is abusive, even if consent is obtained. Children are not deemed mature enough to provide consent for sexual activity.

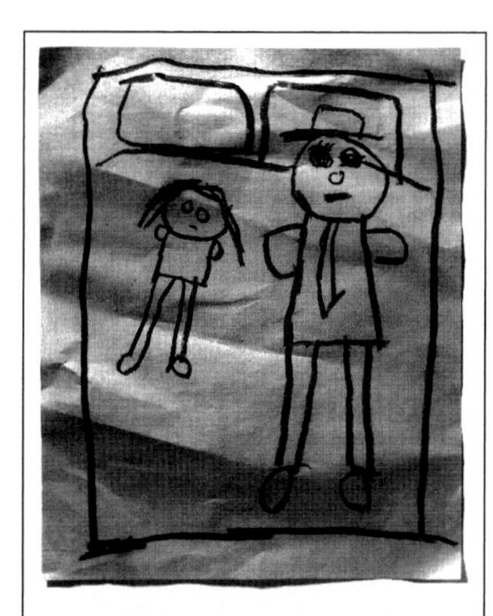
So there really was a monster in her bedroom.
For many kids, there's a real reason to be afraid of the dark.
Last year in Indiana, there were 6,912 substantiated cases of sexual abuse. The trauma can be devastating for the child and for the family. So listen closely to the children around you.
If you hear something you don't want to believe, perhaps you should. For helpful information on child abuse prevention, contact the LaPorte County Child Abuse Prevention Council, 7451 Johnson Road, Michigan City, IN 46360. (219) 874-0007
LaPorte County Child Abuse Prevention Council

***Child Sexual Abuse*** Not all monsters are imaginary. Some are even family members.

No one knows how many children are sexually abused. The number of reported cases, some 150,000 annually, has been rising steadily but may still represent only the tip of the iceberg. Like rape, child sexual abuse is greatly underreported. A nationwide telephone poll revealed that one woman in four (27%) and one man in six (16%) reported some form of sexual abuse during childhood.[64] The sexual abuse of children cuts across all racial, ethnic, and economic boundaries. The average age at which children are first sexually abused ranges between 7 and 10 for boys and 6 and 12 for girls.[65]

As with rape, most child molesters are not strangers. Perhaps 75 to 80% have a relationship with the child or the child's family. Typically they are relatives or step-relatives, family friends, or neighbors. Parents who discover that their child has been abused by a family member are often reluctant to notify authorities. When the molester is a family member, they may feel that such problems are "family matters" that are best kept private. Others may be reluctant to notify authorities for fear that it may shame the family or that they may be held accountable for failing to protect the child.

Sexual molestation ranges from exhibitionism, kissing, fondling, and sexual touching to oral sex and anal intercourse and, in the case of girls, vaginal intercourse. Genital fondling is most common. Intercourse is relatively uncommon, reported by fewer than 5% of females. Thirty-eight percent report genital fondling and 10% report exhibitionism.[66] However, in cases of repeated abuse by a family member, it may begin with fondling during the preschool years, progress to oral sex or mutual masturbation during the early school years, and then to sexual penetration (vaginal or anal intercourse) during preadolescence or adolescence.

Physical force is seldom used by molesters. Children tend not to be worldly-wise and are often taken in by abusers who tell them that they would like to "show them something," "teach them something," or do something with them that they would "like." The molester may seek to gain the child's affection and discourage the child from disclosing the sexual activity by showering him or her with attention and gifts. Or the molester may threaten the child or the child's family to prevent disclosure.

Most abused children suffer one incident of abuse, but some cases persist for months or years. Children who are abused by family members are most likely to suffer repetitive incidents. Boys are more likely than girls to be abused in public places, by strangers, and by people outside the family. Boys are also more likely to be threatened and physically injured.

## Who Molests Children?

Heterosexual men account for the great majority of child molesters. Women and gay males account for but a small percentage. Some child molesters have a type of sexual disorder called **pedophilia,** which involves the presence of recurrent sexual urges or desires for children. Not all molesters fit this pattern. Many have only occasional urges, which they act on when a convenient opportunity arises.

**Talking Glossary**
Pedophilia
**G2101**

**Pedophilia** A type of sexual disorder characterized by sexual attraction to children.

Some pedophiles engage only in **incest.** Others restrict their activity to children outside their own families. Some pedophiles fit the stereotype of a weak, passive, shy, socially inept, and isolated man who feels threatened by mature relationships and turns to children for sexual gratification. However, those who engage in incest with their own children tend to fall on either end of the dominance spectrum: some are very dominant, others are very passive.[67] Some pedophiles were sexually abused as children and may be trying to master the experience by reversing it. Cycles of abuse may be perpetuated from generation to generation as children who are sexually abused later become molesters themselves.

## Health Effects of Child Sexual Abuse

Abused children may suffer genital injuries and psychosomatic problems such as stomachaches and headaches. Molested girls may suffer hormonal and immunological problems.[68] One study found that sexually abused girls produced excess levels of stress hormones (epinephrine and norepinephrine) and the neurotransmitter dopamine, which suggests that their bodies were persistently overstressed.

Molested children may experience short-term and long-term psychological problems, including anger, depression, anxiety, eating disorders, self-destructive behavior, suicide attempts, posttraumatic stress disorder (PTSD), low self-esteem, mistrust of others, and feelings of detachment.[69] They commonly "act out" by displaying aggressive or antisocial behavior, delinquency, and tantrums. Older children often turn to substance abuse (alcohol and drugs).

Some abused children become withdrawn and retreat into fantasy or refuse to leave the house. Regressive behaviors, such as thumb-sucking, fear of the dark, and fear of strangers, are also common. Many survivors of childhood sexual abuse—like many rape survivors—show signs of PTSD, such as flashbacks, nightmares, numbing of emotions, and feelings of estrangement. Sometimes the effects of abuse are "masked" and become known through the development of school problems, fears, or eating or sleeping problems.

Late adolescence and early adulthood seem to be especially difficult periods for survivors of childhood sexual abuse. Unresolved feelings of anger, guilt, and mistrust may prevent the development of intimate relationships. Adolescent survivors are more likely than their peers to become delinquent, suicidal, and sexually active.

Psychological distress can linger into adulthood. Adult survivors who blame themselves for the abuse tend to have more psychological problems, especially depression and low self-esteem, than those who do not. The long-term consequences of child sexual abuse tend to be greater for children who were abused by their fathers or stepfathers, who experienced penetration, who were subjected to threats or force, and who suffered prolonged and severe abuse. Children who were victims of incest often feel a deep sense of betrayal by the offender and perhaps by other family members, especially mothers, whom they see as failing to protect them. Incest survivors may feel powerless to control their bodies or their lives.

PREVENTION

### *Preventing Child Sexual Abuse*

Sexual abuse prevention efforts include communitywide initiatives, such as enactment and enforcement of laws requiring teachers and helping professionals to report cases of suspected child abuse. Many states have enacted laws that require convicted sex offenders to register with the local police. (They are known commonly as "Megan's laws," after a seven-year-old New Jersey girl who was killed by a neighbor with a history of sexual assault.) The laws are intended to let members of the community know of the presence of sex offenders.[70]

Two out of three children participate in school-based programs that help them understand what sexual abuse is and how they can avert it.[71] Many of us were taught never to accept a ride or candy from a stranger, but much child sexual abuse is committed by familiar adults, often a family member or friend. Children need to recognize the difference between acceptable touching, as in an affectionate embrace or pat on the head, and unacceptable or "bad" touching. It is helpful to use dolls so that children can see what is "good" and "bad." Even elementary school children are capable of learning basic concepts of prevention. Better school-based programs help prepare children to handle an actual encounter with a molester. Children are taught to use strategies like running away, yelling, or saying no when they are threatened by an abuser. They are also more likely to report any such incidents to adults.

**Incest** Sexual relations or marriage between people so closely related by blood that it is prohibited by law or culturally taboo.

Children can easily be intimidated by molesters. They may thus be unable to say no to a molester, even though they want to and know that it is the right thing to do. Even if children cannot prevent abuse, they can be encouraged to tell someone about the experience. Most prevention programs emphasize teaching children messages such as "It's not your fault," "Never keep a bad or scary secret," and "Always tell your parents about this, especially if someone says you shouldn't tell them."[72] Children need to be told about the types of threats they might receive for disclosing the abuse. They are more likely to disclose abuse if they are reassured that they will be believed, that their parents will still love them, and that they and their families will be protected from the molester.

Establishing the credibility of children's reports of sexual abuse is a difficult problem. Children tend to be suggestible; they may be led to believe that abuse occurred when it did not by investigators who may unwittingly "plant" ideas in their minds or ask leading questions. Even more controversial are so-called recovered memories of childhood sexual or physical abuse that the person first becomes aware of during adulthood, usually during therapy or hypnosis.[73] The courts face a vexing task of separating true from faulty memories, especially when there is no direct evidence of abuse.

School-based prevention programs focus on protecting the individual child. At the societal level, better screening is needed to monitor the hiring of child care workers. Administrators and teachers in preschool and day-care facilities also need to be educated to recognize the signs of sexual abuse and to report suspected cases. Treatment programs are also needed to help people who recognize that they are sexually attracted to children *before* they molest them.

Smart Quiz Q2104

### think about it!

- **Do you know of anyone who was exposed to childhood sexual abuse? What was the experience like at the time? What were its lingering effects? Was the perpetrator reported to authorities? Why or why not?**

**critical thinking Why do you think that males account for a disproportionate number of child molesters?**

**Sexual harassment** Unwelcome comments, gestures, demands, overtures, or physical contact of a sexual nature.

## SEXUAL HARASSMENT

**Sexual harassment** is a form of sexual coercion that involves unwelcome sexual comments, jokes, overtures, demands for sexual favors, even outright physical contact. The great majority of cases are committed by men against women. In 1986, the U.S. Supreme Court recognized sexual harassment as a form of sex discrimination. Employers can be held accountable if the offending behavior creates a hostile work environment for the employee or interferes with the employee's performance.

Sexual harassment has more to do with the abuse of power than with sexual desire. Relatively few cases of sexual harassment involve unwelcome requests or demands for sexual favors. Most involve sexual taunts, unwelcome sexual gestures, or comments in which sex is used to humiliate, control, or frighten someone, usually a woman. The harasser usually abuses a dominant position to take advantage of the victim's vulnerability. Sexual harassment may also be used as a tactic of social control—a means of keeping women "in their place." This is especially so in settings that are traditional male preserves, such as the firehouse, the construction site, or the military academy or service unit.

Harassers in the workplace can be employers, supervisors, coworkers, or clients. In some cases company clients make unwelcome sexual advances to employees that are ignored or approved of by the boss. If a worker asks a coworker for a date and is refused, it is not sexual harassment. If the coworker persists with unwelcome advances and does not take no for an answer, the behavior crosses the line from a social invitation to harassment (see Figure 21.4).

Under the law, people subjected to sexual harassment can obtain a court order to have the harassment stopped, have their jobs reinstated (when they have lost them by resisting sexual advances), receive back pay and lost benefits, and obtain monetary awards for the emotional strain imposed by the harassment. However, proving charges of sexual harassment is generally difficult because there are usually no corroborating witnesses or evidence. As a result, relatively few women who encounter sexual harassment in the workplace, only about 3%, file formal complaints or seek legal remedies.[74] Like people subjected to other forms of sexual coercion, people who encounter sexual harassment often do not report

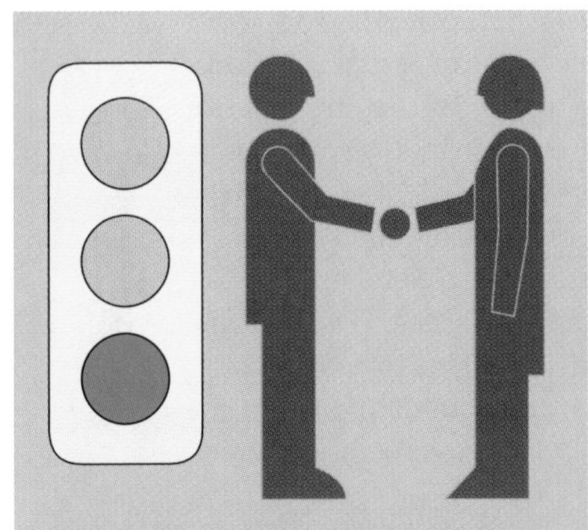

These actions do not constitute sexual harassment. They are typical interactions and common courtesies that happen regularly in an office environment. Some examples:

- Performance counseling
- Touching which could not be perceived in a sexual way, such as placing a hand on a person's elbow
- Counseling on (professional) appearance
- Everyday social interaction such as saying, "Hello, how are you?" or "Did you have a good weekend?"
- Expressing concern or encouragement
- A polite compliment or friendly conversation

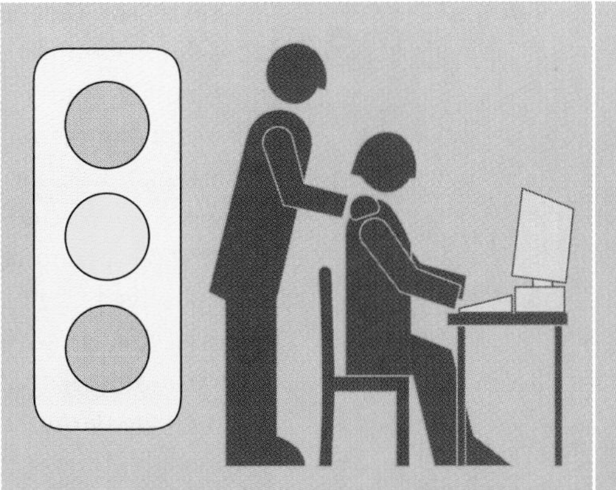

Many of these behaviors fall into gray areas but some are obvious examples of sexual harassment. Examples:

- Violating "personal" space (getting too close)
- Whistling
- Questions about personal life
- Lewd or off-color jokes
- Leering or staring
- Repeated requests for a date after being told no
- (Hanging) suggestive posters or calendars (where they may offend others)
- Foul language
- Unwanted letters or poems
- Sexually suggestive touching
- Sitting or gesturing sexually

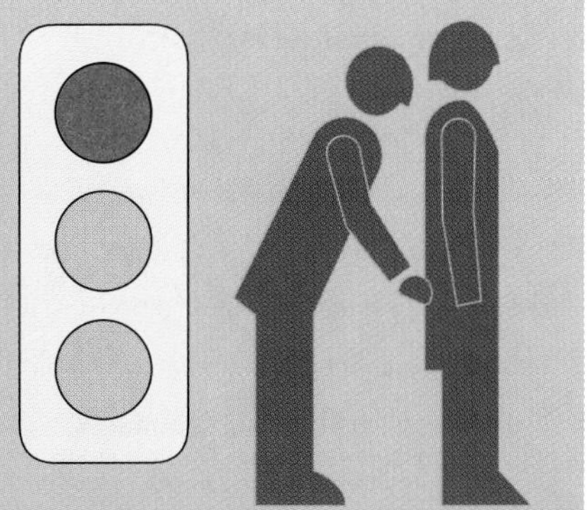

These behaviors are always considered to be sexual harassment. Examples are:

- Sexual favors in return for employment rewards and threats if sexual favors are not provided
- (Hanging or using) sexually explicit pictures, including calendars or posters (where they might offend others
- Sexually explicit remarks
- Using office (or other) status to request a date
- Obscene letters or comments
- Grabbing, forced kissing, fondling
- Sexual assault and rape

**Figure 21.4** ***What Is Sexual Harassment?***

the offense for fear that they will not be believed or will be subjected to retaliation. Some fear that they will lose their jobs or opportunities to advance in their careers.

Sexual harassment is recognized as the most common form of sexual victimization.[76] No one knows precisely how many people suffer sexual harassment, especially since the great majority of incidents go unreported. A *New York Times*/CBS News poll found that 38% of the women sampled reported that they had been the object of sexual advances or remarks from supervisors or other men in positions of power.[77] The number of sexual harassment complaints filed with the U.S. government rose by 50% between 1992 and 1995, to more than 15,000 cases. Overall, as many as half the women in the United States encounter some form of sexual harassment on the job or in college.

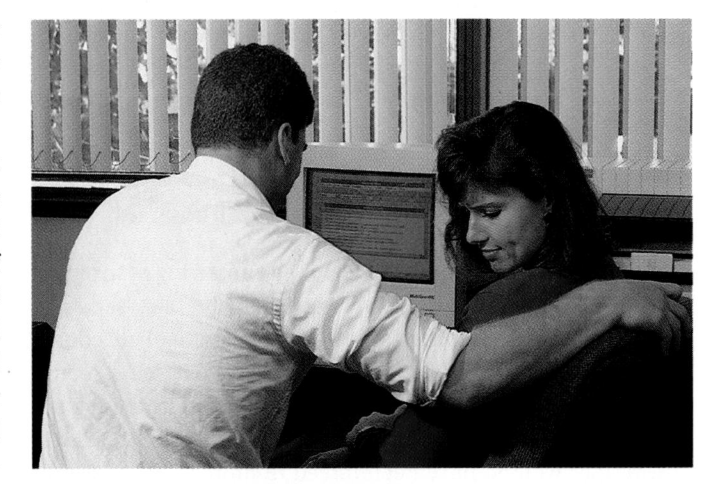

***Is This Sexual Harassment?*** How is sexual harassment defined? Do you believe that this man's behavior crosses the line? Would you think so if you were this woman? What would you do if you were sexually harassed?

**TABLE 21.3**

| Types of Sexual Harassment[75] |
|---|
| Verbal harassment or abuse |
| Subtle pressure for sexual activity |
| Remarks about a person's clothing, body, or sexual activities |
| Leering at or ogling a person's body |
| Unwelcome touching, patting, or pinching |
| Brushing against a person's body |
| Demands for sexual favors accompanied by implied or overt threats concerning one's job or student status |
| Physical assault |

Research overseas finds that about 70% of the women who work in Japan and 50% of those who work in Europe have encountered sexual harassment.[78]

Overall, about 25 to 30% of college students report at least one incident of sexual harassment.[79] Sexual harassment on campus usually involves the less severe forms of harassment, such as sexist comments and sexual remarks by faculty or professors, as well as come-ons, suggestive looks, propositions, and light touching. Relatively few acts involve direct pressure for sexual intercourse.

Sexual harassment may also occur between patients and doctors, or between therapists and clients. These professionals may abuse their power and influence over clients to pressure them into having sexual relations. The harassment may be disguised, expressed in terms of its supposed "therapeutic benefits."

### Health Effects of Sexual Harassment

Sexual harassment is not just annoying or insensitive. Three of four people who are sexually harassed report physical or emotional reactions such as anxiety, irritability, lowered self-esteem, and anger.[80] Some find harassment on the job so unbearable that they feel forced to resign. College women have been forced to drop courses, switch majors, change graduate programs, or even change colleges because they were unable to stop persistent sexual harassment from professors.

One reason that sexual harassment is so stressful is that as with other forms of sexual coercion, the blame unfairly tends to fall on the victim. Harassers may claim that the charges against them are exaggerated or that the person bringing charges "overreacted" or "took me too seriously." In our society, women are expected to be "nice"—to be passive and not "make a scene." The woman who assertively protects her rights may be branded a troublemaker. As one commentator put it, "Women are damned if they assert themselves and victimized if they don't."[81]

## PREVENTION

### *Resisting Sexual Harassment*

What would you do if you were sexually harassed by an employer or a professor? Would you try to ignore it and hope that it would stop? What actions might you take? We offer some suggestions that may be helpful. Recognize, however, that responsibility for sexual harassment always lies with the perpetrator and the organization that permits sexual harassment to take place, not with the person subjected to the harassment.

1. *Convey a professional attitude.* Harassment may be stopped cold by responding to the harasser with a businesslike, professional attitude.
2. *Discourage harassing behavior and encourage appropriate behavior.* Harassment may also be stopped cold by shaping the harasser's behavior. Your reactions to the harasser may encourage businesslike behavior and discourage flirtatious or suggestive behavior. If a harassing professor suggests that you come back after school to review your term paper so that the two of you will be undisturbed, set limits assertively. Tell the professor that you'd feel more comfortable discussing the paper during regular office hours. Remain task-oriented. Stick to business. The harasser should quickly get the message that you wish to maintain a strictly professional relationship. If the harasser persists, use a more direct response: "Professor Jones, I'd like to keep our relationship on a purely professional basis, OK?"
3. *Avoid being alone with the harasser.* If you are being harassed by your professor but need some advice about preparing your term paper, approach him or her after class when other students are around, not privately during office hours. Or bring a friend to wait outside the office while you consult the professor.

4. *Maintain a record.* Keep a record of all incidents of harassment as documentation in the event you decide to lodge an official complaint. The record should include the following: (1) where the incident took place; (2) the date and time; (3) what happened, including the exact words that were used, if you can recall them; (4) how you felt; and (5) the names of witnesses. Some people who have been subjected to sexual harassment have carried a hidden tape recorder during contacts with the harasser. Such recordings may not be admissible in a court of law, but they are persuasive in organizational grievance procedures. A hidden tape recorder may be illegal in your state, however. It is thus advisable to check the law.
5. *Talk with the harasser.* It may be uncomfortable to address the issue directly with a harasser, but doing so puts the offender on notice that you are aware of the harassment and want it to stop. It may be helpful to frame your approach in terms of a description of the specific offending actions (e.g., "When we were alone in the office, you repeatedly attempted to touch me or brush up against me"); your feelings about the offending behavior ("It made me feel like my privacy was being violated. I'm very upset about this and haven't been sleeping well"); and what you would like the offender to do ("So I'd like you to agree never to attempt to touch me again, OK?"). Having a talk with the harasser may stop the harassment. If the harasser denies the accusations, it may be necessary to take further action.
6. *Write a letter to the harasser.* Set down on paper a record of the offending behavior, and put the harasser on notice that the harassment must stop. Your letter might (1) describe what happened ("Several times you have made sexist comments about my body"); (2) describe how you felt ("It made me feel like a sexual object when you talked to me that way"); and (3) describe what you would like the harasser to do ("I want you to stop making sexist comments to me"). Keep a copy of the letter.
7. *Seek support.* Support from people you trust can help you through the often trying process of resisting sexual harassment. Talking with others allows you to express your feelings and receive emotional support, encouragement, and advice. In addition, it may strengthen your case if you have the opportunity to identify and talk with other people who have been harassed by the offender.
8. *File a complaint.* Companies and institutions are required by law to respond reasonably to complaints of sexual harassment. In large organizations, a designated official (sometimes an ombudsman, affirmative action officer, or sexual harassment advisor) is usually charged to handle such complaints. Set up an appointment with this official to discuss your experiences. Ask about the grievance procedures in the organization and your right to confidentiality. Have available a record of the dates of the incidents, what happened, how you felt about it, and so on.

   The two major government agencies that handle charges of sexual harassment are the Equal Employment Opportunity Commission (look under the government section of your phone book for the telephone number of the nearest office) and your state Human Rights Commission (listed in your phone book under state or municipal government). These agencies may offer advice on how you can protect your legal rights and proceed with a formal complaint.
9. *Seek legal remedies.* Sexual harassment is illegal and actionable. If you are considering legal action, consult an attorney familiar with this area of law. You may be entitled to back pay (if you were fired for reasons arising from the sexual harassment), job reinstatement, and punitive damages.

## think about it!

- **Have you or a friend been exposed to sexual harassment? How did you or the friend handle the situation? Are you happy with the way the situation was handled? Why or why not?**
- **Imagine that you are sexually harassed and want to report it, but a friend advises, "Why make such a fuss? Is it really worth it? After all, complaining could backfire." How would you respond?**

**critical thinking** **Agree or disagree and support your answer: Because of all the publicity, people who are intolerant of normal sexual advances, or who want to punish their supervisors, are now crying sexual harassment.**

Smart Quiz
Q2105

# Turning Off Your Anger Alarm[82]

## Take Charge

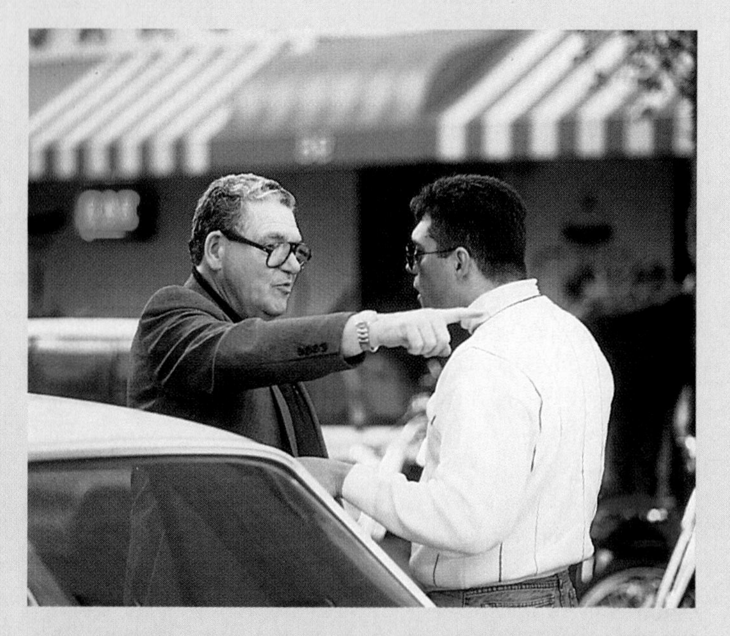

*Anger Control* Anger is linked not only to aggression but also to cardiovascular disorders, such as hypertension and coronary heart disease. What can you do to tone down your anger alarm when faced with frustration or confrontative situations?

Anger can trigger aggression. People who heat up at the slightest provocation may also be jeopardizing their health. People with chronic anger or hostility are at increased risk of developing hypertension and coronary heart disease. Anger floods the body with stress hormones that may eventually damage the cardiovascular system. Mental health professionals help people with anger-control problems identify and correct anger-inducing thoughts that they have in conflict situations, such as thinking that a stranger's rudeness is a personal affront to them that deserves retaliation.

Anger is prompted by a person's reactions to frustrating or provocative situations, not by the situations themselves. People make themselves angry by thinking angering thoughts. By challenging these thoughts, they can learn to turn down their anger alarm, avoid hostile confrontations, and save wear and tear on their cardiovascular systems.

Is anger a problem for you? If so, perhaps you work yourself up when you think other people are treating you unfairly. Perhaps you interpret a stranger's rudeness as a personal affront. Perhaps you demand that others live up to your expectations and get angry with them when they don't. Perhaps you assume that other people are hostile toward you when they are not. Here are some suggestions for toning down your response to angering situations:

1. *Pay attention to your feelings.* When you feel yourself getting hot under the collar, tell yourself to stop and think. Take stock of anger-arousing thoughts.
2. *Pause to consider the evidence.* Are you taking the situation too personally? Are you overreacting? Are you jumping to conclusions about the other person's motives? Are there other ways of viewing the person's behavior, other than as a personal affront?
3. *Try more adaptive thoughts,* such as "I don't have to get upset just because *he's* upset. I can deal with this. Easy does it."
4. *Practice a competing response to anger,* such as calming mental imagery or relaxation exercises. Or disrupt anger by taking a walk around the block, watching TV, or reading. Or, to paraphrase Mark Twain, count to 10 when you're angry. If that doesn't work, count to 100. The time-honored technique of counting to 10 short-circuits impulsive responses to provocations. It gives you time to collect your thoughts and to replace infuriating thoughts with calming thoughts: "Hey, calm down. This is not worth getting bent out of shape over. Stay cool."

5. *Change your response to annoying people.* Don't let them get you steamed. Tell yourself that the other person is being silly and you're not going to let yourself be bothered by it. Or say what's on your mind assertively but not angrily. Let it out and let it go.
6. *Counter anger with empathy.* Rather than saying, "What a despicable person he is to act that way," think, "Maybe she's having a rough day," or, "He's just jealous of me and is acting out like a child." Or, "He must be a very unhappy person to act that way." Or, "She may have reasons—or thinks she has reasons—for acting this way. But that's her problem, not mine. Don't take it personally."
7. *Think through alternative, assertive (not aggressive) solutions to the problem or situation* and formulate a plan of action.
8. *Give yourself a mental pat on the back for coping assertively, not aggressively, in the situation.*

Now, think of the situations in which you have felt angry or acted out in anger. How might you have handled the situation differently? What thoughts can you rehearse to keep your cool if the situation should arise again? Table 21.4 offers calming alternatives to thoughts that trigger anger.

Smart Quiz
Q2106

TABLE 21.4

**Anger Management: Replacing Angering Thoughts with Calming Alternatives**

| Situation | Angering Thoughts | Calming Alternative |
|---|---|---|
| A provocateur says, "So what are you going to do about it?" | "That jerk. Who does he think he is? I'll teach him a lesson he won't forget!" | "He must really have a problem if he acts this way. But that's his problem. I don't have to act at his level." |
| You get caught in a monster traffic jam. | "Why does this always happen to me? I can't stand this." | "This may be inconvenient, but it's not the end of the world. Don't blow it out of proportion. Everyone gets caught in traffic every now and then. Just relax and listen to some music." |
| You're waiting behind someone in the checkout line at the supermarket who has to cash a check. It seems like it's taking hours. | "He has some nerve holding up the line. It's so unfair for someone to make other people wait. I'd like to tell him off!" | "It will only take a few minutes. People have a right to cash their checks in the market. Just relax and read a magazine off the rack while you wait." |
| You're cruising looking for a parking spot when suddenly another car cuts you off and seizes a vacant parking space. | "No one should be allowed to treat me like this. I'd like to punch him out." | "Don't expect other people to always be considerate of your interests. Stop personalizing things." "Relax, there's no sense going to war over this." |
| Your spouse or partner comes home several hours later than expected, without calling ahead. | "It's so unfair. I can't let him (her) treat me like this." | "Make it fair. Explain how you feel without putting him (her) down." |
| You're watching a movie at the theater and someone sitting next to you is talking throughout the picture. | "Don't they have any regard for other people's rights? I'm so angry with these people I could tear their heads off." | "Even if they're inconsiderate, it doesn't mean I have to get angry about it or ruin my enjoyment of the movie. If they don't quiet down when I ask them, I'll just change my seat or call the manager." |
| A person insults you or treats you disrespectfully. | "I just can't walk away from this like nothing happened." | "Of course you can. When did anger ever settle anything? There are better ways of handling this than getting steamed." |

# SUMMING UP

## Questions and Answers

**1. Which industrialized nation has the greatest incidence of homicide among young people?** The United States. Our homicide rate is ten times that of Japan and is the highest among industrialized nations.

### SPOUSE ABUSE

**2. How many women are abused by their spouses?** About one woman in eight suffers a severe beating from her husband or male partner each year. Women are more likely to be beaten, raped, or killed by the men they live with than by strangers or acquaintances.

**3. Who commits spouse abuse?** Women as well as men abuse their spouses. Women are far more likely to be seriously injured, however. Many spouse abusers have problems controlling violent impulses. Many have low self-esteem and are overly dependent on their partners. The use of alcohol or other drugs raises the risk of abuse.

**4. What are the health effects of spouse abuse?** Spouse abuse can cause physical injury, emotional problems, even death. Psychological effects can linger and include posttraumatic stress disorder (PTSD), depression, low self-esteem, substance abuse, even suicide.

### CHILD ABUSE

**5. Who commits child abuse?** Child abuse is found across all socioeconomic and ethnic divisions. However, teenage parents, single parents, poor parents, and poorly educated parents are most likely to abuse or neglect their children.

**6. What kinds of child abuse are there?** These include neglect, physical abuse, sexual abuse, and emotional maltreatment.

**7. What are the health effects of child abuse?** These include serious and sometimes life-threatening physical injuries. Nearly half of all child fatalities due to maltreatment result from neglect. Abused or neglected children may have problems relating to other people, lack empathy, do poorly in school, have low self-esteem, and have suicidal thoughts or make suicide attempts.

### RAPE

**8. What types of rape are there?** Types of rape include stranger rape, acquaintance rape, marital rape, male rape, and rape by females. Women are more likely to be raped by men they know than by strangers.

**9. Why do men rape women?** Although sexual motivation plays a role in many rapes, the use of sex to express aggression, anger, and power is more central to our understanding of rape. Many observers contend that our society breeds rapists by socializing males to be socially and sexually dominant in their relationships with women.

**10. How can rape survivors be helped?** Treatment of rape survivors typically involves helping them through the immediate crisis and then helping to foster long-term adjustment. It would also help if society were less prone to blaming the victim.

### CHILD SEXUAL ABUSE

**11. What is child sexual abuse?** Any form of sexual contact between an adult and a child is abusive, even if force or physical threat is not used, since children are incapable of consenting to sexual activity. Genital fondling is the most common type of abuse.

**12. Who are the child molesters?** Child sexual abuse, like rape and other forms of sexual coercion, cuts across all socioeconomic classes. In most cases, the molesters are close to the children they abuse—relatives, step-relatives, family friends, and neighbors.

**13. What are the health effects of child sexual abuse?** Children who are sexually abused often suffer social and emotional problems that impair their development and persist into adulthood, affecting their self-esteem and their intimate relationships.

**14. How can child sexual abuse be prevented?** In addition to learning to avoid strangers, children need to learn the difference between "good touching," such as an affectionate embrace or a pat on the head, and "bad touching." Children who may not be able to prevent abuse may nevertheless be encouraged to tell someone about it.

## SEXUAL HARASSMENT

**15. What is sexual harassment?** Sexual harassment involves sexual comments, gestures, overtures, demands, or physical contact that are unwelcome to the recipient. Sexual harassment may have more to do with issues of power and control than sexual motives. Sexual harassment may be used as a tactic to keep women "in their place," especially in work settings that are traditional male preserves.

**16. How can sexual harassment be resisted?** Suggestions include conveying a professional attitude, avoiding being alone with the harasser, keeping a record of incidents, and seeking legal remedies.

## Suggested Readings

**Toch, H.** *Violent Men: An Inquiry into the Psychology of Violence.* Washington, DC: American Psychological Association, 1992. Explorations of the psychological underpinnings of violence in men.

**Grauerholz, E., and Koralewski, M. A. (Eds.).** *Sexual Coercion: A Sourcebook on Its Nature, Causes, and Prevention.* Lexington, MA: Lexington Books, 1991. Leading experts discuss the problems of sexual coercion, from rape to child sexual abuse.

**U.S. Department of Justice.** *Crime in the United States: Uniform Crime Reports.* Washington, DC: Author. An annual compilation of crime statistics in the United States.

**Warshaw, R. (1988).** *I Never Called it Rape.* A probing review of the problem of acquaintance rape and date rape.

## DID YOU KNOW THAT

- Lead poisoning is the number-one environmental hazard facing U.S. children? p.601
- Most cases of lead poisoning in children come from ingesting lead dust, not from eating lead paint chips? p.601
- Your new foam mattress, carpeting, and even plastic telephone may be making you sick? p.603
- Supermarkets may sell imported foods that are contaminated with pesticides that are banned in the United States, and it's perfectly legal? p.606
- You are likely to be exposed to greater concentrations of pesticides in the home than outdoors? p.606
- Driving while using a car phone is about as dangerous as driving with a blood alcohol level at the legal limit? p.612
- The world's population is growing by more than 225,000 people *every day?* p.613
- The global temperature has been rising and people are at least partly to blame? p.621
- Excessive heat—not lightning, tornadoes, or hurricanes—is the leading weather-related killer? p.622

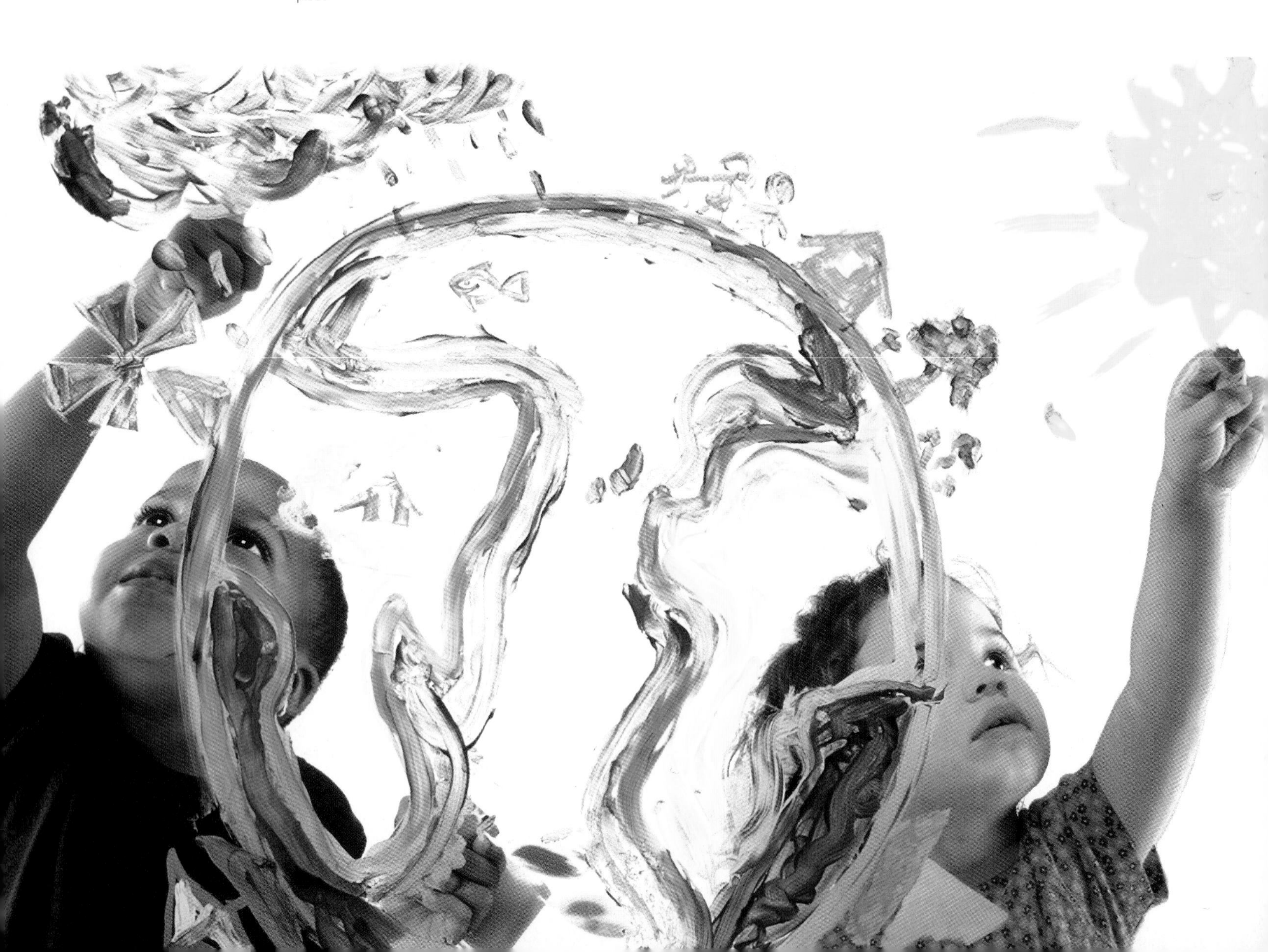

# Health and the Environment

The good earth: *It provides us with air to breathe, food to eat, and water to drink. It protects us from the most harmful ultraviolet rays from the sun.*

*Our health depends on many factors—our genes, dietary and exercise habits, avoidance of tobacco and other harmful substances, and the ability of our bodies to protect us from infectious agents and cancerous growths. Our health also depends on the quality of our environment. The* ***environment*** *refers to the totality of our surroundings—the plants and animals, including people; water, air, and soil; and factors such as climate (temperature, precipitation) and geography (mountains, valleys, oceans). And as sociologists would point out, our relationship to the environment also involves cultural and social factors.*

22

TABLE 22.1

**Types of Environmental Hazards**

| Types of Hazards | Examples |
|---|---|
| Toxic chemical hazards | Toxic chemical hazards include chemical substances that are toxic or poisonous to living organisms. There are thousands of natural and synthetic (human-made) toxins, including heavy metals, petrochemicals, and pesticides, many of which pose health risks to people and other organisms that are exposed to them. |
| Biological hazards | Biological hazards include viruses, bacteria, protozoa, and other disease-causing microorganisms or pathogens. They are also the chief cause of food-borne and water-borne diseases in the United States as well as worldwide. |
| Physical hazards | Examples of physical hazards include radiation, natural disasters (floods, earthquakes, and fires); violence; accidents in the home, in the workplace, or in transit; and noise. Physical hazards often vary according to living conditions—where you live and what you live near. Practicing personal safety, such as wearing seat belts and using other safety equipment, also influences the risks posed by physical hazards. |
| Cultural/social hazards | These include hazards we are exposed to in our culture and society, such as overpopulation, unhealthy learned habits (like smoking and excessive alcohol intake), lack of access to health care, and poverty. Violence can be considered both a physical hazard and a cultural/social hazard. Some environmental hazards may interconnect. The poor, for instance, are more likely to work and live near environmental hazards and to suffer a disproportionate share of their ill effects. Agricultural workers, many of whom are poor immigrants, may be forced into close contact with dangerous pesticides and other hazards in order to make a living. |

Social factors such as the distribution of wealth, access to health care, discrimination, and governmental systems also figure into the relationship between health and the environment. They help create the gaps in health status between different economic and ethnic groups. For instance, a disproportionate share of the nation's toxic waste sites are in areas populated by ethnic minority groups and poor people.

Many environmental health risks are connected to the accelerated rate of change in modern society. As we approach the new millennium, advances in technology are introducing new substances into the environment, some of which may harm the environment and people's health. Today, roughly 65,000 synthetic (manufactured) chemicals are used throughout the world.[1] Most have not been assessed for health risks. Given this state of affairs, many of us aren't sure whether we can turn on our water taps with confidence, breathe the air, or safely consume the foods we buy.

Cultural values, attitudes, and beliefs play an important role in our relationship with the environment. Many indigenous peoples, including Native Americans, respect the environment that sustains them. In industrialized countries such as ours, however, the environment is often taken for granted. Or it is abused and degraded by unchecked industrial development. With the publication of Rachel Carson's now-classic *Silent Spring* in 1962 (a searing indictment of environmental damage caused by hazards such as pesticides), attitudes toward the environment slowly began to shift. Americans who had acted as if the earth were an infinite resource to be plundered without consequences now began to view it as a finite resource that needed our stewardship. Of course, many environmentalists believe that this value is not widespread enough.

**Environment** All of the living and nonliving components that exist where an organism lives.

**Environmental hazard** An environmental factor with potential to cause harm to individuals.

The environment that sustains us also contains hazards—many of them human-made—that threaten our health. In Chapter 11, we discussed *teratogens*—substances that cause birth defects. We saw in Chapter 15 that we are literally immersed in a sea of *pathogens*—viruses, bacteria, and other microorganisms in the air, water, and soil. In Chapter 18, we noted that some forms of cancer may be caused by exposure to certain environmental agents, or *carcinogens.*

This chapter focuses on other **environmental hazards,** such as toxic chemicals, radiation, pollution, overpopulation, and changes in the earth's atmosphere—depletion of the ozone layer and global warming. Environmental hazards are classified by environmental health scientists as shown in Table 22.1.[2] In this chapter we learn how environmental risks threaten our health and how we can eliminate or reduce them.

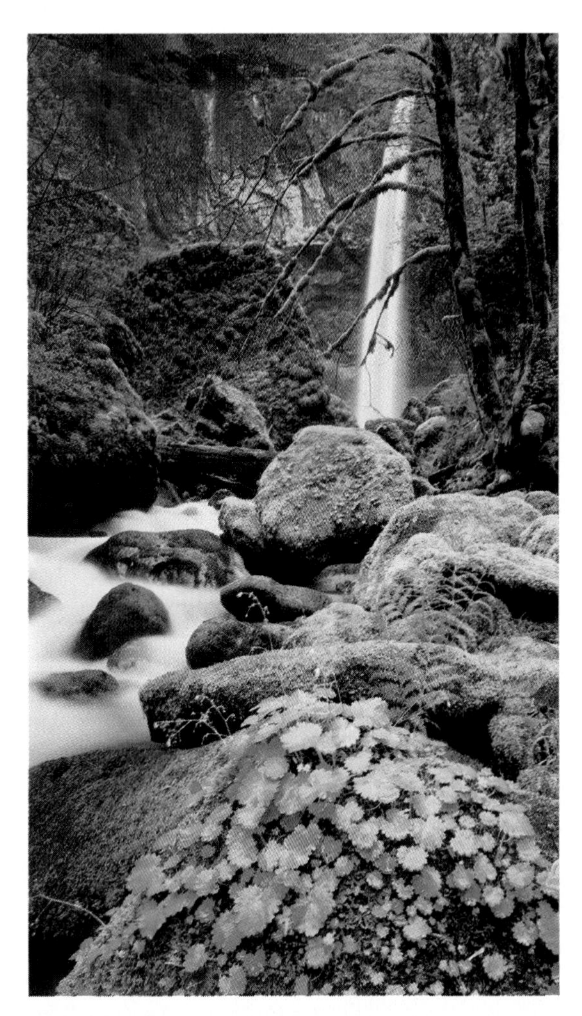

***The Good Earth*** By doing our part and supporting conservation efforts, we can all help preserve the environment.

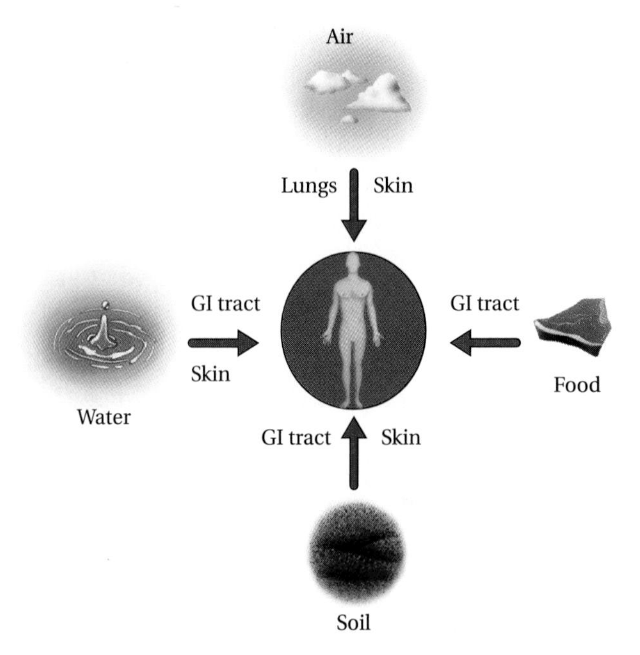


**Figure 22.1** ***Routes of Human Exposure to Environmental Hazards*** Environmental hazards can enter the body through various routes of exposure, including the skin, the gastrointestinal (GI) tract, and the lungs.

# ENVIRONMENTAL TOXINS—NATURAL AND HUMAN-MADE RISKS

Nature produces countless toxins, and humans have invented countless more. A **toxin** is a poisonous substance that impairs an organism's normal functioning. The major environmental toxins that concern us are (1) natural and synthetic **toxins** (metals, pesticides, and some petrochemicals) and (2) radioactive substances (ultraviolet rays, X-rays, radon, among other sources). Environmental toxins enter the body through three major routes—the lungs, skin, and gastrointestinal tract (as the result of eating contaminated food or drinking contaminated water) (see Figure 22.1).

## Health Effects of Environmental Toxins

Environmental toxins can harm our health in various ways. Pesticides are toxic chemicals that not only kill insects but can also harm humans and other animals. Other toxins, especially certain forms of radiation, are **mutagens.** They can cause mutations in the genetic structure of living organisms. Many mutagens are *carcinogens,* or substances that cause cancer. Toxins like lead and mercury are **neurotoxins** (nerve poisons); they can damage the brain and central nervous system (CNS). Many toxins exert a combination of adverse effects.

Talking Glossary
Mutagens
G2201

Though some toxins are metabolized (broken down) by the body and excreted, others can accumulate in the body and cause chronic health problems. **Bioaccumulation** is the process by which high concentrations of toxins build up within the body. Some toxins travel through the bloodstream to affect target organs. (A **target organ** is an organ that is susceptible to damage by certain chemicals.)

Glossary
Bioaccumulation
G2202

**Toxins** Poisonous substances.

**Mutagen** Any substance that causes genetic mutations.

**Neurotoxin** A toxin that produces adverse effects in the brain and central nervous system.

**Bioaccumulation** The process by which toxins accumulate in the bodies of animals.

**Target organ** An organ susceptible to damage by particular chemicals.

# HealthCheck

## How Do You Rate Environmental Health Hazards?

Uncertainty is a fact of life. Even getting out of bed in the morning is somewhat risky. (You could fall.) Driving to work, flying on an airplane, and eating a fat-filled dessert all entail some risk. Our personal appraisal of risk influences the decisions we make. What if we find a wonderful house that's at the right price because it's near a high-voltage power line? If we buy or rent it, are we endangering our health?

This ***HealthCheck*** is about perceptions versus realities. Consider the following environmental problems. Rate them according to the amount of risk you perceive each one to entail: as either high, medium, or low in risk. Then read on to see how they were rated by the U.S. public and by a panel of experts.

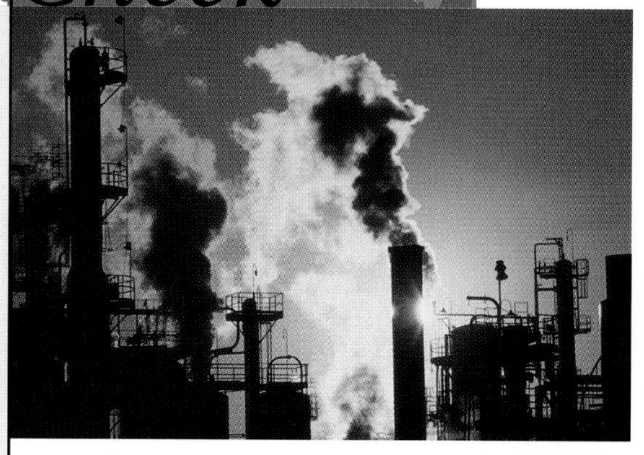

____ Acid rain
____ Chemical leaks from underground storage tanks
____ Coastal water contamination
____ Damaged wetlands
____ Genetic alteration
____ Greenhouse effect
____ Hazardous waste sites
____ Indoor air pollution
____ Indoor radon
____ Industrial air pollution
____ Industrial waterway pollution
____ Microwave oven radiation
____ Nonhazardous waste sites
____ Oil spills
____ Ozone-layer destruction
____ Pesticides
____ Pollution from industrial accidents
____ Radiation from a nuclear accident
____ Radioactive waste
____ Sewage plant water pollution
____ Tap-water contamination
____ Vehicle exhaust
____ Water pollution from farm runoff
____ Water pollution from urban runoff
____ Workplace chemicals
____ X-ray radiation

### Ratings by the Public versus the Experts

The Roper Poll reveals that **perceived risks** may be at odds with **actual risks.** We may *perceive* something as very risky even though scientific evidence suggests that there is little if any *actual* risk. Or we may perceive an actual risk as harmless.

Table 22.2 shows that the public's perception of the risk regarding environmental issues often differed sharply from the judgments of an Environmental Protection Agency (EPA) task force of scientists. For example, the public ranked hazardous waste sites as the single most dangerous environmental health threat. Yet according to the EPA scientists, they pose a medium to low risk. Similarly, the public ranked indoor air pollution relatively low on the list of health hazards. But according to the EPA panel, it ranked high in risk.

Why these discrepancies? In part, scientific information may not be available, or if it is, it may be hard for nonscientists to understand. Then too, many people are uncomfortable with complex issues and scientific data, so they oversimplify or jump to conclusions. People may also perceive risks according to how they affect their own lives, while scientists assess risks according to how they affect large groups of people. Overall, the risk posed by hazardous waste sites to the entire U.S. population is judged by experts to be less than that posed by other hazards. But if you happen to live near a hazardous waste site or know someone who does, your personal estimate of risk may be much higher than the ranking assigned by the experts.

People also react differently to public versus private risks. **Public risks** are those to which we are involuntarily exposed, such as nuclear accidents and pollution. A **private risk**—smoking, not exercising, driving a car—is one that we voluntarily take. We generally react with more fear to public risks, because we perceive them as beyond our control. Yet many private risks are far riskier. Of a total population of 270 million, some 50,000 people die in car accidents each year in the U.S. The average person's chance of getting killed in a car each year is nearly 1 in 5,000. The lifetime risk, assuming we live to age 70, is estimated to be 1 in 70.[4] This is an astonishingly high risk ratio when compared with most other hazards, yet few have proposed banning automobiles. Although the risk of dying in a car accident far outweighs the risks of many pesticides on food, people can choose not to drive cars (though in our society this may be a bit of a stretch), but they cannot choose not to eat. Nor can we escape encircling air pollution.

**Perceived risk** The amount of risk posed by a factor or factors as perceived by individuals.

**Actual risk** The amount of risk posed by a factor or factors as based on scientific evidence.

**Public risk** The risk associated with a factor in the environment to which we are involuntarily exposed.

**Private risk** The risk associated with a factor that we can control voluntarily.

TABLE 22.2

**Public versus Environmental Protection Agency (EPA) Expert Task Force Rankings of Environmental Risks**[3]

| Ranking by American Public | Risk Level According to EPA Task Force |
|---|---|
| 1. Hazardous waste sites (highest) | Medium to low |
| 2. Workplace chemicals | High |
| 3. Industrial waterway pollution | Low |
| 4. Nuclear accident radiation | Not rated by task force |
| 5. Radioactive waste | Not rated by task force |
| 6. Chemical leaks from underground storage tanks | Medium to low |
| 7. Pesticides | High |
| 8. Pollution from industrial accidents | Medium to low |
| 9. Water pollution from farm runoff | Medium |
| 10. Tap-water contamination | High |
| 11. Industrial air pollution | High |
| 12. Ozone-layer destruction | High |
| 13. Coastal water contamination | Low |
| 14. Sewage plant water pollution | Medium to low |
| 15. Vehicle exhaust | High |
| 16. Oil spills | Medium to low |
| 17. Acid rain | High |
| 18. Water pollution from urban runoff | Medium |
| 19. Damaged wetlands | Low |
| 20. Genetic alteration | Low |
| 21. Nonhazardous waste sites | Medium to low |
| 22. Greenhouse effect | Low |
| 23. Indoor air pollution | High |
| 24. X-ray radiation | Not rated by task force |
| 25. Indoor radon | High |
| 26. Microwave oven radiation (lowest) | Not rated by task force |

The kidneys, for example, are especially vulnerable to damage by the toxic metal cadmium. The lungs are susceptible to many toxic particles in air pollution.

Some people, such as infants and children, pregnant women, people with impaired immune systems, and older people, are more sensitive to the effects of certain toxins. The health hazards of toxins are **dose dependent.** That is, their effects depend on the amount that is absorbed relative to body weight. Thus a child who eats the same serving of contaminated fish as an adult, or who inhales an equal amount of airborne toxin, is at greater risk of adverse effects. Additionally, children's major organ systems are not yet fully mature, so they are less able to metabolize and eliminate toxic substances from the body. Pregnant women are at increased risk for various toxins that can cause birth defects or problems after birth. Many toxins cross the placenta and enter the circulatory system of the fetus. Toxins can also pose disproportionate risks to older people. The slowing down of metabolism in later life also means that toxins are eliminated more slowly in older persons.

## Toxic Chemicals

Many naturally occurring and synthetic chemicals pose threats to our health.

**Arsenic** **Arsenic** is a naturally occurring metallic toxin present in small amounts ("traces") in various foods. Arsenic traces in foods are apparently *inert,* or inactive, and not believed to pose a health threat. Yet tobacco contains arsenic, which does pose a health risk to smokers. And as a component of wood preservatives and pesticides, arsenic can be an extremely hazardous carcinogen for workers and others regularly exposed to it. Depending on the amount and route of the exposure, arsenic produces symptoms that can range from rashes and nausea to skin cancer and lung cancer.

**Dose dependent** Effects of drugs or other substances that are dependent on the amount of the substance used.

**Arsenic** A naturally occurring, metal-like toxin commonly found in minute amounts in various foods.

**Asbestos** A mineral previously used for insulation and fireproofing; can cause lung cancer and other respiratory illnesses.

**Aflatoxin** A naturally occurring chemical produced by molds; in high doses, acts as a potent carcinogen.

**Minerals** Iron, selenium, zinc, and other mineral elements are found in the soil and in small amounts in the body. We need traces of these minerals in the foods we eat or in supplements to maintain good health. When taken in excess amounts, or when they react with other elements, they can become toxic. Inhaling high doses of the compound selenium dioxide, for example, which is produced when waste is burned, causes eye, nose, and throat irritation, breathing problems, and nausea, and may lead to cancer.

One common mineral toxin is found at home—asbestos. **Asbestos** is a mineral that was widely used for insulation in building construction and as a fire retardant until the early 1970s, when the health consequences of inhaling asbestos fibers became clear. Tiny fibers of asbestos can become dislodged when the material is installed or when it deteriorates or is disturbed during repairs. If large amounts of asbestos fibers are inhaled and become lodged in the lungs, they can cause serious lung disorders, including lung cancer. More than 9 million American workers are believed to have been exposed to asbestos dust on the job.[5] Many houses and schools still contain asbestos. When it is found, it should be removed, contained, or sealed by a trained asbestos removal contractor. This is *not* a do-it-yourself job, because you may accidentally release dangerous fibers into the air. Your local health department should be able to help you find a qualified contractor.

**Close-up**
Asbestos: Q & A
T2201

**Aflatoxin** **Aflatoxin** is a natural toxin produced by a mold that grows on grains and nuts, including peanuts.[6] In high doses, aflatoxin is a potent carcinogen. But at strictly controlled lower doses in foods such as peanut butter, it is considered safe by the Food and Drug Administration (FDA).

**Talking Glossary**
Aflatoxin
G2203

**Heavy Metals** Heavy metals, such as lead, mercury, and cadmium, are naturally occurring inorganic metallic elements that are usually toxic even in low concentrations. Heavy metals are mined and used in countless products from paints to batteries. Many heavy metals such as lead are potent neurotoxins. Some are also carcinogens.

Lead occurs naturally in ore and soil. Lead gets into air, water, and other soil from industrial emissions, lead-based products like paint, leaded gasoline exhaust (lead is still present in many truck fuels), and incineration. Serious health complications can arise when it is breathed or ingested, especially over time. Lead contamination is one of the most serious environmental health hazards faced by millions of children, pregnant women, and workers in the United States.

**Lead poisoning** is considered the number-one environmental health problem facing U.S. children. Though we are all at risk of lead contamination, children—especially those under six—are at much greater risk, since they absorb up to four times as much lead as adults exposed to the same levels. According to the Centers for Disease Control and Prevention, more than 6 million preschool children in urban areas and some 400,000 pregnant women may have unsafe levels of lead in their bodies. In pregnant women, lead can cause miscarriages, premature birth, low birth weight, and damage to the nervous systems of newborns. Adults exposed to high levels of lead are at risk for developing high blood pressure, kidney and gastrointestinal problems, and hearing damage.[7]

Lead exposure in children, even in small doses, can disrupt normal brain development and lead to lower IQ, reduced attention span, and hearing problems. At higher doses, it can cause permanent brain damage. Lead may lead to subtle and not-so-subtle behavioral problems, especially aggressive and hyperactive behavior in children. Researchers report a link between lead levels in the body and aggressive and delinquent behavior in children.[8]

With the reduction of lead in gasoline and foods, the major sources for exposure are lead-based paint, unglazed pottery, dust and soil, and drinking water. More than one American in ten is serviced by a water system with excess levels of lead.[9] Older houses with lead paint in dilapidated condition, or in which lead paint is disturbed by renovations, are a particular danger. Though lead paint was banned in 1978, old lead-based paint still covers the walls of about one-quarter of the private dwellings in the U.S.

All children under six should be screened for lead, as should adults at risk. The Centers for Disease Control and Prevention has set the safety standard for blood levels at 10 micrograms or less of lead per deciliter of blood. If a child lives in a dwelling containing lead paint, the first screening should be done at the age of 6 months. Children at low risk should be screened at 12 months and retested at age 2.[10]

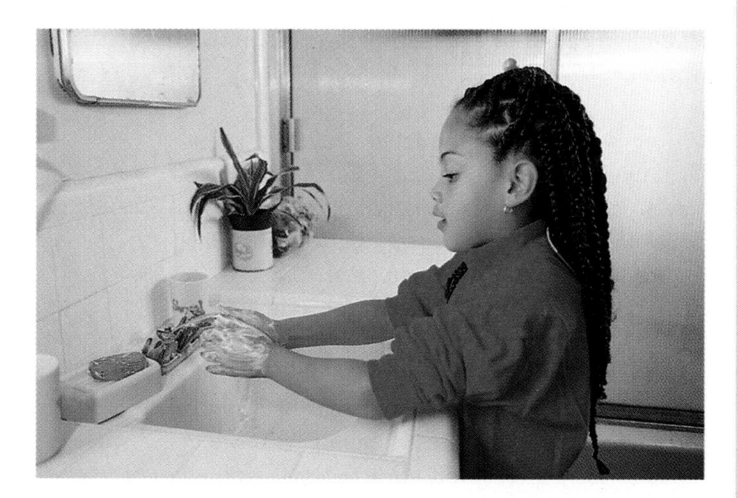

***Getting the Lead Out*** Washing your hands regularly, and encouraging your children to do so, removes not only pathogens but also household dust that may contain lead particles.

PREVENTION

## *Getting the Lead Out*[11]

Most of us know that eating paint chips can produce lead poisoning. But in actuality, lead poisoning by this means is uncommon. Most cases of lead poisoning are caused by ingestion of household dust that is contaminated by lead. When leaded paint flakes or is disturbed by home renovations, it sheds particles that get into dust, furniture and flooring, toys, dishes, and food. Hand-to-mouth contamination occurs when children touch these objects and then bring the dust to their mouths. Three-quarters of the lead consumed by children comes from paint dust in their homes. Another 20% comes from lead in drinking water.

All children are at risk for lead poisoning, but poor children, including a disproportionate number of children of color, are most at risk. They are more likely than affluent children to live in delapidated older housing that was painted with lead-based paint. Inner-city housing is also likely to be located in areas with high levels of lead contamination from industry and truck emissions. Though blood lead levels of young children dropped by 76% from 1978 to the early 1990s—thanks largely to removal of lead from gasolines and household paints—one-third of urban African-American children still have unhealthy blood lead levels. Lead absorption is also highest among children with iron deficiencies, a problem especially prevalent among poor children.

Culturally related practices are also sources of lead poisoning. Mexican Americans in the lower Rio Grande Valley in Texas, for instance, commonly use earthenware pots glazed with a lead oxide compound called *greta.* Although most users understand that the pots are a potential source of lead poisoning, many erroneously believe that certain folk remedies, such as filling the pot with vinegar and letting it stand for a day or two, will rid the cookware of lead. The use of certain cosmetics and ethnic foods may also be sources of lead contamination.

Lead in the soil is yet another hazard.

**Lead poisoning** Toxic metal poisoning, from the ingestion or inhalation of large amounts of lead.

Lead enters the soil largely through emissions from leaded gasoline. Here again, poorer children are at greater risk, because they are more likely to play in yards with little ground cover that might serve as a barrier to prevent soil contamination.

Lead poisoning is a problem not only for poor children. Children in more affluent households may be affected, especially those living in houses built before 1960, when lead paint was used extensively. Despite the risks, most young children—especially poor children—have not been tested for exposure to lead.

***Protecting Yourself and Your Family from Lead Contamination*** There is much we can do to protect ourselves and our children from lead contamination:

- *Have your child tested regularly for lead.* Health officials recommend testing of all preschool children.
- *Vacuum your carpeting and bare floors frequently to remove household dust.* But don't vacuum with children present. All vacuum cleaners emit dust particles into the air as they suck up dirt. Some vacuums emit more dust than others. When purchasing a vacuum, select one that emits a low level of dust (check *Consumer Reports* for a listing of low-emission models).
- *Always use cold water for drinking, cooking, or preparing baby formula.* Lead leaches from pipes more easily into warm water. Let the cold water run for 30 seconds or so before using it. First-drawn water can be used for cleaning and watering plants.
- *Avoid water softeners.* Lead also leaches more readily into softened water.
- *Wash your hands frequently and have your children do the same.* Washing removes household dust.
- *Make sure your children get ample supplies of iron, calcium, and protein.* Lack of these nutrients can increase absorption of lead.
- *Never store, serve, or cook foods or beverages in lead-based crystal or in lead-glazed commercial china or ceramic ware.* Check for the lead content of pottery before purchase.
- *Avoid using imported canned goods, which may contain lead solder.*
- *Workers who are exposed to lead on the job should change their clothing and shoes before returning home.* People with hobbies that expose them to lead products, such as stained-glass making, should pursue these interests away from home.
- *Residents of homes with lead paint should consult with a lead abatement contractor or specialist trained and certified by the Environmental Protection Agency.* Professional lead abatement companies can remove leaded paint or contain it safely by covering it with wallboard or some other impervious material.
- *Have your tap water tested for lead.* The EPA has set a level of 15 parts per billion (ppb) and above as the point at which people should take action to correct lead levels in drinking water, such as by installing filtration devices.
- *Test the soil around your house for lead.* If lead levels are high, the lead should be removed or covered with grass or with a layer of mulch, or blocked with shrubbery or bushes so that children cannot play in the area.

**Petrochemicals** Substances refined from fossil fuels, especially petroleum and natural gas.

**Fossil fuels** Energy sources found in deposits in the earth, including oil, natural gas, and coal.

Mercury is a silver-white metal that changes to liquid at ordinary temperatures and evaporates into the air. The effects of inhaling mercury range from mild tremors to fetal abnormalities and brain damage. Mercury discharged from plants and factories into bodies of water forms the compound methyl mercury, which can contaminate fish. People who eat contaminated fish can develop serious neurological disorders and/or give birth to children with birth defects.

Like lead and mercury, cadmium also accumulates in the environment. Cadmium is widely used in electroplating, batteries, paints (as a pigment), fertilizers, and plastics. It is also one of the many carcinogenic chemicals found in cigarette smoke. Traces of cadmium in the air, water, and soil are widespread. Prolonged exposure to high levels of cadmium can lead to kidney disease and possibly cancer.

**Petrochemicals** **Petrochemicals** are chemicals manufactured from the refinement of **fossil fuels,** especially petroleum and natural gas. Fossil fuels are *nonrenewable energy sources* since their deposits cannot be replenished. Once used, they're gone. Petrochemicals are a distinctly modern invention dating to the 1940s. The U.S. petrochemical industry—the fourth largest in the U.S.—produces about 500 million tons of petrochemicals annually. Petrochemical products include cosmetics, wood preservatives, synthetic resins, plastics, paints, coatings, pharmaceuticals, soaps and detergents, chemical solvents, and agricultural products such as fertilizers and pesticides.

We know how to make desirable products from petrochemicals, but we are less knowledgeable about how to safely dispose of the hazardous wastes created from their manufacture. Another problem is disposal of the **nonbiodegradable** waste when these products are discarded. Petrochemicals and their by-products are among the greatest sources of pollution of the air, water, and soil. You can do your part in protecting the environment by buying as few nonbiodegradable products as possible and recycling whenever possible.

PREVENTION

## Preventing Poisoning at Home

Many household chemicals are dangerous, even deadly, when ingested or absorbed into the body. The dangers are greatest for children. Each year more than 1 million children in the U.S. are accidentally poisoned. More than 90% of poisonings occur in the home.[12] Children are naturally inquisitive and may not realize that the colorful container under the sink isn't filled with fruit drink, but with a toxic detergent. Though manufacturers have been using child-resistant containers since the early 1970s, parents need to ensure that household chemicals are stored safely. Here are some suggestions to help prevent household poisonings:

- *Keep household chemicals out of reach of small children.* This includes detergents, bleaches, cleansers, solvents, dishwashing liquid, and paint products. Don't store these or other household chemicals under the sink, in the medicine cabinet, or anywhere children can reach.
- *Check product labels and follow instructions for use and storage.*
- *Never switch containers.* Never pour household chemicals into other containers, especially non-child-resistant containers.
- *Discard old or outdated medication.*
- *Keep alert.* Keep an eye on children, especially when they explore their surroundings. Child-*resistant* does not mean child-*proof.* Given enough time, even young children may figure out how to open containers.
- *Keep the local poison control hotline number handy.* Check your phone directory for the telephone number of your local poison control hotline. Keep it within reach. If no poison control hotline is available in your community, dial 911 or call the telephone operator in the case of emergency. If you suspect your child has ingested a possible toxic substance, call for help immediately.

**Formaldehyde** **Formaldehyde,** one of the most commonly used petrochemicals, is a colorless gas usually sold to manufacturers in an alcohol solution. Its popularity as a manufacturing component (specifically, as a preservative and finishing agent) stems from its superior ability to bind different substances together to produce new, complex compounds.[13] A very partial list of common formaldehyde-containing products includes particleboard, plywood paneling, fiberboard, plastic telephones, foam mattresses, carpeting, cosmetics, and pharmaceuticals.

Talking Glossary
Formaldehyde
G2204

New products made with formaldehyde release formaldehyde gas—a process called "outgassing"—until it all evaporates. Outgassing can take months after a product reaches the market. Some people have sensitivities to the gas, which leads to respiratory and skin problems. Products such as foam mattresses, carpeting, and even plastic telephones can make people sick for months after they buy them.

Close-up
More on formaldehyde
T2202

People who are sensitive to formaldehyde can develop **allergic contact dermatitis,** which is characterized by red, itchy skin and blisters. Other outgassing symptoms include respiratory infections, eye and sinus irritation, coughing, and runny noses. Formaldehyde has also been found to cause cancer in animals. Because of health concerns, there is a growing market for formaldehyde-free products (ask your furniture retailer). Though the cost of formaldehyde-free products may be higher, many consumers feel it is worth it.

**Organochlorines** **Organochlorines** (also called *chlorinated hydrocarbons*) are a class of petrochemicals in which the element chlorine is added during processing. Roughly 11,000 organochlorines are manufactured or used in industrial production of petrochemicals.[14] They are used to make pesticides, plastics, solvents, refrigerants, and other products.

Talking Glossary
Organochlorines
G2205

Organochlorines pose grave threats. Some of the better known organochlorines include some of the most dangerous pollutants: the pesticide *DDT* (dichlorodiphenyl-trichloroethane), toxic substances called dioxins, insulating and con-

**Nonbiodegradable** Substances that, when disposed of, do not decompose.

**Formaldehyde** A clear, toxic gas used as a preservative and in manufacturing.

**Allergic contact dermatitis** An allergic skin response produced on contact with a chemical substance to which a person is sensitive.

**Organochlorines** A class of petrochemicals, including some pesticides and other toxic substances, with a wide range of industrial uses.

ducting agents called PCBs, and refrigerant and propellant gases called CFCs. Because of the dangers posed by organochlorines and other chlorinated products used in manufacturing, the American Public Health Association has urged banning many industrial uses of chlorine.[15]

Organochlorines are neurotoxins; they can severely damage the nervous system. They're also linked to damage of reproductive organs, birth defects, and immune system disorders. Exposure to organochlorines such as DDT and PCB may increase the risk of breast cancer and other cancers. DDT has been detected in breast tissue and breast milk, from which it can be passed along to nursing babies.[16]

Many organochlorines resist **biodegradation,** so they are hard to remove from the environment. CFCs make their way into the atmosphere, where they can damage the protective **ozone layer** in the upper atmosphere by consuming **ozone** molecules. DDT and dioxin can make their way into the **food chain,** and eventually to us, when they pollute the grass and soil. They contaminate fruits and vegetables that wind up in the bellies of livestock that graze on grass and are in turn eaten by people. These chemicals are stored (bioaccumulate) in the fatty tissues of animals, including humans. From these tissues they are released slowly into the bloodstream, causing chronic damage. Though DDT, PCBs, and CFCs are now banned in the United States, they remain in the environment in large quantities.

**Dioxins** are a group of unwanted chemical by-products formed during the production of some chlorinated petrochemicals, including herbicides (plant-killing chemicals). Their potential hazards came to public attention during the Vietnam war, when a dioxin-containing herbicide called Agent Orange was used to clear the jungles so that enemy troops would be revealed. The Vietnamese, U.S. soldiers, and domestic animals exposed to Agent Orange suffered various health problems. Dioxin is a possible carcinogen, although it would appear to account for a very small percentage of cases of cancer.[17] However, even low levels of dioxin—the levels consumed by average Americans—can cause other health complications, such as birth defects and infertility. Dioxin gets into our food supply when residues from industrial incinerators settle on grass, which is eaten by cows, absorbed into their fat, and passed along to us in meat and dairy products.

**Biodegradation** The process of natural decay and absorption into the environment.

**Ozone Layer** The ozone-rich layer of the earth's upper atmosphere that helps to limit the amount of ultraviolet radiation that reaches the earth.

**Ozone** A highly reactive form of oxygen toxic even at low levels in inhaled air.

**Food chain** The sequence in which organisms feed on smaller or less complex organisms and are consumed by larger or more complex organisms.

**Dioxins** Highly toxic chlorinated hydrocarbons, formed during industrial processes from the heating of substances containing chlorine.

**Polychlorinated biphenyls (PCBs)** Highly toxic organochlorines used in various manufacturing processes, but now banned in the U.S.

**Solvents** Chemical liquids that dissolve other substances.

**Polychlorinated biphenyls,** or **PCBs,** are highly toxic organochlorines that were used in electric transformers as insulators and coolants, as well as in lubricants, pesticides, plastic, inks, and paper. Petrochemical facilities widely discharged PCBs into rivers. Because of mounting suspicions that PCBs cause birth defects and cancer, they were banned in 1979. Like dioxins, however, they persist in the environment today. They are found in old refrigerators and other household appliances, in toxic waste sites, in bodies of water, and in soil. They continue to contaminate food, fish, and wildlife, and are absorbed by people in foods. Fetal exposure to PCBs can result in lower IQ and problems with memory and paying attention during childhood.[18] PCBs can also be passed to infants in the mother's milk and can affect adults' reproductive systems.[19]

**Talking Glossary**
Polychlorinated biphenyls
G2206

**Solvents** **Solvents** are petrochemical liquids that dissolve other substances. Solvents are used as oil and paint thinners (such as turpentine), aerosols, dry-cleaning agents, glues, fingernail polish, typewriter correction fluid, and bleaches. Some solvents contain chlorine (and thus are organochlorines); others contain alcohol (methanol); and still others contain acids (acetone).

*Perchloroethylene* is a solvent used as a dry-cleaning agent and in pesticides. Because it is known to cause cancer in animals, care should be taken to avoid inhaling it, a problem faced by people working in the dry-cleaning business or living near a dry-cleaning plant. As a general safety rule, consumers should air out dry-cleaned clothing for several hours before wearing it. Some brands of nail polish contain *toluene,* another toxic petrochemical linked to chronic liver and kidney damage.

Many widely used chlorinated solvents, including *trichloroethylene* and *methylene chloride,* are also suspected carcinogens. Furniture strippers and other paint solvents often contain methylene chloride. Trichloroethylene is an extremely common solvent used in paint strippers, rug cleaners, spot removers, typewriter correction fluids, and industrial cleaners. It has also been found in the water supplies of numerous communities across the United States.[20]

PREVENTION

## Using Solvents Safely

All toxic substances must be handled with care. When using solvents and other toxic products, follow these precautions:

- *Read the label.* Look for warnings like "danger," "hazardous substance," or "caution." Note whether the ingredients are flammable. Follow directions carefully, including directions for disposal.
- *Wear a face mask when using solvents, especially when the directions include warnings such as "Avoid breathing dust."*
- *Wear plastic or vinyl gloves.*
- *Do not allow children in newly painted rooms or near workplaces where solvents are used.*
- *Do not smoke while using solvents or use them near an open flame.*

According to the California State Department of Health Services, over 60 different solvents are commonly used in consumer products. The most common are ethanol, isopropyl, kerosene, propylene glycol, isobutane, and propane. With *proper use,* none is highly toxic. Nonetheless, about 250 tons per day of these materials are released into California's air, contributing to the pollution problem.

The following solvents pose greater health risks. The first group should not be used. They consist of known or suspected carcinogens. The second group is less toxic but still quite dangerous and should be used only with extreme care:

*Do not use* (known or suspected carcinogens): benzene, carbon tetrachloride, chloroform, ethylene dichloride, perchloroethylene, dioxane.

*Use with extreme care:* toluene, xylene, methylene chloride, styrene, methyl cellosolve, phenol, ketones.

Manufacturers are required by law to provide warning labels and directions for safe use on the packaging of hazardous products and to list known or suspected carcinogens. However, they are not required to provide a detailed listing of ingredients of many common household products. To find out about the safety of many kinds of products, you can contact the U.S. Consumer Product Safety Commission in Washington, D.C.

**Pesticides** Pesticides are chemical poisons used to kill "pests" such as insects, rodents, and weeds. Pesticides have clear benefits; they allow farmers to produce more plentiful crops on smaller acreages. Like other toxins, pesticides may be natural or synthetic.

**Natural pesticides** include toxins produced by certain insects, plants, and even mixtures containing metals and metallic-like elements such as mercury and arsenic. Manufactured or **synthetic pesticides** include insecticides, herbicides, and fungicides, among others. As their names imply, insecticides kill insects, herbicides kill plants, and fungicides kill fungi (molds and mildew).

Close-up
What is a pesticide?
T2203

There are some 40,000 synthetic pesticides in use today, containing about 600 active ingredients. These products range from moth crystals and tick collars to powerful defoliants. Pesticides are most widely used on food crops such as wheat, corn, and soybeans. They are also routinely spread on lawns and gardens to keep them free of pests. Synthetic pesticide use has nearly doubled since the 1960s. Approximately 800 million to 1 billion pounds of pesticides are applied to crops each year.[21] Even with this massive assault, however, about one-third of the world's food crops are lost to pests.[22]

The use of synthetic pesticides presents society with hard choices. When first introduced some 50 years ago, they were hailed as "miracle workers" that would halt the devastation of crops, ease the labor of farming, and eliminate famines and insect-borne plagues. These hopes were borne out to a degree. But during the decades that followed, public attention shifted to the risks posed by pesticides. For example, DDT (like many other synthetic pesticides) does not discriminate between unwanted pests and "good" insects and other forms of wildlife. Pesticides not only kill insects and other pests; they can also harm wildlife, plant life, aquatic life, and people. Agricultural workers and people living near farms face the greatest risk from pesticide exposure, including toxic effects from acute exposure. Yet we are all at risk of some level of exposure. Pesticides contaminate soil, air, plant life, and water and can be absorbed by humans and other animals through the skin, inhaled, or ingested.

Close-up
DDT and breast cancer
T2204

**Organochlorine Pesticides** Some of the better known—and more dangerous—pes-

**Natural pesticides** Toxins produced by insects and plants that are used to eradicate pests.

**Synthetic pesticides** Manufactured or synthesized pest-killing substances, including insecticides, herbicides, and fungicides.

ticides are organochlorines such as DDT, heptachlor, chlordane, and lindane. Lindane (brand name Kwell) is used to kill head lice and pubic lice. The FDA advises parents not to overuse lindane because of possible toxic effects.[23] The other three are known or suspected carcinogens and have been banned for most uses in the United States. They are still manufactured in the U.S. for export, however, and continue to be produced in other countries. As a result, contaminated foods continue to enter the U.S. in what environmentalists call the **circle of poison.** The circle of poison refers to the practice of exporting banned chemicals to other, often poor, countries, where they are then used to produce food products that are in turn sent back to the country that banned and exported the chemicals. Heptachlor and chlordane, for example, have returned to the U.S. in beef and milk products. Consumers are often unaware that they are buying contaminated products from their supermarkets.

Talking Glossary
Organophosphates
G2207

**Organophosphate Pesticides** A second class of potentially dangerous pesticides is the **organophosphates**—chemicals containing phosphorus, oxygen, and sometimes sulfur. In addition to their use as pesticides, organophosphates are used in chemical weapons. Not all organophosphates are highly toxic, but many are, such as parathion. Though strictly regulated in the U.S., parathion continues to be used on many agricultural crops and is a leading cause of farm worker poisoning. Parathion is a neurotoxin that poisons on contact. Symptoms range from dizziness to convulsions and death due to respiratory failure. Parathion is also a suspected carcinogen. Chemical spills of parathion have caused massive fish kills.

Talking Glossary
Synthetic pyrethroid
G2208

**Safer Alternatives to Pesticides** Many pests are now resistant to the organophosphate and organochlorine pesticides. Partly out of necessity, and partly in response to the public outcry over their health risks, pesticide manufacturers are producing fewer toxic and persistent products called *botanicals,* or *biological pesticides.* Chief among them are insecticides based on **synthetic pyrethroid,** which is similar to a natural insecticide present in certain chrysanthemums. The pyrethroids are fairly low in toxicity, are quick-acting on insects, and do not persist in the environment as long as the organochlorines and organophosphates. Also, they are not absorbed into the skin as much. But they *are* moderately to highly toxic when swallowed, so caution in handling remains essential. There is an ever-growing number of synthetic pyrethroid products. Two of the most common are resmethrin and pemethrin. Resmethrin is an indoor flying insect killer. Pemethrin is used in flea sprays and in agriculture.

Gardeners can also buy Dipel, the trade name for a bacterial agent called *Bacillus thuringiensis.* Dipel attacks caterpillars and other insects in the worm stage. Many kinds of insecticidal soaps, especially those manufactured by the company Safer Products, attack aphids and other pests.

**Circle of poison** The practice of exporting banned chemicals to other, often poorer, countries; they are used in products sent back to the original country.

**Organophosphates** Chemical compounds, many of which are toxic, used as pesticides and as chemical weapons.

**Synthetic pyrethroid** A pesticide lethal to insects but with low toxicity to humans.

PREVENTION

## *Minimizing the Risks of Household Pesticides*

Pesticides are poisons. Each year, thousands of farm workers fall ill from exposure to pesticides, and hospitals routinely treat people who mishandle weed killers and other household pesticides. Yet we are all exposed to pesticides in the foods we eat and the air we breathe.

***Health Exposure to Household Pesticides*** You are likely to be exposed to greater concentrations of pesticides in the home than outdoors (where they are dispersed more widely).[24] Some indoor exposure comes from emissions from lawn treatments wafting into the home, but much household exposure comes from the use of an arsenal of powerful pesticides lurking under the sink or stuck on a shelf in the hall closet.[25] Indoor exposure is greatest in cold weather, when houses are sealed tight, and immediately following lawn treatments (including your neighbors' lawns) during spring and summer.

Three of four American households use pesticides, most often to get rid of ants and cockroaches. The average household has three to four pesticides, ranging from pest strips and bait boxes to flea shampoos for the family dog. All told there are more than 20,000 different pesticides containing more than 300 active ingredients used in the home. Household pests are not only pesty but potentially dangerous. Many people are allergic to shedded cockroach parts, and stings and bites from ants and other pests can be life-threatening to some people. Many pests carry disease-causing organisms. But while it makes good health sense to keep our homes free of pests, we need to consider the consequences of overuse

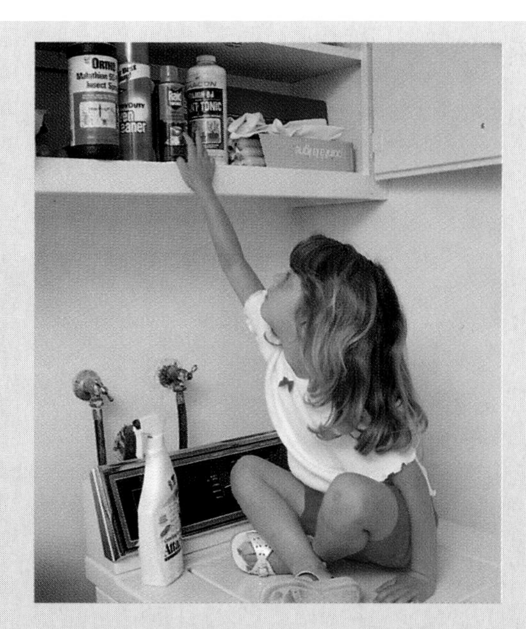

***Preventing Household Poisonings*** Never leave household chemicals in places that are within children's reach or accessible to them.

and unwise use of common pesticides. For example, 140,000 pesticide exposures were reported to poison control centers in 1993. The great majority (93%) involved home use of pesticides. More than half of these incidents involved children under the age of five. The reported exposures may be the tip of the proverbial iceberg, as many more cases (millions perhaps) may involve the effects of chronic exposure that go unrecognized or misdiagnosed.

***Health Risks of Chronic Exposure*** Though most household pesticides have low toxicity, researchers are concerned that chronic exposure may affect bodily systems such as the nervous system and the immune system. Children are at greatest risk of pesticide-related health problems. Yard and household use of pesticides has been linked to an increased risk of some forms of childhood cancer.[26]

**Take Charge**
Protecting children from pesticides and lead poisoning
**C2201**

***Safety Tips for Using Household Pesticides*** If you must use household pesticides, the basic rule to follow is to minimize exposure as much as possible. Be especially careful with infants and young children. Here are some specific tips:[27]

- *Read all application labels carefully, and assume that children are still more sensitive than the labels indicate.*
- *Store pesticides away from children and pets—and you.* Never transfer pesticides to soft-drink bottles or other containers that you or your children might mistake for something to eat or drink.
- *Rinse, peel, and skin fruits whenever possible.* Scrub vegetables thoroughly.
- *If you use pesticides indoors, make certain that there is adequate ventilation and keep children away.* Cover all food when using airborne insecticides. If you hire a pest control company to rid your home of cockroaches, ants, or other pests, closely monitor the workers' activities.
- *Follow a stepwise approach for eliminating pests.* Begin with first-line defenses, such as screens. Next, employ baits (like Combat) or traps. Then, and only if necessary, should you consider using airborne insecticides. Only when absolutely necessary should you consider fumigation or "foggers" to exterminate such pests as termites or fleas. Use a professional exterminator and keep the family away from the fumigated area until it is thoroughly ventilated (at least overnight). Cover all dishes, food, and cooking equipment during the procedure. Make sure the exterminator does not use chlordane-based products. Afterward, thoroughly clean any area where the spray may have settled. If you have questions regarding the safety of the chemicals, call the Food and Drug Administration (FDA).
- *Stay off chemically treated lawns until pesticides have settled into the soil.* Keep children and pets off them as well. If you are applying professional-grade chemicals, hire a licensed firm to do it. You can also consider ways of protecting your lawn without chemicals, or choose to live with a less than perfect lawn that is safe for children and animals.
- When in contact with pesticides, *wear rubber gloves and cover yourself from head to toe in protective clothing.* Most pesticide poisoning occurs through skin contamination. Wear protective eye coverings. If walking in pesticide-covered areas, wear rubber boots. Close windows if pesticides are used in your yard or a nearby yard. Clean and vacuum furniture and flooring where pesticide residue may fall.
- *Use flea collars (pest strips) only with caution, especially if children pet the animal.* Ask your veterinarian about risks posed by flea collars and possible alternatives. Avoid flea collars containing organophosphates.
- *Discontinue pesticide use at the first sign of dizziness, headache, eye, nose, throat, or skin irritation, and immediately consult a health care provider.*

## Radiation—The Benefits, the Risks

**Radiation** (radiant energy) is the release of energy in the form of waves or particles. The wave form of radiation is called **electromagnetic radiation.** Elec-

**Radiation** The emission of energy in the form of particles or waves.

**Electromagnetic radiation** Radiation in the form of electromagnetic waves, including radio waves, X-rays, gamma waves, and microwaves.

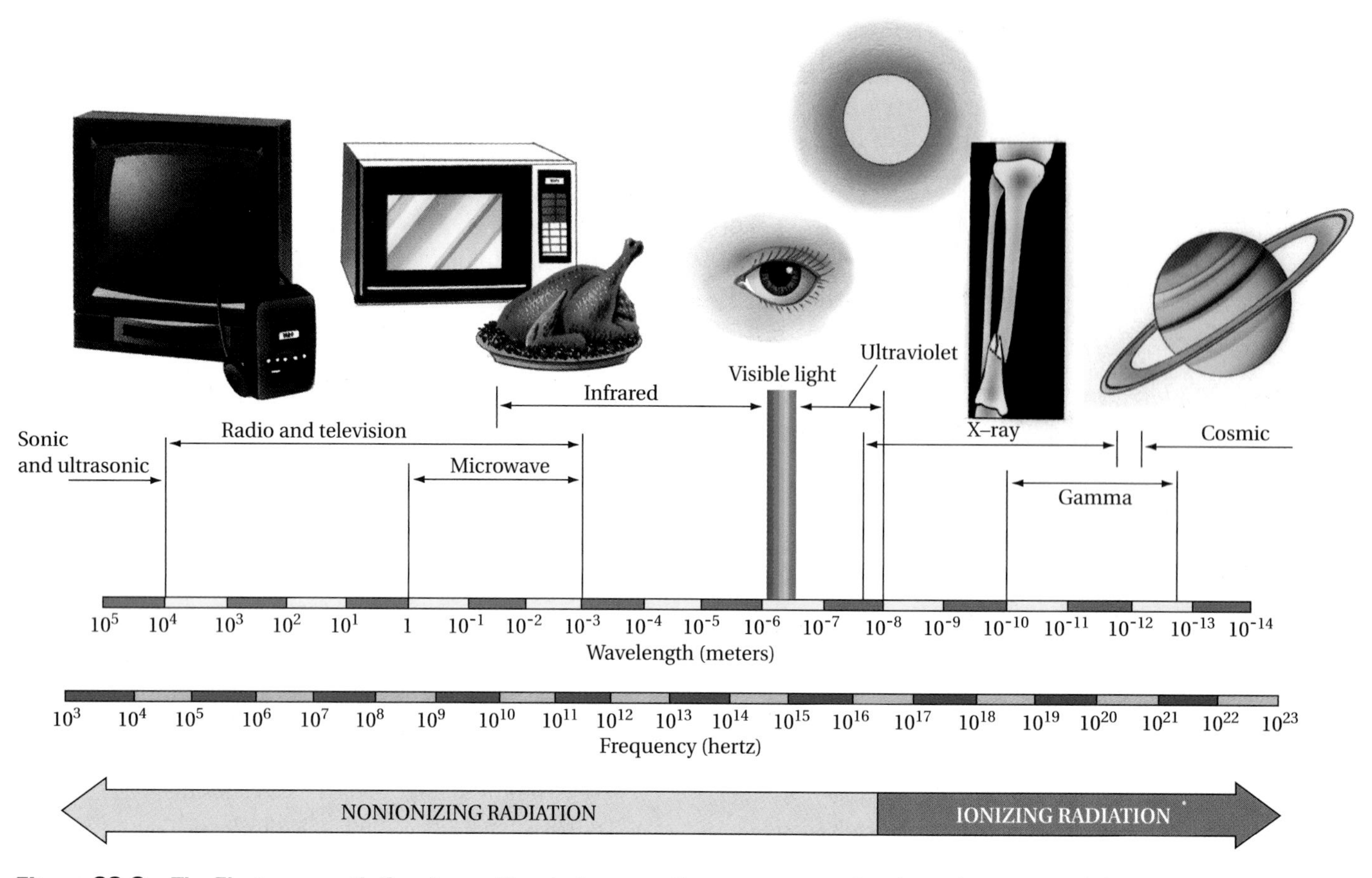


**Figure 22.2** ***The Electromagnetic Spectrum*** The electromagnetic spectrum contains the various types of electromagnetic, or waveform, radiation. We can sense only a small portion of the electromagnetic spectrum, principally within the range of visible light.

tromagnetic radiation includes visible light, ultraviolet light, X-rays, radio waves, microwaves, and other rays of the **electromagnetic spectrum** (see Figure 22.2). We can see only the portion of the electromagnetic spectrum referred to as visible light. Shorter-wave radiation, such as X-rays, is more powerful and poses more potential health risks than longer-wave radiation, such as radio and television signals. The shorter wavelengths pack more energy.

**Particle radiation** involves the emission of bits of atoms—electrons, protons, and neutrons—that spin out at high velocities during the natural decay of radioactive substances, from nuclear bomb blasts, and from nuclear reactor accidents. **Cosmic rays** are another form of particle radiation. They are bursts of energy originating from outer space.

Some elements, such as uranium and radium, are naturally radioactive. They constantly emit waves or particles. Nuclear reactors and accelerators manufacture artificial radioactive substances. These substances are used in medicine, agriculture, food preservation, and consumer products such as smoke detectors.

The word *radiation* may conjure up images of weapons of mass destruction or of nuclear reactor accidents, but the use of artificial radiation has on the whole been positive. Lives have been saved by radiotherapy. Because radiation kills bacteria in food, irradiated food products have longer shelf lives. Radiation has also been used to cause mutations in seeds, making some food crops more resistant to pests. The end of the cold war put a halt to the massive buildup of nuclear weapons. But in its place, we face the "hot" and dangerous task of disposing of this arsenal and of the radioactive wastes used in its assembly. Disposing of radioactive wastes produced by nuclear power plants and hospitals is yet another environmental challenge and potential health risk. There also remain the risks of nuclear power plant and transport accidents.

**Electromagnetic spectrum** The entire range of electromagnetic radiation.

**Particle radiation** Radiation consisting of the emission of subatomic matter, such as protons, neutrons, and electrons.

**Cosmic rays** A form of high-energy, particle radiation originating in outer space.

**Use of Radiation in Dentistry and Medicine** The use of radiation in diagnostic medical procedures, such as X-rays, computerized tomography scans (CAT scans), and other imaging techniques, allows health professionals to probe deep within the body without surgery. Mammograms, or specialized breast X-rays, can detect tumors before they can be felt. Dental X-rays reveal tooth and bone decay, allowing treatment before serious damage results.

**Nuclear medicine** is the branch of medicine that uses radiation to diagnose and treat disease. Ionizing (X-ray) radiation is used to treat certain forms of cancer, including breast cancer. Nonionizing radiation, such as infrared light, has helped speed recovery from muscle injuries. Physicians also inject small amounts, or "traces," of radioactive chemical substances, called **radioisotopes,** into the patient's bloodstream and then follow their movements in the body by means of specialized detecting equipment. Tracers bind to specific tissues or organs, allowing physicians to visualize and detect tumors and other abnormalities. Radioisotopes are also used in the treatment of thyroid disorders and other health problems. Physicians also use injectable radioactive substances to detect blockages in blood vessels in and around the heart.

Talking Glossary
Radioisotopes
G2209

**Ionizing vs. Nonionizing Radiation** **Ions** are electrically charged atoms or groups of atoms. Atoms become positively charged when they lose electrons and negatively charged when they gain electrons.

**Ionizing radiation** is powerful, high-energy radiation that is capable of causing atoms to become electrically charged or ionized. Sources of ionizing radiation include X-rays, **gamma rays,** cosmic rays, radiation emitted from nuclear power plant accidents, and radiation emitted naturally from radioactive substances such as uranium and radium. Ionizing radiation is more hazardous than nonionizing radiation because it emits the more dangerous, shorter wavelengths. Ionizing radiation can change the DNA structure within a cell's chromosomes, which can destroy the cell's ability to replicate. It can also lead to cancer. The cancer risk depends upon the intensity and length of exposure.

Exposure to radiation is measured in **rads** (radiation absorption doses). The average person is exposed to 360 mrads (an mrad is 1/1000 of a rad) of ionizing radiation a year.[28] Most of the radiation to which we are exposed comes from natural sources—rocks and soil, radon, and cosmic rays. X-rays account for about 11% of the average person's exposure to radiation. Acute exposure levels as low as 50 rads can cause **radiation sickness,** which causes nausea, fatigue, anemia, bleeding from the mouth and gums, hair loss, and immune system disorders. Higher doses have more severe effects, including death. A dose of 800 rads is fatal to humans, though some deaths occur with as little as 200 rads. There is no agreed-upon "safe" level of exposure to radiation, but average levels of exposure have minimal health risks. Long-term exposure to higher-than-average levels of radiation may cause serious health problems, including cancer.

In 1986, high levels of ionizing radiation instantly killed 31 people in the immediate vicinity of the Chernobyl nuclear power plant accident in the former Soviet Union—the world's worst such accident. The radiation released was nearly 200 times greater than that from the 1945 atomic bomb blasts at Hiroshima and Nagasaki combined.[29] Nearby people who survived suffered severe damage to skin, bone marrow, and the gastrointestinal tract. Thousands of villages in the area became uninhabitable. Radioactive fallout was spread by the wind to some 20 countries. Grass eaten by lambs in Wales, milk drunk by Poles, and air breathed by Swedes all became contaminated.

**Nonionizing radiation** does not produce ions. Common sources of nonionizing radiation include ultraviolet light (sunlight), electrical appliances, computers and televisions, and high-voltage power lines. Nonionizing radiation is less dangerous than ionizing radiation but can still cause harm. The most plentiful source of nonionizing radiation is sunlight, which can damage the skin, leading to premature wrinkling and skin cancer. The evidence of health

**Nuclear medicine** The medical use of radiation in the diagnosis and treatment of illness.

**Radioisotope** A radioactive form of an element; some are used in medical diagnosis and treatment.

**Ions** Atoms or atomic particles bearing positive or negative charges.

**Ionizing radiation** Powerful, high-energy radiation capable of changing the structure of atoms.

**Gamma rays** High-energy, penetrating ionizing radiation emitted from the nucleus of a radioactive atom.

**Rad** Short for *radiation absorbed dose,* a measure of exposure to radiation; represents the amount of ionizing radiation that a body absorbs per unit mass of matter.

**Radiation sickness** Illness caused by overexposure to radiation; may be fatal at high levels.

**Nonionizing radiation** Radiation that does not cause atoms to become ions, e.g., sunlight and radiation emitted by electrical appliances.

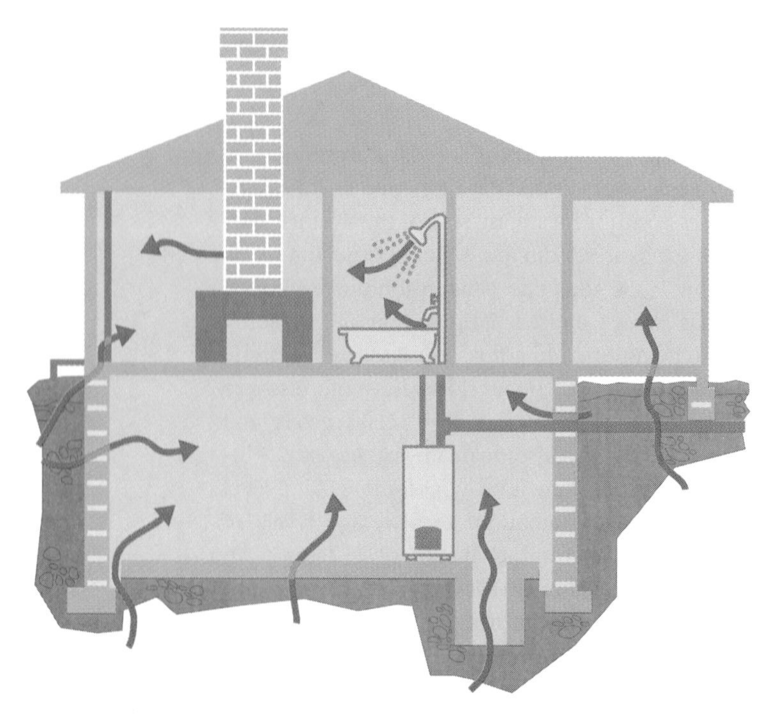

**Figure 22.3** ***How Radon Enters Your Home*** Radon can seep into our homes through cracks in the floor or foundation, through exposed soil, and around pipe fittings. Radon can also enter the water supply in the home and pass into the household air whenever you turn on the shower or faucet. *Source:* Adapted from *Live Longer Live Better,* © 1995 The Reader's Digest Association, Inc. Used by permission of the Reader's Digest Association, Inc.

risks is mixed and inconclusive for other forms of nonionizing radiation, such as the energy emitted from electrical equipment and electric power lines. Let us take a closer look at the effects of two common sources of ionizing radiation—radon and X-rays—and two common sources of nonionizing radiation—ultraviolet light and electromagnetic radiation.

**Radon** Most of our exposure to ionizing radiation comes from natural rather than human-made sources, such as cosmic rays and radioactive elements in the earth. The greatest single source is **radon,** a radioactive gas emitted during the natural decay of the element uranium. Outdoors, radon presents little danger, except for underground miners exposed to high levels on the job. However, radon in the ground can enter our homes, schools, and office buildings through cracks or pores in concrete floors and walls, floor drains, sump pumps, joints, hollow-block walls, stone fireplaces, well water, and dirt floors (see Figure 22.3). Radon gas that becomes trapped in buildings may be inhaled. Tiny radioactive particles of radon may become lodged in the lungs, where they can accumulate and possibly cause lung cancer. Since radon is fat soluble, it can also become lodged in bone marrow, which may lead to leukemia.[30] High levels of radon are found in parts of every state in the United States.[31]

Radon cannot be detected by our senses. The FDA has called for radon testing in every home and for correcting the problem when the gas exceeds a certain threshold level. This level is exceeded in about 6% of U.S. homes.[32] Though the risk of radon exposure to the health of the average person remains uncertain, it is prudent to reduce radon exposure by taking the steps outlined in the nearby ***Prevention*** feature.

**Radon** A radioactive gas emitted from the natural decay of uranium.

**X-ray** High-energy, ionizing radiation; can penetrate most solid objects and project images on photographic film.

**Computerized tomography scan (CAT scan)** A type of X-ray that provides computerized, three-dimensional images of internal body structures by passing X-ray beams through the body at different angles.

PREVENTION

### *Reducing Exposure to Radon*

Nearly 1 American home in 15 contains radon. Because of concern about the possible health risks of radon, the EPA and the Surgeon General recommend that all homes at ground level be tested for radon. Testing is relatively easy and inexpensive. EPA-approved "do-it-yourself" kits are available in local hardware stores. You can also hire EPA-qualified or state-certified radon testers.

Getting rid of radon may be as simple and straightforward as opening basement and first-floor windows and vents, which allows the gas to escape. But this method may lead to loss of heat (or air-conditioning) and security concerns. Other procedures include sealing basements and installing ventilation systems. Your state department of environmental protection can assist you in obtaining testing devices, interpreting results, and determining strategies for reducing radon levels in the home. A phone call will start the process.

**X-Rays** **X-rays** are waves of electromagnetic radiation of very short wavelengths. They penetrate the body and project images of internal structures onto photographic film to reveal abnormalities, such as broken bones, tumors, and tooth decay. The **computerized tomography scan (CAT scan)** combines the X-ray with computer imaging. A CAT scan beams X-rays at the body from different angles. The computer analyzes the results to project a three-dimensional image of the inner structures of the body on a monitor. The dose of radiation emitted by X-ray machines is fairly small, and the risk of harm very low. However, X-rays are not entirely risk-free, especially if the procedure is repeated often. Repeated X-rays can increase the risk of cancer and genetic damage. X-rays are especially risky to pregnant women and should be avoided unless they are essential. Some other cautions are outlined in the accompanying ***Prevention*** feature.

## PREVENTION

### *Practicing X-Ray Safety*

These guidelines can help you ensure that X-rays are used appropriately and safely:[33]

1. *Ask the doctor why an X-ray is needed.* Chest X-rays are no longer considered routine. Chest X-rays and other X-rays should be used only when the results might affect medical treatment or outcomes.
2. *Don't insist that your doctor perform an X-ray test.* An X-ray should only be taken only when your doctor or dentist believes it is necessary. On the other hand . . .
3. *Don't refuse an X-ray procedure because of fear of the harmful effects of ionizing radiation.* Not having an X-ray when it is medically indicated may pose a greater risk than the small exposure to radiation.
4. *Make sure your doctor or medical technician knows when you are pregnant or suspect that you might be.* X-rays can affect the fetus.
5. *If reproductive organs are to be in the direct X-ray beam, request a lead shield.* (Shielding cannot be used when X-rays are taken *of* the reproductive organs.)
6. *Keep a record of X-ray examinations.* Retrieving previous X-rays sometimes eliminates the need for new ones or can provide doctors with information about changes in internal organs over time.

**Ultraviolet (UV) Radiation.** **Ultraviolet (UV) radiation** is radiation in the form of sunlight. Two different types of UV radiation pose threats to our health: UV-A and UV-B. Both types lie in the nonionizing portion of the electromagnetic spectrum. UV-B radiation is the shorter of the two and thus the more hazardous, but both can damage the skin and eyes.

The ozone layer provides a limited amount of protection against UV-B radiation. Sunburns are caused by overexposure to UV-B rays. UV-B rays can cause cataracts if eyes aren't protected with UV-blocking sunglasses. They can also lead to skin cancer (see Chapter 18). The steep rise in skin cancers in recent years may be linked to the increased popularity of sunbathing, perhaps in combination with the thinning of the ozone layer.

**Electromagnetic Fields (EMFs)** **Electromagnetic fields (EMFs)** are forms of nonionizing electromagnetic radiation emitted from electric power lines and electrical appliances and consumer products found in homes and offices. Toasters and televisions, electric blankets and hair dryers, microwave ovens and computer monitors—all produce invisible electromagnetic fields. Electric appliances emit electric fields even when they are turned off, as long as they remain plugged into electrical sockets. They must be turned on, however, to produce EMFs, which are combinations of electric and magnetic fields.

EMFs are strongest at their source and weaken with distance. Magnetic fields are more of a concern for health, because unlike electric fields, they pass through the body. The power of the magnetic field from planet earth is 200 to 300 times greater than the levels emitted from electric power lines and appliances.[34] Yet the earth's magnetic field is relatively constant and doesn't change direction. In contrast, magnetic fields associated with EMFs alternate (change direction) 120 times per second. Some scientists believe this may make a difference in how they affect us.

Just how significant is the health threat posed by EMFs? An expert panel convened by the National Research Council concluded that despite more than 500 **epidemiological studies,** there was still no convincing evidence that exposure to electromagnetic radiation from electric power lines or household appliances causes cancer or other health problems.[35] Moreover, a recent large-scale study showed no evidence linking childhood leukemia to exposure to electric power lines.[36] The National Academy of Sciences does not believe that there is enough evidence of a health hazard from EMFs generated by household appliances, computer monitors, or electric power lines to take action.

**Close-up**
More on EMFs and cancer
**T2205**

Concerns have also been raised about potential health hazards associated with using hand-held cellu-

**Ultraviolet (UV) radiation** Radiation from the sun in the form of sunlight.

**Electromagnetic fields (EMFs)** Alternating electrical and magnetic fields that act as a source of nonionizing radiation.

**Epidemiological studies** Studies of the causes and control of epidemic diseases or of differences in disease rates between populations.

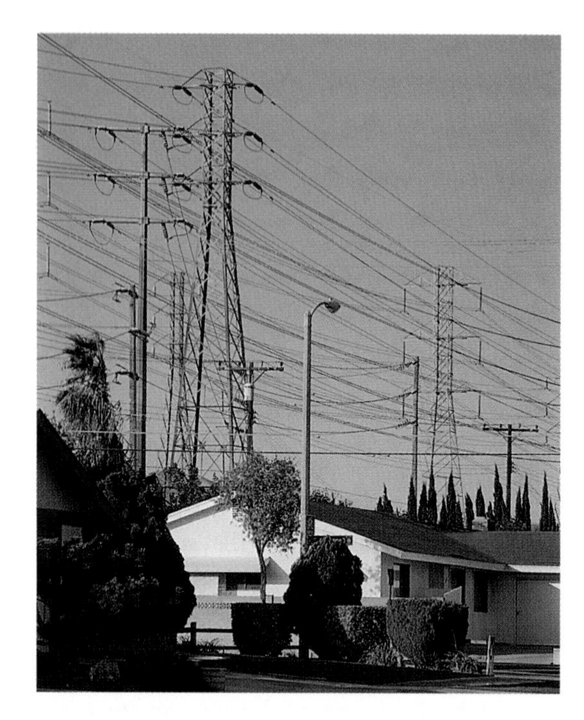

***Electric Power Lines—A Health Risk?*** Despite more than 500 studies, scientists have failed to find convincing evidence that exposure to electromagnetic radiation from electric power lines or household appliances causes cancer or other health problems.

lar phones. These devices operate at frequencies nearly 15 million times higher than electrical appliances in the house. (Portable cordless phones used in the home operate at very low frequencies.) Despite the public outcry for an investigation after a man claimed on a national talk show that his wife had died of brain cancer caused by the use of cellular telephones, the FDA has found no proof that use of cellular phones is harmful. However, the agency did not rule out any possible risk, submitting that it simply did not have enough information to reach a definitive conclusion. Meanwhile, the agency advises users of cellular phones that they might minimize potential risks by keeping conversations short or by using a semiportable phone in which the power supply and antenna are separated from the handset, which itself emits no radio waves. Or use a car phone connected to an antenna mounted on the outside of the car.[37]

**Extremely low-frequency electromagnetic radiation (ELF)** A type of nonionizing radiation emitted by electrical appliances.

**Microwaves** A type of nonionizing radiation, characterized by extremely high-frequency electromagnetic waves; cause molecules to vibrate rapidly, producing heat.

Apart from possible radiation dangers, a recent study found cell phone users were four times more likely to get into an automobile accident when they were using their car phones than when they were not.[38] Driving and using a car phone is about as dangerous as driving with a blood alcohol level at the legal limit. Researchers claim that the danger comes from a loss of concentration, not from fiddling with the phone itself. If you do need to use a car phone, keep conversations brief and avoid unnecessary calls or calls in dangerous driving situations. Better yet, pull off the road if you need to use the phone.

**Extremely Low-Frequency Electromagnetic Radiation (ELFs)** Computer monitors, TVs, radios, microwave ovens, and other home and office appliances emit **extremely low-frequency electromagnetic radiation,** or **ELFs.** Since many of us spend hours each day in close contact with ELF-producing equipment, concerns about health risks are understandable. Though no one has demonstrated a causal link between exposure to ELFs and health problems, research continues. In the meantime, one can reduce exposure to EMFs (including ELFs) by not sitting or standing too close to the TV, microwave oven, computer monitor, or other appliances when they are turned on; by avoiding or limiting use of electric blankets; and by placing one's alarm clock at least three feet from one's head.

**Microwaves** are forms of electromagnetic radiation used in radar, radio and television transmitters, and microwave ovens. In microwave ovens, microwaves cause water molecules in food to vibrate very fast. The vibrations produce heat, which cooks the food. Microwave-cooked food is not radioactive, and microwave ovens, when used and maintained properly, pose no health risks. Still, microwave ovens may leak radiation, so it is best to check the seal on the door regularly.

It remains uncertain whether exposure to ELFs from computer monitors (video display terminals, or VDTs) poses any health risks.[39] A recent review reported reassuring evidence that using monitors during pregnancy did not pose a risk of miscarriages, birth defects, or low birth weights.[40] Nonetheless, it would be prudent to observe these safety precautions:

1. *Select a low-radiation computer monitor—one that meets the Swedish MRII standard for low ELF emissions.*
2. *Sit 28 inches or more from the computer screen (about an arm's length away).* ELF emissions fall off sharply at distances beyond 28 inches.

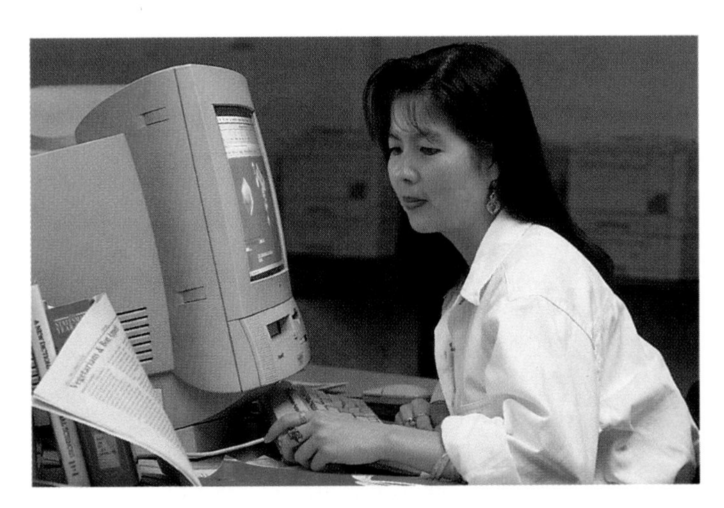

***Keeping Your Distance*** To limit your exposure to ELFs, you should sit at least 28 inches away from your computer screen, which is about an arm's length away (farther away than this young woman is sitting).

3. *Do not sit within five feet of the back or side of other computer terminals.* Greater levels of ELF emissions are found to the sides and rear of computer terminals than in front. Workers in offices where computer operators are stationed side by side or facing one another are most at risk of ELF exposure from other workers' terminals.

Smart Quiz
Q2201

## think about it!

- **What toxic chemicals are lurking in your home right now? Pesticides? Lead? Asbestos? How can you find out? How should you handle them?**
- **Would you question a doctor who wants you to have an X-ray? Why or why not?**
- **What do you do when you are near a lawn or trees that are being sprayed? What *should* you do?**

**critical thinking How has technology improved the quality of life? How has it threatened the environment and health?**

# OVERPOPULATION

The population of planet earth is about 6 billion people—more than double the number of just 40 years ago. If present trends continue, the world population will jump to 9 billion by the year 2041.[41]

The population is growing at a rate of 1.5% annually. This may not sound like much, but it translates into more than 225,000 additional people each and every day! There are more and more people to house and feed when only about 15% of the world's current population, fewer than 1 billion people, have the basic resources—ample and nutritious food, clean water, and basic health care—needed to sustain them. Today, more than a billion people, about one person in four, live in poverty. With projections of more than 3 billion more human inhabitants by the middle of the next century, there is the prospect of widespread famine and epidemics spread by contaminated water supplies and inadequate health care.

Smart Reference
Global fertility and population
R2201

The most explosive growth is taking place in developing countries in Asia, Africa, and Latin America. India, the world's fastest growing country, is expected to surpass the population of the world's currently most populous country, China, by the year 2025.[42] Developing countries account for about 95% of the world's population growth. They also contain the greatest share of poor people.

Industrialized nations, the U.S. and Canada included, are also growing, but at slower rates. Nonetheless, the U.S. population is expected to increase by about 25% by the year 2025. Though industrialized nations account for a minority of the world's population, they consume about 85% of the world's wealth and material goods.[43] The U.S. alone, with only 4% of the world's population, consumes one-quarter of the world's annual production of oil.[44]

## Ecological Threats of Overpopulation

As the world's human population increases, so do demands for food and shelter. The population explosion threatens the earth's **carrying capacity**—the maximum number of organisms it can support without degrading the environment. Sixty percent of the world's people still rely on wood for cooking, posing an ever-growing threat of deforestation. Some damage to wilderness, forested, and jungle areas is caused by pollution from factories and fossil-fuel-burning vehicles and homes. Other damage is caused by ever-expanding human development—the clearing of undeveloped land for agriculture, the cutting of large tracts of timber for housing, and the clear-

**Carrying capacity** The maximum number of organisms that can be supported without degrading the environment.

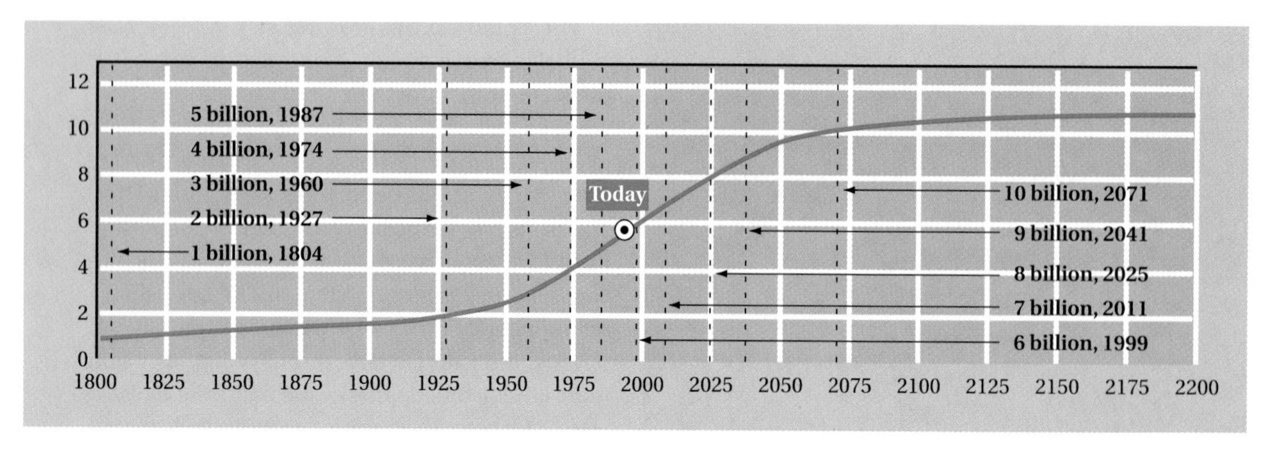


**Figure 22.4** ***World Population Growth*** World population continues to expand, though not quite as fast as experts had expected. Still, world population, now nearly 5.8 billion, is expected to level off by the end of the twenty-first century at 10.73 billion according to a recent United Nations study.

ing of forested areas for roads and houses. The world has lost one-fifth of its rain forests and one-fifth of its topsoil since 1950. Topsoil provides nutrients for plants and holds their roots in place. The depletion of topsoil is mainly caused by human factors such as pollution, the paving of roads and pouring of foundations for housing developments, and failure to allow fields to lie fallow. People in developing nations are caught in the squeeze between protecting the land and the need to feed an ever-growing number of people. Thus many of them do not allow enough time between plantings to let nutrients build back up in the soil.

## Health Threats of Overpopulation

The reduction in rain forests and other wilderness areas has also led to the extinction of tens of thousands of plant and animal species.[45] As tropical rain forests are cleared for development, people are coming into contact with insects and other carriers of once-remote diseases, leading to outbreaks of diseases that people have little or no defense against. At the same time, more poor people around the globe are leaving rural areas and crowding into cities ill equipped to handle their needs, leading to unsanitary conditions that serve as a breeding ground for disease.

There is also some good news to report on the population front. Though population growth worldwide continues to rise, the rate of increase has slowed in recent years (see Figure 22.4). Widespread use of contraceptives has decreased fertility rates.[46] Contraceptive use increased from 9% of total married couples of reproductive age in the 1960s to more than 50% of couples in the 1990s. Still, in today's world, the average woman bears 2.96 children.

Some environmentalists favor a policy of **zero population growth.** That is the level at which birth rates would match death rates. Zero population growth would require that the average woman bear closer to two children than three. Some European nations have achieved zero population growth, and China is turning the corner toward it. Other environmentalists see worldwide zero population growth as more of an ideal than a realistic goal. However, experts agree that massive supplies of affordable contraceptives will be needed, especially in developing countries, if global population is to be stabilized. Concerns about overpopulation are not restricted to poorer nations, however. All of us need to be aware of the impact of population on the environment and to make responsible reproductive choices.

**Zero population growth** The level at which birth rates match death rates.

### think about it!

- **What are the connections between overpopulation and health?**

**critical thinking** **Agree or disagree and support your answer: Overpopulation may be a problem for other countries, but not for the United States and Canada.**

Smart Quiz
Q2202

# POLLUTION

**Pollution** is contamination of the environment. Some forms of pollution occur naturally, as when ash and gases are spewed into the air from volcanic eruptions. Most pollution is caused by human activity, however, such as the discharge of industrial wastes and the burning of fossil fuels to heat our homes, power our cars, and run our factories.

## Air Pollution

Air is a mixture of oxygen (about 20%) and other gases, mostly nitrogen. People spew pollutants into the air from car exhausts, factories, buildings, and homes. This makes breathing hazardous to their own health and to that of other living organisms.

**Outdoor ("Ambient") Air Pollution** By far the greatest source of human-produced air pollution comes from the combustion of nonrenewable fossil fuels—the burning of oil, natural gas, and coal to power motor vehicles, heat our homes and buildings, and provide electrical power. About 80% of the energy used in the U.S. comes from burning fossil fuels.[47] The remainder comes from nuclear, solar, and wind power.

The primary constituents of outdoor air pollution are carbon monoxide, sulfur dioxide, nitrogen dioxide, hydrocarbons, and suspended particles called particulate matter. Nature makes a comparatively minor contribution: Dust, plant pollen, spores, gases from volcanic eruptions (the chief source of sulfuric gas), forest fires ignited by lightning strikes, and emissions from marshes and crops are some of the major sources. The single greatest source of methane, for instance, is rice paddies.

**Carbon monoxide** is a poisonous gas formed from the incomplete combustion of fuels, wood, solid trash, and tobacco smoke. Motor vehicles, especially those with inefficient engines and faulty exhaust systems, contribute almost half of carbon monoxide pollution. The balance comes from the burning of fossil fuels and trash. Carbon monoxide is also a dangerous indoor pollutant.

**Smart Reference**
Electric vehicles
R2202

Coal-burning electric power plants and exhaust from cars, trucks, and other motor vehicles are the chief sources of **sulfur dioxide** and **nitrogen dioxide.** These pollutants are the principal components of acid rain. High levels of sulfur dioxide and nitrogen dioxide irritate the respiratory tract and lungs, increasing the risk of respiratory diseases such as bronchitis and pneumonia.

**Acid rain** is precipitation (rain or snow) that contains residues of industrial wastes and car exhausts. Motor vehicles and smokestacks in fossil-fuel-burning power plants discharge sulfur dioxide and nitrogen dioxide into the atmosphere, where they combine with water molecules to form sulfuric acid and nitric acid. Other pollutants found in acid rain include toxic substances such as aluminum, cadmium, lead, and methyl mercury. The pollutants in acid rain contaminate soil and stunt the growth of trees and other vegetation; kill fish and other aquatic organisms; and make their way into our food supply. About 25,000 lakes in the U.S. are damaged by acid rain.

Though we lack firm evidence of direct effects of acid rain on human health, environmentalists believe that we should stop acid rain now, before damaging health effects on people become evident. We know that acid rain adversely affects the health of other mammals, such as moose living in areas with high concentrations of acid rain.

**Hydrocarbons** are volatile organic compounds consisting of carbon and hydrogen. They are produced by the incomplete combustion of fossil fuels in factories and motor vehicle engines, as well as by the simple evaporation of solvents and fuels into the atmosphere. The catalytic convertors now required on motor vehicles in the U.S. and many other countries reduce hydrocarbon emissions.

**Smart Reference**
Beyond batteries
R2203

Another significant source of air pollution is **particulate matter**—dust, soot, ash, and other tiny solid particles. Some particulate matter dispersed in the air is merely annoying. Other kinds, especially pesticides, asbestos, and lead particles, are hazardous to health.

Tiny particles of pollutants in the air are mainly emitted from coal-burning power plants, auto and truck exhausts, and industrial plants. They can be drawn into the lungs,

**Pollution** Contamination or tainting of the environment.

**Carbon monoxide** An odorless, poisonous flammable gas produced from the burning of carbon with insufficient air.

**Sulfur dioxide** A suffocating gas formed from the burning of sulfur; produced by coal-burning electric power plants and motor vehicle exhaust.

**Nitrogen dioxide** A pollutant created by coal-burning electric power plants and the burning of fossil fuels in engines; irritates the respiratory system.

**Acid rain** Damaging precipitation formed when pollutants such as sulfur dioxide and nitrogen oxide combine with water in the atmosphere.

**Hydrocarbons** Volatile organic compounds consisting of hydrogen and carbon produced by the incomplete combustion of fossil fuels and evaporation of solvents and fuels.

**Particulate matter** Dust, soot, ash, and other tiny solid particles.

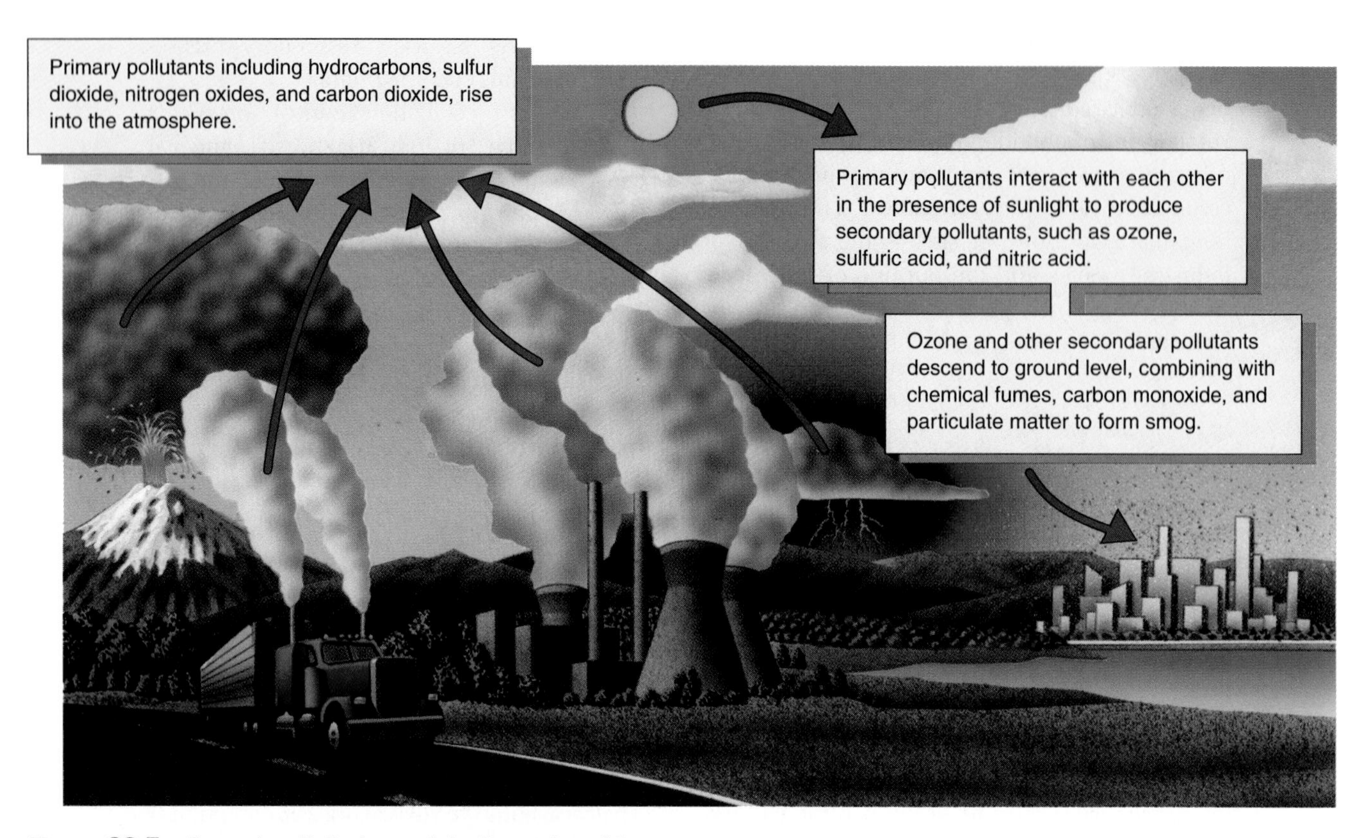

Primary pollutants including hydrocarbons, sulfur dioxide, nitrogen oxides, and carbon dioxide, rise into the atmosphere.
Primary pollutants interact with each other in the presence of sunlight to produce secondary pollutants, such as ozone, sulfuric acid, and nitric acid.
Ozone and other secondary pollutants descend to ground level, combining with chemical fumes, carbon monoxide, and particulate matter to form smog.


**Figure 22.5** ***Secondary Pollution and the Formation of Smog***

causing illness and death from prolonged exposure. These fine particles account for thousands of deaths each year in major metropolitan areas such as New York, Chicago, and Los Angeles.[48]

In the atmosphere, hydrocarbon emissions interact with sunlight and other primary pollutants such as sulfur dioxide and nitrogen oxides to produce **secondary air pollution** in the form of ozone, nitric acid, sulfuric acid, and other pollutants (see Figure 22.5). These secondary pollutants descend to ground level, combining with particulate matter, carbon monoxide, and smoke and chemical gases spewed from auto exhausts and industrial plants to form the unhealthy, foggy haze called *smog*. Smog pollutes the air of many of our major cities.

Ozone is a highly reactive oxygen molecule that occurs naturally in the stratosphere (upper atmosphere) as a by-product of sunlight acting upon normal oxygen. The ozone created in the upper atmosphere protects living things from the most dangerous forms of ultraviolet radiation. Without this protective ozone layer (about 12 to 30 miles above the earth), plants and animals would not be able to survive on land. (Some ultraviolet rays do pass through the ozone layer, however.) It is ironic that the same ozone which preserves life when it is in the upper atmosphere is toxic even in low concentrations when we inhale it at ground level.

**Secondary air pollution** Pollution produced by chemical interactions involving primary pollutants.

**Photosynthesis** The process by which plants use sunlight to produce carbohydrates from carbon dioxide and water.

### Health Effects of Outdoor Air Pollution

Air pollution irritates the lungs and eyes and causes respiratory symptoms such as shortness of breath, coughing, and sore throat. Chronic exposure can weaken the immune system and damage the lungs, which can lead to or aggravate lung disorders such as bronchitis and emphysema. Air pollution is also linked to an increased risk of cancer and heart disease. A study of more than 150 metropolitan areas in the U.S. linked exposure to high levels of air pollution to increased mortality—not as significant a factor in mortality as smoking, but a significant link nonetheless.[49] Even low levels of air pollution can be harmful, impairing lung function and leading to respiratory symptoms.[50] Pollutants can also literally choke the life out of plants, which, through **photosynthesis,** manufacture the oxygen we need to survive.

**Smart Reference**
Smog from space
R2204

Ozone interferes with the lung's ability to defend itself against invading microorganisms, increasing the chances of lung and respiratory infections. It also dampens the body's immune response, which increases susceptibility to pathogens.[51] The people most affected by smog are children, older people, and people with asthma, chronic bronchitis, or emphysema. Yet even robust, healthy people who seem unaffected by high ozone levels may suffer lung damage. Children living in areas with high levels of smog are more likely to have chronic bronchitis and be absent from school due to chest colds and pneumonia than are children in communities with cleaner air.[52] Health officials are concerned that breathing smog regularly early in life may lead to the development of chronic lung problems.

**Depletion of the Ozone Layer—Another Consequence of Pollution** You can't see it, but the ozone layer above the earth's surface has been thinning, so much so that a hole about the size of North America forms seasonally in the ozone layer over the South Pole. In other areas, the ozone layer has thinned to a lesser but still dangerous degree. The depletion of ozone is caused primarily by the release into the atmosphere of petrochemicals called **chlorofluorocarbons,** or **CFCs.** CFCs are organochlorine gases composed of carbon, chlorine, and fluorine. CFCs are used primarily as coolants in refrigerators and air conditioners, as aerosol propellants, and in the manufacture of foam insulation. CFCs release chlorine molecules into the atmosphere that literally eat ozone molecules. Because of this danger, the U.S. banned the use of CFCs in aerosols in 1978. In 1992, 93 nations agreed to stop production of CFCs by developed countries by the end of 1995. Developing nations have until the year 2010 to phase them out.

**Talking Glossary**
Chlorofluorocarbons
G2210

Refrigerator manufacturers have begun using hydrochlorofluorocarbons, or HCFCs, in place of CFCs. They too deplete ozone, but not as much as CFCs. Production of HCFCs is due to be phased out in developed countries by the year 2020. This timetable may accelerate as soon as substitute chemicals can be developed for HCFCs. Production of yet another ozone-depleting chemical, methyl bromide, an agricultural pesticide, is due to be gradually phased out.[53]

Health officials fear that the thinning of the ozone layer may increase the risk of skin cancer and immune system disorders in humans. The good news is that the phasing out of ozone-depleting chemicals should lead the ozone layer to begin to thicken after the year 2000. The bad news is that skin cancers usually develop decades after exposure. Damage caused by the diminishing ozone layer during the latter part of the twentieth century may thus not produce malignant skin tumors until well into the next millennium.

**Indoor Air Pollution** Nearly all of us are aware of the dangers of outdoor air pollution. But what about the air in your own home? Might it too be dangerous to breathe?

Indoor pollutants, such as radon, lead particles, and fumes and gases from petrochemical and pesticide products, pose significant health risks to millions of people. Because homes and offices are often sealed for energy efficiency, indoor pollutants tend to be more concentrated than outdoor pollutants.[54] We can do much to make our homes safe from airborne pollutants such as radon, pesticides, and lead contamination. Just airing out the house once or twice a day during times of the year when windows are usually shut can help remove residues from cleaning sprays, pesticides, and other chemicals used around the house.

## PREVENTION

### *Keeping Your Home Safe from Carbon Monoxide Poisoning*

Carbon monoxide poisoning in the home takes the lives of about 200 people annually in the U.S. and results in 5,000 emergency room visits.[55] Most people killed by carbon monoxide poisoning die in their sleep. One of the most common sources of carbon monoxide poisoning is a faulty or inefficient furnace, space heater, water heater, or wood stove. Here are some tips to keep your home safe from carbon monoxide:

- *Make sure your home heating system is maintained properly.*
- *Adequately ventilate a fireplace or wood stove.*
- *Never build an enclosure around a household heating system that restricts the flow of air.*
- *Never use a stove or oven to heat a home, or use a kerosene heater indoors, unless it is properly vented to the outside.* Also, never barbecue or burn charcoal indoors.

**Chlorofluorocarbons (CFCs)** Chemicals composed of carbon, chlorine, and fluorine; used as coolants, aerosol propellants, solvents, and in Styrofoam. Involved in the depletion of the ozone layer.

- *Never stay in an idling vehicle with the windows shut.* Leaks from the exhaust system can draw carbon monoxide into the passenger compartment. And keep your car's exhaust system in good repair.
- *Install a carbon monoxide detector.* The cost—about $50—is worth the peace of mind. Consult *Consumer Reports* magazine for ratings of various models.

## Water Pollution

Most of the earth (about 70%) is covered with water. But most of this water, 97%, is salt water and unfit to drink. Only 3% of the earth's water is fresh water, and only about 1% of this is drinkable. Still, this 1% would be enough to serve the needs of the world's population were it not for water pollution. As it stands, however, millions of people, mostly in developing nations but also in the U.S. and other industrialized nations, do not have clean water to drink.

The world's fresh water supplies come from two sources: ground water and surface water. **Ground water** comes from rain and snow that collects underground in natural **aquifers** of rock, gravel, and sand. **Surface water** comes from ponds, lakes, rivers, streams, and reservoirs. About half of the drinking water in the U.S. comes from ground water and half from surface water.

**America's Water—Is It Fit to Drink?** All publicly supplied water undergoes some form of purification and treatment. (Private well users must hire their own inspectors to check for contaminants and are advised to do so annually.) Water purification involves several steps, beginning with filtration through sand beds, addition of chemicals that attract suspended particles, filtration to remove the particles, and—finally—disinfection and fluoridation. Chlorine is used widely as a disinfectant to kill harmful microbes. Chlorination itself has not been shown to produce a health hazard.[56] By contrast, the risks of typhoid and cholera from drinking contaminated water are very real and deadly. Fluoridation is used in about half of the nation's public water supply to prevent tooth decay.

**Close-up** More on fluoridated water T2206

**Ground water** Water from snow and rain that collects in underground aquifers.

**Aquifers** Geological formations that hold water.

**Surface water** Water found overground in ponds, lakes, rivers, streams, and reservoirs.

The provision of safe drinking water is one of the great success stories in U.S. public health in this century. The elimination of epidemics spread by contaminated water, such as cholera, typhoid, and dysentery, has saved an incalculable number of lives and is a major contributor to the increase in life expectancy that has occurred since the beginning of the century.[57] Even so, while tap water is safe to drink for the majority of people in most U.S. communities,[58] there is still a long way to go to meet the goal of providing clean drinking water to all Americans.

Water pollution has been greatly reduced since the passage of the Clean Water Act in 1972. Yet many water systems in the U.S. are not up to standards. Large amounts of toxic substances such as lead, mercury, cadmium, and other pollutants, as well as potentially dangerous microbes, are present in the nation's water supply. They contaminate drinking water and threaten fish and wildlife.[59] As many as *one in five* U.S. residents drinks tap water from water systems that violate federal clean water standards. The Centers for Disease Control and Prevention reports that more than 7,000 Americans each year become sick from drinking tap water. This figure represents but the tip of the iceberg, since in most cases people don't realize that it is their drinking water that is making them sick.

A major problem with America's water supply is that many of our water systems depend on outdated water treatment. More than 90% of major water systems in the U.S. rely on chemical removal systems that were installed more than 50 years ago.

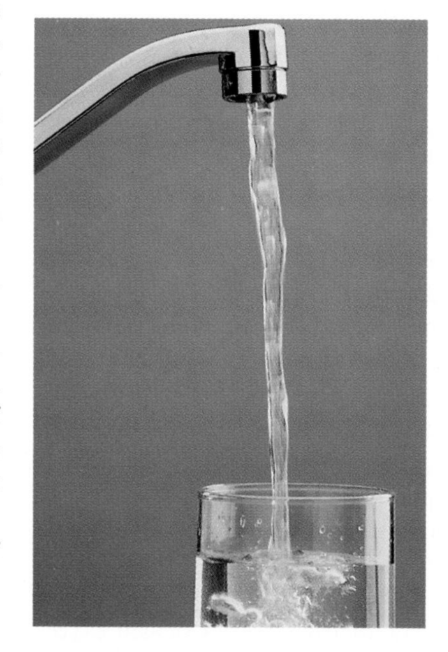

***Is This Water Fit To Drink?*** Is your tap water safe to drink? Does your community's water supply meet clean water standards? What can you and your neighbors do to ensure that the water coming into your homes is safe to drink?

These systems were not designed to filter out many of the chemical contaminants produced today, including many pesticides and industrial waste products. Some systems fail to meet EPA standards intended to safeguard against disease-causing organisms. Another problem is that many water systems fail to safeguard the watershed, the system of aquifers and streams that provide source water for the system. Polluted discharges or runoffs from farms, lawns, and city streets contaminate the watersheds that service many communities.

Another problem with this aging water supply system is that many of the pipes that bring water into the nation's cities and homes are more than a hundred years old and subject to cracking and crumbling. Many were also made with lead, which can leach into the water and make it unsafe to drink.

**What Can Be Done?** The availability of clean drinking water is essential to public health. Ensuring the safety of the water supply is a shared responsibility of government, industry, and a concerned citizenry. Providing clean drinking water to all Americans is an achievable goal, but only if the necessary funds are provided to upgrade existing water systems. Along these lines, water safety experts recognize that several steps are needed:[60]

- *Enacting legislation that imposes tougher clean water standards and requires major water systems to establish multiple barriers of protection to safeguard their watersheds.*
- *Beefing up the enforcement efforts of federal agencies responsible for protecting our water supply.*
- *Making funds available to renovate aging water systems.* Many water suppliers serve fewer than a thousand people and cannot afford the costs of complying with rigorous testing and treatment requirements. To address this problem, the federal government is seeking to make funds available to help smaller water companies comply with the law and waive requirements to test for contaminants that are never found in certain areas.

**What You Can Do to Protect Your Household Water Supply[61]** Is your household water fit to drink? Water suppliers are required to test processed water regularly and to make the results available to the public. To find out about the quality of your local water supply, request a copy of the latest test results from your water supplier. The phone number for your local water supplier appears on your water bill and is also listed in your local phone book.

Testing the water supply at the source is one thing, but what about the water that comes out of your tap? The only way to know whether your tap water is contaminated is to have it tested. Some municipalities will test tap water free of charge. Commercial services will test tap water for a fee of about $25 for lead testing to about $50 or higher depending on how many other substances are tested for. Use a lab that carries state or EPA certification. You should ask for two tests, one for water first drawn in the morning and another for water drawn after it is run for 30 seconds or long enough for it to turn cold. First-drawn water sits in pipes overnight, so it is likely to contain a higher concentration of sediment and contaminants like lead that can leach from pipes. For a listing of certified water-testing laboratories in your area, contact the Environmental Protection Agency (EPA) in Washington, D.C.

If you are concerned about the quality of your household water, you might switch to bottled water for drinking and cooking purposes or install a water-treatment device, such as a specialized water filter. If you do switch to bottled water, check that it has been tested for contaminants or has been filtered through a purification process. If you decide to use a water filter, select one that has been certified by NSF International, a nonprofit group of scientists and engineers that tests water-treatment devices. Water filters help remove certain organisms and chemicals, but you need to check that the filter is the right one for the job. Some filters take out certain chemicals such as lead, rust, and chlorine, but not other chemicals. Some take out harmful microorganisms, such as **cryptosporidium.** Cryptosporidium is a microscopic parasite that causes intestinal problems such as diarrhea. In people with weakened immune systems, such as people with AIDS and those undergoing chemotherapy, cryptosporidium can be far more dangerous, even deadly. This nasty bug is not killed off by chlorine and has turned up in both municipal and private water supplies across the country.

**Talking Glossary**
Cryptosporidium
G2211

**Cryptosporidium** A protozoan parasite that can cause diarrhea and more serious consequences in persons with compromised immune systems.

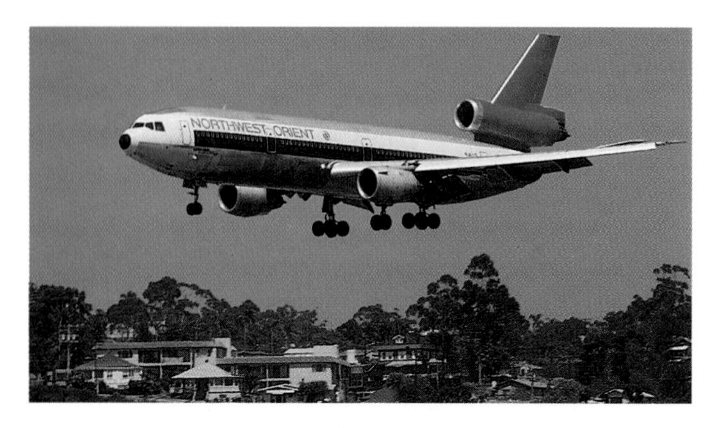

***Noise Pollution*** Noise is more than annoying; it can lead to hearing loss, health problems, and learning problems.

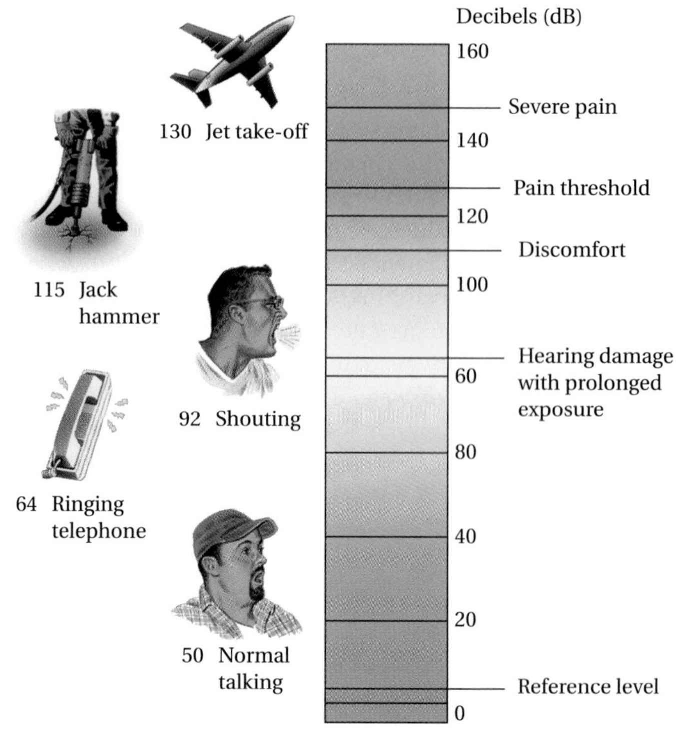


**Figure 22.6** ***Sounds and Decibels*** Permanent hearing loss may occur from prolonged exposure to sound over 85 dB. The threshold level of human hearing is just above 0 dB.

## Noise Pollution—More Than an Annoyance

**Noise** is not just annoying. It can lead to hearing loss, elevated blood pressure, learning problems, and other health problems. A recent study reported that children attending kindergartens in areas with high levels of traffic noise had higher blood pressure readings than children attending schools in quieter areas.[62]

Noise is sound that is loud, discordant, or disagreeable. The loudness of sound is measured in decibels (dB). As seen in Figure 22.6, our threshold for hearing begins at around 1 decibel. Any sound over 35 to 45 decibels can disturb sleep. Sound becomes noise at about 60 decibels. At levels of 85 dB or higher, noise can trigger the body's stress response, inducing elevated blood pressure and indigestion. At about 125 dB and beyond, noise becomes physically painful. Prolonged exposure to noise of about 70 decibels or higher can permanently damage hearing. Note that the sound levels at rock concerts typically exceed 100 decibels. (Many aging rock musicians and frequent concertgoers now suffer from hearing loss.) Unmindful of the dangers, many young people play "Walkman" type personal stereos at similarly dangerous volumes, day after day. Though some cases of extreme noise (like explosions) can instantly rupture the eardrum, most cases of hearing loss are cumulative and occur gradually. You may not realize the damage you are doing to your ears by listening to loud music until many years afterward. Though hearing loss is common among older people in our society, it is not inevitable. Older people in less technologically advanced societies often retain good hearing. Hearing loss in later life in our society is strongly related to years of prior abuse from loud music and noise.

**Noise** Loud, harsh, or noxious sound.

Occupational noise has long been recognized as a serious health problem in the workplace. According to the National Safety Council, between 7 and 10 million people in the U.S. work in settings where noise presents some risk of hearing loss. The Occupational Health and Safety Administration (OSHA) requires employers to monitor noise levels and provide annual hearing tests for employees who are exposed to noise levels of 85 decibels or above. OSHA also mandates that employees be encouraged to wear hearing protection devices. However, these regulations are often not followed, and there are too few OSHA inspectors for the thousands of plants that require monitoring.

PREVENTION

### *Preventing Noise-Induced Hearing Loss*

Taking steps now to avoid exposure to excessive noise can help prevent noise-induced hearing loss later in life:

- *When you can't avoid excessive noise, as in worksites, wear hearing protectors or soft foam or silicone-type earplugs.*
- *Use your fingers (carefully!) as earplugs in an emergency.*

- *Turn down the volume on your stereo, especially when using earphones.*
- *Do not attend ear-splitting concerts.*
- *Sound-protect your home with heavy curtains, acoustical ceiling and wall tiles, double-paned windows, and thick carpeting.* Caulk windows and doors that let in sounds.
- *Don't become a noise polluter.* Don't honk your car horn except in an emergency (no, it is not an emergency if the driver ahead of you takes a moment to get moving when the light turns green). Keep your stereo or portable radio at a level that won't bother your neighbors. Keep the muffler on your car in good working condition.
- *If you live in a particularly noisy area, organize your neighbors to pressure government officials to seek remedies.*

Smart Quiz Q2203

**think about it!**

- **Do you attend ear-splitting concerts? What might be the effects on your hearing, especially later in life?**

**critical thinking** **Agree or disagree and support your answer: The dangers of pollution are much exaggerated.**

**critical thinking** **Agree or disagree and support your answer: A good way to protect oneself from air pollution is to stay indoors.**

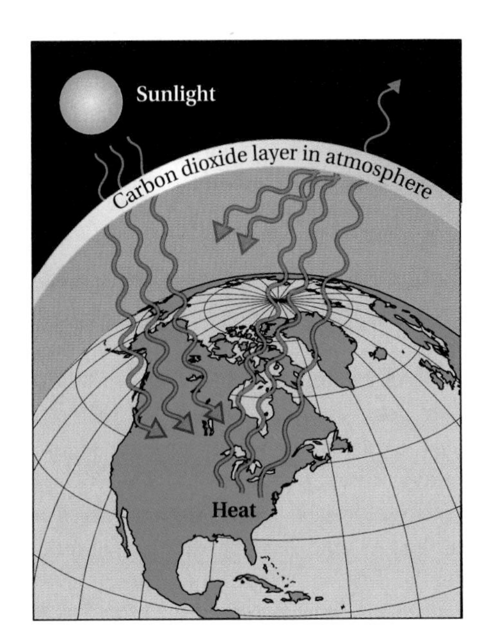


**Figure 22.7** ***The Greenhouse Effect*** The greenhouse effect occurs when carbon dioxide and other gases rise into the atmosphere and trap heat that would normally dissipate into outer space.

## GLOBAL WARMING—YES, IT'S GETTING HOTTER OUT THERE

For years scientists debated whether rising global temperatures during the past century were a natural variation in weather patterns or a sign of the **greenhouse effect** (see Figure 22.7). A greenhouse shields plants from the cold outside but lets in sunlight. Our atmosphere—composed of gases, moisture, and particles—also functions as a greenhouse. It shields the earth from the cold of outer space while letting in sunlight. The greenhouse effect is the gradual rise in atmospheric temperature due to the presence of carbon dioxide and other greenhouse gases that are released by the burning of fossil fuels, such as coal, oil, and natural gas.[63] The gases trap heat in the atmosphere that would normally radiate out into space.

Smart Reference Noxious nutrients R2205

In 1995, a United Nations expert panel on the environment reached the conclusion that yes, **global warming** is occurring, and we humans are at least partly to blame.[64] The average global temperature has risen about 1 degree Fahrenheit during the twentieth century. This may not seem like much, but bear in mind that the difference in average global temperature between today and the depths of the last ice age is only 5 to 9 degrees.[65] The U.N. panel offered a dim forecast of a further increase in global temperatures of between 1.44 degrees and 6.3 degrees Fahrenheit by the year 2100 unless action is taken to curb emissions of heat-trapping gases. Even if we succeed in curtailing these emissions, the global temperature may continue to rise by perhaps 1 to 3.6 degrees during the next century.

### Effects of Global Warming

Why should we be concerned about global warming? The reasons are far-reaching. A warming climate means more extreme

**Greenhouse effect** The rise in atmospheric temperature due to the buildup of heat-trapping gases produced by the burning of fossil fuels.

**Global warming** The rise in atmospheric temperatures worldwide.

weather patterns, causing more droughts and flooding and reduced crop yields, heightening the threat of starvation. Melting of the polar ice caps would raise sea levels in many parts of the world and cause large-scale displacement of populations. Rising temperatures in temperate areas can bring mosquitoes that carry such tropical diseases as malaria, yellow fever, and dengue. Another consequence of global warming is increased frequency of killer heat waves, like the one that took the lives of an estimated 700 Chicagoans in July 1995. Excessive heat—not lightning, tornadoes, or hurricanes—is the leading weather-related killer.[66]

Global warming may be responsible for several thousand deaths each year due to heat stress in the U.S. alone. As one leading expert, Laurence S. Kalkstein of the Center for Climatic Research at the University of Delaware, reported, "Living in heat-trapping brick tenements with black-tar roofs, many poor, elderly, or frail residents of New York, Chicago, and other cities will be unable to adjust to a warming climate."[67] Paradoxically, some scientists believe that the climatic changes associated with global warming may be responsible not only for hotter summers and more severe droughts, but also for a greater frequency of severe snowstorms, such as the record-setting snowstorms that hit the eastern United States in the winter of 1995–96.[68] Global warming increases the flow of warm, moist air over the Atlantic, creating the makings of major winter storms when these warm air masses smack against cold air masses blowing down from Canada. Global warming may be at least partly responsible for the unusual weather that many parts of the U.S. have experienced in recent years.

**Take Charge**
CDC prevention guidelines: Hot weather emergencies **C2202**
CDC prevention guidelines: Other heat-related problems **C2203**

**Smart Reference**
The coming climate **R2206**

### What Can Be Done?

The environmental threats posed by the burning of fossil fuels include not only global warming but also increased air pollution and acid rain. Lessening our dependence on fossil fuels, especially coal and petroleum products like gasoline and home heating oil, could slow or reverse these trends. Knowing what to do is one thing; doing it is quite another. Some progress has been made in reducing fossil fuel consumption. Automobiles today are much more fuel-efficient than they were 20 or 30 years ago. In 1990, a set of amendments to the original Clean Air Act of 1970 established even stricter emission standards. These revised standards require utilities to cut their sulfur dioxide emissions to half of 1980 levels by the year 2005. Coal-burning utilities are required to install new burner technologies that will reduce nitrogen oxide emissions by about 30 to 50%.

It would also be helpful to develop technologies that make greater use of alternative energy sources to further reduce our dependence on fossil fuels. These alternatives might include solar power, wind power, and electric cars. It would help to expand conservation efforts by encouraging people to use more energy-efficient modes of transportation, such as public transportation rather than private automobiles, and to use more foot power (bicycling and walking) in place of motorized vehicles. It would help to work with governments around the world to implement programs of reforestation. These steps could make our environment safer and healthier for all creatures, large and small, who share the good earth.

**think about it!**

- **What are the potential effects of global warming on *your* health? Why?**
- **Which do you find more unpleasant: heat waves or prolonged bouts of cold weather? Why?**

**critical thinking** **Agree or disagree and support your answer: How I and others live our lives can have either a positive or negative impact on the earth.**

**Smart Quiz**
**Q2204**

## THE WASTE CRISIS—WHERE CAN WE DUMP ALL THE GARBAGE?

Americans generate more than 200 million tons of household waste annually. This amounts to more than 4 pounds of discarded packaging, food wastes, old appliances, paper products, yard waste, cans and bottles, and other waste per person each and every day. Every hour, we throw out some 2 million plastic bottles alone.[69] Even with the rise of community recycling programs and increased public awareness about the emerging waste crisis, the amount of waste generated in the U.S. has risen each year for as long as the flow of garbage has been measured. Three key factors contribute to the rising levels of waste:

1. The huge increase in single-person households, each of which is equipped with household products that larger family units typically share.
2. The rise in the use of throwaway products that make cooking and cleaning and diapering babies more convenient but produce more waste.
3. The growth of an "information economy," which is increasingly dependent on paper products—from computer paper to junk mail.[70]

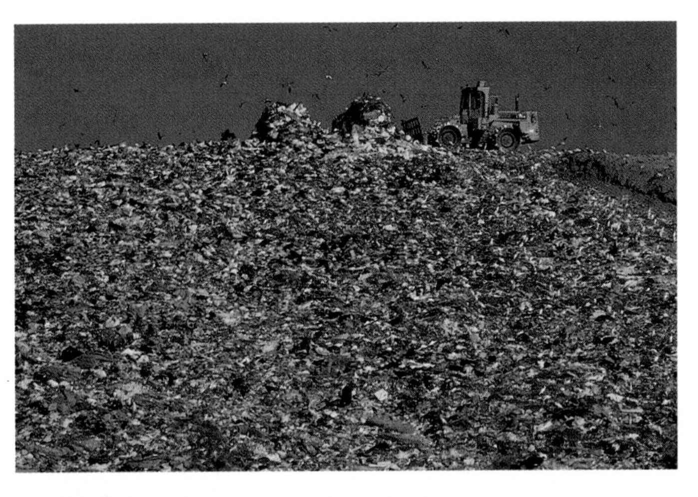

***Mountains of Garbage*** Finding environmentally sound ways of disposing of trash will remain a major challenge well into the new millennium.

## Solid Waste

**Solid waste** includes hazardous and nonhazardous wastes from all sources, everything from discarded newspapers and cans to food wastes and packaging. Solid waste is classified as *hazardous* if it is ignitable, corrosive, reactive, or toxic. Hazardous waste poses risks to health and to the environment. *Municipal solid waste* (MSW) is waste produced by households and light industry. This includes virtually anything we as individuals or business owners toss into the trash. While only about 1% of household waste is toxic, collectively this translates into about 2 million tons of toxic waste in the trash each year.

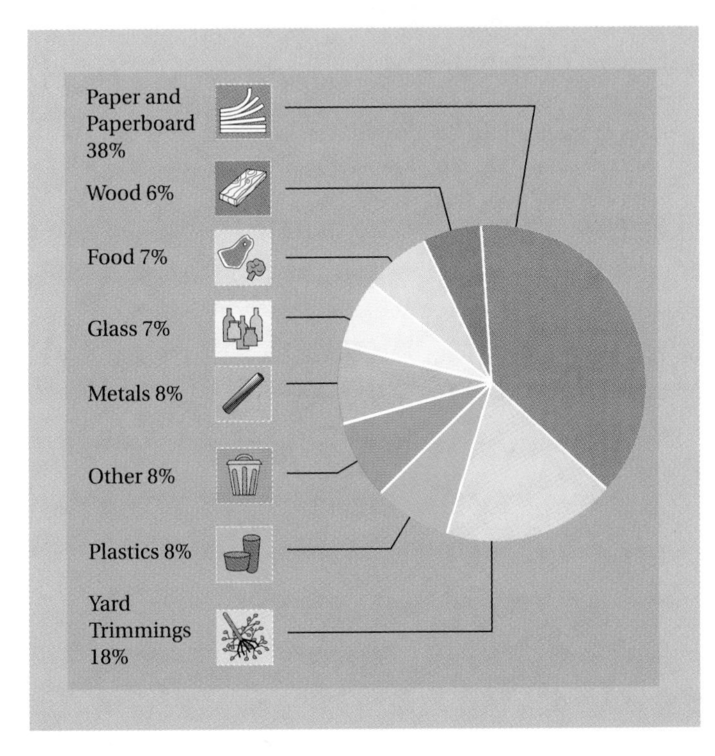


**Figure 22.8** ***What We Throw Out—MSW Materials by Weight*** MSW, or municipal solid waste, consists of what households and light industry discard in the trash. Paper and paperboard is by far the largest contributor. Environmentalists fear that we may simply run out of room to put all this garbage or dispose of it in ways that damage the environment. For this reason it is important for all of us to begin practicing waste prevention. A good place to start is to reduce our reliance on nonrecyclable paper goods.

Figure 22.8 illustrates the sources of municipal solid waste in the U.S. What is the largest contributor to MSW? Hands down, it's discarded paper and paperboard. Yet MSW is but the tip of the iceberg in the solid waste universe. *Industrial solid waste,* the waste material produced by heavy industry, government, agriculture, and sewage and mining, among other sources, consists of more than 13 *billion* tons per year. About 200 million tons of industrial solid waste is considered hazardous.

What happens to all this garbage? Most wastes are buried in **landfills**—underground disposal areas lined with plastic to keep hazardous materials from leaking and contaminating ground water and soil. When filled, landfills are capped over with asphalt or other materials. Thousands of older landfills, however, do leak contaminants into soil and water. Although new landfills are better designed to prevent leaks, a combination of high start-up and operating costs, diminishing number of available sites, and public opposition to placing them in people's neighborhoods—the "Not in My Backyard," or NIMBY, syndrome—has prevented many new sites from opening. According to the national

**Solid waste** Waste in the form of garbage or refuse.

**Landfills** Underground disposal areas for discarding solid waste.

Solid Waste Management Association, an industry group, more than half of U.S. landfills will run out of room by the turn of the century. Many already have.

Waste not buried in landfills is either placed in open dumps (both on water and land), incinerated, buried in underground injection wells, or recovered through recycling and composting. **Incineration** is the burning of solid waste under carefully controlled conditions. Incineration reduces the volume of waste but produces air pollution. Air emissions from incinerators are called *fly ash,* which often contains dioxin, heavy metals, and acid gases. Pollution-control devices like scrubbers reduce but don't eliminate the problem. In the absence of any major new developments in waste management technology, *waste prevention* will surely become a watchword in the new millennium.

## Cleaning Up Hazardous Waste Sites

The nation is littered with toxic waste sites where heavy industry has dumped chemicals and other hazardous wastes into the ground or discharged them into canals, rivers, and streams. The federal government has undertaken to clean up abandoned or uncontrolled hazardous waste sites. In 1980, the U.S. Congress enacted the Superfund Act, funding a large-scale cleanup of these sites. To date, some 1,200 high-priority sites have been identified, though only about 200 have been cleaned up thus far. Another 32,000 sites are considered potentially dangerous, including some municipal landfills. One in four Americans lives within four miles of a Superfund site.[71] As seen in the nearby ***World of Diversity*** feature, a disproportionate number of toxic waste facilities are located in areas with high concentrations of lower-income and nonwhite people.

### think about it!

- **Do you recycle? If not, why not?**
- **Why do you think toxic waste sites are more likely to be located near communities inhabited by ethnic minority groups and poor people?**

Smart Quiz
Q2205

**Incineration** The burning of solid waste; spews pollutants into the air.

**Environmental racism** Racial bias in environmental policy and enforcement.

WORLD OF *diversity*

## Toxic Communities and Environmental Racism[72]

The placement of toxic waste sites is not color-blind. A landmark 1987 nationwide survey by the United Church of Christ Commission for Racial Justice found that race, even more than income, was the most prominent factor in determining the placement of commercially owned toxic waste facilities—landfills, toxic waste dumps, and incinerators. Only about a quarter of the population is African American or Hispanic American, but 60% of the largest toxic waste facilities are located in their communities. Three of five African Americans and Hispanic Americans, and nearly half of all Native Americans, live near poorly monitored toxic waste facilities.

African Americans and Hispanic Americans are also more likely than whites to live in areas with poor air quality. Though race and income are often intertwined, these differences are not explained simply by income or socioeconomic status. Though poor people are more likely than affluent people to live in areas of substandard air quality, even among poor people, African Americans and Hispanic Americans are more likely to breathe polluted air than poor whites are. Why? Largely because air-polluting facilities, such as industrial plants and electric generating facilities, are disproportionately placed in areas with a high percentage of minority residents. Again, race is a more important factor in accounting for the placement of these environmental hazards than income.

Nobody wants environmental hazards in his or her backyard (the "NIMBY" syndrome). Industries therefore typically place these facilities in communities with the least political clout. These are typically poor and minority communities. The residents may be less well organized than their more affluent neighbors. They may lack the resources of time, money, and contacts to affect policy decisions. Or they may be at a disadvantage because they are underrepresented on governing or regulatory bodies.

**Environmental racism** is the term used to refer to racial bias in policy-making and enforcement processes. Environmental racism permits a disproportionate number of environmental hazards in predominantly minority communities and fails to enforce pollution standards evenly, regardless of the race or income of the affected population. For example, studies show that polluters of minority communities are fined only half as much on average as polluters of predominantly white communities.[73]

Terms such as *environmental racism* and *environmental justice* parallel concerns for justice and equality in other spheres of life, including housing and education. As one environmental expert put it, "To know that environmental inequalities exist and to continue to do nothing about them will perpetuate separate societies and will deprive the poor, [African Americans], and other minorities of equitable environmental protection."[74]

# Doing Your Part to Make the Environment Safer and Healthier

## Take Charge

Choose the statement below—1, 2, or 3—that best represents your attitudes about health and the environment:

1. The government will see to it that the environment is safe. I do not need to worry about it.
2. While the environment may contain hazardous substances, once I am in my home I am relatively free from danger.
3. I am responsible for safeguarding my health. Doing so includes being informed about hazardous substances and fighting the pollution and other environmental threats that affect me, my family, and my community.

We hope you endorsed statement 3. Protecting the environment involves you as well as us. Our historical practice of using natural resources on demand and carelessly disposing of waste products has resulted in an environmental emergency as we enter the new millennium.

The effects of environmental pollution may have been a nuisance half a century ago. Today, they are a global crisis. Governments alone cannot save the earth. Each person needs to understand that pollution is a real threat to life—not just human life, but all life. Each of us shares the responsibility to protect the environment for future generations. Each of us, alone and working with others, can come to the aid of the environment by changing his or her environmental behavior. Ask yourself what you can do in your home and community to make the environment safer and healthier for us all. Here are some suggestions:

**Video**
Daily living for a healthy planet
V2201

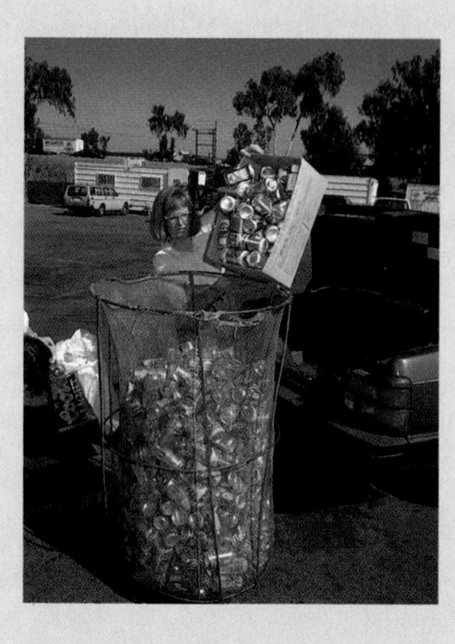

***Green Is Not Just a Color, but a State of Mind*** What can you do in your home and community to make the environment safer and healthier for us all?

### In the Home

- *Reduce unnecessary packaging.* Buy concentrates or large-sized packages whenever possible. A 50-oz. bottle of concentrated laundry detergent, for example, uses 20% less plastic than the 64-oz. bottle of detergent it replaces. A 2-pound box of cereal contains less packaging than two 1-pound boxes.
- *Test your house for radon. Test your water for lead and other contaminants.* Take corrective action if needed.
- *Reduce toxic wastes.* Use less-toxic pesticides and solvents whenever possible. If you must use toxic products, do so sparingly.
- *Sort out discarded solvents, pesticides, and other hazardous materials from other trash.* Many communities collect household hazardous wastes on certain days to help residents safely dispose of them.
- *Switch to reusable products.* Cut down on wasted paper and plastic products—the two largest sources of household waste. Bring your own shopping bag to the supermarket rather than use plastic or paper bags that get tossed away with the garbage. Reuse bags, containers, and other items. Use rechargeable batteries.
- *Use less energy.* Turn off lights and electrical appliances when they are not needed. Turn off the TV when no one is watching. Buy energy-efficient appliances, and keep them in good working condition. Don't overuse your air conditioner, washing machine, dryer, or dishwasher. Don't overheat your home. Use energy-efficient settings on your dishwasher and washing machine. Don't run them with less than a full load. Switch to energy-conserving light bulbs. Use energy-efficient fluorescent lighting, where possible, in place of incandescent lighting. These steps will not only conserve resources but also reduce your energy bills.
- *Use less water.* Take showers rather than baths (which use more water). Take shorter showers. Install water-flow restrictors on faucets. Replace high-water-use toilets with low-water-use models (those with a 1.5 gallon capacity). Avoid excess flushing. Don't leave the water running while shaving or at other times.
- *Do not use aerosol spray cans that use ozone-depleting propellants.* Switch to nonaerosol sprays, such as pumps.

- *Choose recyclable products and containers. Then recycle them!* Sort newspapers, aluminum cans, and glass products and deposit them in your community's recycling bins.

## In Your Community

- *Leave the car at home for short hops around the neighborhood.* Use foot power instead.
- *Use mass transportation rather than the car.* When possible, take the train or the bus and leave the car at home.
- *Carpool to work or school.* Many companies and communities have carpooling programs. Check them out.
- *Take responsibility for your own garbage.* Bring reusable bags to cart away your own garbage from campsites, picnic areas, parks, and the beach.
- *Become more environmentally aware.* Government and consumer watchdog organizations are available to help you learn more about environmental issues. Table 22.3 lists resources at the national level. For a list of local agencies and organizations, check your phone directory or inquire at your town or village hall or city government.
- *Educate others about reducing waste and recycling.* If your community doesn't have a recycling program, establish one. Make your preferences for recyclables known to manufacturers, merchants, and community leaders. Be creative. Find new ways to reduce waste quantity and toxicity.
- *Don't pollute.* Don't litter or dump your trash in roadside containers. Don't pollute the air that others breathe with tobacco smoke or emissions from letting your car idle.
- *Get involved.* Donate your time to your local conservation group. Organize people in your community to confront local environmental hazards, such as nearby dump sites. Join community programs for cleaning parks and recreational areas. Participate in environmental conservation organizations. Vote with your pocketbook: Buy products from companies with good environmental records.
- *Speak your mind.* Tell your legislators—members of Congress, municipal leaders, and state officials—that you expect them to defend and expand laws that preserve and protect the environment. Make known your opinions on pending legislation to your elected representatives through letters and telephone calls.

**Close-up**
Earth day: Get involved
T2207

**Smart Quiz**
Q2206

TABLE 22.3

**Who's Who in Environmental Protection**

| Agency | Telephone No. | What They Do |
|---|---|---|
| Environmental Protection Agency (EPA)* | 202-260-2090 | Committed to safeguarding the environment, it seeks to protect human health and our natural resources by ensuring that environmental protection laws and regulations are implemented and enforced effectively. |
| Food and Drug Administration (FDA) | 301-827-4420 | Seeks to ensure the health and safety of the nation's food supply. It regularly tests foods for the presence of chemical and biological contaminants. It also oversees the approval process for new drugs. |
| National Institute for Occupational Safety and Health (NIOSH) | 800-356-4674 | Through research and prevention, it seeks to provide a safer and healthier workplace for all Americans. |
| Occupational Safety and Health Administration (OSHA) | 202-219-8148 | Enforces worksite safety and health laws and maintains the quality of these standards, in order to ensure a healthy and safe worksite for workers. |
| National Institute of Environmental Health Sciences Public Clearinghouse | 800-643-4794 | Conducts basic research on the effects on human health of environmental factors such as pollution. |
| U.S. Department of Housing and Urban Development (HUD) | 202-708-1422 | Funds lead-removal or abatement programs in public housing. |
| Consumer Product Safety Commission | 800-638-2772 | An independent regulatory commission responsible for ensuring the safety of consumer products around the home. It requires hazardous materials to carry warning labels and issues warnings about household hazards, such as lead paint. |
| Agency for Toxic Substances and Disease Registry (ATSDR) | 404-639-0501 | Evaluates health risks posed by environmental threats, such as toxic waste sites. |

*Many states and municipalities also have environmental protection agencies. Check the municipal government pages in your telephone directory.

# SUMMING UP

## Questions and Answers

**1. What is the environment?** The environment refers to our surroundings—the plants, people, and other animals; water, air, and soil; and factors such as climate and geography.

### ENVIRONMENTAL TOXINS—NATURAL AND HUMAN-MADE RISKS

**2. What kinds of environmental health hazards are there?** Environment health hazards include toxic chemical hazards, biological hazards, physical hazards, and cultural/social hazards.

**3. What are toxins?** Toxins are poisonous substances that impair an organism's normal functioning. The major environmental toxins are natural and synthetic substances such as metals, pesticides, and some petrochemicals; and radioactive substances such as ultraviolet rays, X-rays, and radon.

**4. How do environmental toxins harm health?** Some, like pesticides, poison people directly. Other toxins, like forms of radiation, are mutagens, which can cause mutations in genes; carcinogens, which cause cancer; and neurotoxins, like lead and mercury, which damage the nervous system.

**5. What kinds of toxic chemicals are there?** Many. They include arsenic, minerals such as asbestos, aflatoxin, heavy metals, and petrochemicals.

### OVERPOPULATION

**6. What is happening with population growth around the world?** It's mushrooming. We are expecting it to grow by 50% in less than 50 years.

**7. What health problems are connected with overpopulation?** Overpopulation brings the prospect of widespread famine and epidemics spread by contaminated water supplies and inadequate health care.

### POLLUTION

**8. What is air pollution?** The greatest source of outdoor air pollution is the combustion of fossil fuels. The primary components of outdoor air pollution are carbon monoxide, sulfur dioxide, nitrogen dioxide, hydrocarbons, particulate matter, and ozone. Indoor air pollutants include radon, lead particles, mercury fumes, and fumes and gases from petrochemicals and pesticides. Two consequences of air pollution are acid rain and depletion of the ozone layer.

**9. What is water pollution?** Water pollution consists of toxic substances, such as lead, mercury, and cadmium, and potentially dangerous microbes.

**10. What is noise pollution?** Noise pollution is persistent, loud, disagreeable sound. It causes health problems such as elevated blood pressure and hearing loss.

### GLOBAL WARMING—YES, IT'S GETTING HOTTER OUT THERE

**11. Is global warming occurring?** The scientific consensus is *yes*. The cause appears to be the greenhouse effect, in which gases that are released by the burning of fossil fuels trap heat that would normally be released into outer space in the atmosphere.

**12. What are the effects of global warming?** Global warming leads to more extreme weather patterns, more droughts and flooding, reduced crop yields, mosquitoes, and heat waves.

### THE WASTE CRISIS—WHERE CAN WE DUMP ALL THE GARBAGE?

**13. What factors contribute to the growing mountains of garbage?** Three factors are involved in the United States: the increase in single-person households, use of throwaway products, and growth of a paper-dependent "information economy."

**14. What happens to solid wastes?** Most are buried in landfills. The rest are placed in open dumps, incinerated, buried in underground injection wells, or recovered through recycling and composting.

## References and Suggested Readings

### SMART REFERENCES FROM SCIENTIFIC AMERICAN

**Doyle, R. Global Fertility and Population.** *Scientific American,* 276(3) (March 1997), 26. **R2201**

**Sperling, D. The Case for Electric Vehicles.** *Scientific American,* 275(5) (November 1996), 54–59. **R2202**

**Beardsley, T. Beyond Batteries. "Explorations" from Scientific American's www site,** December 1996. **R2203**

**Sinha, G. Atmospheric Science: Smog from Space.** *Scientific American,* 275(3) (September 1996), 26. **R2204**

**Beardsley, T. When Nutrients Turn Noxious.** *Scientific American,* 276(6) (June 1997), 24. **R2205**

**Karl, T.R., Nicholls, N., and Gregory, J. The Coming Climate.** *Scientific American,* 276(5) (May 1997), 78–83. **R2206**

## SUGGESTED READINGS

**Steinman, D., and Wisner, R. M.** *Living Healthy in a Toxic World.* New York: Berkley Publishing Group, 1996. Practical advice about protecting yourself and your family from everyday poisons, chemicals, and pollution.

**Moeller, D. W.** *Environmental Health.* Cambridge: Harvard University Press, 1992. A leading textbook on relationships between the environment and health.

**MacEachern, D.** *Save Our Planet.* New York: Dell, 1990. Practical suggestions for making changes in our lives that can benefit the environment.

**Olkowski, W., Daar, S., and Olkowski, H.** *Common-Sense Pest Control.* Newtown, CT: Taunton Press, 1991. A single-volume encyclopedia of least-toxic pest control methods for home and garden. A must for every gardener.

**Ehrlich, P. R.** *The Population Explosion.* New York: Ballantine Books, 1990. Population expert Paul Ehrlich's treatise on the dangers of world population growth for humankind as well as the environment.

# Managing Your Health Care

## DID YOU KNOW THAT

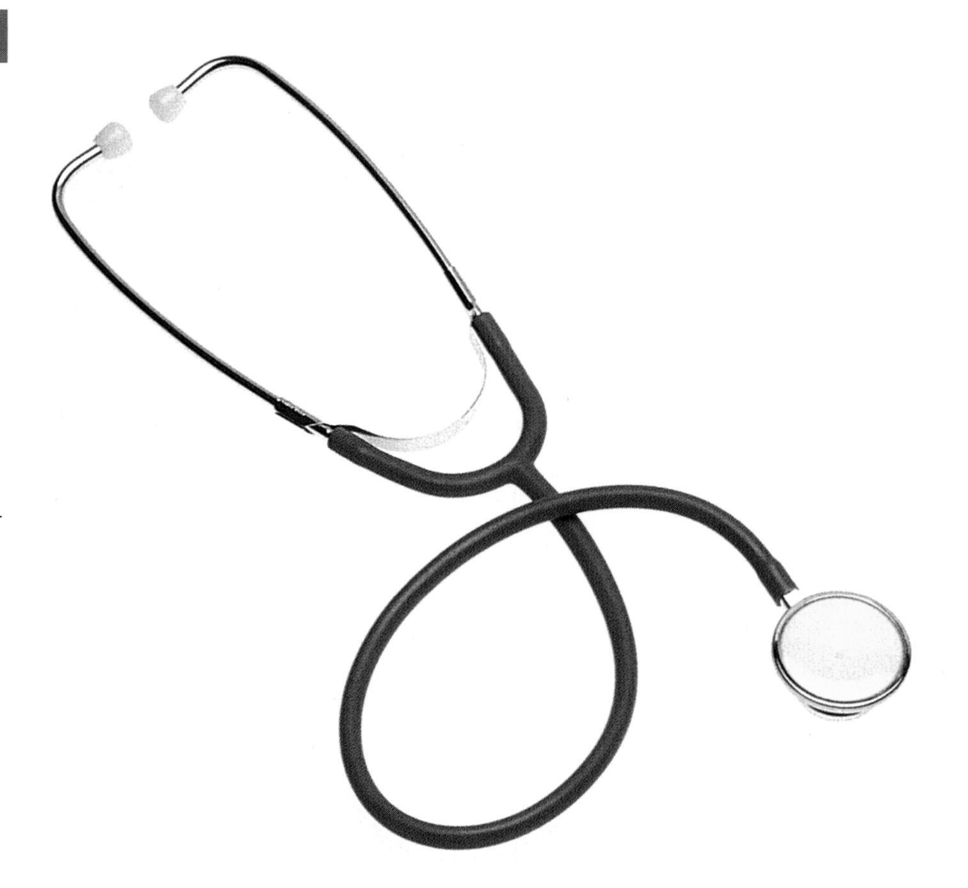

- The health care system isn't really a "system"? p.632
- People in the United States pay twice as much for health care as they pay for national defense? p.632
- Some medical specialists pay more than $100,000 a year for malpractice insurance? p.632
- With each passing year, the percentage of workers being given a choice about their health care coverage between a conventional plan or a managed care plan is shrinking? p.643
- Only about one in four working Americans who receives health insurance through his or her job is covered by a traditional fee-for-service plan? p.644
- Students are not always covered by their parents' insurance plans? p.645
- More than one-half of all Americans with employer-sponsored health coverage belong to HMOs? p.646
- Present evidence shows that HMOs offer about the same quality of care, as judged by outside doctors, as traditional health plans? p.647
- Medicare is the single largest payer for health care in the United States? p.651
- More than one-third of young children in the United States have been inadequately immunized against polio and other preventable diseases? p.654

# 23

*Health care is more complicated today than it once was. The model of the family doctor as a solo practitioner in independent private practice is giving way to an increasingly complex mix of medicine and big business. We have entered an age of managed care—a setup that has one hand on the stethoscope and the other on the pocketbook. With the bewildering array of health care plans available today, it is no wonder that many of us find it difficult to make informed health care choices. This chapter charts your way through the health care maze. You learn to decipher the acronyms that dot the managed care field—terms like HMOs, PPOs, and POS plans. You learn the advantages and disadvantages of managed care compared with conventional health care plans and how to protect yourself from* mis*managed care.*

*More broadly, this chapter is about you, the health care consumer. The responsibility for managing* your *health care does not lie with physicians, government programs, or insurance carriers. It lies with* you. *Each of us has a responsibility to become an active, informed health care consumer. We take an active role in managing our health care by educating ourselves about our health care options, choosing our health care providers wisely, and weighing treatment alternatives carefully.*

## HEALTH CARE IN AMERICA

The U.S. health care system isn't really an organized system. It is more of a loosely coordinated network of health care providers, government support programs, and health insurance and managed care companies. The health care "system" is based on altruistic motives of preventing and caring for people with health problems, but it is also big business. Very big business. Health care is the second largest industry in the United States—only retailing is bigger. Health care costs reached $976 billion by 1994, or about $3,500 for every person in the U.S.[1] Health care costs accounted for about 14% of the nation's gross national product (GNP) in 1995, more than twice the amount spent on national defense. Health care costs, which have risen more than tenfold since 1950, continue to rise, although the rate of increase began to slow during the 1990s (see Figure 23.1). Still, health care costs could top $2 trillion annually early in the new millennium.[2]

Why does health care cost so much? One reason is that more doctors today are practicing defensive medicine to protect themselves from **malpractice** suits. They do so by ordering tests and performing procedures that may not be medically necessary but may shield them from liability. Higher insurance premiums (some specialists pay more than $100,000 annually) are passed along in the form of higher fees to patients. Another reason is that Americans are living longer, and people need more medical care as they age. Another factor is the advent of expensive diagnostic tests, like MRIs and CAT scans, and medical procedures like angioplasty and coronary bypass surgery. A bypass operation can cost $40,000; an angioplasty, $20,000. (Figure 23.2 shows how your health care dollar is spent.)

Still another reason for rising health care costs is the lack of incentives for consumers or health care providers to limit costs. Historically, consumers did not pay for much of their care. Costs were largely borne by employers in the form of medical insurance premiums and by government programs like Medicaid and Medicare, which provided care for older people, the disabled, and the poor.[3] The lack of economic incentives to curtail costs results in unnecessary procedures, duplication of services, and general inefficiency.

**Malpractice** Failure of a professional to render proper treatment, especially when injury or harm occurs as a result.

**Managed care** A system of controlling health care costs by eliminating waste and unnecessary medical procedures.

**Allied health professionals** Individuals trained in one of the allied health fields, such as optometry, dentistry, occupational therapy, podiatry, and psychology.

The health care system is in flux today. Large employers, joined by state and federal governments, are balking at footing the ever-rising health care bill. They are turning to **managed care** companies that promise to contain costs while providing quality health care. Whether or not managed care plans can accomplish these goals, increasing numbers of Americans are joining managed care plans or being pushed into them by their employers. Managed care is even making inroads in government-supported programs like Medicare and Medicaid.

Worries about health care run deep and are not limited to concerns about managed care. People worry about whether they will be able to obtain health insurance or keep it if they are laid off. Over 17% of Americans, about 40 million people, are uninsured.[4] The uninsured include nearly one in seven young people under the age of 18 and more than one in four 18- to 24-year-olds. The problem is worse among ethnic minorities. One out of three Hispanic Americans and one out of four African Americans under the age of 65 have no health insurance, compared with one out of six white Americans.

Let us look at the health care plans available today and what they may mean for you. First, however, let us review the different types of health care providers and facilities that are available in the health care field today and efforts to introduce some needed reforms in the health care system.

### Types of Health Care Providers

Though we typically think of a "health care provider" as a physician, many kinds of health care professionals perform distinct roles. There are physicians and nurses as well as **allied health professionals** such as dentists, optometrists, physical therapists, and pharmacists.

**Physicians** Physicians are medical doctors who hold either an M.D. (Doctor of Medicine) or a D.O. (Doctor of Osteopathy) degree. Osteopaths make up about 5% of the physicians in the U.S., with the rest holding M.D. degrees. D.O.s and M.D.s complete a rigorous four-year medical curriculum followed by internship and residency training. The training for both M.D.s and D.O.s is similar except

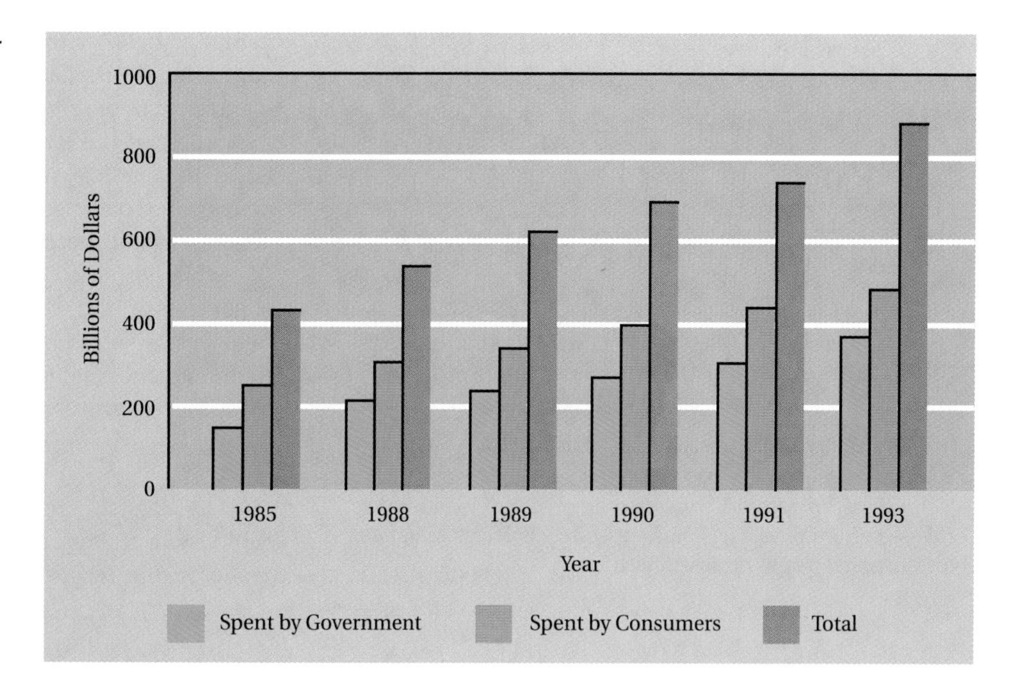


**Figure 23.1** ***National Health Expenditures—Costs Keep Rising*** Health care costs have been rising steadily, giving fuel to the growth of managed care companies, which promise to curb costs while maintaining quality care. But can they accomplish these two, sometimes conflicting, objectives?

that osteopathic training places somewhat greater emphasis on the musculoskeletal system. Both types of physicians employ the usual forms of medical diagnosis and therapy, including drugs, surgery, and radiation.

Once, most physicians were family doctors or general practitioners (G.P.s). Today, most are specialists who treat only one body system or restrict their practice to one specific type of disease or disorder, such as cancer (see Table 23.1). Physicians become specialists through specialized residency training. Once they pass a formal examination in their specialty, they become "board certified." That is, they are credentialed as specialists by a recognized medical specialty board.

General internal medicine, general pediatrics, and family medicine are the medical specialties that provide the bulk of primary care in the United States. At a time when the nation needs more primary care physicians, the percentage of medical students intending to become board certified in these areas has been dropping—to fewer than one

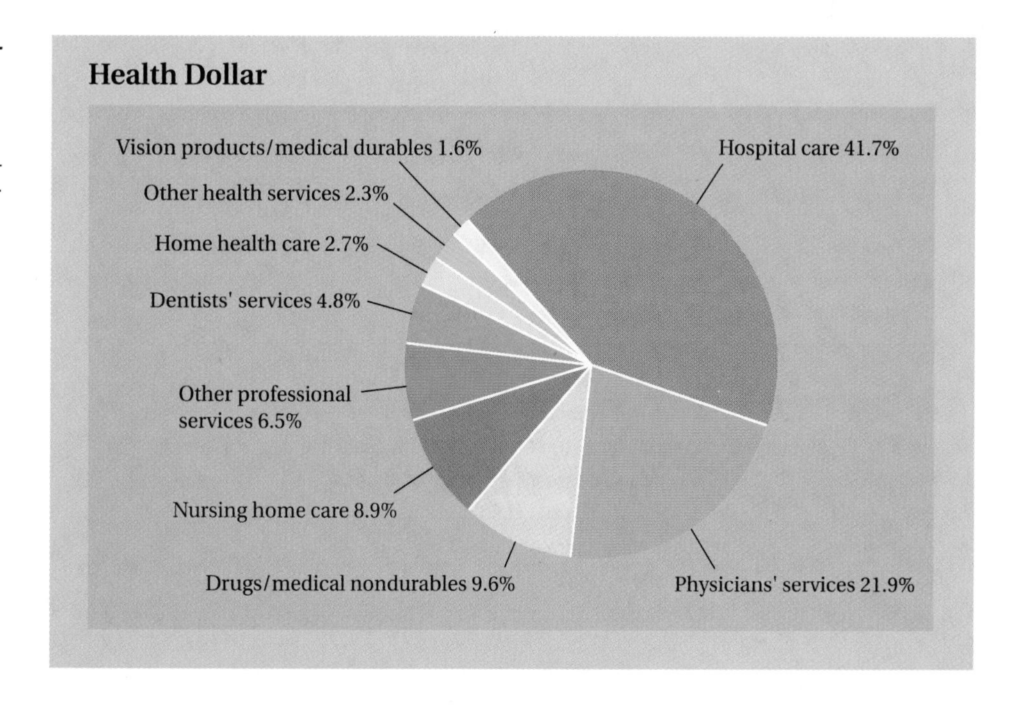


**Figure 23.2** ***Where Our Health Dollar Goes*** The largest piece of the health care pie goes to pay for the costs of hospital care. Perhaps if greater efforts were placed on preventive care, there would be less need for expensive hospitalization.

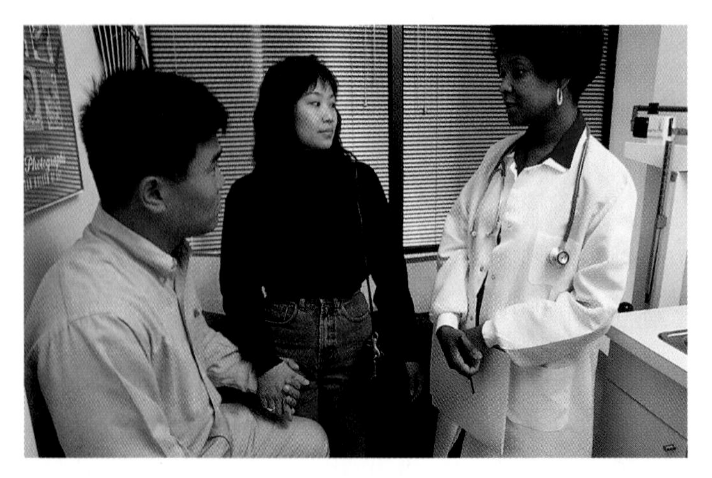

***Health Care Providers*** There are many types of health care providers, from physicians, nurses, and technicians to various types of allied health professionals.

in four by 1990.[5] At the same time, medical knowledge is rapidly expanding. Ever more complicated medical technologies and procedures are emerging, providing the impetus for even more specialists. The medical profession and health care system are challenged to balance the needs for generalists and specialists. A change is blowing in the wind, however. The growth of managed care, which uses primary care physicians as gatekeepers for specialists in order to control costs, is leading to an increased demand for generalists. Demand for specialists still exceeds that for generalists, but the gap is narrowing.[6]

**Nurses** Nurses are the backbone of the health care system and represent the largest professional group in the health industry. Even though the

TABLE 23.1

**Types of Medical Specialists**

| Who They Are | What They Do |
|---|---|
| Allergists | Diagnose and treat allergies |
| Anesthesiologists | Administer anesthetics and monitor the condition of patients under anesthesia |
| Cardiologists | Diagnose and treat heart disease |
| Dermatologists | Diagnose and treat skin diseases |
| Emergency physicians | Diagnose and treat conditions resulting from trauma or sudden illness |
| Endocrinologists | Diagnose and treat conditions and diseases of the glands of internal secretion |
| Family physicians | Diagnose and treat a wide variety of conditions affecting all family members |
| Gastroenterologists | Diagnose and treat digestive disorders involving the stomach, intestines, and related structures |
| Geriatricians | Diagnose and treat conditions affecting older people |
| Gynecologists | Diagnose and treat conditions affecting the female reproductive organs |
| Hematologists | Diagnose and treat blood disorders and diseases |
| Internists | Diagnose and treat conditions involving anatomy and physiology of internal body organs |
| Nephrologists | Diagnose and treat conditions involving the kidneys |
| Neurologists | Diagnose and treat conditions involving the central nervous system |
| Obstetricians | Provide clinical management of pregnancy, labor, delivery, and the period following childbirth |
| Oncologists | Diagnose and treat cancer |
| Ophthalmologists | Diagnose and treat disorders and diseases of the eye |
| Orthopedists | Diagnose and treat conditions involving the musculoskeletal system |
| Pathologists | Examine bodily tissues for presence of disease or abnormalities |
| Otorhinolaryngologists | Diagnose and treat diseases of the ear, nose, and throat |
| Pediatricians | Diagnose and treat diseases of children |
| Proctologists | Diagnose and treat conditions involving the rectum and anus |
| Psychiatrists | Diagnose and treat nervous or mental disorders |
| Radiologists | Use radiation in the diagnosis and treatment of disease |
| Urologists | Diagnose and treat diseases of the urinary system in females and the genitourinary system in males |

numbers of registered nurses (R.N.s) exceeded 2 million in the 1990s, the demand for their services continues to outstrip the supply. Some parts of the country have experienced severe shortages. This shortage is expected to increase sharply in the new millennium as the aging of the population and expanding medical technology put skilled nurses in even greater demand. Not surprisingly, nursing is expected to rank among the 20 hottest professions by the year 2000.[7] As a result of this escalating demand, nurses' salaries are expected to increase significantly into the new millennium.

Though the great majority (about 75%) of registered nurses work in hospitals, about one in four works in a setting such as independent practice, private duty, public health, occupational health, nursing education, student health, extended care, or ambulatory care.[8] Different types of R.N.s vary in terms of their educational backgrounds and nursing duties:

1. *R.N., Associate Degree:* Has completed a two-year program, earning an associate's degree (A.D.). Most of these R.N.s work in hospitals. Though they are crucial to the health care delivery system, their professional options are not as varied as those of R.N.s with bachelor's, master's, or doctoral degrees.
2. *R.N., Diploma:* Has completed a three-year program, usually affiliated with a hospital. Their professional options are similar to those of R.N.s with A.D. degrees.
3. *R. N., Bachelor of Science Degree:* Has completed a four-year program in a college or university and earned a Bachelor of Science in Nursing (B.S.N.) degree. Professional options are greater than for an R.N. with an A.D. or diploma. For example, an R.N. with a B.S.N. is more likely to gain employment as a school nurse.
4. *R.N., Nurse Practitioner:* Has completed a bachelor's and master's program in nursing (or a practitioner program). Nurse practitioners work in different capacities, including family nurse practitioners, who specialize in treating families, and obstetrics-gynecology nurse practitioners, who specialize in women's health.
5. *R. N., Clinical Nurse Specialist:* Has completed a bachelor's and master's degree in nursing, specializing in an area of practice such as cardiovascular disease, pulmonary disease, pediatrics, gerontology, or psychiatry. Roles for clinical nurse specialists are broader and include clinician, manager, educator, consultant, and researcher in their specialty fields.
6. *R.N., Certified Nurse-Midwife:* Has been educated in both nursing and midwifery in either a master's degree or certification program. Certified nurse-midwives may be self-employed or work in birthing centers, nurse-physician practices, or hospitals.
7. *R. N., Nurse Researcher and/or Nurse Educator:* Has completed at least a bachelor's and master's degree and possibly a doctoral degree in nursing. These R.N.s may teach in nursing programs in universities, colleges, or hospital-affiliated programs. A doctorate is usually required for teaching in colleges or universities.

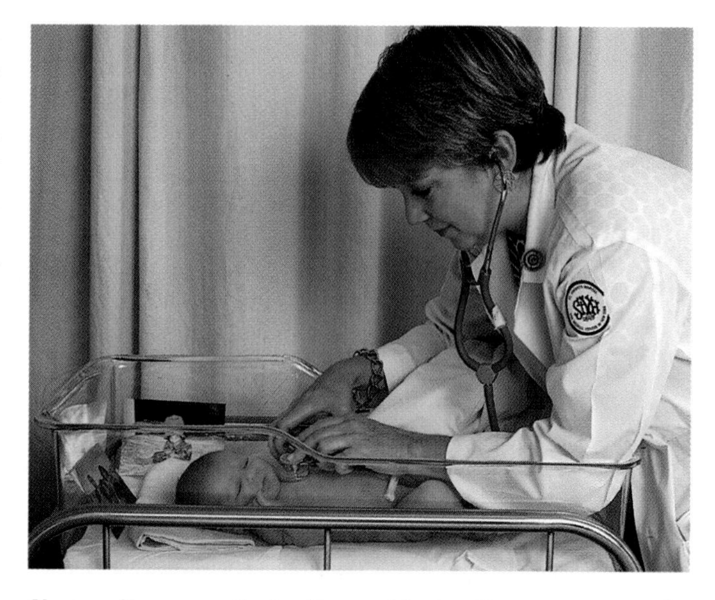

***Nurses*** Nurses are the backbone of the health care system and the largest group of health care professionals in the country. They perform a wide range of services, depending on their educational backgrounds and specified duties.

Many other health care professionals serve in allied fields, such as dentistry. They work cooperatively with physicians and nurses to provide comprehensive health care.

**Dentists** Dentists complete a bachelor's degree and four years of dental school, earning either a Doctor of Medical Dentistry (D.M.D.) or Doctor of Dental Surgery (D.D.S.) degree. Dentists diagnose and treat diseases of the teeth, gums, and oral cavity and provide preventive dental care. They may prescribe drugs and perform surgery as needed in the treatment of dental conditions.

**Technicians** Medical technicians serve a variety of functions, such as drawing blood, taking X-rays, doing laboratory work, or assisting dentists as oral hygienists. Depending on their positions and where they live, they have various kinds of education, training, and college degrees.

**Physicians' Assistants** Physicians' assistants (P.A.s) are typically trained in university settings at the bachelor's level and take a state test for licensure. They work under a physician's supervision and perform certain medical procedures, such as suturing superficial wounds, so as to free up the physician's time. P.A.s typically practice in hospitals, clinics, or physicians' offices.

**Pharmacists** Pharmacists complete at least a bachelor's degree in pharmacy and may have additional training at the master's or doctoral level. Pharmacists dispense medications and advise patients concerning proper use of medications and possible complications, including side effects.

**Psychologists** Psychologists who provide health care services hold a doctoral degree, either a Ph.D. (Doctor of Philosophy) or Psy.D. (Doctor of Psychology) degree. Psychologists employ psychological tests and perform research. Those with training in clinical psychology diagnose psychological disorders and practice psychotherapy.

**Optometrists** Optometrists obtain the Doctor of Optometry (O.D.) degree. They are qualified to perform vision tests and prescribe and fit corrective glasses and contact lenses. Medical conditions affecting the eyes are treated by ophthalmologists, medical doctors who specialize in the treatment of eye diseases.

With so many allied health professions, professional roles and competencies sometimes overlap. Psychiatrists and psychologists diagnose and treat psychological disorders. Optometrists and ophthalmologists conduct eye exams and prescribe glasses and contact lenses. Nurse practitioners perform some of the same procedures or examinations as physicians. Optometrists in 47 states can prescribe drugs, as can some psychologists who have been trained in a special federal program. Such diffusion of roles can confuse consumers. It also occasionally leads to conflicts or "turf battles" between the professions. Optometrists, for example, have clashed with ophthalmologists over the right to use a laser process to correct nearsightedness, a technique that only medical doctors have been permitted to use.[9] The issue of prescription privileges for psychologists remains a hotly contested issue between psychologists and psychiatrists and within the field of psychology itself. Health care consumers need to be acquainted with the backgrounds and roles of the professionals they consult. When in doubt, the best approach is the direct one: Ask your health care providers to discuss the scope of their practices and the types of services they can provide in meeting your health care needs.

## Types of Health Care Facilities

Health care is delivered in many different kinds of facilities ranging from doctor's offices to hospitals.

**Hospitals** Hospitals are the primary institutional settings for delivering health care. There are many types of hospitals, each serving particular health care needs. These include community and municipal hospitals, Veterans Administration hospitals, and long-term care facilities, such as psychiatric hospitals and rehabilitation institutes.

Hospitals vary in their range of services and their capacity to house patients. A small rural or community hospital may be able to provide inpatient care for fewer than 25 patients, may employ only a few nurses and ancillary staff, and may limit its services to the basics, such as medical-surgical, labor and delivery, newborn care, laboratory work, and pharmaceutical services.

Larger hospitals and medical centers are typically located in metropolitan areas and may be affiliated with schools of medicine and nursing. Some offer a wide variety of medical services. In addition to direct care, larger hospitals often have teaching and research functions. They may have hundreds of beds and employ thousands of professionals (e.g., nurses, doctors, laboratory technicians) and ancillary staff (e.g., secretaries, administrators, aides, maintenance workers). They may have coronary care and intensive care units, specialized clinics and diagnostic services, trauma units, social services, and rehabilitation and long-term care facilities.

A large hospital is a highly complex system that is bound to be confusing to the newly admitted patient. It is best to have some familiarity with the structure and organization of your local hospital or medical center before you need it. Most larger hospitals offer tours or brochures to people in the community. It is also helpful to have someone, such as a close friend or family member, as a companion if you need to be hospitalized. This person can act as an advocate for you when dealing with the hospital bureaucracy.

With increasing pressures on hospitals to contain costs, many carry out elective surgery on an outpatient or ambulatory care basis whenever feasible. Advances in surgical procedures have enabled many patients to go home on the same day or on the day following surgery. Minimizing hospital stays reduces costs and appeals to patients who prefer to recuperate in their own homes.

**Extended Care Facilities** Hospitals have increasingly become intensive care facilities that provide treatment for trauma and acute disease. The reasons for this are largely economic. Hospitals are labor-intensive and expensive to operate. Insurance companies and government programs that pay for most hospital services seek lower-cost alternatives to extended stays, such as extended care facilities, hospices, and home health care. The recovery process or maintenance period for serious and prolonged disease or disability also typically occurs in extended care facilities.

**Extended care facilities** include nursing homes and convalescent homes. These institutions provide long-term medical, nursing, or custodial care for patients with chronic physical illness and disability that prevents them from living more independently. **Rehabilitation centers** provide treatment and rehabilitative services for patients suffering from stroke, spinal cord injuries, degenerative diseases, and other disabling conditions. They seek to restore patients to their maximal level of functioning and independence. **Psychiatric hospitals** provide long-term care to people with severe psychological disorders, such as schizophrenia. They also share the goal of moving patients toward more independence and higher levels of functioning. Hospices provide institutional as well as home care that respects the dignity of the terminally ill (see Chapter 20).

**Home Health Care** Many people who suffer serious or prolonged illness or disability prefer to receive medical care in their own homes. **Home health care** can enable infirm older people to remain in their own homes rather than be confined to a nursing home or other institution. People with degenerative diseases that impair their mobility may also be able to function at home under a home health care plan.

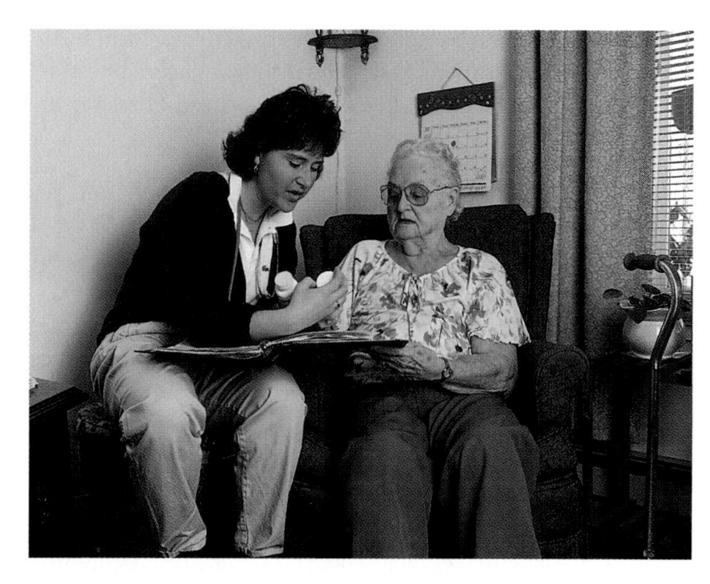

***Home Health Care*** Home health care makes it possible for many infirm older people to remain in their homes rather than be confined to nursing homes or other institutions.

The movement toward home health care is driven not only by preference but by costs. Home health care typically costs far less than comparable treatment in a hospital or residential facility. Home health care services vary with the needs of the patient. They may include visits by a registered nurse to perform such procedures as catheterizations, injections, and dressing changes; regular visits by trained home care aides to provide custodial care, such as bathing, eating, and dressing; and physical therapy services.

Home health care offers many advantages, but lapses in care and outright abuses have been known to occur. The patient or the family needs to investigate the quality of the home health care programs in their area and monitor the services regularly. People seeking home health care should ask for referrals from their family physicians. It would also be prudent to check out the reputation of the home health care agency with the head nurse on a medical or surgical unit

**Extended care facilities** Inpatient facilities providing long-term custodial or medical care, especially for people suffering from chronic diseases or requiring continued rehabilitation.

**Rehabilitation centers** Health care facilities providing comprehensive services to help people with disabilities achieve a maximum level of functioning and a more satisfying and independent life.

**Psychiatric hospitals** Specialized hospitals providing inpatient psychiatric services.

**Home health care** A system of providing health care services to people in their homes.

at your local hospital and with your local health department. Your state health department can tell you whether the agency has been cited for any deficiencies.

**Outpatient Facilities** Most health care services are offered on an outpatient basis and housed in a hospital, clinic, or medical office setting. Most larger hospitals offer outpatient services in clinics tied to specialty areas such as pediatrics, gynecology, oncology, and psychiatry. In medical centers affiliated with medical schools, the clinics may function as part of the medical school department and provide training opportunities to medical students and residents.

Many colleges and universities operate student health centers. These centers are freestanding medical clinics that provide a range of medical services to students and in some cases to faculty members, staff members, and their families. Some of the larger student health centers provide inpatient as well as outpatient services.

Small or large groups of physicians may also form a clinic. Depending on their resources, clinics may offer diagnosis and treatment services for a few or many health care specialties. In larger clinics, there may be hundreds of physicians and nurses treating a wide range of health care problems. Health care providers in clinics consist primarily of physicians, nurses, nurse specialists and nurse practitioners, physician assistants, and support staff.

Community health centers, or public health clinics, primarily serve residents of traditionally underserved communities. Private physicians in these areas may be hard to find or unwilling to accept patients without private insurance or the ability to pay for medical services out of pocket. Community health centers treat patients who are eligible for government-subsidized care, such as Medicaid and Medicare, as well as those with other forms of health coverage. They typically offer a wide range of medical and mental health services at relatively modest cost.

A physician who practices alone or in a small group practice usually specializes in a particular area of practice, such as pediatrics, gynecology, or family practice. Physicians in group practices may use outside support services, such as labs and X-ray facilities, or have their own. They may also employ registered nurses to perform a wide variety of services or form partnerships with nurse practitioners or certified nurse midwives.

PREVENTION

## *Your Health Checkup—What Happens and Why*

People who actively manage their health care obtain regular medical checkups. They also educate themselves so they understand what happens during a medical exam, why it happens, and what is expected of them.

**Meeting and Speaking with Your Health Care Provider** From the start of your conversation, your health care provider or HCP—typically a physician or a nurse—begins an initial assessment of your physical and psychological health status. The HCP judges whether you appear to be taking care of yourself by noting your personal hygiene, grooming, dress, and presence of any body odors. The HCP judges your mental status by observing your general state of alertness, your ability to state your problems and to recall symptoms (their frequency, duration, intensity, location), and your nonverbal behavior (e.g., body posture, facial expression, and voice intensity).

**Taking Your Medical History** The conscientious HCP takes a thorough medical history. This information should be obtained on the first visit and updated regularly. It includes information about past illnesses, hospitalizations and surgical procedures, and family history of illness. Other relevant information, such as marital and family background, educational level, and health habits (smoking, exercise, alcohol intake), is gathered. To ensure the best possible care, you need to cooperate fully by giving information that is as complete and accurate as possible. The information goes into your medical record, which is held by your HCP. Medical records are confidential. They cannot be released without your consent except under special circumstances, such as a court order by a judge. However, you may be required to release certain medical records as a condition of receiving reimbursement from your medical insurance carrier or managed care company, or when you apply for life insurance.

**The Physical Exam** You may be asked to remove your outer clothing and don an examination gown so that your HCP can conduct a thorough physical exam. The exam may vary from one practitioner to another but generally covers the following areas:

1. *Vital signs:* In addition to checking your weight and height, the HCP will record your vital signs, such as body temperature, pulse, and blood pressure. This information gives a general indication of your health status, which is investigated further during the examination.
2. *Heart and lung function:* The HCP will use his or her hands, eyes, ears, and sense of smell to touch, examine visually, listen, and note body odors for indications of

pathology. The HCP will use a stethoscope to listen to your chest and back to evaluate your lung function and breathing. The HCP will thump your chest and back to further assess the condition of your lungs and use the stethoscope to check heart action and blood flow. The HCP may further assess respiratory and cardiac status through a resting electrocardiogram (ECG) or a dynamic (active) ECG. The HCP will assess subtle signs of disturbed heart or lung function by noting symptoms such as a bluish coloring **(cyanosis)** of the nail beds, lips, mouth, and skin.

Talking Glossary
Cyanosis
G2301

3. *Head and neck:* Examining the size, shape, and contour of the head can reveal information about abnormalities of the skull and brain.
4. *Eyes:* The reaction of the pupils to light and the movement of the eyeball can reveal information about neurological problems.
5. *Nose and sinuses:* Signs of inflammation, discharges, obstructions, and nosebleeds can indicate problems relating to allergies, sinus infections, lesions, or underlying structural problems.
6. *Ears:* Examination of the external ear, ear canals, and eardrum can reveal inflammations due to infection, blockages, and deformities.
7. *Mouth and pharynx:* The condition of the lips and mucosal lining of the mouth (color, texture, presence of lesions) can reveal the presence of infections, structural abnormalities, or cancer.
8. *Neck, lymph nodes, thyroid gland, and trachea:* The HCP will examine for **symmetry, edema,** presence of masses or of abnormal shape, tenderness, or mobility. Examination of blood vessels in the neck can reveal cardiovascular problems. Enlarged lymph nodes may indicate infection or malignancy. An enlarged **thyroid gland** indicates a disturbance of thyroid function. Displacement of the **trachea** (windpipe) can be caused by masses in the neck or pulmonary (lung) abnormalities.

Talking Glossary
Edema, Thyroid, Trachea
G2302

9. *Breasts:* The HCP should screen for breast cancer by checking both breasts for symmetry, masses, thickening, retraction or dimpling of skin, discharge from the nipples, tenderness, size, contour, and color. This information can reveal tumors or fibrous conditions. A man's breasts should also be checked, as breast cancer can occur in males.
10. *Abdomen:* By touch and visual inspection, the HCP will examine the abdomen for signs of pathology (including masses, displacement, distention, and irregularities in shape and symmetry) of the interior organs, including the stomach, liver, intestines, pancreas, and bladder. The HCP will ask the patient to report any pain during the examination.
11. *Female genitalia and rectum:* The HCP will examine the external and internal genitalia, taking into account symmetry and shape and looking for signs of infection, such as lesions, thickening, ulcerations, discharges, or unusual odors and color. A Pap smear will be taken to screen for cervical cancer. The **perianal** area is inspected for inflammation, discoloration, lesions, and hemorrhoids. The **rectum** should be examined internally for any abnormalities of the rectal cavity.

Talking Glossary
Perianal
G2303

12. *Male genitalia and rectum:* Examination of the male genitalia should include the external genitals (penis, scrotum), the **groin,** and the prostate gland. Abnormal signs that indicate infection or diseased condition of the organs, such as masses, enlargements, discharges, lesions, swelling, and inflammation, will be noted. The rectum should be examined, during which the prostate gland will be **palpated.** The healthy prostate gland feels firm without bogginess, tenderness, hardness, or **nodules.**

Talking Glossary
Palpate, Nodule
G2304

13. *Musculoskeletal system:* The HCP pays attention to how the patient moves and walks about the room, rises from a chair, gets on and off the examining table, and moves upon request. Information about range of joint movement, muscle strength and tone, and general condition of the bones, muscles, and joints may reveal injury, effects of aging, or disease.
14. *Neurological system and mental functioning:* The HCP evaluates the patient's psychological health by noting whether he or she answers questions coher-

**Cyanosis** A bluish or purplish coloration resulting from deficient oxygenation of the blood.

**Symmetry** A condition of likeness in both halves.

**Edema** Swelling.

**Thyroid gland** An endocrine gland lying on both sides of the windpipe; produces thyroxin, a hormone involved in regulating body metabolism and growth.

**Trachea** The tube that carries air between the larynx and the bronchial tubes; also called the windpipe.

**Perianal** Surrounding the anus.

**Rectum** The terminal portion of the intestine, ending in the *anus,* the opening through which solid waste is excreted.

**Groin** The area between the thigh and the trunk. Also called the *inguinal region.*

**Palpate** To examine by touch.

**Nodules** Small nodes or swellings.

ently, by asking questions about his or her psychological state ("Have you noticed any changes in your mood or emotions lately?"), and by attending to the patient's facial expression and other nonverbal cues for signs of depression, confusion, or belligerence. The HCP also assesses nerve function, sensory function, motor function, and reflexes, looking for signs of neurological impairment.

### Common Diagnostic Tests Used during Physical Checkups

1. *Urinalysis.* Laboratory examination of your urine tells the HCP a great deal about your health, especially the health of your bladder and kidneys. The presence of glucose in your urine suggests that you may have diabetes mellitus. Normal urine is pale yellow to amber, clear to slightly hazy, and mildly aromatic.
2. *Blood analysis.* A blood sample may be taken and analyzed to measure numbers of white and red blood cells, platelets, hemoglobin, **hematocrit,** clotting and bleeding times; blood gas values such as **pH level** (acidity or alkalinity); blood chemistry values such as levels of glucose, cholesterol, chloride, calcium, and other minerals; and **serology** values (e.g., presence of antibodies to hepatitis, syphilis, and HIV). You may be asked not to eat for a certain amount of time before your blood is taken to avoid producing misleading values in your blood test.

Talking Glossary
Hematocrit, Serology
G2305

3. *Stool exam and sigmoidoscopy.* Your HCP may request a stool specimen. It will be analyzed for blood, bacteria, and parasites. After a certain age or when there are signs of abnormalities, such as chronic diarrhea or blood in the stool, your HCP will perform a **sigmoidoscopy. Proctoscopes** and **sigmoidoscopes** allow the examiner to see within the rectum in order to examine the condition of the rectum and other organs.

Talking Glossary
Sigmoidoscopy, Proctoscope, Sigmoidoscope
G2306

4. *Mammography.* After a certain age or with the presence of symptoms or a family history of breast cancer, the HCP will ask a female patient to have a mammogram to detect cancerous lumps or masses that may be too tiny to be discovered manually.
5. *Chest X-ray.* Because of the dangers of radiation, a chest X-ray is no longer a standard part of a medical checkup. It may be ordered when suspicions are raised about abnormalities or pathology in the lungs, heart, diaphragm, aorta, or chest wall. Women who are pregnant or suspect that they might be should not undergo an X-ray because of possible harm to the fetus.

**Hematocrit** The ratio of the volume of red blood cells to a given volume of blood, expressed as a percentage.

**pH level** The degree of acidity or alkalinity of a substance.

**Serology** Laboratory analysis of blood serum.

**Sigmoidoscopy** Use of the sigmoidoscope to examine the colon.

**Proctoscope** Instrument used to examine the rectum.

**Sigmoidoscope** A flexible tubular instrument used for examining the colon.

## Alternative Therapies

Alternative therapies (also called unconventional treatment) involve the use of nontraditional or nonstandard approaches to medical treatment. Medicine is evolving, and some nontraditional techniques of today may enter the mainstream of medical practice tomorrow if they are shown to be effective. Alternative therapies include Eastern therapies such as acupuncture and transcendental meditation, vitamin therapy, chiropractic, nutritional therapies, homeopathy, biofeedback, herbal remedies, massage, and unconventional therapies, such as the use of bee pollen in treating allergy sufferers. Many of these practices are widely accepted in other parts of the world and have been used for many years in Western cultures.

Use of alternative therapies is not limited to a few patients on the fringe. Americans spend billions of dollars each year on alternative medical care. One in ten Americans consults an unconventional practitioner each year.[10] Unconventional practitioners include chiropractors, spiritual and herbal healers, homeopathic practitioners, acupuncturists, and massage therapists. Another 25% use unconventional therapies on their own, such as taking large doses of vitamins or participating in self-help groups. People with back conditions are the most common users of alternative therapies. About one in three back pain sufferers seeks alternative care, usually chiropractic.

Long dismissed by the medical establishment, unconventional therapies are now often recognized as legitimate areas of scientific study. One sign of this recognition was the establishment in 1992 of the Office of Alternative Medicine within the prestigious National Institutes of Health (NIH), the federal agency that oversees biomedical research in the U.S.[11] The OAM serves as a clearinghouse for information on alternative therapies, coordinates studies on alternative treatments under way in other NIH departments, and provides grants to support research on the effectiveness of alternative therapies.

Medical insurance carriers have traditionally picked up little if any of the costs of alternative therapies. Today, however, about half of the alternative medical treatments people use are covered by some form of health insurance. Certain insurers cover treatments such as acupuncture for chronic pain, diet and meditation programs in the treatment of heart disease, and massage therapy.[12] Let us consider some alternative therapies in greater detail.

**Meditation** **Meditation** refers to techniques that induce a relaxed state by focusing the attention on some activity, object, or image. In some cultures, meditation is believed to help people achieve spiritual or creative enlightenment. Meditation stands at the boundary between traditional and alternative medicine. Traditional medicine has increasingly come to accept meditation for some uses, including combating stress and high blood pressure.

**Biofeedback** **Biofeedback** refers to the use of specialized equipment to provide people with information (feedback) about their internal bodily states or activities, such as heart rate, muscle tension, and body temperature. Feedback may be provided in the form of tones that increase or decrease in pitch in relation to changes in internal bodily states. By learning to change the tone in the desired direction (making it rise or fall in pitch, for instance), people can gain control over various bodily functions. They may learn to induce states of relaxation by reducing muscle tension in selected muscle groups or by increasing the frequency of certain brain wave patterns. Biofeedback is now commonly used to treat such conditions as hypertension, headaches, and stress.

**Visualization** **Visualization** involves the use of mental imagery to alter bodily functions such as heart rate and blood pressure. Like meditation, visualization (such as by mentally picturing oneself lying on a warm, tropical beach) can help people achieve a relaxed state, which can calm the nervous system and lower the heart and breathing rates. Visualization is also widely used to treat chronic pain. People in pain may use mental imagery to psychologically detach themselves from their pain.

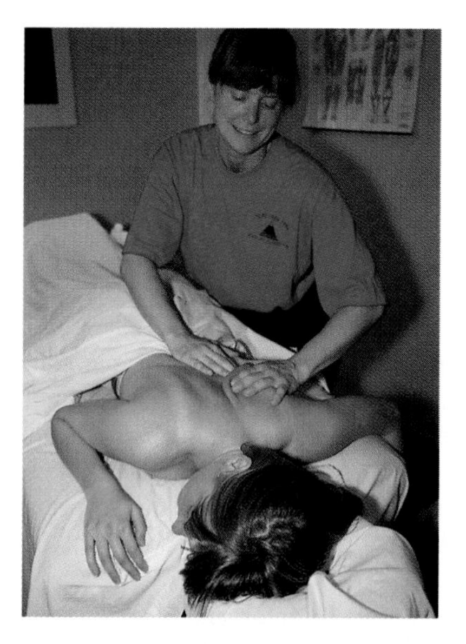

***Massage Therapy*** Therapeutic massage is widely used as a means of combating stress by loosening tight muscles and inducing feelings of relaxation. Researchers are now examining whether it may have other benefits, such as bolstering the body's immune system.

**Therapeutic Massage** Massage has long been recognized as an antidote to stress. It helps loosen tight muscles and eases one into a deeply relaxed state. Now researchers are investigating whether **therapeutic massage** has other health benefits, such as improving immunological functioning, speeding recovery from hard workouts, combating insomnia, and relieving pain. Massage therapy is emerging as a major adjunctive therapy that not only feels great but can help combat stress and may improve the body's ability to fend off colds and viruses.[13]

More than 50 types of massage are practiced today, ranging from Swedish massage, in which the therapist mostly uses gliding, kneading, and rubbing strokes, to sports massage, which focuses mostly on areas of the body that are overworked during exercise. Shiatsu is a Japanese style of massage that stimulates areas that lie along acupuncture pathways that practitioners believe run from the head to the toes. Practitioners believe that massaging these acupuncture points stimulates a healthy flow of energy. Western scientists suspect that the pressure applied on these points might release endorphins, natural chemicals produced in the brain that deaden pain and produce feelings of pleasure. Unlike Swedish massage, during which the client lies unclothed on a padded

**Meditation** A method of focused attention that induces a state of relaxation.

**Biofeedback** A device that provides information about the user's internal bodily states.

**Visualization** The use of mental imagery to achieve a therapeutic benefit.

**Therapeutic massage** The therapeutic use of rubbing and kneading the body to improve circulation, increase suppleness, and promote relaxation.

table covered by a sheet, in shiatsu the client remains clothed and lies on the floor or on a mat.

If you are interested in exploring the health benefits of massage therapy, choose a good massage therapist, preferably someone who is certified by the National Certification Board of Therapeutic Massage and Bodywork. Certification requires completing a course of study and passing a test. Many states and the District of Columbia require massage therapists to be licensed by the state. Some insurance companies cover at least a portion of the expenses for therapeutic massage, but usually only when it is prescribed by a physician and considered medically appropriate (for example, for treating back pain or a pulled muscle).

**Acupuncture** **Acupuncture** has been practiced in Chinese medicine for over 2,000 years. In this technique, thin needles are inserted at certain points on the body and rotated by the acupuncturist. According to traditional Chinese medicine, manipulation of the needles releases the body's natural healing energy. Though Western medicine has scoffed at the notion of acupuncture releasing a natural healing energy, there is some evidence that acupuncture can help treat health problems such as back pain, asthma, arthritis, migraine headaches, and complications from strokes.[14]

If acupuncture helps, it may be because it, like massage, releases endorphins, the body's natural painkillers. Acupuncture may also stimulate release of body chemicals that fight the body's inflammatory response, which could yield benefits in treating arthritis and allergic reactions, including asthma. Though scientific research on the health benefits of acupuncture remains scanty, more than 12 million Americans have turned to acupuncture. Many more might try it if it were covered by insurance.

**Acupuncture** A traditional technique of Chinese medicine believed to release natural healing energies. Thin needles are inserted and rotated at specific points along the body.

Talking Glossary
Homeopathy
G2307

**Homeopathy** An alternative medical approach based on the use of tiny doses of curative substances.

**Reflexology** The practice of massaging parts of the foot to relieve stress or pain in other parts of the body.

**Iridology** The study of how changes in the iris of the eye may be related to disease.

**Herbology** Herbal medicine; the use of natural substances from plants, trees, and flowers to treat disease.

**Chiropractic** A system of health care based on the premise that spinal misalignments play a significant role in many physical problems.

**Homeopathy** **Homeopathy** emphasizes the treatment of the patient rather than the disease. Homeopathic practitioners, some of whom are licensed physicians, emphasize building up the patient's strength through rest, a healthy diet, microscopic doses of drugs, and positive thinking. The goal is to enable the person to resist disease. Homeopathic practitioners use minuscule levels of natural substances as curative remedies. They believe that the healing powers of these substances are unleashed by vigorously shaking the ingredients, which they maintain changes the substance's energy pattern.

Though many traditional doctors subscribe to some tenets of homeopathy, such as the focus on the whole patient, they do not believe that the smaller the dosage of a drug or natural substance, the more potent its effects—shaken or not. The recently created Office of Alternative Medicine of the National Institutes of Health intends to take a critical look at the claims made by homeopathic practitioners.

Close-up
Homeopathy: Real medicine or empty promises?
T2301

Other unconventional treatments include **reflexology** (treatment based on manipulating pressure points on the hands and feet to relieve stress and pain), **iridology** (treatment based on abnormal markings of the iris of the eye), and **herbology** (medicinal uses of plants). Though the medical establishment remains skeptical of these treatments, the use of **chiropractic** (treatment by manipulation of the spinal column) in the treatment of lower back pain has been gaining support, even among some members of the medical professon.[15] The use of chiropractic to treat other medical problems remains more controversial.

Talking Glossary
Reflexology, Iridology, Herbology, Chiropractic
G2308

**A Word of Caution** Alternative therapies should not be used in place of conventional medicine, since alternative medical practitioners may miss underlying pathology. A person with back pain, for instance, may have a hidden problem such as a tumor that can go unrecognized if the person forgoes seeing a medical doctor. As medicine continues to evolve, support may build for some forms of alternative medicine. In the meantime, the age-old adage applies: Let the buyer beware. Many of the claims for the health benefits of alternative medicine are just that—claims, not scientific fact.

## Health Care Reform

The American health care system is massive, largely unmanageable, and plagued by ever-rising costs. One person in four is uninsured or *under*insured. Many people fall through the cracks of the health insurance system. They are not poor enough to qualify for government-subsidized health care programs, and they are not wealthy enough to purchase a health insurance policy on their own. Thus, they face the prospect of not being able to pay for medical care or of going bankrupt in the process. Many either are unemployed or work for small employers who do not provide health insurance benefits.

These concerns about the health care system spurred efforts at reform in the early 1990s. Though the large-scale reforms advanced by the first Clinton administration failed to garner congressional support, some smaller-scale but much-needed reforms have been enacted. A major piece of reform came in 1996, when a bill was signed into law that guaranteed that workers could keep their health insurance if they should change jobs or be laid off. The law also prevents companies from denying coverage to people with pre-existing conditions. However, the bill does not prevent health insurance companies from tagging on higher premiums for people with pre-existing conditions.[16]

Health care reformers hope that additional legislative initiatives will move toward the goal of universal health insurance. In the meantime, major changes are occurring in the health insurance field, largely because employers and governments are balking at paying for ever-rising health care costs.

Smart Quiz
Q2301

### think about it!

- **Have you or your family ever experienced "sticker shock" when you learned of the cost of health care? Describe the situation.**
- **What kinds of health care providers have you used? For what kinds of problems?**
- **What kinds of health care facilities have been used by you or your family? What were the experience and the cost like?**

**critical thinking** **Agree or disagree and support your answer: People should not use alternative therapies until they have been proved to be safe and effective.**

**critical thinking** **Agree or disagree and support your answer: Employers should be required to offer health insurance coverage to all workers, including part-time workers.**

## TYPES OF HEALTH INSURANCE PLANS

Visiting a doctor today can range from $75 to $250 or more for a specialist. In addition to the doctor's fees, there are expensive lab tests and sophisticated diagnostic tests, such as the MRI, which can cost $1,000 or more. Should you require hospitalization or surgery, the costs can quickly exceed the reach of all but the wealthiest among us. Were it not for medical insurance, quality medical care might be limited to the very wealthy.

A variety of programs have been developed to help Americans afford health care. They include (1) private health insurance, including traditional insurance ("fee-for-service") plans and managed care plans; (2) government insurance such as Medicaid and Medicare; and (3) public health programs, such as well-baby clinics (WBCs) and family planning clinics.

Medical care is shifting rapidly from traditional fee-for-service insurance plans to managed care. While few people in 1970 had even heard of managed care, today three of four workers and their families, some 150 million Americans, belong to a managed care plan.[17] The meteoric rise in the utilization of managed care during the 1980s and 1990s was fueled by the steep rise in conventional, fee-for-service insurance premiums—paid largely by employers. In the early 1980s, premiums for fee-for-service Blue Cross and Blue Shield plans shot up 20 to 30% per year. As a result, large companies began shifting their health care coverage from fee-for-service plans to managed care plans that promised to constrain rising costs.[18]

With each passing year, the percentage of workers being given a choice about their health care coverage is shrinking, down from 90% in 1988 to about 50% by 1996. Employees are being forced to enroll in managed care plans or to use physicians from a designated provider list. Many are asked to pay more for doctor visits, to contribute more to annual premiums, and to pay larger **deductibles.** As we look toward the new millennium, the traditional fee-for-service or indemnity plan that provided your parents with free or low-cost health insurance, low deductibles, and a choice of health care providers may well become a statistical rarity.[19] To hold on to their market, many traditional fee-for-service carriers are beginning to offer a range of managed care plans.

**Deductible** The annual amount that the individual must pay for medical expenses before the health insurance plan starts contributing its share.

We have also entered an era of mergers and realignments among health care benefits companies. Health maintenance organizations (HMOs) are merging with other HMOs, and managed care companies are merging with large insurance companies. The largest merger to date occurred in 1996, when Aetna Life and Casualty Company, a major insurance company, purchased U.S. Healthcare, Inc., one of the nation's largest managed health care companies. The combined company became the largest health benefits company in the U.S., serving some 23 million people, or 1 of every 12 Americans. It provides both medical insurance benefits and direct medical services.[20]

What might the shift toward larger health care benefits companies mean to the average consumer? It will probably mean a more limited range of health care options, because these stronger companies will control an increasing share of the market and be better able to dictate fees paid to doctors and hospitals. HMOs and managed care companies have gotten so large, critics say, that they are stifling innovation in health care, dictating where patients can go for care and what kinds of care they will pay for. Fighting this tide, groups of hospitals and doctors, and in some cases coalitions of large employers, have banded together to bypass managed care companies and offer managed care plans of their own.[21] In 1996, the federal government loosened restraints on doctors, allowing them to form networks of their own, set prices, and market their services to employers.[22]

Unless we plan never to get ill or need medical services, chances are that we will be affected by changes in the health care benefits field. These changes will determine what types of health care plans will be available to us, what they will cost, and what benefits they will provide. Even if we are presently covered by a conventional fee-for-service plan through our school or place of employment, a managed care plan may be in the offing.

Let us take a closer look at the two major types of health insurance plans, fee-for-service plans and managed care plans. Knowing these plans' advantages and disadvantages helps us to make informed decisions regarding our health care.

## Fee-for-Service Plans

**Fee-for-service (FFS) plans** Traditional insurance plans in which the insurance carrier pays a percentage of covered medical expenses after deductibles.

**Fee-for-service (FFS) plans** (also called *indemnity plans*) were once the "standard" form of private health insurance. Today, however, only about one in four working Americans who receives health insurance through his or her job is covered by a fee-for-service plan. Under an FSS plan, you can use any licensed physician or other health care provider (such as a psychologist or podiatrist), or use the services of any accredited hospital, and the plan will pay for a certain proportion—usually 80%—of the charges after an annual deductible is met (typically $100 to $500). Coinsurance is the percentage of the bill that the insured person must pay, or copay.

Some plans also impose an annual or a lifetime cap. These are the maximum amounts they will cover for a particular condition within a given year or the person's lifetime. Under a fee-for-service plan, insurance carriers have nonexclusive relationships with physicians and other health care providers. This means that health care providers are free to treat anyone they like regardless of their patients' insurance coverage.

In this traditional "unmanaged" plan, the insurance carrier processes claims and pay bills for services rendered by physicians and other health care providers at rates that reflect customary and reasonable charges. Charges imposed by doctors in excess of the eligible charges (charges that the insurance company deems reasonable) are not covered by the plan. For this reason, it is prudent to check with your insurance carrier to determine the limit on its coverage before undergoing any expensive medical treatments or procedures, such as elective surgery. You may be able to find health care practitioners, including surgeons, whose charges fall within the plan's guidelines. Or you might ask your health care providers whether they are willing to reduce their fees to the level set by your insurance company. Don't be hesitant about asking for a fee reduction if you fear that the costs may exceed your insurance coverage or ability to pay. Plans also vary with respect to their restrictions and limitations, so check the fine print. Such services as dental work and vision tests and eyeglasses are commonly not covered. Limitations may be imposed on treatment for psychological disorders. Plans also limit coverage to treatments they deem medically necessary and effective (certain experimental treatments are excluded).

Indemnity plans are usually purchased by employers for their employees as part of a benefits package. The broader the coverage, the greater the cost. In some cases, employees are required to contribute a portion of the annual premiums.

Individuals or families may also purchase health insurance for themselves, though usually at higher cost than the comparable plans offered to large employers.

Colleges and universities may provide students with opportunities to purchase health insurance, typically at a lower cost than they could obtain on their own. Students may assume that they are automatically covered by their parents' insurance plans. This is not always the case, especially if the student is no longer a minor. Some insurance companies offer parents an option (at higher cost) to cover the health care of their nonminor children who are still students.

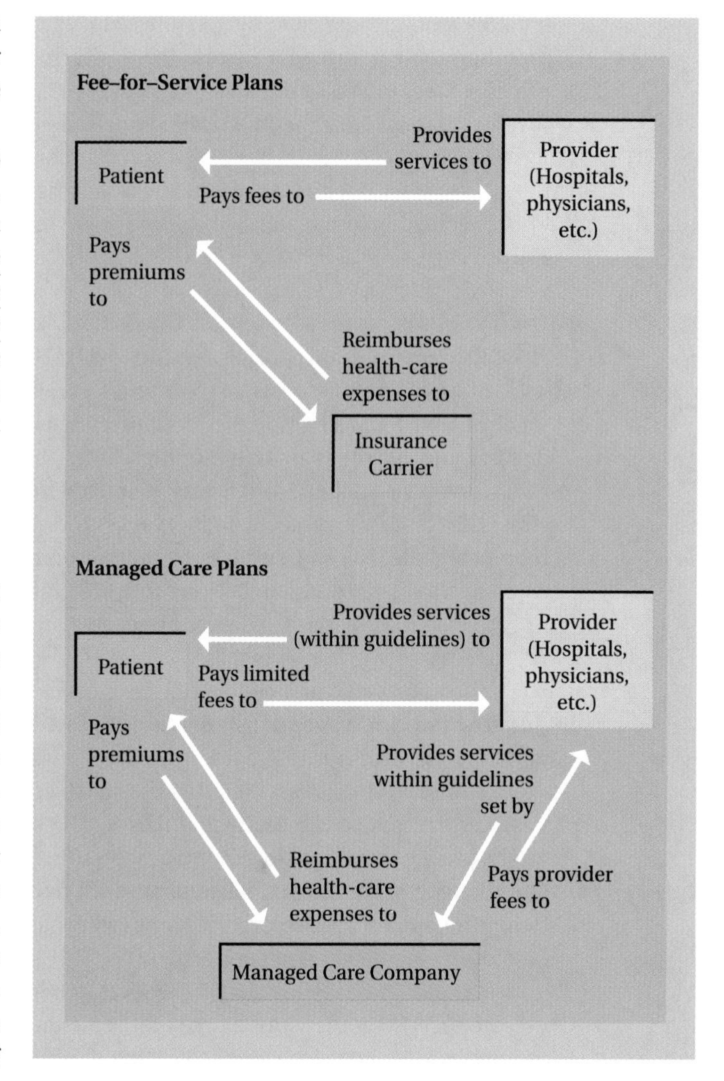


**Figure 23.3** *Samples of Health Insurance Plans*

## Managed Care

A managed care plan is also called a *prepaid* health insurance plan. In such plans, a group of doctors or hospitals, or, more typically, a managed care company, agrees to provide health care services to individuals or groups of employees for a prepaid amount of money (see Figure 23.3). Premiums are usually **capitated.** That is, the managed care company gets a certain amount of money for each member (enrollee) in the plan, regardless of how much medical care the member requires. Large employers usually pay for these annual premiums, though individuals may pay a fixed annual fee plus a modest **copayment** (typically $5 or $10) for doctor's visits with little or no deductible. If members choose to see a doctor who is not on the list of approved providers, they can expect to pay more or all of the bill.

The assumption underlying managed care is that it is possible to reduce costs while maintaining quality care by cutting waste and use of unnecessary or unduly expensive medical tests and procedures. A managed care plan might more accurately be described as a *managed costs* plan, since it attempts to provide health care services while containing costs. Managed care companies employ case managers and health care professionals who serve as "gatekeepers" by overseeing referrals for consultations with specialists, use of expensive diagnostic tests (like MRI), and expensive medical procedures. Managed care companies also monitor the referral practices of doctors in their networks. In some cases, the plans reward doctors with economic incentives (bonuses) for limiting their use of outside specialists and medical tests, and penalize those they consider wasteful.

The most common types of managed care plans are preferred provider organizations (PPOs) and health maintenance organizations (HMOs).

### Preferred Provider Organizations (PPOs)

**Preferred provider organizations,** or **PPOs,** are groups of health care providers who agree, in return for patient referrals, to provide health care to members of a managed care plan for fees that are typically 15 to 20% lower than their customary rates. Physicians treat patients in their own offices as they do under conventional FFS plans and are free to treat

**Capitated** A fixed amount paid per individual in the health plan, regardless of medical services used.

**Copayment** A set amount the individual pays for a medical service provided under HMO coverage.

**Preferred provider organizations (PPOs)** A group of health care providers who agree to provide services to members of a managed care plan for a discounted rate.

patients who are not members of the plan. Plan members select providers from the preferred provider list supplied by the managed care company, which pays for the medical services less required copayments or deductibles. Members may also select doctors or use medical facilities not participating in the plan but will pay more for the privilege.

### Health Maintenance Organizations (HMOs)

A **health maintenance organization** or **HMO** is a prepaid medical service plan that offers medical and surgical services through affiliated doctors and hospitals or freestanding clinics. In 1970, only 3.6 million Americans belonged to HMOs. By 1996, more than 60 million did.[23] Today, more than half of all employees in company-sponsored health insurance plans belong to HMOs, up from fewer than a third as recently as the late 1980s.[24]

As the managed care field continues to evolve, the structure of HMOs and their relationships with participating health care providers are becoming more complex. HMOs vary in terms of where services are provided (individual doctor's office, group practices, or staffed medical care setting) and the type of contractual relationship with participating doctors (exclusive vs. nonexclusive; employee vs. independent contractor).[25]

The traditional HMO is a **staff model HMO.** In this type of HMO, the company operates a community-based clinic or health facility that offers a wide range of medical services from primary care to specialty clinics. The physicians on staff treat only HMO members. The basic drawback of the staff model HMO is that many patients are reluctant to give up their usual doctors or the choice of doctors in their communities. Consequently, HMOs have been shifting away from the staff model toward models that allow members greater flexibility. In one increasingly popular model, the **point of service (POS)** plan, members of the HMO can use health care providers within an approved network or go outside the network for a higher per-visit charge. Providers within the network may have an exclusive or nonexclusive relationship with the HMO.

**Managed Care—The Pros and Cons** Managed care companies are typically for-profit business ventures. When outlays for medical expenses fall below the *capitated* (per-subscriber) level, the managed care company makes money. When outlays exceed the capitated level, the company may lose money. Since the company is motivated to maximize profits, it strives to keep medical expenses down. Many people are understandably concerned that the profit motive may lead companies to cut corners in providing medical care.[26] Even doctor-managed HMOs are not immune to potential conflicts of interest when capitated fees begin slipping below medical expenses. Critics contend that managed care companies restrict the range of medically necessary services in a number of ways, as in denying benefits for some services, making other services less accessible, excluding expensive drugs, and making members and primary care physicians "jump through hoops" to get certain services approved. Adjusting to the constraints of managed care has left many patients and their doctors angry and confused.

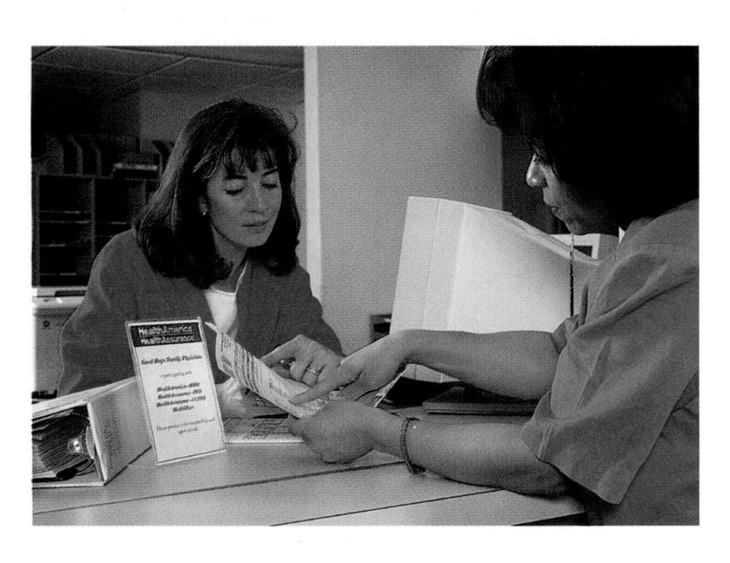

***Managed Care or Managed Costs?*** The growth of health maintenance organizations (HMOs) and other types of managed care plans has been phenomenal. Yet critics contend that managed care companies care more about managing costs than providing needed services.

**Health maintenance organization (HMO)** A prepaid managed care plan: costs are usually based on a fixed amount of money per enrollee.

**Staff model HMO** An HMO that offers comprehensive services only in a center with its own health care professionals.

**Point of service (POS)** An HMO that allows members to choose in-network doctors at low cost or outside doctors at higher cost.

Critics also contend that managed care systems may compromise the integrity of the physician-patient relationship. Plans may offer bonuses to participating physicians for limiting their use of expensive diagnostic tests and referrals to specialists or other ancillary services. Plans may also drop doctors who refer too many patients for expensive tests or procedures. For these reasons, doctors may have conflicting loyalties between their own self-interest and the patient's best interests.[27] Of course, physicians are bound by the ethical principles of their profession to put the patient's interests first and not to withhold needed care. Even so, the appropriateness of many treatments is not a black-and-white issue but falls within the doctor's discretion.

Patients, of course, may not know that available procedures and treatments are being withheld from them. Critics argue that physicians should divulge potential conflicts of interests to their patients, to state regulators, or to both (a few states now require disclosure[28]). The federal government recently placed limits on the bonuses that HMOs can pay doctors for controlling costs for services provided to Medicare and Medicaid patients.[29] Patients should not hesitate to ask their health care providers for full disclosure of financial incentives that might pose a conflict of interest and how they intend to deal with the issue. If the health care provider asks why you want to know, or appears defensive or evasive, you may want to consider finding someone else.

Managed care has defenders as well as critics. Defenders note that managed care plans offer a wider range of services, including preventive care (e.g., annual physical exams, well-baby care, mammograms) and vision examinations, than typical FFS plans do. They offer low or no deductibles and lower out-of-pocket expenses for medical visits (typically a $5 or $10 copayment rather than a 20% contribution under an FFS plan). Plans now offer a wider choice of providers in many cases, including opportunities for members to use out-of-network providers, albeit at a higher cost. Since managed care companies do not receive any higher fees for providing more services under capitation, they stand to benefit by emphasizing preventive services to keep their members well. Supporters of managed care also argue that sufficient controls exist to ensure that necessary medical care is provided, including medical ethics, fear of malpractice suits, and oversight by state regulators. With an eye toward improving quality of care, some companies conduct surveys of patients and reward doctors who are more highly rated by patients.

As with many issues in the public eye, there are two sides to the argument over managed care. Managed care holds the promise of cutting unnecessary expenses without compromising quality medical care. But is it a promise that cannot be kept? Just how are managed care plans shaping up? Are they delivering quality service for lower cost, or are they sacrificing quality for the sake of corporate profits?

**The Scorecard on Managed Care** Evidence on the quality of managed care comes largely from studies on HMOs, the most widely used model of managed care. When HMOs are compared with traditional fee-for-service plans, the HMOs have:[30]

- Lower rates of hospitalization and reduced lengths of stay
- Less use of expensive laboratory tests and procedures
- Greater emphasis on preventive medicine
- Some lower ratings of enrollee satisfaction with services received, but greater satisfaction with costs
- Roughly comparable quality of care as judged by peer reviewers (other doctors who review patient charts to see if the care provided was appropriate)

Overall, the available evidence shows HMOs offer about the same quality of care, as judged by outside doctors, as traditional plans do, but at lower cost.[31] From the standpoint of the consumer, the scorecard on HMOs is mixed. HMO patients are generally *less* satisfied with the services they receive, but *more* satisfied with the costs, than are members of traditional fee-for-service plans. Then, too, the performance of HMOs varies widely from place to place. Some plans may be better than others. Perhaps what is needed is not one type of plan or another, but a more flexible health delivery system that provides people with a freer choice of plans.

Quality of care is one thing. Stemming the rise in health care costs is another. Managed care appears to be slowing the rate of growth in health care costs in the U.S. as well as the costs of health insurance premiums.[32] Still, costs continue to rise.

# HealthCheck

## Choosing a Health Care Plan

Selecting a health care plan has important consequences. Unfortunately, many of us have little or no option when it comes to choosing one. The plan offered by your employer may be the only choice available to you, unless you want to shop around and pay premiums on your own. Some companies do offer a limited range of choices. And self-employed people are on their own when it comes to acquiring medical insurance.

The uninformed way of choosing a health care plan is to be swayed by television commercials that show healthy, vigorous members of a particular plan enjoying the fullness of life. The informed way is to acquire information and carefully weigh the advantages and disadvantages of a variety of plans. Here we offer some suggestions for making an informed choice. First we sort out the advantages and disadvantages of managed care plans vs. fee-for-service plans (see Table 23.2). Then we see how to choose a particular plan.

### Selecting a Fee-for-Service Plan

If you are in the market for a health insurance fee-for-service plan, you may well want to consider the three C's—cost, coverage, and choice—in determining which plan best suits your needs.

**Cost** The bottom line for most people is the bottom line. What are the premiums? What are the deductibles? How much will you be charged for physician visits? What other out-of-pocket expenses will you incur, such as medication costs, fees for second opinions, or fees for consultations with specialists? How much will you have to pay for hospitalization or major surgery? Are your out-of-pocket expenses capped at some amount, so that the plan reverts to 100% coverage above a certain amount? (Hospitalization for a major illness or major surgery can easily top five figures and in some cases six figures.) Are there annual or lifetime caps on some coverages? What is the plan's track record on rate increases? (Avoid companies with a history of large increases.)

**Coverage** Plans vary widely in coverage. While all plans cover basic medical services, some also cover dental care, mental health care, preventive care (such as annual checkups), maternity benefits, and vision testing and eyeglasses. Some also cover dental expenses, but usually at a higher premium. There may be some kinds of exclusions, such as cosmetic surgery and experimental procedures. There may be restrictions on coverage for pre-existing conditions. Ask yourself whether the plan provides the kinds of coverage you think you will need. The more comprehensive the coverage, and the lower the caps on out-of-pocket payments, the better.

**Choice** Does the plan allow you to choose your own doctor or must you select a doctor from a list? If the latter is the case, are you permitted to use a doctor outside the list? If so, at what additional cost?

### Selecting a Managed Care Plan[37]

It matters little whether the waiting room at the local HMO is nicely furnished. Consider the hard facts concerning outcomes and performance. Compare the coverage and the costs for regular medical visits and more intensive care, such as hospitalization and surgery. What happens when you are away from home and need emergency care? What about long-term care? What about exclusions or waiting periods for treatment for pre-existing conditions? What approvals are needed before your primary care provider can refer you to a specialist? What are the fee arrangements if you decide to seek services from outside providers? Does the plan have a history of paying claims promptly? Does the plan exclude treatments you may want because it considers them experimental?

One place to start in evaluating the quality of the plan is to ask whether it is approved by the accrediting organization, the National Committee for Quality Assurance. This nonprofit organization evaluates the plan's doctors, its responsiveness to members, and the services provided.[38] You can find out whether a particular plan is accredited by contacting the National Committee for Quality Assurance at 2000 L Street NW, Suite 500, Washington, DC 20036 (Tel: 202-955-3500).

Even an accredited plan may have a large number of complaints filed against it. To find out, call your state insurance department. Inquire about the nature of complaints, whether their number exceeds the average for plans in your area, and the proportion of complaints that have been upheld.

Another source of information is consumer satisfaction surveys, which ask plan members to judge the services they receive. Consumer satisfaction surveys have been conducted by some large employers, government groups, and some private survey companies. Ask the benefits official at your place of employment if a consumer survey of the members of the plans in your area has been conducted and is available for your review. Another resource is the book *Consumers' Guide to Health Plans,* which is based on consumer satisfaction surveys of some 90,000 patients in 250 HMOs. It is available from the Center for the Study of Services, 733 15th St. NW, Suite 820, Washington, DC 20005.

TABLE 23.2

**Comparing Fee-for-Service and Managed Care Plans[36]**

| Advantages | Disadvantages | Assessing Your Needs |
|---|---|---|
| **Fee-for-Service (Indemnity) Plan** | | |
| Greater choice of primary physicians, specialists, and treatment facilities. | Out-of-pocket expenses for medical visits and procedures typically exceed copayments required under managed care. | How important to you is flexibility in choice of your primary care physician and specialists? |
| Fewer restrictions placed on use of specialist services and expensive diagnostic tests. | Typically requires higher deductibles and offers narrower coverage for preventive care, eye care, and dental care. | Are you willing to pay more by way of out-of-pocket expenses and deductibles to have more of a choice in selecting your own doctors? |
| Allows usual relationship with primary care providers, even if they are not in any provider network. | Allowable charges may not fully cover costs for medical visits and procedures. | Can you afford the deductibles? The annual premiums? The out-of-pocket expenses for medical visits? |
| | Typically has more exclusions and limitations than managed care plans. | Can you accept the exclusions and limitations in the plan or do you need broader coverage? |
| **Managed Care Plan** | | |
| Typically offers broader coverage for preventive care such as screening tests, vaccinations, well-child visits, and annual physicals. | Limited freedom of choice in selecting primary care physicians, specialists, or hospital facilities. | How willing are you to accept the limitations of managed care in terms of choice of doctors and referrals to specialists—or to pay the extra costs for going outside the provider network? |
| Typically offers more comprehensive services, including dental care, eye care, prenatal services for pregnant women, and health education and lifestyle management classes for stress reduction, weight control, etc. | Staffed HMOs may have less convenient hours available than private physicians in some areas or longer waiting times for appointments. | What services are provided by the managed care plan that are not offered in a fee-for-service plan? How important are these services to you? |
| Lower copayment for medical visits. | The effort to control costs may lead company to engage in "cherry-picking" by offering services only to healthier groups who are likely to use fewer and cheaper services. | Do you have an allegiance to doctors who are not part of the provider network or HMO? |
| Little or no deductible. | Choices of approved health care providers and facilities may be limited to a provider list. | Do you have confidence in the doctors included in the network or HMO? |
| May offer a choice of providers from an HMO network or outside health care providers (though at a higher cost). | Choosing treatment providers outside provider list may incur substantially greater costs relative to FFS plans. | How troublesome are the claims forms in fee-for-service plan vs. the managed care plan? |
| May conduct regular consumer evaluations to improve quality of care. | Quality of care may suffer because of financial incentives to limit use of specialists and expensive tests and procedures. | What are the differences between these plans in waiting periods for examinations or reimbursement of out-of-pocket expenses? |
| A fixed monthly fee that covers all services. | Use of outside specialists or special diagnostic tests must be preapproved. | Do you have confidence that the managed care plan will approve emergency care or specialized care? How might you go about finding out? |
| Oversight procedures may avoid medically unnecessary and possibly dangerous diagnostic tests or procedures. | Primary care physicians may opt out of the plan or be dropped ("deselected") by the plan, forcing patients to find new doctors. | |
| Minimal claim forms or none. | Patient's former physician may not be affiliated with the plan. | |
| May reduce costs to patients for medical treatment. | May rely too heavily on generalists in treating conditions that should be followed by specialists, such as shifting cancer care from oncologists to primary care physicians. | |
| | May limit or restrict phone calls to primary care physicians. | |

Visit the HMO if it is housed in a central location, or visit practitioners affiliated with the plan who see patients in their private offices. Get a feel for the facility. Consider how responsive the physicians and support staff are to patients, how long they keep patients waiting, and whether the waiting room appears overcrowded, which may indicate a pattern of overbooking appointments. Table 23.3 offers some pointers to consider when evaluating an HMO.

**TABLE 23.3**

**Looking under an HMO's Hood**[39]

Besides asking about location and cost, here is a checklist of some points to consider when shopping for a managed care plan:

- What percentage of the plan's network doctors are board certified and what percentage leave each year?
- Has the plan been audited by the National Committee for Quality Assurance or other organization, and if so, can you inspect the report?
- What's in the sample benefits contract?
- How many complaints filed with the state insurance department against the plan have been upheld?
- Must primary care physicians receive permission from the HMO before making referrals to specialists? And for women, does that rule include gynecologists?
- How easy is it to file an appeal when medical treatment is denied?
- What portion of the plan's premium dollars is spent on medical care?
- What financial incentives do doctors receive for holding down the cost of medical care?
- What type of preventive care, like immunizations, does the plan offer?
- What kind of preauthorization is needed for hospitalization?
- Is a prescription drug you regularly take on the plan's list of medications approved for payment?

Even if all Americans belonged to HMOs, medical economists estimate that there would be only a 10% cost savings in total health care expenditures.[33] The cost savings achieved by HMOs will not, in themselves, rein in the ever-increasing cost of health care in the U.S.

The American Medical Association has issued a bill of rights for members of HMOs and other managed care plans. Though the "bill of rights" doesn't carry the force of law, it does govern what is expected of physicians who participate in these plans (see Table 23.4).

Americans are clearly worried about their health insurance. Many people fear that their health benefits will be reduced or that their health care will become unaffordable.[34] They fear having a more limited choice of physicians and being forced by their employers to join managed care plans. Will the health care delivery system in the new millennium appease these concerns or add fuel to them?

**TABLE 23.4**

**A Health Care Bill of Rights for Managed Care Patients**[35]

- Your physician is obligated to put your interests first.
- Your physician is obligated to advocate for care that he or she believes will materially benefit your health.
- Your physician is obligated to disclose all treatment alternatives to you, even those not covered by the plan. You can then decide whether to appeal for coverage of a desired treatment or seek the treatment outside the plan.
- Adequate means should be established for appealing disputes regarding medically necessary care.
- The plan must reveal any limitations or restrictions of benefits to prospective members before they decide to join.
- The plan must neither encourage nor allow substandard care.
- Any incentives that limit care to patients must be disclosed by administrators upon initial enrollment in the plan and at least annually thereafter.
- Limits should be placed on the financial incentives that health care providers within the plan receive for limiting care.

## WORLD OF *diversity*

### Serving the Underserved

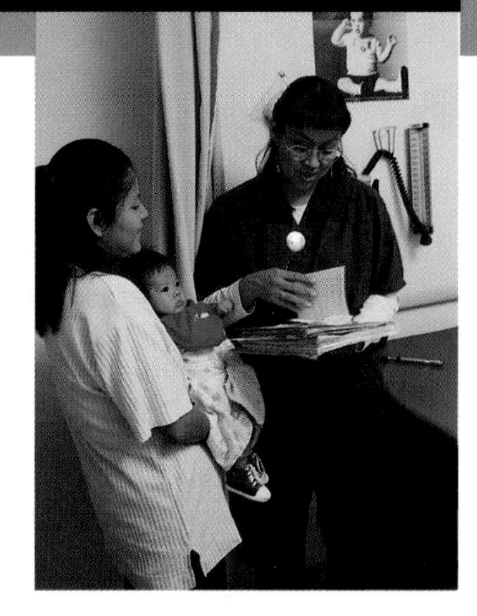

Many groups in our society have limited access to medical care, especially poor people, ethnic minority groups, and people living in remote areas. For the very poor, the Medicaid program ordinarily picks up the tab for medical services. But barriers such as transportation problems, language differences, unwillingness of providers to treat Medicaid patients, and perceptions of callous treatment from providers limit access to health care. Many Medicaid recipients face long delays for appointments and hours in doctors' waiting rooms.

The working poor also have limited access to health care services. Low-paid workers may not be financially eligible for Medicaid, but they may also lack private health insurance because it is not offered by their employers and they cannot afford it on their own. Largely because of disparities in health insurance coverage, low-income families actually pay more than twice the share of family income for health care than do high-income families.[48] Recent immigrants, migrant workers, and the working poor employed in small businesses are most likely to be uninsured or underinsured.

Not only the uninsured or underinsured have difficulty obtaining medical care. About 75% of the people who are unable to obtain care *have* health insurance.[49] The major barrier to obtaining care for people with and without insurance is clear—cost. To the insured, factors such as deductibles, copayments, and restrictions on medical services block access to care.

People living in remote areas may have to travel 75 miles or more to see a doctor, and even further if they require specialists or hospitalization. Consider the situation faced by many Native Americans. Although they are eligible for free health care through the Indian Health Service (IHS), many live in rural areas in which there are few providers. Many are also poor and cannot afford to travel to obtain health care.

Poverty and race are important factors in access to health care.[50] African Americans make up about 12% of the U.S. population but account for about 17% of those who are uninsured. African Americans are also less likely than non-Hispanic white Americans to carry private health insurance. Greater unemployment among African Americans figures prominently into this disparity, since health insurance is often tied to employment. African Americans are also more likely than whites to work for small companies and in some industries that are less likely to provide health insurance to workers, such as service trades. Disparities also exist in the quality of care. Even when health insurance or government programs like Medicare and Medicaid are available, African Americans and poor people tend to receive lower-quality care than do white and affluent people.

The new millennium may see increased use of managed care programs for the poor and underserved. Managed care plans offer the promise of reducing costs to patients and expanding use of preventive services. *Healthy People 2000* stated the goal of reducing disparities in access to health care among different ethnic and socioeconomic groups in the United States. But unless safeguards are able to ensure quality care, managed care programs could increase rather than decrease the disparity in health care status that now exists.[51]

## Government-Sponsored Health Care Programs

Two major government programs, Medicare and Medicaid, provide health care services to the poor, to people with disabilities, and to older people.

**Medicare** **Medicare** is the nation's health care program for older people and people with disabilities. The program pays 80% (after deductibles) of most medical expenses for eligible individuals. The Medicare program is the single largest payer in the health care system in the U.S., footing about 20% of the nation's annual health bill.[40] Even so, Medicare coverage is limited. It doesn't cover prescription drugs, dentures, or glasses. It carries a high deductible for hospitalization. Many Medicare recipients

**Medicare** A federal program providing health care coverage for older Americans and people with disabilities.

turn to private insurers to purchase **Medigap policies** to fill the gaps in their Medicare coverage.

Medicare is a contributory program. Beneficiaries pay for a portion of the costs in the form of monthly premiums, an annual deductible, and copayments of 20% of most doctor's bills. Employees also make regular payroll contributions during their working careers.

Medicare has been a great benefit for older people and for people with disabilities, but concerns are mounting about the financial security of the program. Costs for maintaining the program have been rising steadily (see Figure 23.4). The program covers some 37 million Americans and is the second costliest government program, after Social Security. Though some of the costs for the program are offset by contributions from beneficiaries, most of the costs are borne by current workers through payroll deductions and by employers through matching contributions. The Medicare system, already on shaky fiscal ground, faces a financial shock wave early in the new millennium as millions of baby-boomers reach retirement age and become eligible for benefits. Future generations of Americans and their employers may be saddled with huge increases in payroll deductions and employer contributions to meet future expenses.

Legislators and public health officials have considered various alternatives to balance the Medicare budget. Yet little has been done, largely because none of the choices is politically palatable. They include reducing benefits, raising the eligibility age even higher (by present law it will rise to age 66 in 2009 and to age 67 in 2027), requiring higher contributions by more affluent beneficiaries, or increasing the tax burden on younger Americans.

One effort to control Medicare costs ties reimbursement to hospitals to criteria based on **diagnostic related groups,** or **DRGs.** The DRG is a classification system based on a patient's age, diagnosis, and the procedures used. It is used to predict the use of hospital services, including length of stay, for patients with specific medical conditions. It sets a fixed fee that hospitals can collect for these patients. If costs exceed those called for by the designated DRG, the hospital absorbs the shortfall. If costs are less than the allowable costs, the hospital brings in more money.

HMOs are making significant inroads in signing up Medicare recipients. The Medicare program contracts with HMOs to provide recipients with medical services on a fixed cost basis per patient. Medicare subscribers who switch to HMOs continue to pay their regular monthly premiums for doctors' services. Though only about 10% of Medicare subscribers had signed up for HMOs by the mid-1990s, interest has been growing, largely because HMOs typically offer expanded services at lower

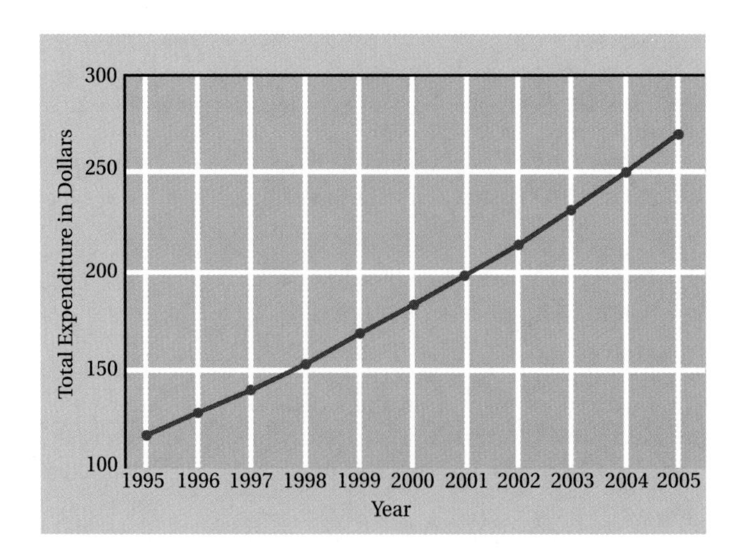


**Figure 23.4** ***Medicare Costs on the Rise*** Medicare costs have been rising steadily and are expected to continue to rise as increasing numbers of Americans become senior citizens. The gap between expenditures and income has also been climbing, raising concerns about the financial security of the Medicare program.

**Medigap policy** An insurance policy with a private carrier that fills gaps in Medicare coverage.

**Diagnostic related groups (DRGs)** Classifications used to determine reimbursement rates to hospitals for particular medical conditions.

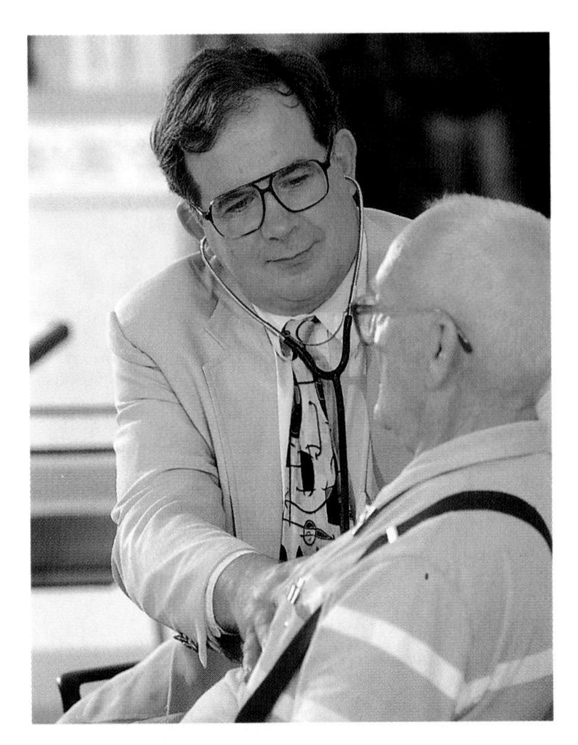

***Medicare—Approaching a Crisis?*** Medicare, the nation's health care program for older Americans, faces a potential financial shock wave as millions of baby-boomers reach retirement age during the early twenty-first century.

costs, such as doctors' visits with no annual deductible (it's $100 under regular Medicare), $5 or $10 copayments for each medical visit (compared with 20% under Medicare), annual physicals, and unlimited hospitalization with no deductibles (Medicare coverage is limited to the first 90 days and requires a deductible).[41] It remains unclear how well Medicare recipients will be served by HMOs. The question is whether costs will be controlled at the expense of quality care.

**Medicaid** Created in 1965 as part of the same legislative package that created Medicare, **Medicaid** provides medical care to the poor. Unlike Medicare, Medicaid is a noncontributory program. That is, people do not pay premiums to receive benefits. Medicaid is funded by federal and state governments. The federal government funds about 65% of the costs, and the states contribute the balance.[42] By 1993, Medicaid provided benefits to more than 32 million people, up from 10 million just four years earlier.[43] Teaching hospitals, community health centers, and inner-city physicians provide the bulk of services to Medicaid patients.

Like Medicare, the costs for Medicaid have been rising rapidly, from about $50 billion in the late 1980s to more than $100 billion by the mid-1990s. In an attempt to curtail rising costs, some states have cut Medicaid benefits. Others have moved Medicaid beneficiaries into managed care plans, typically HMOs. By the mid-1990s, about 8 million Medicaid beneficiaries were enrolled in managed care plans, with the number doubling in 1994 alone. HMOs package health care programs for Medicaid recipients on a fixed per-person basis that promises to reduce the costs for medical services. However, as HMOs expand into Medicaid, concerns have been raised that they will simply sign up Medicaid recipients but withhold needed care to minimize their costs. This is especially threatening to the most vulnerable populations, such as the disabled and chronically ill, who consume the lion's share of medical services under Medicaid. These fears may be well founded, since older people and poor people with chronic medical conditions like diabetes and hypertension fare more poorly under managed care than under conventional insurance plans.[44] By contrast, the average patient does about as well in either type of plan.

## Public Health Programs

Public health programs emphasize preventive health care. They are relatively poorly funded in this country, because most medical resources are focused on treatment rather than prevention. Examples of public health programs include Child Health Clinics (CHCs), family planning clinics, the Women's, Infants and Children (WIC) program, and immunization programs. Public health programs typically offer services on a **sliding scale.** Fees are based on the ability to pay. Public health programs probably do more to decrease human suffering and with less state and federal support than any other sector of the health care system. Perhaps the role of public health will be expanded in the future as governments seek ways of delivering quality health care to the most people for the lowest cost.

**Medicaid** A federal program that provides health care benefits to the poor.

**Sliding scale** A system for adjusting fees according to the individual's income level.

## PREVENTION

### Treatment Yes, Prevention Maybe

A national survey underscores the underemphasis on prevention in the American health care system. It found that more than half of American women 50 to 69 years of age had never had a mammogram, more than a third of women over the age of 17 had not had a breast exam within the previous two years, one in five had not had a Pap smear within the past four years, and more than a third of children aged two to five had been inadequately immunized against polio, DPT, or MMR[45] (see Figure 23.5). A UCLA study found that 40% of women over 40 had not had their breasts examined by a doctor during the previous year.[46] Though people without health insurance were less likely to have had regular preventive services, most of the people failing to get these services *did* carry health insurance. Table 23.5 lists nine essential screening tests—what they involve and when you should be tested.

One reason that many insured people do not receive preventive care is that many insurance plans do not cover it. For other insured people, copayments and deductibles are impediments to preventive care. Yet some people just put off regular medical exams or fail to go to the doctor unless they feel sick. Yet for many health problems, including cancer, delays in detection and treatment can have serious, even deadly, consequences.

### think about it!

- **Do you have health insurance? What kind? Did you choose your insurance plan? Why or why not?**
- **Are there deductibles or copayments in your health insurance plan? If so, how have they affected your health-related behavior?**
- **Would you ask your health care provider if he or she has incentives for not referring you to a specialist or ordering costly tests or procedures? If not, why not?**

**critical thinking** **Agree or disagree and support your answer: Managed care causes health care providers a conflict of interest.**

**critical thinking** **What factors should you consider in choosing a health care plan?**

**critical thinking** **Are there any barriers in your efforts to secure adequate health care? What are they? What can you do about them?**

Smart Quiz
Q2302

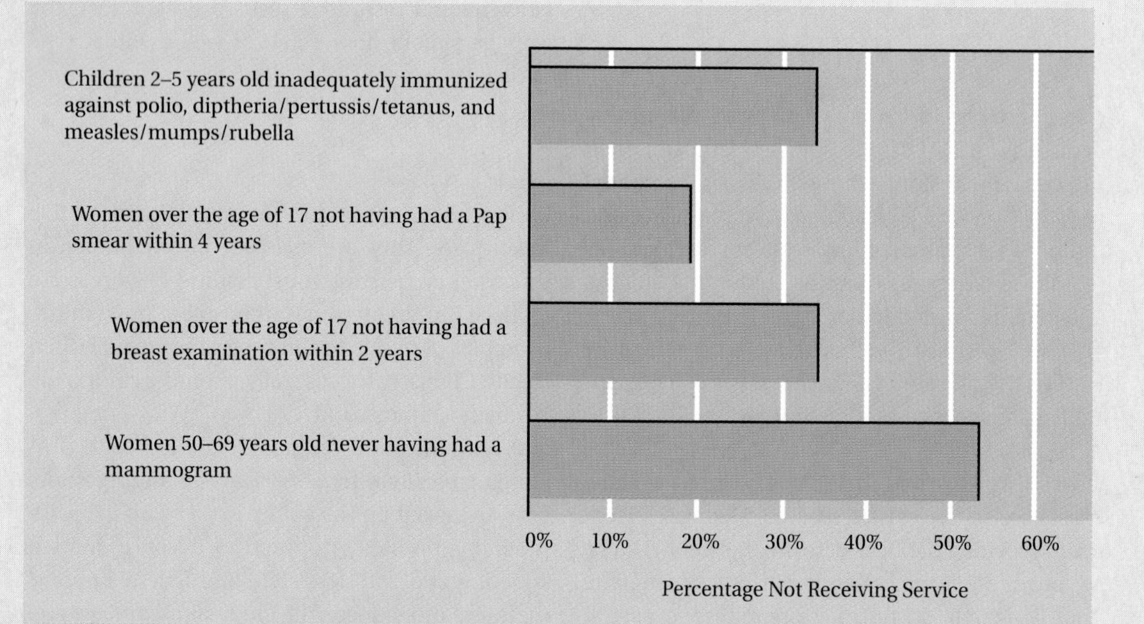


**Figure 23.5** ***People Not Receiving Specific Preventive Services*** Many people do not receive the preventive care they need. How about you? Are your vaccinations up to date? Do you have regular medical checkups with a qualified health care provider? Do you follow the guidelines for cancer screening described in Chapter 18? If you are a woman, do you perform monthly breast self-exams? If you are a man, do you perform monthly testicular self-exams? These tests are described in Chapter 9. If the answer to any of these questions is no, it's time to conduct a careful self-review of your health care needs. Practicing good preventive care can reduce your risk of developing serious, even life-threatening illnesses, or help catch them at their earliest and most treatable stages.

TABLE 23.5

## Nine Essential Screening Tests[47]

| Type of Test | What It Involves | When You Should Be Tested |
|---|---|---|
| Cholesterol screening | A small amount of blood is analyzed to provide readings of total blood cholesterol (milligrams per deciliter, with readings over 200 considered borderline and over 240 high), LDL ("bad") cholesterol, HDL ("good") cholesterol, ratio of HDL to total cholesterol, and triglycerides (other blood fats). | Experts differ in their recommendations, with some favoring early testing (beginning in one's twenties) and others favoring testing beginning in one's forties. People with a history of heart disease or high cholesterol should consult their doctors about the need for early testing. |
| Mammogram and clinical breast exam | In a clinical breast exam, the examiner feels the breast, looking for suspicious lumps. A mammogram is a specialized breast X-ray that can detect small lumps that cannot yet be felt upon examination. | The American Cancer Society recommends that women should have annual mammograms beginning at age 40. Women over forty should have an annual clinical breast exam, while women under forty should have one every three years beginning at age 20. |
| Colon cancer | In a *fecal occult blood test,* a stool sample is taken and analyzed for the presence of blood, a possible sign of cancer. The interior of the colon can be examined for the presence of precancerous polyps by use of a flexible device, called a *sigmoidoscope,* that is inserted into the rectum. A more thorough analysis, called a *colonoscopy,* is used with people at high risk of colon cancer. | Fecal blood tests should be conducted annually beginning at age 50. The sigmoidoscopy is recommended for people 50 years of age or older once every three to five years. |
| Pap smear | A sample of cells is gently scraped from the surface of the woman's cervix and analyzed in a lab for signs of cervical cancer. | Most physicians recommend annual Pap smears for women by the time they reach their late teens, or earlier if they become sexually active. |
| Blood pressure | An inflatable cuff is wrapped around the upper arm to measure the systolic pressure when the heart beats and diastolic pressure when the heart relaxes between beats. | People with normal blood pressure should be evaluated once every other year. People with a family history of hypertension or other risk factors, such as obesity, should be tested annually. |
| Bone density | The most accurate test is a specialized type of X-ray device, called a *dual X-ray absorptiometry,* or DXA, which is sensitive enough to detect bone loss as low as 1 percent. | Recommended for postmenopausal women to help them evaluate the need for hormone replacement therapy to help prevent osteoporosis. |
| HIV | Blood, saliva, and urine tests used to detect antibodies to HIV, the virus that causes AIDS. The Western blot test (run on a blood sample) confirms the presence of the virus itself. | When concerned about possible exposure to HIV through needle sharing or unprotected sexual contact with partners of unknown HIV status. |
| Skin cancer | A full head-to-toe examination by a doctor, preferably a dermatologist, who looks for moles that are irregularly shaped or asymmetrical, are larger than a pencil eraser, have unusual coloration, or have changed or grown since the previous visit. Suspicious moles may be removed and biopsied to see if they are cancerous. | The American Cancer Society recommends a skin exam every three years for people age 20 to 30, and thereafter annually. Annual skin exams are most important for people at higher risk of melanoma, the most dangerous form of skin cancer. This includes people with pale skin, those with lots of moles, those with a family history of melanoma, and those with a history of two or more blistering sunburns during childhood or adolescence. |
| Prostate cancer | A manual rectal exam can help detect abnormalities in the prostate, including prostate cancer. A blood test called the PSA test measures the levels of a protein, prostate-specific antigen (PSA), that seeps out of the prostate gland when it is cancerous or enlarged. The PSA test can often detect the presence of cancer before abnormalities can be felt during a physical exam. | Most physicians recommend an annual rectal exam for men beginning at about age 40. The PSA test is usually recommended for men by age 50. |

# Taking an Active Role in Managing Your Health Care

## Take Charge

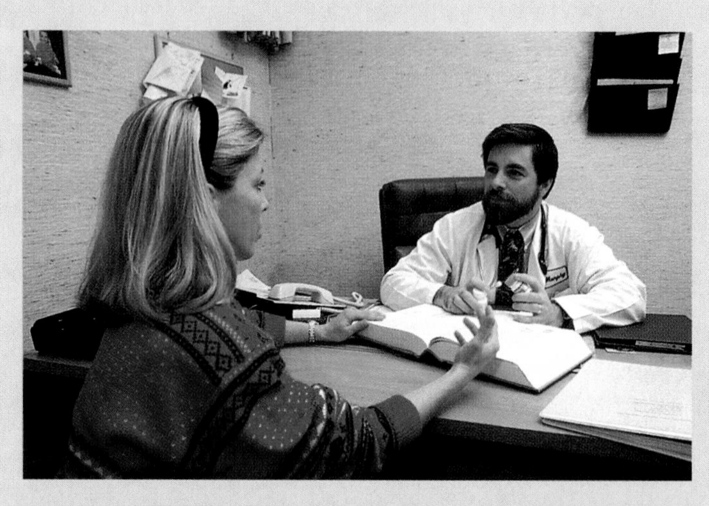

***Taking an Active Role*** People who take an active role in managing their health care ask questions—lots of questions—to ensure they have the information they need to make informed health care choices.

Some people are passive health care consumers. They wait until they get sick to seek health care or learn about health care options. They may carry an insurance card but know little about the range of health services covered by their plan. Passive health care consumers typically do not get the best possible health care. They indirectly participate in the escalation of health care costs because they do not use services such as regular physical examinations that might prevent the development of serious and costly medical conditions or reduce their severity.

Passive health care consumers may think of the health care system as too complicated to understand. Their attitudes and beliefs undercut their motivation to manage their own health care—"I prefer to just leave medical matters in the hands of my doctor," "I do not really care what it costs, my insurance will cover it anyway," and, "I basically believe that all health care providers are competent and have my best interests at heart."

By contrast, people who take an active role in managing their health care ask questions—plenty of them—of their health care providers to help ensure that they get the best-quality care and understand the treatment alternatives available. They believe that *they,* not their health care providers or their insurance carriers, are ultimately responsible for managing their own health care. They take steps to protect themselves from mismanaged care.

What about you? Are you an active or a passive health care consumer? Take a moment to evaluate whether you are actively managing your own health care by answering the questions in the ***HealthCheck*** feature (p. 659). Then ask yourself what changes you can make in your attitudes and behavior to get the most out of your health care.

### Talking to Your Doctor—Being Seen *and* Heard[52]

Hearing "The doctor will see you now" is not only an invitation to be seen. It is also an invitation to be *heard.* People who take an active role in managing their health care let their doctors know what is ailing them and gather as much information as they need to make informed decisions regarding treatment. Many people feel that their doctors don't give them the time they need to discuss their complaints or concerns.

Consumers' biggest complaint about health care is that they feel rushed by their physicians. One of four patients responding to a *Health* magazine/Roper Poll said that his or her typical appointment lasts ten minutes or less. Though your doctor's time is certainly valuable (as is yours), you have the right to be heard and to ask your doctor to take the time to explain your condition and recommended treatment in language you can understand. When communicating with your doctor:

- *Describe your symptoms and complaints as clearly and as fully as possible.* Don't hold back, cover up, or distort your symptoms. After all, your health is at stake. By the same token, don't embellish your symptoms or repeat yourself. If your doctor interrupts you, say something like, "Doctor, if I may just finish. I'd like you to have the full picture." If your doctor seems more interested in ushering you through the door than hearing you out, think about finding another doctor.
- *Don't accept a treatment recommendation you don't want.* If your doctor's rationale for the treatment plan leaves you shaking your head, seek another opinion. Don't feel pressured to accept a treatment plan that doesn't feel right.
- *Insist on explanations in plain language.* Patients' major complaint about patient-doctor communication is that the doctor does not explain things clearly—a problem cited by more than one in three (34%) people in the *Health* magazine/Roper Poll. You can't make informed choices regarding treatment options if your doctor lacks the ability or interest to help you understand them.

- *Don't be swayed by a doctor who says your problems are "in your head."* Doctors may not take complaints seriously when there are no findings on physical examination or laboratory tests, especially if symptoms seem vague, like feelings of fatigue. If your doctor is stumped, you may need to consult another doctor.

## Avoiding Mismanaged Care[53]

Successful managed care is a two-way responsibility. Managed care organizations should provide quality medical care and disclose service limitations and any incentives for limiting patient care. Consumers are responsible for leading a healthy lifestyle, consuming medical resources wisely, and exercising personal initiative to help make managed care work. Consumers who take an active role in managing their health care—including managing their managed care plans—can take several steps to protect themselves against mismanaged care:

- *Discuss coverage for hospital stays.* If you're planning major surgery, find out in advance what costs your managed care company will cover and how long a period of hospitalization you'll be permitted. Discuss with your physician whether your coverage is reasonable for your type of surgery.
- *Insist on your right to see a specialist.* Though it is a sensitive point, inquire whether your doctor participates in any incentive program or feels pressured to minimize referrals to specialists. If your doctor doesn't provide straightforward answers, it's time to shop around for another doctor. If you feel that your condition calls for a specialist, and one is not available to you as a member of the managed care plan, demand one. If you must go outside your plan to obtain a specialist's services, have the specialist cite his or her medical findings that justify the need for these services. Use this document to appeal the denial for coverage.
- *Learn what to do in case of emergencies.* If you are faced with a medical emergency, your first concern is to get proper care, not to haggle over costs with your managed care company. But before an emergency arises, you should take the time to learn about the provisions in your plan for obtaining emergency care. Most plans require that you first contact a participating doctor, who will then direct you to an emergency room covered by the plan. However, many HMOs refuse to pay for emergency services if they later decide that the patient's condition did not require them. It may not matter even if the plan's own doctors advised the patient to go to the nearest emergency room. The hospital may then seek payment from the patient.[54]
- *If you are refused coverage.* If you are refused coverage for medical services not covered by your plan, including emergency care, file an appeal. (The appeals process is typically laid out in the plan's handbook.) Document the need for services. Include supporting documents from physicians who referred you or provided the services. If the managed care company still refuses to pay, file an appeal. If an appeal doesn't succeed, your employer's benefits manager may be able to intercede on your behalf. You may also file a formal complaint with your state department of insurance, which establishes a paper trail supporting your case. As a last resort, you may wish to consult a lawyer.

## Sort through the Hype on Health Claims

Every now and then we hear claims touting some new miracle drug, vitamin, or hormone that promises to enhance our health and vitality, prevent disease, or even reverse the effects of aging. Some of these claims are outright hoaxes or forms of **medical quackery.** Some take promising scientific leads and exaggerate or distort the evidence. While the federal Food and Drug Administration (FDA) regulates health claims for drugs and medications, many of the substances found in your health food store or neighborhood supermarket purporting to have disease-preventive or anti-aging effects are classified as foods and are not regulated as drugs. It's basically "buyer beware" when it comes to sorting through claims of health food products and alternative therapies.

**Close-up**
Health claims: Separating fact from fiction
T2302

Active health care consumers do not take health claims at face value. They recognize that health care products not only may not work as promised but could possibly be harmful. Advertisers and marketers have a vested interest in getting you to buy their products or use their services, and they may put self-promotion before truth. To protect yourself, seek information from objective, third-party sources to evaluate any products or services claiming health benefits. A good place to start is your local library. Consult a librarian to help you find critical reviews that sort through the scientific evidence, such as those found in popular magazines like *Consumer Reports* or health newsletters published by leading universities or public interest organizations like the Society for Science in the Public Interest. You may also wish to consult with your personal physician or other health providers, or your college health instructor, to sort out the facts from the hype concerning health claims. If you feel you have been defrauded by an unscrupulous health care provider, file a complaint with your state attorney general or consumer protection agency.

**Close-up**
More on medical quackery
T2303

**Close-up**
Top health frauds
T2304

## Get Involved in the Health Care Debate

Health care issues, such as universal health insurance, are not only of interest to politicians and lobbyists for the health care industry. They concern us all. People who take

**Medical quackery** Medical fraud or fakery; use of products or practices lacking any legitimate basis for claims of medical effectiveness.

responsibility for managing their health care don't stand idly by and accept whatever politicians and pressure groups decide is in their best interest. As individuals and as groups, we can become involved in the health care debate taking place in the halls of Congress and in state legislatures. Strategies for getting involved include the following:

1. *Lobby.* Anyone can lobby. You can lobby informally by talking about health care issues with friends and family and writing letters to newspaper and magazine editors and to state and national legislators. Organizing a group of people who share your convictions and are willing to make them known to legislators can carry an even greater impact. Opinions expressed in letters and telephone calls will be heard and can have a substantial impact. Here are some guidelines for writing to your legislators:

   - *Find out who your state legislators and members of Congress are.* You can call 1-202-225-3121 (toll call) for a listing of members of Congress. For a listing of state and local officials, use the state and municipal pages in your telephone book.
   - *Address legislators properly and send correspondence to the correct addresses.* Here is a partial listing of the addresses of federal legislators:

     Senator __________
     United States Senate
     Washington, DC 20510

     Representative__________
     U.S. House of Representatives
     Washington, DC 20515

     Honorable__________
     Senate Majority Leader
     U.S. Senate
     Washington, DC 20510

     Honorable__________
     Speaker of the House
     U.S. House of Representatives
     Washington, DC 20515

   Date your letter. Give your full name, address, and telephone number. Identify yourself as a registered voter (if you are) and give your district number if you are writing to a state senator or assemblyperson. Identify the legislative bill and its number, or the issue you are addressing. Explain your position/opinion from the perspective of a voter and a health care consumer (and as a future provider, if appropriate). Be accurate, clear, and brief in your writing. Don't be emotional, vague, or threatening. Explain what you want your legislator to do (vote for a specific bill, identified by number) and what you are willing to do in return (vote for your legislators, work for them, or promote their candidacy to your friends and family members). Indicate at the bottom of the letter what organizations you are sending copies of the letter to, and do so.

2. *Join organizations that support your views.* Many advocacy organizations have taken positions on health care reform. Ask for their literature and decide which organizations best speak for you.
3. *Vote.* Educate yourself about the positions taken by the candidates and vote. If you do not exercise your right to vote, you live with the choices of the people who do.

In making this chapter work best for you, remember that the best health care system is a partnership between caring health care professionals and consumers who are actively involved in managing their own health care. What have you learned that you can put into practice beginning today to protect your health and get the most out of your health care?

Smart Quiz
Q2303

# Health*Check*

## *Are You an Active Health Care Consumer?*

Circle the statement that best represents your beliefs and attitudes concerning your health care:

| | | |
|---|---|---|
| I avoid thinking about my health care until a health care need arises. | or | I make an effort to think about my health care needs and plan ahead to meet these needs. |
| I don't know how to locate a personal physician and other health care providers in my area. | or | I have established a relationship with a primary health care provider and other health care providers, such as a dentist, an eye care specialist, and (if I'm a woman) a gynecologist. |
| I'm not aware of the major hospitals, clinics, and other medical facilities in my area or, if I am aware of them, I don't know what services they provide. | or | I not only know where the major health care facilities in my area are located but also know what services they offer and how to get there in case of emergency. |
| I don't keep a list of phone numbers handy for hospitals and doctors I could call in case of medical need. | or | I keep handy a list of phone numbers and know whom I would call in the case of a medical emergency or other medical needs. |
| I usually skip regular medical examinations, either because I don't have the time or don't know how to go about arranging for a physical. | or | I have regular medical exams and have established a relationship with a primary health care provider who knows my health record. |
| I lack the means of paying for health care and have not made arrangements in case I need medical services. | or | I maintain health care coverage. |
| To be honest, I tend to ignore symptoms for as long as possible in the hope that they will disappear. | or | I pay attention to any changes in my body and bring any symptoms or complaints to the attention of my primary health care provider. |
| I sometimes use emergency services, such as ambulances, police, and emergency units, when they are not necessary. | or | I always work through my primary health care provider when I am in need of health care, including emergency care. |
| I really don't know what I would do or where I would go in the case of a medical emergency. | or | I know how to handle a medical emergency—whom I would call and where I would go to get emergency care. |
| I sometimes or often fail to keep medical appointments or arrive late for them. | or | I keep appointments and arrive on time. |
| I sometimes or often fail to call to cancel appointments ahead of time. | or | I always call to cancel appointments if necessary. |
| I sometimes hold back information from my health care provider or believe that doctors should just know what's bothering me without my having to tell them. | or | I readily offer information to my health care provider and describe my symptoms as clearly as possible. |
| I sometimes or often give incomplete information on medical histories due to embarrassment, forgetfulness, or inattention. | or | I give complete information and do not withhold, embellish, or distort information about my health. |
| I sometimes or often fail to pay attention to the instructions I receive from my doctor. | or | I listen carefully to instructions, take notes, and ask for explanations of my medical condition. |

| | | |
|---|---|---|
| I generally don't ask my physician to explain medical terms I don't understand. | or | I always ask my doctor to explain any terms I don't understand. |
| I generally accept everything my doctor tells me without questioning. | or | I assertively ask questions when I don't understand or agree with the treatment plan. |
| I sometimes or often fail to follow instructions that I have agreed to follow, such as not filling prescriptions or not taking medications according to schedule. | or | I carefully follow instructions which I agreed to; if I'm not sure of the directions to follow, I call my doctor (or pharmacist) and ask for clarification. |
| I sometimes or often fail to keep follow-up appointments or neglect to call to update my health care provider on my condition. | or | I reliably keep follow-up appointments and make update calls when indicated. |
| I simply stop following a treatment that has troubling effects or no effects and don't bother to inform my health care provider. | or | If a treatment doesn't appear to be working or produces negative effects, I call my health care provider for a consultation before making any changes in the treatment plan. |
| I don't examine medical bills carefully, especially those that are paid by my insurance company. | or | I carefully examine bills for any errors or duplication of services charged and bring any discrepancies to the attention of my health care provider. |
| I don't question any charges for medical services, even if I think they are excessive or inappropriate. | or | I question my health care provider about any charges that appear excessive or inappropriate. |
| I generally neglect filling out insurance claim forms for as long as possible. | or | I promptly complete insurance forms and drop them in the mail as soon as possible. |
| I generally don't keep records of my medical treatments and insurance claims. | or | I keep full and complete records of my medical visits and copies of insurance claim statements. |

*Interpreting Your Score:* Statements in the left-hand column reflect a passive approach to managing your health care. Statements in the right-hand column represent an active approach. The more statements you circled in the right column, the more active a role you are taking in managing your health care. For any statements in the left column you circled, consider how you can change your behavior to become an active rather than a passive health care consumer.

# SUMMING UP

## Questions and Answers

### HEALTH CARE IN AMERICA

**1. What is the U.S. health care system?** In truth, it's less of a system than it is a loosely coordinated network of health care providers, government support programs, and health insurance companies.

**2. Why does health care cost so much?** Reasons include the practice of defensive medicine (as physicians try to protect themselves from malpractice suits), the fact that Americans are living longer, the advent of expensive diagnostic tests and medical procedures, and the lack of incentives for consumers or health care providers to constrain costs.

**3. How are employers attempting to control health care costs?** One way is by turning to managed care companies. Managed care is even making inroads in Medicare and Medicaid programs.

**4. What kinds of health care providers are there?** These include physicians (M.D.s and D.O.s), nurses, dentists, technicians, physicians' assistants, pharmacists, psychologists, and optometrists.

**5. What kinds of health care facilities are there?** These include hospitals, extended care facilities, home health care, and outpatient facilities.

**6. What are "alternative therapies"?** These are unconventional treatments, many of which have *not* been shown to be effective. They include acupuncture, meditation, vitamin therapy, chiropractic, nutritional therapies, homeopathy, biofeedback, herbal remedies, and massage.

### TYPES OF HEALTH INSURANCE PLANS

**7. What kinds of health insurance plans are there?** They include private health insurance (traditional "fee-for-service" plans and managed care plans), government insurance such as Medicaid and Medicare, and public health programs such as well-baby clinics (WBCs) and family planning clinics. In traditional "unmanaged" plans, the insurance carrier processes claims and pays bills for services at customary rates.

**8. What are the trends in health insurance?** Medical care is shifting rapidly from indemnity (fee-for-service) insurance plans to managed care. Fewer and fewer workers are given a choice about their health care coverage.

**9. What is managed care?** In these plans, doctors, hospitals, or a health benefits company agree to provide health care services to employees for a prepaid amount of money. The assumption is that costs can be contained while quality care is maintained. Some managed care plans reward doctors for limiting their use of outside specialists and medical tests and penalize them when they are "wasteful." Managed care plans include preferred provider organizations (PPOs) and health maintenance organizations (HMOs).

**10. What are Medicare and Medicaid?** These are government programs that provide health care to poor people, to people with disabilities, and to older people.

**11. Who is underserved by health care today?** Underserved people include poor people, ethnic minority groups, and people living in remote areas. Barriers to health care include transportation problems, language differences, unwillingness of providers to treat people on Medicaid, and insensitive treatment by providers.

## Suggested Readings

*How to Find the Best Doctors, Hospitals, and HMOs for You and Your Family.* New York: Castle Connolly Medical Ltd., 1995. A guide to finding the best health care providers.

**McCall, T. B.** *Examining Your Doctor: A Patient's Guide to Avoiding Harmful Medical Care.* Secaucus, NJ: Citadel Press, published by Carol Publishing Group, 1996. A step-by-step approach to evaluating the competence of your doctors and the quality of the care they provide.

**Tyberg, T., and Rothaus, E.** *Hospital Smarts: The Insider's Survival Guide to Your Hospital, Your Doctor, The Nursing Staff—And Your Bill.* New York: Hearst Books, 1995. Written by two physicians, it provides information to help you navigate through a hospitalization, including such topics as patients' rights, questions to ask your doctor, and deciphering your hospital bill.

**Vickery, D. M., and Fries, J. F.** *Take Care of Yourself.* Reading, MA: Addison Wesley, 1994 (5th ed.). A best-selling health guide that provides useful information on more than 120 common health problems, as well as information about choosing a health plan, getting the most from your health care, and avoiding serious illness. Includes decision charts showing when to see a doctor.

**Raymond, A. G.** *The HMO Health Care Companion.* New York: HarperCollins, 1994. A consumer's guide to choosing and using HMOs, and getting the most of the care and coverage they provide.

# Appendix A Hotlines to Health

## CHILD AND ADOLESCENT HEALTH

**National Clearinghouse on Family Support and Children's Mental Health**
Research and Training Center on Family Support and Children's Mental Health
P.O. Box 751
Portland, OR 97207-0751
(800) 628-1696
*Offers a series of fact sheets about children's mental health and maintains a state-by-state resource directory for services for children.*

**Children and Adolescent Service System Program (CASSP) Technical Assistance Center**
Georgetown University Child Development Center
3307 M Street NW
Washington, DC 20007-3935
(202) 687-5000
*Offers information packets and other publications on issues relating to children and adolescents with serious mental health problems.*

**Federation for Families of Children's Mental Health**
1021 Prince Street
Alexandria, VA 22314
(703) 684-7710
*A national parent-run organization that provides information and referrals within a network of federation chapters throughout the country involved with the mental health needs of children and adolescents.*

**Attention Deficit Information Network**
475 Hillside Avenue
Needham, MA 02194
(617) 455-9895
*Offers information on the latest research on attention-deficit disorder and its treatment.*

**Children with Attention Deficit Disorders (CHADD)**
499 NW 70th Avenue, Suite 308
Plantation, FL 33317
(305) 587-3700
*Publishes newsletters for parents and professionals on attentional disorders and offers information on support groups for families.*

**National Down Syndrome Society Hotline**
666 Broadway
8th Floor, Suite 810
New York, NY 10012-2317
(800) 221-4602
*Provides free information packets about Down syndrome and offers referrals to local support programs for children with Down syndrome.*

**Boys Town National Hotline (Child Abuse)**
13940 Gutowski Road
Boys Town, NE 68010
(800) 448-3000
(800) 448-1833 (TDD)
*Offers a 24-hour hotline and provides a range of services, including short-term intervention and counseling and referrals to local community resources for abused, neglected, and troubled children and adolescents.*

**Childhelp/IOF Foresters National Child Abuse Hotline**
15757 N. 78 Street
Scottsdale, AZ 85260
(800) 4-A-CHILD (422-4453)
(800) 2-A-CHILD (222-4453) (TDD)
*A national child abuse hotline offering information and referrals to prevention and treatment services in the caller's geographic area as well as telephone crisis counseling to both child abuse victims and abusers.*

**National Clearinghouse on Child Abuse and Neglect Information**
P.O. Box 1182
Washington, DC 20013-1182
(800) 394-3366
*A national clearinghouse for information about child abuse and neglect, it distributes a free publications catalog upon request.*

**Covenant House Nineline**
Covenant House
346 W. 17 Street
New York, NY 10011
(800) 999-9999
*Operates a 24-hour crisis line for youths, teens, and families and offers locally based referrals throughout the United States. Offers help to young people with problems such as drugs, child abuse, and homelessness.*

**National Youth Crisis Hotline**
P.O. Box 178408
San Diego, CA 92177-8408
(800) HIT-HOME (448-4663)
(619) 292-5683
*This 24-hour hotline offers short-term counseling services and referrals to youths needing drug treatment, shelters, and counseling programs. Offers help to young people dealing with problems involving pregnancy, abuse, and suicidal thinking.*

**National Center for Missing and Exploited Children**
2101 Wilson Boulevard, Suite 550
Arlington, VA 22201
(800) 843-5678
*Operates a hotline for people to report missing children and sightings of missing children.*

**Learning Disabilities Association of America**
4156 Library Road
Pittsburgh, PA 15234
(412) 341-8077
*An information and referral service within a network of state chapters and local support groups that offers assistance to children and their families coping with learning disabilities.*

**National Center for Learning Disabilities**
381 Park Avenue South, Suite 1401
New York, NY 10016
(212) 545-7510
*An information and referral service, the center also publishes a magazine,* Their World, *which focuses on the true stories of children and their families coping with learning disabilities.*

**The Orton Dyslexia Society**
Chester Building, Suite 382
8600 LaSalle Road
Baltimore, MD 21286-2044
(410) 296-0232
(800) 222-3123
*A national organization that serves as a clearinghouse of information about dyslexia and referrals to local resources.*

## ALCOHOL- AND DRUG-RELATED PROBLEMS

**Adcare Hospital Helpline**
107 Lincoln Street
Worcester, MA 01605
(800) ALCOHOL (252-6465)
(800) 345-3552
*Operates a 24-hour hotline offering information and referral for alcohol and other drug abuse problems.*

**Alcoholics Anonymous World Services, Inc.**
475 Riverside Drive
New York, NY 10115
(212) 870-3400
*Provides information about Alcoholics Anonymous. People seeking telephone numbers for local Alcoholics Anonymous chapters should use their local phone directory.*

**Adult Children of Alcoholics (ACOA)**
P.O. Box 3216
Torrance, CA 90510
(310) 534-1815
*Offers help to people recovering from growing up in an alcoholic family.*

**Al-Anon Family Group Headquarters**
Box 182, Madison Square Station
New York, NY 10159
(800) 356-9996
*A national organization providing assistance to families and friends of alcoholics. The national headquarters offers literature and refers people needing assistance to local meetings.*

**National Council on Alcoholism**
12 West 21 Street, 7th Floor
New York, NY 10010
(212) 206-6770
(800) 622-2255
*Provides information on alcoholism and referrals to affiliates around the country offering treatment services.*

**Mothers Against Drunk Driving**
511 E. John Carpenter Freeway, Suite 700
Irving, TX 75062
(214) 744-6233
*A national organization committed to stopping drunk driving, it provides support groups for victims of drunk driving and their families, among other services.*

**Hazelden Foundation–Alcohol/Medication Addiction**
P.O. Box 11
Center City, Minnesota 55012-0011
(800) 257-7800
*From a leading alcohol addiction treatment center, information and publications about drug and alcohol addiction, and referrals for all types of mental health problems.*

**National Council on Alcoholism and Drug Dependence, Inc.**
12 W. 21 Street
New York, NY 10016
(800) 622-2255
*A 24-hour referral hotline, it offers referrals to local affiliates for counseling as well as written information on alcoholism and drug dependence.*

**National Clearinghouse for Alcohol and Drug Information**
P.O. Box 2345
Rockville, MD 20847-2345
(301) 468-2600
Touch Tone: (800) 788-2800
Rotary: (800) 729-6686
TTY/TD: (800) 487-4889
*Provides information on a wide range of topics concerned with alcohol- and drug-related problems as well as referral services.*

**National Institute on Drug Abuse Hotline**
5600 Fishers Lane
Rockville, MD 20857
(800) 662-HELP (662-4357) (English)
(800) 66-AYUDA (662-9832) (Spanish)
(800) 228-0427 (TDD)
*From the federal agency at the forefront of drug treatment, it provides callers with information on alcohol and drug abuse and availability of treatment services throughout the U.S.*

**National Cocaine Hotline**
Phoenix House
164 W. 74 Street
New York, NY 10023
(800) COCAINE (262-2463)
*A 24-hour national hotline, it provides referrals to drug rehabilitation centers and answers to questions about cocaine and other drugs.*

**"Just Say No" International**
2000 Franklin Street, Suite 400
Oakland, CA 94612
(800) 258-2766
*An organization representing some 13,000 clubs that provides materials, technical assistance, and training directed toward helping young people lead drug-free lives.*

**American Council for Drug Education**
164 W. 74th Street
New York, NY 10023
(800) 488-DRUG (488-3784)
*Operates a clearinghouse of information relating to alcohol and substance abuse and provides referrals through (800) COCAINE (262-2463).*

**Families Anonymous (FA)**
P.O. Box 3475
Culver City, CA 90231-3475
(310) 313-5800
(800) 736-9805
*Offers a 12-step program for parents and other family members of people with drug- and alcohol-related problems.*

**Narcotics Anonymous**
P.O. Box 9999
Van Nuys, CA 91409
(818) 773-9999
*A peer-support organization that offers help to narcotic addicts.*

**Nar-Anon Family Groups**
P.O. Box 2562
Palos Verdes Peninsula, CA 90274
(310) 547-5800
*Similar to Al-Anon, it offers information and sponsors support groups and meetings for families of people on drugs.*

**Cocaine Anonymous (CA)**
3740 Overland Avenue
Los Angeles, CA 90034
(310) 559-5833
(800) 347-8998
*A national referral line that links callers to local numbers where they can speak to people trained to help cocaine abusers and provide them with referrals to treatment facilities. Applies the AA 12-step approach to persons addicted to cocaine.*

**Co-Anon Family Groups**
P.O. Box 64742-66
Los Angeles, CA 90064
(818) 377-4317
*Similar to Al-Anon, it offers information and listings of meetings for families of cocaine addicts.*

## CHRONIC AND DEGENERATIVE DISEASES

**American Heart Association**
7272 Greenville Avenue
Dallas, TX 75231
(800) AHA-USA1 (242-8721)
(214) 373-6300
*Offers information about cardiovascular disease and referrals to heart care specialists.*

**American Heart Association Stroke Connection**
7272 Greenville Avenue
Dallas, TX 75231-4596
(800) 553-6321
*Provides literature about strokes and listings of more than 1,000 stroke support groups throughout the U.S.*

**National Stroke Association**
1565 Clarkson Street
Denver, CO 80218
(800) STROKES (787-6537)
*Provides information about stroke prevention, treatment, and rehabilitation as well as referral information for stroke survivors and their families.*

**American Lung Association**
1740 Broadway
New York, NY 10019
(212) 315-8700
(800) LUNG-USA (586-4872)
*Offers a wide range of information about lung diseases and smoking cessation, including referrals for smoking cessation programs and counseling services.*

**Lung Line**
**National Jewish Center for Immunology and Respiratory Medicine**
1400 Jackson Street
Denver, CO 80206
(800) 222-5864
(800) 552-LUNG (552-5864) (LUNG FACTS)
*Registered nurses provide answers to questions about smoking and asthma, emphysema, chronic bronchitis, allergies, juvenile rheumatoid arthritis, smoking, and other respiratory and immune system disorders. LUNG FACTS is a 24-hour, 7-days-a-week automated information service on lung diseases and immunological disorders that you can access using a touch-tone telephone.*

**Office on Smoking and Health**
4770 Buford Highway NE
Mailstop K50
Atlanta, GA 30341
(770) 488-5705
*Offers information about smoking patterns, health consequences of smoking, and smoking cessation.*

**National Institute for Allergy and Infectious Diseases (NIAID)**
Building 31, Room 7A-50
Bethesda, MD 20892
(301) 496-5717
*From the federal agency within NIH that oversees the nation's fight against allergic and infectious disease, it offers educational materials on these health problems.*

**Asthma and Allergy Foundation of America**
1125 15 Street NW, Suite 502
Washington, DC 20005
(800) 727-8462
*A 24-hour hotline, it provides information about asthma and allergies, as well as referrals to physicians.*

**American Liver Foundation**
1425 Pompton Ave.
Cedar Grove, NJ 07009
(800) 223-0179
*Provides information and fact sheets about liver disease and referrals to physicians specializing in liver disease and related support groups.*

**American Cancer Society Response Line**
19 West 56 Street
New York, NY 10019
(800) 227-2345
*Offers publications and information about cancer from the country's leading cancer organization. Also refers callers to local chapters for support services.*

**National Cancer Institute (NCI)**
**National Institutes of Health**
**Cancer Information Service (CIS), Office of Cancer Communications**
31 Center Drive, MSC 2850
Building 31, Room 10A-07
Bethesda, MD 20892-2580
(800) 4-CANCER (422-6237)
*The federal government's cancer research agency, the NCI provides brochures and booklets about various types of cancer and state-of-the-art treatment and clinical trial information. Answers cancer-related questions from the public, cancer patients and families, and health professionals.*

**Y-Me National Organization for Breast Cancer Information Support Program**
212 W. Van Buren
Chicago, IL 60607
(800) 221-2141
*Offers counseling and treatment information to breast cancer patients as well as referrals to treatment providers and information about peer-support groups and self-help counseling.*

**American Institute for Cancer Research**
1759 R Street NW
Washington, DC 20009
(800) 843-8114
*Maintains a Nutrition Hotline staffed by registered dieticians and offers free educational publications about diet, nutrition, and cancer prevention.*

**Cancer Care, Inc.**
1180 Avenue of the Americas
New York, NY 10036
(212) 302-2400
*Helps cancer patients and their families and friends cope with the impact of cancer at no cost. Offers information about cancer support services including homemaking services, hospices, child care services, treatment centers, and other community resources as well as guidance for caring for patients at home.*

**Candlelighters Childhood Cancer Foundation**
7910 Woodmont Avenue, Suite 460
Bethesda, MD 20814
(800) 366-2223
*Provides information and support to children with cancer and their families.*

**Leukemia Society of America**
600 Third Avenue
New York, NY 10016
(212) 573-8484
*Offers literature about leukemia, as well as information about treatment providers and family support groups.*

**Skin Cancer Foundation**
245 Fifth Avenue, Suite 2402
New York, NY 10016
(212) 725-5176
*Provides information on how to protect your skin from the sun and identify the early signs of skin cancer.*

**American Diabetes Association**
1660 Duke Street
Alexandria, VA 22314
(800) 232-3472
*Offers a range of services to people with diabetes and their families as well as providing general information to the public about diabetes.*

**National Digestive Diseases Information Clearinghouse**
2 Information Way
Bethesda, MD 20892-3570
(301) 654-3810
*A federal agency, the clearinghouse collects and disseminates information on digestive diseases to patients and health professionals in the form of fact sheets and information packets.*

**Juvenile Diabetes Foundation International Hotline**
120 Wall Street, 19th Floor
New York, NY 10005
(800) 223-1138
*Provides answers to questions about juvenile diabetes and referrals to local chapters, physicians, and clinics.*

**National Headache Foundation**
428 W. St. James Place, 2nd Floor
Chicago, IL 60614
(800) 843-2256
*Provides literature about headaches and treatment options.*

**American Association of Kidney Patients**
100 South Ashley Driver, Suite 280
Tampa, FL 33602
(800) 749-2257
*Provides information about renal diseases and helps renal patients and their families cope with renal conditions.*

**American Foundation for Urologic Disease**
(800) 242-2383
*Offers educational materials about urologic diseases and responds to requests for referrals and support group information.*

**National Kidney Foundation**
30 East 33 Street
New York, NY 10016
(800) 622-9010
*Offers information about kidney disease and referrals to treatment providers.*

**American Parkinson Disease Association**
1250 Hylan Boulevard, Suite 4B
Staten Island, NY 10305
(800) 223-2732
*Offers information about Parkinson's disease and referrals to treatment providers.*

**National Parkinson Foundation, Inc.**
1501 NW 9th Avenue
Bob Hope Road
Miami, FL 331362
(800) 327-4545
*Offers educational materials about Parkinson's disease and information about physician referrals and support groups.*

**Arthritis Foundation Information Line**
(800) 283-7800
*Offers publications and information about arthritis and referrals to local organizations.*

**The National Osteoporosis Foundation (NOF)**
1150 17 Street NW, Suite 500
Washington, DC 20036-4603
(202) 223-2226
*A leading resource for people with osteoporosis, the NOF offers up-to-date, medically sound information on the causes, prevention, detection, and treatment of osteoporosis.*

**National Institute of Arthritis and Musculoskeletal and Skin Diseases (NIAMS) Clearinghouse (NAMSIC)**
1 AMS Circle
Bethesda, MD 20892-3675
(301) 496-8188
*A government institute within NIH, it offers publications on more than 600 different diseases and disorders related to arthritis as well as musculoskeletal and skin diseases.*

**National Multiple Sclerosis Association of America**
706 Haddonfield Road
Cherry Hill, NJ 08002
(800) 532-7667
*Provides specialists to answer questions about MS.*

**Crohn's and Colitis Foundation of America, Inc.**
386 Park Avenue South, 17th Floor
New York, NY 10016
(800) 932-2423
(800) 343-3637 (warehouse)
*Offers educational materials about Crohn's disease and ulcerative colitis and referrals to local support groups and medical specialists.*

**Cystic Fibrosis Foundation**
6931 Arlington Road
Bethesda, MD 20814
(800) 344-4823
*Offers information about cystic fibrosis and offers referrals to local treatment providers.*

**Epilepsy Foundation of America (EFA)**
4351 Garden City Drive
Landover, MD 20785-2267
(800) 332-1000
*Provides information about epilepsy as well as referrals to local chapters of the organization.*

**Huntington's Disease Society of America**
140 W. 22 Street, 6th Floor
New York, NY 10011
(800) 345-4372 (Patients and family members)
*Offers information about Huntington's disease and referrals to physicians, support groups, and local chapters of the organization.*

**The Lupus Foundation of America, Inc.**
1300 Piccard Drive, Suite 200
Rockville, MD 20850
(800) 558-0121
(301) 670-9292
*Provides information about lupus and services provided by the organization.*

## MENTAL HEALTH AND PSYCHOLOGICAL DISORDERS

**National Mental Health Association Information Center**
1021 Prince Street
Alexandria, VA 22314-2971
(800) 969-NMHA (969-6642)
*A referral and information service for people seeking help for mental health problems.*

**National Alliance for the Mentally Ill**
200 N. Glebe Road, Suite 1015
Arlington, VA 22203
(800) 950-6264
*An advocacy group representing mentally ill people and their families, it provides information to consumers and professionals about issues affecting the mentally ill. Also offers a self-help phone line for people suffering from emotional problems.*

**National Mental Health Consumer Self-Help Clearinghouse (NMHCSHC)**
1211 Chestnut Street, 11th Floor
Philadelphia, PA 19107
(800) 688-4226
(800) 553-4539
*Serves as a clearinghouse for information about mental health self-help programs as well as providing an information and referral service to consumers needing assistance with mental health problems.*

**National Institute of Mental Health (NIMH)**
5600 Fisher's Lane, Room 702
Rockville, MD 20857
(301) 443-4513
*The government agency within NIH that focuses on mental health, it provides publications and pamphlets on mental health and has specialists who can answer questions about mental health.*

**Rehabilitation and Research Training Center**
Boston University Psychiatric Rehabilitation Center
930 Commonwealth Avenue
Boston, MA 02215
(617) 353-3550
*Maintains an electronic bulletin board to help people in need of psychiatric rehabilitation get in contact with rehabilitation facilities.*

**National Empowerment Center**
20 Ballard Road
Lawrence, MA 01843
(800) 769-3728
*Maintains a national directory of mutual support groups and drop-in centers.*

**American Academy of Child and Adolescent Psychiatry**
36-15 Wisconsin Avenue NW
Washington, DC 20016
(800) 333-7636
*An organization representing child and adolescent psychiatrists, it distributes fact sheets on mental illnesses affecting youngsters.*

**National Anxiety Foundation**
3135 Custer Drive
Lexington, KY 40517
(606) 272-7166
*Offers information about anxiety disorders, such as panic disorder and obsessive-compulsive disorder, as well as listing referrals to treatment providers.*

**Panic Disorder**
(800) 64-PANIC (647-2642)
*This is a resource center that provides information about panic disorder but does not offer referral services.*

**Obsessive Compulsive Foundation**
P.O. Box 70
Milford, CT 06460-0070
(203) 878-5669
*Provides information about obsessive-compulsive disorder and information for ordering related videotapes and books. Sponsors more than 250 support groups nationwide.*

**Depression/Awareness, Recognition, and Treatment Information (D/ART)**
5600 Fishers Lane, Room 10-85
Rockville, MD 20857
(301) 443-4140
(800) 421-4211 for a free brochure
*Offers information about depression, eating disorders, manic depression, and related topics.*

**National Depressive & Manic Depressive Association**
730 N. Franklin Street, Suite 501
Chicago, IL 60610
(800) 82-NDMDA (826-3632)
*Provides literature on depression and manic depression as well as referral sources to obtain help for depression and related disorders and information about support groups throughout the U.S.*

**National Foundation for Depressive Illness**
P.O. Box 2257
New York, NY 10116
(800) 248-4344
*Offers a referral list upon request and information about the signs of depressive illness and treatment options.*

**National Sleep Foundation**
729 15 Street NW, 4th Floor
Washington, DC 20005
(202) 785-2300
*Offers information about sleep disorders, such as insomnia, sleep apnea, narcolepsy, night terrors, and drowsy driving, as well as a listing of accredited sleep centers organized by geographic area.*

**National Association of Anorexia Nervosa and Associated Disorders (ANAD)**
P.O. Box 7
Highland Park, IL 60035
(847) 831-3438
*A referral and information service, it offers information packets and maintains a listing of free support groups across the country.*

**American Anorexia/Bulimia Association, Inc. (AABA)**
293 Central Park West, Suite 1R
New York, NY 10024
(212) 501-8351
*An information and referral service, it provides educational materials and referrals for professionals and support groups nationwide regarding bulimia and related conditions.*

**National Eating Disorders Association**
6655 S. Yale Avenue
Tulsa, OK 74136
(918) 481-4044
*A nonprofit organization that provides referrals to clinicians specializing in eating disorders and sends educational materials, packets, and information on support groups.*

**Overeaters Anonymous World Service**
P.O. Box 44020
Rio Rancho, NM 87174
(505) 891-2664
*Offers a program for recovery from compulsive overeating and provides a list of meeting groups worldwide and some general information about the organization.*

**National Resource Center on Homelessness and Mental Illness**
262 Delaware Avenue
Delmar, NY 10254
(800) 444-7415
*Maintains a compendium of information about homelessness and mental illness as well as offering technical assistance and information about services and housing for the homeless and mentally ill population.*

## HIV/AIDS AND OTHER STDs

**National AIDS Information Hotline**
**Centers for Disease Control and Prevention**
(800) 342-AIDS (342-2437)
*Information about HIV/AIDS and referral resources nationwide, 24 hours a day.*

**Canadian AIDS Hotline**
**AIDS Committee of Toronto**
(800) 267-6600

**CDC National AIDS Clearinghouse**
P.O. Box 6003
Rockville, MD 20849-6003
(800) 458-5231
*A national clearinghouse of information on HIV and AIDS, it distributes up-to-date information and educational materials, as well as making referrals nationally to AIDS organizations for publications and HIV/AIDS-related services.*

**CDC National STD Hotline**
c/o American Social Health Association
P.O. Box 13827
Research Triangle Park (RTP), NC 27709
(800) 227-8922
(800) 344-7432 (Spanish) (7 days/week, 8 A.M. to 2 A.M. Eastern time)
(800) 243-7889 (TDD) (M–F 10 A.M. to 10 P.M. Eastern time)
*A 24-hour helpline, it answers questions about STD prevention and transmission as well as providing referrals to community clinics that offer free or low-cost examination and treatment.*

**AIDS Clinical Trials Information Service**
P.O. Box 6421
Rockville, MD 20849-6421
(800) 874-2572
(800) 243-7012 (TDD)
*Offers up-to-date information about federally and privately sponsored clinical trials for people with HIV/AIDS.*

**Sex Information and Education Council of the United States (SIECUS)**
130 W. 42 Street, Suite 2500
New York, NY 10036
(212) 819-9770
*A national clearinghouse for information about sexuality, SIECUS provides bibliographies on topics concerning human sexuality and can direct callers to agencies, hotlines, and other resources to help them with their personal questions regarding AIDS or other sexual topics.*

## AGING AND AGING-RELATED DISORDERS

**National Institute on Aging (NIA Information Center)**
P.O. Box 8057
Gaithersburg, MD 20898-8057
(800) 222-2225
*Provides publications about healthy aging, with information about health promotion, medical care, the body, safety, nutrition, and planning for later years.*

**American Geriatric Society**
770 Lexington Avenue, Suite 300
New York, NY 10021
(212) 308-1414
*Offers information about aging, including a newsletter and journal, and referrals to geriatric specialists.*

**Alzheimer's Association**
919 N. Michigan Avenue, Suite 1000
Chicago, IL 60611-1676
(800) 272-3900
*A national organization that offers information about AD and referrals to local chapters and support groups.*

**Alzheimer's Disease Education and Referral Center**
P.O. Box 8250
Silver Spring, MD 20907-8250
(800) 438-4380
*Maintains and distributes information about AD and current research in the field as well as providing referrals to treatment centers, support groups, and family support services.*

**Alzheimer's Disease and Related Disorders Association**
919 N. Michigan Avenue, Suite 1000
Chicago, IL 60611-1676
(800) 621-0379
*Offers assistance and information to Alzheimer's families through its 188 chapters nationwide.*

## FOOD AND NUTRITION

**American Dietetic Association Hotline**
National Center for Nutrition and Dietetics—American Dietetics Association
216 W. Jackson Boulevard
Chicago, IL 60606
(800) 366-1655
*Offers information about food and nutrition.*

**National Dairy Council**
10255 W. Higgins Road, Suite 900
Rosemont, IL 60018-5616
(800) 426-8271
*An industry trade group, it provides educational materials on dairy foods and nutrition.*

**Calcium Information Center**
(800) 321-2681
*Provides information on calcium nutrition and its role in health promotion as well as related information on osteoporosis; provides answers to specific questions about calcium.*

**Center for Food Safety and Applied Nutrition (FDA)**
200 Sea Street SW
Washington, DC 20204
(301) 827-4420
*A service of the FDA, it distributes the* FDA Consumer, *the official magazine of the U.S. Food and Drug Administration, containing the latest findings on diet and nutrition, benefits and side effects of new medications, and related health information (subscription only).*

**Center for Science in the Public Interest**
1875 Connecticut Avenue NW, Suite 300
Washington, DC 20009-5728
(202) 332-9110
*A public interest group, it focuses on health and nutrition issues, offering a range of books, posters, visual aids, and other literature, including a newsletter,* Nutrition Action, *which is available on a subscription basis.*

**Food and Drug Administration**
Office of Regulatory Affairs
Consumer Affairs and Information Staff
5600 Fishers Lane (HFC-110)
Rockville, MD 20857
(301) 443-4166
*The federal agency responsible for ensuring the safety of the foods we eat and the drugs we use, it offers publications and materials of interest to consumers and professionals.*

## FITNESS

**Aerobics and Fitness Foundation of America**
15250 Ventura Boulevard, Suite 200
Sherman Oaks, CA 91403
(800) 233-4886
*Provides information about safe, healthful exercise programs and activities as well as information on certification for aerobics teachers and professionals.*

**President's Council on Physical Fitness and Sports**
200 Independence Avenue SW
HHH Building, Room 738-H
Washington, DC 20201
(202) 690-9000
*Offers literature to help people make physical fitness and exercise a part of their lifestyle.*

## SERVICES FOR PEOPLE WITH DISABILITIES

**American Council of the Blind**
1155 15 Street NW, Suite 720
Washington, DC 20005
(800) 424-8666
(202) 467-5081
*Offers educational materials and information about blindness and referrals to clinics and other services for the blind and visually impaired.*

**The Lighthouse National Center for Vision and Aging**
111 E. 59 Street
New York, NY 10022
(800) 334-5497 (voice, TDD)
*Offers educational materials and information about age-related vision loss to the general public and professionals.*

**American Speech–Language–Hearing Association**
10801 Rockville Pike
Rockville, MD 20852
(800) 638-8255
*Provides information about speech/language disorders and hearing impairments and referrals to certified audiologists.*

**Dial A Hearing Screening Test**
(800) 222-3277
*Answers questions about hearing problems and provides referrals to local telephone numbers. Offers a two-minute telephone hearing screening test. Also makes referrals to ear, nose, and throat specialists and organizations providing information on ear-related problems.*

**National Institute on Deafness and Other Communication Disorders Information Clearinghouse**
1 Communication Avenue
Bethesda, MD 20892-3456
(800) 241-1044
(800) 241-1055 (TT)
*A federal agency that collects and distributes information and educational materials on hearing, balance, smell, taste, voice, speech, and language.*

**Stuttering Foundation of America**
P.O. Box 11749
Memphis, TN 38111-0749
(800) 992-9392
*Provides information about stuttering problems and referrals to speech-language pathologists.*

**Americans with Disabilities Act Hotline**
(800) 514-0301
(800) 514-0383 (TTY)
(202) 514-6193 (electronic bulletin board)
*Sponsored by the U.S. Department of Justice, it provides a 24-hour recording of information on the Americans with Disabilities Act. The recording also allows callers to request related publications.*

**United Cerebral Palsy Association**
1660 L Street NW, Suite 700
Washington, DC 20036
(800) 872-5827
*Offers information about cerebral palsy and responds to requests for referrals to local affiliates.*

**Health Resource Center**
(800) 544-3284
(202) 939-9320
*Operates a national clearinghouse on postsecondary education for individuals with disabilities.*

**American Paralysis Association**
500 Morris Avenue
Springfield, NJ 07081
(800) 225-0292
*Provides information about the latest developments in spinal cord injury research.*

**American Paralysis Association Spinal Cord Injury Hotline**
(800) 526-3456
*Sponsored by American Paralysis Association, the hotline provides literature on spinal cord injuries and makes referrals to organizations and support groups for people with spinal cord injuries.*

**National Rehabilitation Information Center**
8455 Colesville Road, Suite 935
Silver Spring, MD 20910
(800) 346-2742
*Offers information on rehabilitation issues and concerns.*

**National Spinal Cord Injury Association**
8300 Colesville Road, Suite 551
Silver Spring, MD 20910
(800) 962-9629 (for members and individuals with spinal cord injuries; no vendors)
(800) 935-2722 (in MA; nonmembers, public, professionals)
*Offers peer-counseling services to people with spinal cord injuries through local chapters and organizations as well as providing information about spinal cord injuries.*

**National Head Injury Foundation, Family Helpline**
Brain Injury Association
1776 Massachusetts Ave. NW, Suite 100
Washington, DC 20036
(800) 444-6443
*Provides information and educational materials about brain injury and locations of rehabilitative facilities, community services, and programs for the prevention of traumatic brain injury.*

## WOMEN'S HEALTH ISSUES

**Endometriosis Association**
(800) 992-3636
*Provides information about endometriosis.*

**PMS Access**
(800) 222-4767
*Provides information about controlling and treating PMS.*

**Women's Sports Foundation**
Eisenhower Park
East Meadow, NY 11554
(800) 227-3988
*Offers information about women's sports, physical fitness, and sports medicine.*

**ASPO/Lamaze (American Society for Psychoprophylaxis in Obstetrics)**
1200 19 Street NW, Suite 300
Washington, DC 20036
(800) 368-4404
*Provides information about prepared childbirth and how to locate an ASPO-certified childbirth educator in your area.*

**International Childbirth Education Association**
P.O. Box 20048
Minneapolis, MN 55420
(800) 624-4934 (book center orders)
(612) 854-8600 (in MN) (general information)
*Provides referrals to local chapters and support groups and operates a mail-order service for books on childbirth.*

**Planned Parenthood Federation of America, Inc.**
810 Seventh Avenue
New York, NY 10019
(800) 230-PLAN (230-7526)
*Offers information about family planning as well as reproductive and sexual health.*

**La Leche League International**
1400 N. Meacham Road
Schaumberg, IL 60173
(800) LA-LECHE (525-3243)
(847) 519-7730
*Provides breast-feeding information and mother-to-mother support for women who wish to breast-feed.*

## DEATH AND DYING

**National Hospice Organization (NHO)**
1901 N. Moore Street, Suite 901
Arlington, VA 22209
(800) 658-8898 (referrals)
(703) 243-5900
*Provides information and educational materials to the public about hospice care and referrals.*

**The Living Bank**
P.O. Box 6725
Houston, TX 77265
(800) 528-2971
*A 24-hour hotline, it operates a national registry and referral service for people wanting to donate their tissues and vital organs for transplantation.*

**United Network for Organ Sharing**
(800) 243-6667
*A 24-hour hotline, it provides information and referrals for organ donation and transplantation and provides organ donor cards.*

**Choice in Dying**
200 Varick Street, 10th Floor
New York, NY 10014
(800) 989-WILL (989-9455)
(212) 366-5540
*Provides information about living wills and related issues.*

## MISCELLANEOUS

**National Marrow Donor Program**
3433 Broadway NE, Suite 500
Minneapolis, MN 55413
(800) MARROW-2 (627-7692)
*Offers information about bone marrow donation and transplantation and lists of local donor centers.*

**American Dental Association (Catalog Sales)**
P.O. Box 776
St. Charles, IL 60174
(800) 947-4746
*Distributes educational materials on dental health topics, such as dentures, tooth decay, smoking, diet, oral care, and fluoridation.*

**National Health Information Center**
P.O. Box 1133
Washington, DC 20013-1133
(800) 336-4797
*Helps people make contact with health organizations throughout the U.S.*

**Agency for Health Care Policy and Research Clearinghouse**
P.O. Box 8547
Silver Spring, MD 20907
(800) 358-9295
(410) 381-3150 (outside the United States)
*The government agency responsible for monitoring health care services in the U.S., it offers free publications on topics relating to health care utilization, costs, and expenditures as well as clinical practice guidelines.*

**American Trauma Society (ATS)**
8903 Presidential Parkway, Suite 512
Upper Marlboro, MD 20772-2656
(800) 556-7890
*Answers questions about trauma and medical emergencies.*

**American Red Cross Public Inquiries Office**
8111 Gatehouse Road
Falls Church, VA 22042
(703) 206-7090
*Offers information and publications about disaster preparedness and response as well as other activities of the national organization ranging from CPR classes to lifeguard training.*

**Office of Minority Health Resource Center**
P.O. Box 37337
Washington, DC 20013-7337
(800) 444-6472
*Provides information and referrals focused on the health-related issues of minorities.*

**Impotence Information Center**
P.O. Box 9
Minneapolis, MN 55440
(800) 843-4315
(800) 543-9632
*Provides information about the causes of erectile dysfunction and available treatments.*

**National Domestic Violence Hotline**
(800) 799-7233
*A 24-hour hotline that provides help to victims of domestic violence and referrals to local agencies.*

**National Coalition Against Domestic Violence (NCADV)**
119 Constitution Avenue NE
Washington, DC 20002
(800) 799-7233
(202) 544-7358
*A national organization of shelters and support services for battered women and their children.*

**National Lead Information Hotline**
(800) LEAD-FYI (532-3394) (hotline)
(800) 424-LEAD (424-5323) (clearinghouse)
(800) 526-5456 (TDD)
*Offers information on lead poisoning and prevention.*

**New York Public Interest Research Group Fund**
NYPIRG Publications
9 Murray Street, 3rd Floor
New York, NY 10007-2272
(212) 349-6460
*The informative booklet on lead poisoning prevention,* Get the Lead Out, *is available upon request.*

**American Leprosy Missions (Hansen's Disease)**
1 ALM Way
Greenville, SC 29601
(800) 543-3131
*Offers information and educational materials about leprosy.*

**American SIDS Institute**
6065 Roswell Road, Suite 876
Atlanta, GA 30328
(800) 232-7437
*A 24-hour service, the hotline provides answers to questions from families and physicians about sudden infant death syndrome (SIDS), distributes related information, and makes referrals to other organizations.*

**SIDS Alliance**
1314 Bedford Avenue, Suite 210
Baltimore, MD 21208
(800) 221-7437
*Offers educational materials and referrals about SIDS.*

**National Association for Sickle Cell Disease**
200 Corporate Point, Suite 495
Culver City, CA 90230-7633
(800) 421-8453
*Provides information about the disease and opportunities for genetic counseling.*

**National Organization for Rare Disorders**
P.O. Box 8923
New Fairfield, CT 06812
(800) 999-6673
*Offers information about rare disorders and referrals to organizations providing help to people with specific disorders.*

# Appendix B Scoring Keys

## CHAPTER 2

### Life Orientation (Optimism)

In order to arrive at your total score for the test, first *reverse* your score on items 3, 8, 9, and 12. That is, change a 4 a 0, a 3 to a 1, leave a 2 the same, and change a 1 to a 3 and a 0 to a 4. Now add the scores for items 1, 3, 4, 5, 8, 9, 11, and 12. (Items 2, 6, 7, and 10 are "fillers"; that is, your responses are not scored as part of the test.) Your total score can range from 0 to 32.

Following are the norms for the test. The average (mean) score for men was 21.03 (standard deviation = 4.56), and the mean score for women was 21.41 (standard deviation = 5.22). Scores above 26 may be considered quite optimistic, and scores below 16, quite pessimistic. Scores between 16 and 26 are within a broad average range, and higher scores within this range are relatively more optimistic.

## CHAPTER 3

### Type A Scale

"Yes" answers suggest a Type A personality pattern. The more "yes" answers, the stronger the Type A pattern. In evaluating whether or not you are a Type A, don't be concerned with the precise number of "yes" answers. We have no normative data for you. Yet you should have little trouble spotting yourself as "hard core" or "moderately afflicted"—that is, if you are honest with yourself.

## CHAPTER 4

### "Are You Depressed?" Scale

If you answered "yes" to at least five of the statements, including either item 1 or 2, and if these complaints have persisted for at least 2 weeks, then professional help is strongly recommended. If you answered "yes" to the third statement, we suggest that you immediately consult a health professional. Contact your college or university counseling or health center. Or talk to your instructor.

## CHAPTER 8

### Scale on Endorsement of Traditional or Liberal Marital Roles

Below each of the scoring codes (AS, AM, DM, and DS) there is a number. Underline the numbers beneath each of your answers. Then add the underlined numbers to obtain your total score.

The total score can vary from 10 to 40. A score of 10–20 shows moderate to high traditionalism concerning marital roles, while a score of 30–40 shows moderate to high liberalism. A score between 20 and 30 suggests that you are a middle-of-the-roader.

Your endorsement of a traditional or a liberal marital role is not a matter of right or wrong. However, if you and your potential or actual spouse endorse significantly different marital roles, you may have certain role conflicts. It may be worthwhile to have a frank talk with your partner about your goals and values to determine whether the two of you have major disagreements and are willing to work to resolve them.

## CHAPTER 8

### Rathus Assertiveness Schedule (RAS)

To compute your score, first change the signs (plus to minus; minus to plus) for those items followed by an asterisk (*). For example, if the response to an asterisked item was 2, place a minus sign (−) before the 2. If the response to an asterisked item was −3, change the minus sign to a plus sign (+). Then add up the scores of the 30 items.

Scores on the assertiveness schedule can vary from +90 to −90. The table (next column) shows you how your score compares to those of 764 women and 637 men from 35 college campuses across the United States. For example, if you are a woman and your score was 26, it exceeded that of 80% of the women in the sample. A score of 15 for a male exceeds that of 55 to 60% of the men in the sample.

**Percentiles for Scores on the RAS**[1]

| Women's Scores | Percentile | Men's Scores |
|---|---|---|
| 55 | 99 | 65 |
| 48 | 97 | 54 |
| 45 | 95 | 48 |
| 37 | 90 | 40 |
| 31 | 85 | 33 |
| 26 | 80 | 30 |
| 23 | 75 | 26 |
| 19 | 70 | 24 |
| 17 | 65 | 19 |
| 14 | 60 | 17 |
| 11 | 55 | 15 |
| 8 | 50 | 11 |
| 6 | 45 | 8 |
| 2 | 40 | 6 |
| −1 | 35 | 3 |
| −4 | 30 | 1 |
| −8 | 25 | −3 |
| −13 | 20 | −7 |
| −17 | 15 | −11 |
| −24 | 10 | −15 |
| −34 | 5 | −24 |
| −39 | 3 | −30 |
| −48 | 1 | −41 |

## CHAPTER 9

### *HealthCheck* on Menopause

Every item on this HealthCheck is false. They all represent myths about menopause, not realities. To which myths did you fall prey?

**1.** *Menopause is abnormal.* Of course not. Menopause is a normal development in women's lives.

**2.** *The medical establishment considers menopause a disease.* No longer. Menopause is described as a "deficiency syndrome" today. The term refers to the decline in secretion of estrogen and progesterone. Of course, the term *deficiency* also has negative meanings.

**3.** *After menopause, women need complete replacement of estrogen.* Not necessarily. Some estrogen continues to be produced by the adrenal glands, fatty tissue, and the brain.

[1] Source of data: Nevid, J. S., & Rathus, S. A. Multivariate and Normative Data Pertaining to the RAS with the College Population. *Behavior Therapy, 9* (1978), 675.

**4.** *Menopause is accompanied by depression and anxiety.* Not necessarily. Studies that have followed healthy women through menopause have found that menopause is not significantly related to depression, anxiety, stress, anger, or job dissatisfaction. Much of a woman's response to menopause reflects its meaning to her, not physical changes. Women who adopt the commonly held belief that menopause signals the beginning of the end of life may develop a sense of hopelessness about the future. Women whose entire lives have centered around childbearing and child rearing are more likely to suffer a sense of loss. Moreover, there is a harmful tendency—even among some health professionals—to consider depression and other complaints of middle-aged women as menopausal rather than to explore other biological and social factors.

**5.** *At menopause, women suffer debilitating hot flashes.* Many women do not have hot flashes. Among those who do, the flashes are often relatively mild.

**6.** *A woman who has had a hysterectomy will not undergo menopause.* It depends on whether or not the ovaries (the major producers of estrogen) were also removed. If they were not, menopause should proceed normally.

**7.** *Menopause signals an end to a woman's sexual appetite.* Not at all. Many women feel liberated by the severing of the ties between sex and reproduction.

**8.** *Menopause ends a woman's childbearing years.* Not necessarily! Postmenopausal women do not produce ova. However, ova from donors have been fertilized in laboratory dishes. The developing embryos have been implanted in the uteruses of postmenopausal women and carried to term.

**9.** *A woman's general level of activity is lower after menopause.* Many postmenopausal women become peppier and more assertive.

**10.** *Men are not affected by their wives' experience of menopause.* Many men are, of course. Men could become still more understanding if they learned about menopause and if their wives felt freer to talk to them about it.

## CHAPTER 10

### Reasoning about Abortion Scale

First tally your scores for the following items: 1, 3, 7, 8, 9, 11, 13, 14, 17, and 20. This score represents your support for a *pro-choice* point of view: ______.

Now tally your scores for the remaining items: 2, 4, 5, 6, 10, 12, 15, 16, 18, and 19. This score represents your support for a *pro-life* point of view: ______.

Now subtract your *pro-choice* score from your *pro-life* score. Write the difference, including the sign, here: ______. A positive score indicates agreement with a pro-life philosophy. A negative score indicates agreement with a pro-choice philosophy. The higher your score, the more strongly you agree with the philosophy you endorsed. Scores may range from −40 to +40.

One sample of 230 undergraduate students (115 of each gender) obtained a mean score of −7.48 and a median score of −13.33.[2] This indicates that the students tended to be pro-choice in their attitudes. Another sample of 38 graduate students (31 women and 7 men) obtained mean scores of −11 to −12 and median scores of −17 to −18 on two separate occasions. Scores for other samples may vary.

## CHAPTER 14

### Why Do You Smoke?

How to score:

**1.** Enter the number you have circled for each question in the spaces below, putting the number you have circled to question A over line A, to question B over line B, etc.

**2.** Add the three scores on each line to get your totals. For example, the sum of your scores over lines A, G, and M gives you your score on *Stimulation;* lines B, H, and N give the score on *Handling,* etc.

| | | | | | | | Totals |
|---|---|---|---|---|---|---|---|
| ______ | + | ______ | + | ______ | = | ______ | |
| A | | G | | M | | | **Stimulation** |
| ______ | + | ______ | + | ______ | = | ______ | |
| B | | H | | N | | | **Handling** |
| ______ | + | ______ | + | ______ | = | ______ | |
| C | | I | | O | | | **Pleasurable Relaxation** |
| ______ | + | ______ | + | ______ | = | ______ | |
| D | | J | | P | | | **Crutch: Tension Reduction** |
| ______ | + | ______ | + | ______ | = | ______ | |
| E | | K | | Q | | | **Craving: Psychological Addiction** |
| ______ | + | ______ | + | ______ | = | ______ | |
| F | | L | | R | | | **Habit** |

Scores can vary from 3 to 15. Any score of 11 or above is high; any score of 7 or below is low.

What kind of smoker are you? What do you get out of smoking? What does it do for you? This test is designed to provide you with a score on each of six factors relating to smoking. Your smoking may be characterized by only one of these factors or by a combination of two or more factors. In any event, this test will help you identify what you use smoking for and what kind of satisfaction you think you get from smoking.

The six factors measured by this test describe different ways of experiencing or managing certain kinds of feelings. Three of these feeling states represent the positive feelings people get from smoking: a sense of increased energy or stimulation; the satisfaction of handling or manipulating things; the enhancing of pleasurable feelings accompanying a state of well-being. The fourth relates to a decreasing of negative feeling states such as anxiety, anger, shame, and so forth. The fifth is a complex pattern of increasing and decreasing "craving" for a cigarette, representing the psychological addiction to smoking. The sixth is habit smoking, which takes place in an absence of feeling—purely automatic smoking.

A score of 11 or above on any factor indicates that this factor is an important source of satisfaction for you. The higher your score (15 is the highest), the more important a particular factor is in your smoking and the more useful the discussion of that factor can be in your efforts to quit.

[2] Parsons, N. K., Richards, H. C., & Kanter, G. D. Validation of a Scale to Measure Reasoning About Abortion. *Journal of Counseling Psychology, 37* (1990), 107–112.

## CHAPTER 20

### The Death Concern Scale

Scores on the Death Concern Scale[3] vary from 30 to 120. Calculate your total score by summing the scores for each of the 30 items. Place your total score here: ______

*Low scorers (30–67)* Low scorers admit to little if any concern about death. A low score may reflect a personal philosophy in which death is viewed as meaningful and acceptable within the scheme of things. A low score can also suggest that you are really reluctant to consider and accept the reality of death. A third possibility is that you tend not to think about things that do not immediately affect you, and death, perhaps, may seem a long way off. Upon reflection, you should have little difficulty deciding which possibility applies to you.

*Average scorers (68–80)* Average scorers show some concern about death, but they are not excessively anxious about it.

*High scorers (81–120)* High scorers probably experienced a great deal of anxiety when they first saw the title of the questionnaire. They are likely to be highly apprehensive about death and to show anxiety whenever the topic is raised. Perhaps they have had more than their share of illnesses or have become sensitized by the deaths of loved ones. High scorers may be generally anxious people for whom fear of death is not an isolated concern. People who find themselves preoccupied with death sometimes benefit from discussing their concerns with a counselor.

[3] Source: Rathus, S. A., & Nevid, J. S. *Adjustment and Growth: The Challenges of Life* (6th ed.). Fort Worth: Harcourt Brace College Publishers, 1995, p. 530. Reprinted with Permission.

# Appendix C    Nutritional Guidelines

## Fast Food Facts

The first part of this appendix provides nutritional information on items served at some popular fast food restaurants. Percent Daily Values are based on a 2,000 calorie diet. Your daily values may be higher or lower depending on your calorie needs.

| | | 2,000 Calories | 2,500 Calories |
|---|---|---|---|
| Total Fat | Less than | 65g | 80g |
| Saturated Fat | Less than | 20g | 25g |
| Cholesterol | Less than | 300mg | 300mg |
| Sodium | Less than | 2,400mg | 2,400mg |
| Carbohydrates | | 300g | 375g |
| Dietary Fiber | | 25g | 30g |

### Burger King

| | SERVING SIZE (grams) | CALORIES | CALORIES FROM FAT | TOTAL FAT (grams) | % DAILY VALUE | SATURATED FAT (grams) | % DAILY VALUE | CHOLESTEROL (milligrams) | % DAILY VALUE | SODIUM (milligrams) | % DAILY VALUE | CARBOHYDRATES (grams) | % DAILY VALUE | DIETARY FIBER (grams) | % DAILY VALUE | SUGARS (grams) | PROTEIN (grams) | % DAILY VALUE | | | |
|---|---|---|---|---|---|---|---|---|---|---|---|---|---|---|---|---|---|---|---|---|---|
| | | | | | | | | | | | | | | | | | | VITAMIN A | VITAMIN C | CALCIUM | IRON |
| WHOPPER® Sandwich | 270 | 640 | 350 | 39 | 60 | 11 | 55 | 90 | 30 | 870 | 36 | 45 | 15 | 3 | 12 | 8 | 27 | 10 | 15 | 8 | 25 |
| WHOPPER® with Cheese Sandwich | 294 | 730 | 410 | 46 | 77 | 16 | 80 | 115 | 38 | 1350 | 56 | 46 | 15 | 3 | 12 | 8 | 33 | 15 | 15 | 25 | 25 |
| DOUBLE WHOPPER® Sandwich | 351 | 870 | 500 | 56 | 86 | 19 | 95 | 170 | 57 | 940 | 39 | 45 | 15 | 3 | 12 | 8 | 46 | 10 | 15 | 8 | 40 |
| DOUBLE WHOPPER® with Cheese Sandwich | 375 | 960 | 570 | 63 | 97 | 24 | 120 | 195 | 65 | 1420 | 59 | 46 | 15 | 3 | 12 | 8 | 52 | 15 | 15 | 25 | 40 |
| WHOPPER JR.® Sandwich | 164 | 420 | 220 | 24 | 37 | 8 | 40 | 60 | 20 | 530 | 22 | 29 | 10 | 2 | 8 | 5 | 21 | 4 | 8 | 6 | 20 |
| WHOPPER JR.® with Cheese Sandwich | 177 | 460 | 250 | 28 | 43 | 10 | 50 | 75 | 25 | 770 | 32 | 29 | 10 | 2 | 8 | 5 | 23 | 8 | 8 | 15 | 20 |
| Hamburger | 126 | 330 | 140 | 15 | 23 | 6 | 30 | 55 | 18 | 530 | 22 | 28 | 9 | 1 | 4 | 4 | 20 | 2 | 0 | 4 | 15 |
| Cheeseburger | 138 | 380 | 170 | 19 | 29 | 9 | 45 | 65 | 22 | 770 | 32 | 28 | 9 | 1 | 4 | 5 | 23 | 6 | 0 | 10 | 15 |
| Double Cheeseburger | 210 | 600 | 320 | 36 | 55 | 17 | 85 | 135 | 45 | 1060 | 44 | 28 | 9 | 1 | 4 | 5 | 41 | 8 | 0 | 20 | 25 |
| Double Cheeseburger with Bacon | 218 | 640 | 350 | 39 | 60 | 18 | 90 | 145 | 48 | 1240 | 52 | 28 | 9 | 1 | 4 | 5 | 44 | 8 | 0 | 20 | 25 |
| BK BIG FISH™ Sandwich | 255 | 700 | 370 | 41 | 63 | 6 | 30 | 90 | 30 | 980 | 41 | 56 | 19 | 3 | 12 | 4 | 26 | 2 | 2 | 6 | 15 |
| BK BROILER® Chicken Sandwich | 248 | 550 | 260 | 29 | 45 | 6 | 30 | 80 | 27 | 480 | 20 | 41 | 14 | 2 | 8 | 4 | 30 | 6 | 10 | 6 | 30 |
| Chicken Sandwich | 229 | 710 | 390 | 43 | 66 | 9 | 45 | 60 | 20 | 1400 | 58 | 54 | 18 | 2 | 8 | 4 | 26 | 0 | 0 | 10 | 20 |
| CHICKEN TENDERS® (6 piece) | 88 | 230 | 110 | 12 | 18 | 3 | 15 | 35 | 12 | 530 | 22 | 14 | 5 | 2 | 8 | 0 | 16 | 0 | 0 | 0 | 4 |
| Barbecue Dipping Sauce | 28 | 35 | 0 | 0 | — | 0 | — | 0 | — | 400 | 17 | 9 | 10 | 0 | — | 7 | 0 | — | — | — | — |
| Sweet & Sour Dipping Sauce | 28 | 45 | 0 | 0 | — | 0 | — | 0 | — | 50 | 2 | 11 | 4 | 0 | — | 10 | 0 | — | — | — | — |
| Broiled Chicken Salad* | 302 | 200 | 90 | 10 | 15 | 4 | 20 | 60 | 20 | 110 | 5 | 7 | 2 | 3 | 12 | 5 | 21 | 100 | 25 | 15 | 20 |
| Garden Salad* | 215 | 100 | 45 | 5 | 8 | 3 | 15 | 15 | 5 | 110 | 5 | 7 | 2 | 3 | 12 | 5 | 6 | 110 | 50 | 15 | 6 |
| Side Salad* | 133 | 60 | 25 | 3 | 5 | 2 | 10 | 5 | 17 | 55 | 2 | 4 | 1 | 2 | 8 | 3 | 3 | 50 | 20 | 8 | 4 |
| French Fries (Medium, Salted) | 116 | 370 | 180 | 20 | 31 | 5 | 25 | 0 | — | 240 | 10 | 43 | 14 | 3 | 12 | 0 | 5 | 0 | 6 | 0 | 6 |
| Onion Rings | 124 | 310 | 130 | 14 | 22 | 2 | 10 | 0 | — | 810 | 34 | 41 | 14 | 6 | 24 | 6 | 4 | 0 | 0 | 10 | 8 |
| CROISSAN'WICH® w/Sausage, Egg & Cheese | 176 | 600 | 410 | 46 | 71 | 16 | 80 | 260 | 87 | 1140 | 48 | 25 | 8 | 1 | 4 | 3 | 22 | 8 | 0 | 15 | 20 |
| Biscuit with Sausage | 151 | 590 | 360 | 40 | 62 | 13 | 65 | 45 | 15 | 1390 | 58 | 41 | 14 | 1 | 4 | 2 | 16 | 0 | 0 | 6 | 20 |
| Biscuit with Bacon, Egg and Cheese | 171 | 510 | 280 | 31 | 48 | 10 | 50 | 225 | 75 | 1530 | 64 | 39 | 13 | 1 | 4 | 3 | 19 | 8 | 0 | 15 | 15 |
| Dutch Apple Pie | 113 | 300 | 140 | 15 | 23 | 3 | 15 | 0 | — | 230 | 10 | 39 | 13 | 2 | 8 | 22 | 3 | 0 | 10 | 0 | 8 |
| Chocolate Shake (Medium) | 284 | 320 | 60 | 7 | 11 | 4 | 20 | 20 | 7 | 230 | 10 | 54 | 18 | 3 | 12 | 48 | 9 | 6 | 0 | 20 | 10 |

**without dressing*

## Domino's Pizza

| | SERVING SIZE (grams) | CALORIES | CALORIES FROM FAT | TOTAL FAT (grams) | % DAILY VALUE | SATURATED FAT (grams) | % DAILY VALUE | CHOLESTEROL (milligrams) | % DAILY VALUE | SODIUM (milligrams) | % DAILY VALUE | CARBOHYDRATES (grams) | % DAILY VALUE | DIETARY FIBER (grams) | % DAILY VALUE | SUGARS (grams) | PROTEIN (grams) | % DAILY VALUE | | | |
|---|---|---|---|---|---|---|---|---|---|---|---|---|---|---|---|---|---|---|---|---|---|
| | | | | | | | | | | | | | | | | | | VITAMIN A | VITAMIN C | CALCIUM | IRON |
| 14" Large Pizza Hand-Tossed Crust (2 Slices) | 137 | | | | | | | | | | | | | | | | | | | | |
| Plain Cheese | | 319 | 88 | 10 | 15 | 4 | 22 | 18 | 6 | 622 | 26 | 44 | 15 | 2 | 8 | 2 | 14 | 9 | 9 | 26 | 19 |
| Pepperoni | | 374 | 133 | 15 | 23 | 6 | 32 | 29 | 10 | 800 | 33 | 44 | 15 | 2 | 9 | 2 | 16 | 9 | 9 | 26 | 21 |
| Mushrooms | | 321 | 88 | 10 | 15 | 4 | 22 | 18 | 6 | 622 | 26 | 45 | 15 | 2 | 9 | 2 | 14 | 9 | 10 | 26 | 20 |
| Green Peppers | | 321 | 88 | 10 | 15 | 4 | 22 | 18 | 6 | 623 | 26 | 45 | 15 | 2 | 9 | 2 | 14 | 10 | 29 | 26 | 20 |
| Italian Sausage | | 363 | 119 | 13 | 20 | 6 | 29 | 27 | 9 | 759 | 32 | 46 | 15 | 2 | 10 | 2 | 15 | 9 | 9 | 27 | 21 |
| Ham and Pineapple | | 343 | 94 | 11 | 16 | 5 | 23 | 25 | 8 | 779 | 32 | 47 | 16 | 2 | 9 | 4 | 16 | 9 | 11 | 26 | 21 |
| Extra Cheese | | 364 | 119 | 13 | 20 | 7 | 34 | 27 | 9 | 739 | 31 | 44 | 15 | 2 | 8 | 2 | 17 | 10 | 9 | 38 | 20 |
| Deep-Dish Crust (2 Slices) | 175 | | | | | | | | | | | | | | | | | | | | |
| Plain Cheese | | 464 | 177 | 20 | 30 | 7 | 36 | 23 | 8 | 978 | 41 | 55 | 18 | 3 | 11 | 4 | 18 | 9 | 5 | 33 | 22 |
| Pepperoni | | 519 | 221 | 25 | 38 | 9 | 46 | 35 | 12 | 1154 | 48 | 55 | 18 | 3 | 12 | 4 | 21 | 9 | 5 | 34 | 24 |
| Mushrooms | | 466 | 177 | 20 | 30 | 7 | 36 | 23 | 8 | 978 | 41 | 55 | 18 | 3 | 12 | 4 | 18 | 9 | 5 | 33 | 23 |
| Green Peppers | | 466 | 177 | 20 | 30 | 7 | 36 | 23 | 8 | 978 | 41 | 55 | 18 | 3 | 12 | 4 | 18 | 10 | 15 | 33 | 23 |
| Italian Sausage | | 508 | 208 | 23 | 36 | 9 | 42 | 32 | 11 | 1114 | 46 | 56 | 19 | 3 | 12 | 4 | 20 | 10 | 5 | 34 | 24 |
| Ham and Pineapple | | 488 | 183 | 20 | 31 | 7 | 37 | 30 | 10 | 1134 | 47 | 57 | 19 | 3 | 12 | 6 | 21 | 9 | 7 | 34 | 24 |
| Extra Cheese | | 509 | 208 | 23 | 36 | 9 | 46 | 32 | 11 | 1094 | 46 | 55 | 18 | 3 | 11 | 4 | 21 | 11 | 5 | 45 | 23 |
| BREADSTICKS (1 Piece) | 22.14 | 78 | 30 | 3 | 1 | 1 | — | 0 | — | 158 | 7 | 11 | 4 | — | — | — | 2 | — | — | 1 | — |
| HOT BUFFALO WINGS (10 Wings) | 249 | 449 | 215 | 24 | 37 | 7 | 32 | 256 | 85 | 3544 | 148 | 5 | 2 | 2 | 8 | 2.1 | 55 | 27 | 19 | 5 | 17 |



## KFC

| | SERVING SIZE (grams) | CALORIES | CALORIES FROM FAT | TOTAL FAT (grams) | % DAILY VALUE | SATURATED FAT (grams) | % DAILY VALUE | CHOLESTEROL (milligrams) | % DAILY VALUE | SODIUM (milligrams) | % DAILY VALUE | CARBOHYDRATES (grams) | % DAILY VALUE | DIETARY FIBER (grams) | % DAILY VALUE | SUGARS (grams) | PROTEIN (grams) | VITAMIN A | VITAMIN C | CALCIUM | IRON |
|---|---|---|---|---|---|---|---|---|---|---|---|---|---|---|---|---|---|---|---|---|---|
| ORIGINAL RECIPE® Chicken-Breast | 153 | 400 | 220 | 24 | 38 | 6 | 31 | 135 | 45 | 1116 | 47 | 16 | 5 | 1 | 4 | 0 | 29 | — | — | 4 | 6 |
| ORIGINAL RECIPE® Chicken-Drumstick | 61 | 140 | 80 | 9 | 13 | 2 | 10 | 75 | 25 | 422 | 18 | 4 | 1 | 0 | — | 0 | 13 | — | — | — | 4 |
| EXTRA TASTY CRISPY™ Chicken-Breast | 168 | 470 | 250 | 28 | 42 | 7 | 35 | 80 | 27 | 930 | 39 | 25 | 8 | 1 | 4 | 0 | 31 | — | — | 4 | 6 |
| EXTRA TASTY CRISPY™ Chicken-Drumstick | 67 | 190 | 100 | 11 | 17 | 3 | 14 | 60 | 20 | 260 | 11 | 8 | 3 | 0 | — | 0 | 13 | — | — | — | 4 |
| TENDER ROAST® Chicken—Breast with Skin | 139 | 251 | 97 | 11 | 17 | 23 | 15 | 151 | 50 | 830 | 35 | 1 | — | 0 | — | 0 | 37 | — | — | — | — |
| TRC—Breast without Skin | 118 | 169 | 39 | 4 | 7 | 1 | 6 | 112 | 37 | 797 | 33 | 1 | — | 0 | — | 0 | 31 | — | — | — | — |
| TRC—Drumstick with Skin | 55 | 97 | 39 | 4 | 5 | 1 | 6 | 85 | 28 | 271 | 11 | 0 | — | 0 | — | 0 | 15 | — | — | — | — |
| TRC—Drumstick without Skin | 38 | 67 | 22 | 2 | 4 | 1 | 3 | 63 | 21 | 259 | 11 | 0 | — | 0 | — | 0 | 11 | — | — | — | — |
| CHUNKY CHICKEN Pot Pie | 368 | 770 | 378 | 42 | 65 | 13 | 65 | 70 | 3 | 2160 | 90 | 69 | 23 | 5 | 20 | 8 | 29 | 80 | 2 | 10 | 10 |
| ORIGINAL RECIPE Chicken Sandwich | 206 | 497 | 201 | 22 | 34 | 5 | 24 | 52 | 17 | 1213 | 50 | 46 | 15 | 3 | 12 | 2 | 29 | — | — | 10 | 15 |
| VALUE BBQ Flavored Chicken Sandwich | 149 | 256 | 74 | 8 | 12 | 1 | 5 | 57 | 19 | 782 | 33 | 28 | 9 | 2 | 7 | 18 | 17 | — | 6 | 6 | 23 |
| Mashed Potatoes with Gravy | 136 | 120 | 50 | 6 | 9 | 1 | 5 | 0 | — | 440 | 18 | 17 | 6 | 2 | 8 | 0 | 1 | — | — | — | 2 |
| Cole Slaw | 142 | 180 | 80 | 9 | 14 | 2 | 8 | 5 | 2 | 280 | 12 | 21 | 7 | 3 | 12 | 20 | 2 | — | 60 | 4 | 4 |
| Biscuit | 56 | 180 | 80 | 10 | 14 | 3 | 12 | 0 | — | 560 | 23 | 20 | 7 | 0 | — | 2 | 4 | — | — | 2 | 6 |
| Corn on the Cob with Savory | 143 | 190 | 25 | 3 | 5 | 1 | 2 | 0 | — | 20 | 1 | 34 | 11 | 4 | 16 | 2 | 5 | 25 | 10 | — | 4 |
| Green Beans | 132 | 45 | 15 | 2 | 2 | 1 | 2 | 5 | 2 | 730 | 30 | 7 | 2 | 3 | 12 | 3 | 1 | 4 | 4 | 4 | 4 |

## McDonald's

| | SERVING SIZE (grams) | CALORIES | CALORIES FROM FAT | TOTAL FAT (grams) | % DAILY VALUE | SATURATED FAT (grams) | % DAILY VALUE | CHOLESTEROL (milligrams) | % DAILY VALUE | SODIUM (milligrams) | % DAILY VALUE | CARBOHYDRATES (grams) | % DAILY VALUE | DIETARY FIBER (grams) | % DAILY VALUE | SUGARS (grams) | PROTEIN (grams) | % DAILY VALUE | | | |
|---|---|---|---|---|---|---|---|---|---|---|---|---|---|---|---|---|---|---|---|---|---|
| | | | | | | | | | | | | | | | | | | VITAMIN A | VITAMIN C | CALCIUM | IRON |
| Hamburger | 106 | 270 | 90 | 10 | 15 | 3.5 | 18 | 30 | 10 | 530 | 22 | 34 | 11 | 2 | 9 | 7 | 12 | 2 | 4 | 15 | 15 |
| Cheeseburger | 120 | 320 | 130 | 14 | 22 | 6 | 30 | 45 | 14 | 770 | 32 | 35 | 12 | 2 | 9 | 7 | 15 | 6 | 4 | 15 | 15 |
| QUARTER POUNDER® | 172 | 430 | 190 | 21 | 32 | 8 | 40 | 70 | 23 | 730 | 30 | 37 | 12 | 2 | 8 | 8 | 23 | 2 | 4 | 15 | 25 |
| QUARTER POUNDER® with Cheese | 200 | 530 | 270 | 30 | 46 | 13 | 63 | 95 | 32 | 1200 | 50 | 38 | 13 | 2 | 8 | 9 | 28 | 10 | 4 | 15 | 25 |
| BIG MAC® | 215 | 530 | 250 | 28 | 43 | 10 | 49 | 80 | 26 | 880 | 37 | 47 | 16 | 3 | 13 | 8 | 25 | 6 | 4 | 20 | 25 |
| ARCH DELUXE™ | 247 | 570 | 280 | 31 | 48 | 11 | 55 | 90 | 30 | 1110 | 46 | 43 | 14 | 4 | 17 | 9 | 29 | 10 | 10 | 8 | 25 |
| ARCH DELUXE™ with Bacon | 255 | 610 | 310 | 34 | 53 | 12 | 60 | 100 | 33 | 1250 | 52 | 43 | 14 | 4 | 17 | 9 | 33 | 10 | 10 | 8 | 25 |
| CRISPY CHICKEN DELUXE™ | 232 | 530 | 230 | 26 | 40 | 4 | 20 | 60 | 19 | 1140 | 48 | 47 | 16 | 4 | 15 | 6 | 27 | 6 | 8 | 6 | 15 |
| FISH FILET DELUXE™ | 236 | 510 | 180 | 20 | 30 | 4.5 | 23 | 50 | 17 | 1120 | 46 | 59 | 20 | 5 | 18 | 6 | 24 | 6 | 4 | 8 | 15 |
| GRILLED CHICKEN DELUXE™ | 213 | 330 | 50 | 6 | 9 | 1 | 5 | 50 | 16 | 970 | 40 | 42 | 14 | 4 | 15 | 6 | 27 | 4 | 8 | 6 | 15 |
| CHICKEN McNUGGETS® (6 Piece) | 106 | 290 | 150 | 17 | 26 | 3.5 | 18 | 60 | 21 | 510 | 21 | 15 | 5 | 0 | 0 | 0 | 18 | — | — | 2 | 6 |
| Barbeque Sauce (1 pkg.) | 28 | 45 | 0 | 0 | 0 | 0 | 0 | 0 | 0 | 250 | 10 | 10 | 3 | 0 | 0 | 10 | 0 | — | 6 | — | — |
| Honey Mustard (1 pkg.) | 14 | 50 | 40 | 4.5 | 7 | 0.5 | 3 | 10 | 3 | 85 | 4 | 3 | 1 | 0 | 0 | 3 | 0 | — | — | — | — |
| Small French Fries | 68 | 210 | 90 | 10 | 15 | 1.5 | 9 | 0 | 0 | 135 | 6 | 26 | 9 | 2 | 10 | 0 | 3 | — | 15 | — | 2 |
| Large French Fries | 147 | 450 | 200 | 22 | 33 | 4 | 19 | 0 | 0 | 290 | 12 | 57 | 19 | 5 | 21 | 0 | 6 | — | 30 | 2 | 6 |
| Garden Salad | 177 | 35 | 0 | 0 | 0 | 0 | 0 | 0 | 0 | 20 | 1 | 7 | 2 | 2 | 8 | 3 | 2 | 120 | 40 | 4 | 6 |
| Grilled Chicken Salad Deluxe | 213 | 110 | 10 | 1 | 2 | 0 | 0 | 45 | 16 | 240 | 10 | 5 | 2 | 2 | 6 | 2 | 21 | 110 | 25 | 4 | 8 |
| EGG McMUFFIN® | 137 | 290 | 110 | 12 | 19 | 4.5 | 23 | 235 | 78 | 710 | 30 | 27 | 9 | 1 | 6 | 3 | 17 | 10 | 2 | 15 | 15 |
| SAUSAGE McMUFFIN® | 112 | 360 | 210 | 23 | 35 | 8 | 41 | 45 | 15 | 740 | 31 | 26 | 9 | 1 | 6 | 2 | 13 | 4 | — | 15 | 10 |
| SAUSAGE McMUFFIN® with Egg | 163 | 440 | 250 | 28 | 44 | 10 | 50 | 255 | 86 | 810 | 34 | 27 | 9 | 1 | 6 | 3 | 19 | 10 | — | 15 | 15 |
| Hot Fudge Sundae | 179 | 290 | 45 | 5 | 8 | 4.5 | 24 | 5 | 2 | 200 | 8 | 53 | 18 | 2 | 7 | 45 | 8 | 10 | 2 | 25 | 2 |
| Baked Apple Pie | 77 | 260 | 120 | 13 | 20 | 3.5 | 17 | 0 | 0 | 200 | 8 | 34 | 11 | <1 | 4 | 13 | 3 | — | 40 | 2 | 6 |
| Lowfat Chocolate Shake—Small | 414 ml | 340 | 50 | 5 | 8 | 3.5 | 17 | 25 | 8 | 270 | 11 | 62 | 21 | 1 | 4 | 56 | 12 | 4 | 4 | 40 | 4 |

## Subway®

| | SERVING SIZE (grams) | CALORIES | CALORIE % REDUCTION | CALORIES FROM FAT | TOTAL FAT (grams) | TOTAL FAT % REDUCTION | % DAILY VALUE | SATURATED FAT (grams) | % DAILY VALUE | CHOLESTEROL (milligrams) | % DAILY VALUE | SODIUM (milligrams) | % DAILY VALUE | CARBOHYDRATES (grams) | % DAILY VALUE | DIETARY FIBER (grams) | % DAILY VALUE | SUGARS (grams) | PROTEIN (grams) | PERCENT OF RDA | | | |
|---|---|---|---|---|---|---|---|---|---|---|---|---|---|---|---|---|---|---|---|---|---|---|---|
| | | | | | | | | | | | | | | | | | | | | VITAMIN A | VITAMIN C | CALCIUM | IRON |
| 6″ COLD SUBS | | | | | | | | | | | | | | | | | | | | | | | |
| Veggie Delite | 182 | 237 | | 25 | 3 | | 5 | 0 | — | 0 | — | 593 | 25 | 44 | 15 | 3 | 12 | 2 | 9 | 12 | 25 | — | 17 |
| Turkey Breast | 239 | 289 | | 36 | 4 | | 6 | 1 | 5 | 19 | 6 | 1403 | 58 | 46 | 15 | 3 | 12 | 2 | 18 | 12 | 25 | 4 | 17 |
| Ham | 239 | 302 | | 45 | 5 | | 8 | 1 | 5 | 28 | 9 | 1319 | 55 | 45 | 15 | 3 | 12 | 3 | 19 | 12 | 25 | 4 | 17 |
| Roast Beef | 239 | 303 | | 45 | 5 | | 8 | 1 | 5 | 20 | 7 | 939 | 39 | 45 | 15 | 3 | 12 | 3 | 20 | 12 | 25 | 3 | 17 |
| SUBWAY CLUB® | 253 | 312 | | 45 | 5 | | 8 | 1 | 5 | 26 | 9 | 1352 | 56 | 46 | 15 | 3 | 12 | 3 | 21 | 12 | 25 | 3 | 22 |
| B.L.T. | 198 | 327 | | 95 | 10 | | 15 | 3 | 15 | 16 | 5 | 957 | 40 | 44 | 15 | 3 | 12 | 2 | 14 | 12 | 25 | 3 | 17 |
| Cold Cut Trio | 253 | 378 | | 118 | 13 | | 20 | 4 | 20 | 64 | 21 | 1412 | 59 | 46 | 15 | 3 | 12 | 2 | 20 | 13 | 27 | 6 | 22 |
| Tuna* | 253 | 391 | 28 | 135 | 15 | 53 | 23 | 2 | 10 | 32 | 11 | 940 | 39 | 46 | 15 | 3 | 12 | 2 | 19 | 15 | 25 | 4 | 17 |
| Tuna | 253 | 542 | | 291 | 32 | | 49 | 5 | 25 | 36 | 12 | 886 | 37 | 44 | 15 | 3 | 12 | 2 | 19 | 13 | 25 | 4 | 17 |
| SUBWAY SEAFOOD & CRAB®* | 253 | 347 | 19 | 89 | 10 | 47 | 15 | 2 | 10 | 32 | 11 | 884 | 37 | 45 | 15 | 3 | 12 | 2 | 20 | 13 | 25 | 3 | 17 |
| SUBWAY SEAFOOD & CRAB® | 253 | 430 | | 174 | 19 | | 29 | 3 | 15 | 34 | 11 | 860 | 36 | 44 | 15 | 3 | 12 | 2 | 20 | 12 | 25 | 3 | 17 |
| 6″ HOT SUBS | | | | | | | | | | | | | | | | | | | | | | | |
| Roasted Chicken Breast | 253 | 348 | | 54 | 6 | | 9 | 1 | 5 | 48 | 16 | 978 | 40 | 47 | 16 | 3 | 12 | 3 | 27 | 12 | 25 | 4 | 17 |
| Steak & Cheese ▲ | 264 | 398 | | 88 | 10 | | 15 | 6 | 30 | 70 | 23 | 1117 | 47 | 47 | 16 | 3 | 12 | 4 | 30 | 18 | 30 | 10 | 28 |
| SUBWAY MELT™ ▲ | 258 | 382 | | 107 | 12 | | 18 | 5 | 25 | 42 | 14 | 1746 | 72 | 46 | 15 | 3 | 12 | 3 | 23 | 16 | 25 | 10 | 17 |
| Meatball | 267 | 419 | | 145 | 16 | | 25 | 6 | 30 | 33 | 11 | 1046 | 43 | 51 | 17 | 3 | 12 | 4 | 19 | 14 | 27 | 4 | 22 |
| CONDIMENTS & EXTRAS | | | | | | | | | | | | | | | | | | | | | | | |
| Light Mayonnaise (1 tsp.) | 5 | 18 | | 18 | 2 | | 3 | — | — | 2 | 1 | 33 | 1 | — | — | — | — | — | — | — | — | — | — |
| Bacon (2 Slices) | 8 | 45 | | 36 | 4 | | 6 | 1 | 5 | 8 | 3 | 182 | 8 | — | — | — | — | — | 2 | — | — | — | — |
| Cheese (2 Triangles) | 11 | 41 | | 27 | 3 | | 5 | 2 | 10 | 10 | 3 | 201 | 8 | — | — | — | — | — | 2 | 3 | — | 6 | — |
| Mayonnaise (1 tsp.) | 5 | 37 | | 36 | 4 | | 6 | 1 | 5 | 3 | 1 | 27 | 1 | — | — | — | — | — | — | — | — | — | — |
| Olive Oil Blend (1 tsp.) | 5 | 45 | | 45 | 5 | | | 1 | 5 | — | — | — | — | — | — | — | — | — | — | — | — | — | — |

**Values are only suggested serving sizes. Individual amounts may vary.**

***Standard Sandwiches include:*** *Wheat Bread • Meat/Poultry or Seafood • Onions • Lettuce • Tomatoes • Pickles • Green Peppers • Olives*

***Free upon request:*** *Cheese • Olive Oil Blend • Mayonnaise • Light Mayonnaise • Mustard • Vinegar • Salt • Pepper • Hot Peppers*

* Made with Light Mayonnaise.
Values do not include cheese or condiments unless indicated ▲.

## Taco Bell

| | SERVING SIZE (grams) | CALORIES | % CALORIE REDUCTION | CALORIES FROM FAT | TOTAL FAT (grams) | % FAT REDUCTION | % DAILY VALUE | SATURATED FAT (grams) | % DAILY VALUE | CHOLESTEROL (milligrams) | % DAILY VALUE | SODIUM (milligrams) | % DAILY VALUE | CARBOHYDRATES (grams) | % DAILY VALUE | DIETARY FIBER (grams) | % DAILY VALUE | SUGARS (grams) | PROTEIN (grams) | % DAILY VALUE: VITAMIN A | VITAMIN C | CALCIUM | IRON |
|---|---|---|---|---|---|---|---|---|---|---|---|---|---|---|---|---|---|---|---|---|---|---|---|
| Taco | 78 | 170 | | 90 | 10 | | 15 | 4 | 20 | 30 | 10 | 280 | 12 | 11 | 4 | 1 | 4 | 0 | 10 | 4 | 0 | 6 | 4 |
| Soft Taco | 99 | 210 | | 90 | 10 | | 15 | $4\frac{1}{2}$ | 23 | 30 | 10 | 530 | 22 | 20 | 7 | 2 | 8 | 1 | 12 | 4 | 4 | 8 | 6 |
| TACO SUPREME® | 113 | 220 | | 120 | 13 | | 20 | 6 | 30 | 45 | 15 | 290 | 12 | 13 | 4 | 2 | 8 | 2 | 11 | 6 | 6 | 8 | 6 |
| SOFT TACO SUPREME® | 135 | 260 | | 120 | 14 | | 22 | 7 | 35 | 45 | 15 | 540 | 23 | 22 | 7 | 2 | 8 | 2 | 13 | 4 | 6 | 10 | 6 |
| Bean Burrito | 198 | 380 | | 110 | 12 | | 18 | 4 | 20 | 10 | 3 | 1140 | 48 | 55 | 18 | 12 | 48 | 2 | 13 | 30 | 2 | 15 | 15 |
| BURRITO SUPREME® | 248 | 440 | | 170 | 18 | | 28 | 8 | 40 | 45 | 15 | 1220 | 51 | 50 | 17 | 8 | 32 | 3 | 19 | 30 | 8 | 15 | 10 |
| BIG BEEF BURRITO SUPREME® | 291 | 520 | | 210 | 23 | | 35 | 10 | 50 | 70 | 23 | 1450 | 60 | 52 | 17 | 9 | 36 | 3 | 26 | 30 | 8 | 15 | 15 |
| Light Chicken Burrito | 177 | 310 | 29 | 70 | 8 | 50 | 12 | 2 | 10 | 25 | 8 | 980 | 41 | 41 | 14 | 3 | 12 | 3 | 18 | 40 | 4 | 20 | 6 |
| Chicken Burrito | 177 | 400 | | 140 | 16 | | 25 | 5 | 25 | 55 | 18 | 720 | 30 | 45 | 15 | 1 | 4 | 2 | 19 | 25 | 4 | 20 | 20 |
| LIGHT CHICKEN BURRITO SUPREME® | 248 | 430 | 28 | 120 | 13 | 50 | 20 | 3 | 15 | 55 | 18 | 1410 | 59 | 52 | 17 | 3 | 12 | 4 | 25 | 35 | 10 | 15 | 8 |
| Chicken BURRITO SUPREME® | 248 | 550 | | 230 | 26 | | 40 | 9 | 45 | 95 | 32 | 730 | 30 | 50 | 17 | 1 | 4 | 2 | 30 | 25 | 15 | 20 | 20 |
| Light Chicken Soft Taco | 120 | 180 | 39 | 45 | 5 | 55 | 8 | $1\frac{1}{2}$ | 8 | 25 | 8 | 660 | 28 | 21 | 7 | 2 | 8 | 3 | 13 | 20 | 8 | 10 | 4 |
| Chicken Soft Taco | 120 | 250 | | 100 | 11 | | 17 | $3\frac{1}{2}$ | 18 | 45 | 15 | 380 | 16 | 23 | 8 | 0 | 0 | 1 | 15 | 15 | 8 | 10 | 10 |
| Taco Salad with Salsa | 539 | 840 | | 470 | 52 | | 80 | 15 | 75 | 75 | 25 | 1670 | 70 | 62 | 21 | 13 | 52 | 8 | 32 | 150 | 40 | 25 | 35 |
| Taco Salad w/Salsa without Shell | 454 | 420 | | 190 | 21 | | 32 | 11 | 55 | 75 | 25 | 1420 | 59 | 29 | 10 | 13 | 52 | 8 | 26 | 150 | 35 | 25 | 25 |
| Steak FAJITA WRAP™ | 220 | 460 | | 190 | 21 | | 32 | 6 | 30 | 35 | 12 | 1130 | 47 | 48 | 16 | 3 | 12 | 2 | 20 | 4 | 4 | 15 | 10 |
| Chicken FAJITA WRAP™ | 220 | 460 | | 190 | 21 | | 32 | 6 | 30 | 45 | 15 | 1220 | 51 | 49 | 16 | 3 | 12 | 4 | 18 | 4 | 6 | 15 | 6 |
| Veggie FAJITA WRAP™ | 220 | 420 | | 170 | 19 | | 29 | 5 | 25 | 20 | 7 | 920 | 38 | 51 | 17 | 3 | 12 | 2 | 11 | 8 | 4 | 15 | 6 |
| Steak FAJITA WRAP™ Supreme | 255 | 510 | | 230 | 25 | | 38 | 8 | 40 | 45 | 15 | 1140 | 48 | 50 | 17 | 3 | 12 | 4 | 21 | 4 | 10 | 15 | 10 |
| Chicken FAJITA WRAP™ Supreme | 255 | 500 | | 230 | 25 | | 38 | 8 | 40 | 55 | 18 | 1230 | 51 | 51 | 17 | 3 | 12 | 5 | 19 | 4 | 10 | 15 | 8 |
| Veggie FAJITA WRAP™ Supreme | 255 | 460 | | 210 | 23 | | 35 | 8 | 40 | 30 | 10 | 930 | 39 | 53 | 18 | 3 | 12 | 4 | 11 | 8 | 10 | 15 | 6 |
| Nachos | 99 | 310 | | 160 | 18 | | 28 | $3\frac{1}{2}$ | 18 | 5 | 2 | 540 | 23 | 34 | 11 | 3 | 12 | 2 | 2 | 6 | 0 | 10 | 0 |
| BIG BEEF NACHOS SUPREME | 191 | 430 | | 210 | 24 | | 37 | 7 | 35 | 40 | 13 | 720 | 30 | 43 | 14 | 9 | 36 | 3 | 12 | 4 | 6 | 10 | 10 |
| NACHOS BELLGRANDE® | 305 | 740 | | 350 | 39 | | 60 | 10 | 50 | 40 | 13 | 1200 | 50 | 83 | 28 | 17 | 68 | 4 | 16 | 6 | 6 | 20 | 15 |
| Cinnamon Twists | 28 | 140 | | 50 | 6 | | 9 | 0 | 0 | 0 | 0 | 190 | 8 | 19 | 6 | 0 | 0 | 0 | 1 | 4 | 0 | 0 | 2 |

## Wendy's

| | SERVING SIZE (grams) | CALORIES | CALORIES FROM FAT | TOTAL FAT (grams) | % DAILY VALUE | SATURATED FAT (grams) | % DAILY VALUE | CHOLESTEROL (milligrams) | % DAILY VALUE | SODIUM (milligrams) | % DAILY VALUE | TOTAL CARBOHYDRATES (grams) | % DAILY VALUE | DIETARY FIBER (grams) | % DAILY VALUE | SUGARS (grams) | PROTEIN (grams) | % DAILY VALUE | | | |
|---|---|---|---|---|---|---|---|---|---|---|---|---|---|---|---|---|---|---|---|---|---|
| | | | | | | | | | | | | | | | | | | VITAMIN A | VITAMIN C | CALCIUM | IRON |
| Plain Single | 133 | 360 | 140 | 16 | 25 | 6 | 30 | 65 | 22 | 460 | 19 | 31 | 10 | 2 | 8 | 5 | 25 | 0 | 0 | 10 | 25 |
| Single with Everything | 219 | 420 | 180 | 20 | 31 | 7 | 35 | 70 | 23 | 810 | 34 | 37 | 12 | 3 | 12 | 9 | 26 | 6 | 10 | 10 | 30 |
| Big Bacon Classic | 287 | 610 | 290 | 33 | 51 | 13 | 65 | 105 | 35 | 1510 | 63 | 45 | 15 | 3 | 12 | 11 | 36 | 15 | 25 | 25 | 35 |
| Jr. Hamburger | 117 | 270 | 90 | 10 | 15 | 3 | 15 | 30 | 10 | 560 | 23 | 34 | 11 | 2 | 8 | 7 | 15 | 2 | 2 | 10 | 20 |
| Jr. Cheeseburger | 129 | 320 | 120 | 13 | 20 | 6 | 30 | 45 | 15 | 770 | 32 | 34 | 11 | 2 | 8 | 7 | 17 | 6 | 2 | 15 | 20 |
| Jr. Bacon Cheeseburger | 170 | 410 | 190 | 21 | 32 | 8 | 40 | 60 | 20 | 910 | 38 | 34 | 11 | 2 | 8 | 7 | 22 | 8 | 15 | 15 | 20 |
| Jr. Cheeseburger Deluxe | 179 | 360 | 150 | 16 | 25 | 6 | 30 | 45 | 15 | 840 | 35 | 36 | 12 | 3 | 12 | 9 | 18 | 10 | 10 | 15 | 20 |
| Grilled Chicken Sandwich | 177 | 290 | 60 | 7 | 11 | 1.5 | 8 | 55 | 18 | 720 | 30 | 35 | 12 | 2 | 8 | 8 | 24 | 4 | 10 | 10 | 15 |
| Breaded Chicken Sandwich | 208 | 440 | 160 | 18 | 28 | 3 | 15 | 60 | 20 | 840 | 35 | 44 | 15 | 2 | 8 | 6 | 28 | 4 | 10 | 10 | 15 |
| Chicken Nuggets | | | | | | | | | | | | | | | | | | | | | |
| 6 piece | 94 | 280 | 180 | 20 | 31 | 5 | 25 | 50 | 17 | 600 | 25 | 12 | 4 | 0 | 0 | N/A | 14 | 0 | 0 | 2 | 4 |
| Barbeque Sauce | 28 | 50 | 0 | 0 | 0 | 0 | 0 | 0 | 0 | 100 | 4 | 11 | 4 | N/A | — | N/A | 1 | 6 | 0 | 0 | 4 |
| Honey | 14 | 45 | 0 | 0 | 0 | 0 | 0 | 0 | 0 | 0 | 0 | 12 | 4 | 0 | 0 | 12 | 0 | 0 | 0 | 0 | 0 |
| Sweet & Sour Sauce | 28 | 45 | 0 | 0 | 0 | 0 | 0 | 0 | 0 | 55 | 2 | 11 | 4 | N/A | — | N/A | 0 | 0 | 0 | 0 | 2 |
| Sweet Mustard Sauce | 28 | 50 | 10 | 1 | 2 | 0 | 0 | 0 | 0 | 140 | 6 | 9 | 3 | N/A | — | N/A | 1 | 0 | 0 | 0 | 0 |
| CHILI | | | | | | | | | | | | | | | | | | | | | |
| Small | 227 | 210 | 60 | 7 | 11 | 2.5 | 13 | 30 | 10 | 800 | 33 | 21 | 7 | 5 | 20 | 5 | 15 | 8 | 6 | 8 | 15 |
| Large | 340 | 310 | 90 | 10 | 15 | 4 | 20 | 45 | 15 | 1190 | 50 | 32 | 11 | 7 | 28 | 8 | 23 | 10 | 10 | 10 | 25 |
| Deluxe Garden Salad | 271 | 110 | 50 | 6 | 9 | 1 | 5 | 0 | 0 | 320 | 13 | 10 | 3 | 4 | 16 | 5 | 7 | 110 | 60 | 20 | 8 |
| Grilled Chicken Salad | 338 | 200 | 70 | 8 | 12 | 1.5 | 8 | 50 | 17 | 690 | 29 | 10 | 3 | 4 | 16 | 5 | 25 | 110 | 60 | 20 | 10 |
| Side Salad | 155 | 60 | 25 | 3 | 5 | 0.5 | 3 | 0 | 0 | 160 | 7 | 5 | 2 | 2 | 8 | 2 | 4 | 50 | 30 | 10 | 4 |
| FRENCH FRIES | | | | | | | | | | | | | | | | | | | | | |
| Small | 91 | 260 | 120 | 13 | 20 | 2.5 | 13 | 0 | 0 | 85 | 4 | 33 | 11 | 3 | 12 | 0 | 3 | 0 | 8 | 2 | 4 |
| Medium | 130 | 380 | 170 | 19 | 29 | 4 | 20 | 0 | 0 | 120 | 5 | 47 | 16 | 5 | 20 | 0 | 5 | 0 | 10 | 2 | 6 |
| Biggie | 159 | 460 | 200 | 23 | 35 | 5 | 25 | 0 | 0 | 150 | 6 | 58 | 19 | 6 | 24 | 0 | 6 | 0 | 15 | 2 | 8 |
| BAKED POTATO | | | | | | | | | | | | | | | | | | | | | |
| Plain | 284 | 310 | 0 | 0 | 0 | 0 | 0 | 0 | 0 | 25 | 1 | 71 | 24 | 7 | 28 | 5 | 7 | 0 | 60 | 2 | 20 |
| Bacon & Cheese | 380 | 540 | 160 | 18 | 28 | 4 | 20 | 20 | 7 | 1430 | 60 | 78 | 26 | 7 | 28 | 5 | 17 | 10 | 60 | 20 | 25 |
| Broccoli & Cheese | 411 | 470 | 120 | 14 | 22 | 3 | 15 | 5 | 2 | 470 | 20 | 80 | 27 | 9 | 36 | 6 | 9 | 35 | 120 | 20 | 25 |
| Cheese | 383 | 570 | 210 | 23 | 35 | 9 | 45 | 30 | 10 | 640 | 27 | 78 | 26 | 7 | 28 | 5 | 14 | 15 | 60 | 40 | 25 |
| Chili & Cheese | 439 | 620 | 220 | 24 | 37 | 9 | 45 | 40 | 13 | 780 | 33 | 83 | 28 | 9 | 36 | 7 | 20 | 20 | 60 | 35 | 30 |
| Sour Cream & Chives | 314 | 380 | 60 | 6 | 9 | 4 | 20 | 15 | 5 | 40 | 2 | 74 | 25 | 8 | 32 | 6 | 8 | 30 | 80 | 8 | 25 |
| FROSTY™ Dairy Dessert, Small | 243 | 340 | 90 | 10 | 15 | 5 | 25 | 40 | 13 | 200 | 8 | 57 | 19 | 3 | 12 | 47 | 9 | 8 | 0 | 30 | 6 |
| Medium | 324 | 460 | 120 | 13 | 20 | 7 | 35 | 55 | 18 | 260 | 11 | 76 | 25 | 4 | 16 | 63 | 12 | 10 | 0 | 40 | 6 |

## High-Fiber Foods

| Food | Dietary fiber (grams) |
|---|---|
| **Fruits** | |
| Apple with skin, 1 medium | 3 |
| Banana, 1 medium | 2 |
| Strawberries, 1 cup | 3 |
| Pear with skin, $\frac{1}{2}$ large | 3 |
| Prunes, 3 | 3 |
| Raisins, $\frac{1}{4}$ cup | 3 |
| Raspberries, $\frac{1}{2}$ cup | 3 |
| Blueberries, $\frac{1}{2}$ cup | 2 |
| Orange, 1 medium | 2 |
| **Breads** | |
| Whole-wheat, rye, or pumpernickel, 1 slice | 1 to 2 |
| Muffins (bran, oat, corn), 1 | 1 to 2 |
| Triscuits or Rye Krisp, 3 | 3 |
| Whole-wheat English muffin, 1 | 2 to 4 |
| Corn tortillas, 1 small | 1 to 2 |
| Whole-wheat bagel, 1 small | 1 to 2 |
| **Grains** | |
| Brown rice, $\frac{1}{2}$ cup | 2 |
| Wild rice, $\frac{1}{2}$ cup | 4 |
| Barley, whole grain, $\frac{1}{2}$ cup | 2 |
| Whole-wheat pasta, $\frac{1}{2}$ cup | 2 |
| Bulgur, $\frac{1}{3}$ cup | 2 |
| **Legumes** | |
| Cooked dried beans (kidney, pinto, black northern, navy), $\frac{1}{2}$ cup | 6 |
| Cooked dried peas, $\frac{1}{2}$ cup | 4 |
| Cooked lentils, $\frac{1}{2}$ cup | 4 |
| Cooked lima beans, $\frac{1}{2}$ cup | 4 |
| **Vegetables** | |
| Canned corn, $\frac{1}{2}$ cup | 3 |
| Broccoli, brussels sprouts, carrots, parsnip, spinach, $\frac{1}{2}$ cup | 2 |
| Potato with skin, 1 medium | 2 |

*Note:* Dietary fiber is found only in foods of plant origin. Since the outer layer is high in fiber, leave the skin on your fruits and vegetables. Also look for breakfast cereals that are high in fiber, such as all-bran cereals.

## Lean Cuts of Meat

| | |
|---|---|
| Beef | Roasts/steaks: Round, loin, sirloin, chuck |
| Pork | Roasts/chops: tenderloin, center loin, ham |
| Veal | All cuts except ground |
| Lamb | Roasts/chops: Leg, loin, foreshanks |
| Chicken and turkey | Light and dark meat, without the skin |
| Fish and shellfish | Most are low in fat; those marinated or canned in oil are higher |

## Added Sugar in Common Foods

| Food groups | Added sugars (teaspoons) |
|---|---|
| **Bread, cereal, rice, and pasta** | |
| Bread, 1 slice | 0 |
| Muffin, 1 medium | 1 |
| Cookies, 2 medium | 1 |
| Danish pastry, 1 medium | 1 |
| Doughnut, 1 medium | 2 |
| Ready-to-eat cereal, sweetened, 1 ounce | * |
| Pound cake, fat-free, 1 ounce | 2 |
| Angel food cake, $\frac{1}{12}$ tube cake | 5 |
| Cake, frosted, $\frac{1}{16}$ average | 6 |
| Pie, fruit, 2 crust, $\frac{1}{6}$ 8-inch pie | 6 |
| **Fruit** | |
| Fruit, canned in juice, $\frac{1}{2}$ cup | 0 |
| Fruit, canned in light syrup, $\frac{1}{2}$ cup | 2 |
| Fruit, canned in heavy syrup, $\frac{1}{2}$ cup | 4 |
| **Milk, yogurt, and cheese** | |
| Milk, plain, 1 cup | 0 |
| Chocolate milk, 2%, 1 cup | 3 |
| Lowfat yogurt, plain, 8 ounce | 0 |
| Lowfat yogurt, fruit, 8 ounce | 5 |
| Ice cream, ice milk, or frozen yogurt ($\frac{1}{2}$ cup) | 7 |
| Chocolate shake, 10 fl. ounce | 3 |
| **Other** | |
| Sugar, jam, or jelly, 1 teaspoon | 1 |
| Syrup or honey, 1 tablespoon | 3 |
| Chocolate bar, 1 ounce | 3 |
| Fruit sorbet, $\frac{1}{2}$ cup | 3 |
| Gelatin dessert, $\frac{1}{2}$ cup | 4 |
| Sherbet, $\frac{1}{2}$ cup | 5 |
| Cola, 12 fl. ounce | 9 |
| Fruit drink, 12 fl. ounce | 12 |

*Note:* Four grams of sugar = 1 teaspoon.

### Cholesterol Content of Some Common Foods

|  |  |
|---|---|
| Liver (3 ounces) | 331 milligrams |
| Egg (1 yolk) | 213 milligrams |
| Beef or chicken (3 ounces, cooked) | 76 milligrams |
| Whole milk (1 cup) | 33 milligrams |
| Skim milk (1 cup) | 4 milligrams |

### Dietary Sources of Common Antioxidant Nutrients

| Nutrient | Sources |
|---|---|
| Vitamin C | Citrus fruits, broccoli, tomatoes, green peppers, potatoes |
| Vitamin E | Wheat germ, whole grains, oatmeal, peanuts, brown rice, vegetable oils |
| Beta-carotene | Carrots, broccoli, sweet potatoes, spinach, squash, peaches, cantaloupe |

# Appendix D Emergency First Aid

Throughout this text, we have stressed the importance of seeking qualified health professionals to deal with health problems and emergencies. Most readers will not fall into that category. Nevertheless, people become ill or have accidents when health professionals are not nearby. If you are present at such a time, you should think about getting the person to a health professional as soon as possible. But *sometimes, as soon as possible is not soon enough.* In such cases, it may be necessary, even life-saving, to practice first aid.

This appendix lists a number of kinds of health emergencies which may require first aid. In each case, there is a list of signs or symptoms that will help you determine what the problem is. Then there are specific instructions as to what you can do.

## BREATHING EMERGENCIES

### 1. *If the person is not breathing and is unconscious:*

#### Signs

The person's chest doesn't rise and fall.

You cannot hear or feel the person breathing.

The person's skin appears to be pale or has a bluish tint.

#### What to Do

Send someone to call for an ambulance (dial 911 or your local emergency operator).

Tilt the person's head back and lift his or her chin.

Check for breathing in this position for about 5 seconds.

### 1A. *If the person is* not *breathing and has* no *pulse:*

Pinch the person's nose shut, open your mouth, and make a seal around the person's mouth with your own. (For an infant or small child, cover both his or her mouth and nose with your mouth.)

Provide two slow breaths, making sure that the person's chest gently rises.

Feel for a pulse along the groove beside the windpipe in the neck for 5 to 10 seconds.

### 1B. *If the person is not breathing but* has *a pulse:*

Provide "rescue" breaths:

In the case of an adult, give one breath every 5 seconds.

In the case of an infant or child, give one breath every 3 seconds.

Continue to give rescue breaths as long as the person has a pulse, even if he or she is not breathing. If the person vomits, turn him or her on the side, wipe the mouth clean, and continue with rescue breathing.

### 2. *In case of drowning (if the person is not breathing and has been underwater—drowning can occur in the home as well as in a pool or at the beach):*

#### What to Do

Send someone to call for an ambulance (dial 911 or your local emergency operator).

Tilt the person's head back and lift his or her chin.

Check for breathing in this position for about 5 seconds.

If the airway seems to be clear, give two slow breaths.

If the breaths do not go in, tilt the head again and try to give the breaths again.

If the breaths still do not go in, try the Heimlich maneuver (abdominal thrusts) several times. Then lift the jaw and the tongue and sweep any objects out of the mouth. Repeat the breaths and the abdominal thrusts until the breaths go in or until the person breathes on his or her own.

## BURNS

There are different degrees of burns. First aid for each is similar, but more serious burns also require medical attention.

#### Kinds of Burns

| | |
|---|---|
| First degree: | Skin is red (medical help optional) |
| Second degree: | Skin is blistered (medical help optional) |
| Third degree: | Skin is charred (medical help required) |

#### What to Do

If necessary, send someone to call for an ambulance. In the case of fire, have someone call the fire department (dial 911 or your local emergency operator).

If the person is on fire, try to put it out and remove any burning clothing.

Next, cool down the burn. Use cool or cold water. It is preferable not to use ice except on small surface burns. If an area cannot be dunked in water, you can apply wet towels, cloths, or sheets. Keep fabrics cool by repeatedly spraying them or dunking them in water.

Loosely cover the burn to prevent infection. Use sterile dressings or a clean cloth. Do *not* use plastic, especially on the face.

#### For Sunburn

Cool down the burn.

Prevent additional damage by using a sunscreen or staying out of the sun.

Protect unbroken blisters with loose bandages.

Prevent infection by keeping broken blisters clean. When in doubt, seek medical advice.

## CARDIAC EMERGENCIES (CHEST PAIN AND CARDIAC ARREST)

The two main kinds of cardiac (heart) emergencies are a heart attack and cessation (stoppage) of beating. A heart attack is mainly symptomized by chest pain and shortness of breath. When the heart stops beating, people lose consciousness. Chest pain may also have other causes, but it is wise to follow the first-aid procedures described here.

#### Signs of Chest Pain

Pain or pressure in the chest. It may vary from discomfort to intense, crushing pain that is not relieved by changing position, resting, or pain medication. The pain may spread to the jaw, upper abdomen, or down the left shoulder and arm.

The person may have trouble breathing. The person may feel extreme shortness of breath, and breathing may be faster than usual.

The pulse may be irregular, or faster or slower than normal.

The person may sweat more than usual, leaving the skin moist. The skin may be pale or bluish in appearance from oxygen deprivation.

#### What to Do for Chest Pain

Send someone to call for an ambulance (dial 911 or your local emergency operator).

Have the person discontinue activity and rest. Loosen restrictive clothing. Help the person find a comfortable position (sitting may make breathing easier).

Ask if the person has prescribed medication (such as nitroglycerine). If so, help him or her get it and take it.

Pay close attention to the person's breathing and pulse.

### Signs of Cardiac Arrest (Heart Stoppage)

Loss of consciousness

Lack of response to talking and prodding

Lack of breathing and pulse

### What to Do for Cardiac Arrest

Send someone to call for an ambulance (dial 911 or your local emergency operator).

Check to see if the person is breathing.

**1.** ***If the person is not breathing:***

Tilt his or her head back, pinch his or her nose, and give two slow breaths. The breaths should make the chest rise gently.

Feel for a pulse along the groove beside the windpipe in the neck.

**2.** ***If there is no pulse, try the following:***

a

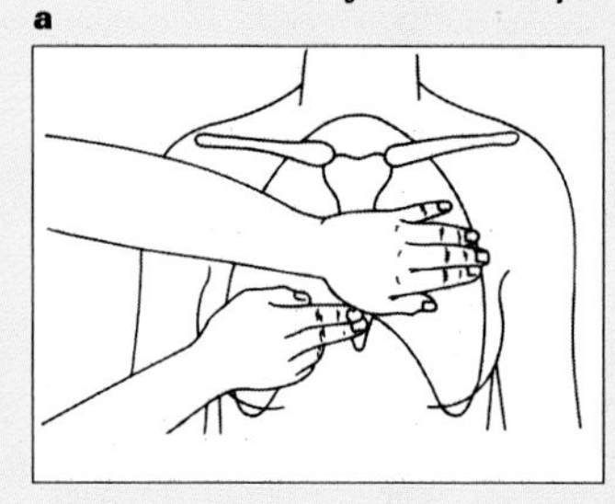

**a.** Position your hand over the breastbone in the center of the chest.

**b.** Position your shoulders over your hands (so that your weight is on your hands) and compress (press down on) the chest about 15 times in 10 seconds.

b

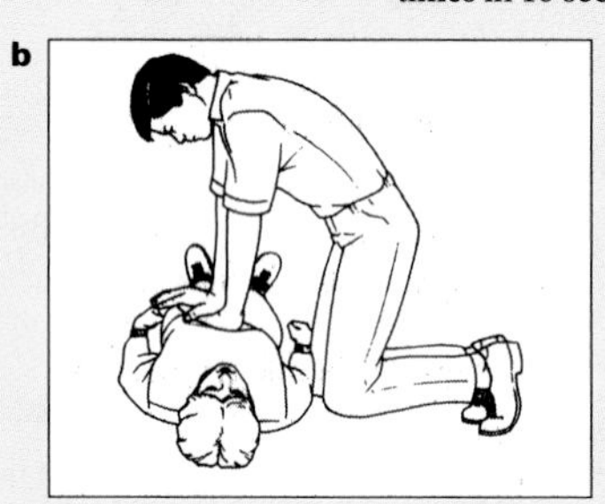

c

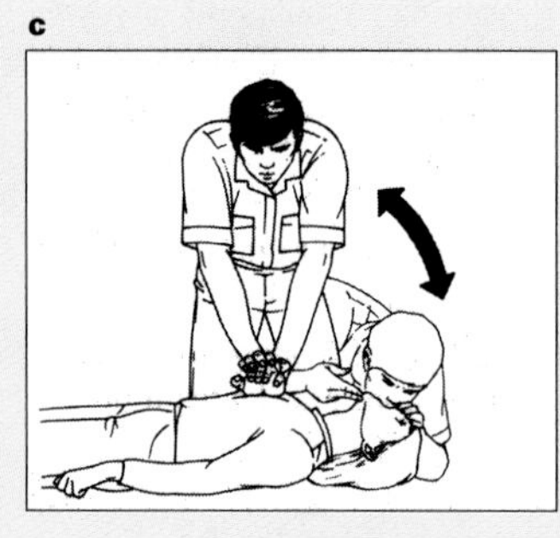

**c.** Give two slow breaths.

Repeat the procedure three times (that is, three sets of 15 compressions followed by two breaths).

To learn more about cardiopulmonary resuscitation (CPR), contact your local health department or hospital center for information about classes in your area.

## CHOKING

### Signs

Clutching the throat with the hands.

Inability to speak, breathe, or cough with any force.

High-pitched wheezing.

### What to Do

Send someone to call for an ambulance (dial 911 or your local emergency operator).

Use the Heimlich maneuver. That is, stand behind the person. Place the thumb side of one fist against the center of the person's abdomen, just above the navel. Grasp your fist with your other hand. Now give quick, repeated upward thrusts.

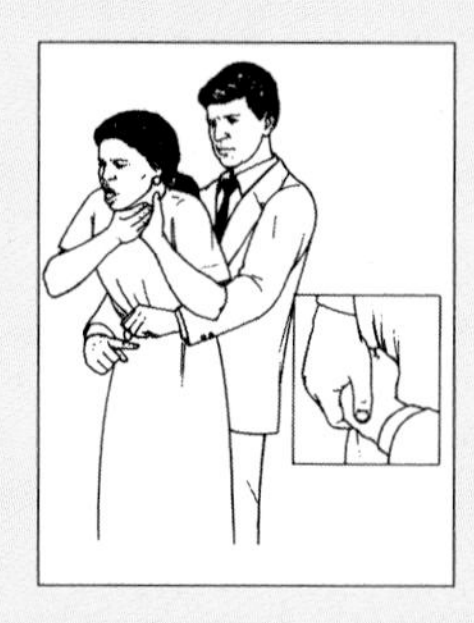

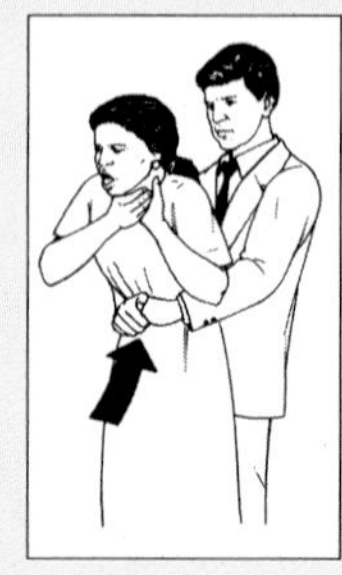

Repeat Heimlich maneuver until the object (usually poorly chewed food or, in the case of a child, a toy) is coughed up and the person breathes on his or her own.

If the person loses consciousness, check the mouth for food or any object and try to sweep it out. Use the Heimlich maneuver as best you can.

## FROSTBITE

### Signs

Lack of feeling in the area (fingers, toes, cheek, etc.)

Skin looks waxy or discolored—white, gray, yellow, or blue)

Skin is cold to the touch

### What to Do

Send someone to call for an ambulance (dial 911 or your local emergency operator).

Gently warm the area, preferably by soaking it in warm (not hot!) water of about 100 to 105°F until it looks reddened, feels warm, and feeling returns.

To help prevent infection, loosely bandage the area with a dry, sterile dressing.

In addition, handle the area gently. Avoid rubbing. Keep frostbitten fingers or toes separated with dry, sterile gauze (but do not attempt to pry fingers or toes apart). Do not break blisters.

## INJURIES TO MUSCLES, BONES, AND JOINTS

These kinds of injuries include bruises, sprains, strains, dislocations, and fractures (breaks of bones). They can be difficult to tell apart (even for a health professional), but first aid for all of them is the same.

### Signs

Pain

Swelling and bruising

### What to Do

Rest the injured limb or part. Immobilize it, if necessary.

Avoid movements or activities that cause pain.

Apply ice or a cold pack to the injured area to reduce swelling and pain. Place the ice in a cloth or towel to prevent direct contact with the skin.

Send someone to call for an ambulance (dial 911 or your local emergency operator) if serious injury is suspected or the injured person cannot move. Other reasons for calling an ambulance: There is a deformity; it feels or sounds as if the bones are rubbing together; a "snapping" or "popping" sound was heard when the injury occurred; there is an open wound around the injury; the injured area is numb; the injury involves the head, neck, or back; or the person has trouble breathing.

## POISONING

Poisons are substances that cause illness or injury if they enter the body. Poisons can get into the body by means of swallowing them, breathing them in, touching them, or injecting them.

### Signs

Trouble breathing (e.g., shallow, rapid breathing)

Nausea, vomiting, diarrhea

Pain in the chest or abdomen

Sweating

Seizures

Burns on the lips, tongue, or skin

*Note:* Some people with intense allergic reactions may look as though they have been poisoned. However, people with allergic reactions also often have tightness in the chest; swelling of the face, neck, and tongue; or rashes or hives.

In the case of poisoning, there may also be signs in the environment. For example, if someone is lying on the floor and having seizures, a spilled container or open medicine cabinet suggests that one should think of the possibility of poisoning. Unusual odors, smoke, and overturned or damaged plants are also suggestions that poisoning may have occurred.

### What to Do

Look around the scene of the problem for clues as to what substance may be responsible for the poisoning.

When in doubt, call for an ambulance (dial 911 or your local emergency operator) and call your local Poison Control Center (PCC). You will usually find the phone number of a nearby PCC inside the front cover of your telephone directory.

Do *not* give the poisoned person anything to eat or drink unless you are told to do so by a medical professional or a staff member of a Poison Control Center.

And . . .

Write the telephone number of your Poison Control Center here, and dog-ear the page:

Poison Control Center: ____________

# Glossary

## A

**ABCDE model** Levinger's view describes five stages of romantic relationships: attraction, building, continuation, deterioration, and ending.

**Abortion** Termination of a pregnancy before the fetus achieves viability outside the womb.

**Abstinence syndrome** A cluster of withdrawal symptoms that is characteristic of abrupt cessation of use of a particular drug.

**Acculturated** The state of adapting to a host culture.

**Acculturation** The process by which immigrant or native peoples adapt to the host or mainstream culture.

**Acetylcholine (ACh)** A neurotransmitter involved in the process of muscle contraction.

**Acid rain** Damaging precipitation formed when pollutants such as sulfur dioxide and nitrogen oxide combine with water in the atmosphere.

**Acquaintance rape** Rape committed by an acquaintance of the victim.

**Acquired immunity** Immunity produced when the body makes its own antibodies against infectious agents; may be acquired naturally by contracting an infection or by vaccination.

**Acquired immunodeficiency syndrome (AIDS)** A condition caused by the human immunodeficiency virus (HIV); characterized by destruction of the immune system, leaving the body vulnerable to various "opportunistic" diseases.

**Acrophobia** Fear of heights.

**Active euthanasia** Intentional administration of lethal drugs or other means of producing a painless death in a person with an incurable and painful disease or condition.

**Active immunity** Immunity acquired through developing antibodies by contracting an infection or in response to vaccination.

**Actual risk** The amount of risk posed by a factor or factors as based on scientific evidence.

**Acupuncture** A traditional technique of Chinese medicine believed to release natural healing energies. Thin needles are inserted and rotated at specific points along the body.

**Acute infection** Infection in which pathogens cause an immediate set of symptoms; usually short-term.

**Adipose tissue** The body tissue in which fat is stored.

**Adjustment disorder** A mild psychological disorder characterized by a maladaptive reaction to a stressful event or experience.

**Adrenal cortex** The outer part of the adrenal glands, which produces corticosteroids.

**Adrenal glands** Endocrine glands that lie just above the kidneys and produce various stress hormones.

**Adrenal medulla** The inner part of the adrenal glands; produces adrenaline and noradrenaline.

**Adrenaline** Also called epinephrine. A hormone produced by the adrenal medulla; accelerates heart and respiration rate and leads to the release of energy reserves.

**Adrenocorticotrophic hormone (ACTH)** A hormone produced by the pituitary gland; activates the adrenal cortex to secrete corticosteroids.

**Aerobic exercise** Physical activity requiring sustained elevation in oxygen utilization.

**Aflatoxin** A naturally occurring chemical produced by molds; in high doses, acts as a potent carcinogen.

**Afterburner effect** Increased rate of metabolization of fat after exercise stops.

**Age of viability** The age at which a fetus can sustain independent life.

**Ageism** Attitudes of prejudice and discrimination toward older persons.

**Aging** The progressive changes and declines in functioning that begin after sexual maturation and continue until death.

**Agoraphobia** A phobia characterized by fear of public places.

**Alarm reaction** The body's initial response to stress; activation of the sympathetic nervous system and release of stress hormones.

**Alcohol** An intoxicating liquid that contains ethyl alcohol; other forms of alcohol include methyl (wood) alcohol and rubbing alcohol.

**Alcohol abuse** A pattern of misuse of alcohol in which heavy or continued drinking becomes associated with health problems and/or impaired social functioning.

**Alcohol dependence** An addiction to alcohol. Characterized by a loss of control over alcohol use, physiological dependence, and a withdrawal syndrome following abrupt cessation of drinking. Also called *alcoholism*.

**Alcoholic cardiomyopathy** A potentially fatal condition involving the deterioration of the heart muscle due to heavy alcohol consumption.

**Alcoholic hepatitis** An inflammation of the liver caused by chronic alcoholism.

**Allergens** Commonly occurring, normally harmless antigens that trigger an allergic reaction.

**Allergic contact dermatitis** An allergic skin response produced on contact with a chemical substance to which a person is sensitive.

**Allergic rhinitis** (hay fever) A common allergy caused when airborne allergen particles (pollen, dust, mold, animal dander, etc.) enter the noses and throats of allergic persons.

**Allergy** A hypersensitivity disorder of the immune system; ordinarily harmless substances cause an allergic response in sensitive people.

**Allied health professionals** Individuals trained in one of the allied health fields, such as optometry, dentistry, occupational therapy, podiatry, and psychology.

**Alpha waves** A brain wave pattern associated with states of relaxation.

**Alveoli** The air cells of the lungs where gases are exchanged during respiration.

**Alzheimer's disease (AD)** An irreversible brain disease involving gradual loss of mental abilities, especially memory, as well as personality changes.

**Amenorrhea** The absence of menstruation.

**Amino acids** Organic compounds from which proteins are made.

**Amniocentesis** A procedure for drawing off and examining fetal cells in the amniotic fluid to determine the presence of various disorders in the fetus.

**Amniotic fluid** Fluid within the amniotic sac that suspends and protects the fetus.

**Amniotic sac** The sac containing the fetus.

**Amphetamine psychosis** An acute psychotic reaction induced by the ingestion of amphetamines that mimics acute episodes of paranoid schizophrenia.

**Amphetamines** A class of synthetic stimulants.

**Anabolic steroids** Synthetic versions of the male sex hormone testosterone.

**Anaerobic exercise** Short bursts of intense muscle activity not requiring sustained elevation in oxygen utilization.

**Anal intercourse** A sexual practice involving insertion of the penis into the rectum of either a male or female partner.

**Analgesic drugs** Drugs that relieve pain, such as aspirin and ibuprofen.

**Anaphylaxis** A severe allergic reaction; treated with injections of adrenaline.

**Androgens** Male sex hormones.

**Anemia** A condition involving a lack of hemoglobin in the blood, causing such symptoms as weakness, paleness, heart palpitations, shortness of breath, and lack of vigor.

**Anencephaly** A fatal congenital defect in which a child is born without a brain or with only a rudimentary brain.

**Aneurysm** A ballooning out of an artery wall.

**Anger rape** A vicious rape motivated by anger and resentment toward women.

**Angina** Heart pain arising from insufficient blood flow to the heart.

**Anilingus** Oral–anal sexual stimulation.

**Anorexia nervosa** An eating disorder characterized by the maintenance of an unhealthily low body weight, an intense fear of gaining weight, a distorted body image, and, in females, an absence of menstruation.

**Antagonists** Drugs that block or neutralize the actions of other drugs.

**Anti-inflammatories** Drugs that combat inflammation.

**Antibiotics** Drugs that inhibit the growth of bacterial organisms.

**Antibody** A specialized type of protein produced by white blood cells; attaches itself to invading microbes and other foreign bodies, inactivates them, and marks them for destruction.

**Antibody-mediated immunity** Antibodies, along with other white cells, disarm and dispose of antigens.

**Antidepressants** Drugs that combat depression by altering the availability of neurotransmitters in the brain.

**Antigen** Substance recognized by the immune system as foreign; induces the production of antibodies.

**Antihistamine** A drug that blocks the actions of histamine, a substance released in the body during an allergic reaction.

**Antimicrobial drugs** Drugs targeted against pathogens; include antibiotics, antivirals, antifungals, antihelminthics, and antiprotozoals.

**Antioxidants** Agents believed to contribute to health by reducing the buildup of free radicals in the body.

**Antisocial personality disorder** A personality disturbance characterized by disregard of social norms and conventions, impulsivity, callousness, and failure to live up to interpersonal and vocational commitments.

**Anxiety** An emotional state characterized by heightened arousal, feelings of nervousness or tension, and a sense of apprehension or foreboding about the future.

**Anxiety disorders** Psychological disorders involving excessive or inappropriate anxiety reactions.

**Aorta** The main artery in the body; carries oxygen-rich blood from the left ventricle to smaller blood vessels for delivery throughout the body.

**Aquifers** Geological formations that hold water.

**Areola** The dark ring on the breast that encircles the nipple.

**Arrhythmia** An irregular heart rhythm.

**Arsenic** A naturally occurring, metal-like toxin commonly found in minute amounts in various foods.

**Arteries** Vessels that carry blood from the heart and that connect to capillaries.

**Arteriosclerosis** ("hardening of the arteries") A condition in which the walls of arteries become thicker and harder and lose elasticity.

**Arthritis** Inflammation of a joint, typically accompanied by pain, stiffness, and swelling.

**Artificial insemination** Introduction of sperm into a woman's reproductive tract through means other than sexual intercourse.

**Artificial pacemaker** A small device that transmits electrical impulses to the heart to maintain a normal heartbeat.

**Artificially acquired active immunity (AAAI)** Immunity that develops after an artificial, or intentional, exposure to antigens contained in vaccines or toxoids.

**Asbestos** A mineral previously used for insulation and fireproofing; can cause lung cancer and other respiratory illnesses.

**Assertiveness training** A behavior therapy program aimed at helping inhibited or unassertive people learn to express their feelings and stand up for their rights.

**Asthma** Chronic, noninfectious lung disease characterized by a temporary obstruction and spasms of the bronchial airways or bronchi.

**Asymptomatic** Without symptoms.

**Atherosclerosis** A form of arteriosclerosis characterized by the thickening of artery walls and narrowing of the arterial passageways due to the buildup of fatty deposits or plaque.

**Atrial fibrillation** Too-rapid contractions of the atria; disrupts the coordination of the ventricles.

**Atrial flutter** Overly rapid atrial contractions, but at a somewhat slower and more regular rate than is the case in atrial fibrillation.

**Atrium** The upper chamber in each half of the heart.

**Autoimmune disorders** "Self-against-self" diseases in which the immune system mistakenly attacks the body's own cells.

**Autoimmune response** The production of antibodies that attack naturally occurring substances in the body that are (incorrectly) recognized as being foreign or harmful.

**Autonomic nervous system (ANS)** The part of the peripheral nervous system that "automatically" controls processes such as heart rate, respiration, and endocrine functioning.

**Autonomy** Self-direction or independence.

**Autopsy** The surgical examination and dissection of a dead body to ascertain the cause and circumstances of death.

**Axon** The thin, tubelike part of the neuron along which the nervous impulse travels for transmission to the adjoining neuron.

## B

**B-Cells** Immune cells that produce antibodies.

**Bacteria** Microscopic, single-celled organisms that live in air, soil, food, plants, animals, and humans.

**Bacterial vaginosis (BV)** Vaginitis usually caused by the *Gardnerella vaginalis* bacterium.

**Ballistic stretching** Stretching that involves repetitive bouncing motions.

**Barbiturates** A class of depressant drugs with sedating or calming effects.

**Barium enema** An enema administers radioactive barium to facilitate X-rays of the lower intestinal tract.

**Basal body temperature (BBT) method** A fertility awareness method of contraception that relies on prediction of ovulation by tracking a woman's temperature during the menstrual cycle.

**Basal cell carcinoma (BSC)** A form of nonmelanoma skin cancer; easily curable if treated early.

**Basal metabolic rate (BMR)** The minimum amount of energy needed to maintain bodily functions, apart from digestion.

**Behavior modification** Psychological interventions that apply learning principles to help people change their behavior.

**Behavior therapy** A therapy based on the systematic application of learning techniques to help people change problem behaviors.

**Benign** Noncancerous.

**Benzodiazepines** A class of minor tranquilizers, including such drugs as Valium, Librium, and Halcion.

**Bereavement** The state of deprivation brought about by the loss of a close friend or loved one.

**Beriberi** A deficiency disorder caused by a lack of the vitamin thiamine. Characterized by difficulties with memory and concentration, fatigue, lethargy, insomnia, loss of appetite, and irritability.

**Beta-carotene** A type of carotenoid from which the body manufactures vitamin A, found in rich supply in carrots, sweet potatoes, and spinach.

**Bioaccumulation** The process by which toxins accumulate in the bodies of animals.

**Biodegradation** The process of natural decay and absorption into the environment.

**Bioelectrical impedance analysis** A method of measuring body fat by analyzing the changes in electrical conductance (impedance) as a mild electric current is passed through the body.

**Biofeedback** A device that provides information about the user's internal bodily states.

**Biofeedback training (BFT)** The use of physiological monitoring equipment to help people develop the ability to gain some control over internal functions.

**Biomarkers** Physiological measures of aging, such as aerobic capacity and muscle strength.

**Bipolar disorder** A mood disorder characterized by mood swings between severe depression and mania.

**Bisexuals** People who are erotically attracted to, and have interest in developing romantic relationships with, both men and women.

**Blackouts** An episode involving a loss of consciousness.

**Blood** The circulatory system fluid that carries nutrients and oxygen to cells as well as substances such as hormones and antibodies; also removes waste products and carbon dioxide.

**Blood alcohol level (BAL)** The amount of alcohol in the bloodstream, as measured in percent.

**Blood plasma** The liquid part of the blood.

**Board-certified** A physician who has met the criteria required for certification in a medical specialty area by a recognized medical specialty board.

**Body mass index (BMI)** A measure of obesity that takes into account both weight and height. It is calculated by dividing body weight (in kilograms) by the square of the person's height (in meters).

**Bone marrow** Soft material within bones.

**Bones** Living tissues that support and move the body; consist of a matrix of the protein collagen and the mineral calcium.

**Bradycardia** An abnormally slow heart rate.

**Brain death** Complete cessation of brain activity as evidenced by an absence of brain wave activity.

**Braxton-Hicks contractions** So-called false labor contractions, these are relatively painless.

**Breast self-examination** A self-administered breast exam in which the woman feels for lumps or abnormalities.

**Breech presentation** Emergence of the baby feet first from the uterus.

**Bronchi** The tubes leading from the windpipe to the interior of the lungs.

**Bronchial tubes** The passageways through which air travels from the windpipe to the lungs.

**Bronchitis** An inflammation of the bronchial tubes; characterized by excess mucus production, a phlegmy cough, fever, and impaired breathing.

**Bronchodilators** Drugs that dilate (open) clogged airways and ease shortness of breath.

**Bulimia nervosa** An eating disorder characterized by repeated episodes of binge eating followed by purging and by persistent fears of gaining weight.

**Burnout** Physical and mental fatigue or exhaustion caused by excessive work-related stress.

**Caesarean section** A method of childbirth in which the fetus is delivered through a surgical incision in the abdomen.

**Caffeine** A mild stimulant found in coffee, tea, colas, and chocolate.

**Calcium** A mineral essential to the growth and maintenance of bones.

**Calendar method** A fertility awareness (rhythm) method of contraception that relies on prediction of ovulation by tracking menstrual cycles.

**Calorie** A measure of food energy, which is equivalent to the amount of energy required to raise the temperature of 1 gram of water by 1 degree Celsius.

**Cancer** Diseases characterized by the development of malignant tumors, which may invade surrounding tissues and spread to other sites in the body.

**Candidiasis** Vaginitis caused by a yeastlike fungus, *Candida albicans*.

**Capillaries** Tiny vessels that carry blood from the smallest arteries directly to cells.

**Capitated** A fixed amount paid per individual in the health plan, regardless of medical services used.

**Carbohydrates** Organic compounds forming the structural parts of plants that are important sources of nutrition for animals and humans.

**Carbon monoxide** An odorless, poisonous flammable gas produced from the burning of carbon with insufficient air.

**Carcinogenesis** The process by which cancer arises and develops.

**Carcinogenic** Cancer-causing.

**Carcinogens** Cancer-causing substances.

**Carcinoma** Cancer originating in the epithelial tissues of the body.

**Cardiac arrest** A condition in which the heart stops beating; results shortly in death.

**Cardiac output** The amount of blood the heart pumps per minute.

**Cardiomyopathy** A disease of the heart muscle or myocardium.

**Cardiopulmonary resuscitation (CPR)** Emergency medical treatment used to restore coronary and pulmonary functioning following cardiac arrest.

**Cardiorespiratory endurance** The ability of the cardiorespiratory system to deliver oxygen to working muscles at a rate sufficient to sustain vigorous activity over an extended period.

**Cardiorespiratory system** The system of heart, lungs, arteries, capillaries, and veins that circulates blood through the body and delivers oxygen to all body tissue, including muscle.

**Cardiovascular disease (CVD)** A disease of the heart or blood vessels.

**Carotenoids** Types of plant pigments (beta-carotene is one) that may have disease-preventive benefits.

**Carrying capacity** The maximum number of organisms that can be supported without degrading the environment.

**Cartilage** A flexible, tough type of connective tissue that often covers the end of bones and acts as a "lining" for the joints.

**Cataracts** A clouding of the eyes, which reduces vision; a common result of aging.

**Celibacy** Abstinence from sexual activity.

**Cell senescence** A condition in which cells stop dividing and become dormant; eventually leads to cell death.

**Cell-mediated immunity** White blood cells destroy antigens without the aid of antibodies.

**Cellular death** Complete death of cellular tissue resulting from the stoppage of blood flow.

**Central nervous system** One of the two major parts of the nervous system; consists of the brain and spinal cord.

**Cephalic presentation** Emergence of the baby head first from the uterus.

**Cephalocaudal** From the head downward.

**Cerebral hemorrhage** Rupture of a blood vessel in the brain.

**Cerebral palsy** A muscular disorder characterized by spastic paralysis; caused by damage to the central nervous system usually occurring prior to or during birth.

**Cervicitis** Inflammation of the cervix.

**Cervix** The lower end of the uterus.

**Chancre** A sore or ulcer.

**Chancroid** An STD caused by the *Hemophilus ducreyi* bacterium. Also called soft chancre.

**Chattel** A movable piece of personal property, such as furniture or livestock.

**Chemotherapy** The use of drugs to combat disease; the use of anticancer drugs to treat malignancies.

**Chewing tobacco** Tobacco leaves that have been prepared for chewing or sucking when lodged between the cheek and gum.

**Chiropractic** A system of health care based on the premise that spinal misalignments play a significant role in many physical problems.

**Chlamydia** Bacteria that cause infections of the eyes and urogenital tract.

**Chlorofluorocarbons (CFCs)** Chemicals composed of carbon, chlorine, and fluorine; used as coolants, aerosol propellants, solvents, and in Styrofoam. Involved in the depletion of the ozone layer.

**Cholera** An infection of the small intestine that produces diarrhea and vomiting; can lead to life-threatening loss of fluids and electrolytes.

**Cholesterol** A natural, fatlike substance found in humans and animals.

**Chorion** The membrane that envelops the amniotic sac and fetus.

**Chorionic villus sampling (CVS)** A test for prenatal abnormalities involving analysis of material snipped from the chorion, the membrane containing the amniotic sac and fetus.

**Chromosomes** Rodlike structures found in the nuclei of every living cell that carry the genetic code in the form of genes.

**Chronic bronchitis** An inflammation of the lining of the bronchial tubes, producing chronic coughing.

**Chronic fatigue syndrome (CFS)** A long-term condition involving extreme fatigue and a variety of other symptoms.

**Chronic infection** Long-term infection.

**Chronic obstructive pulmonary disease (COPD)** General term applying to chronic lung diseases, especially emphysema and chronic bronchitis, which result in impaired lung function.

**Chronic stress** Persistent or recurrent stress.

**Cilia** Tiny hairlike projections on the surface of cells in the nose, respiratory tract, and other sites that sweep away invading organisms.

**Circle of poison** The practice of exporting banned chemicals to other, often poorer, countries; they are used in products sent back to the original country.

**Circulatory system** The network of blood vessels that carries blood throughout the body.

**Circumcision** Surgical removal of the foreskin of the penis.

**Cirrhosis of the liver** A disease of the liver in which scar tissue replaces healthy liver tissue.

**Claustrophobia** Fear of enclosed spaces.

**Clinical breast examination** A breast exam performed by a health care provider to detect lumps or abnormalities.

**Clinical psychologists** Psychologists who specialize in the diagnosis and treatment of psychological disorders.

**Clinical social workers** Social workers trained to work with people with psychological problems.

**Clitoridectomy** Surgical removal of the clitoris.

**Clitoris** A female sex organ consisting of a shaft and glans located above the urethral opening. It is extremely sensitive to sexual sensations.

**Coagulation** The process of blood clotting.

**Cocaine** An addictive stimulant drug derived from coca leaves that increases mental alertness and induces a euphoric rush.

**Cocaine psychosis** An acute psychotic reaction induced by the use of cocaine, often involving paranoid delusions.

**Codeine** Another narcotic drug derived from the opium poppy that is used medically to deaden pain and to suppress coughing.

**Codependent** A person involved in a close relationship with a drug-dependent person who plays a part in enabling or maintaining the other person's chemical dependency.

**Cognitive therapy** A therapy that helps clients identify and correct dysfunctional thinking patterns.

**Cohabitation** Living together as though married but without legal sanction.

**Coitus** Sexual intercourse.

**Coitus interruptus** A method of contraception in which the penis is withdrawn from the vagina before ejaculation.

**Collagen** A fibrous protein that is the major structural component of skin, cartilage, tendon, and connective tissues.

**Collectivists** People who define themselves in terms of belonging to certain groups.

**Colonoscopy** The visual examination of the colon through the use of a colonoscope, an elongated instrument for viewing inner surfaces of the body.

**Colony-stimulating factors (CSFs)** Proteins found in blood serum that stimulate the bone marrow to produce more white blood cells and other blood cells.

**Colostomy bag** A bag worn outside of the body to collect fecal waste following surgical removal of the bowel.

**Combination pill** A birth-control pill that contains synthetic estrogen and progesterone.

**Common cold** A mild, short-lived, contagious viral infection of the upper respiratory tract.

**Competencies** Skills or abilities needed to perform tasks.

**Complex carbohydrates** A class of carbohydrates that includes starches and fibers.

**Computerized axial tomography scan (CAT scan)** An X-ray machine that passes a narrow X-ray beam through the body at different angles and generates a computer-enhanced image of internal structures.

**Conception** The inception of pregnancy that results from the fertilization of an ovum.

**Conditional positive regard** Judging a person's value in terms of the acceptability of the person's behavior at a given time.

**Condom** A sheath made of animal membrane or latex that covers the penis during coitus and serves as a barrier to sperm following ejaculation.

**Conflict** A state of tension resulting from two opposing motives occurring simultaneously.

**Congenital heart defects** Heart defects present at birth.

**Congenital syphilis** A syphilis infection that is present at birth.

**Congestive heart failure** A condition in which the heart is unable to pump out as much blood as it receives, leading to a backing up or pooling of blood in the veins, lungs, and extremities.

**Contagious** Describes a person who harbors an infectious organism and is capable of transmitting it to others.

**Contraception** Methods or devices that prevent conception.

**Cool-down** Reduced pace of activity, such as stretching, performed for 5 to 10 minutes before the end of exercise sessions.

**Copayment** A set amount the individual pays for a medical service provided under HMO coverage.

**Corona** The ridge that separates the glans from the body of the penis.

**Coronary angiography** *(angiogram)* Rapid-sequence X-rays detect a radioactive dye as it passes through the coronary arteries; provides information on blockages restricting blood flow to the heart.

**Coronary artery bypass graft (CABG) surgery** A surgical technique that grafts pieces of vein from elsewhere in the body to direct the flow of blood around a blocked or narrowed coronary artery.

**Coronary heart disease (CHD)** A disease usually caused by damage to coronary arteries; the heart's blood supply becomes insufficient.

**Coroner** A public official with responsibility for investigating deaths not clearly resulting from natural causes.

**Corpus luteum** The follicle that has released an ovum and then produces copious amounts of progesterone and estrogen during the luteal phase of a woman's cycle.

**Corticosteroids** Steroids or steroidal hormones that help the body cope with stress by making stored energy available.

**Corticotrophin-releasing hormone (CRH)** A substance produced by the hypothalamus that causes the pituitary gland to release adrenocorticotrophic hormone (ACTH).

**Cosmic rays** A form of high-energy, particle radiation originating in outer space.

**Counselors** Professionals who counsel people with psychological problems and disabilities.

**Couples therapy** Therapy for married or unmarried couples that focuses on improving their relationships.

**Crack** A hardened form of cocaine that comes in the form of pebbles ("rocks") that can be smoked.

**Critical period of vulnerability** A period of time during which an embryo or fetus is vulnerable to the effects of a teratogen.

**Critical thinking** The adoption of a questioning attitude characterized by a careful weighing of evidence and thoughtful analysis of the claims and arguments of others.

**Cryosurgery** Surgery using freezing temperatures produced by liquid nitrogen or carbon dioxide in order to destroy cancerous tissue.

**Cryptosporidium** A protozoan parasite that can cause diarrhea and more serious consequences in persons with compromised immune systems.

**Culture method** A body fluid specimen containing unidentified bacteria is placed in a plate with special nutrients that allow bacteria to multiply. The bacterial strain can be identified by its shape and growth pattern.

**Cunnilingus** Oral stimulation of the female genitals.

**Cyanosis** A bluish or purplish coloration resulting from deficient oxygenation of the blood.

**Cystitis** An inflammation of the urinary bladder.

**Cytokines** Chemicals involved in growth regulation; help coordinate the immune response.

# D

**Daily hassles** Minor annoyances of daily life that are common sources of stress.

**Date rape** A type of acquaintance rape in which the assailant is the person's date.

**Death** The irreversible cessation of vital life functions.

**Decongestant** Medication that eases stuffy noses and reduces mucus buildup.

**Deductible** The annual amount that the individual must pay for medical expenses before the health insurance plan starts contributing its share.

**Defense mechanism** According to Freud, a way in which the mind distorts reality to keep anxiety-evoking or troubling ideas or impulses away from consciousness.

**Defibrillator** An electrical device that stops heart fibrillation by applying electrical countershocks to the heart through electrodes placed on the chest.

**Deliriant** A substance that induces delirium, or a state of gross mental confusion, excitability, and disorientation.

**Delirium tremens (DTs)** A withdrawal syndrome in chronic alcoholics characterized by extreme restlessness, sweating, disorientation, and hallucinations.

**Delta-9-tetrahydrocannabinol (THC)** The psychoactive ingredient in marijuana and hashish.

**Delusions** False, unshakable beliefs.

**Dementia** A psychological disorder involving a deterioration of mental functioning involving memory, reasoning, use of language, judgment, and ability to carry out purposeful actions.

**Dendrites** The rootlike structures at the end of neurons that receive nerve impulses from adjoining neurons.

**Deoxyribonucleic acid (DNA)** The molecule that makes up genes and chromosomes.

**Depo-Provera** A synthetic form of progesterone that works as a contraceptive by inhibiting ovulation.

**Depressants** Drugs such as barbiturates, tranquilizers, opiates, and alcohol that lower the rate of nervous system activity.

**Designated driver** A person who, chosen as the driver for a group, is expected to abstain from alcohol.

**Designer drugs** Synthetic drugs manufactured in illicit labs that are chemical analogues (drugs having similar properties and effects) of illegal drugs.

**Detoxification** The process of eliminating drugs from a person's body, usually under supervised conditions where withdrawal symptoms can be monitored and controlled.

**DHEA** A hormone produced by the adrenal glands; appears to play an important role in the production of other hormones and in the immune system.

**Diabetes mellitus** A metabolic disease involving insufficient production of insulin or a failure of cells to utilize the insulin produced.

**Diagnostic related groups (DRGs)** Classifications used to determine reimbursement rates to hospitals for particular medical conditions.

**Diaphragm** A muscular wall separating the chest cavity from the abdomen. For each inbreath, the diaphragm contracts, which causes the lungs to expand and take in air.

**Diaphragm** A shallow rubber cup or dome, fitted to the contour of a woman's vagina, that is coated with a spermicide and inserted before coitus to prevent conception.

**Diaphragmatic breathing** Deep and regular breathing that can be monitored by the movement of the diaphragm with each inbreath and outbreath.

**Dietary fiber** Complex carbohydrates that form the structural parts of plants, such as cellulose and pectin, that cannot be broken down by human digestive enzymes.

**Digital Rectal Examination (DRE)** A test used to screen for colorectal and prostate cancer; the physician inserts a gloved finger into the rectum to feel for abnormal growths.

**Digital subtraction angiography (DSA)** An angiogram that detects blockages in the major blood vessels in the neck and brain.

**Digitalis** A drug, such as digoxin, that improves the heart's pumping ability by increasing the force of cardiac contractions.

**Dilate** To open or widen.

**Dilation and curettage (D&C)** An operation in which the cervix is dilated and uterine contents gently scraped away.

**Dilation and evacuation (D&E)** An abortion method in which the cervix is dilated before vacuum aspiration.

**Dioxins** Highly toxic chlorinated hydrocarbons, formed during industrial processes from the heating of substances containing chlorine.

**Diphtheria** Acute upper-respiratory-tract bacterial infection of the tonsil area transmitted by inhaled droplets.

**Disease** A disruption of bodily functions linked to an identifiable group of signs and symptoms.

**Distillation** A process of boiling out the alcohol from the fermentation process and then condensing the vapors back into a liquid form.

**Distress** Emotional or physical pain or suffering.

**Diuretics** Agents that increase the rate of excretion of urine from the body; used in treating congestive heart failure, hypertension, and other cardiovascular problems.

**Diverticulosis** Inflammation of small pockets or sacs that may form in the wall of the colon and that become filled with stagnant feces, causing pain and discomfort. In severe cases, can be life-threatening.

**Dizygotic (DZ) twins** Twins that develop from two separate fertilized eggs and thus have half their genes in common, like any other two siblings. Also called fraternal twins.

**Doctor-assisted suicide** Suicide, usually of a person suffering from an incurable and painful disease, in which a physician helps to administer a lethal drug.

**Donor IVF** A variation of in vitro fertilization in which the ovum is taken from one woman, fertilized, and then injected into the uterus or Fallopian tube of another woman.

**Dopamine** A neurotransmitter believed to play a role in schizophrenia.

**Dose dependent** Effects of drugs or other substances that are dependent on the amount of the substance used.

**Dose-response relationship** The relationship between the dosage level of a drug and its effects on the user.

**Douche** To rinse or wash the vaginal canal by inserting a liquid and allowing it to drain out.

**Down syndrome** A chromosomal abnormality that leads to mental retardation; caused by an extra chromosome on the twenty-first pair.

**Dream analysis** A technique used in psychoanalysis that attempts to extract the symbolic meaning of dreams in a way that reveals unconscious material.

**Drug** A chemical agent that affects biological function.

**Drug abuse** Repeated use of a drug even when it is causing or aggravating personal, occupational, or health problems.

**Drug addiction** A state of physiological dependence on a drug that is accompanied by a lack of control over its use.

**Drug misuse** Use of a drug for the wrong reason.

**Dying** The state of approaching death.

**Dysmenorrhea** Pain or discomfort during menstruation.

**Dyspareunia** Painful intercourse.

**Dysthymia** A depressive disorder involving states of chronic, mild depression.

## E

**Eating disorders** Disturbances of eating behavior, including anorexia nervosa and bulimia nervosa.

**Ebola** A highly fatal viral disease spread to humans by monkeys.

**Echocardiogram** A device that uses reflected sound waves ("echoes") to create an image of the internal structure and movement of the heart.

**Eclectic therapy** In psychotherapy, the use of techniques or principles from different therapeutic approaches.

**Ectoparasites** Parasites that live on the outside of the host's body (endoparasites live within the body).

**Edema** Swelling.

**Efface** To become thin.

**Ego identity** The sense of who one is and what one stands for.

**Ejaculatory ducts** Ducts through which sperm pass through the prostate gland and into the urethra.

**Elastin** A protein in connective tissue that is the basic component in elastic fibers.

**Elder abuse** Abuse of the elderly, including physical abuse, verbal abuse, neglect, or financial exploitation.

**Elder bias** Discrimination against the elderly in medical practice and other institutional settings.

**Electrocardiogram (ECG or EKG)** A device for recording and graphing the electrical activity of the heart.

**Electrodesiccation** Destruction of cancerous tissues or growths by use of heat.

**Electroencephalogram (EEG)** A device that uses electrodes on the scalp to measure and display brain wave activity.

**Electrolyte** A substance that conducts electricity.

**Electromagnetic fields (EMFs)** Alternating electrical and magnetic fields that act as a source of nonionizing radiation.

**Electromagnetic radiation** Radiation in the form of electromagnetic waves, including radio waves, X-rays, gamma waves, and microwaves.

**Electromagnetic spectrum** The entire range of electromagnetic radiation.

**Electromyographic (EMG) biofeedback** Changes in muscle tension in selected muscles are relayed to the user in the form of audio or video signals.

**Electroshock therapy (ECT)** A therapy for severe depression involving the administration of brief pulses of electricity to the patient's brain.

**Electrostimulation** The use of electric current to block pain signals.

**Embalming** A process of replacing the blood and bodily fluids of a dead body with chemicals to prevent decay.

**Embolism** An obstruction of a blood vessel, usually caused by a blood clot.

**Embryo** The stage of prenatal development that begins with the implantation of a fertilized ovum in the uterus and concludes with the development of the major organ systems at about two months after conception.

**Embryonic stage** The stage of prenatal development that lasts from implantation through the eighth week; the major organ systems differentiate.

**Embryonic transfer** A method of conception in which a woman volunteer is artificially inseminated by the male partner of the intended mother. The embryo is later transferred to the uterus of the intended mother.

**Emerging infectious diseases** Infections seemingly new to the human scene and those that have reemerged or appear in new strains.

**Emphysema** A lung disease involving destruction of the walls of the air sacs (alveoli) in the lungs.

**Endocardium** The inner layer of the heart.

**Endocrine system** The system of glands that secrete hormones directly into the bloodstream, rather than by means of ducts.

**Endogenous microorganisms** Organisms that normally live within the body; disturbances in their growth can cause infection.

**Endometriosis** A condition caused by the growth of endometrial tissue in the abdominal cavity or elsewhere outside the uterus.

**Endometrium** The innermost layer of the uterus.

**Endorphins** Naturally occurring hormones that directly stimulate pleasure centers in the brain.

**Environment** All of the living and nonliving components that exist where an organism lives.

**Environmental hazard** An environmental factor with potential to cause harm to individuals.

**Environmental health** The relationship between organisms and their physical environment that allows them to survive and flourish.

**Environmental racism** Racial bias in environmental policy and enforcement.

**Epicardium** The outermost layer of the wall of the heart.

**Epidemic** The rapid spread or increased prevalence of a disease within a group or population.

**Epidemiological studies** Studies of the causes and control of epidemic diseases or of differences in disease rates between populations.

**Epididymis** A tube that lies against the back wall of each testicle and serves as a storage facility for sperm.

**Epididymitis** Inflammation of the epididymis.

**Episiotomy** A surgical incision in the perineum that widens the birth canal, preventing random tearing during childbirth.

**Epithelial tissue** Tissue that covers the outer surface of the body and lines internal body surfaces.

**Epstein-Barr virus (EBV)** A virus that causes infectious mononucleosis.

**Erythrocytes** Red blood cells; carry oxygen to cells.

**Essential amino acids** Amino acids essential to survival that must be obtained from the food we eat since the body is unable to manufacture them on its own.

**Estrogen** A generic term for female sex hormones that promote the development of female secondary sex characteristics and regulate the menstrual cycle.

**Ethanol** Another term for ethyl alcohol, the psychoactive substance in alcohol.

**Ethnic group** A group of people who are united by their cultural heritage, race, language, and common history.

**Eustress** "Good stress," which motivates and energizes us.

**Euthanasia** Causing a painless death in a person suffering from an incurable and painful disease or condition.

**Excitement phase** The first phase of the sexual response cycle, characterized by erection in the male, vaginal lubrication in the female, and muscle tension and heart rate increases in males and females.

**Exercise** A structured sequence of movements performed consistently over a period of time that contribute to fitness.

**Exercise electrocardiogram** *(stress test)* An electrocardiogram taken when the heart is stressed during exercise.

**Exhaustion stage** The final stage of the response to prolonged stress, characterized by depletion of bodily resources and a lowering of resistance to illness.

**Exit events** Life events involving loss of significant others through death, divorce or separation, termination of relationships, or relocation.

**Exogenous microorganisms** Organisms that do not normally inhabit the host.

**Expectorant** A cough remedy ingredient that helps to expel phlegm.

**Extended care facilities** Inpatient facilities providing long-term custodial or medical care, especially for people suffering from chronic diseases or requiring continued rehabilitation.

**External locus of control** The perception that one's future is determined by forces beyond one's control.

**Extremely low-frequency electromagnetic radiation (ELF)** A type of nonionizing radiation emitted by electrical appliances.

## F

**Fallopian tubes** Tubes that extend from the upper uterus toward the ovaries and conduct ova to the uterus.

**False positive** An erroneous positive test result or clinical finding.

**Family therapy** Therapy that helps troubled families learn to communicate better and resolve conflicts.

**Fat cells** Body cells that store fat.

**Fats** Organic compounds that form the basis of fatty tissue of animals, including humans, and are also found in some plants.

**Fatty liver** A condition involving an accumulation of fat in the liver, causing enlargement of the organ.

**Fauna** Animal life, including microscopic organisms, living within a particular area.

**Fear** Anxiety experienced in response to a specific threat or object.

**Fecal Occult Blood Test (FOBT)** A test for blood in the stool, used to detect the presence of precancerous or cancerous polyps.

**Fee-for-service (FFS) plans** Traditional insurance plans in which the insurance carrier pays a percentage of covered medical expenses after deductibles.

**Fellatio** Oral stimulation of the male genitals.

**Female orgasmic disorder** Inability or persistent difficulty achieving orgasm.

**Female sexual arousal disorder** Persistent difficulty in becoming sexually aroused, denoted by a lack of vaginal lubrication in response to sexual stimulation.

**Fermentation** A process by which yeast is used to convert sugar into ethyl alcohol and carbon dioxide.

**Fertilization** In humans, the union of an ovum and a sperm cell, resulting in the formation of a zygote.

**Fetal alcohol syndrome (FAS)** A cluster of symptoms caused by maternal drinking in which the child shows developmental lags and facial deformities.

**Fight-or-flight reaction** Corresponds to the alarm reaction; mobilization of the body's resources to fend off a threat by fighting or fleeing.

**Fitness** The ability to perform moderate to vigorous levels of physical activity without undue fatigue.

**Flexibility** The ability of the joints to move through their entire range of motion without undue stress. Flexibility is measured by the length and amount of stretch in the tissues surrounding the joints.

**Flora** Plant life indigenous to specific environments.

**Flushing response** A physiological reaction to the ingestion of alcohol that is characterized by reddening and warming of the face, and sometimes nausea and other unpleasant reactions.

**Folic acid** A B vitamin, also known as folate, that helps prevent neural tube defects and may play a role in preventing heart disease.

**Follicle** A capsule within an ovary that contains an ovum.

**Follicle-stimulating hormone (FSH)** A pituitary hormone that stimulates development of follicles in the ovaries.

**Food allergies** Hypersensitivities to certain foods.

**Food chain** The sequence in which organisms feed on smaller or less complex organisms and are consumed by larger or more complex organisms.

**Forcible rape** Sexual intercourse with a nonconsenting person achieved by force or threat of force.

**Foreplay** Physical interactions that are sexually stimulating and set the stage for intercourse.

**Foreskin** The loose skin that covers the penile glans.

**Formaldehyde** A clear, toxic gas used as a preservative and in manufacturing.

**Fossil fuels** Energy sources found in deposits in the earth, including oil, natural gas, and coal.

**Fracture** A broken bone.

**Free association** A technique used in psychoanalysis in which the patient is encouraged to verbalize any thoughts that come to mind, free of any conscious efforts to censure or edit them.

**Free radicals** Metabolic waste products produced during normal oxidation that may damage cell membranes and genetic material.

**Freebase cocaine** A form of cocaine in which the drug is first heated with ether to separate its more potent component (the "free base") and then smoked.

**Frostbite** Skin damage produced by prolonged exposure to cold air.

**Frustration** The negative feeling state experienced when one's efforts to pursue one's goals are thwarted.

**Fungi** Primitive plant organisms such as yeasts and molds.

## G

**Gamete intrafallopian transfer (GIFT)** A method of conception in which sperm and ova are inserted into a Fallopian tube to encourage conception.

**Gamma globulin** Antibody-rich serum from the blood of another person or animal used to induce passive immunity.

**Gamma rays** High-energy, penetrating ionizing radiation emitted from the nucleus of a radioactive atom.

**Gamma-aminobutyric acid (GABA)** An inhibitory neurotransmitter believed to play a role in anxiety.

**Gate theory of pain** Explains that the perception of pain involves a gating mechanism in the central nervous system that allows or blocks pain messages to the brain.

**Gateway drug** A drug serving as a stepping-stone or gateway to use of other, usually harder, drugs.

**Gay males** Male homosexuals.

**Gender** The state of being male or female.

**Gender identity** The psychological sense of being male or female.

**Gender reassignment surgery** Surgery that modifies a person's genitalia into a likeness of the genitalia of the opposite sex.

**Gender roles** Complex clusters of ways in which males and females are expected to behave in a given culture.

**Gender typing** The process by which children acquire behavior that is deemed appropriate to their gender.

**Gender-role stereotypes** Fixed, conventional ideas about the roles performed by men and women.

**Gene therapy** The alteration of a person's genetic material to fight disease.

**General adaptation syndrome (GAS)** Describes the body's three-stage response to persistent or intense stress.

**General anesthesia** The use of drugs to put people to sleep and eliminate pain, as during childbirth.

**General paresis** Mental illness caused by neurosyphilis; characterized by gross confusion.

**Generalized anxiety disorder** A disorder characterized by a high level of anxiety that is not limited to particular situations, and general feelings of worry, dread, and foreboding.

**Genes** The basic units or building blocks of heredity that contain the genetic code.

**Genital warts** Caused by the human papilloma virus; takes the form of warts around the genitals and anus.

**Germ cell** A cell from which a new organism develops.

**Germinal stage** Prenatal development from conception through implantation in the uterus.

**Gerontology** The study of aging and the elderly.

**Gestational diabetes** Diabetes developed during pregnancy.

**Giardiasis** A diarrheal disease caused by a protozoan parasite.

**Glans** The head of the penis or clitoris.

**Glaucoma** An eye disease involving a buildup of fluid pressure inside the eyeball; can damage the eye, impair vision, and sometimes cause blindness.

**Global warming** The rise in atmospheric temperatures worldwide.

**Glucose** A form of sugar produced by digestion; transported by blood to cells.

**Goals** The ends toward which we strive that result in satisfaction of needs.

**Gonorrhea** Caused by the *gonococcus* bacterium; characterized by a discharge and burning urination. Can give rise to PID and infertility.

**Gradual exposure** A behavior therapy technique for overcoming phobias involving actual exposure to increasingly fearful stimuli or situations.

**Greenhouse effect** The rise in atmospheric temperature due to the buildup of heat-trapping gases produced by the burning of fossil fuels.

**Grief** Emotional suffering, sorrow, or distress resulting from loss or other misfortune.

**Groin** The area between the thigh and the trunk. Also called the inguinal region.

**Ground water** Water from snow and rain that collects in underground aquifers.

**Group therapy** Therapy in which clients are treated together.

**Gynecologist** A physician who treats women's diseases, especially of the reproductive tract.

## H

**Hallucinations** False sense perceptions, such as "hearing voices" or seeing things that are not there.

**Hallucinogenic drugs** Psychoactive drugs that alter sensory processes and induce hallucinations.

**Hangover** The unpleasant after effects of drinking too much alcohol, characterized by such symptoms as headache and nausea.

**Hashish** Also known as "hash," the resin of the cannabis plant, which contains the most potent concentration of THC.

**Health** Soundness of body and mind; a state of vigor and vitality that permits one to function effectively physically, psychologically, and socially.

**Health maintenance organization (HMO)** A prepaid managed care plan that offers medical services through affiliated doctors and hospitals or freestanding clinics. Costs are usually based on a fixed amount of money per enrolled member.

**Heart attack** The common term for a myocardial infarction.

**Heart murmur** Abnormal heart sound resulting from some disturbance in the normal flow of blood through the heart.

**Heart rate** The number of heartbeats per minute.

**Heart transplant** The replacement of a diseased heart with a healthy donor heart.

**Heat cramps** Painful muscle spasms resulting from hard work in hot temperatures without an adequate supply of fluids and salt.

**Heat exhaustion** An acute reaction to excessive heat, characterized by dizziness, cold skin, weak pulse, nausea, weakness, and headache, leading to collapse.

**Heat stress** A condition in which body temperature rises, sometimes to dangerous levels; may result in heat cramps, heat exhaustion, hyperthermia, and heat stroke.

**Heat stroke** A dangerous, potentially life-threatening reaction to excessive heat characterized by extremely high fever.

**Hegar's sign** Softness of a section of the uterus between the uterine body and the cervix indicates that a woman is pregnant.

**Helper T-cells** White blood cells that search for antigens and signal other lymphocytes to gather at the site of infection.

**Hematocrit** The ratio of the volume of red blood cells to a given volume of blood, expressed as a percentage.

**Hemoglobin** Iron-containing pigment in red blood cells that gives blood its reddish color; transports oxygen to tissues.

**Hemophiliacs** Persons with a hereditary blood coagulation disorder characterized by excessive bleeding.

**Hepatitis** An inflammation of the liver caused by various viruses or exposure to toxins.

**Hepatitis A** A type of hepatitis, or inflammation of the liver, caused by the hepatitis A virus.

**Herbology** Herbal medicine; the use of natural substances from plants, trees, and flowers to treat disease.

**Heroin** A naturally occurring opiate derived from morphine that has strong addictive properties.

**Herpes simplex virus type 1 (HSV-1)** The virus that causes oral herpes; characterized by cold sores or fever blisters on the lips or mouth.

**Herpes simplex virus type 2 (HSV-2)** The virus that causes genital herpes.

**Heterosexuals** People who are erotically attracted to, and who prefer to have romantic relationships with, members of the opposite gender.

**High-density lipoprotein (HDL)** Cholesterol considered good because it sweeps away cholesterol deposits from artery walls for elimination from the body, thereby lowering the risk of cardiovascular disease.

**Histamines** Substances released during allergic reactions that stimulate secretion of mucus, dilate blood vessels, and produce allergy symptoms.

**Hodgkin's disease** A rare type of lymphoma (cancer of the lymphatic system) characterized by enlargement of the lymph nodes.

**Holistic medicine** An approach to treatment that focuses on the whole person, including physical, emotional, spiritual, and social aspects, not just the disease.

**Home health care** A system of providing health care services to people in their homes.

**Homeopathy** An alternative medical approach based on the use of tiny doses of curative substances.

**Homeostasis** The maintenance of a steady state.

**Homogamy** The practice of marrying people who are similar in social background and standing.

**Hormone therapy** The use of hormones to retard the growth of cancerous cells.

**Hormone-replacement therapy (HRT)** The use of artificial female sex hormones in postmenopausal women.

**Hormones** Substances secreted by endocrine glands that are involved in the regulation of a wide range of bodily processes, including reproduction and growth.

**Hospice** An approach to treating dying patients that focuses on support and understanding, rather than curative treatment; also refers to houses or facilities that provide palliative (supportive) care to dying patients.

**Host** Person, plant, or animal that provides a hospitable environment for a pathogen.

**Human chorionic gonadotropin (HCG)** A hormone produced by women shortly after conception which stimulates the corpus luteum to continue to produce progesterone. The presence of HCG in a woman's urine indicates that she is pregnant.

**Human growth hormone (hGH)** A hormone produced by the pituitary gland; involved in regulating growth and development during childhood and adolescence.

**Human immunodeficiency virus (HIV)** A sexually transmitted virus that destroys the immune system.

**Hydrocarbons** Volatile organic compounds consisting of hydrogen and carbon produced by the incomplete combustion of fossil fuels and evaporation of solvents and fuels.

**Hydrostatic weighing** A method of measuring body weight by weighing a person both underwater and out of water and comparing the results.

**Hymen** A fold of tissue across the vaginal opening that is usually present at birth and remains at least partly intact until a woman engages in coitus.

**Hypertension** High blood pressure; generally, a blood pressure reading of 140 (systolic)/90 (diastolic) or higher. A major risk factor in heart disease and stroke.

**Hyperthermia** A bodily state characterized by unusually high fever.

**Hypnotics** Types of drugs that have sleep-inducing effects.

**Hypothalamus** A structure in the lower middle part of the brain, involved in regulating a range of processes, including motivation, emotion, and body temperature.

**Hypothermia** Extreme loss of heat in the body characterized by an unusually low body temperature.

**Hysterectomy** Surgical removal of the uterus.

**Hysterotomy** An abortion method in which the fetus is removed by caesarean section.

## I

**Ideal self** The mental image corresponding to what we believe we ought to be like.

**Identity crises** In Erikson's view, periods of serious soul-searching and self-examination that contribute to achieving ego identity.

**Immune response** The sequence of events that occurs when the immune system detects antigens.

**Immune system** The body's system for identifying and eliminating disease-causing agents, such as bacteria and viruses, and for disposing of diseased, mutated, or worn-out cells.

**Immunity** Protection against specific infections and diseases.

**Immunoglobulin E (IgE)** An antibody produced in response to allergens. Triggers mast cells to release an inflammatory chemical, histamine, which causes reactions such as itching and sneezing.

**Immunosuppression** Weakened or suppressed immune system.

**Immunotherapy** Treatment of disease involving efforts to boost the functioning of the immune system.

**Impaired glucose tolerance (IGT)** Indicates excessive levels of glucose in the blood after eating a carbohydrate-rich meal, but not high enough to be indicative of diabetes.

**Impetigo** A contagious bacterial skin disease, primarily affecting the skin around the mouth and nose.

**In vitro fertilization (IVF)** A method of conception in which mature ova are surgically removed from an ovary and placed in a laboratory dish along with sperm.

**Incest** Sexual relations or marriage between people so closely related by blood that it is prohibited by law or culturally taboo.

**Incineration** The burning of solid waste; spews pollutants into the air.

**Incubation period** The time between the entrance of the pathogen and the first symptoms.

**Individualists** People who define themselves in terms of their own personal identities.

**Individuation** The process of developing a psychological identity separate and distinct from others.

**Induced abortion** The purposeful termination of a pregnancy before the embryo or fetus is capable of sustaining independent life.

**Infarct** An area of dead or dying tissue as the result of an insufficient blood supply to the tissue.

**Infection** The contamination and injury caused by multiplying pathogens.

**Infectious diseases** Diseases caused by direct or indirect contact with an infectious agent. Also called communicable diseases.

**Infectious mononucleosis** A viral disease caused by the Epstein-Barr virus; acute stage characterized by fever, sore throat, and enlarged lymph nodes and spleen.

**Infertility** Inability to conceive a child.

**Inflammation** The nonspecific defense reaction to pathogen-induced tissue damage; the swelling or redness that occurs around an injured area..

**Influenza (flu)** An acute viral lower-respiratory-tract infection.

**Inhalants** Chemical fumes that are inhaled for their psychoactive effects.

**Injecting drug user (IDU)** A person who injects psychoactive drugs.

**Innate immunity** Immunity acquired by transfer of mother's antibodies to the fetus, through her bloodstream and, later, via breast milk.

**Insoluble fibers** Types of dietary fiber that are not dissolvable in water.

**Insomnia** Difficulty falling asleep, remaining asleep, or achieving restorative sleep.

**Insulin** A hormone produced by the pancreas that plays an essential role in the metabolism and regulation of blood sugar (glucose).

**Insulin-dependent diabetes mellitus (IDDM) (juvenile or Type 1 diabetes)** Diabetes that usually develops in childhood or young adulthood; the person requires daily doses of insulin.

**Integumentary system** The skin, along with its attachments, including hair and nails.

**Interferons** Proteins manufactured by the body that have antiviral and antitumor effects.

**Interleukin-2 (IL-2)** A naturally occurring growth factor that helps the immune system destroy cancer cells.

**Internal locus of control** The perception that the control over rewards and punishments resides within the individual.

**Intimacy** Feelings of closeness and connectedness characterized by sharing of inmost thoughts and feelings.

**Intoxication** A state of drunkenness brought on by the use of alcohol or other intoxicating drugs.

**Intra-amniotic infusion** An abortion method in which a substance is injected into the amniotic sac to induce premature labor.

**Intracytoplasmic injection** A method of conception involving the injection of sperm directly into an ovum.

**Intrauterine device (IUD)** A small object that is inserted into the uterus and left in place to prevent conception.

**Intravenous drug user (IVDU)** An injecting drug user (IDU) who injects drugs intravenously (into a vein).

**Ionizing radiation** Powerful, high-energy radiation capable of changing the structure of atoms.

**Ions** Atoms or atomic particles bearing positive or negative charges.

**Iridology** The study of how changes in the iris of the eye may be related to disease.

**Iron** An essential mineral, a metallic element that forms part of the makeup of hemoglobin.

**Irritable bowel syndrome (IBS)** An oversensitivity of the digestive system, resulting in attacks of diarrhea, nausea, gas, and abdominal pain after eating certain foods or during times of stress.

**Ischemia** An insufficiency of blood supply to a part of the body.

**Isokinetic exercise** Exercise in which muscles contract against a selected resistance through the full range of motion; requires use of an exercise machine.

**Isometric exercise** Contraction of a muscle which is not accompanied by any joint movement and in which the muscle remains the same length (does not shorten) even as tension increases.

**Isotonic exercise** Exercise in which muscles are repeatedly contracted under constant resistance throughout the full range of motion of the joint.

## J

**Job stress** Pressures, demands, or dissatisfaction associated with work.

## K

**Keratinocytes** Cells in the outer layer of the skin that are regularly shed and renewed.

**Killer T-cells** White blood cells with a receptor that matches a specific antigen; killer T-cells lock onto that antigen and kill it.

## L

**Labia majora** Large folds of skin that run downward from the mons along the sides of the vulva.

**Labia minora** Hairless, light-colored membranes located between the labia majora.

**Laetrile** A drug derived from apricot pits; its alleged anticancer effects are unproved.

**Lamaze method** A childbirth method in which women learn to relax and to breathe in patterns that conserve energy and lessen pain.

**Landfills** Underground disposal areas for discarding solid waste.

**Laparoscopy** A method of sterilization in which a laparoscope is inserted through a small incision just below the navel and used to close off the Fallopian tubes.

**Latent infection** "Hidden" or inactive infection in which pathogens are not active enough to produce symptoms.

**Lead poisoning** Toxic metal poisoning, from the ingestion or inhalation of large amounts of lead.

**Legionnaire's disease** A severe type of bacterial pneumonia caused by the *Legionella* bacterium.

**Lesbians** Female homosexuals.

**Leukemia** Cancer forming in the blood and blood-forming tissues of the body.

**Leukocytes** White blood cells; combat infection.

**Life changes** Positive or negative changes in life circumstances that are stressful because they impose on us a demand to adjust.

**Life expectancy** The statistical average number of years that people in a given population can expect to live.

**Life transitions** Changes in our roles or life situations caused by anticipated or unexpected events.

**Ligaments** Tough fibrous tissue that connects bone to bone.

**Lipoprotein** A compound or complex of fat and protein by which fats are transported through the bloodstream.

**Liver** The largest organ in the body. Performs a vital role in many metabolic processes, including the metabolism of alcohol.

**Living will** A document prepared when a person is well directing to termination of life-sustaining treatment under certain conditions.

**Local anesthesia** Anesthesia that eliminates pain in a specific area of the body, as during childbirth.

**Lochia** A reddish vaginal discharge that may persist for a month after delivery.

**Longevity** The maximum number of years an organism can expect to live under the best circumstances.

**Low-density lipoprotein** (LDL) Cholesterol considered bad because it forms fatty deposits that can stick to artery walls and restrict the flow of blood to vital body organs, setting the stage for heart attacks and strokes.

**Lumpectomy** A breast cancer treatment in which the tumor and surrounding tissue are surgically removed but the breast is spared.

**Lupus erythematosus** A chronic autoimmune disease involving inflammation of the connective tissue; can affect many body organs and systems.

**Luteal phase** The third phase of the menstrual cycle, named after the corpus luteum, which begins to secrete large amounts of progesterone and estrogen following ovulation.

**Luteinizing hormone (LH)** A hormone that helps regulate the menstrual cycle by triggering ovulation.

**Lyme disease** An infectious disease spread by ticks; caused by the bacterium *Borrelia burgdorferi*.

**Lymph** The clear fluid found in lymphatic vessels.

**Lymph nodes** Lymphatic glands located throughout the body; produce and store lymphocytes and filter out infectious agents.

**Lymphatic system** The system of vessels, nodes, ducts, organs, and cells that manufacture and store lymphocytes and help destroy infectious agents.

**Lymphocytes** White blood cells that defend the body against antigens.

**Lymphoma** Cancer forming in the cells of the lymphatic system.

**Lysergic acid diethylamide (LSD)** A hallucinogenic drug, more commonly known by its abbreviation.

## M

**Macrophages** Phagocytes that enter body tissues and scavenge for worn-out cells and cellular debris.

**Magnetic resonance imaging (MRI)** The use of magnets to create a computerized image of internal body structures.

**Major depression** A severe form of depression characterized by downcast mood, negative thinking, and other related features, such as changes in sleeping patterns and appetite, and without a history of manic episodes..

**Malaria** Potentially deadly protozoal disease transmitted by mosquitoes.

**Male erectile disorder** Persistent difficulty achieving or maintaining an erection sufficient to allow the man to engage in or complete sexual intercourse.

**Male orgasmic disorder** Inability or persistent difficulty achieving orgasm.

**Malignant** Cancerous growths capable of invading surrounding tissue and spreading to other sites.

**Malignant melanoma** A potentially deadly form of cancer that forms in melanin-forming cells, most commonly found in the skin but sometimes in other parts of the body.

**Malpractice** Failure of a professional to render proper treatment, especially when injury or harm occurs as a result.

**Mammary glands** Milk-secreting glands.

**Mammogram** X-ray of the breast.

**Mammography** Procedure for taking X-rays of the breast (mammograms).

**Managed care** A system of controlling health care costs by eliminating waste and unnecessary medical procedures.

**Manic episodes** Episodes of extremely inflated mood and excitability.

**Marijuana** A drug, derived from the *Cannabis sativa* plant, with relaxant and mild hallucinogenic effects.

**Mast cell** Cell that lines the mucous membranes and connective tissue, such as skin and body-lining tissue; secretes histamines in response to allergens.

**Mastectomy** Surgical removal of the breast.

**Masturbation** Sexual self-stimulation.

**Matching hypothesis** The concept that people tend to develop romantic relationships with people who are similar to themselves in attractiveness.

**Maximal oxygen consumption ($VO_2$ max)** The maximum amount of oxygen the body is able to take in and consume.

**Maximum heart rate** The fastest rate that the heart should beat during exercise.

**MDMA** Known popularly as "ecstasy," a designer drug that is an amphetamine analogue.

**Measles** Highly contagious viral infection of the respiratory tract, characterized by red spots.

**Medicaid** A federal program that provides health care benefits to the poor.

**Medical examiner** An official, trained as a physician, who performs autopsies in deaths suspected of resulting from unnatural causes.

**Medical quackery** Medical fraud or fakery; use of products or practices lacking any legitimate basis for claims of medical effectiveness.

**Medicare** A federal program providing health care coverage for older Americans and people with disabilities.

**Medigap policy** An insurance policy with a private carrier that fills gaps in Medicare coverage.

**Meditation** A method of focused attention that induces a state of relaxation.

**Megadoses** Extremely high doses of a drug or substance.

**Melanin** Pigment that gives color to skin and hair and other body tissues.

**Melanoma** Cancer of the melanin-containing cells of the skin.

**Melatonin** A hormone produced by the pineal gland that is believed to play a role in regulating the sleep-wake cycle.

**Memory cells** T-cells or B-cells that recognize and dispose of reintroduced antigens, sometimes years after initial infection.

**Menopause** The cessation of menstruation.

**Menstrual phase** The fourth phase of the menstrual cycle, during which the endometrium is sloughed off in the menstrual flow.

**Menstruation** The cyclical bleeding that stems from the shedding of the uterine lining (endometrium).

**Mercury** A silver-white metallic element that is liquid at ordinary temperatures.

**Mescaline** A hallucinogenic drug derived from the peyote cactus.

**Mesoderm** The central layer of the embryo from which the bones and muscles develop.

**Metastases** Secondary tumors that arise from the primary growth and spread to another part of the body.

**Methadone** A synthetic opiate that is used as a substitute for heroin in the treatment of heroin addiction.

**Methaqualone** A type of sedative drug with addictive properties; can induce coma when ingested in large doses.

**Microorganism** Any microscopic entity capable of carrying on life processes.

**Microwaves** A type of nonionizing radiation, characterized by extremely high-frequency electromagnetic waves; cause molecules to vibrate rapidly, producing heat.

**Migraine headache** A type of severe headache characterized by piercing or throbbing sensations on one side of the head.

**Minerals** Inorganic elements obtained from the food we eat that are essential to survival.

**Minilaparotomy** Tubal sterilization in which a small incision is made in the abdomen to provide access to the Fallopian tubes.

**Minipill** A birth-control pill that contains synthetic progesterone but no estrogen.

**Miscarriage** The sudden, involuntary expulsion of the embryo or fetus from the uterus before it is capable of independent life. Also called spontaneous abortion.

**Monoclonal antibodies** Manufactured antibodies capable of identifying antigens on cancer cells.

**Monozygotic (MZ) twins** Twins that develop from the same fertilized egg cell and thus share identical genes. Also called identical twins.

**Mons veneris** A mound of fatty tissue that covers the joint of the pubic bones, below the abdomen and above the clitoris.

**Mood disorders** Mood disturbances that affect a person's ability to function effectively or are unduly prolonged or severe.

**Morbidity** Prevalence of disease.

**Morning sickness** A symptom of pregnancy; may include nausea, food aversions, and vomiting.

**Morphine** A narcotic drug, one of the most powerful derivatives of the opium poppy.

**Mortality** Death rate.

**Motility** Self-propulsion. A measure of the viability of sperm cells.

**Mourning** The ways of expressing grief in accordance with the customs of a particular culture.

**Mucous membranes** Membranous linings of bodily passageways or cavities.

**Mucus** Thick, sticky fluid containing immune cells secreted by the mucous membranes.

**Multiple sclerosis (MS)** A central nervous system disorder; the myelin coating that insulates nerve cells is damaged or destroyed.

**Muscle atrophy** A deterioration or loss of muscle tone.

**Muscle endurance** The ability to contract muscles repeatedly over time.

**Muscle hypertrophy** Increase in the size of muscle cells, resulting in increased muscle size.

**Muscle strength** The amount of force, or power, that one or more muscles can apply in a single contraction.

**Muscle tone** The degree of firmness in a muscle. A certain amount of muscle tone is needed for a muscle to perform.

**Muscles** Cells grouped in long, slender bundles called muscle fibers that contract to move an organ or part of the body.

**Musculoskeletal system** The system of bones, muscles, and linking connective tissue, such as tendons, ligaments, and cartilage.

**Mutagen** Any substance that causes genetic mutations.

**Mutate** To undergo mutation, a change in genetic structure.

**Mutations** A change in a cell's genetic structure that replicates in each cell division.

**Mutuality** A phase in building a relationship in which a couple come to regard themselves as "we."

**Myelin** A fatlike substance that coats the axons of certain neurons and helps smooth transmission of nervous impulses.

**Myocardial infarction (MI)** A condition involving damage or death of heart tissue due to an insufficient blood flow to the heart; usually the result of a blockage in one or more coronary arteries.

**Myocardium** The middle layer of the heart, consisting of the heart muscle.

**Myotonia** Muscle tension.

## N

**Naloxone** A drug that blocks the actions of opiates such as heroin, so that such drugs no longer produce a high when they are used.

**Narcotics** Drugs, primarily opiates, that have sleep-inducing and pain-relieving effects with a high potential for addiction.

**Natural childbirth** A method of childbirth in which women use no anesthesia but are given other strategies for coping with discomfort.

**Natural killer (NK) cells** White blood cells that can destroy viruses and tumor cells.

**Natural pesticides** Toxins produced by insects and plants that are used to eradicate pests.

**Naturally acquired active immunity (NAAI)** Immunity that follows illness; results from the natural production of antibodies against specific pathogens.

**Near-death experiences (NDEs)** Experiences reported by people who came close to dying or who were considered "clinically dead" but survived.

**Need** A state of want, or a condition arising from a deficiency status, such as hunger or thirst.

**Need for achievement** A psychological need to accomplish extrinsic goals, such as success and esteem.

**Neonate** A newborn child.

**Neural tube** The area in the embryo from which the nervous system will develop.

**Neurons** Nerve cells.

**Neurosyphilis** Syphilitic infection of the central nervous system; can cause brain damage and death.

**Neurotoxin** A toxin that produces adverse effects in the brain and central nervous system.

**Neurotransmitters** Chemical substances that transfer impulses from one neuron to another.

**Nicotine** A stimulant drug found naturally in tobacco.

**Nitrogen dioxide** A pollutant created by coal-burning electric power plants and the burning of fossil fuels in engines; irritates the respiratory system.

**Nitrosamines** Cancer-causing chemical substances formed in the stomach following ingestion of nitrates and nitrites.

**Nodules** Small nodes or swellings.

**Noise** Loud, harsh, or noxious sound.

**Nonbiodegradable** Substances that, when disposed of, do not decompose.

**Non-Hodgkin's lymphomas** All forms of lymphoma other than Hodgkin's disease.

**Noninsulin-dependent diabetes mellitus (NIDM) (adult-onset or Type II diabetes)** Diabetes that usually develops in middle or later life; involves a breakdown in the body's use of insulin.

**Nonionizing radiation** Radiation that does not cause atoms to become ions, e.g., sunlight and radiation emitted by electrical appliances.

**Nonmelanoma skin cancers** Skin cancers other than melanoma, including basal cell and squamous cell carcinomas.

**Noradrenaline** A hormone produced by the adrenal medulla; has chemical properties similar to adrenaline. In the nervous system, noradrenaline functions as a neurotransmitter.

**Nosocomial infections** Infections acquired in hospitals.

**Nuclear medicine** The medical use of radiation in the diagnosis and treatment of illness.

**Nutrients** Essential substances in food that our bodies need but are incapable of producing on their own.

**Nutrition** The process by which plants and animals ingest and utilize food.

**Obesity** A condition of excess body fat.

**Obsessive-compulsive disorder (OCD)** An anxiety disorder characterized by obsessions (nagging, intrusive thoughts or images) and/or compulsions (repetitive behaviors that the person feels compelled to perform).

**Ocular herpes** A herpes infection of the eye.

**Oncogenes** Genes involved in normal processes of cell growth and regulation, may give rise to cancerous growths if subjected to mutations or viral influences.

**Oncologists** Medical doctors who specialize in the diagnosis and treatment of cancer.

**Oncology** The branch of medical science dealing with the study of cancer.

**Oophorectomy** Surgical removal of one or both ovaries.

**Ophthalmia neonatorum** A gonorrheal infection of the eyes of newborns; contracted by passing through an infected birth canal.

**Opiates** Narcotics defived from the opium poppy or synthesized to have opiatelike properties and effects.

**Opium** A narcotic drug derived from the opium poppy.

**Opportunistic infections** Infections caused by organisms that flourish because of a weakness in the immune system.

**Optimism** The tendency to look on the more favorable aspects of events or future possibilities.

**Oral contraceptive** A contraceptive consisting of sex hormones that is taken by mouth.

**Organochlorines** A class of petrochemicals, including some pesticides and other toxic substances, with a wide range of industrial uses.

**Organophosphates** Chemical compounds, many of which are toxic, used as pesticides and as chemical weapons.

**Orgasmic phase** The third phase of the sexual response cycle, characterized by the rhythmic contractions of orgasm.

**Osteoarthritis** A chronic degenerative form of arthritis linked to wear and tear on the joints.

**Osteoporosis** A degenerative condition characterized by the loss of bone density, which makes bones more brittle and prone to break.

**Ovaries** Organs that produce ova and the hormones estrogen and progesterone.

**Over-the-counter (OTC) drugs** Drugs available for sale without a prescription.

**Overloading** The gradual increasing of the burden placed on the body to achieve a training effect.

**Overweight** A body weight exceeding desirable weight for a person of a given age, height, and body frame, usually based on the criterion of 20% above desirable weight.

**Ovulation** The release of an ovum from an ovary.

**Ovulation method** A fertility awareness method of contraception that relies on prediction of ovulation by tracking the viscosity of the cervical mucus.

**Ovulatory phase** The second stage of the menstrual cycle during which a follicle ruptures and releases a mature ovum.

**Oxytocin** A pituitary hormone that stimulates uterine contractions.

**Ozone** A highly reactive form of oxygen toxic even at low levels in inhaled air.

**Ozone Layer** The ozone-rich layer of the earth's upper atmosphere that helps to limit the amount of ultraviolet radiation that reaches the earth.

**Palliative care** Treatment focused on the relief or reduction of pain and suffering rather than cure.

**Palpate** To examine by touch.

**Pancreas** A gland located near the stomach that secretes a digestive fluid into the intestines and manufactures the hormone insulin.

**Pandemic** An epidemic affecting a whole country, a continent, or the entire world.

**Panic disorder** An anxiety disorder characterized by episodes of sheer terror, called panic attacks, and by the fear of such attacks occurring again.

**Pap test or Pap smear** The scraping of a "smear" of cells from the vagina and cervix for microscopic examination to reveal cancer.

**Parasites** Organisms that live within or on the surface of other organisms; they do not benefit their host.

**Parasitic worms** *(helminths)* Multicellular parasites or worms.

**Parasympathetic branch** The branch of the autonomic nervous system involved in processes such as digestion that preserve and replenish energy stores.

**Particle radiation** Radiation consisting of the emission of subatomic matter, such as protons, neutrons, and electrons.

**Particulate matter** Dust, soot, ash, and other tiny solid particles.

**Passive carriers** Persons who harbor infectious organisms, do not exhibit symptoms, but are capable of infecting others.

**Passive euthanasia** The withholding or withdrawal of life-sustaining treatment to hasten death.

**Passive immunity** Temporary immunity created by introducing antibodies from another person or animal; also present at birth for about six months.

**Pathogenic** Disease-causing.

**Pathogens** Disease-causing organisms, including bacteria, viruses, fungi (yeasts and molds), and animal parasites such as insects and worms.

**Patriarchy** A form of social organization in which the father or eldest male runs the group or family. More broadly, government, rule, or domination by men.

**Peak days** The days during the menstrual cycle during which a woman is most likely to be fertile.

**Peak experience** A moment of intense joy and personal satisfaction arising from self-actualization.

**Pediculosis** A parasitic infestation by pubic lice *(Pthirus pubis);* causes itching.

**Pedophilia** A type of sexual disorder characterized by sexual attraction to children.

**Pellagra** A deficiency disorder caused by a lack of the vitamin niacin. Characterized by skin eruptions, diarrhea, neurological disturbances, and psychological problems involving anxiety, depression, and memory deficits for recent events.

**Pelvic inflammatory disease (PID)** Inflammation of the pelvic region that can be caused by organisms such as gonococcus bacterium; may lead to infertility.

**Penis** The male organ that becomes erect during sexual arousal and through which sperm and urine pass.

**Perceived risk** The amount of risk posed by a factor or factors as perceived by individuals.

**Percutaneous transluminal coronary angioplasty (PTCA)** *(balloon angioplasty)* Widening a blocked artery by inflating a tiny balloon within the artery, compressing the blockage against the artery wall.

**Performance anxiety** Anxiety stemming from an overconcern with the quality of one's performance.

**Perianal** Surrounding the anus.

**Pericardial cavity** The moistened sac that contains the heart.

**Perineum** The area between the vulva and the anus.

**Peripheral nervous system** One of the two major parts of the nervous system; consists of the nerves that connect the brain and spinal cord to the internal organs, skin, and muscles.

**Personality** The constellation of traits, attitudes, dispositions, and behavioral patterns that constitutes our individuality.

**Pertussis** *(whooping cough)* Acute upper-respiratory childhood disease caused by the bacterium *B. pertussis*.

**Petrochemicals** Substances refined from fossil fuels, especially petroleum and natural gas.

**pH level** The degree of acidity or alkalinity of a substance.

**Phagocytes** A major class of white blood cells that seek out and destroy antigens in the bloodstream.

**Pharmacology** The study of drugs and their role in medicine.

**Pharmacy** The discipline relating to the preparation and dispensing of drugs.

**Pharyngeal gonorrhea** A gonorrheal infection characterized by a sore throat.

**Phencyclidine (PCP)** Commonly called "angel dust," a deliriant drug with unpredictable and sometimes dangerous effects.

**Phenylketonuria** A genetic disorder involving inability to break down the amino acid phenylalanine. Abbreviated PKU.

**Phobia** An excessive or irrational fear.

**Photoaging** Skin wrinkling caused by exposure to ultraviolet rays.

**Photosynthesis** The process by which plants use sunlight to produce carbohydrates from carbon dioxide and water.

**Physical activity** Any demand made on muscles beyond the resting state.

**Physical health** Soundness of body.

**Physiological dependence** A state of bodily need for a drug, evidenced by the appearance of characteristic withdrawal symptoms upon abrupt cessation of use of the drug.

**Phytochemicals** Naturally occurring plant chemicals.

**Pinworm** A helminth that causes an infection of the intestines and rectum.

**Pituitary gland** A brain structure dubbed the "master gland" that secretes hormones involved in growth, regulation of the menstrual cycle, and childbirth.

**Placenta** An organ connected to the fetus by the umbilical cord. The placenta serves as a relay station between mother and fetus, allowing the exchange of nutrients and wastes.

**Plaque** Fatty deposits that accumulate along the inner walls of arteries.

**Plateau phase** The second phase of the sexual response cycle, characterized by increases in vasocongestion, muscle tension, heart rate, and blood pressure in preparation for orgasm.

**Platelets** Round or oval disks in the blood that help blood clot when there is a wound or injury.

**Pneumonia** Acute infectious disease of the respiratory tract; causes fluids to collect in air sacs in the lungs.

**Point of service (POS)** An HMO that allows members to choose in-network doctors at low cost or outside doctors at higher cost.

**Polio** Poliomyelitis, a viral disease affecting the spinal cord and the brain; can lead to muscular degeneration, paralysis, and deformity.

**Pollution** Contamination or tainting of the environment.

**Polyabusers** People with drug abuse problems involving two or more drugs.

**Polychlorinated biphenyls (PCBs)** Highly toxic organochlorines used in various manufacturing processes, but now banned in the U.S.

**Polyps** Bulging masses of tissue, which may become cancerous.

**Postpartum** Following birth.

**Postpartum depression (PPD)** Persistent and severe mood changes during the postpartum period, involving feelings of despair and apathy and characterized by changes in appetite and sleep, low self-esteem, and difficulty concentrating.

**Posttraumatic stress disorder (PTSD)** A psychological disorder involving a maladaptive reaction to a traumatic experience. Onset may be delayed until months or years after the traumatic event.

**Potentiate** Relating to drugs, to enhance a drug's effects or potency.

**Power rape** A rape motivated primarily by the desire to exercise power or control over the victim.

**Preferred provider organizations (PPOs)** A group of health care providers who agree to provide services to members of a managed care plan for a discounted rate.

**Premature ejaculation** A sexual dysfunction in which ejaculation occurs too rapidly or with minimal sexual stimulation.

**Premenstrual syndrome (PMS)** Physical and psychological symptoms that afflict many women during the days before their menstrual period.

**Prenatal anoxia** Oxygen deprivation.

**Prepuce** The fold of skin covering the glans of the clitoris (or penis).

**Presbycusis** Hearing loss, especially in the higher frequencies, that accompanies aging.

**Presbyopia** Loss of elasticity in the lens of the eye; diminishes ability to focus on small, close objects.

**Preterm** Born before 37 weeks of gestation.

**Primary care physician** A physician who provides a patient with regular, ongoing medical care and makes recommendations to specialists when the need arises.

**Primary tumor** The original site of a tumor or growth.

**Private risk** The risk associated with a factor that we can control voluntarily.

**Proctoscope** Instrument used to examine the rectum.

**Prodromal stage** The initial stage of a disease before the onset of acute symptoms.

**Progesterone** A steroid hormone involved in regulation of the menstrual cycle.

**Progressive muscle relaxation** A form of relaxation training that achieves the reduction of muscle tension through a series of tensing and relaxing exercises involving selected muscle groups.

**Proliferative phase** The first phase of the menstrual cycle during which the endometrium proliferates.

**Prophylactic** An agent that protects against disease.

**Prostaglandins** Hormones that play a role in the transmission of pain messages to the brain; also stimulate uterine contractions.

**Prostate gland** The gland that lies beneath the bladder and secretes prostatic fluid, which gives semen its characteristic odor and texture.

**Prostate-specific antigen (PSA)** An enzyme produced in the epithelial cells of the prostate gland. Abnormally high blood levels of PSA may indicate prostate cancer.

**Prostatitis** Inflammation of the prostate gland.

**Proteins** Organic molecules that form the basic building blocks of body tissues.

**Protozoa** Self-contained single-cell parasites that thrive in water.

**Proximodistal** From the central axis of the body outward.

**Pseudoephedrine** A sympathomimetic drug used as a nasal decongestant.

**Psilocybin** A hallucinogenic drug derived from certain types of mushrooms.

**Psychedelics** Hallucinogenic drugs that have been used in religious ceremonies among Native American peoples and others for their mind-expanding and hallucinogenic effects.

**Psychiatric hospitals** Specialized hospitals providing inpatient psychiatric services.

**Psychiatrists** Physicians who specialize in the practice of psychiatry.

**Psychoactive drugs** Drugs that act on the brain to affect mental processes.

**Psychoanalysis** The type of therapy developed by Sigmund Freud that helps people achieve insight into unconscious processes and conflicts that are believed to give rise to psychological problems.

**Psychoanalyst** A practitioner of psychoanalysis, the method of therapy that focuses on probing the childhood roots of emotional problems.

**Psychological dependence** A pattern of compulsive or habitual use of a drug indicating impaired control over the use of the drug but without physiological signs of dependence.

**Psychological disorder** A disturbance of psychological functioning resulting in emotional distress or impaired functioning (also called a mental disorder or mental illness).

**Psychological hardiness** A cluster of traits, characterized by commitment, challenge, and control, that buffer the effects of stress.

**Psychological health** Soundness of mind, characterized by a cluster of characteristics such as accurate perceptions, clear thinking, emotional stability, and adaptive behavior.

**Psychoneuroimmunology** The scientific study of interrelationships among stress and the body's nervous system, immune system, and endocrine system.

**Psychotherapy** Therapy involving a systematic interaction between a patient and a therapist based on the application of psychological principles.

**Psychotic disorder** A psychological disorder involving symptoms that indicate a break with reality, such as hallucinations and delusions.

**Psychotropics** Psychoactive drugs used in the treatment of psychological or mental disorders.

**Public risk** The risk associated with a factor in the environment to which we are involuntarily exposed.

**Pulmonary artery** The artery carrying deoxygenated blood from the right ventricle of the heart to the lungs.

**Pus** A yellowish liquidy substance that results from inflammation.

## Q

**Quality-adjusted life years (QALY)** Years of healthy life.

## R

**Rabies** A viral disease that primarily affects the central nervous system; can lead to paralysis and death if not treated immediately.

**Rad** Short for *radiation absorbed dose,* a measure of exposure to radiation; represents the amount of ionizing radiation that a body absorbs per unit mass of matter.

**Radiation** The emission of energy in the form of particles or waves.

**Radiation sickness** Illness caused by overexposure to radiation; may be fatal at high levels.

**Radiation therapy** Use of high-energy X-rays to eradicate or shrink cancerous growths.

**Radical hysterectomy** The surgical removal of cervix, uterus, Fallopian tubes, ovaries, part of the vagina, and possibly nearby lymph nodes.

**Radical prostatectomy** Surgical removal of the entire prostate gland.

**Radioisotope** A radioactive form of an element; some are used in medical diagnosis and treatment.

**Radionuclide imaging** A specialized scanning device detects blockages of blood flow in and around the heart by tracking the movement of radioactive substances injected into the bloodstream.

**Radon** An invisible, odorless radioactive gas emitted from the natural decay of uranium; may pass from the soil into our homes.

**Rational suicide** Suicide based on a rational decision that life is not worth living in light of current suffering.

**Rational-emotive therapy** A cognitive therapy that focuses on helping people dispute and correct irrational thinking.

**Reaction time** Time it takes to respond to a stimulus.

**Receptors** The sites on receiving neurons where neurotransmitters "dock."

**Recessive trait** A trait that is not expressed when the gene or genes involved have been paired with dominant genes.

**Reciprocity** Mutual exchange.

**Rectum** The terminal portion of the intestine, ending in the anus, the opening through which solid waste is excreted.

**Reflexology** The practice of massaging parts of the foot to relieve stress or pain in other parts of the body.

**Refractory period** A period of time following a response (e.g., orgasm) during which an individual is no longer responsive to stimulation (e.g., sexual stimulation).

**Rehabilitation centers** Health care facilities providing comprehensive services to help people with disabilities achieve a maximum level of functioning and a more satisfying and independent life.

**Relapse** The recurrence of a disorder or problem behavior.

**Relapse prevention training** Psychological techniques aimed at preventing relapse.

**Relaxation response** A state of relaxation brought about by meditation that is characterized by a slowing down of metabolism and a lowering of blood pressure in people with hypertension.

**Relaxation training** Techniques aimed at helping people learn to relax.

**REM sleep** The stage of sleep characterized by rapid eye movements under the sleeper's closed eyelids; associated with dreaming.

**Remission** A lessening of severity or abatement of the symptoms of a disease.

**Repetition maximum (RM)** The maximum amount of force a person is able to exert in one repetition.

**Repression** A defense mechanism, described as motivated forgetting, by which the unconscious mind banishes troubling ideas or impulses from awareness.

**Resistance stage** The body attempts to conserve its resources in an attempt to cope with prolonged stress. Also called the adaptation stage.

**Resistance training** Muscle training involving repeated movement or lifting against an opposing force or weight.

**Resolution phase** The fourth phase of the sexual response cycle, during which the body gradually returns to its prearoused state.

**Respiratory distress syndrome** A cluster of breathing problems, including weak and irregular breathing, to which preterm babies are especially prone.

**Resting heart rate** The number of times per minute the heart beats at rest.

**Resting metabolic rate (RMR)** The minimum energy that the body requires to maintain bodily functions including digestion.

**Reye's syndrome** A potentially fatal brain disease that can follow a viral infection, most commonly in children.

**Rh incompatibility** A condition in which antibodies produced by a pregnant woman are transmitted to the fetus and may cause brain damage or death.

**Rheumatic fever** An inflammatory disease that may follow a streptococcal infection; may damage the heart valves and kidneys.

**Rheumatoid arthritis** Chronic inflammatory form of arthritis; the membranes lining the joints become inflamed, resulting in swelling, stiffness, and pain.

**Rhinoviruses** A class of small RNA viruses that are the major causes of the common cold.

**RICE principle** A program of rest, ice, compression, and elevation used in the treatment of exercise-related injuries.

**Rickets** A bone disorder in children resulting from a lack of vitamin D. Can lead to skeletal deformities and disturbances in growth.

**Rickettsiae** Bacterialike organisms that grow inside insects and other parasites; transmitted to humans via bites by lice, fleas, ticks, and mites.

**Rigor mortis** The stiffening of the muscles that occurs several hours after death.

**Ringworm** A fungal skin infection characterized by red patches, itching, and scaling.

**Risk assessment** A procedure for assessing the relative health risk of various hazards.

**Risk factors** Factors that indicate an increased risk of developing a particular disease or disorder.

**Rocky Mountain spotted fever** A tick-borne disease caused by *Rickettsia rickettsii;* produces fever, skin eruptions, and pain in the joints, bones, and muscles.

**Rubella** A viral infection that can cause mental retardation and heart disease in an embryo. Also called German measles.

## S

**Sadistic rape** A savage rape in which the victim is subjected to painful and humiliating experiences and events, sometimes including ritualized acts of torture.

**Sarcoma** Cancer originating in connective tissues of the body.

**Scabies** A parasitic infestation caused by a tiny mite *(Sarcoptes scabiei);* causes itching.

**Scarlet fever** A contagious streptococcal infection characterized by sore throat, scarlet rash, and fever.

**Schistosomiasis** A water-borne infection caused by a worm called a fluke.

**Schizophrenia** An enduring psychotic disorder involving disturbances in thought processes, perception, emotion, and behavior.

**Scrotum** The pouch of loose skin that contains the testes.

**Scurvy** A deficiency disorder resulting from a lack of vitamin C. Characterized by swollen and bleeding gums, weakness, loss of energy, and loosening of teeth.

**Seasonal affective disorder (SAD)** A type of major depression involving episodes of severe depression during the fall and winter months, followed by elevated mood in spring and summer.

**Sebaceous glands** Glands in the skin that produce oily secretions.

**Sebum** A fatty secretion of the sebaceous glands of the skin.

**Second-hand smoking** Ingestion of tobacco smoke from other people's lit cigarettes.

**Secondary air pollution** Pollution produced by chemical interactions involving primary pollutants.

**Secondary tumors** *(metastases)* Cancerous growths that arise from the primary tumor, and spread to other locations.

**Sedative** A central nervous system depressant that has calming and relaxing effects.

**Seizure** A sudden attack involving a disruption of brain electrical rhythms, as in the type of convulsive seizure occurring during epileptic attacks.

**Self-actualization** A tendency to strive to realize one's potential.

**Self-assertiveness** Expression of one's feeling and beliefs in a way that is true to oneself.

**Self-concept** One's perception of oneself.

**Self-disclosure** The revelation of personal, perhaps intimate, information.

**Self-esteem** A sense of self-worth or self-approval.

**Self-help group** A group of people with a common psychological problem whose members help each other cope.

**Semen** The whitish fluid that constitutes the ejaculate, consisting of sperm and glandular secretions.

**Seminal vesicles** Small glands that lie behind the bladder and secrete fluids that combine with sperm in the ejaculatory ducts.

**Sensation-seeking** The tendency to seek exciting or highly stimulating activities that heighten one's physical sensations.

**Serial monogamy** A pattern of involvement in one exclusive relationship after another, as opposed to engaging in multiple sexual relationships at the same time.

**Serology** Laboratory analysis of blood serum.

**Serotonin** A neurotransmitter involved in regulating motor functions that is also linked to depression.

**Set point theory** The theory that an individual's body weight is genetically set at a given weight range, or set point, that the body works to maintain.

**Sexual differentiation** The process by which males and females develop distinct reproductive anatomy.

**Sexual dysfunctions** Persistent difficulties with sexual interest, arousal, or response.

**Sexual harassment** Unwelcome comments, gestures, demands, overtures, or physical contact of a sexual nature.

**Sexual orientation** The direction of one's sexual interests toward members of the same gender, the opposite gender, or both genders.

**Sexual response cycle** The four-phase model of sexual response.

**Sexually transmitted diseases** *(STDs)* Diseases that are communicated through sexual contact.

**Shigellosis** An STD caused by the *Shigella* bacterium.

**Shin splints** Injuries that involve tears in muscle fibers.

**Shyness** A quality of timidness or reserve around other people.

**Sickle-cell anemia** An inherited blood disorder that afflicts mainly African Americans. Deformed sickle-shaped blood cells obstruct small blood vessels, decreasing their capacity to carry oxygen.

**Sigmoidoscope** A flexible tubular instrument used for examining the colon.

**Sigmoidoscopy** Insertion of a hollow flexible lighted tube (the sigmoidosope) into the lower colon to detect polyps.

**Simple carbohydrates** A class of carbohydrates consisting of small molecules, including various sugars.

**Skeletal muscles** The muscles attached to the bones of the skeleton.

**Skinfold thickness** The thickness of the folds of skin, usually of the underarms, waist, or back, that is used to estimate the percentage of body fat.

**Sleep apnea** A condition characterized by a temporary cessation of breathing during sleep.

**Sliding scale** A system for adjusting fees according to the individual's income level.

**Small talk** A superficial kind of conversation that stresses breadth of topic coverage rather than in-depth discussion.

**Smallpox** A devastating viral disease, now eradicated, that produced high fever and skin eruptions.

**Smegma** A secretion that accumulates under the foreskin or around the clitoris.

**Smoker's face** A characteristic wrinkling of the face around the lips and eyes due to smoke.

**Snuff** A powdered form of tobacco that can be inhaled through the nose or sucked when placed inside the cheek.

**Social health** The ability to relate effectively to family members, intimate partners, friends, and work associates.

**Social phobia** Fear of social interactions.

**Socialization** The process of guiding people into socially acceptable behavior patterns by means of information, rewards, and punishments.

**Socioeconomic status (SES)** Relative position in terms of education and economic standing.

**Sodium** A metallic element that functions as an electrolyte in the body.

**Solid waste** Waste in the form of garbage or refuse.

**Soluble fibers** Types of dietary fiber that are dissolvable in water.

**Solvents** Chemical liquids that dissolve other substances.

**Soma** A cell body.

**Somatic nervous system** The part of the peripheral nervous system that involves the voluntary control of skeletal muscles and feeds information from the sense organs to the brain.

**Specific phobias** Phobias involving specific objects or situations, such as fear of enclosed spaces (claustrophobia) or of small animals or insects.

**Speculum** A medical instrument used to enlarge openings of body canals or cavities to allow inspection of the inner areas.

**Sperm** The male germ cell.

**Spina bifida** A congenital defect in which the child is born with a hole in the tube that surrounds the spinal cord.

**Spiritual health** Finding a higher level of meaning in life by connecting to social, religious, or aesthetic experiences beyond oneself.

**Spleen** A lymphatic organ that produces lymphocytes, destroys worn-out red blood cells, and acts as a reservoir for blood.

**Sprains** Sudden joint twists that stretch or tear ligaments, the tough fibrous tissue connecting bone to bone.

**Squamous cell carcinoma** Another form of nonmelanoma skin cancer; easily curable if treated early.

**Staff model HMO** An HMO that offers comprehensive services only in a center with its own health care professionals.

**Staining method** Colored dyes are mixed with bacteria-laden cells. The way a stain binds to cells helps with bacterial identification.

**Staphylococci** A type of bacteria that causes infections such as food poisoning, urinary tract infections, and toxic shock syndrome.

**Starch** A complex carbohydrate that forms an important part of the structure of plants such as corn, rice, wheat, potatoes, and beans.

**Static stretching** Stretching in which muscles are fully extended and then gradually stretched to the limit of the joint movement.

**Statutory rape** Sexual intercourse with a person who is below the age of consent, even if the person cooperates.

**Sterilization** Surgical procedures that render people incapable of reproduction without affecting sexual response.

**Stillbirth** The birth of a dead fetus.

**Stimulants** Psychoactive drugs that increase the level of activity of the central nervous system.

**Strains** Stretches ("muscle pulls") or actual tears in muscle fibers or surrounding tissue.

**Stranger rape** Rape committed by an assailant previously unknown to the victim.

**Strep throat** A bacterial infection caused by streptococcal bacteria; characterized by a painful and reddish sore throat, fever, ear pain, and enlarged lymph nodes. May occur without noticeable symptoms.

**Streptococci** A type of bacteria, some of which cause various infections, including strep throat and certain types of pneumonia.

**Stress** In human terms, stress refers to pressures that require a person to adjust.

**Stress fractures** Microscopic breaks in bones caused by repeated and excessive pressure or pounding.

**Stress test** A method of evaluating cardiorespiratory fitness by measuring oxygen consumption and heart functioning in response to increasingly stressful physical demands during exercise, usually on a treadmill or stationary bicycle.

**Stressors** Sources of stress.

**Stroke** Destruction of brain tissue resulting from the blockage of a blood vessel or bleeding in the brain. Also called cerebrovascular accident (CVA).

**Sugar** A simple carbohydrate present in different forms in many of the foods we eat.

**Sulfur dioxide** A suffocating gas formed from the burning of sulfur; produced by coal-burning electric power plants and motor vehicle exhaust.

**Suppressant** A cough remedy ingredient that inhibits the coughing reflex.

**Suppressor genes** Genes that curb cell division and suppress tumor development.

**Suppressor T-cells** Immune cells that regulate the activities of T- and B-lymphocytes; prevent damage to healthy cells.

**Surface contact** A probing phase of building a relationship in which people seek common ground and check out feelings of attraction.

**Surface water** Water found overground in ponds, lakes, rivers, streams, and reservoirs.

**Surfactants** Substances that prevent the walls of the airways from sticking together.

**Surrogate mother** A woman who is impregnated through artificial insemination with the sperm of a prospective father, carries the baby to term, and then gives it to the prospective parents.

**Symmetry** A condition of likeness in both halves.

**Sympathetic branch** The branch of the autonomic nervous system that accelerates bodily processes and releases stores of energy needed for physical exertion; activated as part of the alarm reaction to stress.

**Sympathetic pregnancy** The experiencing of signs of pregnancy by the father.

**Sympathomimetic** An agent that activates the sympathetic nervous system.

**Synaptic cleft** The gap or junction between neurons through which nerve impulses pass.

**Synergistic effect** As applied to drug interactions, the action of two or more drugs operating together to enhance the overall effect to a level greater than the sum of the effects of each drug operating by itself.

**Synthetic pesticides** Manufactured or synthesized pest-killing substances, including insecticides, herbicides, and fungicides.

**Synthetic pyrethroid** A pesticide lethal to insects but with low toxicity to humans.

**Syphilis** A sexually transmitted disease caused by the Treponema pallidum bacterium; may progress from a chancre to a skin rash to damage to the cardiovascular and central nervous systems.

**Systematic desensitization** A behavior therapy technique for overcoming phobias by means of a series of imagined encounters with feared objects or stimuli while the person remains deeply relaxed.

## T

**T-cells** Lymphocytes that mature in the thymus and aid the body's response to antigens.

**Tachycardia** An abnormally rapid heart rate.

**Tar** The sticky residue in tobacco smoke, containing many carcinogens and other toxins.

**Tardive dyskinesia** A potentially irreversible disorder involving involuntary movement that arises from long-term use of certain antipsychotic drugs such as Thorazine and Mellaril.

**Target heart rate range** The range of heartbeats per minute during vigorous exercise that is sufficient to overload the heart but not so intense as to be anaerobic. Range is between 60 and 85% of the person's maximum heart rate.

**Target organ** An organ susceptible to damage by particular chemicals.

**Tay-Sachs disease** A fatal neurological disorder that primarily afflicts Jews of Eastern European origin.

**Tendinitis** Inflammation of tendons.

**Tendons** Fibrous connective tissue that connects muscles to bones and other body parts.

**Teratogens** Environmental influences or agents that can damage an embryo or fetus.

**Terminal knobs** The structures at the end of axon terminals containing sacs of neurotransmitters.

**Terminals** The small branching structures at the tips of axons.

**Testes** The male gonads, which produce sperm and the male sex hormone testosterone.

**Testosterone** The male sex hormone that fosters the development of male sex characteristics and is connected with the sex drive.

**Tetanus** An acute infection caused when bacteria-laden spores enter the body through breaks in the skin.

**Thanatologist** A scholar of thanatology, the interdisciplinary study of death and dying.

**Therapeutic massage** The therapeutic use of rubbing and kneading the body to improve circulation, increase suppleness, and promote relaxation.

**Thermal biofeedback** Temperature devices called thermistors relay changes in temperature in selected areas of the user's body.

**Thermogenesis** The production of heat, generally within the body.

**Thrombus** A blood clot that blocks a blood vessel or cavity of the heart.

**Thymus** A lymphatic organ in which T-cells mature.

**Thyroid gland** An endocrine gland lying on both sides of the windpipe; produces thyroxin, a hormone involved in regulating body metabolism and growth.

**Tibia** The inner and larger of the two bones in the leg, extending from the knee to the ankle.

**Tobacco** A member of a family of plants containing nicotine, its leaves are prepared for smoking, chewing, or use as snuff.

**Tolerance** A feature of drug dependence in which the user comes to need larger amounts of the drug to achieve the same effect.

**Toxemia** A life-threatening condition during pregnancy that is characterized by high blood pressure.

**Toxic shock syndrome (TSS)** A rare and sometimes fatal bacterial infection linked to tampon use.

**Toxicity** The quality or degree of being poisonous.

**Toxins** Poisonous chemical substances that damage cells, tissues, and organs.

**Trachea** The tube that carries air between the larynx and the bronchial tubes; also called the windpipe.

**Trachoma** A chronic form of conjunctivitis (inflammation of the mucous membrane of the eyelids) caused by a strain of chlamydia.

**Training** (also called conditioning) The body's gradual adjustment to increasingly demanding levels of repetitive and progressive movements.

**Training effect** The benefits to the heart, lungs, muscles, and bones produced by overloading.

**Trans-fatty acid** A type of fatty acid produced in the hardening process of margarine that can raise blood cholesterol levels.

**Transcendental meditation (TM)** An adaptation of an Indian meditation technique involving the repetition of a mantra with each outbreath.

**Transference** A relationship a person develops with a therapist or other figure that represents a reenactment of an earlier conflicted relationship.

**Transition** The process during which the cervix becomes nearly fully dilated and the head of the fetus begins to move into the birth canal.

**Transsexual** A person who has a gender-identity disorder and who feels trapped in the body of the wrong gender.

**Transvaginal sonography (TVS)** Imaging technique using ultrasonic sound waves to assess a woman's inner reproductive organs.

**Transverse position** A crosswise birth position.

**Trichomoniasis** Vaginitis caused by the protozoan *Trichomonas vaginalis*.

**Triglycerides** Common fats found in the bloodstream, derived from fats and carbohydrates in food.

**Tubal ligation** The Fallopian tubes are surgically blocked to prevent the meeting of sperm and ova.

**Tuberculosis (TB)** Bacterial infection that usually affects the lungs and sometimes other parts of the body, including the brain, kidneys, or spine.

**Tumor** A mass of excess body tissue or growth, which may or may not be cancerous.

**Tumor necrosis factor (TNF)** A naturally occurring body protein that can be lethal to cancer cells.

**Type A personality** A personality type characterized by impatience, time urgency, competitiveness, and hostility.

**Typhus** A group of infectious diseases especially prevalent among people living in unsanitary conditions; characterized by weakness, severe headache, and fever.

## U

**Ulcers** Open sores or lesions occurring in the skin or within body cavities such as the lining of the stomach and the small intestine.

**Ultrasound** The use of high-pitched sound waves bounced off the fetus to reveal its form.

**Ultrasound imaging** High-frequency sound waves are used to produce an image of organs or tissues.

**Ultraviolet (UV) radiation** Radiation from the sun in the form of sunlight.

**Ultraviolet A (UVA)** A form of ultraviolet radiation from sunlight that can damage the skin and eyes.

**Ultraviolet B (UVB)** A more dangerous form of ultraviolet radiation from sunlight that is principally responsible for sunburns.

**Umbilical cord** A tube that connects the fetus to the placenta.

**Unconditional positive regard** Unconditional acceptance of the intrinsic merit or worth of another person regardless of the person's behavior at the moment.

**Unconscious** Outside of awareness; in Freud's theory, unconscious conflicts of a sexual or aggressive nature lie at the root of psychological problems.

**Urethral opening** The opening through which urine passes from the female's body.

**Urethritis** An inflammation of the bladder or urethra.

**Urethritis** Inflammation of the urethra.

**Urogenital tract** Organs constituting the urinary and reproductive organs.

**Uterus** The hollow, muscular, pear-shaped organ in which a fertilized ovum implants and develops until birth.

## V

**Vaccination** A means of introducing a weakened or partial form of an infectious agent into the body so as to produce immunity without producing the full-blown illness.

**Vaccine** A substance containing killed or weakened bacterium, virus, or toxoid that stimulates the production of antibodies against these substances.

**Vacuum aspiration** Removal of the uterine contents by suction. An abortion method used early in pregnancy.

**Vagina** The tubular female sex organ that contains the penis during sexual intercourse and through which a baby is born.

**Vaginal ring** A contraceptive device shaped like a diaphragm that is worn in the vagina; slowly releases either a combination of estrogen and progestin or progestin only.

**Vaginismus** A sexual dysfunction characterized by involuntary contraction of the muscles surrounding the vagina, preventing penile penetration or rendering penetration painful.

**Vaginitis** Any type of vaginal infection or inflammation.

**Values** The worth or importance placed on objects or goals; standards of worth.

**Varicose veins** Abnormally enlarged or swollen veins, usually in the lower extremities.

**Vas deferens** A tube that conducts sperm from the testicle to the ejaculatory duct of the penis.

**Vasectomy** A sterilization procedure in which both vas deferens are severed, preventing sperm from reaching the ejaculatory duct.

**Vasocongestion** The swelling of the genital tissues with blood, which causes erection of the penis and engorgement of the area surrounding the vaginal opening.

**Vasodilators** Agents that expand (dilate) blood vessels, allowing blood to flow more freely.

**VDRL** A test for the presence of antibodies to *Treponema pallidum* in the blood.

**Vectors** Animal or insect carriers of infectious agents.

**Veins** Blood vessels that carry blood back to the heart.

**Vena cavae** The largest veins; carry blood directly into the heart.

**Ventricle** The lower chamber in each half of the heart.

**Ventricular fibrillation** Irregular contractions of the two ventricles of the heart; impairs the heart's ability to pump blood effectively.

**Very low calorie diet (VLCD)** A protein-sparing, low-calorie diet typically consisting of 800 calories or less.

**Virus** Particles consisting of a core of nucleic acid and a coat of protein; incapable of replicating outside living cells.

**Viscosity** Stickiness, consistency.

**Visualization** The use of mental imagery to achieve a therapeutic benefit.

**Vitamin deficiency syndromes** Deficiency disorders arising from deficiencies of various vitamins.

**Vitamins** Organic substances required in minute amounts to serve a variety of vital roles in metabolism, growth, and maintenance of bodily processes.

**Vulva** The external sexual structures of the female.

## W

**Warm-up** Mild exercise and stretching performed for 10 to 15 minutes prior to vigorous exercise.

**Wellness** A state of optimum health, characterized by active efforts to maximize one's physical health and well-being.

**Wernicke-Korsakoff's syndrome** A deficiency syndrome resulting from a lack of the vitamin thiamine; appears most often in alcoholics who neglect their diets. Characterized by memory loss and confusion.

**White blood cells** (*leukocytes*) Specialized immune cells in the blood, these are the front-line soldiers in the body's war against invading pathogens.

**Workaholics** People who are consumed by their work to the exclusion of personal relationships and leisure pursuits.

## X

**X-ray** High-energy, ionizing radiation; can penetrate most solid objects and project images on photographic film.

## Z

**Zero population growth** The level at which birth rates match death rates.

**Zero tolerance laws** Laws prohibiting underage persons from driving if they have any detectable level of alcohol in their blood.

**Zygote** A fertilized ovum.

**Zygote intrafallopian transfer (ZIFT)** A method of conception in which an ovum is fertilized in a laboratory dish and then placed in a Fallopian tube.

# References


## CHAPTER 1

1. Esterling, B. A., et al. Defensiveness, Trait Anxiety, and Epstein-Barr Viral Capsid Antigen Antibody Titers in Healthy College Students. *Health Psychology, 12* (1993), 132–139; Herbert, T. B., and Cohen, S. Depression and Immunity: A Meta-Analytic Review. *Psychological Bulletin, 113* (1993), 472–486; Kemeny, M. E., et al. Repeated Bereavement, Depressed Mood, and Immune Parameters in HIV Seropositive and Seronegative Gay Men. *Health Psychology, 13* (1994), 14–24.
2. Maier, S. F., Watkins, L. R., and Fleshner, M. Psychoneuroimmunology: The Interface between Behavior, Brain, and Immunity. *American Psychologist, 49* (1994), 1004–1017; O'Leary, A. Stress, Emotion, and Human Immune Functions. *Psychological Bulletin, 108* (1990), 383–382; Kiecolt-Glaser, J. K., et al. Marital Quality, Marital Disruption, and Immune Function. *Psychosomatic Medicine, 49* (1987), 13–34; Kiecolt-Glaser, J. K., et al. Marital Discord and Immunity in Males. *Psychosomatic Medicine, 50* (1988), 213–229; Kiecolt-Glaser, J. K., et al. Stress and the Transformation of Lymphocytes in Epstein-Barr Virus. *Journal of Behavioral Medicine, 7* (1984), 1–12.
3. U.S. Department of Health and Human Services (USDHHS). *Healthy People 2000: National Health Promotion and Disease Prevention Objectives.* Boston, MA: Jones and Bartlett, 1992.
4. USDHHS. *Healthy People 2000,* p. 253.
5. Published by the Public Health Service of the U.S. Department of Health and Human Services.
6. National Center for Health Statistics (NCHS), Centers for Disease Control and Prevention. *Births and Deaths for 1995,* 1996.
7. NCHS, 1996.
8. NCHS, 1996.
9. National Center for Health Statistics (NCHS). *Monitoring Health Care in America: Quarterly Fact Sheet,* Centers for Disease Control and Prevention, September 1995.
10. Redelmeier, D. A., and Tibshirani, R. J. Association between Cellular Telephone Calls and Motor Vehicle Collisions. *New England Journal of Medicine, 336* (1997), 453–458.
11. Anderson, N. B. Behavioral and Sociocultural Perspectives on Ethnicity and Health: Introduction to the Special Issue. *Health Psychology, 14* (1995), 589–591.
12. Angell, M. Privilege and Health—What Is the Connection? *New England Journal of Medicine, 329* (1993), 126–127; Guralnik, J. M., et al. Educational Status and Active Life Expectancy among Older Blacks and Whites. *New England Journal of Medicine, 329* (1993), 110–116; Penn, N. E., et al. Panel VI. Ethnic Minorities, Health Care Systems, and Behavior. *Health Psychology, 14* (1995), 641–648. Pappas, G., et al. The Increasing Disparity of Mortality between Socioeconomic Groups in the United States, 1960 and 1986. *New England Journal of Medicine, 329* (1993), 103–109.
13. Flack, J. M., et al. Panel I: Epidemiology of Minority Health. *Health Psychology, 14* (1995), 592–600.
14. Leary, W. E. Black Hypertension May Reflect Other Ills. *The New York Times,* October 21, 1991, p. C3.
15. Anderson, 1995.
16. Ayanian, J. Z. Heart Disease in Black and White. *New England Journal of Medicine, 329* (1993), 656–658.
17. Peterson, E. D., et al. Racial Variation in the Use of Coronary-Revascularization Procedures. *New England Journal of Medicine, 336* (1997), 480–486.
18. Andersen, B. L. Psychological Interventions for Cancer Patients to Enhance the Quality of Life. *Journal of Consulting and Clinical Psychology, 60* (1992), 552–568; Bal, D. G. Cancer in African Americans. *Ca-A Cancer Journal for Clinicians, 42* (1992), 5–6.
19. Baquet, C. R., et al. Socioeconomic Factors and Cancer Incidence among Blacks and Whites. *Journal of the National Cancer Institute, 83* (1991), 551–557.
20. U.S. Department of Health and Human Services (USDHHS). *Health, United States 1995. HHS Issues Annual Report, with Special Profile of Women's Health.* Press Release, June 18, 1996.
21. Ayanian, J. Z., et al. The Relation between Health Insurance Coverage and Clinical Outcome among Women with Breast Cancer. *New England Journal of Medicine, 329* (1993), 326–331.
22. Anderson, 1995.
23. Heart Disease Higher in Mexican-Americans. *Newsday,* March 18, 1997, p. A17.
24. Ziv, T. A., and Lo, B. Denial of Care to Illegal Immigrants—Proposition 187 in California. *New England Journal of Medicine, 332* (1995), 1095–1098.
25. Cohen, L. A. Diet and Cancer. *Scientific American,* November 1987, pp. 42–48, 53–54.
26. Curb, J. D., and Marcus, E. B. Body Fat and Obesity in Japanese Americans. *American Journal of Clinical Nutrition, 53* (1991), 1552S–1555S.
27. National Institutes of Health. *Backgrounder: What Is the Women's Health Initiative?* Internet posting, updated February 28, 1996.
28. Doctors Tie Male Mentality to Shorter Life Span. *The New York Times,* June 14, 1995, p. C14.
29. USDHHS, 1996.
30. USDHHS, 1996.
31. Lurie, N., et al. Preventive Care for Women: Does the Sex of the Physician matter? *New England Journal of Medicine, 329* (1993), 478–482.
32. Hall, J. A., et al. Performance Quality, Gender, and Professional Role: A Study of Physicians and Nonphysicians in 16 Ambulatory-Care Practices. *Medical Care, 28* (1990), 489–501.
33. Adler, N. E., et al. Socioeconomic Status and Health: The Challenge of the Gradient. *American Psychologist, 49* (1994), 15–24; Abraham, L. K. *Mama Might Be Better Off Dead: The Failure of Health Care in Urban America.* Chicago: University of Chicago Press, 1993; Rogers, D. E., and Ginzberg, E. *Medical Care and the Health of the Poor.* Boulder, CO: Westview Press, 1993; Shweder, R. A. It's Called Poor Health for a Reason. *The New York Times,* March 9, 1997, p. E5.
34. Winkleby, M., Fortmann, S., and Barrett, D. Social Class Disparities in Risk Factors for Disease: Eight-Year Prevalence Patterns by

Level of Education. *Preventive Medicine, 19* (1991), 1–12; Ford, E. S., et al. Physical Activity Behaviors in Lower and Higher Socioeconomic Status Populations. *American Journal of Epidemiology, 133* (1991), 1246–1256.
35. Johnson, K. W., et al. Panel II: Macrosocial and environmental influences on minority health. *Health Psychology, 14* (1995), 601–612; Myers, H. F., et al. Behavioral Risk Factors Related to Chronic Diseases in Ethnic Minorities. *Health Psychology, 14* (1995), 622–631.
36. Cohen, S., Tyrrell, D. A. J., and Smith, A. P. Negative Life Events, Perceived Stress, Negative Affect, and Susceptibility to the Common Cold. *Journal of Personality and Social Psychology, 64* (1993), 131–140.
37. Adler et al., 1994.
38. Abraham, 1993; Rogers and Ginzberg, 1993.
39. Adapted from Rathus, S. A., and Nevid, J. S. *Adjustment and Growth: The Challenges of Life,* 6th ed. Ft. Worth, TX: Harcourt Brace College Publishers. Copyright © 1995 by Holt, Rinehart and Winston, reprinted with permission of the publisher.
40. Procon: Should Patients Be Allowed to See Their Doctors' Reports Cards? *Health,* November/December 1995, p. 28; Schneider, E. C., and Epstein, A. M. Influence of Cardiac-Surgery Performance Reports on Referral Practices and Access to Care—A Survey of Cardiovascular Specialists. *New England Journal of Medicine, 335* (1996), 251–256; Krieger, L. M. Cardiac-Surgery Performance Reports. *New England Journal of Medicine, 336* (1997), 442–443 (Letter).
41. How Good Is Your Doctor? *Consumer Reports on Health,* April 1996, pp. 42–43.
42. How Good Is Your Doctor? 1996.
43. How to Maintain Your Own Medical Record. *Consumer Reports on Health,* March 1996, p. 32.

### CHAPTER 2

1. Moyers, B. *Healing and the Mind.* New York: Doubleday, 1993, p. 2.
2. Rathus, S. A., and Nevid, J. S. *Adjustment and Growth: The Challenges of Life,* 6th ed. Fort Worth, TX: Harcourt Brace College Publishers. Copyright © 1995 by Holt, Rinehart and Winston, reprinted by permission of the publisher.
3. McClelland, D. C. Achievement and Entrepreneurship: A Longitudinal Study. *Journal of Personality and Social Psychology, 1* (1965), 389–392.
4. Dweck, C. S. Self-Theories and Goals: Their Role in Motivation, Personality, and Development. In R. A. Dienstbier (Ed.), *Nebraska Symposium on Motivation,* vol. 38. Lincoln, NE: University of Nebraska Press, 1990, pp. 199–235.
5. Cohn, L. D., Macfarlane, S., Yanez, C., and Imai, W. K. Risk-Perception: Differences between Adolescents and Adults. *Health Psychology, 14* (1995), 217–222.
6. Berger, E. M., University of Minnesota, Minneapolis.
7. Goleman, D. *Emotional Intelligence.* New York: Bantam Books, 1995.
8. Manning, M. M., and Wright, T. L. Self-Efficacy Expectancies, Outcome Expectancies, and the Persistence of Pain Control in Childbirth. *Journal of Personality and Social Psychology, 45* (1983), 421–431.
9. Condiotte, M. M., and Lichtenstein, E. Self-Efficacy and Relapse in Smoking Cessation Programs. *Journal of Consulting and Clinical Psychology, 49* (1981), 648–658; Marlatt, G. A., and Gordon, J. R. Determinants of Relapse: Implications for the Maintenance of Behavior Change. In P. O. Davidson and S. M. Davidson (Eds.), *Behavioral Medicine: Changing Health Lifestyles.* New York: Brunner/Mazel, 1980.
10. Rosenbaum, M., and Hadari, D. Personal Efficacy, External Locus of Control, and Perceived Contingency of Parental Reinforcement among Depressed, Paranoid, and Normal Subjects. *Journal of Personality and Social Psychology, 49* (1985), 539–547.
11. Steinmetz, J. L., Lewinsohn, P. M., and Antonuccio, D. O. Prediction of Individual Outcome in a Group Intervention for Depression. *Journal of Consulting and Clinical Psychology, 51* (1983), 331–337.
12. Feltz, D. L. Path Analysis of the Causal Elements in Bandura's Theory of Self-Efficacy and an Anxiety-Based Model of Avoidance Behavior. *Journal of Personality and Social Psychology, 42* (1982), 764–781.
13. Kobasa, S. C. Stressful Life Events, Personality, and Health: An Inquiry into Hardiness. *Journal of Personality and Social Psychology, 37* (1979), 1–11; Kobasa, S. C., Maddi, S. R., and Kahn, S. Hardiness and Health: A Prospective Study. *Journal of Personality and Social Psychology, 42* (1982), 168–177; Kobasa, S. C., and Puccetti, M. C. Personality and Social Resources in Stress Resistance. *Journal of Personality and Social Psychology, 45* (1983), 839–850.
14. Goleman, 1995.
15. Scheier, M. F., and Carver, C. S. Optimism, Coping, and Health: Assessment and Implications of Generalized Outcome Expectancies. *Health Psychology, 4* (1985), 219–247.
16. Gil, K. M., et al. The Relationship of Negative Thoughts to Pain and Psychological Distress. *Behavior Therapy, 21* (1990), 349–362.
17. Carver, C. S., and Gaines, J. G. Optimism, Pessimism, and Postpartum Depression. *Cognitive Therapy and Research, 11* (1987), 449–462.
18. Scheier, M. F., et al. Dispositional Optimism and Recovery from Coronary Artery Bypass Surgery: The Beneficial Effects on Physical and Psychological Well-Being. *Journal of Personality and Social Psychology, 57* (1989), 1024–1040.
19. Scheier, M. F., and Carver, C. S. Optimism, Coping, and Health: Assessment and Implications of Generalized Outcome Expectancies. *Health Psychology, 4* (1985), 219–247.
20. Kuiper, N. A., and Martin, R. A. (1993). Humor and Self-Concept. *Humor International Journal of Humor Research, 6* (1993), 251–270; Martin, R. A., et al. Humor, Coping with Stress, Self-Concept, and Psychological Well-Being. *Humor International Journal of Humor Research, 6* (1993), 89–104.
21. Kaplan, H. R. *Lottery Winners.* New York: Harper & Row, 1978.
22. Lykken, D. T. Cited in Goleman, D. A Set Point for Happiness. *The New York Times,* July 21, 1996, p. E2.
23. Ginsburg, G., and Bronstein, P. Family Factors Related to Children's Intrinsic/Extrinsic Motivational Orientation and Academic Performance. *Child Development, 64* (1993), 1461–1474; Gottfried, A. E., Fleming, J. S., and Gottfried, A. W. Role of Parental Motivational Practices in Children's Academic Intrinsic Motivation and Achievement. *Journal of Educational Psychology, 86* (1994), 104–113.
24. Dweck, C. S. Self-Theories and Goals: Their Role in Motivation, Personality, and Development. In R. A. Diensthier (Ed.), *Nebraska Symposium on Motivation,* vol. 38. Lincoln, NE: University of Nebraska Press, 1990, pp. 199–235.
25. Greene, B. African American Women. In L. Comas-Diaz and B. A. Greene (Eds.), *Women of Color and Mental Health.* New York: Guilford Press, 1993; Lewis-Fernández, R., and Kleinman, A. Culture, Personality, and Psychopathology. *Journal of Abnormal Psychology, 103* (1994), 67–71.
26. Triandis, H. C. Cross-Cultural Studies of Individualism and Collectivism. In J. J. Berman (Ed.), *Nebraska Symposium on Motivation, 1989. Cross-Cultural Perspectives.* Lincoln, NE: University of Nebraska Press, 1990.
27. Markus, H., and Kitayama, S. Culture and the Self: Implications for Cognition, Emotion, and Motivation. *Psychological Review, 98*(2) (1991), 224–253.
28. Draguns, J. G. Personality and Culture: Are They Relevant for the Enhancement of Quality of Mental Life? In P. R. Dasen, J. W. Berry, and N. Sartorius (Eds.), *Health and Cross-Cultural Psychology: Toward Applications.* Newbury Park, CA: Sage, 1988; Triandis, H. C. *Culture and Social Behavior.* New York: McGraw-Hill, 1994.
29. Griffith, J. Relationship between Acculturation and Psychological Impairment in Adult Mexican-Americans. *Hispanic Journal of Behavioral Sciences, 5* (1983), 431–459.
30. Caetano, R. Acculturation and Drinking Patterns among U.S. Hispanics. *British Journal of Addiction, 82* (1987), 789–799.
31. Burnam, M. A., et al. Acculturation and Lifetime Prevalence of Psychiatric Disorders among Mexican Americans in Los Angeles. *Journal of Health and Social Behavior, 28* (1987), 89–102; Sorenson, S. B. and Golding,

J. M. Suicide Ideation and Attempts in Hispanics and Non-Hispanic Whites: Demographic and Psychiatric Disorder Issues. *Suicide and Life-Threatening Behavior, 18* (1988), 205–218.

32. Pumariega, A. J. Acculturation and Eating Attitudes in Adolescent Girls: A Comparative Correlational Study. *Journal of the American Academy of Child Psychiatry, 25* (1986), 276–279.
33. Salgado de Snyder, V. N., Cervantes, R. C., and Padilla, A. M. Gender and Ethnic Differences in Psychosocial Stress and Generalized Distress among Hispanics. *Sex Roles, 22* (1990), 441–453; Neff, J. A., and Hoppe, S. K. Race/Ethnicity, Acculturation, and Psychological Distress: Fatalism and Religiosity as Cultural Resources. *Journal of Community Psychology, 21* (1993), 3–20; Zamanian, K., et al. Acculturation and Depression in Mexican-American Elderly. *Gerontologist, 11* (1992), 109–121.
34. Blatt, S. The Destructiveness of Perfectionism. *American Psychologist, 50* (1995), 1003–1020.
35. Ellis, A., and Dryden, W. *The Practice of Rational Emotive Therapy.* New York: Springer, 1987.

### CHAPTER 3

1. Lazarus, R. S. The Trivialization of Distress. In B. L. Hammonds, and C. J. Scheirer (Eds.), *Psychology And Health: The Master Lecture Series.* Washington, DC: American Psychological Association, 1984.
2. Are You Being Worked to Death? *Consumer Reports on Health,* July 1996, p. 78.
3. Freudenberger, H. J. Burnout: Past, Present, and Future Concerns. In *Professional Burnout in Medicine and the Helping Professions.* New York: Haworth Press, 1989.
4. Miller, T. Q., et al. Reasons for the Trend toward Null Findings in Research on Type A Behavior. *Psychological Bulletin, 110* (1991), 469–485.
5. Adapted from Nevid, J. S., Rathus, S. A., and Greene, B. V. *Abnormal Psychology in a Changing World.* Upper Saddle River: Prentice-Hall, Inc., 1997, p. 176. Reprinted by permission of Prentice-Hall, Inc.
6. Friedman, M., and Ulmer, D. *Treating Type A Behavior and Your Heart.* New York: Fawcett Crest, 1984; Krantz, D. S., Dembroski, T. M., and MacDougall, J. M. Unique and Common Variance in Structured Interview and Jenkins Activity Survey Measures of the Type A Behavior Pattern. *Journal of Personality and Social Psychology, 4* (1982), 303–313.; Musante, L., et al. Component Analysis of the Type A Coronary-Prone Behavior Pattern in Male and Female College Students. *Journal of Person-ality and Social Psychology, 45* (1983), 1104–1117.
7. Turk, Dennis C., and Nash, Justin M. Chronic Pain: New Ways to Cope. In D. Goleman and J. Gurin (Eds.), *Mind/Body Medicine: How to Use Your Mind for Better Health,* Yonkers, NY: Consumer Reports Books, 1993.
8. Kolko, D. J., and Rickard-Figueroa, J. L. Effects of Video Games on the Adverse Corollaries of Chemotherapy in Pediatric Oncology Patients: A Single-Case Analysis. *Journal of Consulting and Clinical Psychology, 53* (1985), 223–228; Redd, W. H., et al. Cognitive/Attentional Distraction in the Control of Conditioned Nausea in Pediatric Cancer Patients Receiving Chemotherapy. *Journal of Consulting and Clinical Psychology, 55* (1987), 391–395.
9. Kabat-Zinn, John. Mindfulness Meditation: Health Benefits of an Ancient Buddhist Practice. In D. Goleman and J. Gurin (Eds.), *Mind/Body Medicine: How to Use Your Mind for Better Health.* Yonkers, NY: Consumer Reports Books, 1993.
10. Kabat-Zinn, 1993.
11. Esterling, B. A., et al. Defensiveness, Trait Anxiety, and Epstein-Barr Viral Capsid Antigen Antibody Titers in Healthy College Students. *Health Psychology, 12* (1993), 132–139; Herbert, T. B., and Cohen, S. Depression and Immunity: A Meta-Analytic Review. *Psychological Bulletin, 113* (1993), 472–486; Kemeny, M. E. Emotions and the Immune System. In B. Moyers, *Healing and the Mind.* New York: Doubleday, 1993.
12. DeAngelis, T. Firefighters' PTSD at Dangerous Levels. *APA Monitor, 26*(2) (1995), 36–37.
13. North, C. S., Smith, E. M., and Spitznagel, E. L. Posttraumatic Stress Disorder in Survivors of a Mass Shooting. *American Journal of Psychiatry, 151* (1994), 82–88.
14. Andersen, B. L., Kiecolt-Glaser, J. K., and Glaser, R. A Biobehavioral Model of Cancer Stress and Disease Course. *American Psychologist, 49* (1994), 389–404; Glaser, R., and others. Stress-Related Activation of Epstein-Barr Virus. *Brain, Behavior, and Immunity, 5* (1991), 219–232; Maier, S. F., Watkins, L. R., and Fleshner, M. Psychoneuroimmunology: The Interface between Behavior, Brain, and Immunity. *American Psychologist, 49* (1994), 1004–1017.
15. Kiecolt-Glaser, J. K., et al. Slowing of Wound Healing by Psychological Stress. *Lancet, 346* (1995), 1194–1196.
16. Jenkins, C. D., et al. Quantifying and Predicting Recovery after Heart Surgery. *Psychosomatic Medicine, 56* (1994), 203–212; Levenson, J. L., and Bemis, C. The Role of Psychological Factors in Cancer Onset and Progression. *Psychosmatics, 32* (1991), 124–132; MacLean, W. E., et al. (1992). Psychological Adjustment of Children with Asthma: Effects of Illness Severity and Recent Stressful Life Events. *Journal of Pediatric Psychology, 17* (1992), 159–171.
17. Riley, V. Psychoneuroendocrine Influences on Immunocompetence and Neoplasia. *Science, 212* (1981), 1100–1109.
18. Jenkins, C. D. Epidemiology of Cardiovascular Diseases. *Journal of Consulting and Clinical Psychology, 56* (1988), 324–332.
19. LaCroix, A. Z., and Haynes, S. G. Gender Differences in the Stressfulness of Workplace Roles: A Focus on Work and Health. In R. Barnett, G. Baruch, and L. Biener (Eds.), *Gender and Stress.* New York: The Free Press, 1987, pp. 96–121.
20. Stone, A. A., et al. Daily Events Are Associated with a Secretory Immune Response to an Oral Antigen in Men. *Health Psychology, 13* (1994), 440–446.
21. Jemmott, J. B., et al. Academic Stress, Power Motivation, and Decrease in Secretion Rate of Salivary Secretory Immunoglobulin. A. *Lancet,* June 25, 1983, pp. 1400–1402; Kiecolt-Glaser, J. K., et al. Stress and the Transformation of Lymphocytes in Epstein-Barr Virus. *Journal of Behavioral Medicine, 7* (1984), 1–12.
22. Mind over Matter, *Connecticut Magazine,* September 1992, p. 81.
23. Fleming, R., et al. Mediation of Stress at Three Mile Island by Social Support. *Journal of Human Stress, 8* (1982), 14–22.
24. House, J. S., Robbins, C., and Metzner, H. L. The Association of Social Relationships and Activities with Mortality: Prospective Evidence from the Tecumseh Community Health Study. *American Journal of Epidemiology, 116* (1982), 123–140.
25. Berkman, L. F., and Syme, S. L. Social Networks, Host Resistance, and Mortality: A Nine-Year Follow-up Study of Alameda County Residents. *American Journal of Epidemiology, 109* (1979), 186–204; Berkman, L. F., and Breslow, L. *Health and Ways of Living: The Alameda County Study.* New York: Oxford University Press, 1983.
26. Does Stress Kill?, *Consumer Reports on Health,* July 1995, p. 75.
27. Reprinted from Rathus, S. A., and Fichner-Rathus, L. *Making the Most of College* (2nd ed.). Englewood Cliffs, NJ: Prentice Hall, 1994.
28. Esterling, B. A., et al. Emotional Disclosure through Writing or Speaking Modulates Latent Epstein-Barr Virus Antibody Titers. *Journal of Consulting and Clinical Psychology, 62* (1994), 130–140; Glaser, R. et al. Stress and the Memory T-cell Response to the Epstein-Barr Virus in Healthy Medical Students. *Health Psychology, 12* (1993), 435–442; Pennebaker, J. W., Kiecolt-Glaser, J. K., and Glaser, R. Disclosure of Traumas and Immune Function: Health Implications for Psychotherapy. *Journal of Consulting and Clinical Psychology, 56* (1988), 239–245.
29. Martin, R. A., and Lefcourt, H. M. Sense of Humor as a Moderator of the Relation between Stressors and Moods. *Journal of Personality and Social Psychology, 45* (1983), 1313–1324.
30. Fischman, J. Getting Tough. *Psychology Today, 21* (1987), 26–28.

31. Benson, H. *The Relaxation Response.* New York: Morrow, 1975.
32. Benson, H., Manzetta, B. R., and Rosner, B. Decreased Systolic Blood Pressure in Hypertensive Subjects Who Practiced Meditation. *Journal of Clinical Investigation, 52* (1973), 8; Brody, J. E. Relaxation Method May Aid Health. *The New York Times,* August 7, 1996, p. C10.
33. *Prevention,* December, 1995, p. 70.
34. Friedman and Ulmer, 1984.

**CHAPTER 4**

1. Adapted from Rathus, S. A., and Nevid, J. S. *Adjustment and Growth: The Challenges of Life,* 6th ed. Fort Worth, TX: Harcourt Brace College Publishers, 1995.
2. Kessler, R. C. The National Comorbidity Survey: Preliminary Results and Future Directions. *International Journal of Methods in Psychiatric Research, 4* (1994), 114.1–114.13.
3. Myers, D. G. *The Pursuit of Happiness.* New York: William Morrow, 1992, p. 43.; Robins, L. N., et al. Lifetime Prevalence of Specific Psychiatric Disorders in Three Sites. *Archives of General Psychiatry, 41* (1984), 949–958.
4. National Advisory Mental Health Council. Basic Behavioral Science Research for Mental Health: A National Investment. *American Psychologist, 50* (1995), 485–493.
5. Neighbors, H. W. Improving the Mental Health of Black Americans: Lessons from the Community Health Movement. In D. P. Willis (Ed.), *Health Policies and Black Americans.* New Brunswick, NJ: Transaction, 1990.
6. Ogur, B. Long Day's Journey into Night: Women and Prescription Drug Abuse. *Women and Health, 11* (1986), 99–115.
7. McGrath, E., Keita, G. P. Strickland, B. R., and Russo, N. F. *Women and Depression: Risk Factors and Treatment Issues.* Washington DC: American Psychological Association, 1990.
8. Bianchi, S. M., and Spain, D. *Women, Work and Family in America.* Washington D.C.: Population Reference Bureau, 1997.
9. Shumaker, S. A., and Hill, D. R. Gender Differences in Social Support and Physical Health. *Health Psychology, 10* (1991), 102–111.
10. Kessler, R. C., et al. Lifetime and 12-Month Prevalence of DSM-III-R Psychiatric Disorders in the United States: Results from the National Comorbidity Survey. *Archives of General Psychiatry, 51* (1994), 8–19.
11. Westermeyer, J. The Role of Ethnicity in Substance Abuse. In B. Stimmel (Ed.), *Cultural and Sociological Aspects of Alcoholism and Substance Abuse.* New York: Haworth Press, 1984, pp. 9–18.
12. Timpson, J., et al. Depression in a Native Canadian in Northwestern Ontario: Sadness, Grief or Spiritual Illness? Canada's Mental Health, 36 (1988) (2–3), p. 6.
13. Goleman, D. More than 1 in 4 U.S. Adults Suffers from a Psychological Disorder Each Year. *The New York Times,* March 17, 1993, pp. C13.; U.S. Department of Health and Human Services (DHHS). *Healthy People 2000,* Pub. No. (PHS) 91–50212. Washington, DC: U.S. Government Printing Office. p. 208.
14. Goleman, 1993.
15. Gilbert, S. Harnessing the Power of Light, *Good Health Magazine, The New York Times,* April 26, 1992.
16. Brody, J. E. Myriad Masks Hide an Epidemic of Depression *The New York Times,* September 30, 1992, p. C12. Copyright © 1992 by The New York Times Co. Reprinted by permission.
17. Gottesman, I. I. *Schizophrenia Genetics: The Origins of Madness.* New York: W. H. Freeman, 1991; Kety, S., et al. Mental Illness in the Biological and Adoptive Relatives of Schizophrenic Adoptees: Replication of the Copenhagen Study in the Rest of Denmark. *Archives of General Psychiatry, 51* (1994), 442–455.
18. Clum, G. A., Clum, G. A., and Surls, R. A Meta-Analysis of Treatments for Panic Disorder. *Journal of Consulting and Clinical Psychology, 61* (1993), 317–326.
19. Davis, K. L., et al. Dopamine in Schizophrenia: A Review and Reconceptualization. *American Journal of Psychiatry, 148* (1991), 1474–1486.
20. Clum et al., 1993; Klosko, J. S., et al. A Comparison of Alprazolam and Behavior Therapy in Treatment of Panic Disorder. *Journal of Consulting and Clinical Psychology, 58* (1990), 77–84.
21. Blatt, S. J., et al. Impact of Perfectionism and Need for Approval on the Brief Treatment of Depression: The National Institute of Mental Health Treatment of Depression Collaborative Research Program Revisited. *Journal of Consulting and Clinical Psychology, 63* (1995), 125–132.
22. Burns, D. D. *Feeling Good: The New Mood Therapy.* New York: Morris, 1980; Nevid, J. S., Rathus, S. A., and Greene, B. *Abnormal Psychology in a Changing World* (3rd ed.). Upper Saddle River, NJ: Prentice-Hall, Inc., 1997.
23. Nevid et al., 1997.
24. Keith, S. J., Regier, D. A., and Rae, D. S. Schizophrenic Disorders. In L. N. Robins and D. A. Regier (Eds.), *Psychiatric Disorders in America: The Epidemiologic Catchment Area Study.* New York: The Free Press, 1991, pp. 33–52.
25. Meehan, P. J., et al. Attempted Suicide among Young Adults: Progress toward a Meaningful Estimate of Prevalence. *American Journal of Psychiatry, 149* (1991), 41–44.
26. Blumenthal, S. J. *Suicide and Suicide Prevention* (Comm. Pub. No. 98–497). Washington DC: U.S. Government Printing Office, 1985.
27. Tolchin, M. When Long Life Is Too Much: Suicide Rises among Elderly. *The New York Times,* July 19, 1989, pp. A1, A15.
28. Rich, C. L., Ricketts, J. E., Thaler, R. C., and Young, D. Some Differences between Men and Women Who Commit Suicide. *American Journal of Psychiatry, 145* (1988), 718–722.
29. Centers for Disease Control. *Youth Suicide in the U.S., 1970–1980, Healthy People 2000,* 1992.
30. Resnick, M. Cited in Young Indians Prone to Suicide, Study Finds. *The New York Times,* March 25, 1992, p. D24.
31. *Closing the Gap* Series, Office of Mental Health, State of New York.
32. Shneidman, E. S. *Definition of Suicide.* New York: Wiley, 1985; Shneidman, E. S. A Psychological Approach to Suicide. In G. R. Vanderbos and B. K. Bryant (Eds.), *Cataclysms, Cries, and Catastrophes: Psychology in Action* (Master Lecture Series, vol. 6. Washington, DC: American Psychological Association, 1987, pp. 151–183.
33. Cordes, C. Common Threads Found in Suicide. *APA Monitor, 16* (1985), 11; Gelman, D. The Mystery of Suicide. *Newsweek,* April 18, 1994, pp. 44–49.
34. Rathus, S. A., and Nevid, J. S. *Adjustment and Growth: The Challenges of Life* (6th ed.). Forth Worth, TX: Harcourt Brace College Publishers, 1995; Griffith, J. A. Community Survey of Psychological Impairment among Anglo- and Mexican Americans and Its Relationship to Service Utilization. *Community Mental Health Journal, 21* (1985), 28–41.
35. Shneidman, 1985.
36. U.S. Department of Health and Human Services (USDHHS). *National Household Survey on Drug Abuse: Highlights 1991.* Publication No. (SMA) 93–1979. Washington, DC: U.S. Government Printing Office, 1993.
37. Sackheim, H. A., Prudic, J., and Devanand, D. P. Treatment of Medication-Resistant Depression with Electroconvulsive Therapy. In A. Tasman et al. (Eds.), *Review of Psychiatry,* vol. 9. Washington, DC: American Psychiatric Press, 1990.
38. Devanand, D. P., et al. Does ECT Alter Brain Structure? *American Journal of Psychiatry, 151* (1994), 957–970; Potter, W. Z., and Rudorfer, M. V. "Electroconvulsive Therapy—A Modern Medical Procedure." *New England Journal of Medicine, 328* (1993), 882–883.
39. Doyne, E. J., Chambless, D. L., and Bentler, L. E. Aerobic Exercise as Treatment for Depression in Women. *Behavior Therapy, 14* (1983), 434–440; Folkins, C. H., and Sime, W. E. Physical Fitness Training and Mental Health. *American Psychologist, 36* (1981), 373–389; Klein, D., et al. A Comparative Outcome Study of Group Psychotherapy versus Exercise Treatments for Depression. *International Journal of Mental Health, 13*

(1985), 148–175; McCann, I. L., and Holmes, D. S. Influence of Aerobic Exercise on Depression. *Journal of Personality and Social Psychology, 46* (1984), 1142–1147.

40. Dimsdale, J. E., and Moss, J. Plasma Catecholamines in Stress and Exercise. *Journal of the American Medical Association, 243* (1980), 340–342; Carr, D. B., et al. Physical Conditioning Facilitates the Exercise-Induced Secretion of Beta-Endorphins and Beta-Lipotropin in Women. *New England Journal of Medicine, 305* (1981), 560–563.


### CHAPTER 5

1. Blumenthal, D. Making Sense of the Cholesterol Controversy. *FDA Consumer, 24,* June 1990, p. 12(4); Burros, M. Tough New Warning on Diet Is Issued by Cancer Society. *The New York Times,* September 17, 1996, p. A16.
2. Brody, J. E. Study Finds a Three-Decade Gain in American Eating Habits, But a Long Way to Go. *The New York Times,* September 5, 1996, p. A14; Popkin, B. M. A Comparison of Dietary Trends among Racial and Socioeconomic Groups in the United States. *New England Journal of Medicine, 335* (1996), 716–720.
3. U.S. Department of Agriculture, Human Nutrition Information Service. *Dietary Guidelines for Americans: Eat Food with Adequate Starch and Fiber.* Home and Garden Bulletin No. 232–234. Washington, DC: U.S. Government Printing Office, April 1986.
4. Brody, J. E. Fiber's Benefits Back in War on Heart Ills. *The New York Times,* February 14, 1996, p. C8; Rimm, E. B., et al. Vegetable, Fruit and Cereal Fiber Intake and Risk of Coronary Heart Disease among Men. *Journal of the American Medical Association, 274* (1996), 447–451.
5. Jenkins, D. J. A., et al. Low Glycemic Index Carbohydrate Foods in the Management of Hyperlipidemia. *American Journal of Clinical Nutrition, 42* (1985), 604–617; USDA, *Dietary Guidelines for Americans: Eat Food with Adequate Starch and Fiber,* 1986; Brody, Fiber's Benefits Back in War on Heart Ills. *The New York Times,* February 14, 1996.
6. It's Back! Fiber Is Good for the Heart. *Harvard Health Letter,* August 1996, pp. 6–7.
7. Adapted from American Cancer Society publication, Eating Smart (No. 87–250M–Rev 3/89–No. 2042).
8. U.S. Department of Agriculture, Human Nutrition Information Service. *The Food Guide Pyramid. Home and Garden Bulletin,* No. 252. Washington, DC: U.S. Government Printing Office, 1992.
9. Shapiro, L. A Food Lover's Guide to Fat. *Newsweek,* December 5, 1994, pp. 50–55.
10. U.S. Department of Agriculture, Health Nutrition Information Services. *Nutritive Value of Foods.* Publication No. G–72. Washington, DC: U.S. Government Printing Office, 1991.
11. Willett, W. C., et al. Relation of Meat, Fat, and Fiber Intake to the Risk of Colon Cancer in a Prospective Study among Women. *New England Journal of Medicine, 323* (1990), p. 1664.
12. Should You Be Choosing Butter over Margarine? *Tufts University Diet & Nutrition Letter,* 8(9), November 1990, pp. 1–2.
13. Should You Be Choosing Butter over Margarine?, 1990.
14. Adapted from U.S. Department of Agriculture, Human Nutrition Information Service. *Hints to Reduce Fat and Cholesterol in Your Diet.* Home and Garden Bulletin No. 232–3, 1986. Washington, DC: U.S. Government Printing Office; and other sources.
15. U.S. Department of Agriculture, Human Nutrition Information Service. *Dietary Guidelines for Americans: Avoid Too Much Fat, Saturated Fat, and Cholesterol.* Home and Garden Bulletin No. 232–3. Washington, DC: U.S. Government Printing Office, 1986.
16. Brody, J. E. A Closer Look at the Actual Health Effects of Eggs. *The New York Times,* January 11, 1995, C1, C11.
17. Blumenthal, 1990.
18. Block, G. Rosenberger, W. F., and Patterson, B. H. Calories, Fat and Cholesterol: Intake Patterns in the U.S. Population by Race, Sex and Age. *American Journal of Public Health, 78* (1988), 1150–1154.
19. Beyond Beta Carotene. *UC Berkeley Wellness Letter,* June 1995, p. 2.
20. Olestra: Just Say No. *UC Berkeley Wellness Letter,* February 1996, p. 1.
21. Hurley, J., and Schmidt, S. A Wok on the Wild Side. *Nutrition Action HealthLetter,* Center for Science in the Public Interest, September 1993, pp. 10–12; Hurley, J., and Schmidt, S. Mexican Food: Oilé. *Nutrition Action HealthLetter,* Center for Science in the Public Interest, July/August 1994, pp. 4–8; Hurley, J., and Liebman, B. "When in Rome . . . ," *Nutrition Action HealthLetter,* Center for Science in the Public Interest, January/February 1994, pp. 5–8.
22. Hamilton, E. M. N., Whitney, E. N., and Sizer, F. S. *Nutrition: Concepts and Controversies,* 5th ed. St. Paul, MN: West Publishing, 1991.
23. National Research Council (NRC). Subcommittee on the Tenth Edition of the RDAs. (1989). *Recommended Dietary Allowances/Subcommittee on the Tenth Edition of the RDAs, Food and Nutrition Board, Commission on Life Sciences, National Research Council (10th Revised Edition).* National Academy Press: Washington, DC.
24. Adapted from Combs, G. F., Jr. *The Vitamins: Fundamental Aspects in Nutrition and Health.* San Diego: Academic Press, Inc., 1992; Vitamin E. *FDA Consumer, 24,* November 1990, p. 31; Kurtzweil, P. Vitamin D (Part 2). *FDA Consumer, 24,* October 1990, p. 31.
25. Garland, C. R., et al. Serum 25-Hydroxyvitamin D and Colon Cancer: Eight-Year Prospective Study. *The Lancet II, 8673* (1989), 1175–1178.
26. Scheer, J. Fight Free Radicals with Vitamin E; Research Shows That Vitamin E Offers Protection from Cellular Oxidation, Nitrosamines and Atherosclerosis. *Better Nutrition, 52,* April 1990, p. 8; Cowley, G. et al. Vitamin Revolution. *Newsweek,* June 7, 1993, pp. 46–49.
27. Can Taking Supplements Help You Ward Off Disease? *Tufts University Diet & Nutrition Letter,* 9(2), April 1991, pp. 3–6.
28. Vitamin E in the Diet . . . *Consumer Reports on Health,* August 1995, p. 89.
29. Brody, J. E. Health Factor in Vegetables Still Elusive. *The New York Times,* February 21, 1995, p. C1. Bricklin, M. (with M. Trott). Why We're Pro-Antioxidant. *Prevention,* July 1993, pp. 37–39.
30. Brody, J. E., 1995; Kolata, G. New Study Finds Vitamins Are Not Cancer Preventers. *The New York Times,* July 21, 1994, p. A20.
31. Kolata, G. Studies Find Beta Carotene, Used by Millions, Doesn't Forestall Cancer or Heart Disease. *The New York Times,* January 19, 1996, p. A16.
32. Cowley et al., 1993.
33. Brody, J. E. New Respect for Vitamin E after Years of Faddish Aura. *The New York Times,* May 26, 1993, p. C11.
34. Stampfer, M. J., et al. Vitamin E Consumption and the Risk of Coronary Disease in Women. *New England Journal of Medicine, 328* (1993), 1441.
35. Rimm, E. B., et al. Vitamin E Consumption and the Risk of Coronary Heart Disease in Men. *New England Journal of Medicine, 328* (1993), 1450.
36. Antioxidants: Disappointment and Hope. *Harvard Heart Letter,* 7(2), October 1996, p. 1.
37. Liebman, B. Beyond Beta-Carotene. *Nutrition Action Newsletter,* January/February 1995, Antioxidants: Disappointment and Hope. *Harvard Heart Letter,* 7(2), October 1996, pp. 8–9; No support for Beta Carotene Supplements. *Harvard Heart Letter, 6,* No. 10 (1996), p. 7; How Much Vitamin C Is Enough? *Tufts University Diet & Nutrition Letter, 14*(8), October 1996, p. 8; Facts and Fiction about Vitamin E. *Harvard Health Letter, 22*(1), November 1996, pp. 1–3.
38. Kolata, G., 1996, p. 16.
39. Kolata, 1996.
40. Napier, K. Too Many Vitamins? *Harvard Health Letter,* January 1996, pp. 1–3; Brody, J. E., Sorting Out the Benefits . . . , 1995, p. C8; Brody, J. E., Health Factor in Vegetables Still Elusive, 1995, p. C1; Hamilton et al., 1991.
41. How Much Vitamin C Is Enough? *Tufts University Diet & Nutrition Letter, 14*(8), October 1996, p. 8.
42. Hall, S. S. The Power of Garlic. *Health,* July/August 1994, pp. 82–87; *Self,* October 1995, p. 78; Liebman, B. Beyond Beta-

Carotene, January/February 1995, pp. 8–9; Brody, J. E., Reasons for Garlic's Benefits Are Uncovered. *The New York Times,* July 27, 1994, p. C8; Brody, J. E., Fish Stories and the Hoopla over Fish Oils. *The New York Times,* August 3, 1994, p. C10; Seligmann, J., and Cowley, G. Sex, Lies and Garlic. *Newsweek,* November 6, 1995, pp. 65–68; Phytochemicals: Drugstore in a Salad? *Consumer Reports on Health,* December 1995, pp. 133–135.

43. Gaby, S. K., and Singh, V. N. Vitamin C. In S. K. Gaby, A. Bendich, V. N. Singh, and L. J. Machlin (eds.), *Vitamin Intake and Health: A Scientific Review.* New York: Marcel Dekker, 1991.
44. Gaby and Singh, 1991; NRC, 1989.
45. The Latest Elixir of Life: Vitamin C. *Tufts University Diet & Nutrition Letter, 10*(5), July 1992, p. 1.
46. Was Linus Pauling Right? *UC Berkeley Wellness Letter, 12*(3), December 1995, p. 2.
47. For Men of Childbearing Age. *Tufts University Diet & Nutrition Letter, 10*(4), June 1992, p. 1.
48. Gaby and Singh, 1991; Vitamin C Boosts "Good" HDL. *Consumer Reports on Health,* February 1995, p. 21.
49. The Amazing Story of Niacin. *Tufts University Diet & Nutrition Letter, 9*(2), April 1991, p. 1.
50. Folic Acid for Fighting Birth Defects? *Tufts University Diet & Nutrition Letter, 10*(9), November 1992, pp. 1–2.
51. Folic Acid for All. *Nutrition Action Health-Letter, 19*(10), December 1992, p. 4; Centers for Disease Control. *Morbidity and Mortality Weekly Review, 41,* September 11, 1992.
52. Folic Acid for Fighting Birth Defects?, 1992.
53. Kolata, G. Vitamin to Protect Fetuses Will Be Required in Foods. *The New York Times,* March 1, 1996, p. A1.
54. Folate Finds. *Prevention,* February 1996, p. 26.
55. Morrison, H. I., et al. Serum Folate and Risk of Fatal Coronary Heart Disease. *Journal of the American Medical Association, 275* (1996), 1893–1896.
56. NRC, 1989.
57. Adapted from NRC, 1989; Combs, 1992; and other sources.
58. NIH Consensus Conference: Osteoporosis. *Journal of the American Medical Association, 252* (1984), 799–802.
59. Brody, J. E. The War on Brittle Bones Must Start Early in Life. *The New York Times,* June 15, 1994, p. C7.
60. U.S. Department of Health and Human Services. Publication (FDA) 85–2198. Washington, DC: U.S. Government Printing Office, 1986.
61. Special Report: Iron Overkill. *UC Berkeley Wellness Letter, 12*(10), July 1996, pp. 4–5.
62. The Many Reasons to Cut Back on Salt. *UC Berkeley Wellness Letter, 11*(10), July 1995, pp. 1–2.
63. NBC Nightly News, July 1, 1996.
64. Purdum, T. S. Meat Inspections Facing Overhaul, First in 90 Years. *The New York Times,* July 7, 1996, pp. A1, A11.
65. Brody, J. E. *Jane Brody's The New York Times Guide to Personal Health.* New York: Times Books, 1982, p. 548.
66. How to Avoid Food Poisoning. *Nutrition Action Healthletter,* July/August 1996, pp. 6–8.
67. Portions reprinted from Hecht, A. The Unwelcome Dinner Guest: Preventing Food-Borne Illness. *FDA Consumer,* January/February 1991. Tips for Keeping Food Safe. *Tufts University Diet & Nutrition Letter, 14*(4), June 1996, P. 5; Don't Judge a Burger by Its Color. Other sources include *Tufts University Diet & Nutrition Letter, 13*(6), August 1995, p. 1.
68. Can I Get Good Poisoning from Fresh Fruits and Vegetables? *Health,* January/February 1997, p. 18.
69. U.S. Department of Agriculture, U.S. Department of Health and Human Services. *Dietary Guidelines for Americans* (3rd ed.). Home and Garden Bulletin No. 232. Washington, DC: U.S. Government Printing Office, 1990.
70. Burros, M. In an About-face, U.S. Says Alcohol Has Health Benefits. *The New York Times,* January 3, 1996, pp. A1, C2.
71. U.S. Department of Agriculture, Human Nutrition Information Service. *Dietary Guidelines for Americans.* Home and Garden Bulletins 232–1 and 232–2. Washington, DC, U.S. Government Printing Office, 1986; U.S. Department of Agriculture, Human Nutrition Information Service, *The Food Guide Pyramid.* Home and Garden Bulletin, No. 252. Washington, DC: U.S. Government Printing Office, 1992.
72. U.S. Department of Agriculture, *The Food Guide Pyramid,* 1992.
73. U.S. Department of Agriculture. *Dietary Guidelines for Americans,* 1986; U.S. Department of Agriculture, *The Food Guide Pyramid,* 1992.
74. Burros, M. A Vegetarian Future? It Could Come. *The New York Times,* July 8, 1992, p. C3.
75. Angier, N. Chemists Learn Why Vegetables Are Good for You. *The New York Times,* April 13, 1993, p. C1.
76. Can Fast Food Be Good Food? *Consumer Reports,* August 1994, pp. 493–498; Best Deals at the Drive-in. *Prevention,* July 1995, p. 56; McAlternatives. *UC Berkeley Wellness Letter, 12*(10), July 1996, p. 8; Fast Food: Fatter than Ever. *Consumer Reports on Health,* August 1996, pp. 85–88 and other sources.
77. Adapted from the *Tufts University Diet & Nutrition Letter, 10,* What the New Food Labels Will (and Won't) Dish Up, February 1993, pp. 3–6. Reprinted with permission.

**CHAPTER 6**

1. Beck, M. An Epidemic of Obesity. *Newsweek,* August 1, 1994, pp. 62–63; Burros, M. Despite Awareness of Risks, More in U.S. Are Getting Fat. *The New York Times,* July 17, 1994, pp. A1, A18.
2. Manson, J. E., et al. Cited in Brody, J. E. Just How Perilous Can 25 Extra Pounds Be? *The New York Times,* September 20, 1995, p. C11.
3. Lane, E. Losing Weight Isn't Enough. *New York Newsday,* December 6, 1994, p. A6.
4. U.S. Department of Health and Human Services. *Healthy People 2000* Boston, MA: Jones and Bartlett, 1992.
5. Losing Weight: What Works, What Doesn't. *Consumer Reports,* June 1993, pp. 347–352.
6. Jeffery, R. W. Population Perspectives on the Prevention and Treatment of Obesity in Minority Populations. *American Journal of Clinical Nutrition, 53* (1991), 1621S–1624S.
7. Toufexis, A., et al. Dieting: The Losing Game. *Time,* January 20, 1986, pp. 54–60.
8. Blumenthal, D. Dieting Reassessed. *The New York Times Magazine, Part 2: The Good Health Magazine,* October 9, 1988, pp. 24–25, 53–54.
9. Brody, J. E. For Most Trying to Lose Weight, Dieting Only Makes Things Worse. *The New York Times,* November 23, 1992, pp. A1, A12; Wilson, G. T. Behavioral Treatment of Childhood Obesity: Theoretical and Practical Implications. *Health Psychology, 13* (1994), 371–372.
10. Fallon, A. E., and Rozin, P. Sex Differences in Perceptions of Desirable Body Shape. *Journal of Abnormal Psychology, 94* (1985), 102–105.
11. Cohn, L. D., et al. Body-Figure Preferences in Male and Female Adolescents. *Journal of Abnormal Psychology, 96* (1987), 276–279.
12. Fallon and Rozin, 1985.
13. *Data Fact Sheet: Obesity and Cardiovascular Disease.* Bethesda, MD: National Heart, Lung, and Blood Institute (NHLBI), National Institutes of Health. March 1993.
14. U.S. Department of Agriculture, Human Nutrition Information Service. *Nutrition and Your Health: Dietary Guidelines for Americans* (3rd ed.). Home and Garden Bulletin No. 232. Washington, DC: U.S. Government Printing Office, 1990.
15. Losing Weight: What Works, What Doesn't, 1993.
16. Williamson, D. F., Kahn, H. S., Remington, P. L., and Ands, R. F. The 10-year Incidence of Overweight and Major Weight Gain in U.S. Adults. *Archives of Internal Medicine, 150* (1990), 665–672.
17. Data derived from the National Research Council. Reprinted from U.S. Department of Agriculture, 1990.
18. Losing Weight: What Works, What Doesn't, 1993.
19. *Data Fact Sheet: Obesity and Cardiovascular Disease,* 1993.
20. American Dietetic Association. Position of the American Dietetic Association: Nutrition for Physical Fitness and Athletic Perfor-

mance of Adults. *Journal of the American Dietetic Association, 87* (1987), 933–939.
21. Nieman, D. C. *The Sports Medicine Fitness Course.* Palo Alto, CA: Bull Publishing Co., 1986.
22. Waist-Hip Ratio Seen as an Index of Health. *The New York Times,* January 27, 1993, p. C16.
23. Waist-Hip Ratio Seen as an Index of Health, 1993.
24. Stunkard, A. J., et al. An Adoption Study of Human Obesity. *New England Journal of Medicine, 314* (1986), 193, 198; Stunkard, A. J., et al. A Separated Twin Study of the Body Mass Index. *New England Journal of Medicine, 322* (1990), 1483–1487.
25. Angier, N. Researchers Link Obesity in Humans to Flaw in a Gene. *The New York Times,* December 1, 1994; p. A1; Brownell, K. D. Get Slim with Higher Taxes. *The New York Times,* December 15, 1994, p. A29; Seligmann, J. A Gene That Says, "No More." *Newsweek,* December 12, 1994, p. 86.
26. Brownell, K. D. Dieting and the Search for the Perfect Body: Where Physiology and Culture Collide. *Behavior Therapy, 22* (1991), 1–12.
27. Leibel, R. L., Rosenbaum, M., and Hirsch, J. Changes in Energy Expenditure Resulting from Altered Body Weight. *New England Journal of Medicine, 332* (1995), 621–628.
28. Leibel et al., 1995.
29. Braitman, L. E., Adlin, E. V., and Stanton, J. L., Jr. Obesity and Caloric Intake. *Journal of Chronic Diseases, 38* (1985), 727–732.
30. Brownell, K. D., and Wadden, T. A. Etiology and Treatment of Obesity: Understanding a Serious, Prevalent, and Refractory Disorder. *Journal of Consulting and Clinical Psychology, 60* (1992), 505–517.
31. Brownell and Wadden, 1992.
32. The Sedentary Society. *Harvard Heart Letter, 6* (August 1996), pp. 3–4.
33. More on the Pitfalls of Television Watching. *Tufts University Diet & Nutrition Letter,* June 1992, *10*(4), p. 8.
34. Ernst, N. D., and Harlan, W. R. Obesity and Cardiovascular Disease in Minority Populations: Executive Summary. *American Journal of Clinical Nutrition, 53* (1991), 1507s–1511s; Stunkard, A. J., and Sørensen, T. I. A. Obesity and Socioeconomic Status—A Complex Relation. *New England Journal of Medicine, 329* (1993), 1036–1037.
35. McMurtrie, B. Overweight Fatten Ranks. *New York Newsday,* July 19, 1994, p. A26.
36. Hazuda, H. P., et al. Obesity in Mexican American Subgroups: Findings from the San Antonio Heart Study. *American Journal of Clinical Nutrition, 53* (1991), 1529S–1534S.
37. Burros, 1994; McMurtrie, 1994.
38. Curb, J. D., and Marcus, E. B. Body Fat and Obesity in Japanese-Americans. *American Journal of Clinical Nutrition, 53* (1991), 1552S–1555S.
39. Broussard, B. A., et al. Prevalence of Obesity in American Indians and Alaska Natives. *American Journal of Clinical Nutrition, 53* (1991), 1535–1542; Young, T. K., and Sevenhuysen, G. Obesity in Northern Canadian Indians: Patterns, Determinants, and Consequences. *American Journal of Clinical Nutrition, 49* (1989), 786–793.
40. Jeffery, 1991.
41. U.S. Department of Agriculture. *Nutritive Values of Food.* Washington DC: U.S. Government Printing Office, 1991; U.S. Department of Agriculture, Human Nutrition Information Service *Dietary Guidelines for Americans: If You Drink Alcoholic Beverages, Do So in Moderation.* Home and Garden Bulletin No. 232–7. Washington, DC: U.S. Government Printing Office, April 1986.
42. Adapted from Nevid, J. S., Rathus, S. A., and Green, B. *Abnormal Psychology in a Changing World* (3rd ed.). Upper Saddle River, NJ: Prentice-Hall, 1997, p. 283. Reprinted with permission.
43. *Diagnostic and Statistical Manual of Mental Disorders* (4th ed.). Washington, DC: American Psychiatric Association, 1994.
44. Herzog, D. B., Keller, M. B., and Lavori, P. W. Outcome in Anorexia and Bulimia Nervosa: A Review of the Literature. *Journal of Nervous and Mental Disease, 176* (1988), 131–143.
45. French, S. A., Perry, C. L., Leon, G. R., and Fulkerson, J. A. Dieting Behaviors and Weight Change History in Female Adolescents. *Health Psychology, 14* (1995), 548–555.
46. Adapted from Boskind-White, M., and White, W. C. *Bulimarexia: The Binge-Purge Cycle.* New York: W. W. Norton, p. 29, 1983. Reprinted with permission from Nevid et al., 1997, p. 485.
47. Fairburn, C. G., Cooper, Z., and Cooper, P. J. The Clinical Features and Maintenance of Bulimia Nervosa. In K. D. Brownell and J. P. Foreyt (Eds.), *Handbook of Eating Disorders.* New York: Basic Books, 1986, pp. 389–404.
48. French et al., 1995.
49. Strauss, J., and Ryan, R. M. Autonomy Disturbances in Subtypes of Anorexia Nervosa. *Journal of Abnormal Psychology, 96* (1987), 254–258.
50. Kassett, J. A., et al. Psychiatric Disorders in the First-Degree Relatives of Probands with Bulimia Nervosa. *American Journal of Psychiatry, 146* (1989), 1468–1471.
51. Halmi, K. A., Eckert, E., LaDu, T. J., and Cohen, J. Treatment Efficacy of Cyproheptadine and Amitriptyline. *Archives of General Psychiatry, 43* (1986), 177–181.
52. Fluoxetine Bulimia Nervosa Collaborative Study Group. Fluoxetine in the Treatment of Bulimia Nervosa: A Multicenter, Placebo-Controlled, Double-Blind Trial. *Archives of General Psychiatry, 49* (1992), 139–147; McCann, U. D., and Agras, W. S. Successful Treatment of Nonpurging Bulimia Nervosa with Desipramine: A Double-Blind, Placebo-Controlled Study. *American Journal of Psychiatry, 147* (1990), 1509–1513.
53. Kolata, G. The Burdens of Being Overweight: Mistreatment and Misconceptions. *The New York Times,* November 22, 1992, pp. A1, A38.
54. Rosenthal, E. Commercial Diets Lack Proof of Their Long-Term Success. *The New York Times,* November 24, 1992, pp. A1, C11.
55. The Dietary Guidelines Become More User Friendly. *Tufts University Diet & Nutrition Letter, 11*(8), pp. 4–5.
56. Brownell and Wadden, 1992.
57. Wilson, G. T. Behavioral Treatment of Childhood Obesity: Theoretical and Practical Implications. *Health Psychology, 13* (1994), 371–372.
58. Adapted from Nevid et al., 1997. Reprinted with permission.
59. Losing Weight: What Works, What Doesn't, 1993.
60. Brownell and Wadden, 1992.
61. Brody, J. E. Study Finds a Liquid Diet Works (But Not for the 50% Who Quit). *The New York Times,* May 15, 1992, p. B7.
62. National Task Force on the Prevention and Treatment of Obesity. Very Low-Calorie Diets. *Journal of the American Medical Association, 270* (1993), 967–974; Wadden, T. A., Foster, G. D., and Letizia, K. A. One-year Behavioral Treatment of Obesity: Comparison of Moderate and Severe Caloric Restriction and the Effects of Weight Maintenance Therapy. *Journal of Consulting and Clinical Psychology, 62* (1994), 165–171.
63. Craighead, L. W., and Agras, W. S. Mechanisms of Action in Cognitive-Behavioral and Pharmacological Interventions for Obesity and Bulimia Nervosa. *Journal of Consulting and Clinical Psychology, 59* (1991), 115–125.
64. Kolata, G. Appetite Suppressants Aid Obese. *The New York Times,* July 5, 1992, p. B1.
65. Losing Weight: What Works, What Doesn't, 1993.
66. Abenhaim, L., et al. Appetite-Suppressant Drugs and the Risk of Primary Pulmonary Hypertension. *New England Journal of Medicine, 335* (1996), 609–616.
67. The Real Risk of the New Diet Pill. *Health,* November/December 1996, p. 18.
68. Leary, W. E. U.S. Panel Endorses Bypass Surgery for Obesity. *The New York Times,* March 27, 1991, p. B12.
69. Leary, 1991.
70. You Needn't Starve to Keep Off Lost Pounds. *Tufts University Diet & Nutrition Letter, 12*(7), February 1990, p. 7.

### CHAPTER 7

1. National Sporting Goods Association. Exercise Walking Remains America's Favorite Participant Sport. Press Release May 1992; Thomas, D. Q., and Rippee, N. E. *Is Your Aerobic Class Killing You?* Pennington, NJ: A Cappella Books, 1992, p. 3.

2. Myers, C., *Walking: A Complete Guide to the Complete Exercise.* New York: Random House, 1992, p. 4.
3. Brody, J., Unkindest Cut: Children's Fitness. *The New York Times,* February 3, 1993, p. C13.
4. Pierce, E. F., et al., Fitness Profiles and Activity Patterns of Entering College Students. *Journal of American College Health, 41* (1995), 59–62.
5. Bouchard, C., Shephard, R. J., and Stephens, T. (Eds.), *Physical Activity, Fitness, and Health: Consensus Statement,* 1993, p. 61. Proceedings of the Second International Consensus Symposium on Physical Activity, Fitness, and Health, Toronto, Ontario, Canada, May 1992. Champaign, IL: Human Kinetics Publishers, p. 15.
6. Bouchard et al., 1993.
7. Simon, H. B. *Staying Well: Your Complete Guide to Disease Prevention.* Boston: Houghton Mifflin, 1992, p. 418.
8. Leary, W. E., Exercise Helps Severe Hypertension Patients, Study Finds. *The New York Times,* November 30, 1995, p. A22.
9. Castelli, W., In with the Good, *Runner's World,* December 1987.
10. Kokkinos, P. et al. Miles Run per Week and High-Density Lipoprotein Cholesterol Levels in Healthy, Middle-aged Men. *Archives of Internal Medicine, 155,* p. 415; Gentle Exercise Is Good . . . , *Consumer Reports on Health,* July 1995, p. 77.
11. Brody, J. E. Study Says a Blood Fat Alone Isn't a Heart Threat. *The New York Times,* April 29, 1993, p. B9; NIH Consensus Development Panel on Triglyceride, High-Density Lipoprotein, and Coronary Heart Disease. *Journal of the American Medical Association, 269*(4) (1993), 505–510.
12. Does Exercise Boost Immunity? *Consumer Reports on Health,* April 1995, p. 37.
13. Paffenbarger, R. S., Lee, I-Min, and Wing, A. L., The Influence of Physical Activity on the Incidence of Site-Specific Cancers in College Alumni. In M. M. Jacobs (Ed.), *Exercise, Calories, Fat, and Cancer.* New York: Plenum Press, 1992, pp. 7–15; Bouchard et al., 1993.
14. Does Exercise Boost Immunity?, 1995.
15. Brody, J. E. Regimen of Moderate Exercise Tied to Drop in Breast Cancer. *The New York Times,* September 21, 1994, p. C10.
16. Chrischilles, E., Sherman, T., and Wallace, R. Cost and Health Effects of Osteoporotic Fractures. *Bone, 15* (1994), 377–386.
17. LeFavi, B. Exercise Isn't Only Prevention: Now It's Part of the Treatment. *Muscle and Fitness,* June 1992, p. 158.
18. Robinson, T. L., Snow-Harter, C., et al. Gymnasts Exhibit Higher Bone Mass than Runners Despite Similar Prevalence of Amenorrhea and Oligomenorrhea. *Journal of Bone Mineral Research, 10* (1995), 26–35.
19. Kohl, H. W., et al., Musculoskeletal Strength and Serum Lipid Levels in Men and Women. *Medicine and Science in Sports and Exercise, 24*(10) (1992), 1080–1087.
20. Pate, R. R., et al. Physical Activity and Public Health: A Recommendation from the Centers for Disease Control and Prevention and the American College of Sports Medicine. *Journal of the American Medical Associations, 273* (1995), 402–407. Reprinted with permission of the *Journal of the American Medical Association.*
21. Pate et al., 1995, p. 404.
22. Gentle Exercise Is Good, 1995, p. 77.
23. Jaret, P. The Great Fitness Debate. *Health,* September 1994, p. 64.
24. State Surveys Find Few Adults Exercise Enough. *The New York Times,* August 10, 1996, p. A12.
25. Gentle Exercise Is Good, 1995, p. 77; *Physical Activity and Health At-A-Glance: A Report of the Surgeon General,* Washington, D.C.: U.S. Government Printing Office, 1996.
26. The President's Council on Physical Fitness and Sports and Centers for Disease Control and Prevention, National Center for Chronic Disease Prevention and Health Promotion Division of Nutrition and Physical Activity. *Morbidity and Mortality.* In *Physical Activity and Health: A Report of the Surgeon General,* 1996.
27. Brody, J. E. Trying to Reconcile Exercise Findings. *The New York Times,* April 23, 1995, sec. 1, p. A22; Lee, I., et al. Exercise Intensity and Longevity in Men: The Harvard Alumni Health Study. *Journal of the American Medical Association, 273* (1995), 1179–1184.
28. American College of Sports Medicine. *Guidelines for Exercise Testing and Prescription* (4th ed.). Philadelphia: Lea & Febiger, 1991: Pate et al., 1995.
29. Bouchard, C., and Shephard, R. J. Physical Activity, Fitness, and Health: The Model and Key Concepts. In C. Bouchard et al., 1993.
30. Blair, S., et al. Physical Fitness and All-cause Mortality: A Prospective Study of Health Men and Women. *Journal of the American Medical Association, 262* (1989), 2395–2401.
31. Pollock, M. L., and Wilmore, J. H., *Exercise in Health and Disease* (2nd ed.). Philadelphia: W. B. Saunders, 1990.
32. Leon, A. S., et al. Leisure Time Physical Activity Levels and Risk of Coronary Heart Disease and Death: The Multiple Risk Factor Intervention Model. *Journal of the American Medical Association, 258* (1987), 2388–2395.
33. Arnheim, D. D., and Prentice, W. E. *Principles of Athletic Training* (8th ed.). St. Louis: Mosby Year Book Inc., 1993.
34. American College of Sports Medicine. Recommended Quantity and Quality of Exercise. Position Stand Pamphlet.
35. Pierce, E. F., et al., Fitness Profiles and Activity Patterns of Entering College Students.
36. American College of Sports Medicine. Recommended Quantity and Quality of Exercise. Position Stand Pamphlet.
37. National Heart, Lung, and Blood Institute, National Institutes of Health, and American Heart Association. *Exercise and Your Heart: A Guide to Physical Activity,* NIH Pub. No. 93–1677, August 1993, p. 6.
38. An IQ Test for "Losers." *Tufts University Diet and Nutrition Letter,* March 1992, p. 1.
39. Can Fat Be Fit? *UC Berkeley Wellness Letter,* November 1995, p. 3.
40. Brody, J. E. Exercise Can Improve Many Aspects of a Disabled Person's Life. *The New York Times,* January 25, 1990, p. B11.
41. Does Exercise Boost Immunity?, 1995.
42. Does Exercise Boost Immunity?, 1995.
43. Anderson, O. Exercise Overload. *American Health,* January/February 1991, p. 27; Yessis, M. Work Hard, Rest Easy. *Muscle and Fitness,* December 1992, p. 59.
44. Kunz, J. R. M., and Finkel, A. (Eds.). *The American Medical Association Family Medical Guide, Revised and updated.* New York: Random House, 1987, p. 543.
45. American College of Sports Medicine. *Prevention of Heat Injuries during Running.* Position Stand Pamphlet.
46. National Heart, Lung, and Blood Institute, National Institutes of Health. *Exercise and Your Heart: A Guide to Physical Activity.* NIH Publication No. 93–1677, Revised August 1993.
47. National Sporting Goods Association Press Release, April 1992.
48. Starzinger, P. H., Sneaking Around, *American Health,* March 1993, pp. 56–60.
49. U.S. Department of Health and Human Services. *Healthy People 2000. National Health Promotion and Disease Prevention Objectives.* Washington, DC: U.S. Government Printing Office, 1991.
50. Schieber, R. A., Branche-Dorsey, C. M., Ryan, G. W., et al. Risk Factors for Injuries from In-Line Skating and the Effectiveness of Safety Gear. *The New England Journal of Medicine, 335* (1996), 1630–1635; U.S. Study Tells Skaters Where to Put the Pads. *The New York Times,* November 18, 1996, p. A20.
51. *Exercise and Your Heart: A Guide to Physical Activity,* 1993.
52. Safe Winter Workouts. *Consumer Reports on Health,* February 1995, p. 20.
53. Nutrition and Exercise: What Your Body Needs. *UC Berkeley Wellness Letter,* May 1993, p. 4.
54. Gillin, J. C. The Long and the Short of Sleeping Pills. *New England Journal of Medicine, 324* (1991), 1735–1736.
55. Poppy, J. Easy Does It. *Health,* October 1995, p. 42.
56. Aeni, A., Hoffman, M. D., and Clifford, P. S. Energy Expenditure with Indoor Exercise Machines. *Journal of the American Medical Association, 275* (1996), 1424–1427; The Best Indoor Exercise Machine. *Harvard Heart Letter,* August 1996, p. 8.
57. Making Fitness Stick, *Consumer Reports on Health,* February 1995, p. 20.

58. Gauvin, L. Cited in Sheehan, G. Too Legit to Quit. *Runner's World,* March 1992, p. 16.
59. Making Fitness Stick, 1995.
60. Poppy, 1995.
61. Sullivan, D., 1995, *Self,* September 1995, pp. 164–168; and other sources.
62. Chartrand, S. Growing Problems with Repetitive Stress Injuries. *The New York Times,* March 31, 1996.

### CHAPTER 8

1. Levinger, G. Development and Change. In H. H. Kelley et al. (Eds.), *Close Relationships.* New York: W. H. Freeman, 1983.
2. Michael, R. T., Gagnon, J. H., Laumann, E. O., and Kolata, G. *Sex in America: A Definitive Survey.* Boston: Little, Brown, 1994.
3. Nevid, J. S. Sex Differences in Factors of Romantic Attraction. *Sex Roles, 11* (1984), 401–411.
4. Buss, D. M. *The Evolution of Desire: Strategies of Human Mating.* New York: Basic Books, 1994.
5. Based on information in Sprecher, S., Sullivan, Q., and Hatfield, E. Mate Selection Preferences: Gender Differences Examined in a National Sample. *Journal of Personality and Social Psychology, 66*(6) (1994), 1074–1080.
6. Adapted from Rathus, S. A., and Nevid, J. S. *Behavior Therapy.* New York: Doubleday, 1977.
7. Michael, R. T., et al., 1994, pp. 45–47.
8. Griffin, E., and Sparks, G. G. Friends Forever: A Longitudinal Exploration of Intimacy in Same-Sex Friends and Platonic Pairs. *Journal of Social and Personal Relationships, 7* (1990), 29–46; Cappella, J. N., and Palmer, M. T. (1990). Attitude Similarity, Relational History, and Attraction: The Mediating Effects of Kinesic and Vocal Behaviors. *Communication Monographs, 5* (1990), 161–183; Laumann, E. O., et al. *The Social Organization of Sexuality: Sexual Practices in the United States.* Chicago: University of Chicago Press, 1994.
9. Feingold, A. Sex Differences in the Effects of Similarity and Physical Attractiveness on Opposite-Sex Attraction. *Basic and Applied Social Psychology, 12* (1991), 357–367.
10. Berscheid, E. Some Comments on Love's Anatomy: Or, Whatever Happened to Old-fashioned Lust? In R. J. Sternberg and M. L. Barnes (Eds.), *The Psychology of Love* (pp. 359–374). New Haven, CN: Yale University Press, 1988; Simpson, J. A., Campbell, B., and Berscheid, E. The Association between Romantic Love and Marriage: Kephart (1967) Twice Revisited. *Personality and Social Psychology Bulletin,* 1986, 363–372.
11. Sternberg, R. J. *The Triangle of Love: Intimacy, Passion, Commitment.* New York: Basic Books, 1988.
12. Adapted from Sternberg, 1988.
13. Cited in Steinhauer, J. No Marriage, No Apologies. *The New York Times,* July 6, 1995, pp. C1, C7.
14. Steinhauer, 1995.
15. Riche, M. Postmarital Society. *American Demographics,* November 23–26, 1988, 60.
16. Adapted from Laumann, E. O. Gagnon, J. H., Michael, R. T., and Michaels, S. *The Social Organization of Sexuality: Sexual Practices in the United States.* Chicago: University of Chicago Press, 1994.
17. Oppenheim Mason, K., with the assistance of D. R. Denison and A. J. Schacht. *Sex-Role Attitude Items and Scales from U.S. Sample Surveys.* Rockville, MD: National Institute of Mental Health, 1975, pp. 16–19.
18. Adapted by permission from Knox, D. *Choices in Relationships* p.164. Copyright © 1988 by West Publishing Company. All rights reserved.
19. Sengupta, S. Survey Finds 90's College Freshmen More Conservative than Predecessors. *The New York Times,* January 13, 1997, p. A14.
20. Kilborn, P. T. Shifts in Families Reach a Plateau, Study Says. *The New York Times,* November 27, 1996, p. 18.
21. Reprinted from Rathus, S. A. A 30-Item Schedule for Assessing Assertive Behavior. *Behavior Therapy, 4* (1973), 398–406.

### CHAPTER 9

1. Adelson, A. Study Attacks Women's Roles in TV. *The New York Times,* November 19, 1990, p. C18.
2. Hyde, J. S., and Plant, E. A. Magnitude of Psychological Gender Differences: Another Side to the Story. *American Psychologist, 50* (1995) 159–161; Voyer, D., Voyer, S., and Bryden, M. P. Magnitude of Sex Differences in Spatial Abilities: A Meta-Analysis and Consideration of Critical Variables. *Psychological Bulletin, 117* (1995), 250–270.
3. Feingold, A. Gender Differences in Personality: A Meta-Analysis. *Psychological Bulletin, 116* (1994), 429–456.
4. Ahmed, R. A. Women in Egypt and the Sudan. In L. L. Adler (Ed.), *Women in Cross-Cultural Perspective.* New York: Praeger, 1991, pp. 107–134.
5. Ahmed, 1991; Rosenthal, A. M. Female Genital Torture. *The New York Times,* November 12, 1993, p. A33.
6. Kaplan, D. A. Is It Torture or Tradition? *Newsweek,* December 20, 1993, p. 124.
7. Rosenthal, A. M. The Possible Dream. *The New York Times,* June 13, 1995, p. A25.
8. Boston Women's Health Book Collective. *The New Our Bodies, Ourselves.* New York: Simon & Schuster, 1992.
9. Morrison, E. S., et al. *Growing Up Sexual.* New York: Van Nostrand Reinhold, 1980, pp. 66–70.
10. Gruber, V. A., and Wildman, B. G. The Impact of Dysmenorrhea on Daily Activities. *Behaviour Research and Therapy, 25* (1987), 123–128.
11. Rubinow, D. R., and Schmidt, P. J. The Treatment of Premenstrual Syndrome—Forward into the Past. *New England Journal of Medicine, 332* (1995), 1574–1575.
12. Liberman, U. A., et al. Effect of Oral Alendronate on Bone Mineral Density and the Incidence of Fractures in Postmenopausal Osteoporosis. *New England Journal of Medicine, 333* (1995), 1437–1443.
13. Colditz, G. A., et al. The Use of Estrogens and Progestins and the Risk of Breast Cancer in Postmenopausal Women. *New England Journal of Medicine, 332* (1995), 1589–1593.
14. Stampfer, M. J., et al. Ten-Year Follow-Up Study of Estrogen Replacement Therapy in Relation to Cardiovascular Disease and Mortality. Paper presented at the 24th annual meeting of the Society for Epidemiologic Research, Buffalo, New York, June 11–14, 1991.
15. Mixture May Rival Estrogen in Preventing Heart Disease. *The New York Times,* August 15, 1996, p. A18.
16. Touchette, N. HIV-1 Link Prompts Circumspection of Circumcision. *The Journal of NIH Research, 3* (1991), 44–46.
17. Brody, J. E. Hormone Replacement Therapy for Men: When Does it Help? *The New York Times,* August 30, 1995, p. C8.
18. Masters, W. H., and Johnson, V. E. *Human Sexual Response.* Boston: Little, Brown, 1966.
19. Adapted from Laumann, E. O., Gagnon, J. H., Michael, R. T., and Michaels, S. *The Social Organization of Sexuality: Sexual Practices in the United States.* Chicago: University of Chicago Press, 1994, Table 3.3, p. 86.
20. Laumann et al., 1994.
21. Leitenberg, H., Detzer, M. J., and Srebnik, D. Gender Differences in Masturbation and the Relation of Masturbation Experience in Preadolescence and/or Early Adolescence to Sexual Behavior and Sexual Adjustment in Young Adulthood. *Archives of Sexual Behavior, 22* (1993), 87–98.
22. Laumann et al., 1994.
23. Laumann et al., 1994.
24. Voeller, B. AIDS and Heterosexual Anal Intercourse. *Archives of Sexual Behavior,* 20 (1991), 233–276.
25. Janus, S. S., and Janus, C. L. *The Janus Report on Sexual Behavior.* New York: Wiley, 1993; Laumann et al., 1994.
26. Bell, A. P., Weinberg, M. S., and Hammersmith, S. K. *Sexual Preference: Its Development in Men and Women,* Bloomington, IN: University of Indiana Press, 1981.
27. Bailey, J. M., and Pillard, R. C. A Genetic Study of Male Sexual Orientation. *Archives of General Psychiatry, 48* (1991), 1089–1096.
28. Collaer, M. L., and Hines, M. Human Behavioral Sex Differences: A Role for Gonadal Hormones during Early Development? *Psychological Bulletin, 118* (1995), 55–107.
29. LeVay, S. A Difference in Hypothalamic Structure between Heterosexual and Homosexual Men. *Science, 253* (1991), 1034–1037.

30. Rathus, S. A., Nevid, J. S., and Fichner-Rathus, L. *Human Sexuality in a World of Diversity,* 3rd ed. Boston: Allyn & Bacon, 1997.
31. Adapted from Laumann et al., 1994, Tables 10.8A and 10.8B, pp. 370 and 371.
32. *Diagnostic and Statistical Manual of Mental Disorders,* 4th ed. Washington, DC: American Psychiatric Association, 1994.
33. Woolf, S. H. Current Concepts: Screening for Prostate Cancer with Prostate-Specific Antigen—An Examination of the Evidence. *New England Journal of Medicine, 333* (1995), 1401–1405.
34. Vazi, R., Best, D., Davis, S., and Kaiser, M. Evaluation of a Testicular Cancer Curriculum for Adolescents. *Journal of Pediatrics, 114* (1989), 150–162.
35. Carlile, T. Breast Cancer Detection. *Cancer, 47* (1981), 1164–1169.
36. *For Men Only: Testicular Cancer and How to Do TSE (A Self-Exam),* rev. ed. Atlanta: American Cancer Society, 1990.

### CHAPTER 10

1. Howards, S. S. Current Concepts: Treatment of Male Infertility. *New England Journal of Medicine, 332* (1995), 312–317.
2. Highlights of a new report from the National Center for Health Statistics (NCHS). *Contraceptive Use in the United States: 1982–90.* February 14, 1995.
3. White, E., et al. Breast Cancer among Young U.S. Women in Relation to Oral Contraceptive Use. *Journal of the National Cancer Institute,* April 6, 1994; Malone, K. E., et al. Oral Contraceptives in Relation to Breast Cancer. *Epidemiologic Reviews, 15* (1993), 80–97; Schlesselman, J. J. Net Effect of Oral Contraceptive Use on the Risk of Cancer in Women in the United States. *Obstetrics & Gynecology, 85* (1995), 793–801; The Pill: A Clean Bill of Health. *UC Berkeley Wellness Letter, 13*(3), December 1996, p. 1.
4. Mishell, D. R., Jr. Medical Progress: Contraception. *New England Journal of Medicine, 320* (1989), 777–787.
5. Brody, J. E. The Known and Potential Benefits of the Pill. *The New York Times,* October 2, 1996, p. C11; Hatcher, R. A., et al. *Contraceptive Technology 1992–1994* (16th rev. ed.). New York: Irvington Publishers, 1994.
6. Hatcher et al., 1994.
7. Cates, W., Jr., and Stone, K. M. Family Planning, Sexually Transmitted Diseases, and Contraceptive Choice: A Literature Update—Part II. *Family Planning Perspectives, 24* (1992), 122–127.
8. Adapted from Centers for Disease Control pamphlet, *Condoms and Sexual Transmitted Diseases . . . Especially AIDS* (HHS Publication FDA 90–4329), and other sources.
9. Feature adapted from CDC pamphlet, *Condoms and Sexually Transmitted Diseases . . . Especially AIDS,* and the American Social Health Association pamphlet, *Condoms, Contraceptives, and Sexually Transmitted Disease.*
10. Altman, L. K. New Caution, and Some Reassurance, on Vasectomy. *The New York Times,* February 21, 1993, sec. 4, p. 2.
11. Giovannucci, E., et al. A Prospective Cohort Study of Vasectomy and Prostate Cancer in U.S. Men. *Journal of the American Medical Association, 269* (1993), 873–877; Giovannucci, E., et al. A Retrospective Cohort Study of Vasectomy and Prostate Cancer in U.S. Men. *Journal of the American Medical Association, 269* (1993), 878–882.
12. Perlman, et al. To the Editor. *Journal of the American Medical Association, 270* (1993), 706–707.
13. Walt, V. Some 2nd Thoughts on Depo. *New York Newsday,* July 26, 1993, p. 13.
14. Laird, J. A Male Pill? Gender Discrepancies in Contraceptive Commitment. *Feminism and Psychology, 4*(3), 1994, 458–468.
15. Abortion Rate in 1994 Hits a 20-year low. *The New York Times,* January 5, 1997.
16. Sagan, C., and Dryan, A. The Question of Abortion: A Search for Answers. *Parade Magazine,* April 22, 1990, pp. 4–8.
17. Adapted from Parsons, N. K., Richards, H. C., and Kanter, G. D. Validation of a Scale to Measure Reasoning about Abortion. *Journal of Counseling Psychology, 37* (1990), 107–112. Copyright © 1990 by the American Psychological Association. Adapted with permission.
18. Population Council (1995). Cited in Brody, J. E. Abortion Method Using Two Drugs Gains in a Study. *The New York Times,* August 31, 1995, pp. A1, B12.
19. Smolowe, J. New, Improved and Ready for Battle. *Time,* June 14, 1993, p. 51.
20. Hausknecht, R. U. Methotrexate and Misoprostol to Terminate Early Pregnancy. *New England Journal of Medicine, 333* (1995), 537–540.
21. Knox, D. *Choices in Relationships.* St. Paul: West Publishing Co., 1988, p. 455.
22. Armsworth, M. W. Psychological Response to Abortion. *Journal of Counseling and Development, 69* (1991), 377–379.
23. Major, B., and Cozzarelli, C. Psychosocial Predictors of Adjustment to Abortion. *Journal of Social Issues, 48* (1992), 121–142.
24. Adapted from Bumiller, E. Japan's Abortion Agony: In a Country That Prohibits the Pill, Reality Collides with Religion. *Washington Post,* October 25, 1990.
25. Angier, N. Future of the Pill May Lie Just over the Counter. *The New York Times,* 1993, sec. 4, p. 5.

### CHAPTER 11

1. Samuels, M., and Samuels, N. *The Well Pregnancy Book.* New York: Harper & Row, 1986.
2. Leary, W. E. Screening of All Newborns Urged for Sickle Cell Disease. *The New York Times,* April 28, 1993, p. C11.
3. Hubbard, R., and Wald, E. *Exploding the Gene Myth.* Boston: Beacon Press, 1993.
4. *Fetal Heart Rate Patterns.* Technical Bulletin. No. 207. Washington, DC: American College of Obstetricians and Gynecologists, 1995.
5. U.S. Says 349,000 Caesareans in 1991 Were Not Necessary. *The New York Times,* April 23, 1993, p. A16.
6. Singh, G. K., and Yu, S. M. Cited in Pear, R. Infant Mortality Rate Drops but Racial Disparity Grows. *The New York Times,* July 10, 1995, p. B9.
7. Singh and Yu, 1995.
8. McLaughlin, F. J., et al. Randomized Trial of Comprehensive Prenatal Care for Low-income Women: Effect on Infant Birth Weight. *Pediatrics, 89* (1992), 128–132.
9. Barr, H. M., et al. Prenatal Exposure to Alcohol, Caffeine, Tobacco, and Aspirin. *Developmental Psychology, 26* (1990), 339–348; McLaughlin et al., 1992.
10. McLaughlin et al., 1992.
11. Data from Department of Health, City of New York, 1990.
12. Campbell, S. B., and Cohn, J. F. Prevalence and Correlates of Postpartum Depression in First-time Mothers. *Journal of Abnormal Psychology, 100* (1991), 594–599.
13. Oakley, G. P., and Erickson, J. D. Vitamin A and Birth Defects. *New England Journal of Medicine, 333* (1995), 1414–1415.
14. Rothman, K. J., et al. Teratogenicity of High Vitamin A Intake. *New England Journal of Medicine, 333* (1995), 1369–1373.
15. Niccols, G. A. Fetal Alcohol Syndrome: Implications for Psychologists. *Clinical Psychology Review, 14* (1994), 91–111. Streissguth, A. P. A Long-Term Perspective of FAS. *Alcohol Health and Research World, 18* (1994), 74–81.
16. Coles, C. Critical Periods for Prenatal Alcohol Exposure: Evidence from Animal and Human Studies. *Alcohol Health and Research World, 18*(1) (1994), 22–29.
17. Niccols, 1994.
18. Jacobson, J. L., and Jacobson, S. W. Prenatal Alcohol Exposure and Neurobehavioral Development: Where Is the Threshold? *Alcohol Health and Research World, 18*(1) (1994), 30–36.
19. Astley, S. J., et al. Analysis of Facial Shape in Children Gestationally Exposed to Marijuana, Alcohol, and/or Cocaine. *Pediatrics, 89* (1992), 67–77.
20. Floyd, R. L., Rimer, B. K., Giovino, G. A., Mullen, P. D., and Sullivan, S. E. A Review of Smoking in Pregnancy: Effects on Pregnancy Outcomes and Cessation Efforts. *Annual Review of Public Health, 14* (1993), 379–411.
21. Day, N. L., and Richardson, G. A. Comparative Teratogenicity of Alcohol and Other Drugs. *Alcohol Health and Research World, 18*(1), (1994), 42–48.
22. Schoendorf, K. C., and Kiely, J. L. Relation-

ship of Sudden Infant Death Syndrome to Maternal during and after Pregnancy. *Pediatrics, 90* (1992), 905–908.

23. Barr et al., 1990.
24. Floyd et al., 1993.

### CHAPTER 12

1. U.S. Department of Health and Human Services (USDHSS). *NIDA Capsules: Highlight of an Attitudes and Knowledge Survey about Illegal Drug Use.* No. 19. Public Health Service, Alcohol, Drug Abuse and Mental Health Administration, National Institute on Drug Abuse. Rockville, MD: National Institute on Drug Abuse, 1992.
2. *Diagnostic and Statistical Manual of Mental Disorders,* 4th ed. Washington, DC: American Psychiatric Association, 1994.
3. Ridker, P. M., et al. Inflammation, Aspirin, and the Risk of Cardiovascular Disease in Apparently Healthy Men. *New England Journal of Medicine, 336* (1997), 973–979.
4. National Institute on Aging, U.S. Department of Health and Human Services, Public Health Service, National Institutes of Health, 1995.
5. Schneider, N. G. Nicotine Gum in Smoking Cessation: Rationale, Efficacy, and Proper Use. *Comprehensive Therapy, 13* (1987), 32–37.
6. Goldstein, A. *Addiction: From Biology to Drug Policy.* New York: W. H. Freeman, 1994, p. 2.
7. Gawin, F. H. Cocaine Addiction: Psychology and Neurophysiology. *Science, 251* (1991), 1581.
8. U.S. Department of Health and Human Services (USDHSS). *NIDA Capsules: Summary of Findings from the 1991 National Household Survey on Drug Abuse.* No. 20. Public Health Service, Alcohol, Drug Abuse and Mental Health Administration, National Institute on Drug Abuse. Rockville, MD: National Institute on Drug Abuse, 1991.
9. Pihl, R. O., and Peterson, J. B. Etiology. *Annual Review of Addictions Research and Treatment, 2* (1992), 153–175, p. 155.
10. Azar, B. Several Genetic Traits Linked to Alcoholism: *APA Monitor, 26* (5) (1995), 21–22; Haney, M., et al. Cocaine Sensitivity in Roman High and Low Avoidance Rats Is Modulated by Sex and Gonadal Hormone Status. *Brain Research, 645* (1–2) (1994), 179–185; Pomerleau, O. F., Collins, A. C., Shiffman, S., and Pomerleau, C. S. Why Some People Smoke and Others Do Not: New Perspectives. *Journal of Consulting and Clinical Psychology, 61* (1993), 723–731.
11. Weiss, R. D., Mirin, S. M., and Bartel, R. L. *Cocaine,* 2/e. Washington, DC: American Psychiatric Press, Inc., 1993.
12. Goldstein, 1994, p. 140.
13. Weiss, Mirin, and Bartel, p. 71.
14. Weiss, Mirin, and Bartel, pp. 100–101.
15. Ellickson, P. L., Hays, R. D., and Bell, R. M. Stepping Through the Drug Use Sequence: Longitudinal Scalogram Analysis of Initiation and Regular Use. *Journal of Abnormal Psychology, 101* (1992), 441–451.
16. Ellickson et al., 1992.
17. Johnston, L., O'Malley, P., and Bachman, J. *Illicit Drug Use, Smoking, and Drinking by America's High School Students, College Students, and Young Adults.* DHHS Publication No. (ADM) 91–1813. Rockville, MD: Alcohol, Drug Abuse and Mental Health Administration, 1991.
18. U.S. Department of Health and Human Services (USDHHS). *National Household Survey on Drug Abuse: Highlights 1991.* DHHS Publication No. (SMA) 93–1979. Washington, DC: U.S. Government Printing Office, 1993a, p. 9.
19. Johnston, L. D., O'Malley, P. M., and Bachman, J. G. *National Survey Results on Drug Use from The Monitoring the Future Study, 1975–1995, Vol. I. Secondary School Students.* U.S. Department of Health and Human Services, Public Health Service, National Institutes of Health: National Institute on Drug Abuse, 1996.
20. Johnston, et al., 1996, vol. I.
21. NBC Nightly News, December 3, 1996.
22. NBC Nightly News, August 21, 1996.
23. Johnston, L. D., O'Malley, P. M., and Bachman, J. G. *National Survey Results on Drug Use from the Monitoring the Future Study, 1975–1994. Volume II. College Students and Young Adults.* U.S. Department of Health and Human Services, Public Health Service, National Institutes of Health: National Institute on Drug Abuse, 1996, Tables 23 (p. 160) and 25 (p. 162).
24. U.S. Department of Health and Human Services (USDHSS). *NIDA Capsules: Research on Drugs and the Workplace.* No. 24, Public Health Service, Alcohol, Drug Abuse and Mental Health Administration, National Institute on Drug Abuse. Rockville, MD: National Institute on Drug Abuse, 1990a.
25. USDHHS, 1990a.
26. Joyce, T., Racine, A. D., and Mocan, N. The Consequences and Costs of Maternal Substance Abuse in New York City: A Pooled Time-Series, Cross-Section Analysis. *Journal of Health Economics, 11* (1992), 297–314.
27. U.S. House of Representatives. *On the Edge of the American Dream: A Social and Economic Profile in 1992.* A report by the Chairman, Select Committee on Narcotics Abuse and Control. Washington, DC. U.S. Government Printing Office, 1992.
28. U.S. House of Representatives, 1992.
29. U.S. House of Representatives, 1992.
30. U.S. Department of Health and Human Services (USDHHS), Substance Abuse and Mental Health Services Administration. *National Household Survey on Drug Abuse: Population Estimates 1992.* DHHS Publication No. (SMA) 93–2053, Washington, DC: U.S. Government Printing Office, October 1993b.
31. U.S. Department of Health and Human Services (USDHSS). *NIDA Capsules: Substance Abuse among Blacks in the U.S.* No. 34. Public Health Service, Alcohol, Drug Abuse and Mental Health Administration, National Institute on Drug Abuse. Rockville, MD: National Institute on Drug Abuse, 1990b.
32. USDHHS, 1990b.
33. Anthony, J. C., Warner, L. A., and Kessler, R. C. Comparative Epidemiology of Dependence on Tobacco, Alcohol, Controlled Substances, and Inhalants: Basic Findings from the National Comorbidity Survey. *Experimental and Clinical Psychopharmacology, 2* (1994), 244–268.
34. Lillie-Blanton, M., Anthony, J. C., and Schuster, C. R. Probing the Meaning of Racial/Ethnic Group Comparisons in Crack Cocaine Smoking. *Journal of the American Medical Association, 269* (1993), 993–997.
35. Ling, G. S. F., et al. Separation of Morphine Analgesia from Physical Dependence. *Science,* 226 (1984), 462–464; U.S. Department of Health and Human Services (USDHSS). *NIDA Capsules: Heroin.* No. 11. Public Health Service, Alcohol, Drug Abuse and Mental Health Administration, National Institute on Drug Abuse. Rockville, MD: National Institute on Drug Abuse, 1986a.
36. Goldstein, 1994, p. 138.
37. USDHHS, 1991.
38. Goldstein, 1994, p. 141.
39. U.S. House of Representatives, 1992, p. 3.
40. Grounds for Breaking the Coffee Habit? *Tufts University Diet & Nutrition Letter, 7*(10) (1990), pp. 3–6.
41. Goldstein, 1994, p. 180.
42. Light Coffee Drinkers Are Hooked, Too. *Tufts University Diet & Nutrition Letter, 10*(10) (1993), pp. 1–2.
43. Hatch, E. E., and Bracken, M. B. Caffeine Use During Pregnancy: How Much Is Safe? *Journal of the American Medical Association, 270,* (1993), 46–47; Hilchey, T. Women Reassured on Coffee Intake. *The New York Times,* February 3, 1993, p. A11; Mills, J. L., et al. Moderate Caffeine Use and the Risk of Spontaneous Abortion and Intrauterine Growth Retardation. *Journal of the American Medical Association, 269* (1993), 593–597.
44. Data from *Tufts University Diet & Nutrition Letter,* February 1990, vol. 7, no. 12, p. 4.
45. National Institute of Drug Abuse. *NIDA Capsule. Methamphetamine Abuse.* Doc. C–89–06, 1995.
46. USDHHS, 1993a, p. 9.
47. Weiss and Mirin, 1987.
48. Gawin, F. H., et al. Desipramine Facilitation of Initial Cocaine Abstinence. *Archives of General Psychiatry, 46* (1989), 117–121.
49. Gawin et al., 1989.
50. Goldstein, 1994, p. 158.
51. Weiss and Mirin, 1987.
52. USDHHS, 1991.

53. National Institute of Drug Abuse. *NIDA Capsule. LSD (Lysergic Acid Diethylamide).* Doc. C–92–01, 195, 1995.
54. USDHHS, 1991.
55. U.S. Department of Health and Human Services (USDHSS). *NIDA Capsules: LSD (Lysergic Acid Diethylamide).* No. 39. Public Health Service, Alcohol, Drug Abuse and Mental Health Administration, National Institute on Drug Abuse. Rockville, MD: National Institute on Drug Abuse, 1992.
56. USDHHS, 1992.
57. USDHHS, 1992.
58. National Institute of Drug Abuse. *NIDA Capsule. PCP (Phencyclidine).* Doc. C–86–08, 1995.
59. USDHHS, 1991.
60. USDHHS, 1991; USDHHS, 1993a.
61. Goldstein, 1994, p. 174.
62. U.S. Department of Health and Human Services (USDHSS). *NIDA Capsules: Marijuana Update.* No. 12. Public Health Service, Alcohol, Drug Abuse and Mental Health Administration, Rockville, MD: National Institute on Drug Abuse, 1989.
63. Goldstein, 1994, pp. 169–170.
64. Cowley, G. Can Marijuana be Medicine? *Newsweek,* February 3, 1997, pp. 22–27; Conant, M. This Is Smart Medicine. *Newsweek,* February 3, 1997, p. 26.
65. Kassirer, J. P. Federal Foolishness and Marijuana. *Journal of the American Medical Association, 336* (1997), 366–367 [Editorial].
66. Johnston et al., 1996, vol. I.
67. U.S. Department of Health and Human Services (USDHSS). *NIDA Capsules: Designer Drugs.* No. 10. Public Health Service, Alcohol, Drug Abuse and Mental Health Administration, National Institute on Drug Abuse. Rockville, MD: National Institute on Drug Abuse, 1986b.
68. Yesalis, C., et al. Anabolic-Androgenic Steroid Use in the United States. *Journal of the American Medical Association, 270* (1993), 1217–1221.
69. Pope, H., and Katz, D. Affective and Psychotic Symptoms Associated with Anabolic Steroid Use. *American Journal of Psychiatry, 145* (1988), 487–490.
70. Vital Statistics, 1994. *Health Magazine,* January/February, 1994, p. 14.
71. Pope, H., and Katz, D. Homicide and Near-Homicide by Anabolic Steroid Users. *Journal of Clinical Psychiatry, 51* (1990), 28–31.
72. Yesalis et al., 1993; USDHHS, 1991.
73. National Institute of Drug Abuse. *NIDA Capsule. Anabolic Steroid Use by Students, 1995.* Doc. C–93–03.
74. U.S. House of Representatives, 1992.
75. U.S. House of Representatives, 1992.
76. U.S. Department of Health and Human Services (USDHSS). *NIDA Capsules: Drug Abuse Treatment.* No. 27. U.S. Department of Health and Human Services (USDHSS), Public Health Service, Alcohol, Drug Abuse and Mental Health Administration, National Institute on Drug Abuse. Rockville, MD: National Institute on Drug Abuse, 1988.
77. Goldstein, 1994.
78. Treaster, J. B. It's Not Legalization, but a User–Friendly Drug Strategy. *The New York Times,* December 19, 1993, sec. 4, p. 5.
79. Gawin, F. H., et al., 1989.
80. Adapted from Goldstein, 1994.
81. Tolchin, M. U.S. Imposes New Alcohol Test Rules. *The New York Times,* February 4, 1994, p. A15.


### CHAPTER 13


1. U.S. Department of Health and Human Services (USDHHS). *Alcohol Research: Promise for the Decade.* USDHHS, Public Health Service, Alcohol, Drug Abuse, and Mental Health Administration, National Institute on Alcohol Abuse and Alcoholism, Pub. No. ADM–92–1990. Washington, DC, USDHHS, 1991a; Leary, W. E. Responses of Alcoholics to Therapies Seem Similar. *The New York Times,* December 18, 1996, p. A17.
2. Goldstein, A. *Addiction: From Biology to Drug Policy.* New York: W. H. Freeman, 1994, p. 120.
3. USDHHS, 1991a.
4. U.S. Department of Education. *Youth & Alcohol: Selected Reports to the Surgeon General.* Washington, DC: U.S. Government Printing Office, 1993, p. 11.
5. Statistical Abstracts of the United States, 1991.
6. USDHHS, 1991a.
7. Alcohol's Toll. *Addiction & Recovery, 10* (1990), p. 52.
8. *Seventh Special Report on Alcohol and Health.* Rockville, MD: National Clearinghouse for Alcohol and Drug Abuse Information, 1990.
9. Pihl, R. O., Peterson, J., and Finn, P. (1990). Inherited Predisposition to Alcoholism: Characteristics of Sons of Male Alcoholics. *Journal of Abnormal Psychology, 99* (1990), 291–301; Pollock, V. E. (1992). Meta-Analysis of Subjective Sensitivity to Alcohol in Sons of Alcoholics. *American Journal of Psychiatry, 149* (1992), 1534–1538.
10. Schafer, J., and Brown, S. Marijuana and Cocaine Effect Expectancies and Drug Use Patterns. *Journal of Consulting and Clinical Psychology, 59* (1991), 558–565; Thombs, D. L. (1991). Expectancies versus Demographics in Discriminating between College Drinkers: Implications for Alcohol Abuse Prevention. *Health Education Research, 6* (1991), 491–495.
11. Brown, S. A. Expectancies versus Background in the Prediction of College Drinking Patterns. *Journal of Consulting and Clinical Psychology, 53* (1985), 123–130.
12. "Beer Belly" More than a Figure of Speech. *Tufts University Diet & Nutrition Letter, 10*(5), July 1992, p. 1.
13. Engs, R. C., and Hanson, D. J. Gender Differences in Drinking Patterns and Problems among College Students: A Review of the Literature. *Journal of Alcohol and Drug Education, 35* (1990), 36–47.
14. Anthony, J. C., and Helzer, J. E. Syndromes of Drug Abuse and Dependence. In L. N. Robins and D. A. Regier (Eds.), *Psychiatric Disorders in America: The Epidemiologic Catchment Area Study.* New York: The Free Press, 1991, pp. 116–154.
15. Gordon, C. M., and Carey, M. P. Alcohol's Effects on Requisites for Sexual Risk Reduction in Men: An Initial Experimental Investigation. *Health Psychology, 15* (1996), 56–60.
16. Ray, O., and Ksir, C. Behavioral Effects of Blood Alcohol Levels. In *Drugs, Society, and Human Behavior,* 5th ed. St. Louis: Times Mirror/Mosby College Publishing, 1990. Reprinted with permission.
17. Collins, J. J., and Messerschmidt, P. M. (1993). Epidemiology of Alcohol-Related Violence. *Alcohol Health and Research World, 17* (1993), 93–100; Martin, S. E. The Epidemiology of Alcohol-Related Interpersonal Violence. *Alcohol Health and Research World, 16* (1992), 230–237.
18. National Commission on Drug-Free Schools. *Toward a Drug-Free Generation: A Nation's Responsibility.* Washington, DC: U.S. Department of Education, 1990.
19. U.S. Department of Education, 1993.
20. U.S. Department of Health and Human Services (USDHHS). Public Health Service, Alcohol, Drug Abuse, and Mental Health Administration. *Alcohol Practices and Potentials of American Colleges and Universities.* Washington, DC: U.S. Government Printing Office, 1991b.
21. Parker, R. N. The Effects of Context on Alcohol and Violence. Special Issue: Alcohol, Aggression, and Injury. *Alcohol: Health and Research World, 17* (1993), 117–122; Pihl, R. O., and Peterson, J. B. Alcohol, Drug Use and Aggressive Behavior. In S. Hodgins (Ed.), *Mental Disorder and Crime* (pp. 263–283). Newbury Park, CA: Sage, 1993; and other sources.
22. U.S. Department of Education, 1993, p. 2.
23. McGinnis, J. M., and Foege, W. H. Actual Causes of Death in the United States. *Journal of the American Medical Association, 270* (1993), 2207–2212; Scott, B. M., Denniston, R. W., and Magruder, K. M. (1992). Alcohol Advertising in the African-American Community. *The Journal of Drug Issues, 22* (1992), 455–469.
24. McGinnis and Foege, 1993.
25. NIAAA Report Links Drinking and Early Death. *The Addiction Letter, 6,* October 1990, p. 5.
26. Blot, W. J., et al. Smoking and Drinking in Relation to Oral and Pharyngeal Cancer. *Cancer Research, 48* (1988), 3282–3287.
27. Roselle, G. A. Alcohol and the Immune System, and Grossman, C. J., and Wilson, E. J.

The Immune System. *Alcohol World: Health & Research, 16.* National Institute on Alcohol Abuse and Alcoholism, NIH Publication No. 93–3466, 1992.

28. Hanna, E., et al. Dying to Be Equal: Women, Alcohol, and Cardiovascular Disease. *British Journal of Addiction, 87* (1992), 1593–1597.
29. Alcohol's Toll, 1990.
30. Klatsky, A. L., Freidman, G. D., and Siegelaub, A. B. Alcohol and Mortality: A Ten-year Kaiser-Permanente Experience. *Annals of Internal Medicine, 95* (1981), 139–145; Gordon, T., and Doyle, J. T. Drinking and Mortality: The Albany Study. *American Journal of Epidemiology, 125* (1987), 263–270.
31. Stampfer, M., and Hennekens, C. Alcohol Consumption and Cardiovascular Disease in Women. *New England Journal of Medicine, 319* (1988), 267–273.
32. Uncorking the Facts about Alcohol and Your Health. *Tufts University Diet & Nutrition Letter, 13,* August 1995, pp. 4–7.
33. Gaziano, J. M. Moderate Alcohol Intake, Increased Levels of High-Density Lipoprotein and Its Subfractions, and Decreased Risk of Myocardial Infarction. *New England Journal of Medicine, 329* (1993), 1829–1834.
34. California Medication Association. Most Alcoholics Are Not Skid Row Drunks. *HealthTips,* May 1990, p. 3.
35. Langenbucher, J. W., and Chung, T. Onset and Staging of DSM-IV Alcohol Dependence Using Mean Age and Survival-Hazard Methods. *Journal of Abnormal Psychology, 104* (1995), 346–354.
36. NIAAA. *Children of Alcoholics.* Rockville, MD: National Institute on Alcohol Abuse and Alcoholism, 1993.
37. Hill, S. Y. Introduction: The Biological Consequences. In *Alcoholism and Alcohol Abuse among Women: Research Issues.* Rockville, MD: National Institute on Alcohol Abuse and Alcoholism, 1980.
38. Schoenborn, C. A. Exposure to Alcoholism in the Family: United States, 1988. USDHHS, Public Health Service, Centers for Disease Control, National Center for Health Statistics. Washington, DC: U.S. Government Printing Office, 1991.
39. NIAAA. *Alcohol-Induced Medical Consequences in Women.* Rockville, MD: National Institute on Alcohol Abuse and Alcoholism, 1993.
40. Adapted from *Newsweek,* February 20, 1989, p. 52.
41. Adapted from Rice, F. P. *The Adolescent* (7th ed.). Boston: Allyn & Bacon, 1992.
42. Maier, T. Drug Hailed as a "Magic Bullet" Has Skeptics. *Newsday,* February 21, 1995, p. B23.
43. Henslin, J. M. *Sociology.* Boston: Allyn & Bacon, 1993.
44. Schoenborn, 1991.
45. McCarty, D., et al. Alcoholism, Drug Abuse, and the Homeless. *American Psychologist, 46* (1991), 1139–1148.
46. National Highway Traffic Safety Administration. *Fatal Accident Reporting System: 1987.* Washington, DC: U.S. Department of Transportation, 1988.
47. U.S. Department of Education, 1993, p. 1.
48. Centers for Disease Control and Prevention (CDC). Factors Potentially Associated with Reductions in Alcohol-Related Traffic Fatalities—1990 and 1991. *Mortality and Morbidity Weekly Report, 41* (1992), 893–899.
49. National Commission on Drug-Free Schools, 1990.
50. Eigen, L. D. Alconol Practices, Policies, and Potentials of American Colleges and Universities: An OSAP White Paper. Rockville, MD: U.S. Department of Health and Human Services, 1991, p. 4.
51. Eigen, 1991; Phillips, J. C., and Heesacker, M. College Students Admission of Alcoholism and Intention to Change Alcohol-Related Behavior. *Journal of College Student Development, 33* (1992), 403–410.
52. Eigen, 1991, p. 6.
53. U.S. Department of Health and Human Services (USDHHS). *HHS News: National High School Senior Survey, 1990.* Washington, DC: USDHHS, January 24, 1991.
54. Johnston, L. D., Bachman, J. G., and O'Malley, P. M. *Monitoring the Future: a Continuing Study of the Lifestyles and Values of Youth.* Ann Arbor, MI: University of Michigan News and Information Services, January 25, 1992.
55. Eigen, 1991.
56. Rappaport, R. J. (1993). Preventing and Responding to Alcohol Overdose on the College Campus. *Journal of College Student Development, 34* (1993), 69–70.
57. Rappaport, 1993.
58. A Time-Honored Campus Tradition: Binge Drinking *Tufts University Diet & Nutrition Letter, 10*(6), August 1992, p. 2.
59. Adler, J., with D. Rosenberg. The Endless Binge. *Newsweek,* December 19, 1994, pp. 72–73.
60. Eigen, 1991.
61. Cooper, M. L. Alcohol and Increased Behavioral Risk for AIDS. *Alcohol World: Health & Research, 16,* National Institute on Alcohol Abuse and Alcoholism, NIH Publication No. 93–3466; 1992, pp. 64–72.
62. Kruger, T. E., and Jerrells, T. R. Potential Role of Alcohol in Human Immunodeficiency Virus Infection. *Alcohol World: Health & Research, 16,* National Institute on Alcohol Abuse and Alcoholism, NIH Publication No. 93–3466, 1992, pp. 57–63.
63. Butcher, A. H., Manning, D. T., and O'Neal, E. C. HIV-related Sexual Behaviors of College Students. *Journal of American College Health, 40* (1991), 115–118.
64. Celis, W. Drinking by College Women Raises New Concern. *The New York Times,* February 16, 1994, p. A18.
65. National Institute on Drug Abuse. *National Household Survey on Drug Abuse, Main Findings, 1990.* Rockville, MD: Alcohol, Drug Abuse and Mental Health Administration, 1990.
66. U.S. Department of Education, 1993; and others.
67. National Institute on Drug Abuse. *National Survey Results on Drug Use from Monitoring the Future Study, 1975–1992. Volume II: College Students and Young Adults.* Rockville, MD: National Institutes of Health, 1993.
68. Devor, E. J. A Developmental-Genetic Model of Alcoholism: Implications for Genetic Research. *Journal of Consulting and Clinical Psychology, 62* (1994), 1108–1115.
69. Newlin, D. B., and Thomson, J. B. Alcohol Challenge with Sons of Alcoholics: A Critical Review and Analysis. *Psychological Bulletin, 108* (1990), 383–402; Pihl, R. O., Peterson, J., and Finn, P. (1990). Inherited Predisposition to Alcoholism: Characteristics of Sons of Male Alcoholics. *Journal of Abnormal Psychology, 99* (1990), 291–301; Goleman, D. Scientists Pinpoint Brain Irregularities in Drug Addicts. *The New York Times,* June 26, 1990, pp. C1, C7.
70. Goleman, 1990, pp. C1, C7.
71. Pickens, R. W., et al. Heterogeneity in the Inheritance of Alcoholism: A Study of Male and Female Twins. *Archives of General Psychiatry, 48* (1991), 19–28; Prescott, C. A., et al. Genetic and Environmental Influences on Lifetime Alcohol-Related Problems in a Volunteer Sample of Older Twins. *Journal of Studies on Alcohol, 55* (1994), 184–202.
72. McGue, M., Pickens, R. W., and Sivkis, D. S. Sex and Age Effects on the Inheritance of Alcohol Problems: A Twin Study. *Journal of Abnormal Psychology, 101* (1992), 3–17; Svikis, D. S., Velez, M. L., and Pickens, R. W. Genetic Aspects of Alcohol Use and Alcoholism in Women. *Alcohol Health & Research World, 18* (1994), 192–196.
73. Study Finds Students at Small Colleges Drink More. *The New York Times,* September 20, 1992, p. 33.
74. Adapted from Nevid, J. S., Rathus, S. A., and Green, B. *Abnormal Psychology in a Changing World* (3rd ed.). Upper Saddle River, NJ: Prentice-Hall, 1997, pp. 348–349.
75. Grant, B. F., et al. Prevalence of DSM-IV Alcohol Abuse and Dependence: United States, 1992. *Alcohol Health & Research World, 18* (1994), 243–248; Caetano, R. Findings from the 1984 National Survey of Alcohol Use among U.S. Hispanics. In W. B. Clark and M. E. Hilton (Eds.), *Alcohol in America: Drinking Practices and Problems.* Albany: State University of New York Press, 1991, pp. 293–307. Lex, B. W. Review of Alcohol Problems in Ethnic Minority Groups. *Journal of Consulting and Clinical Psychology, 55* (1987), 293–300; Kessler, R. C., et al. Lifetime and 12-month Prevalence of DSM-III-R Psychiatric Disorders in the United States: Results from the National

Comorbidity Survey. *Archives of General Psychiatry, 51* (1994), 8–19. Anthony, J. D., and Helzer, J. E. (1991). Syndromes of Drug Abuse and Dependence. In L. N. Robins and D. A. Regier (Eds.), *Psychiatric Disorders in America: The Epidemiologic Catchment Area Study.* New York: The Free Press, 1991, pp. 116–154. Herd, D. (1991). Drinking Patterns in the Black Population. In W. B. Clark and M. E. Hilton (Eds.), *Alcohol in America: Drinking Practices and Problems.* Albany: State University of New York Press, pp. 308–328. Berlin, I. N. Effects of Changing Native American Cultures on Child Development. *Journal of Community Psychology, 15* (1987), 299–306; Darrow, S. L., et al. Sociodemographic Correlates of Alcohol Consumption among African-American and White Women. *Women & Health, 18* (1992), 35–51; Johnson, R. C., and Nagoshi, C. T. Asians, Asian-Americans and Alcohol. *Journal of Psychoactive Drugs, 22* (1990), 45–52; Ellickson, P. L., Hays, R. D., and Bell, R. M. Stepping through the Drug Use Sequence: Longitudinal Scalogram Analysis of Initiation and Regular Use. *Journal of Abnormal Psychology, 101* (1992), 441–451; Park, J. Y., et al. The Flushing Response to Alcohol Use among Koreans and Taiwanese. *Journal of Studies on Alcohol, 45* (1984), 481–485. Newlin, D. B. The Skin-Flushing Response: Autonomic, Self-Report, and Conditioned Response to Repeated Administrations of Alcohol in Asian Men. *Journal of Abnormal Psychology, 98* (1989), 421–425, Moncher, M. S., Holden, G. W., and Trimble, J. E. Substance Abuse among Native-American Youth. *Journal of Consulting and Clinical Psychology, 58* (1990), 408–415.

76. Sanchez-Craig, M., and Wilkinson, D. A. Treating Problem Drinkers Who Are Not Severely Dependent on Alcohol. *Drugs and Society, 1* (1986/87), 39–67; Marlatt, G. A., et al. Harm Reduction for Alcohol Problems: Moving Beyond the Controlled Drinking Controversy. *Behavior Therapy, 24* (1993), 461–504.
77. Elkins, R. A. An Appraisal of Chemical Aversion (Emetic Therapy) Approaches to Alcoholism Treatment. *Behaviour Research & Therapy, 29* (1991), 387–413.
78. Cowley, G. A New Assault on Addiction. *Newsweek,* January 30, 1995, p. 51; Volpi-celli, J. R., et al. Naltrexone and the Treatment of Alcohol Dependence. *Alcohol Health & Research World, 18* (1994), 272–278.
79. Anton, R. F. Medications for Treating Alcoholism. *Alcohol Health & Research World, 18* (1994), 265–271.
80. Chaloupka, F. J., Saffer, H., and Grossman, M. Alcohol-Control Policies and Motor-Vehicle Fatalities. *Journal of Legal Studies, 22* (1993), 161–186.
81. Burrell, L. F. Student Perceptions of Alcohol Consumption. *Journal of Alcohol and Drug Education, 37* (1992), 107–113.
82. Hoxie, P., et al. *Alcohol and Fatal Recreational Boating Accidents.* U.S. Department of Transportation System Center, Report No. DOT–TSC–CD88–1, 1988.
83. Bar, J. S., and Carey, M. M. Biases in the Perceptions of the Consequences of Alcohol Use among College Students. *Journal Studies on Alcohol, 54* (1993), 54–60.

### CHAPTER 14

1. *Newsweek,* July 4, 1994, p. 45; U.S. Department of Health and Human Services (USDHHS), Public Health Service, National Institutes of Health, National Cancer Institute. *Strategies to Control Tobacco Use in the United States: A Blueprint for Public Health Action in the 1990's.* (NIH Publication No. (92–3316). Washington, DC: National Cancer Institute, 1991a; NBC Nightly News, May 3, 1996.
2. Darnton, J. Report Says Smoking Causes a Global Epidemic of Death. *The New York Times,* September 21, 1994, p. B8.
3. Smoking Will Be World's Biggest Killer. *Newsday,* September 17, 1996, p. A21.
4. Cigarettes: A Constant Pain in the Budget. *Newsweek,* July 18, 1994, p. 65.; Hilts, P. J. Sharp Rise Seen in Smokers' Health Care Costs. *The New York Times,* July 8, 1994, p. A12.
5. Sardella, S. APA Backs Tobacco Tax to Fund Health Reform. *APA Monitor,* January 1994, p. 6.
6. USDHHS, 1991a.
7. USDHHS. *Reducing the Health Consequences of Smoking: 25 Years of Progress. A Report of the Surgeon General* (DHHS Publication No. [CDD] 89–8411). Public Health Service, Centers for Disease Control, Center for Chronic Disease Prevention and Health Promotion, Office on Smoking and Health. Washington, DC, 1989.
8. Angier, N. Cigarettes Trigger Lung Cancer Gene, Researchers Find. *The New York Times,* August 21, 1990, p. C3.
9. USDHHS, 1989; Taylor, C. B., Killen, J. D., and Editors of Consumer Reports Books. *The Facts about Smoking.* Yonkers, NY: Consumer Reports Books, 1991; *Prevention Pipeline,* March–April 1994, vol. 7, no. 2, p. 104.
10. Grady, D. So, Smoking Causes Cancer: This Is News? *The New York Times,* October 28, 1996, sec. 4, p. 3.
11. Bartecchi, C. E., MacKenzie, T. D., and Schrier, R. W. The Human Costs of Tobacco Use (First of Two Parts). *New England Journal of Medicine, 330* (1994), 907–912.
12. Brody, J. Study Finds Stunted Lungs in Young Smokers. *The New York Times,* September 26, 1996, p. B10.
13. Cholesterol and Smoking. *Heart Corps, 2* January–February 1990, p. 11.
14. Hayano, J., et al. Short- and Long-Term Effects of Cigarette Smoking on Heart Rate Variability. *American Journal of Cardiology, 65* (1991), 84.
15. USDHHS. *The Health Benefits of Smoking Cessation: A Report of the Surgeon General* (DHHS Pub. No. CDC 90–8416). Rockville, MD: Centers for Disease Control, Office on Smoking and Health, 1990.
16. USDHHS, 1990; USDHHS. *Healthy People 2000: National Health Promotion and Disease Prevention Objectives* (DHHS Pub. No. PHS 91–50212). Washington, DC: Public Health Service, 1991b; Mayer, J. P. Hawkins, B., and Todd, R. A Randomized Evaluation of Smoking Cessation Intervention for Pregnant Women at a WIC Clinic. *American Journal of Public Health, 80* (1990), 76–79.
17. Passive Smoke's Carcinogen Is Passed in Womb. *USA Today,* March 17, 1993, p. A1.
18. Feng, T. Substance Abuse in Pregnancy. *Current Opinions in Obstetrics and Gynecology, 5* (1993), 16–23; Schoendorf, K. C., and Kiely, J. L. Relationship of Sudden Infant Death Syndrome to Maternal Smoking during and after Pregnancy. *Pediatrics, 90* (1992), 905–908; Malloy, M. H., Hoffman, H. J., and Peterson, D. R. Sudden Infant Death Syndrome and Maternal Smoking. *American Journal of Public Health, 82* (1992), 1380–1382.
19. Brody, J. E. Can't Stop Smoking? Then Lessen the Risks. *The New York Times,* February 17, 1993, p. C12.
20. Hilts, P. J. Major Flaw Cited in Cigarette Data. *The New York Times,* May 2, 1994, pp. A1, A15.
21. USDHHS, 1989.
22. Smoking Triples Death Risk: Study. *Newsday,* February 17, 1993, p. 13.
23. Smoking May Go to Your Belly, *Tufts University Diet & Nutrition Letter,* April, 1990; Smoking and Body Fat. *HeartCorps, 2,* January–February 1990.
24. U.S. Department of Health and Human Services, Public Health Service, National Institutes of Health. *Why Do You Smoke?* (NIH publication No. 87–1822). Bethesda, MD: National Cancer Institute, 1987.
25. USDHHS. *Smoking Addiction. A Report of the Surgeon General, 1988.* [DHHS Pub. No. (CDC) 88–8406.] Washington, DC: Centers for Disease Control, Office on Smoking and Health, 1988.
26. USDHHS, 1991a.
27. Adapted from Taylor and Killen, 1991, pp. 38–39.
28. Benowitz, N. L., and Jacob, P., III. Nicotine Renal Excretion Rate Influences Nicotine Intake during Cigarette Smoking. *Journal of Pharmacological and Experimental Therapeutics, 234* (1985), 153–155.
29. Taylor and Killen, 1991.
30. Are Cigars Safer than Cigarettes? *Health,* November/December 1996, p. 128; Taylor and Killen, 1991.
31. USDHSS, 1989.
32. Smokeless Tobacco Is Ranked by Nicotine Levels for First Time. *The New York Times,* May 5, 1994, p. B12; Taylor and Killen, 1991; USDHHS, 1989.

33. Taylor and Killen, 1991, pp. 125–126.
34. USDHHS, 1989.
35. Altman, L. K. Passive Smoking Tied to Risk of Cancer in Autopsy Study. *The New York Times,* October 7, 1992, p. C13; Glantz, S. A., and Parmley, W. W. Passive Smoking and Heart Disease: Epidemiology, Physiology, and Biochemistry. *Circulation, 83* (1991), 1–12; USDHHS, 1991a. Grady, D. Study Finds Secondhand Smoke Doubles Risk of Heart Disease. *The New York Times,* May 20, 1997, pp. A1, A18.
36. Brownson, R. C., et al. Passive Smoking and Lung Cancer in Nonsmoking Women. *American Journal of Public Health, 82* (1992), 1525–1530; National Research Council, Board of Environmental Studies and Toxicology, Committee on Passive Smoking. *Environmental Tobacco Smoke: Measuring Exposures and Assessing Health Effects.* Washington, DC: National Academy Press, 1986; Fontham, E.T.H., et al. Environmental Tobacco Smoke and Lung Cancer in Nonsmoking Women: A Multicenter Study. *Journal of the American Medical Association, 271* (1994), 1752–1759.
37. Second-hand Smoke: Is It a Hazard? *Consumer Reports,* January 1995, pp. 27–33.
38. Martinez, F. D., et al. Increased Incidence of Asthma in Children of Smoking Mothers. *Pediatrics, 89* (1992), 21–26; Janerich, D. T., et al. Lung Cancer and Exposure to Tobacco Smoke in the Household. *New England Journal of Medicine, 323* (1990), 632–636.
39. USDHHS, 1989, 1991a; Smoking Declines at a Faster Pace. *The New York Times,* May 22, 1992, p. A17.
40. Hilts, P. J. Long-Term Decline in Smoking in U.S. Is Apparently Over. *The New York Times,* May 20, 1994, p. A16.
41. Feder, B. J. Increase in Teen-Age Smoking Sharpest Among Black Males. *The New York Times,* May 24, 1996, p. A20.
42. Feder, 1996.
43. Shenon, P. Asia's Having One Huge Nicotine Fit. *The New York Times,* May 15, 1994, sec. 4, pp. 1, 16.
44. Darnton, 1994, p. B8.
45. USDHSS, 1991a.
46. Smoke Rises. *The New York Times,* December 27, 1993, p. A16.
47. McCord, C., and Freeman, H. P. Excess Mortality in Harlem. *New England Journal of Medicine, 322* (1990), 173–177.
48. USDHHS, 1991a.
49. USDHHS, 1992; Escobedo, L. G., and Remington, P. L. Birth Cohort Analysis of Prevalence of Cigarette Smoking among Hispanics in the United States. *Journal of the American Medical Association, 261* (1989), 66–69; Rogers, R. G., and Crank, J. Ethnic Differences in Smoking Patterns: Findings from NHIS. *Public Health Reports, 103* (1988), 387–393.
50. Marín, G., et al. The Role of Acculturation in the Attitudes, Norms, and Expectancies of Hispanic Smokers. *Journal of Cross Cultural Psychology, 20* (1989), 399–415.
51. Centers for Disease Control and Prevention. Cigarette Smoking among Adults—United States, 1991. *Morbidity and Mortality Weekly Report, 42*(12) (1993), 230–233.
52. USDHHS, 1989.
53. Chung, C. S. *A Report on the Hawaii Behavioral Risk Factor Surveillance System for 1986.* Unpublished Manuscript. School of Public Health, University of Hawaii, 1986.
54. Chen, M. S. *Lay-Led Smoking Cessation Approach for Southeast Asian Men.* Paper Presented at the Program on Smoking Cessation Strategies for Minorities, National Heart, Lung & Blood Institute, National Institutes of Health, Bethesda, MD, February 1991.
55. USDHHS, 1991a.
56. Marín, G., Marín, B. V., et al. Cultural Differences in Attitudes and Expectancies between Hispanic and Non-Hispanic White Smokers. *Hispanic Journal of Behavioral Sciences, 12* (1990), 422–436.
57. Nevid, J. S., and Javier, R. A. *"SI, PUEDO" Smoking Cessation Program for Hispanic Smokers.* Fourth National Forum on Cardiovascular Health, Pulmonary Disorders, and Blood Resources, Minority Health Issues for an Emerging Majority, National Heart, Lung, and Blood Institute, National Institutes of Health, June 1992. Nevid, J. S. Smoking Cessation with Ethnic Minorities: Themes and Approaches. *Journal of Social Distress and the Homeless, 5* (1996), 1–16; Nevid, J. S., and Javier, R. A. Preliminary Investigation of a Culturally-Specific Smoking Cessation Intervention for Hispanic Smokers. *American Journal of Health Promotion,* in press; Nevid, J. S., Javier, R. A., and Moulton, J. (1996). Factors Predicting Participant Attrition in a Community-Based Culturally-Specific Smoking Cessation Program for Hispanic Smokers. *Health Psychology, 15* (1996), 226–229.
58. *The G.A.I.N.S. Project.* American Indian Health Care Association, St. Paul, Minnesota; Johnson, K. M., and Lando, H. Smoking Cessation Strategies for Minorities. Paper Presented at the program *Smoking Cessation Strategies for Minorities.* National Heart, Lung & Blood Institute, National Institutes of Health, Bethesda, MD, February 1991.
59. Chen, M. S., 1991.
60. Lepera, P. ACS Runs Uptown out of Town. *Cancer News, 44: 2* (1990), 20.
61. *The Heart, Body & Soul Project.* A Collaborative Program between the Clergy United for Renewal of East Baltimore (CURE) and the Johns Hopkins Medical Institutions, Center for Health Promotion; Levine, D., et al. Church-Based Smoking Cessation Strategies in Urban Blacks. Paper Presented at the program *Smoking Cessation Strategies for Minorities.* National Heart, Lung & Blood Institute, National Institutes of Health, Bethesda, MD, February 1991.
62. American Lung Association. *Don't Let Your Dreams Go up in Smoke . . . ,* April 1990.
63. USDHHS, 1989; 1991a; *Morbidity and Mortality Weekly Report,* November 12, 1993. vol. 42, no. 44.
64. USDHHS, 1989.
65. Brody, J. E. Smokers Have Higher Breast Cancer Death Risk. *The New York Times,* May 25, 1994, p. C12.
66. Califano, J. A. The Wrong Way to Stay Slim. *New England Journal of Medicine, 333* (1995), 1214–1216.
67. Audrain, J. E., Klesges, R. C., and Klesges, L. M. Relationship between Obesity Status and the Metabolic Effects of Smoking in Women. *Health Psychology, 14* (1995), 116–123.
68. Ogden, J. Effects of Smoking Cessation, Restrained Eating, and Motivational States on Food Intake in the Laboratory. *Health Psychology, 13* (1994), 114–121.
69. Botvin, G. J., et al. Smoking Prevention among Urban Minority Youth: Assessing Effects on Outcome and Mediating Variables. *Health Psychology, 11* (1992), 290–299.
70. USDHHS, 1990; Rosenberg, L., Palmer, J. R., and Shapiro, S. Decline in the Risk of Myocardial Infarction among Women Who Stop Smoking. *New England Journal of Medicine, 322* (1990), p. 213–219; Novello, A. C. Preface. In *The Health Benefits of Smoking Cessation: A Report of the Surgeon General 1990.* (pp. V–XII). U.S. Department of Health and Human Services, Public Health Service, Centers for Disease Control, Center for Chronic Disease Prevention and Health Promotion, Office on Smoking and Health. [DHHS Pub. No. (CDC) 90–8416. Washington, DC: U.S. Government Printing Office.
71. Adapted from Rathus, S. A., and Nevid, J. S. *Adjustment and Growth: The Challenges of Life,* 6th ed. Fort Worth, TX: Harcourt Brace Jovanovich, pp. 243–244. Copyright © 1995 by Holt, Rinehart and Winston, reprinted by permission of the publisher.
72. The Last Draw for Smokers. *UC Berkeley Wellness Letter, 13* October 1996, pp. 2–3.
73. Kolata, G. Nicotine Patch Study Sees 25% Success Rate. *The New York Times,* June 22, 1994, p. A14; U.S. Department of Health and Human Services. *Nurses: Help Your Patient Stop Smoking.* Public Health Service, National Institutes of Health National Heart, Lung, and Blood Institute, Smoking Education Program, NIH Publication No. 02–2962. Washington, DC: National Heart, Lung and Blood Institute, January 1993.
74. Marlatt, G. A., and Gordon, J. R. *Relapse Prevention: Maintenance Strategies in the Treatment of Addictive Behaviors.* New York:

Guilford Press, 1985; Curry, S., Marlatt, G. A., and Gordon, J. R. Abstinence Violation Effect: Validation of an Attributional Construct with Smoking Cessation. *Journal of Consulting and Clinical Psychology, 55* (1987), 145–149.

### CHAPTER 15

1. *WHO: Infectious Diseases Leading Cause of Premature Death Worldwide.* Reuters News Service, June 6, 1996.
2. Price, J. H. Update: Toxic Shock Syndrome. *The Journal of School Health, 51* (1981), 143–145.
3. Petitti, D., and Reingold, A. Tampon Characteristics and Menstrual Toxic Shock Syndrome. *Journal of the American Medical Association, 259* (1988), 686–687; Reingold, A. L., et al. Toxic Shock Syndrome Surveillance in the United States, 1980 to 1981. *Annals of Internal Medicine, 96* (1982), 875–880.
4. Lipman, M. M. Chronic Fatigue Syndrome: Sick and Tired of Being Sick and Tired. *Consumer Reports on Health,* July 1996, p. 83; and other sources.
5. National Institutes of Allergy and Infectious Disease (NIAID), *Report of the Task Force on Microbiology and Infectious Diseases.* NIH Publication No. 92–3320, April 1992.
6. NIAID, *Report of the Task Force on Microbiology and Infectious Diseases,* 1992, p. 46; World Health Organization, as cited in N. D. Kristof, Malaria Makes a Comeback, and Is More Deadly Than Ever. *The New York Times,* January 8, 1997, pp. A1, A10.
7. Hoeprich, P. D., and Jordan, M. C. *Infectious Diseases* (4th ed.). Philadelphia: J. B. Lippincott, 1989.
8. Hoeprich and Jordan, 1989, p. 742.
9. NIAID. Schistosomiasis: Cytokines the Key? *Dateline: NIAID Newsletter,* May 1992, pp. 7, 10.
10. Rosenberg, S. A., *The Transformed Cell: Unlocking the Mysteries of Cancer.* New York: G. P. Putnam, 1992.
11. National Cancer Institute (NCI) and National Institute of Allergy and Infectious Diseases (NIAID). *The Immune System—How It Works.* NIH Publication No. 94–3229, Revised December 1993.
12. Mizel, S. B. and Jaret, P. *In Self-Defense: The Human Immune System–The New Frontier in Medicine.* San Diego: Harcourt Brace Jovanovich, 1985.
13. Henig, R. M. *A Dancing Matrix: Voyages along the Viral Frontier.* New York: Alfred A. Knopf, 1993.
14. Cutts, F. T., Orenstein, W., and Benier, R. H. Causes of Low Preschool Immunization Coverage in the United States. *Annual Review of Public Health, 13* (1992), 385–398.
15. CDC. *Notifiable Diseases: Summary of Reported Cases, by Month, United States, 1994.*
16. Hoeprich and Jordan, 1989, p. 320.
17. U.S. Department of Health and Human Services (USDHHS). *Healthy People 2000: National Health Promotion and Disease Prevention Objectives.* Washington, DC: U.S. Government Printing Office, 1991, p. 513.
18. Bromberg, K. Whooping Cough (Pertussis). In Hoeprich and Jordan, 1989, p. 346.
19. Progress toward Poliomyelitis Eradication—India, December 1995 and January 1996. *Morbidity and Mortality Weekly Report,* vol. 45, no. 18, May 10, 1996, 370–373.
20. The National Vaccine Advisory Committee. The Measles Epidemic: The Problems, Barriers, and Recommendations. *Journal of the American Medical Association, 266* (1991), 1547–1552.
21. Measles—United States, 1995. *Morbidity and Mortality Weekly Report,* vol. 45, no. 15. April 19, 1996, 305–307.
22. Stapleton, J. T., and Lemon, S. M. Hepatitis A. In Hoeprich and Jordan, 1989, p. 765.
23. NIAID. *Hepatitis.* August 1992.
24. Brody, J. E. There Is Bad News and Good about a Hidden Viral Epidemic: Hepatitis C. *The New York Times,* January 22, 1997, p. C9; Experts Warn of a Tripling of Deaths from Hepatitis C by 2017. *The New York Times,* March 27, 1997, p. A21.
25. NIAID. *Hepatitis.* August 1992.
26. Katzenstein, L. Allergies: Nothing to Sneeze At. *American Health,* May 1993, pp. 44–49; How to Fight Hay Fever. *Consumer Reports on Health,* July 1996, p. 82.
27. NIAID. *What You Need to Know about Asthma,* March 1990.
28. Scientists Say Gene Is Linked to Asthma. *The New York Times,* June 7, 1994, p. C14; Cookson, W. O. C. M., and Moffatt, M. R. Asthma–An Epidemic in the Absence of Infection? *Science, 275* (1997), 41–42.
29. Adams, P. F., and Benson, V. Current Estimates from the National Health Interview Survey, National Center for Health Statistics. *Vital Health Statistics, 10*(181), 1991; American Lung Association. *When You Can't Breathe, Nothing Else Matters,* 1996; Centers for Disease Control and Prevention. U.S. Department of Health and Human Services, Public Health Service, National Center for Health Statistics. *Vital and Health Statistics, Current Estimates From the National Health Interview Survey, 1994.* DHHS Publication No. PHS 96–1521, December 1995; Canadian Lung Association, *Asthma,* 1996; National Institute of Allergy and Infectious Diseases, National Institutes of Health. *NIAID Fact Sheet: Asthma and Allergy Statistics,* June 1996; Kolata, G. Identifying Asthma Risk in Children. *The New York Times,* January 19, 1995, p. A21.
30. Altman, L. K. Rise of Asthma Deaths Is Tied to Ignorance of Many Physicians. *The New York Times,* May 4, 1993, C3.
31. Lehrer, M., et al. Relaxation and Music Therapies for Asthma among Patients Prestabilized on Asthma Medication. *Journal of Behavioral Medicine, 17* (1994), 1–24.
32. Canadian Lung Association Home Page, *Asthma Management,* 1996.
33. U.S. Department of Health and Human Services, *Check Your Asthma IQ.* NIH Publication No. 90–1128, January 1990.
34. NINDS. *Multiple Sclerosis—Research Highlights,* 1996.
35. Brody, J. Common Sense on Averting the Common Cold. *The New York Times,* January 20, 1993, p. C12.
36. Spake, A. How (and Why) Colds Become Supercolds. *Self,* January 1996, p. 38.
37. NIAID. *The Common Cold.* NIH Pub No. 85–167, October 1985.
38. *American Medical Association Encyclopedia of Medicine;* Public Citizens Health Research Group, Allan M. Weinstein, M.D.; *The Washington Post,* Cold Remedies Are a Hot Market. Reprinted in *New York Newsday,* April 13, 1993, p. 61; Brody, Jane E., Keeping Your Wits in the Jungle of Cold Remedies. *The New York Times,* January 20, 1993, p. C14.
39. How to Pick a Pain Reliever. *Consumer Reports on Health,* March 1996, pp. 30–32.
40. Huyghe, P. Clear Choices: How to Find the Pain Reliever That's Right for You. *Health,* October 1995, pp. 75–77.
41. Should I Bring a Fever Down or Let It Run Its Course? *Health,* November/December 1995, p. 128.
42. *What Is Influenza (Flu) and How Is It Caused?* American Lung Association, 1995.
43. *Influenza Prevention.* American Lung Association, 1995.
44. Leary, W. E. In Animal Tests, New Pill Seems to Stop Flu. *The New York Times,* January 29, 1997, p. A12.
45. NIAID. *Flu.* NIH Pub. No. 87–187, September 1987.
46. Thompson, D. S. (Ed.) *Every Woman's Health: The Complete Guide to Body and Mind,* New York: Simon & Schuster, p. 739.
47. National Foundation for Infectious Diseases Health Alert. *Guard against Flu/Pneumonia.* Washington, DC.
48. NIAID. *Backgrounder: Tuberculosis.* April 1993.
49. NIAID, *Tuberculosis: What Health Care Workers Should Know,* NIH Publication No. 93–3511, October 1993.
50. NIAID. *Backgrounder: Tuberculosis.* April 1993; Specter, M. Neglected for Years, TB Is Back with Strains That Are Deadlier. *The New York Times,* October 11, 1992, p. A1.
51. NIAID. *Tuberculosis: What Health Care Workers Should Know,* October 1993; and other sources.
52. NIAID. *Backgrounder: Tuberculosis.* April 1993.
53. Brody, J. E. For Time Outdoors, Ways to Avoid Lyme Disease. *The New York Times,* June 26, 1991, p. C9.

54. Rosenthal, E. Flaws Are Seen in Diagnosis and Control of Lyme Disease. *The New York Times,* June 15, 1993, p. A1; Centers for Disease Control and Prevention. *Notifiable Diseases—Summary of Reported Cases, by Month, United States, 1994.*
55. Logigian, E. L., et al. Chronic Neurologic Manifestations of Lyme Disease. *New England Journal of Medicine, 323* (1990), 1438–1444; Arthritis Foundation, 1993, Document ID: lhf00609; Steere, A. C., et al. Association of Chronic Lyme Arthritis with HLA–DR4 and HLA–DR2 Alleles. *New England Journal of Medicine, 323* (1990), 219–223.
56. Krause, P. J., et al. Concurrent Lyme Disease and Babesiosis: Evidence of Increased Severity and Duration of Illness. *Journal of the American Medical Association, 275* (1996), 1657–1660; Garrett, L. Ticks' One-Two Punch. *Newsday,* June 5, 1996, p. A35.
57. Blumenthal, D. Keeping the Bugs Off, While Saving Your Skin. *The New York Times,* June 29, 1991, p. 48.
58. Lyme Disease: Hard to Catch. *UC Berkeley Wellness Letter, 11 (11),* August 1995, pp. 4–5.
59. NIAID. *Backgrounder: Infectious Mononucleosis.* April 1992.
60. Lederberg, J., Shope, R. E., and Oaks, S. C., Jr. (Eds.), *Emerging Infections: Microbial Threats to Health in the United States.* Washington: National Academy of Sciences Press, 1992; National Center for Infectious Diseases. *New, Reemerging, and Drug Resistant Infections,* 1996; Henderson, D. A. Strategies for the Twenty-first Century, Control or Eradication? In D. Walker (Ed.) *Global Infectious Diseases: Prevention, Control, and Eradication.* Vienna: Springer-Verlag, 1992.
61. Grant, S. Stowaway Species Taking Their Toll on Life, Property. *Hartford Courant,* May 30, 1993, p. A1.
62. Henig, 1993.
63. NIAID. *Report of the Task Force on Microbiology and Infectious Diseases.* NIH Publication No. 92-3320, April 1992.
64. Lemonick, M. D. Guerrilla Warfare. *Time* Special Issue, *The Frontiers of Medicine,* Fall 1996, pp. 59–62.
65. Adapted from Centers for Disease Control and Prevention, *Hantavirus Illness in the United States, March 9, 1995;* Frequently-Asked-Questions about Ebola, Frequently-Asked-Questions about Hantavirus Pulmonary Syndrome, Hantavirus Pulmonary Syndrome, and Frequently-Asked-Questions about Dengue Hemorrhagic Fever, all from *Outbreak,* on-line information service that addresses emerging diseases; and other sources.
66. Adapted from Poppy, J. Cold Wars. *Health,* November/December 1995, pp. 103–109; and other sources.
67. NIAID. *Flu,* September 1987; Hoeprich and Jordan, 1989, pp. 344–345.
68. NIAID. *Flu.* 1987.

**CHAPTER 16**

1. Gayle, J., et al. Surveillance for AIDS and HIV Infection among Black and Hispanic Children and Women of Childbearing Age, 1981–1989. *Morbidity and Mortality Weekly Report: Progress in Chronic Disease Prevention, 39,* 23–29. Washington, DC: U.S. Department of Health and Human Services, 1990.
2. Cannistra, S. A., and Niloff, J. M. Cancer of the Uterine Cervix. *New England Journal of Medicine, 334* (1996), 1030–1038.
3. Shelton, D. STDs: A Hidden Epidemic. *American Medical News,* American Medical Association, December 9, 1996.
4. Shelton, 1996.
5. Cannistra and Niloff, 1996.
6. Centers for Disease Control. Progress toward Achieving the 1990 Objectives for the Nation for Sexually Transmitted Diseases. *Morbidity and Mortality Weekly Report 39* (1990), 53–57.
7. Reinisch, J. M. *The Kinsey Institute New Report on Sex: What You Must Know to Be Sexually Literate.* New York: St. Martin's Press, 1990.
8. Adapted from Rathus, S. A. *Psychology* (5th ed.). Fort Worth: Harcourt Brace College Publishers, 1993.
9. Rolfs, R. T., and Nakashima, A. K. Epidemiology of Primary and Secondary Syphilis in the United States: 1981 through 1989. *Journal of the American Medical Association, 264* (1990), 1432–1437.
10. Rolfs, R. T., Goldberg, M., and Sharrar, R. G. Risk Factors for Syphilis: Cocaine Use and Prostitution. *American Journal of Public Health, 80* (1990), 853–857.
11. Centers for Disease Control. Evaluation of Surveillance for *Chlamydia Trachomatis* Infections in the United States, 1987 to 1991. *Mortality and Morbidity Weekly Report, 42* (SS–3) (1993), 21–27.
12. Yarber, W. L., and Parillo, A. V. Adolescents and Sexually Transmitted Diseases. *Journal of School Health, 62* (1992), 331–338.
13. Graham, J. M., and Blanco, J. D. Chlamydial Infections. *Primary Care: Clinics in Office Practice, 17* (1990), 85–93.
14. Reinisch, 1990.
15. Shelton, 1996.
16. Sherman, K. J., et al. Sexually Transmitted Diseases and Tubal Pregnancy. *Sexually Transmitted Diseases, 17* (1990), 115–121.
17. Quinn, T. C., et al. Epidemiologic and Microbiologic Correlates of Chlamydia Trachomatis Infection in Sexual Partnerships. *Journal of the American Medical Association, 276* (1996), 1737–1742.
18. Reinisch, 1990.
19. Hilton, E., et al. Ingestion of Yogurt Containing *Lactobacillus Acidophilus* as Prophylaxis for Candidal Vaginitis. *Annals of Internal Medicine, 116* (1992), 353–357.
20. Reinisch, 1990.
21. Grodstein, F., Goldman, M. G., and Cramer, D. W. Relation of Tubal Infertility to History of Sexually Transmitted Diseases. *American Journal of Epidemiology, 137* (1993), 577–584.
22. Boston Women's Health Book Collective. *The New Our Bodies, Ourselves.* New York: Simon & Schuster, 1992.
23. Centers for Disease Control and Prevention. *HIV/AIDS Surveillance Report: U.S. HIV and AIDS Cases Reported through June 1996, 8*(1), 1996.
24. Hammond, T. The Estimated Prevalence of HIV in the United States: Signs of Decline. *American Journal of Public Health,* May 1996.
25. World Health Organization. Cited in Rise in STDs Concerns Group. *Newsday,* September 12, 1995, p. B27.
26. CDC, 1996.
27. CDC, 1996.
28. CDC, 1996.
29. Simons, M. French Medical Group Asks Doctors with H.I.V. to Halt Surgery. *The New York Times,* January 22, 1997, p. A5; Taylor, R. Dentist-to-Patient HIV-1 Transmission.: More Heat, No Light. *Journal of NIH Research,* July 1993, p. 50.
30. Allen, J. R., and Setlow, V. P. Heterosexual Transmission of HIV: A View of the Future. *Journal of the American Medical Association, 266* (1991), 1695–1696.
31. Caceres, C. F., and van-Griensven, G. J. P. Male Homosexual Transmission of HIV-1. *AIDS, 8*(8) (1994), 1051–1061.
32. CDC, 1996.
33. Schreiber, G. B., et al. The Risk of Transfusion-Transmitted Viral Infections. *New England Journal of Medicine, 334* (1996), 1685–1690.
34. Genes That Protect against AIDS. *The New York Times,* August 14, 1996, p. A18.
35. Kubic, M. New Ways to Prevent and Treat AIDS. *FDA Consumer,* January–February 1997.
36. Chesney, M. A. Cited in Freiberg, P. New Drugs Give Hope to AIDS Patients. *APA Monitor, 27*(6) (1996), 28.
37. Cooper, D. A., et al. Zidovudine in Persons with Asymptomatic HIV Infection and CD4 Cell Counts Greater than 400 per Cubic Millimeter. *New England Journal of Medicine, 329* (1993), 297–303; Kinloch-de Loes, S., et al. (1995). A Controlled Trial of Zidovudine in Primary Human Immunodeficiency Virus Infection. *New England Journal of Medicine, 333* (1995), 408–413.
38. Hammer, S. M., et al. A Trial Comparing Nucleoside Monotherapy with Combination Therapy in HIV-Infected Adults with CD4 Cell Counts from 200 to 500 per Cubic Millimeter. *New England Journal of Medi-*

*cine, 335* (1996), 1081–1090; Katzenstein, D. A., et al. The Relation of Virologic and Immunologic Markers to Clinical Outcomes after Nucleoside Therapy in HIV-Infected Adults with 200 to 500 CD4 Cells per Cubic Millimeter. *New England Journal of Medicine, 355* (1996), 1091–1098.

39. Corey, L., and Holmes, K. K. Therapy for HIV Infection—What Have We Learned? *New England Journal of Medicine, 335* (196), 1142–1144; Deeks, S. G., et al. HIV-1 Protease Inhibitors: A Review for Clinicians. *Journal of the American Medical Association, 277* (1997), 145–153.
40. Balter, M. (1996). AIDS Research: New Hope in HIV Disease. *Science, 274* (1996), 1988–1989.
41. Chartrand, S. Mixers for "Cocktails" Used to Delay AIDS. *The New York Times,* August 12, 1996, p. D2.
42. Altman, L. K. Experiment to See if AIDS Can Be Cured Is Delayed a Year. *The New York Times,* January 23, 1997.
43. Reported by the Associated Press, February 28, 1997.
44. Kolata, G. AIDS Patients Slipping through Safety Net. *The New York Times,* September 15, 1996, p. A24; Balter, 1997; Pear, R. Expense Means Many Can't Get Drugs for AIDS. *The New York Times,* February 16, 1997, pp. A1, A36.
45. Connor, E. M., et al. Reduction of Maternal-Infant Transmission of Human Immunodeficiency Virus Type 1 with Zidovudine Treatment. *New England Journal of Medicine, 331* (1994), 1173–1180.
46. Brody, J. E. Genital Herpes Drug Found Safe for Daily Use. *The New York Times,* July 7, 1993, p. C11.
47. Brody, 1993.
48. Goldberg, L. H., et al. Long-Term Suppression of Recurrent Genital Herpes with Acyclovir. *Archives of Dermatology, 129* (1993), 582–587.
49. Blakeslee, S. An Epidemic of Genital Warts Raises Concern but Not Alarm. *The New York Times,* January 22, 1992, p. C12.
50. Blakeslee, 1992.
51. Cannistra and Niloff, 1996; Ochs, R. Cervical Cancer Comeback. *New York Newsday,* January 11, 1994, pp. 55, 57.
52. Ochs, 1994.
53. MacDonald N. E., et al. High-Risk STD/HIV Behavior among College Students. *Journal of the American Medical Association, 263* (1990), 3155–3159.

### CHAPTER 17

1. The Virtual Heart, *Mayo Clinic Family Health Book* (Interactive Edition). Rochester, MN: Mayo Foundation for Medical Education and Research, 1992.
2. *The Heart: A Virtual Exploration.* Franklin Science Museum, Philadelphia, PA, 1995.
3. Reprinted with permission of the American Heart Association, National Center, 7320 Greenville Avenue, Dallas, TX 75231.
4. News Releases and Fact Sheets. Highlights of a new report from the National Center for Health Statistics (NCHS), *Monitoring Health Care in America: Quarterly Fact Sheet,* March 1996; Heart Disease: Still the Leading Cause of Death in the U.S. *Reuters News Service,* April 8, 1996.
5. McGovern, P. G., et al. Recent Trends in Acute Coronary Heart Disease. *New England Journal of Medicine, 334* (1996), 884–890; Traven, N. D., et al. Coronary Heart Disease Mortality and Sudden Death: Trends and Patterns in 35- to 44-year-old White Males, 1970–1990. *American Journal of Epidemiology, 142* (1995), 45–52; Hunink, M. G. M., et al. Decline in Mortality from Coronary Heart Disease, 1980–1990. *Journal of the American Medical Association, 277* (1997), 535–542.
6. Sources: Giel, D. Fitness and Exercise Issues for Black Americans. *The Physician and Sportsmedicine, 16* (September 1988), no. 9; Klag, M. J. Cited in Leary, W. E. Social Links Are Seen in Black Stress. *The New York Times,* February 6, 1991, p. A16; Lubell, A. Can Exercise Help Treat Hypertension in Black Americans? and Prescribing Exercise to Black Americans, *The Physician and Sportsmedicine,* 16 (September 1988) no. 9; USDHHS, Public Health Service, *Health United States 1990,* DHHS Pub. No. (PHS), 91–1231; Weiss, R. Medicinal Meditation: Study Shows Hypertension Eased in Older Blacks. *Newsday,* November 21, 1995, p. B29.
7. Leary, W. E. Social Links Are Seen in Black Stress. *The New York Times,* February 6, 1991, p. A16; Livingston, I. L. Stress, Hypertension, and Young Black Americans: The Importance of Counseling. *Journal of Multicultural Counseling and Development, 2* (1993), 132–142; Krieger, N., and Sidney, S. Racial Discrimination and Blood Pressure: The CARDIA Study of Young Black and White Adults. *American Journal of Public Health, 86* (1996), 1370–1378; Gillum, R. R. The Epidemiology of Cardiovascular Disease in Black Americans. *New England Journal of Medicine, 335* (1996), 1597–1599.
8. American Heart Association. *Congenital Heart Defects,* 1995.
9. Strokes Cost $41 Billion a Year, Study Says. *The New York Times,* January 28, 1996, p. A23.
10. Health ResponseAbility Systems, *Collective Work & Database,* 1994.
11. American Heart Association. *Stroke—Signals and Action,* 1995.
12. Aggressive Heart Care May Not Extend Life. *The New York Times,* September 5, 1995, p. C3.
13. Johannesson, M., et al. Cost Effectiveness of Simvastatin Treatment to Lower Cholesterol Levels in Patients with Coronary Heart Disease. *New England Journal of Medicine, 336* (1997), 332–336.
14. Study Casts Doubt on Ability of Diet to Lower Cholesterol. *The New York Times,* April 29, 1993, p. B9.
15. Study Finds Cholesterol-Lowering Drug May Save Lives. *The New York Times,* November 17, 1994, p. B11.
16. Brody, J. E., Benefit to Health in Men Is Seen from Cholesterol-Cutting Drug. *The New York Times,* November 16, 1995, p. A1, B4.
17. Brody, J. E. The Safety of 2 Classes of Cholesterol-Cutting Drugs Is Debated. *The New York Times,* January 3, 1996, p. C8.
18. Apelman, V., et al. Randomized Trial of Excimer Laser Angioplasty Versus Balloon Angioplasty for Treatment of Obstructive Coronary Artery Disease. *The Lancet, 347* (1996), 79–84.
19. Bittl, J. A., and Thomas, P. Beyond the Balloon, *Harvard Health Letter, 20,* January 1996, p. 4; The Writing Group for the Bypass Angioplasty Revascularization Investigation (BARI) Investigators. Bypass Surgery and Angioplasty in Patients with Multivessel Coronary Disease. *Journal of the American Medical Association, 277* (1997), 715–721.
20. Alderman, E. L., et al. Comparison of Coronary Bypass Surgery with Angioplasty in Patients with Multivessel Disease. *New England Journal of Medicine, 335* (1996), 217–225; Hlatky, M. A., et al. Medical Care Costs and Quality of Life after Randomization to Coronary Angioplasty or Coronary Bypass Surgery. *New England Journal of Medicine, 336* (1997), 92–99.
21. Vikanski, L. Aspirin's Cardio-Protective Effects Reaffirmed, *Medical Tribune,* May 19, 1994.
22. Anger Fizzles. *Prevention,* February 1996, p. 24.
23. Smith, S. C., Jr., et al. Preventing Heart Attack and Death in Patients with Coronary Disease. *Circulation, 92* (1995), part 1, July, pp. 2–4; Averting Coronary Death. *Consumer Reports on Health,* December 1995, p. 142.
24. NBC Nightly News, January 23, 1997.
25. *Mayo Clinic Family Health Book* (Interactive Edition), 1992.
26. Why Heart Attacks Happen. *Harvard Heart Letter,* January 1996, pp. 5–7.
27. Experts Split on 2 Ways to Treat Heart Attack. *Newsday,* March 22, 1995, p. C 11.
28. 26 Revelations That Will Do Your Heart a World of Good. From the *Harvard Health Letter,* Harvard Medical School, 1995.
29. 26 Revelations That Will Do Your Heart a World of Good, 1995.
30. The National Institute of Neurological Disorders and Stroke t-PA Stroke Study Group. Tissue Plasminogen Activator for Acute Ischemic Stroke. *New England Journal of Medicine, 333* (1995), 1581–1587; Chen, 1996; American Medical Association Science News. *New Drug for Stroke Only as Good as Systems That Go Along with It,* January 29, 1997.
31. Chen, 1996, p. 63; American Medical Association Science News. *Acting on Warning*

*Signs of Stroke Is Latest in Treatment,* January 29, 1997.

32. Jenkins, C. D. Epidemiology of Cardiovascular Diseases. *Journal of Consulting and Clinical Psychology, 56* (1988), 324–332; Stunkard, A. J., and Sørensen, T. I. A. Obesity and Socioeconomic Status—A Complex Relation. *New England Journal of Medicine, 329* (1993), 1036–1037; Ernst, N. D., and Harlan, W. R. Obesity and Cardiovascular Disease in Minority Populations: Executive Summary. *American Journal of Clinical Nutrition, 53* (1991), 1507S–1511S, and other sources.
33. Peterson, E. D., et al. Racial Variation in the Use of Coronary-Revascularization Procedures—Are the Differences Real? Do They Matter? *New England Journal of Medicine, 336* (1997), 480–486.
34. Editors of the University of California at Berkeley Wellness Letter, *The Wellness Engagement Calendar 1996,* New York: Rebus, Inc., 1996.
35. Adapted from The National High Blood Pressure Education Program Working Group. National High Blood Pressure Education Program Working Group Report on Primary Prevention of Hypertension. *Archives of Internal Medicine, 153* (1993), 186–210, and other sources.
36. Risk Factors for Heart Disease. A Publication of the American Heart Association, 1995.
37. Grover, S. A., Coupal, L., and Hu, X. P. Identifying Adults at Increased Risk of Coronary Disease. How Well Do the Current Cholesterol Guidelines Work? *Journal of the American Medical Association, 274* (1995), pp. 801–806; Cowley, G. What's High Cholesterol? *Newsweek,* November 14, 1994, p. 53; Cholesterol Ratios Come of Age. *Consumer Reports on Health, 8,* June 1996, p. 70, and other sources.
38. High Cholesterol: Does Age Matter? *Consumer Reports on Health, 7,* August 1995, pp. 90–91; Cholesterol Through the Ages. *Consumer Reports on Health, 8,* January 1996, p. 10.
39. Brody, J. E. Study Says a Blood Fat Alone Isn't a Heart Threat. *The New York Times,* April 29, 1993, p. B9; NIH Consensus Development Panel on Triglyceride, High-Density Lipoprotein, and Coronary Heart Disease. *Journal of the American Medical Association, 269*(4) (1993), 505–510.
40. Criqui, M. H., et al. Plasma Triglyceride Level and Mortality from Coronary Heart Disease. *New England Journal of Medicine, 328* (1993), 1220–1225; Brody, J. E. Study Says a Blood Fat Alone Rarely Hurts Heart. *The New York Times,* April 29 1993, p. B9.
41. Brody, J. E. The Leading Killer of Women: Heart Disease. *The New York Times,* November 10, 1993, p. C17.
42. Risk Factors for Heart Disease. A Publication of the American Heart Association, 1995.
43. Stampfer, M. J., et al. *Ten-Year Follow-up Study of Estrogen Replacement Therapy in Relation to Cardiovascular Disease and Mortality.* Paper presented at the 24th annual meeting of the Society for Epidemiologic Research, Buffalo, New York, June 11–14, 1991; Study Finds Estrogen Hormone Helps Postmenopausal Women. *The New York Times,* January 1, 1996, p. A 1,2.
44. Estrogen Replacement: More Important than Ever. *Consumer Reports on Health, 7,* November 1995, pp. 121–123.
45. Colditz, G. A., et al. The Use of Estrogens and Progestins and the Risk of Breast Cancer in Postmenopausal Women. *New England Journal of Medicine, 332* (1995), 1589–1593.
46. Estrogen Replacement: More Important than Ever, 1995, p. 121.
47. Estrogen and Breast Cancer. *Consumer Reports on Health, 7,* August 1995, p. 94.
48. Heart Disease: Women at Risk. *Consumer Reports,* May 1993, pp. 300–304.
49. Heart Disease: Women at Risk, 1993.
50. Editors of the University of California at Berkeley Wellness Letter, *The Wellness Engagement Calendar 1996,* New York: Rebus, Inc.
51. Waist-Hip Ratio Seen as an Index of Health. *The New York Times,* January 27, 1993, p. C16.
52. National Cancer Institute. Cited in Lung Cancer Is Said to Overtake Heart Trouble as Smokers' Peril, *The New York Times,* August 22, 1991, p. B10.
53. Miller, T. Q., et al. Reasons for the Trend toward Null Findings in Research on Type A Behavior. *Psychological Bulletin, 110* (1991), 469–485.
54. Angier, N. If Anger Ruins Your Day, It Can Shrink Your Life. *The New York Times,* December 13, 1990, p. B23; Talan, J. Study: Mental Stress Tied to Heart Attacks. *Newsday,* June 5, 1996, p. A35; Coronary Disease: Taking Emotions to Heart. *Harvard Health Letter, 21,* October 1996, pp. 1–3.
55. Markovitz, J. H., et al. Psychological Predictors of Hypertension in the Framingham Study: Is There Tension in Hypertension? *Journal of the American Medical Association, 270* (1993), 2439–2443.
56. Jian, W., et al. Mental Stress–Induced Myocardial Ischemia and Cardiac Events. *Journal of the American Medical Association, 275* (1966), 1651–1656; Are Mental Stress Tests in Cardiology's Future? *Harvard Heart Letter, 7,* October 1996, p. 3.
57. Fizzle Anger. *Prevention,* February 1996, p. 24.
58. Anger Doubles Risk of Attack for Heart Disease Patients. *The New York Times,* March 19, 1994, p. A8; Anger and Heart Attacks Revisited. *Harvard Heart Letter, 6,* February 1996, p. 4.
59. Talan, J. Is Panic Attack a False Alarm? *Newsday,* May 24, 1994, pp. B27, B33.
60. Krantz, D. S., et al. Environmental Stress and Biobehavioral Antecedents of Coronary Heart Disease. *Journal of Consulting and Clinical Psychology, 56* (1988), 333–341.
61. Rotating Work Shifts May Hurt Women's Hearts. *The New York Times,* December 1, 1995, p. A28.
62. Adapted from Eat Right to Lower Your High Blood Cholesterol. U.S. Department of Health and Human Services, Public Health Service, National Institutes of Health, NIH Pub. No. 92–2972, Reprinted March 1992.
63. Boosting Your Good Cholesterol. *UC Berkeley Wellness Letter,* March 1996, p. 6.
64. Heart Disease: The Vitamin B Breakthrough. *Health,* January/February 1997, p. 95.
65. Alcohol and the Heart: Consensus Emerges. *Harvard Heart Letter, 6,* January 1996, pp. 1–3.

### CHAPTER 18

1. CancerNet from the National Cancer Institute, *National Cancer Program: Pathways to Progress* (revised). May 1995.
2. Crossette, B. Noncommunicable Diseases Seen as World Health Challenge. *The New York Times,* September 16, 1996, p. A7.
3. Sources: National Cancer Institute, National Institutes of Health, *Cancer Facts: What Is Cancer,* March 1993; National Cancer Institute, National Institutes of Health. *Cancer Facts, Sites and Types: Questions and Answers about Metastatic Cancer,* April 1996; Weinberg, R. A. How Cancer Arises. *Scientific American, 275* (1996), pp. 62–70.
4. Nash, J. M. The Enemy Within. *Time* Special Issue, *The Frontiers of Medicine,* Fall 1996, pp. 15–23.
5. Ries, L. A. G., et al. (Eds.) *SEER Cancer Statistics Review, 1973–1991: Tables and Graphs.* National Cancer Institute, NIH Pub. No. 94–2789, Bethesda, MD, 1994.
6. Brody, J. E. Decline Seen in Death Rates from Cancer as a Whole. *The New York Times,* November 14, 1996, p. A21; Bailar, J. C., III, and Gornik, H. L. Cancer Undefeated. *The New England Journal of Medicine, 336* (1997), 1569–1574.
7. National Cancer Institute, National Institutes of Health, *Cancer Rates and Risks* (4th ed.). Cancer Statistics Branch, Division of Cancer Prevention and Control, National Cancer Institute, 1996.
8. *Cancer Facts, Sites and Types: Racial Differences in Breast Cancer Survival.* National Cancer Institute, November 1994.
9. *Cancer Facts: What Are the Signs and Symptoms of Cancer?* National Cancer Institute, National Institutes of Health, March 1993; *Cancer Facts, Sites and Types.* National Cancer Institute, National Institutes of Health, March 1993.
10. Earp, J. A. L., et al. The North Carolina Breast Cancer Screening Program: Foundations and Design of a Model for Reaching Older, Minority, Rural Women. *Breast Cancer Research and Treatment, 35* (1995), 7–22.

11. Trichopoulos, D., Li, F. P., and Hunter, D. J. What Causes Cancer? *Scientific American, 275* (1996), pp. 80–87.
12. Trichopoulos, Li, and Hunter, 1996.
13. Evidence Mounts on Cervical Cancer, Smoking. *CNN Health Briefs, Reuters News Service,* April 23, 1996.
14. Whittemore A. S., et al. Prostate Cancer in Relation to Diet, Physical Activity, and Body Size in Blacks, Whites, and Asians in the United States and Canada. *Journal of the National Cancer Institute, 87* (1995), 652–660.
15. Hunter, D. J., et al. Cohort Studies of Fat Intake and the Risk of Breast Cancer—A Pooled Analysis. *New England Journal of Medicine, 334* (1996), 356–361.
16. Clark, L. C., et al. Effects of Selenium Supplementation for Cancer Prevention in Patients with Carcinoma of the Skin: A Randomized Controlled Trial. *Journal of the American Medical Association, 276* (1996), 1957–1963.
17. NIAAA, *Alcohol Alert No. 21,* July 1993.
18. Takada, A., Takase, S., and Tsutsumi, M. Alcohol and Hepatic Carcinogenesis. In R. Yirmiya and A. N. Taylor (Eds.), *Alcohol, Immunity, and Cancer.* Boca Raton, FL: CRC Press, 1993. pp. 187–209; Villa, E., Melegari, M., and Manenti, F. Alcohol, Viral Hepatitis, and Hepatocellular Carcinoma. In R. R. Watson (Ed.), *Alcohol and Cancer.* Boca Raton, Fl: CRC Press, 1992. pp. 151–165; Stinson, F. S., and Debakey, S. F. Alcohol-Related Mortality in the United States, 1979–1988. *British Journal of Addiction, 87* (1992), 777–783.
19. Fuchs, C. S., et al. Alcohol Consumption and Mortality among Women. *New England Journal of Medicine, 332* (1995), 1245–1250.
20. Marks, R., and Motley R. J. Skin Cancer: Recognition and Treatment. *Drugs, 50* (1995), 48–61.
21. U.S. Department of Health and Human Services, Public Health Service, Centers for Disease Control and Prevention. *Colorectal Cancer: The Importance of Early Detection. At-A-Glance 1996;* Yong, L. C, et al. Prospective Study of Relative Weight and Risk of Breast Cancer: The Breast Cancer Detection Demonstration Project Follow-up Study, 1979 to 1987–1989. *American Journal of Epidemiology, 143* (1996), 985–995; Tough New Warning on Diet Is Issued by Cancer Society. *The New York Times,* September 17, 1996, p. A16; Trichopoulos, Li, and Hunter, 1996.
22. Trichopoulos, Li, and Hunter, 1996; Study: Viruses May Cause 15 Percent of Cancers. A Report by the Cancer Research Campaign. *Reuters News Service,* August 1, 1996; Schiffman, M. H, et al. Epidemiologic Evidence Showing That Human Papillomavirus Infection Causes Most Cervical Intraepithelial Neoplasia. *Journal of the National Cancer Institute 85* (1993), 958–964; Brisson, J., et al. Risk Factors for Cervival Intraepithelial Neoplasia: Differences Between Low- and High-Grade Lesions. *American Journal of Epidemiology 140* (1994), 700–710; HIV Alters DNA. Causing Rare Cancer. *Science News, 145,* April 16, 1994, p. 244; Roving Mates Called Factor in Cancer. *The New York Times,* September 7, 1996, p. A10.
23. Sources on genetic defects and cancer: Gailani, M. R., et al. The Role of the Human Homologue of *Drosophilia Patched* in Sporadic Basal Cell Carcinomas. *Nature Genetics, 14* (1996) 78–81; Support for Cancer Link. *The New York Times,* September 3, 1996, p. C3; American Cancer Society, *Breast Cancer Facts & Figures 1996.* American Cancer Society, Inc., December 1995 (rev.); Friend, S. H. Breast Cancer Susceptibility Testing: Realities in the Post-Genomic Era. *Nature Genetics, 13* (1996), 16–17; Smith, J. R., et al. Major Susceptibility Locus for Prostate Cancer on Chromosome 1. *Science, 274* (1996), 1371–1374; Healy, B. BRCA Genes—Bookmaking, Fortunetelling, and Medical Care. *New England Journal of Medicine, 336* (1997), 1448–1449.
24. Angier, N. Scientists Zero In on a Gene Linked to Prostate Cancer. *The New York Times,* November 21, 1996, p. A26.
25. Lynch, Henry T. Cited in National Cancer Institute. Cancer News, Caution Guides Genetic Testing for Hereditary Cancer Genes, *Journal of the National Cancer Institute, 88* (1996), Issue 2, p. 70.
26. Adapted from Do You Have a Cancer Gene? Copyright May 13, 1996, *U.S. News & World Report.* Reprinted with permission.
27. Trichopoulos, Li, and Hunter, 1996.
28. Breast Cancer, Stress Link Disputed in New Study. *CNN Health Briefs, Reuters News Service,* March 15, 1996.
29. Maunsell, E., Brisson, J., and Deschenes, L. Social Support and Survival among Women with Breast Cancer. *Cancer, 76* (1995), 631–637.
30. American Cancer Society, Inc. *Cancer Facts & Figures—1996.* American Cancer Society, Inc., Applied Research Branch, 1996.
31. Miller, B. A., Feuer, E. J., and Hankey, B. F. The Significance of the Rising Incidence of Breast Cancer in the United States. In V. T. Devita, S. Hellman, and S. A. Rosenberg (Eds.), *Important Advances in Oncology.* Philadelphia, PA: J. B. Lippincott Co., 1994, pp. 193–207.
32. NBC Nightly News. Your Body, Your Health. September 11, 1996.
33. Statistics on numbers of cancer cases, mortality rates, survival rates, and signs and symptoms for breast cancer and other types of cancer were compiled from several sources: Twelve major cancers, *Scientific American,* September 1996, pp. 126–132; National Center for Health Statistics. *Monitoring Health Care in America, Quarterly Fact Sheet: Spotlight on Cancer.* U.S. Department of Health and Human Services, June 1996; Cancer Statistics Branch, Division of Cancer Prevention and Control, National Cancer Institute, *Cancer Rates and Risks* (4th ed.), 1996. American Cancer Society. *Cancer Facts & Figures—1996,* and other American Cancer Society publications.
34. Kosary, C. L., et al. *SEER Cancer Statistics Review, 1973–1992: Tables and Graphs.* National Cancer Institute, NIH Publication No. 95–2789, 1995; Fewer Women Dying from Breast Cancer. *The New York Times,* October 4, 1996, p. A22; Rennie, J., and Rusting, R. Making Headway Against Cancer. *Scientific American, 275* (1996, September), pp. 56–59.
35. American Cancer Society, *Breast Cancer Facts and Figures 1996.* American Cancer Society, Inc., December 1995 (rev.); CancerNet, National Cancer Institute, National Institutes of Health. *Questions and Answers About Mammography and Breast Cancer,* August 1995 (rev.).
36. NBC Nightly News, September 11, 1996.
37. As Weight Goes Up, So Does Breast Cancer Risk. *Tufts University Diet & Nutrition Letter, 14* (5), July 1996, pp. 1–2.
38. White, E., et al. Breast Cancer among Young U.S. Women in Relation to Oral contraceptive Use, *Journal of the National Cancer Institute,* April 6, 1994; Malone, K. E., et al. Oral Contraceptives in Relation to Breast Cancer. *Epidemiologic Reviews, 15* (1993), 80–97; Schlesselman, J. J. Net Effect of Oral Contraceptive Use on the Risk of Cancer in Women in the United States. *Obstetrics & Gynecology, 85* (1995), 793–801.
39. Brody, J. E. The Known and Potential Benefits of the Pill. *The New York Times,* October 2, 1996, p. C11.
40. Colditz, G. A., et al. The Use of Estrogens and Progestins and the Risk of Breast Cancer in Postmenopausal Women. *New England Journal of Medicine, 332* (1995), 1589–1593; Brinton, B. A., and Schairer, C. Estrogen Replacement Therapy and Breast Cancer Risk. *Epidemiologic Reviews, 15* (1993), 66–79; Davison, N. E. Is Hormone Replacement Therapy a Risk? *Scientific American, 275* (1996), p. 101.
41. Arriagada, R., et al. Conservative Treatment versus Mastectomy in Early Breast Cancer: Patterns of Failure with 15 Years of Follow-up Data. *Journal of Clinical Oncology, 14* (1996), 1558–1564; Guenther, J. M., et al. Feasibility of Breast-Conserving Therapy for Younger Women with Breast Cancer. *Archives of Surgery, 131* (1996), 632–636.
42. Slim Breast-Cancer Risks. *Prevention,* July 1994, p. 30.
43. Lowering Breast Cancer Risk. *Harvard Health Letter, 21*(11), September 1996, pp. 7–8.
44. Cable News Network (March 23, 1997). American Cancer Society. *Report of Workshop on Guidelines for Breast Cancer Detection.* Chicago, March 7–9, 1997.

45. White, E., Urban, N., and Taylor, V. Mammography Utilization, Public Health Impact and Effectiveness in the United States. In G. S. Omenn et al. (Eds.), *The Annual Review of Public Health, 14.* Palo Alto, CA: Annual Reviews, Inc., 1993, pp. 605–634. CDC. *Implementation of the Breast and Cervical Cancer Mortality Prevention Act: 1992. Progress Report to Congress,* 1994.
46. Kolata, G. Mammogram Talks Prove Indefinite. *The New York Times,* January 24, 1997, pp. A1, A15.
47. Lubin J. H., et al. Lung Cancer in Radon-Exposed Miners and Estimation of Risk from Indoor Exposure. *Journal of the National Cancer Institute, 87* (1995), 817–826; New Study Questions Radon Danger in Houses. *The New York Times,* July 17, 1996, p. A15.
48. Fry, W. A., Menck, H. R., and Winchester, D. P. The National Cancer Data Base Report on Lung Cancer. *Cancer, 77* (1996), 1947–1955.
49. Nicholson, P. W., and Harland, S. J. Inheritance and Testicular Cancer. *British Journal of Cancer, 71* (1995), 421–426.
50. *Colorectal Cancer: The Importance of Early Detection: At-a-Glance.* U.S. Department of Health and Human Services, Public Health Service, Centers for Disease Control and Prevention, 1996.
51. Thune, I., and Lund, E. Physical Activity and Risk of Colorectal Cancer in Men and Women. *British Journal of Cancer, 73* (1996), 1134–1140; Lee, U-M., et al. Physical Activity and Risk of Developing Colorectal Cancer among College Alumni. *Journal of the National Cancer Institute, 83* (1991), 1324–1329.
52. *Colorectal Cancer: The Importance of Early Detection: At-a-Glance.* U.S. Department of Health and Human Services, Public Health Service, Centers for Disease Control and Prevention, 1996. Marshall, J. B. Colorectal Cancer Screening: Present Strategies and Future Prospects. *Postgraduate Medicine, 99* (1996), 253–264; Lang, S. S. The Most Misunderstood Women's Cancer. *Good Housekeeping,* August 1996, pp. 56, 58.
53. American Cancer Society. *Prostate Cancer Information,* 1995; American Cancer Society. *Description of Prostate Cancer,* 1996; National Cancer Institute. *Surge in Prostate Cancer Incidence Rates Due to More PSA Testing, Study Says,* May 16, 1996; U.S. Department of Health and Human Services, Public Health Service. Centers for Disease Control and Prevention. *Prostate Cancer: Can We Reduce Mortality While Preserving Quality of Life? At-A-Glance,* 1995; National Cancer Institute. *NCI Seeks Answers on Prostate Cancer: Causes, Detection, Prevention, and Treatment,* 1996; American Cancer Society, *Prostate Cancer Incidence,* 1996; American Cancer Society. *Prostate Cancer Survival,* 1996; Prostate Cancer: Should You Get a PSA Test? *UC Berkeley Wellness Letter, 11(10),* July 1995, pp. 4–5.
54. Prostate Cancer: Should You Get a PSA Test? *UC Berkeley Wellness Letter, 11(10),* July 1995, pp. 4–5; *Prostate Cancer Survival.* American Cancer Society, 1996; The Swedish Prostate Cancer Paradox. *Journal of the American Medical Association, 277* (1997), 497–498; Johansson, J. E., et al. Fifteen-year Survival in Prostate Cancer: A Prospective Population-Based Study in Sweden. *Journal of the American Medical Association, 277* (1997), 467–471.
55. *Prostate Cancer: Can We Reduce Mortality While Preserving Quality of Life? At-A-Glance,* U.S. Department of Health and Human Services, Public Health Service. Centers for Disease Control and Prevention, 1995; Prostate Cancer: Should You Get a PSA Test? *UC Berkeley Wellness Letter, 11(10),* July 1995, pp. 4–5.
56. Gerber, G. S., et al. Results of Radical Prostatectomy in Men with Clinically Localized Prostate Cancer: Multi-Institutional Pooled Analysis. *Journal of the American Medical Association, 276* (1996), 615–619.
57. *Prostate Cancer Survival.* American Cancer Society, 1996; Menon, M., Parulkar, B. G., and Baker, S. Should We Treat Localized Prostate Cancer? An Opinion. *Urology, 46* (1995), 607–616.
58. Albertsen, P. C. Commentary: African-Americans and Prostate Cancer. *The Cancer Journal from Scientific American, 2*(4), July/August 1996; Vijayakumar, S., et al. Prostate-Specific Antigen Levels in African-Americans Correlate with Insurance Status as an Indicator of Socioeconomic Status. *Cancer Journal from Scientific American, 2* (1996), 225–233; Ross, R. K., Bernstein, L., and Lobo, R. A. 5-alpha-reductase Activity and Risk of Prostate Cancer among Japanese and US White and Black Males. *Lancet 339* (1992), 887–889; *Prostate Cancer Risk Factors.* American Cancer Society, 1996.
59. Mettlin, C. J. The National Cancer Data Base Report on Prostate Cancer. American College of Surgeons Commission on Cancer and the American Cancer Society. *Cancer, 76* (1995), 1104–1112; Fowler, J. E., Jr., and Terrell, F. Survival in Blacks and Whites after Treatment for Localized Prostate Cancer. *Journal of Urology, 156* (1996), 144–145.
60. Jaroff, L. The Man's Cancer. *Time,* April 1, 1996.
61. Coughlin, S. S. Smoking Increases Risk of Death from Prostate Cancer. *American Journal of Epidemiology, 143* (1996), 1002–1006; *Prostate Cancer Risk Factors.* American Cancer Society. 1996.
62. Pasta Perfect. *Nutrition Action Healthletter,* 23, April 1996, p. 12; Prostate Protector. *Prevention,* 1996, p. 25; *Journal of the National Cancer Institute,* December 6, 1995.
63. National Skin Cancer Prevention Education Program, *Skin Cancer At-A-Glance,* U.S. Department of Health and Human Services, Public Health Service, Centers for Disease Control and Prevention, 1996.
64. Marks R., and Motley, R. J. Skin Cancer. Recognition and Treatment. *Drugs, 50* (1995), 48–61.
65. Elder, D. E., Skin Cancer. Melanoma and Other Specific Nonmelanoma Skin Cancers. 75 (1995), 245–256; Rhodes, A. R. Public Education and Cancer of the Skin. What Do People Need to Know about Melanoma and Nonmelanoma Skin Cancer? *Cancer, 75* (1995), 613–636; National Skin Cancer Prevention Education Program, *Skin Cancer At-a-Glance.* U.S. Department of Health and Human Services, Public Health Service, Centers for Disease Control and Prevention, 1996.
66. Trichopoulos, Li, and Hunter, 1996.
67. Melanoma Awareness Low. *Newsday,* May 7, 1996, p. B27.
68. Sun Lamps Beat the Skin. *UC Berkeley Wellness Letter, 11(11),* August 1995, p. 5.
69. Black, H. S., et al. Evidence that a Low-Fat Diet Reduces the Occurrence of Nonmelanoma Skin Cancer. *International Journal of Cancer, 62* (1995), 165–169; Saving Your Skin. *Harvard Health Letter, 21(1),* November 1994, p. 8.
70. Boring, C. C., et al. Cancer Statistics, 1994. *Ca—A Cancer Journal for Clinicians, 44* (1994), 7–26.
71. van Nagell, J. R, Jr. Ovarian Cancer Screening. *Cancer, 76* (1995), 2086–2091.
72. NIH Consensus Conference. Ovarian Cancer: Screening, Treatment, and Follow-up. *Journal of the American Medical Association, 273* (1995), 491–497.
73. Odds in Your Hands. *Prevention,* June 1996, p. 30.
74. *What's New in Cancer Prevention?* Centers for Disease Control and Prevention, 1996.
75. Schiffman M. H, et al. Epidemiologic Evidence Showing That Human Papillomavirus Infection Causes Most Cervical Intraepithelial Neoplasia. *Journal of the National Cancer Institute 85* (1993), 958–964; Brisson J., et al. Risk Factors for Cervical Intraepithelial Neoplasia: Differences Between Low- and High-Grade Lesions. *American Journal of Epidemiology 140* (1994), 700–710.
76. Alvi, A. Oral Cancer: How to Recognize the Danger Signs. *Postgraduate Medicine, 99* (1996), 149–52, 155–6
77. Brown, A. E., and Langdon, J. D. Management of Oral Cancer. *Annual Review of the College of Surgeons of England, 77* (1995), 404–408.
78. National Cancer Institute, National Institutes of Health. *Cancer Facts: Therapy. Questions and Answers about Gene Therapy,* August 1993.
79. Reuters News Service. Researchers Have Discovered a Highly Precise and Potent Way to Target Prostate Cancer. January 31, 1997.

80. Gene Therapy for Lung Cancer Shows Promise, a Study Finds. *The New York Times,* August 29, 1996, p. D18.
81. *Biological Therapies: Using the Immune System to Treat Cancer.* National Cancer Institute, October 1995; University of Pennsylvania, OncoLink. Exciting Cancer Advances with Interferon and New Cytokines Reported at ASCO Meeting, May 20, 1996; Old, L. J., Immunotherapy for Cancer. *Scientific American, 275* (September 1996), 136–143.
82. Atkins, M. B. Commentary: Interleukin-2 Therapy: A Decade of Slow but Steady Progress. *The Cancer Journal from Scientific American, 2*(2), March/April 1996; Atzpodien, J., et al. Combination with Inteferon-Alpha and 5-fluorouracil for Metastatic Renal Cell Cancer. *European Journal of Cancer,* 29A [suppl 5] (1993), S6–S8; Yang, J. C., et al. Randomized Comparison of High-Dose and Low-Dose Intravenous Interleukin-2 for the Therapy of Metastatic Renal Cell Carcinoma: An Interim Report. *Journal of Clinical Oncology, 12* (1994), 1572–1576.
83. Marks and Motley, 1995.
84. Breast Conservation Is a Safe Method in Patients with Small Cancer of the Breast. Long-Term Results of Three Randomized Trials on 1,973 Patients. *European Journal of Cancer, 31a* (1995), 1574–1579.
85. National Cancer Institute, National Institutes of Health. *Cancer Facts: Unconventional Methods, Laetrile.* November 1992.
86. National Cancer Institute, National Institutes of Health. *Cancer Facts: Unconventional Methods, Holistic Medicine.* April 1993.
87. Aulas, J. Alternative Cancer Treatments. *Scientific American, 275* (September 1996), 162–163.
88. Adapted from Buhle, E. L., Jr., *Coping with Survival—Parts 1, 2.* Hospital of the University of Pennsylvania, August 1995 (rev.), CancerNet from the National Cancer Institute, *National Cancer Program: Pathways to Progress,* May 1995 (rev.); National Cancer Institute. *Advanced Cancer—Living Each Day* NIH Publication No. 93–856, 1993, and other sources.
89. CDC. *National Diabetes Fact Sheet,* November 1995; *More Diabetes Information* July 1995 (rev.); *Diabetes: A Serious Public Health Problem. At-A-Glance,* 1996; National Institute of Diabetes and Digestive and Kidney Disease (NIDDK), National Institutes of Health. *Diabetes Statistics.* NIH Publication No. 96–3926, October 1995; NIDDK, National Institutes of Health. *Diabetes Overview.* NIH Publication No. 96–3873, October 1995, updated 6 August 1996; NIDDK. Do Your Level Best: Why it Is Important to Take Care of Your Diabetes, 1996; Wollard, K. The Dynamics and Dangers of Diabetes. *Newsday,* September 17, 1996, p. B22.
90. NIDDK, National Institutes of Health. *Diabetes Overview.* NIH Publication No. 96–3873, October 1995, updated 6 August 1996; Newman J. M., et al. Diabetes-Associated Mortality in Native Americans. *Diabetes Care, 16* (1993), 297–299.
91. Leary, W. E. Panel Urges F.D.A. Approval of New Type of Diabetes Drug. *The New York Times,* December 12, 1996, p. A25; Leary, W. E. New Class of Diabetes Drug is Approved. *The New York Times,* January 31, 1997, p. A24.
92. American Lung Association. *Chronic Bronchitis,* 1996; National Jewish Center for Immunology and Respiratory Medicine. *Management of Chronic Obstructive Pulmonary Disease (COPD),* American Lung Association. *Emphysema,* 1996.
93. Adapted from Health ResponseAbility Systems. *Skin Cancer, Melanoma,* 1993; What's Your UV-Risk score? *Consumer Reports on Health,* June 1996, p. 70, and other sources.
94. Naylor, M. F., et al. High Sun Protection Factor Sunscreens in the Suppression of Actinic Neoplasia. *Archives of Dermatology, 131* (1995), 170–175.
95. Adapted from American Cancer Society publications, *Eating Smart* (No. 87–250M–Rev. 3/89; No. 2042) and *Eat Right* (No. 88–25MM–No. 2099), *Cancer Facts & Figures—1996;* Burros, M. Tough New Warning on Diet Is Issued by Cancer Society. *The New York Times,* September 17, 1996, p. A16; and other sources.
96. Cable News Network. Study: Grapes Inhibit Cancer Growth. January 10, 1997; Meishiang, J., et al., Cancer Chemopreventive Activity of Resveratrol, a Natural Product Derived from Grapes. *Science,* Volume 275, January 10, 1997, pp. 218–220
97. Paffenbarger, R. S., Lee, I-Min, and Wing, A. L., The Influence of Physical Activity on the Incidence of Site-Specific Cancers in College Alumni. In *Exercise, Calories, Fat, and Cancer,* Jacobs, M. M. (Ed.), New York: Plenum Press, 1992, pp. 7–15.; Bouchard, C. R., Shephard, J., and Stephens, T. (Eds.), *Physical Activity, Fitness, and Health: Consensus Statement,* 1993, p. 77; Exercise and Cancer Prevention. *UC Berkeley Wellness Letter,* September 1996, p. 3, and other sources.
98. Berg, K. Metabolic Disease: Diabetes Mellitus. In V. Seefeldt (Ed.), *Physical Activity and Well-Being.* America Alliance of AHPERD, 1986; Blair, S. N., Kohl, H. W., and Gordon, N. F. How Much Exercise is Good for Health? In *Annual Review of Public Health,* G. S. Omenn (Ed.), Palo Alto, CA: Annual Reviews Inc., vol. 13, 1992, p. 112.


### CHAPTER 19


1. Gerber, J., Wolf, J., and Klores, W., et al. *Lifetrends: The Future of Baby Boomers and Other Aging Americans.* New York: Stonesong Press (Macmillan), 1989, p. 2.; Hayflick, L. *How and Why We Age.* New York: Ballantine, 1994, pp. 54–59; Administration on Aging (AoA). *Demographic Changes.* National Aging Information Center, January 1997.
2. Gerber et al., 1989, p. 4.
3. Rathus, S. A. and Nevid, J. S. *Adjustment and Growth: The Challenges of Life* (6th ed.). Fort Worth, TX: Harcourt Brace College Publishers, 1995, p. 440. Copyright © 1995 by Holt, Rinehart and Winston, Inc., reprinted by permission of the publisher.
4. Hayflick, 1994, p. 15.
5. Gerber et al., 1989; p. 6; Hess, B. B., Markson, E. W., and Stein, P. J. *Sociology* (4th ed.). New York: Macmillan, 1993, p. 233.
6. Hayflick, 1994, p. 101.
7. Doctors Tie Male Mentality to Shorter Life Span. *Newsday,* June 14, 1995, p. C14.
8. Hayflick, 1994, p. 58.
9. Barringer, F. Prospects for the Elderly Differ Widely by Sex. *The New York Times,* November 10, 1992, pp. A1, A21.
10. Henslin, J. *Sociology: A Down-to-Earth Approach* (2nd ed.). Needham, MA: Allyn & Bacon, 1995.
11. How Long Will You Live? *Consumer Reports on Health,* May 1995, p. 51. Data drawn from U.S. Department of Health and Human Services, 1995.
12. Henslin, 1995, p. 349.
13. Wray, L. A. Public Policy Implications of an Ethnically Diverse Elderly Population. *Journal of Cross-Cultural Gerontology, 6* (1991), 243–257.
14. Poppy, J. How Old Are You Really? *Health,* November/December 1992, pp. 45–56.
15. U.S. Department of Health & Human Services, *Healthy People 2000;* and other sources.
16. Kart, C. W. *The Realities of Aging: An Introduction to Gerontology* (3rd ed.). Boston: Allyn & Bacon, 1990, p. 222.
17. Evans. W., and Rosenberg, I. H. *Biomarkers: The 10 Determinants of Aging You Can Control.* New York: Simon & Schuster, 1991, p. 28.
18. Evans and Rosenberg, 1991.
19. Thornton, H. A. *A Medical Handbook for Senior Citizens and Their Families.* Dover, MA: Auburn House, 1989.
20. Thornton, 1989, p. 130.
21. Brody, J. E. For Millions, Little or No Sense of Smell Means Diminished Life Quality and Special Problems. *The New York Times,* February 1, 1990, p. B10.
22. Evans and Rosenberg, 1991, p. 244.
23. National Institute on Aging, *In Search of the Secrets of Aging.*
24. Kotre, J., and Hall, E. *Seasons of Life: Our Dramatic Journey from Birth to Death,* Boston: Little, Brown, 1990, p. 328.
25. Evans and Rosenberg, 1991, p. 44.
26. Evans and Rosenberg, 1991, p. 47.
27. Size up your bones . . . now! *Prevention,* February 1996, p. 76.
28. Brody, J. Hip Fracture: A Potential Killer that

Can Be Avoided. *The New York Times,* December 9, 1992, C16.

29. Anderson, J. W. and Gustafsson, N. J., Type II Diabetes: Current Nutrition Management Concepts, *Geriatrics, 41* (1986), 28–38.
30. Study Finds Estrogen Hormone Helps Postmenopausal Women. *The New York Times,* January 1, 1996, p. A12; *How Can I Prevent Osteoporosis?* Published by the National Osteoporosis Foundation, Washington DC.
31. Exercise for the Ages. *Consumer Reports on Health,* July 1996, pp. 73, 75, 76.
32. Study Finds Estrogen Hormone Helps Postmenopausal Women. *The New York Times,* January 1, 1996, p. A12.
33. Estrogen and Breast Cancer. *Consumer Reports on Health, 7*(8), August 1995, p. 94; Col, N. F., et al. Patient-Specific Decisions about Hormone Replacement Therapy in Postmenopausal Women. *Journal of the American Medical Association, 277* (1997), 1140–1147.
34. Schaie, K. W. The Course of Adult Intellectual Development. *American Psychologist, 49* (1994), 304–313.
35. Havighurst, R. J. *Developmental Tasks and Education* (3rd ed.). New York: McKay, 1972.
36. Beck, M. The New Middle Age. *Newsweek,* December 7, 1992, pp. 50–56.
37. Sheehy, G. New Passages: Mapping Your Life across Time. New York: Random House, 1995.
38. Margoshes, P. For Many, Old Age Is the Prime of Life. *APA Monitor, 26*(5) (1995), 36–37.
39. Tavris, C. Life Stages No Longer Dictated. *American Health,* July–August, 1989, pp. 50–58.
40. Schlossberg, N. *Overwhelmed: Coping with Life's Ups and Downs.* Boston: Lexington Books, 1990.
41. Purifoy, F. E., Grodsky, A., and Giambra, L. M. The Relationship of Sexual Daydreaming to Sexual Activity, Sexual Drive, and Sexual Attitudes for Women across the Life-span. *Archives of Sexual Behavior, 21* (1992), 369–375.
42. Katchadourian, H. A. *Fifty: Midlife in Perspective.* New York: Freeman, 1987.
43. Reinisch, J. M. *The Kinsey Institute New Report on Sex: What You Must Know to Be Sexually Literate.* New York: St. Martin's Press, 1990.
44. Reinisch, 1990, p. 227.
45. Adapted from Reinisch, 1990.
46. Smith J. R., Ning, Y., and Pereira-Smith, O. M. Why Are Transformed Cells Immortal? Is the Process Reversible? *American Journal of Clinical Nutrition, 55* (1992) (6 Suppl):1215S–1221S; Hensler, P. J., et al. A Gene Involved in Control of Human Cellular Senescence on Human Chromosome 1q. *Molecular and Cell Biology, 14* (1994), 2291–2297.
47. Hayflick, 1994, pp. 132–133.
48. Weksler, M. E. Immune Senescence. *Annals of Neurology, 35* (1994), Suppl. pp. S35–37; Currie, M. S. Immunosenescence. *Comprehensive Therapeutics, 18* (11) (1992), 26–34.
49. Makinodan T., Lubinski, J., and Fong, T. C. Cellular, Biochemical, and Molecular Basis of T-Cell Senescence. *Archives of Pathology and Laboratory Medicine, 111* (1987), 910–914.
50. National Institute on Aging. *In Search of the Secrets of Aging.*
51. National Institute on Aging, *In Search of the Secrets of Aging;* Harman, D. Free Radical Theory of Aging. *Mutation Research, 275* (1992), 257–66; Harman, D. Free Radical Involvement in Aging. Pathophysiology and Therapeutic Implications. *Drugs and Aging 3* (1993), 60–80.
52. Meydani, S. N., et al. Vitamin E Supplementation and In Vivo Immune Response in Healthy Elderly Subjects: A Randomized Controlled Trial. *New England Journal of Medicine, 277* (1997), 1380–1386.
53. National Institute on Aging, *In Search of the Secrets of Aging.*
54. Hayflick, 1994, p. 244.
55. Walford, R. *Maximum Life Span.* New York: Simon & Schuster, 1983.
56. Lesnikov, V. A., and Pierpaoli, W. Pineal Cross-Transplantation (Old-to-Young and Vice Versa) as Evidence for an Endogenous "Aging Clock." *Annals of the New York Academy of Medicine, 719* (1994), 456–460.
57. DHEA—The Promise of Youth and Health. *UC Berkeley Wellness Letter, 12*(4), January 1996, pp. 1–2.
58. Rudman, D., et al. Effects of Human Growth Hormone in Men over 60 Years Old. *New England Journal of Medicine, 321* (1989); Weiss, R. Human Growth Hormone Therapy. *Health, 7*(7), November–December 1993; Growth Hormone Fails to Reverse Effects of Aging, Researchers Say. *The New York Times,* April 15, 1996, p. A13.
59. The Breathtaking Promises of Melatonin. *UC Berkeley Wellness Letter, March 1996,* 12 (6), pp. 1–2.
60. U.S. Senate Special Committee on Aging. *Aging America: Trends and Projections,* 1991.
61. Pistetsky, D. S. *The Duke University Medical Center Book of Arthritis.* New York: Fawcett Columbine, 1992, p. 22.
62. Willis, D. P. (Ed.). *Health Policies and Black Americans.* New Brunswick, NJ: Transaction, 1990, p. 171.
63. Pistetsky, D. S., 1992, p. 14; Osteoarthritis: Old Scourge, New Hope. *Consumer Reports on Health, 8 (1),* January 1996, p. 3; More Is More: More Exercise Might Mean Less Arthritis Pain. *Prevention.* February 1996, pp. 30–31.
64. Rheumatoid Arthritis: Promising Drugs of the Future. *Harvard Health Letter, 21,* March 1996, p. 7.
65. U.S. Senate Special Committee on Aging, *Aging America: Trends and Projections,* 1991, p. 114.
66. National Institute on Aging, *Special Report on Aging, 1992,* NIH publication # 92–3409.
67. Podolsky, D., and Silberner, J. How Medicine Mistreats the Elderly. *U.S. News & World Report,* January 18, 1993, pp. 72–79.
68. Kart, 1990, p. 129.
69. Cited in Solomon, D. H., et al. *A Consumer Guide to Aging.* Johns Hopkins University Press, 1992, p. 78.
70. Rao, S. M., Huber, S. J., and Bornstein, R. A. Emotional Changes with Multiple Sclerosis and Parkinson's Disease. *Journal of Consulting and Clinical Psychology, 60* (1992), 369–378; Teri, L. Clinical Problems in Older Adults. *Clinician's Research Digest* (Supp 9), November 1992; Teri, L., and Wagner, A. Alzheimer's Disease and Depression. *Journal of Consulting and Clinical Psychology, 60* (1992), 379–391; Solomon, 1992.
71. Blazer, D., et al. The Association of Age and Depression among the Elderly: An Epidemiologic Exploration. *Journal of Gerontology, 46* (1991), 210–215; Dean, A., Kolody, B., Wood, P., and Matt, G. E. The Influence of Living Alone on Depression in Elderly Persons. *Journal of Aging and Health, 4* (1992), 3–18; Williamson, G. M., and Schulz, R. Physical Illness and Symptoms of Depression among Elderly Outpatients. *Psychology and Aging, 7* (1992), 343–351.
72. Goleman, D. Depression in the Old Can Be Deadly but the Symptoms Are Often Missed. *The New York Times,* September 6, 1995, p. C10; Simonsick, E., et al. Depressive Symptomatology and Hypertension: Associated Morbidity and Mortality in Older Adults. *Psychosomatic Medicine, 57* (1995), 427–435.
73. Goleman, D., September 6, 1995, p. C.10; Health-Related Quality of Life in Primary Care Patients with Mental Disorders: Results from the PRIME-MD 1000 Study. *Journal of the American Medical Association, 274* (1995), 1511–1517.
74. Goleman, 1995, p. C10.
75. Kaszniak, A. W., and Scogin, F. R. Assessment of Dementia and Depression in Older Adults. *The Clinical Psychologist, 48* (1995), 17–24.
76. Elderly's Suicide Rate Is Up 9% over 12 Years. *The New York Times,* January 12, 1996, p. A12.
77. Flint, A. J. Epidemiology and Comorbidity of Anxiety Disorders in the Elderly. *American Journal of Psychiatry, 151* (1994), 640–649.
78. Strollo, P. J., and Rogers, R. M. Obstructive Sleep Apnea. *New England Journal of Medicine, 334* (1996), 99–104.
79. Monane, M. Insomnia in the Elderly. Roundtable Conference: Low-Dose Benzodiazepine Therapy in the Treatment of Insomnia. *Journal of Clinical Psychiatry, 53* (1992) (6, Suppl). 23–28; Vitiello, M. V., et al. Sleep in Alzheimer's Disease and the Sundown Syndrome. *Neurology, 42* (1992) (7, Suppl 6), 83–94.
80. Morin et al., 1993; Murtagh, D. R. R., and

Greenwood, K. M. Identifying Effective Psychological Treatments for Insomnia: A Meta-Analysis. *Journal of Consulting and Clinical Psychology, 63* (1995), 79–89.

81. Binstock, R. H., Post, S. G., and Whitehouse, P. J. (Eds.), *Dementia and Aging: Ethics, Values, and Policy Choices.* Baltimore, MD: Johns Hopkins University Press, 1992, p. 2.; Loebel, J. P., Dager, S. R., and Kitchcell, M. A. Alzheimer's Disease. In D. L. Dunner (Ed.), *Current Psychiatric Therapy* (pp. 59–65). Philadelphia: W. B. Saunders, 1993.
82. Cooke, R. Memory's Foe: Progress Seen in Battle vs. Brain Killer. *New York Newsday,* November 8, 1994, p. A16; Kolata, G. Landmark in Alzheimer Research: Breeding Mice with the Disease. *The New York Times,* February 9, 1995, p. A20.
83. Office of Technology Assessment, 1990, p. 11 cited in Binstock et al., *Dementia and Aging,* p. 2; Evans, D. A., Prevalence of Alzheimer's Disease in a Community Population of Older Persons. *Journal of the American Medical Association, 262* (1989), 2551–2556.
84. Update on Alzheimer's Disease. Part I. *The Harvard Mental Health Letter, 11*(6), February 1995, 1–5.
85. Fisher, L. M. Athena Neurosciences Makes Itself Heard in Fight against Alzheimer's. *The New York Times,* February 15, 1995, p. D8.
86. Plomin, R., Owen, M. J., and McGuffin, P. The Genetic Basis of Complex Human Behaviors. *Science, 264* (1994), 1733–1739; Alzheimer's Gene Is Main Factor in Only 10% of Cases. *The New York Times,* February 17, 1997, p. A13; Bergem, A. L. M., et al. Heredity in Late-Onset Alzheimer Disease and Vascular Dementia. *Archives of General Psychiatry, 54* (1997), 264–270.
87. Weiner, M. F. What New Treatments for Alzheimer's Disease Are Being Explored? *The Harvard Mental Health Letter, 13*(1), July 1996, p. 8; The Race for Alzheimer's Treatments. *Harvard Health Letter, 22*(7), May 1997, pp. 1–3; National Institute on Aging. New Findings on Alzheimer's Disease Offer Clues on Causes, Diagnosis, and Treatments. National Institute on Aging, Bethseda, MD, March 11, 1997.
88. FDA Approves Second Drug for Alzheimer's. *The New York Times,* November 27, 1996, p. C8; The Race for Alzheimer's Treatments. *Harvard Health Letter, 22*(7), May 1997, pp. 1–3.
89. Sano, M., et al. Controlled Trial of Selegiline, Alpha-Tocopherol, or Both as Treatment for Alzheimer's Disease. *New England Journal of Medicine, 336* (1997), 1216–1222.
90. Estrogen May Help Alzheimer's Sufferers Keep Their Memory. *Cable News Network,* November 29, 1996.
91. Can Ordinary Pain Relievers Prevent Alzheimer's? *UC Berkeley Wellness Letter, 13*(9), June 1997, pp. 1–2.
92. Wolfe, S., et al. *Worst Pills, Best Pills: The Older Adult's Guide to Avoiding Drug-Induced Death or Illness.* Washington, DC: Public Citizen's Health Research Group, p. 7.
93. Robertson, N. The Intimate Enemy. *Modern Maturity,* February/March 1992, pp. 27–41.
94. Teague, M. L. *Health Promotion Programs: Achieving High-Level Wellness in the Later Years.* Indianapolis, IN: Benchmark Press, 1987, p. 138.
95. U.S. Department of Health and Human Services, *Healthy People 2000,* p. 286.
96. Kolata, G. New Era of Robust Elderly Belies the Fears of Scientists. *The New York Times,* February 27, 1996, pp. A1, C3.
97. Kolata, 1996.
98. Henslin, 1995, p. 367.
99. Pillemer, K., and Hudson, B. A Model Abuse Prevention Program for Nursing Assistants. *Gerontologist, 33*(1) (1993), 128–131.
100. Cohen, A. C., et al. Factors Determining the Decision to Institutionalize Dementing Individuals: A Prospective Study. *The Gerontologist, 22* (1993), 714–720.
101. Adapted from Kramer, J. B. Serving American Indian Elderly in Cities: An Invisible Minority. *Aging Magazine* (1992), pp. 363–364; Wray, L. A. Public Policy Implications of an Ethnically Diverse Population. *Journal of Cross-Cultural Gerontology, 6* (1991), 243–257.
102. Brody, J. E. More of the Elderly Seek the Benefits of Exercise. *The New York Times,* October 4, 1995, p. C11.
103. Kushi, L. H., et al. Physical Activity and Mortality in Postmenopausal Women *Journal of the American Medical Association, 277* (1997), 1287–1292.
104. How to Age Gracefully—Without Frailty or Falls. *Consumer Reports on Health, 8*(2), February 1996, p. 18.
105. Brody, J. E. Up in Age Often Means Down in Nutrition. *The New York Times,* May 11, 1994, C11; Has Growing Older Placed You At Nutritional Risk? *Tufts University Diet and Nutrition Letter, 10,* No. 3, May 1992.
106. Brody, 1994, p. C11.
107. LaGory, M., and Fitzpatrick, K. The Effects of Environmental Context on Elderly Depression. *Journal of Aging and Health, 4* (1992), 459–479.
108. Talan, J. Smart Moves for the Aging Mind. *New York Newsday,* February 7, 1995, p. B25.
109. Healthy Habits: Why Bother? *Consumer Reports on Health, 7*(5), May 1995, pp. 49–51.
110. Brody, J. E. Good Habits Outweigh Genes as Key to a Healthy Old Age. *The New York Times,* February 28, 1996, p. C9.

### CHAPTER 20

1. Kübler-Ross, E. *On Death and Dying.* New York: Macmillan, 1969, p. 8.
2. *Mayo Clinic Family Health Book,* PC 1.0 Version. Copyright 1994 by Mayo Foundation for Medical Education and Research and IVI Publishing, Inc.
3. Rathus, S. A., and Nevid, J. S. *Adjustment and Growth: The Challenges of Life.* (6th Ed.). Ft. Worth: Harcourt Brace, 1995, p. 447. Reprinted with permission.
4. Dickstein, L. S. Death Concern: Measurement and Correlates. *Psychological Reports, 30* (1972), p. 565. Reprinted with permission.
5. Sutherland, C. *Within the Light.* New York: Bantam Books, 1993, pp. ii, 46–47.
6. Sutherland, C. *Reborn in the Light.* New York: Bantam Books, 1995.
7. Many sources contain personal accounts of near-death experiences, including the following: Brinkley, D. *Saved by the Light.* New York: Villard Books, 1994; Eadie, B. J. *Embraced by the Light.* New York: Bantam Books, 1992; Moody, R. A. *Life after Death.* New York: Bantam Books, 1975; Ring, K. *Life at Death.* New York: Quill, 1980; Sutherland, C. *Within the Light.* New York: Bantam Books, 1993.
8. *Project on Death in America Mission Statement,* 1995; Wilkes, P. The Next Pro-Lifers. *The New York Times Magazine,* July 21, 1996, pp. 22–27, 42, 45, 50, 51.
9. Cunningham, R. *Hospice: A Special Kind of Caring.* Hospice Federation of Massachusetts, 1996.
10. Wilkes, 1996.
11. Cunningham, 1996.
12. Hospice Care Often Starts Too Late. *The New York Times,* July 24, 1996, p. C8.
13. *The Basics of Hospice.* National Hospice Organization, Arlington, VA, 1996.
14. A.M.A. Keeps Its Policy Against Aiding Suicide. *The New York Times,* June 26, 1996, p. C9.
15. Attitudes toward Euthanasia Sharply Divided, Survey Finds. *Reuters News Service,* June 28, 1996.
16. Battin, M. Assisted Suicide: Can We Learn Anything from Germany? *Hastings Center Report,* March–April 1992; pp. 44–51; Smith G., II. Reviving the Swan, Extending the Curse of Methuselah, or Adhering to the Kevorkian Ethic? *Cambridge Quarterly of Healthcare Ethics, 2* (1993), 49–56.
17. Battin, 1992.
18. Attitudes toward Euthanasia Sharply Divided, Survey Finds, 1996.
19. Foley, K. M. Medical Issues Related to Physician Assisted Suicide. Testimony to Judiciary Subcommittee on the Constitution, April 29, 1996.
20. Quill, T., Cassel, C., and Meier, D. Care of the Hopelessly Ill—Proposed Clinical Criteria for Physician Assisted Suicide. *New England Journal of Medicine, 327* (1992), 1380–1384.
21. Sacks, M., and Kemperman, I. Final Exit as a Manual for Suicide in Depressed Patients. *American Journal of Psychiatry* (Letters), 149 (1992), 842.
22. Cundiff, D. *The Alternative to Euthanasia. Lecture Outline.* LA County Medical Center, Internet posting, 1996.

23. Battin, M. P. *Ethical Issues in Suicide.* Upper Saddle River, NJ: Prentice Hall, 1996.
24. Depression: a Major Factor in Assisted Suicide, Study Shows. *The Boston Globe,* June 28, 1996.
25. Wilkes, 1996.
26. Humphry, D. *Why I Believe in Voluntary Euthanasia: The Case for Rational Suicide,* 1995.
27. Foley, 1996.
28. Sacks and Kemperman, 1992.
29. Wilkes, 1996.
30. Pace, E. Lester Cruzan Is Dead at 62; Fought to Let His Daughter Die. *The New York Times,* August 19, 1996, p. B12.
31. *Choices in Dying. Website,* 1996; Annas, G. J., and Grodin, M. A. There's No Right to Assisted Suicide. *The New York Times,* January 8, 1997, p. A 15.
32. Chambers, C., et al. Relationship of Advance Directives to Hospital Charges in a Medicare Population. *Archives of Internal Medicine, 154* (1994), 541–547; Logue, B. *Last Rights: Death Control and the Elderly in America.* Oxford: Maxwell Macmillan, 1993.
33. Miller, P. Death with Dignity and the Right to Die: Sometimes Doctors Have a Duty to Hasten Death. *Journal of Medical Ethics, 13* (1987), 81–85.
34. Logue, B. *Last Rights: Death Control and the Elderly in America.* Oxford: Maxwell Macmillan, 1993; Lewin, T. Suits Accuse Medical Community of Ignoring "Right to Die" Orders. *The New York Times,* June 2, 1996, pp. A1, A28.
35. Emanuel, L., and Emanuel, E. Decisions at the End of Life Guided by Communities of Patients. *Hastings Center Report,* September–October, 1993, pp. 6–14. Lambert, P., Gibson, J., and Nathanson, P. The Values History: An Innovation in Surrogate Medical Decision-Making. *Law, Medicine and Health Care, 18* (1990), 202–212; Lynne, J., and Teno, J. The Patient Self-Determination Act—The Need for Empirical Research on Formal Advance Directives. *Hastings Center Report,* January–February 1993, 20–24.
36. Lambert, et al., 1990; Lynne and Teno, 1993.
37. Emanuel and Emanuel, 1993.
38. Molloy, D., et al. The Canadian Experience with Advance Treatment Directives. *Humane Medicine, 9* (1993), 70–76.
39. Bureau of Elder and Adult Services, State of Main, 1996.
40. Seneff, M. G., Wagner, D. P, Wagner, R. P., Zimmerman, J. E., and Knaus, W. A. Hospital and 1-Year Survival of Patients Admitted to Intensive Care Units with Acute Exacerbation of Chronic Obstructive Pulmonary Disease. *Journal of the American Medical Association, 274* (1995), 1852–1857.
41. Emanuel and Emanuel, 1993.
42. Emanuel and Emanuel, 1993; Stelter, K, Elliott, B., and Bruno, C. Living Will Completion in Older Adults. *Archives of Internal Medicine, 152* (1992), 954–959.
43. Adapted from Manitoba Senior Citizens Handbook, *Coping with Death,* January 1995, and other sources.
44. Adapted from 20/20. ABC News, August 30, 1996; *The Funeral Help Program,* a service of the Alzheimer's Research Foundation, Inc., of Virginia, 1996, and other sources; Martin, D. Deathstyles of the Rich and Famous. *The New York Times,* January 12, 1997, Section 4, p. 2.
45. MI Risk Increases Sharply after Death of a Loved One. *Reuters News Services,* April 30, 1996.
46. Parkes, C. M, and Weiss, R. S. *Recovery from Bereavement.* New York: Basic Books, 1983.
47. Adapted from Sinclair, R. alt.support.grief, a Usenet Newsgroup, vol.1/issue 2, May 1995.
48. Source: Wilson, J. *How to Heal: Talking with a Bereavement Counselor,* 1996.
49. Adapted from the American Academy of Child and Adolescent Psychiatry (AACAP), *Children and Grief,* No. 8, AACAP Homepage, October 1992, updated May 1996.
50. Adapted from Shioda, E. *Japanese Customs: Network Sophia Part Two (All About Japan),* 1996. Reprinted with permission of Ms. Etsuko Shioda.
51. *Life Transitions: What's Right for Me?* American Association of Retired Persons, 1995.
52. Adapted from Living Will: How to Exercise Your Last Rights. *Consumer Reports on Health,* June 1996, p. 68, and other sources.
53. Adapted from Time Publishing Ventures, Inc., 1995.
54. Mayo Foundation for Medical Education and Research and IVI Publishing. *Mayo Clinic Family Health Book* (PC 1.0 Version), 1994.


## CHAPTER 21


1. Kristof, N. D. Japanese Say No to Crime: Tough Methods, at a Price. *The New York Times,* May 14, 1995, pp. A1, A8.
2. Cracking Down on Teen-Age Homicide. *The New York Times,* July 13, 1996, p. A18.
3. Homicide Trends Show Record Rate of Firearm-Related Deaths. Reuters News Service. June 7, 1996.
4. Butterfield, F. Major Crimes Fell in '95, Early Data by F.B.I. Indicate. *The New York Times,* May 6, 1996, pp. A1, B8; Butterfield, F. Serious Crime Decreased for Fifth Year in a Row. *The New York Times,* January 5, 1997, p. A10.
5. NBC Nightly News. December 4, 1996.
6. Koss, M. P., et al. *No Safe Haven: Male Violence against Women at Home, at Work, and in the Community.* Washington, DC. American Psychological Association, 1994; Holtzworth-Munroe, A. Marital Violence. *The Harvard Mental Health Letter, 12* (1995), pp. 4–6; O'Leary, K. D. Assessment and Treatment of Partner Abuse. *Clinician's Research Digest,* Supplemental Bulletin 12 (1995, July), pp. 1–2.
7. Koss et al., 1994.
8. Margolin, G., and Burman, B. Wife Abuse versus Marital Violence: Different Terminologies, Explanations, and Solutions. *Clinical Psychology Review, 13* (1993), 59–73; Magdol, L., et al. Gender Differences in Partner Violence in a Birth Cohort of 21-year-olds: Bridging the Gap between Clinical and Epidemiological Approaches. *Journal of Consulting and Clinical Psychology, 65* (1997), 68–78.
9. Margolin and Burman, 1993.
10. Murphy, C. M., Meyer, S. L., and O'Leary, K. D. Dependency Characteristics of Partner Assaultive Men. *Journal of Abnormal Psychology, 103* (1994), 729–735; Else, L., et al. Personality Characteristics of Men Who Physically Abuse Women. *Hospital and Community Psychiatry, 44* (1993), 54–58; Hotaling, G. T., and Sugarman, D. B. An Analysis of Risk Markers in Husband to Wife Violence: The Current State of Knowledge. *Violence and Victims, 1* (1986), 101–124; Murphy, C. M., and O'Farrell, T. J. Factors Associated with Marital Aggression in Male Alcoholics. *Journal of Family Psychology, 8* (1994), 321–335.
11. Astin, M. C. et al. Posttraumatic Stress Disorder and Childhood Abuse in Battered Women: Comparisons with Maritally Distressed Women. *Journal of Consulting and Clinical Psychology, 63* (1995), 308–312; Cascardi, M., and O'Leary, K. D. Depressive Symptomatology, Self-Esteem, and Self-Blame in Battered Women. *Journal of Family Violence, 7* (1992), 249–259; Cascardi, M., et al. Characteristics of Women Physically Abused by Their Spouses and Who Seek Treatment Regarding Marital Conflict. *Journal of Consulting and Clinical Psychology, 63* (1995), 616–623.; O'Leary, 1995.
12. DeAngelis, T. New Threat Associated with Child Abuse. *APA Monitor, 26* (4), April 1995a, pp. 1, 38; DeAngelis, T. Research Documents Trauma of Abuse. *APA Monitor,* April 1995b, *26*(4), p. 34.
13. Koss et al., 1994.
14. Gardiner, S. Out of Harm's Way: Intervention with Children in Shelters. Special Issue: Feminist Perspectives in Child and Youth Care Practices. *Journal of Child and Youth Care, 7* (1992), 41–48.
15. Daro, D., and Wiese, D. *Current Trends in Child Abuse Reporting and Fatalities: Ncpca's 1994 Annual Fifty State Survey.* Chicago, IL: National Committee to Prevent Child Abuse, 1995.
16. Cappelleri, J. C., Eckenrode, J., and Powers, J. L. The Epidemiology of Child Abuse: Findings from the Second National Incidence and Prevalence Study of Child Abuse and Neglect. *American Journal of Public Health, 83* (1993), 1622–1624.
17. Belsky, J. Etiology of Child Maltreatment: a Developmental-Ecological Analysis. *Psychological Bulletin, 114,* 1993, 413–434; Kaplan, S. J. Physical Abuse and Neglect. In M. Lewis (Ed.), *Child and Adolescent Psychiatry: A Comprehensive Textbook* (pp. 1010–1019).

Baltimore: Williams and Wilkins, 1991; Pogge, D. L. Risk Factors in Child Abuse and Neglect. *Journal of Social Distress and the Homeless, 1* (1992), 237–248; Cappelleri et al., 1993; DeAngelis, 1995a,b.

18. Belsky, 1993.
19. Milner, J. S. Social Information Processing and Physical Child Abuse. *Clinical Psychology Review, 13* (1993), 275–294; Pogge, 1992.
20. Pogge, 1992.
21. New York City Board of Education. *Child Abuse and Neglect Prevention Training Manual: Working Together to Make a Difference.* New York: Office of the Chief Executive for Instruction, Office of Student Progress, and Guidance Services Unit, 1984.
22. Daro and Wiese, 1995.
23. Adapted from Alpert, J. L., and Green, D. Child Abuse and Neglect: Perspectives on a National Emergency. *Journal of Social Distress and the Homeless, 1* (1992) pp. 228–229; reprinted with permission from Nevid, J. S., Rathus, S. A., and Greene, B. V. *Abnormal Psychology in a Changing World* (3rd ed). Upper Saddle River, NJ: Prentice-Hall, 1997, p. 542.
24. Cicchetti, D., and Olson, K. The Developmental Psychopathology of Child Maltreatment. In M. Lewis and S. M. Miller (Eds.), *Handbook of Developmental Psychopathology* (pp. 261–279), 1990. New York: Plenum; Conger, R. E. Child Abuse and Self-Esteem in Latency-Aged Children. *American Journal of Forensic Psychology, 10* (1992), 41–45; Stone, N. M. Parental Abuse as a Precursor to Childhood Onset Depression and Suicidality. *Child Psychiatry and Human Development, 24* (1993), 13–24, others.
25. Daro and Wiese, 1995.
26. Rorty, M., Yager, J., and Rossotto, E. Childhood Sexual, Physical and Psychological Abuse in Bulimia Nervosa. *American Journal of Psychiatry, 151* (1994), 1122–1126; Coons, P. M. Confirmation of Childhood Abuse in Child and Adolescent Cases of Multiple Personality Disorder and Dissociative Disorder Not Otherwise Specified. *Journal of Nervous and Mental Disease, 182* (1994), 461–464. Weaver, T. L., and Clum, G. A. Psychological Distress Associated with Interpersonal Violence: A Meta-Analysis. *Clinical Psychology Review, 15* (1995), 115–140; others.
27. Wolfe, D. A., Sas, L., and Wekerle, C. Factors Associated with the Development of Posttraumatic Stress Disorder among Child Victims of Sexual Abuse. *Child Abuse and Neglect, 18* (1994), 37–50; DeAngelis, 1995b.
28. U.S. Bureau of Justice Statistics. *National Crime Victimization Survey.* Washington, DC: U.S. Department of Justice, 1995.
29. U.S. Finds Heavy Toll of Rapes on Young. *The New York Times,* June 23, 1994, p. A12.
30. Koss, M. P., Gidycz, C. A., and Wisniewski, N. The Scope of Rape: Incidence and Prevalence of Sexual Aggression and Victimization in a National Sample of Higher Education Students. *Journal of Consulting and Clinical Psychology, 55* (1987), 162–170.
31. Calhoun, K. S., and Atkeson, B. M. *Treatment of Rape Victims: Facilitating Social Adjustment.* New York: Pergamon Press, 1991; Koss, M. P. Rape: Scope, Impact, Interventions, and Public Policy Responses. *American Psychologist, 48* (1993), 1062–1069.
32. Schafran, L. H. Rape Is Still Underreported. *The New York Times,* August 25, 1995, p. A19.
33. Adapted from Koss, M. P. Stranger and Acquaintance Rape: Are There Differences in the Victim's Experience? *Psychology of Women Quarterly, 12* (1988), 1–24.
34. Tang, C. S., et al. Sexual Aggression and Victimization in Dating Relationships among Chinese College Students. *Archives of Sexual Behavior, 18* (1995), 461–474.
35. Muehlenhard, C. L., and Linton, M. A. Date Rape and Sexual Aggression in Dating Situations: Incidence and Risk Factors. *Journal of Counseling Psychology, 34* (1987), 186–196.
36. Trenton State College. *Sexual Assault Victim Education and Support Unit (SAVES-U) Newsletter,* Spring 1991.
37. Celis, W. Students Trying to Draw Line between Sex and an Assault. *The New York Times,* January 2, 1991, pp. A1, B8.
38. Gibbs, N. When Is It Rape? *Time,* June 3, 1991, pp. 48–54.
39. Dixon, J. Feminist Reforms of Sexual Coercion. In E. Grauerholz and M. A. Koralewski (Eds.), *Sexual Coercion: A Sourcebook on Its Nature, Causes, and Prevention* (pp. 161–171). Lexington, MA: Lexington Books, 1991.
40. Sarrel, P., and Masters, W. Sexual Molestation of Men by Women. *Archives of Sexual Behavior, 11* (1982), 117–131.
41. Barbaree, H. E., and Marshall, W. L. The Role of Male Sexual Arousal in Rape: Six Models. *Journal of Consulting and Clinical Psychology, 59* (1991), 621–630; Hall, G. C. N., and Hirschman, R. Toward a Theory of Sexual Aggression: A Quadripartite Model. *Journal of Consulting and Clinical Psychology, 59* (1991), 662–669. Groth, A. N., and Birnbaum, H. J. *Men Who Rape: The Psychology of the Offender.* New York: Plenum Press, 1979; Groth, A. N. and Hobson, W. The Dynamics of Sexual Assault. In L. Schlesinger and E. Revitch (Eds.), *Sexual Dynamics of Antisocial Behavior.* Springfield, IL: Thomas, 1983.
42. Froth and Hobson, 1983, p. 165.
43. Dietz, P. E., Hazelwood, R. R., and Warren, J. The Sexually Sadistic Criminal and His Offenses. *Bulletin of the American Academy of Psychiatry and the Law, 18* (1990), 163–178.
44. Groth and Birnbuam, 1979.
45. For example, Lisak, D. Sexual Aggression, Masculinity, and Fathers. *Signs, 16* (1991), 238–262.
46. Malamuth, N. M. Rape Proclivity among Males. *Journal of Social Issues, 37* (1981), 138–157.
47. Muehlenhard, C. L., and Falcon, P. L. Men's Heterosocial Skill and Attitudes toward Women as Predictors of Verbal Sexual Coercion and Forceful Rape. *Sex Roles, 23* (1990), 241–259.
48. Levy, D. S. Why Johnny Might Grow Up Violent and Sexist. *Time,* September 16, 1991, pp. 16–19.
49. Eskenazi, G. The Male Athlete and Sexual Assault. *The New York Times,* June 3, 1990, pp. L1, L4.
50. Powell, E. *Talking Back to Sexual Pressure.* Minneapolis, MN: CompCare Publishers, 1991.
51. Burt, M. R. Cultural Myths and Supports for Rape. *Journal of Personality and Social Psychology, 38* (1980), 217–230.
52. Brady, E. C., et al. Date Rape: Expectations, Avoidance Strategies, and Attitudes toward Victims. *Journal of Social Psychology, 131* (1991), 427–429; Margolin, L., Miller, M., and Moran, P. B. When a Kiss Is Not Just a Kiss: Relating Violations on Consent in Kissing to Rape Myth Acceptance. *Sex Roles, 20* (1989), 231–243.
53. Malamuth, 1981; Malamuth, N. M. The Attraction to Sexual Aggression Scale: Part 2. *Journal of Sex Research, 26* (1989), 324–354.
54. Items taken from Burt, M. R. (1980). Cultural Myths and Support for Rape. *Journal of Personalty and Social Psychology, 38* (1980), 217–230. Copyright © 1980 by the American Psychological Association. Reprinted by permission.
55. Calhoun and Atkeson, 1991; McArthur, M. J. Reality Therapy with Rape Victims. *Archives of Psychiatric Nursing, 4* (1990), 360–365; Kimerling, R., and Calhoun, K. S. Somatic Symptoms, Social Support, and Treatment Seeking among Sexual Assault Victims. *Journal of Consulting and Clinical Psychology, 62* (1994), 333–340; Foa, E. B., Riggs, D. S., and Gershuny, B. S. Arousal, Numbing, and Intrusion: Symptom Structure of PTSD Following Assault. *American Journal of Psychiatry, 152* (1995), 115–120, others.
56. Waigandt, A., et al. The Impact of Sexual Assault on Physical Health Status. *Journal of Traumatic Stress, 3* (1990), 93–102.
57. Siegel, J. M., et al. Reactions to Sexual Assault: A Community Study. *Journal of Interpersonal Violence, 5* (1990), 229–246. Reprinted by permission of Sage Publications, Inc.
58. Boston Women's Health Book Collective, 1984; Rathus and Fichner-Rathus, 1994: Reprinted with permission from Rathus, S. A., Nevid, J. S., and Fichner-Rathus, L. *Human Sexuality in a World of Diversity* (3rd ed.). Boston: Allyn and Bacon, 1997.
59. Gidycz, C. A., and Koss, M. P. A Comparison of Group and Individual Sexual Assault Victims. *Psychology of Women Quarterly, 14* (1990) 325–342; Bart, P. B., and O'Brien, P. B. *Stopping Rape: Successful Survival Strategies.* Elmsford, NY: Pergamon Press, 1985, others.

60. Brody, J. E. How to Outwit a Rapist: Rehearse. *The New York Times,* April 28, 1992, p. C13.
61. Thompson, M. E. Self-Defense against Sexual Coercion: Theory, Research, and Practice. In E. Grauerholz and M. A. Koralewski (Eds.), *Sexual Coercion: A Sourcebook on its Nature, Causes, and Prevention* (pp. 111–121). Lexington, MA: Lexington Books, 1991.
62. Thompson, M. E., 1991.
63. Powell, 1991, p. 239.
64. Finkelhor, D., et al. Sexual Abuse in a National Survey of Adult Men and Women: Prevalence, Characteristics, and Risk Factors. *Child Abuse and Neglect 14* (1990), 19–28.
65. Knudsen, D. D. Child Sexual Coercion. In E. Grauerholz and M. A. Koralewski (Eds.), *Sexual Coercion: A Sourcebook on its Nature, Causes, and Prevention* (pp. 17–28). Lexington, MA: Lexington Books, 1991.
66. Knudsen, 1991.
67. Ames, M. A., and Houston, D. A. Legal, Social, and Biological Definitions of Pedophilia. *Archives of Sexual Behavior, 19* (1990), 333–342.
68. De Bellis, M. D., et al. Urinary Catecholamine Excretion in Sexually Abused Girls. *Journal of the American Academy of Child and Adolescent Psychiatry, 33* (1994), 320–327.
69. Finkelhor, 1990; DeAngelis, 1995b; Jackson, J., et al. Young Adult Women Who Report Childhood Intrafamilial Sexual Abuse: Subsequent Adjustment. *Archives of Sexual Behavior, 19* (1990), 211–221; Hoagwood, K. Blame and Adjustment among Women Sexually Abused as Children. *Women and Therapy, 9* (1990), 89–110; Rowan, A. B., et al. Posttraumatic Stress Disorder in a Clinical Sample of Adults Sexually Abused as Children. *Child Abuse and Neglect, 18* (1994), 51–61; Wolfe, D. A., Sas, L., and Wekerle, C. Factors Associated with the Development of Posttraumatic Stress Disorder among Child Victims of Sexual Abuse. *Child Abuse and Neglect, 18* (1994) 37–50; Beitchman, J. H., et al. A Review of the Long-Term Effects of Child Sexual Abuse. *Child Abuse and Neglect, 16* (1992), 101–118; others.
70. Weber, B. First Arrests in New York under Sex-Offender Law. *The New York Times,* July 6, 1996, p. B24.
71. Goleman, D. Abuse-Prevention Efforts Aid Children. *The New York Times,* October 6, 1993, p. C13.
72. Waterman, J., et al. Challenges for the Future. In K. MacFarlane, et al. (Eds.), *Sexual Abuse of Young Children: Evaluation and Treatment* (pp. 315–332). New York: Guilford, 1986.
73. Loftus, E. F., and Ketcham, K. *The Myth of Repressed Memory: False Memories and Allegations of Sexual Abuse.* New York: St. Martin's Press, 1994.
74. Goleman, D. Sexual Harassment: It's about Power, Not Lust. *The New York Times,* October 22, 1991, pp. C1, C12.
75. Powell, 1991, p. 110.
76. Fitzgerald, L. F. Sexual Harassment: Violence against Women in the Workplace. *American Psychologist, 48* (1993), 1070–1076.
77. Kolbert, E. Sexual Harassment at Work Is Pervasive, Survey Suggests. *The New York Times,* October 11, 1991, pp. A1, A17.
78. Castro, J. Sexual Harassment: A Guide. *Time,* January 20, 1992, p. 37.
79. McKinney, K., and Maroules, N. Sexual Harassment. In E. Grauerholz and M. A. Koralewski (Eds.), *Sexual Coercion: A Sourcebook on Its Nature, Causes and Prevention* (pp. 29–44). Lexington, MA: Lexington Books, 1991.
80. Gruber, J. E., and Bjorn, L. Women's Responses to Sexual Harassment: an Analysis of Sociocultural, Organizational, and Personal Resource Models. *Social Science Quarterly, 67* (1986), 814–826; Loy, P. H., and Stewart, L. P. The Extent and Effects of the Sexual Harassment of Working Women. *Sociological Focus, 17* (1984), 31–43.
81. Powell, 1991, p. 114.
82. Adapted from Nevid et al., 1997.

### CHAPTER 22

1. Setterberg, F., and Shavelson, L. *Toxic Nation: The Fight to Save our Communities from Chemical Contamination.* New York: John Wiley & Sons, 1993, p. 28.
2. Miller, E. W., and Miller, R. M. *Environmental Hazards: Toxic Waste and Hazardous Material.* Santa Barbara, CA: ABC-CLIO, Inc., 1991, p. 52.
3. Adapted from Upton, A., and Graber, E. *Staying Healthy in a Risky Environment: The New York University Family Center Medical Guide.* New York: Simon & Schuster, 1993, p. 42. Used with permission.
4. Lehr, Jay H. A New Measure of Risk. In J. H. Lehr (Ed.), *Rational Readings on Environmental Concern.* New York: Van Nostrand Reinhold, 1992, p. 685.
5. *Mayo Clinic Family Health Book: Interactive Edition,* Mayo Clinic, 1994.
6. Harte, J., et al. *Toxics A to Z: A Guide to Everyday Pollution Hazards.* Berkeley, CA: University of California Press, 1991, p. 51.
7. Grady, D. Unexpected Dangers Found in Low Levels of Lead. *The New York Times,* April 17, 1996, p. C9; Hu, H., et al. The Relationship of Bone and Blood Level to Hypertension: The Normative Aging Study. *Journal of the American Medical Association, 275* (1996), 1171–1176; Kim, R., et al. A Longitudinal Study of Low-Level Lead Exposure and Impairment of Renal Function: The Normative Aging Study. *Journal of the American Medical Association, 275* (1996), 1177–1181.
8. Needleman, H. L., et al. Bone Lead Levels and Delinquent Behavior. *Journal of the American Medical Association, 275* (1996), 363–370.
9. Wald, M. L. High Levels of Lead Found in Water Serving 30 Million. *The New York Times,* May 12, 1993, p. A12.
10. National Research Council, *Measuring Lead Exposure in Infants, Children, and Other Sensitive Populations,* NRC Publications, 1993; Braithwaite, R. L., and Taylor, S. E. E. *Health Issues in the Black Community.* San Francisco: Jossey-Bass, 1992, 178–191; EPA. *Fact Sheet on Lead,* June 1993; Wald, 1993; The News on Lead. *UC Berkeley Wellness Letter,* November 1993, pp. 4–5; Brody, J. Lead Is Public Enemy No. 1 in American Children, *The New York Times,* May 4, 1993, p. C3.
11. Urbinato, D. Monitoring Lead in Drinking Water. *EPA Journal,* Summer 1994, p. 19; Schwartz, J., and Levin, R. Lead: Example of the Job Ahead. *EPA Journal,* March/April 1992, pp. 42–44; Brody D. J., et al. Blood Lead Levels in the U.S. Population. *Journal of the American Medical Association, 272* (1994), 277–91; *Blood Lead Levels in the U.S. Population,* U.S. Department of Health & Human Services press release, July 26, 1994; and other sources.
12. NBC Television Network. *Today,* March 23, 1996.
13. Dashefsky, H. S. *Environmental Literacy: Everything You Need to Know about Saving Our Planet.* New York: Random House, 1993, p. 102.
14. Moberg, D. Sunset for Chlorine? *E Magazine,* July/August 1993, pp. 26–31.
15. Sunset for Chlorine. *UC Berkeley Wellness Letter, 11,* September 1995, p. 5.
16. Krieger, N., et al. Breast Cancer and Serum Organochlorines: A Prospective Study among White, Black, and Asian Women. *Journal of the National Cancer Institute,* April 20, 1994; Wolff, M. S., et al. Blood Levels of Organochlorine Residues and Risk of Breast Cancer. *Journal of the National Cancer Institute,* April 21, 1993.
17. Lane, E. Dioxin May Pose a Wider Threat. *New York Newsday,* September 13, 1994, p. A19.
18. Brody, J. E. Study Finds Lasting Damage from Prenatal PCB Exposure. *The New York Times,* July 12, 1996, p. A14.
19. James, R. C. et al. Polychlorinated Biphenyl Exposure and Human Disease. *Journal of Occupational Medicine 35*(2) (1993), 136–148; EPA Office of Toxic Substances, *Hazardous Substance Fact Sheet on PCBs,* July 1988.
20. Campos-Outcalt, D. Trichloroethylene: Environmental and Occupational Exposure. *American Family Physician, 46* (1992), 495–500.
21. Schneider, K. Pesticide Plan Could Uproot U.S. Farming. *The New York Times,* October 10, 1993, E6.
22. Harte et al., 1991, p. 113.

23. Parents Are Warned on Use of Lice Drug. *The New York Times,* April 5, 1996, p. A19.
24. Whitemore, R. W., et al. Non-occupational Exposures to Pesticides for Residents of Two U.S. cities. *Archives of Environmental Contamination & Toxicology,* 26 (1994), 47–59.
25. Grossman J. What's Hiding under the Sink: Dangers of Household Pesticides. *Environmental Health Perspectives, 103,* (6) (1995), 550–554.
26. Leiss, J. K., and Savitz, D. A. Home Pesticide Use and Childhood Cancer: A Case-Control Study. *American Journal of Public Health, 85* (1995), 249–252.
27. Lang L. Are Pesticides a Problem? *Environmental Health Perspectives, 101, No. 7* (1993), 578–583, and other sources.
28. *Mayo Clinic Family Health Book: Interactive Edition,* 1994.
29. Specter, M. 10 Years Later, through Fear, Chernobyl Still Kills in Belarus. *The New York Times,* March 31, 1996, pp. A1, A6.
30. Henshaw, D. L., et al. Radon as a Causative Factor in Induction of Myeloid Leukemia and Other Cancers. *Lancet, 1* (1990) 1008–1012.
31. EPA. *Technical Support Document of the 1992 Citizen's Guide to Radon.* EPA Doc. No. 400-R-92-011. Washington, DC: Environmental Protection Agency, 1992; Lubin, J. H., et al. Lung Cancer in Radon-Exposed Miners and Estimation of Risk from Indoor Exposure. *Journal of the National Cancer Institute, 87* (1995), 817–827; Warner, K. E., Courant, P. N, and Mendez, D. Effects of Residential Mobility on Individual Versus Population Risk of Radon-Related Lung Cancer. *Environmental Health Perspectives, 103, No. 12* (1995), 1144–1149.
32. Radon: Worth Learning About. *Consumer Reports,* July 1995, p. 464.
33. Department of Health, Education and Welfare. *X-rays: Get the Picture on Protection.* HEW Pub. No. (FDA) 79-8088; Wagner, H. N, and Ketchum. L. *Living with Radiation: The Risk, the Promise.* Baltimore: Johns Hopkins University Press, 1989, p. 102.
34. Taubes, G. Electrical Emissions: Dangerous or Not? *The New York Times,* June 22, 1993, pp. C1, C8.
35. Leary, W. E. Panel Sees No Proof of Health Hazards from Power Lines. *The New York Times,* November 1, 1996, pp. A1, A29.
36. Linet, M.S., et al. Residential Exposure to Magnetic Fields and Acute Lymphoblastic Leukemia in Children. *New England Journal of Medicine, 337* (1997), 1–7.
37. Special Risks in Daily Life. *Consumer Reports,* May 1994, p. 359, and other sources.
38. Redelmeier, D. A., and Tibshirani, R. J. Association between Cellular-Telephone Calls and Motor Vehicle Collisions. *New England Journal of Medicine, 336* (1997), 453–458; also as reported by Associated Press, February 13, 1997.
39. For example, Bergqvist, U., Wolgast, E., and Nilsson, B. The Influence of VDT Work on Musculoskeletal Disorders. *Ergonomics, 38* (1995), 754–762.
40. Parazzini, F., et al. Video Display Terminal Use During Pregnancy and Reproductive Outcome—A Meta-Analysis. *Journal of Epidemiology and Community Health, 47* (1993), 265–268.
41. Tuckwell, H. C., and Koziol, J. A. World and Regional Populations. *Biosystems, 31* (1993), 59–63; Crossette, B. World Is Less Crowded than Expected, the U.N. Reports. *The New York Times,* November 17, 1996, p. A3.
42. Raven, P. H., and Johnson, G. B. *Biology* (3rd ed.). St. Louis, MO: Mosby Year Book, 1992, p. 535.
43. Raven and Johnson, 1992, p. 535.
44. Kennedy, P. *Preparing for the Twenty-First Century.* New York: Random House, 1993, p. 25.
45. Kennedy, p. 97.
46. Crossette, 1996; Segal, S. J. Trends in Population and Contraception. *Annals of Medicine, 25* (1993), 51–56.
47. Hilchey, T. Government Survey Finds Decline in a Building Block of Acid Rain. *The New York Times,* September 7, 1993, p. C4.
48. Hilts, P. J. Fine Particles in Air Cause Many Deaths, Study Suggests. *The New York Times,* May 9, 1996, p. B10.
49. Pope, C. A., 3rd. Particulate Air Pollution as a Predictor of Mortality in a Prospective Study of U.S. Adults. *American Journal of Respiratory and CriticalCare Medicine, 151* (1995), 669–674.
50. Brunekreef, B., Dockery, D. W., and Krzyzanowski, M. Epidemiologic Studies on Short-Term Effects of Low Levels of Major Ambient Air Pollution Components. *Environmental Health Perspectives, 103 Suppl 2* (1995), 3–13.
51. Jakab G. J., et al. The Effects of Ozone on Immune Function. *Environmental Health Perspectives, 103 Suppl. 2* (1995), 77–89; Breslin, K. The Impact of Ozone. *Environmental Health Perspectives, 103* (7–8) (1995), 660–664.
52. Study Cites Smog Impact on Youths. *The New York Times,* August 15, 1995, p. C12.
53. Stevens, W. K. 100 Nations Move to Save Ozone Shield. *The New York Times,* December 10, 1995, p. A20.
54. Upton and Graber, 1993, p. 555.
55. *Consumer Reports 1996 Buying Guide.* Yonkers, NY: Consumers Union, 1995, p. 139; Safe at Home. *Consumer Reports,* July 1995, p. 459.
56. Sunset for Chlorine? *UC Berkeley Wellness Letter, 11,* September 1995, p. 5.
57. Sunset for Chlorine?, 1995.
58. Is Our Water Safety Going Down the Drain? *UC Berkeley Wellness Letter, 11,* September 1995, p. 1.
59. Adler, R. The Clean Water Act: Has It Worked? *EPA Journal,* Summer 1994, pp. 10–14; The Safe Drinking Water Act in Retrospect. *EPA Journal,* Summer 1994, p. 15.
60. The Safe Drinking Water Act in Retrospect, 1994, p. 15.
61. Sharp, D. A Clean Drink of Water. *Health,* September 1995, p. 89.
62. Regecova V., and Kellerova, E. Effects of Urban Noise Pollution on Blood Pressure and Heart Rate in Preschool Children. *Journal of Hypertension, 13* (1995), 405–412.
63. Piver, W. T. Global Atmospheric Changes. *Environmental Health Perspectives, 96* (1991), 131–137.
64. Stevens, W. K. Global Warming Experts Call Human Role Likely. *The New York Times,* September 10, 1995, p. A1.; Harte, J., and Lashof, D. Bad Weather? Just Wait. *The New York Times,* January 10, 1996, p. A15.
65. Stevens, W. K. Blame Global Warming for the Blizzard. *The New York Times,* January 14, 1996, p. E4.
66. Keeping Your Cool. *UC Berkeley Wellness Letter,* August 1996, p. 5.
67. Consequences of Climate Change. *Environmental Health Perspectives, 103* (12) (1995), p. 1085.
68. Begley, S. He's Not Full of Hot Air. *Newsweek,* January 22, 1996, pp. 24–29.
69. Environmental Protection Agency (EPA), *Characterization of Municipal Solid Waste in the United States: 1992 Update Executive Summary,* EPA Pub. No. 530–S–92–019, July 1992, p. ES–3; EPA, *Let's Reduce and Recycle: Curriculum for Solid Waste Awareness,* EPA Pub. No. 530–SW–90005, August, 1990.
70. Packaging in the '90s. *Garbage,* December/January 1993, p. 27.
71. Environmental Protection Agency. *The Superfund Program: Ten Years of Progress,* EPA Pub. No. 540/8–91/003, June 1991; EPA News Release, September 1993.
72. Commission for Racial Justice, United Church of Christ. *Toxic Wastes and Race in the United States: A National Report on the Racial and Socioeconomic Characteristics of Communities with Hazardous Waste Sites.* New York: United Church of Christ, 1987. Mohai, P., and Bryant, B. Race, Poverty, and the Environment. *EPA Journal,* March/April 1992, pp. 6–8; Wernette, D. R., and Nieves, L. A. Breathing Polluted Air: Minorities Are Disproportionately Exposed. *EPA Journal,* March/April 1992, pp. 16–17; Children at Risk from Ozone Air Pollution—United States, 1991–1993. *MMWR, 44* (1995, April 28), 309–312.
73. A Place at the Table: A Sierra Roundtable of Race, Justice, and the Environment. *Sierra,* May/June, 1993, p. 51.
74. Wernette and Nieves, 1992, p. 17.


### CHAPTER 23


1. Pear, R. Health Costs Are Growing More Slowly, Report Says. *The New York Times,* May 18, 1996, p. A13.
2. National Leadership Coalition for Health Care Reform, 1991. *A Comprehensive*

*Reform Plan for the Health Care System,* p. 2; Vincenzino, J. V. Health Care Costs: Market Forces and Reform. *Statistical Bulletin of the Metropolitan Insurance Company, 76 (January–March 1995), 29–35.*
3. Naslund, M. J. The Economics of Health Care Reform. *Urology, 44* (1994), 299–304.
4. National Center for Health Statistics (NCHS). *Monitoring Health Care in America: Quarterly Fact Sheet,* Centers for Disease Control and Prevention, September 1995.
5. Budetti, P. P. Achieving a Uniform Federal Primary Care Policy. *Journal of the American Medical Association, 269* (1993), 496–501; Colwill, J. M. Where Have All the Primary Care Applicants Gone? *New England Journal of Medicine, 326* (1992), 387–393; Petersdorf, R. G. *Statement of the Association of American Medical Colleges to the Physician Payment Review Commission.* Washington, DC: Association of American Medical Colleges, 1991.
6. Demand for Generalists up as Specialists Lose Ground. *The New York Times,* September 4, 1996, p. C9.
7. Two Magazines Rate Nursing as Top Career. *American Nurse, 22* (9), (1990), p. 3.
8. Workplace Issues. *American Nurse, 23*(2) (1991), p. 13.
9. Rabinovitz, J. Optometrists Clash with Eye Surgeons over Laser Process. *The New York Times,* April 8, 1996, pp. A1, B6.
10. Eisenberg, D. M., et al. Unconventional Medicine in the United States: Prevalence, Costs, and Patterns of Use. *New England Journal of Medicine, 328* (1993), 246–252.
11. Burstein, P. Medicine Man: An Eclectic Doctor Puts Alternative Therapies to the Test. *American Health,* October 1993, pp. 30–32.
12. Griffin, K. Alternative Care: Finally Some Coverage. *Health,* October 1995, p. 106.
13. Griffin, K. Hands on Healing. *Health,* October 1995, pp. 59–63.
14. Podolsky, D. No to an Ancient Art. *U.S. News and World Report,* May 13, 1996, pp. 78–80.
15. Putting Chiropractic to the Test. Harvard Health Letter, 21 (June 1996), p. 8; White, A. A. Assendelft, W. J. J., et al. The Relationship between Methodological Quality and Conclusions in Reviews of Spinal Manipulation. *Journal of the American Medical Association, 274* (1995), 1942–1948.
16. Purdum, T. S. Clinton Signs Bill to Give Portability in Insurance. *The New York Times,* August 22, 1996, p. B 12.
17. Toner, R. Harry and Louise Were Right, Sort Of. *The New York Times,* November 24, 1996, sec. 4, pp. 1, 3; Meyer, M. Bound and Gagged. *Newsweek,* March 17, 1997, p. 45.
18. Miller, R. H., and Luft, H. S. Managed Care Plans: Characteristics, Growth, and Premium Performance. *Annual Review of Public Health, 15* (1994a), 437–459.
19. Gable, J., et al. The Health Insurance Picture in 1993: Some Rare Good News. *Health Affairs,* Spring (1), 1994, pp. 327–336.
20. Eaton, L. Aetna to Buy U.S. Healthcare in Big Move to Managed Care. *The New York Times,* April 2, 1996, pp. A1, D8.
21. Freudenheim, M. Managed Care Empires in the Making. *The New York Times,* April 2, 1996, pp. D1, D8; NBC Nightly News, December 11, 1996.
22. Pear, R. Doctors May Get Leeway to Rival Large Companies. *The New York Times,* April 8, 1996, pp. A1, B9.
23. Pear, R. Elderly and Poor Do Worse under H.M.O. Plans' Care. *The New York Times,* October 2, 1996, p. A10; Parrish, M. It Could Happen to You. *Health,* May/June 1996, pp. 115–123.
24. Pear, R. H.M.O.'s Refusing Emergency Claims, Hospitals Assert. *The New York Times,* July 9, 1995, pp. A1, A22; Gable et al., 1994
25. Miller and Luft, 1994a, pp. 1512–1513.
26. Randall V. R. Impact of Managed Care Organizations on Ethnic Americans and Underserved Populations. *Journal of Health Care for the Poor and Underserved, 5* (1994), 224–236; 237–9; Ethical Issues in Managed Care: Council on Ethical and Judicial Affairs, American Medical Association. *Journal of the American Medical Association, 273* (1995), 330–335.
27. Ethical Issues in Managed Care, 1995.
28. Freudenheim, M. H.M.O.'s Cope with a Backlash on Cost Cutting. *The New York Times,* May 19, 1996, pp. A1, A22.
29. Pear, R. U.S. Limits H.M.O.'s in Linking Bonuses to Cost Controls. *The New York Times,* December 21, 1996, pp. A1, A24.
30. Miller and Luft, 1994a, pp. 451–542; Miller, R. H., and Luft, H. S. Managed Care Plan Performance since 1980. *Journal of the American Medical Association, 271* (1994b), 1512–1519.
31. The New HMOs: Get Ready. *Health,* May/June 1996, p. 117.
32. Miller and Luft, 1994a, pp. 454–455; Pear, R. Health Costs Are Growing More Slowly, Report Says. *The New York Times,* May 18, 1996, p. A13.
33. Managed Competition: An Analysis of Consumer Concerns. *International Journal of Health Services, 24* (1994), 11–24.
34. Davis, K. et al. Health Insurance: The Size and Shape of the Problem. *Inquiry, 32* (1995, Summer), 196–203.
35. Ethical Issues in Managed Care: Council on Ethical and Judicial Affairs, American Medical Association. *Journal of the American Medical Association, 273* (1995), 330–335.
36. Blendon, R. J., et al. Americans Compare Managed Care, Medicare, and Fee for Service. *Journal of American Health Policy, 4* (1994), 42–47; Hurley, R. E., and Freund, D. A. *Managed Care in Medicaid: Lessons for Policy and Program Design.* Ann Arbor, MI: Health Administration Press, 1993; Rodwin, M. A. Conflicts in Managed Care. *New England Journal of Medicine, 332* (1995), 604–607; Rodwin, M. A. *Medicine, Money and Morals: Physicians' Conflicts of Interest.* New York: Oxford University Press, 1993; Emanuel, E. J., and Dubler, N. N. Preserving the Physician-Patient Relationship in the Era of Managed Care. *Journal of the American Medical Association, 273* (1995), 323–329; Health Maintenance Organizations. Health ResponseAbility Systems, Inc. Doc. lhf00161.
37. Gottlieb, M. Picking a Health Plan: A Shot in the Dark. *The New York Times,* January 14, 1996, pp. 1, 9, and other sources.
38. Gottlieb, 1996.
39. Gottlieb, 1996.
40. Iglehart, J. K. Health Policy Report: The American Health Care System, Medicare. *New England Journal of Medicine, 327* (1992), 1467–1472.
41. Friedman, S. HMOs Get in on the Medicare Act. *Newsday,* March 9, 1996, p. B9.
42. Iglehart, J. K. Health Policy Report: Medicaid and Managed Care. *New England Journal of Medicine, 332* (1995), 1727–1731.
43. *Medicaid—Summary, by State and Other Areas: 1992 and 1993.* U.S. Health Care Financing Administration, unpublished data.
44. Pear, R. Elderly and Poor Do Worse under H.M.O. Plans' Care. *The New York Times,* October 2, 1996, p. A10.
45. Himmelstein, D. U., and Woolhandler, S. Care Denied: US Residents Who Are Unable to Obtain Needed Medical Services. *American Journal of Public Health, 85* (1995), 341–344.
46. Griffin, K. 8 Medical Tests You Shouldn't Ignore. *Health,* May/June 1996, pp. 107–112.
47. Adapted from Griffin, 1996, and other sources.
48. Rasell, V. E., Bernstein, J., and Tang, K. *The Impact of Health Care Financing on Family Budgets.* Economic Policy Institute Briefing Paper. Washington, DC: Economic Policy Institute, 1993.
49. Himmelstein and Woolhandler, 1995.
50. Short, P. F., Cornelius, L. J., and Goldstone, D. E. Health Insurance of Minorities in the United States. *Journal of Health Care for the Poor and Underserved, 1* (1990, Summer), pp. 9–24; Leary, W. E. Health Care Lagging among Blacks and the Poor. *The New York Times,* September 12, 1996, p. A18.
51. Randall, V. R. Impact of Managed Care Organizations on Ethnic Americans and Underserved Populations. *Journal of Health Care for the Poor and Underserved, 5* (1994), 224–236; 237–9.
52. Schlosberg, S. The Doctor Will Hear You Now. *Health,* November/December 1995, pp. 76–80; Communication Breakdown: Who's to Blame? *Health,* November/December 1995, p. 79.
53. Cebrun, A. J. Consumer Responsibility in the HMO Environment. *Journal of Health Care for the Poor and Underserved, 5* (1994), 178–181, 182–184, and other sources.
54. Pear, 1995.

# Illustration Credits

## FIGURE CREDITS

**CHAPTER 1** **Fig. 1.2** Meeting the Nation's Health Goals for the Year 2000. *The New York Times,* April 12, 1995, p. C13. Copyright © 1995 by The New York Times Co. Reprinted by permission.

**CHAPTER 3** **p. 74 Excerpt** From *Abnormal Psychology in a Changing World: 3/e* by Nevid/Rathus/Greene, © 1997. Reprinted by permission of Prentice-Hall, Inc., Upper Saddle River, NJ.

**CHAPTER 4** **p. 83 HealthCheck** From *Abnormal Psychology in a Changing World: 3/e* by Nevid/Rathus/Greene. Copyright © 1997. Reprinted by permission of Prentice-Hall, Inc., Upper Saddle River, NJ. **Fig. 4.1** From *Schizophrenia Genesis* by Gottesman © 1991 by Irving I. Gottesman. Used with permission of W.H. Freeman and Company. **Table 4.3** Nevid, J.S., Rathus, S.A., and Greene, B. *Abnormal Psychology in a Changing World (3rd ed.),* Upper Saddle River, NJ: Prentice-Hall Inc., 1997, pp. 300–301. **Table 4.4** Nevid, J.S., Rathus, S.A., and Greene, B. *Abnormal Psychology in a Changing World (3rd ed.),* Upper Saddle River, NJ: Prentice-Hall, Inc., 1997, p. 140.

**CHAPTER 6** **Fig. 6.3** Reprinted with permission from the University of California at Berkeley Wellness Letter, © Health Letter Associates, 1996.

**CHAPTER 7** **Table 7.1** Physical Activity and Public Health. *The Journal of the American Medical Association, 273* (5), February 1, 1995, p. 404. **Fig. 7.4** Adapted from P.J. Tyne and Mitchell, *Total Stretching.* Chicago: Contemporary Books, Inc. 1983; and Warming Up to Exercise, *The New York Times,* October 16, 1996. Copyright © 1996 by The New York Times Co. Reprinted by permission.

**CHAPTER 10** **Table 10.1** Hatcher, R.A. et al. *Contraceptive Technology 1992–1994 (16th rev. ed.).* New York: Irvington Publishers, 1994. Reprinted by permission; and Reinisch (1990). Copyright © 1990 by The Kinsey Institute for Research in Sex, Gender, and Reproduction. From the *Kinsey Institute New Report on Sex* by June Reinisch, Ph.D. with Ruth Beasley, M.L.S. Reprinted by permission of St. Martin's Press Incorporated.

**CHAPTER 11** **Fig. 11.3** From the *World of Children* by Claire Etaugh and Spencer A. Rathus, copyright © 1994 by Holt, Rinehart and Winston, reproduced by permission of the publisher.

**CHAPTER 12** **Fig. 12.1** Reprinted from *Live Longer Live Better,* copyright © 1995 The Reader's Digest Association, Inc. Used by permission of The Reader's Digest Association, Inc.

**CHAPTER 13** **Fig. 13.3** From *Introduction to Psychology, Eleventh Edition* by Rita L. Atkinson, Richard C. Atkinson, Edward E. Smith, and Daryl J. Bem, copyright © 1993 by Harcourt Brace & Company, reprinted by permission of the publisher. **Fig. 13.5** Source: USDHHS in Grant, B.F., Dufour, M.C., and Harford, T.C., (1988). *Seminars in Liver Disease, 8* (1), p. 16, Thieme Medical Publishers. **Fig. 13.6** From *Abnormal Psychology in a Changing World: 3/e* by Nevid/Rathus/Greene, p. 350, © 1997. Reprinted by permission of Prentice-Hall, Upper Saddle River, NJ.

**CHAPTER 14** **Table 14.1** Adapted from *Adjustment and Growth: The Challenges of Life, Sixth Edition* by Spencer A. Rathus and Jeffrey S. Nevid, copyright © 1995 by Holt, Rinehart and Winston, reprinted by permission of the publisher.

**CHAPTER 17** **Fig. 17.5** USDHHS Public Health Service. Health: United States 1990. DHHS Pub. No (PHS) 91-1232, 1991. **Fig. 17.7** Figure adapted from "Tools for Unclogging Arteries" (© 1996 Harriet Greenfield) in *Harvard Health Letter,* January 1996, p. 4. **Fig 17.8** Centers for Disease Control and Prevention. Protective Effect of Physical Activity on Coronary Heart Diseases. *Morbidity and Mortality Weekly Report,* 36/326 (1987), 426–430. **Fig. 17.9** Reprinted by permission of Prevention Magazine. Copyright © 1997 Rodale Press, Inc. All rights reserved. For subscription information, call 1-800-666-2503.

**CHAPTER 18** **Figs. 18.2 and 18.3** *Cancer Facts & Figures—1996,* The American Cancer Society, Inc. Reprinted by permission of the American Cancer Society, Inc. **Fig. 18.4** Breast Health Program of New York, Leslie Strong, M.D. in *Self,* October 1996, p. 193.

**CHAPTER 19** **Fig. 19.3** Source: World Health Organization O.E.C.D. Census Bureau. *The New York Times,* September 22, 1996, Sec. 4, p. 5. Copyright © 1996 by The New York Times Co. Reprinted by permission. **Fig. 19.8** Source: National Center for Health Statistics. *Monthly Vital Statistics Report. Vol. 39,* No. 7, Supplement (November 18, 1990). **Fig. 19.9** Adapted from Selkoe, Dennis J. Aging Brain, Aging Mind. *Scientific American* (September 1992), p. 138. Copyright © 1992 by Scientific American, Inc. All rights reserved.

**CHAPTER 20** **Fig. 20.1** Copyright © 1996 Choice in Dying, Inc. Reprinted by permission of Choice in Dying, 200 Varick St., New York, NY 10014 (212) 366-5540.

**CHAPTER 22** **Table 22.2** Reprinted with the permission of Simon & Schuster from *Staying Healthy in a Risky Environment—The New York University Medical Center Family Guide* by Arthur C. Upton, M.D., Medical Editor and Eden Graber, M.S., Editor. Copyright ©1993 by Graber Productions, Inc. **Fig. 22.4** Source: United Nations. Crossette, B. The world is less crowded than expected, the U.N. reports. *The New York Times,* November 17, 1996, p. A3. Copyright © 1996 The New York Times Co. Reprinted by permission.

**CHAPTER 23** **Fig. 23.3** Randall, V.R. Impact of Managed Care Organizations on Ethnic Americans and Underserved Populations. *J. of Health Care for the Poor and Underserved. 1994; 5* (3): 224–236. **Fig. 23.5** Himmelstein, D.U. and Woolhandler, S. Care Denied: U.S. Residents Who Are Unable to Obtain Needed Medical Services. *American Journal of Public Health, 85* (3) (March 1995), 343. Copyright © 1995 the American Public Health Association.

**APPENDIX C** **High-Fiber Foods** Adapted from the American Cancer Society publication,

*Eating Smart* (No. 87-250M-Rev. 11/95- No. 2042).

**APPENDIX D** **Figures** From *First Aid Fast,* pp. 25, 31. Courtesy of the American Red Cross. All rights reserved in all countries.

## PHOTO CREDITS

**COVER:** Rod Walker/Workbook/Co-op Stock

**CHAPTER 1** **p. 2** © Lois Greenfield; **p. 4** Tony Freeman/Photo Edit; **p. 5** Sotographs/Gamma Liaison; **p. 8** Nathan Benn/Stock, Boston; **p. 10** Tom McCarthy/The Picture Cube; **p. 15** Richard Pasley/Stock, Boston; **p. 16** Ken Fisher/Tony Stone Images; **p. 18** B. Bachman/The Image Works; **p. 21** Treë; **p. 22** National Institute of Health; **p. 24** Richard Hutchings/Photo Edit.

**CHAPTER 2** **p. 30** © Lois Greenfield; **p. 32** Peter Southwick; **p. 34** Bob Daemmrich/The Image Works; **p. 35** Joe Sohm/Stock, Boston; **p. 37** Shackman/Monkmeyer; **p. 38** David Madison/Tony Stone Images; **p. 39** Michael Newman/Photo Edit; **p. 40** Donna Day/Tony Stone Images; **p. 42** Jose Pelaez/The Stock Market; **p. 44** CNRI/SPL/Science Source/Photo Researchers; **p. 47** Ronnie Kaufman/The Stock Market; **p. 49** Don Mason/The Stock Market.

**CHAPTER 3** **p. 52** © Lois Greenfield; **p. 54** Aaron Strong/Gamma Liaison; **p. 55** Robert Brenner/Photo Edit; **p. 56** Superstock; **p. 59** Kolvoord; **p. 60** Hershkowitz/Monkmeyer; **p. 62** Joel Gordon; **p. 67** Phylus Picardi/Stock, Boston; **p. 68** Steve Gooch/The Daily Oklahoman/Saba; **p. 72** William Johnson/Stock, Boston; **p. 73** PBJ Pictures/Gamma Liaison; **p. 75** Zigy Kaluzny/Tony Stone Images.

**CHAPTER 4** **p. 78** © Lois Greenfield; **p. 82** Bonnie Kamin/Offshoot Stock; **p. 84** Treë; **p. 88** NIH/Science Source/Photo Researchers; **p. 89** Collins/Monkmeyer; **p. 92** Joel Gordon; **p. 95** (top) Michael A. Donato/The Image Bank; (bottom) Richard Howard/Offshoot Stock; **p. 96** David Young-Wolff/Photo Edit; **p. 97** Paul S. Howell/Gamma Liaison.

**CHAPTER 5** **p. 106 and 107** Treë; **p. 108** Felicia Martinez/Photo Edit; **p. 109 & p. 111** Treë; **p. 112** Ken Mengay/Gamma Liaison; **p. 117** Tony Maxwell/The Picture Cube; **p. 122** Charles Thatcher/Tony Stone Images; **p. 126** Paul S. Howell/Gamma Liaison; **p. 129 & p. 131** Treë; **p. 135** Michael Newman/Photo Edit; **p. 136** Don Mason/The Stock Market; **p. 139** Treë.

**CHAPTER 6** **p. 142** © Lois Greenfield; **p. 144** (top) Lincoln Russell/Stock, Boston; (bottom) Jill Greenburg Copyright 1996 the Walt Disney Co. Reprinted by permission of Discover Magazine; **p. 148** (top) Elena Dorfman/Offshoot Stock; **p. 148** Frank Siteman/The Picture Cube; **p. 150** David Stoecklein/The Stock Market; **p. 151** Joel Gordon; **p. 152** Jon Feingersh/The Stock Market; **p. 155** Treë; **p. 157** William Thompson/The Picture Cube; **p. 158 & p. 160** Offshoot Stock; **p. 164** Michael Siluk/The Picture Cube.

**CHAPTER 7** **p. 166 and 167** © Lois Greenfield; **p. 168** Levinson/Monkmeyer Press; **p. 169** Glenn McLaughlin/The Stock Market; **p. 175** Raoul Hackel/Stock, Boston; **p. 177** (top) Michael Newman/Photo Edit; (bottom) John Keating/Photo Researchers; **p. 185** Lori Adamski Peek/Tony Stone Images; **p. 188** Willie L. Hill, Jr./The Image Works; **p. 192** Vision/Photo Researchers; **p. 194** T. Petillot/Explorer/Photo Researchers; **p. 197** David Young-Wolff/Photo Edit.

**CHAPTER 8** **p. 201** © Lois Greenfield; **p. 203** Arvind Garg/Gamma Liason; **p. 204** Joseph Nettis/Stock, Boston; **p. 206** Strauss/Curtis/Offshoot Stock; **p. 209** Bruce Ayres/Tony Stone Images; **p. 213** Reprinted with special permission of King Features Syndicate; **p. 214** Michael Keller/The Stock Market; **p. 218** John Curtis/Offshoot Stock; **p. 220** Cathy © **1968** Cathy Guisewite. Reprinted with permission of Universal Press Syndicate. All Rights Reserved.

**CHAPTER 9** **p. 222** © Lois Greenfield; **p. 225** (left) AP/Wide World Photos; (right) UPI/Corbis-Bettmann; **p. 226** (top) David Young-Wolff/Photo Edit; (bottom) L. Kolvoord/The Image Works; **p. 236** Skjold/The Image Works; **p. 237** Tony Arruza/The Image Works; **p. 246** W. Hill, Jr./The Image Works; **p. 249** Bonnie Kamin; **p. 251** Superstock.

**CHAPTER 10** **p. 256** © Lois Greenfield; **p. 258** D.W. Fawcett/Science Source/Photo Researchers; **p. 261** J. Griffen/The Image Works; **p. 263** Joel Gordon; **p. 266** (top) Hank Morgan/Science Source/Photo Researchers; (left & right) Joel Gordon; **p. 269** Joel Gordon; **p. 274** Joel Gordon; **p. 277** John Chiasson/Gamma Liaison; **p. 282** Kevin Horan/Stock, Boston.

**CHAPTER 11** **p. 286** © Lois Greenfield; **p. 289** Myrleen Ferguson/Photo Edit; **p. 293** Petit Format/Nestle/Science Source/Photo Researchers; **p. 296** Courtesy of the author; **p. 298** S.I.U./Science Source/Photo Researchers; **p. 299** Roger Tully/Tony Stone Images; **p. 304** (top) A. Ramey/Photo Edit; (center) Anne Nielsen/Gamma Liaison.

**CHAPTER 12** **p. 310** © Lois Greenfield; **p. 312** Chris Brown/Stock, Boston; **p. 319** Mark Richards/Photo Edit; **p.324** David Maung/Impact Visuals; **p. 328** Michael Newman/Photo Edit; **p. 330** Treë; **p. 332** Joel Gordon; **p. 334** Rousseau/The Image Works; **p. 335** Stacy Rosenstock/Impact Visuals; **p. 336** Dick Luria/Photo Researchers; **p. 341** Marc Muench/Tony Stone Images.

**CHAPTER 13** **p. 343** Stuart McClymont/Tony Stone Images; **p. 346** (top) Tony Freeman/Photo Edit; (bottom) Bruce Ayers/Tony Stone Images; **p. 348** Tom Raymond/Tony Stone Images; **p. 350** Stephen R. Brown/The Picture Cube; **p. 355** Jeff Greenberg/Photo Edit; **p. 358** Tony Freeman/Photo Edit; **p. 361** Jeff Greenberg/The Picture Cube; **p. 365** Mary Kate Denny/Photo Edit; **p. 370** Tony Freeman/Photo Edit.

**CHAPTER 14** **p. 374** Joel Gordon; **p. 376** Reprinted by permission of the American Cancer Society, Inc.; **p. 380** Martin Rodgers/Tony Stone Images; **p. 382** Ryan J. Hulvat/Design Conceptions; **p. 383** Richard Hutchings/Science Source/Photo Researchers; **p. 386** Lee Snider/The Image Works; **p. 390** Topham/The Image Works; **p. 394** Joel Gordon.

**CHAPTER 15** **p. 396** Dr. Dennis Kunkel/Phototake, NYC; **p. 401** Dr. Tony Brain/Science Photo Library/Photo Researchers; **p. 403** NIBSC/Science Photo Library/Photo Researchers; **p. 406** Henry Horenstein/The Picture Cube; **p. 407** Biology Media/Science Photo Library/Photo Researchers; **p. 411** Michael Newman/Photo Edit; **p. 415** Bachmann/The Image Works; **p. 417** UPI/Corbis-Bettmann; **p. 418** Bruce Ayers/Tony Stone Images; **p. 421** (top) L. Mulvehill/The Image Works; (bottom) Kent Wood/Photo Researchers; **p. 423** Christophe Simon/AFP/Corbis-Bettmann; **p. 426** Gilles Mingasson/Gamma Liaison.

**CHAPTER 16** **p. 430** Alvis Upitis/The Image Bank; **p. 432** Patrick Clark/Monkmeyer; **p. 436** NIH/Science Photo Library/Photo Researchers; **p. 443** Robert Becker/Custom Medical Stock Photo; **p. 445** Susan Van Etten/Photo Edit; **p. 446** AP/Wide World Photos; **p. 448** Biophoto Associates/Photo Researchers; **p. 449** Science Photo Library/Custom Medical Library/Photo Researchers; **p. 450** James Wilson/Woodfin Camp & Associates.

**CHAPTER 17** **p. 454 and 455** © Lois Greenfield; **p. 458** (left) Superstock; (right) Biophoto Associates/Science Source/Photo Researchers; **p. 459** Biophoto Associates/Science Source/Photo Researchers; **p. 462** Michelle Bridwell/Photo Edit; **p. 464** Bruce Ayers/Tony Stone Images; **p. 466** Doug Plummer/Photo Researchers; **p. 470** AP/Wide World Photos; **p. 471** Robert E. Daemmrich/Tony Stone Images; **p. 477** M. Bernson/The Image Works; **p. 479** Reproduced with permission. "Busy people don't have time for the weight. Exercise", © 1997 American Heart Association.

**CHAPTER 18** **p. 482** Jeff Smith/The Image Bank; **p. 489** Richard Vogel/Gamma Liason; **p. 493** Mulvehill/The Image Works; **p. 494** Darryl Estrine; **p. 497** Tom McCarthy/Photo Edit; **p. 499** (left) Dr. P. Marazzi/Science Photo Library/Photo Researchers;(right) James Stevenson/Science Photo Library/Photo Researchers; **p. 506** Tony Freeman/Photo Edit; **p. 508** Tony Freeman/Photo Edit; **p. 510** Richard Hutchings/Photo Researchers.

**CHAPTER 19** **p. 514** Eddie Adams/The Stock Market; **p. 520** Erika Stone; **p. 521** David Young-Wolff/Photo Edit; **p. 524** SPL/Custom Medical Stock Photo; **p. 526** E. Catarina/Stills Press/Retna Ltd.; **p. 531** Bernard Wolf/Monkmeyer; **p. 535** Sybil Shackman/Monkmeyer; **p. 537** Ira Wyman/Sygma; **p. 542** Ken Fisher/Tony Stone Images; **p. 543** Sondra Dawes/The Image Works.

**CHAPTER 20** **p. 545** © Lois Greenfield; **p. 549** AP/Wide World Photos; **p. 552** Yoav Levy/Phototake; **p. 553** Alon Reininger/Contact Press Images; **p. 555** Detroit News/GP/Gamma Liaison; **p. 556** Rob Nelson/Black Star; **p. 560** Skjold/The Image Works; **p. 563** Eric Roth/The Picture Cube; **p. 565** Jon Burbank/The Image Works.

**CHAPTER 21** **p. 569** © Lois Greenfield; **p. 572** Tom & DeeAnn McCarthy/The Stock Market; **p. 575** Joel Gordon; **p. 579** Steve McCurry/Magnum Photos; **p. 581** Rhoda Sidney/Monkmeyer; **p. 584** Courtesy of LaPorte County Child Abuse Prevention Council; **p. 587** John Coletti/The Picture Cube; **p. 590** George Goodwin/The Picture Cube.

**CHAPTER 22** **p. 594** Charles Thatcher/Tony Stone Images; **p. 597** David Muench/Tony Stone Images; **p. 598** Alan Oddie/Photo Edit; **p. 601** David Young-Wolff/Photo Edit; **p. 607** Felicia Martinez/Photo Edit; **p. 612** Tony Freeman/Photo Edit; **p. 613** Stanley Rowin/The Picture Cube; **p. 618** Superstock; **p. 620** Michael J. Howell/The Picture Cube; **p. 623** W. Hill, Jr./The Image Works; **p. 626** David Young-Wolff/Photo Edit.

**CHAPTER 23** **p. 630** Joel Gordon; **p. 634** Ken Lax/Photo Researchers; **p. 635** Erika Stone; **p. 637** Dean Abramson/Stock, Boston; **p. 641** Jeff Greenberg/The Picture Cube; **p. 646** Blair Seitz/Photo Researchers; **p. 651** Joel Gordon; **p. 653** Seth Resnick/Gamma Liasion; **p. 656** Wojnarowicz/The Image Works.

# INDEX

Page numbers in *italics* refer to illustrations